Updates in Hypertension and Cardiovascular Protection

Series editors:
Giuseppe Mancia
Milan, Italy

Enrico Agabiti Rosei
Brescia, Italy

The aim of this series is to provide informative updates on both the knowledge and the clinical management of a disease that, if uncontrolled, can very seriously damage the human body and is still among the leading causes of death worldwide. Although hypertension is associated mainly with cardiovascular, endocrine, and renal disorders, it is highly relevant to a wide range of medical specialties and fields – from family medicine to physiology, genetics, and pharmacology. The topics addressed by volumes in the series *Updates in Hypertension and Cardiovascular Protection* have been selected for their broad significance and will be of interest to all who are involved with this disease, whether residents, fellows, practitioners, or researchers.

More information about this series at http://www.springer.com/series/15049

Reuven Zimlichman • Stevo Julius
Giuseppe Mancia
Editors

Prehypertension and Cardiometabolic Syndrome

European Society of Hypertension

Springer

Editors
Reuven Zimlichman
Sackler Faculty of Medicine
Tel Aviv University
Tel Aviv
Israel

Stevo Julius
Department of Internal Medicine
University of Michigan
Ann Arbor
MI
USA

Giuseppe Mancia
Emeritus Professor of Medicine
University of Milano-Bicocca
Milan
Italy

ISSN 2366-4606 ISSN 2366-4614 (electronic)
Updates in Hypertension and Cardiovascular Protection
ISBN 978-3-319-75309-6 ISBN 978-3-319-75310-2 (eBook)
https://doi.org/10.1007/978-3-319-75310-2

Library of Congress Control Number: 2018956308

This Springer imprint is published by the registered company Springer Nature Switzerland AG
The registered company address is: Gewerbestrasse 11, 6330 Cham, Switzerland

Foreword

This book aims to give information on several pathophysiological and clinical aspects related to the concept of prehypertension. Although the definition of prehypertension in guidelines may be somewhat different, a large amount of clinical and epidemiological data indicates that individuals, not taking antihypertensive treatment, with systolic/diastolic blood pressure slightly below 140/90 mmHg, are at increased risk for sustained hypertension and cardiovascular diseases. The book will provide an up-to-date overview on epidemiological studies supporting the high risk for developing not only hypertension but also organ damage. Information is given on the relation between prehypertension and structural and functional changes in the heart as well as in the large and small arteries, with evidence of increased left ventricular mass, arteriosclerotic changes, and remodeling of small arteries, thus leading to increased cardiovascular and renal events risk. Prehypertensive subjects often present also additional cardiovascular risk factors. The evidence from recent studies supports the rationale for treating prehypertensives not only with lifestyle modification but also with antihypertensive medications, especially those with high normal blood pressure and high–very high cardiovascular risk. The book will be of great use to all researchers and practitioners interested in the prevention and treatment of hypertension, which represents a fundamental step in the reduction of the large cardiovascular disease burden worldwide.

Enrico Agabiti Rosei
Department of Internal Medicine
University of Brescia
Brescia, Italy

Preface

Prehypertension is identified as the blood pressure range from 120/80 to 139/89 mmHg, although its definition has frequently changed over the years with the changing subdivision of the blood pressure spectrum from the lowest to the highest values. The importance of prehypertension for research as well as for public health has long been appreciated for a variety of important reasons. First, within this blood pressure range lays a large fraction of the population. Second, compared to lower blood pressure values, prehypertensive individuals more frequently exhibit also overweight or obesity, glucose intolerance, and dyslipidemias, which make prehypertension an extremely frequent, if not a regular, component of the metabolic syndrome. Third, this clustering of risk factors makes the cardiovascular risk of prehypertension substantially higher than that of individuals with optimal blood pressure values, the risk being made, in many cases, greater by the presence of incipient or even more advanced asymptomatic damage of the heart, the kidney, and the large and small arteries. Finally, prehypertension owes its name to the high probability of a progression of the blood pressure values to a frank hypertensive condition, a phenomenon so frequent as to allow, from the middle age on, most prehypertensives to predict for themselves a hypertensive future. All this makes this condition important for investigating the factors that initially cause the cardiovascular alterations as well as the specific and interactive hemodynamic and metabolic mechanisms participating in the dynamic process that leads to the progressive elevation of blood pressure and organ damage. It is also an especially good setting to test lifestyle or drug-based strategies to effectively prevent this process, with benefits potentially much greater than those offered by later interventions, when the damage is established and likely to be at least in part irreversible.

This book provides a series of chapters on the most recent pathophysiological, epidemiological, diagnostic, and therapeutic research in the prehypertension area, written by a number of well-known experts. We hope this will be of interest to both clinicians and investigators, the former to update their information on the status of evidence-based prevention and treatment strategies in this cardiovascular area and the latter for even more clearly focusing on the gaps in knowledge and device means to fill them by appropriate investigations.

Tel Aviv, Israel — Reuven Zimlichman
Ann Arbor, MI, USA — Stevo Julius
Milan, Italy — Giuseppe Mancia

Contents

Part I

Epidemiology and Statistics

High-Normal Blood Pressure in Children and Adolescents

1

Mieczysław Litwin, Janusz Feber, and Zbigniew Kułaga

1.1 Introduction

Elevated blood pressure (BP) is regarded as the most important, but reversible risk factor for the development of cardiovascular (CV) disease. Epidemiological studies based on data from prospective decade-long observations of cohorts of adults provided strong evidence that systolic blood pressure (SBP) above 140 mmHg significantly increased the risk of CV disease and CV events such as stroke, coronary heart disease, heart failure and chronic kidney disease (CKD). However, the chosen threshold of SBP of 140 mmHg may be artificial, as there is a linear relationship between SBP and CV disease, i.e. the risk of CV disease is increased even at BP levels lower than 140 mmHg. In fact, subjects with SBP above 120 mmHg but still below 140 mmHg had a higher probability of developing arterial hypertension than those with an SBP below 120 mmHg. Although the problems related to CV risk and BP within the high-normal/prehypertensive range is quite well described regarding adults, only recent paediatric studies shed some light on the risk of high-normal/prehypertensive BP in children and adolescents. The aim of this review is to discuss the significant impact of even a mild increase of BP within the high-normal range concerning the development of CV disease and other hypertensive-related complications in children and adolescents.

M. Litwin (✉)
Department of Nephrology and Arterial Hypertension,
The Children's Memorial Health Institute, Warsaw, Poland
e-mail: M.Litwin@IPCZD.PL

J. Feber
Department of Pediatric Nephrology, The Children's Hospital of Eastern Ontario,
Ottawa, ON, Canada

Z. Kułaga
Department of Public Health, The Children's Memorial Health Institute, Warsaw, Poland

R. Zimlichman et al. (eds.), *Prehypertension and Cardiometabolic Syndrome*,
Updates in Hypertension and Cardiovascular Protection,
https://doi.org/10.1007/978-3-319-75310-2_1

1.2 Idea of Prehypertension

The association between systolic and diastolic BP and the development of CV disease and CV events in adults is continuous and graded. This concept is based on 10 years of observational data, which has shown that adults with high-normal BP had significantly greater cumulative incidence of CV events and CV disease than those with normal and optimal BP values. This cumulative incidence of CV disease increased with age and was particularly high among older subjects [1]. As already noted in earlier reports from the Framingham study, adults with BP in a high-normal range had a characteristic intermediary phenotype when compared to those with normal and optimal BP, namely a steady increase in body mass index (BMI), serum cholesterol and age, from an optimal to a high-normal BP range [1]. Further reports also showed that adults with high-normal BP suffer from autonomic dysfunction, visceral obesity and higher uric acid and metabolic abnormalities, typical of metabolic syndrome (MS) [2].

Thus, the threshold of 140/90 mmHg defining arterial hypertension in adults means that the CV risk is significantly greater for those with BP above 140/90, as compared to those with BP below this threshold. However, young adults with BP values in the high-normal range of 130–139/85–89 mmHg also had a greater incidence of arterial hypertension than their peers with lower/normal BP values. These findings indicate that high-normal BP status is an early and transitory stage of hypertensive disease, before the development of sustained arterial hypertension. The idea of a progressive increase of BP from normal through high-normal to hypertensive values is similar to the contemporary view of development of type 2 diabetes from a prediabetic state to fully blown diabetes. As the process of transition from pre-disease to disease state is potentially reversible, the detection and/or treatment of high-normal BP in the early stages may prevent CV complications at a later stage. This notion has led to the concept of "prehypertension" and its use in the classification of BP status in adults [3], implying that prehypertension should be treated as the first stage of hypertension. While this may apply for adults, the situation in children is more complicated due to different BP classifications (based on percentiles or Z-scores rather than absolute BP values) and relatively few longitudinal population data on CV risk associated with BP levels [4].

1.3 Classification of Blood Pressure Status in Children and Adolescents: Definition of High-Normal Blood Pressure/Prehypertension in Children and Adolescents

In contrast to classification of BP status in adults, the definition of arterial hypertension in children and adolescents is not based on the estimation of risk of CV events but rather on statistical distribution of BP values in general population. Thus, the definition of arterial hypertension in children is based on BP percentiles or *Z*-scores and not absolute blood pressure values. The currently used BP threshold defining arterial hypertension is the systolic and/or diastolic BP equal to or higher than the

95th percentile for age, sex and height [5]. The need for using BP percentile values rather than absolute BP values for children and adolescents is based on the BP changing with the development of the child. In adolescents, the situation is even more complicated as younger adolescents would fall within the child category with BP assessments recorded in percentiles, whereas older adolescents (≥16 years of age) may be considered as adults with BP measured in absolute values and criteria adopted by adult hypertension guidelines.

Although CV events and CV disease is rare in childhood, it is clear that elevated BP in childhood and adolescence evolves into arterial hypertension in adulthood. Thus, in 2004, the 4th Task Force Report adopted the JNC VII classification of BP status into paediatric guidelines [6]. According to the 4th Task Force Report, optimal blood pressure has been defined as blood pressure below the 90th percentile for age, sex and height and/or below 120/80 mmHg. The BP values between the 90th and 95th percentile, or above 120/80 mmHg but below the 95th percentile, have been classified as prehypertension. However, this classification, both for adults and children has not been fully accepted in the European Union because the term "prehypertension" implies a pre-disease state and suggests the need for treatment. Thus, the European Society of Hypertension (ESH) in its first paediatric guidelines on diagnosis and treatment of arterial hypertension in children and adolescents proposed to use the term high-normal blood pressure for blood pressure values regarded as prehypertensive in the US classification system [7]. While the use of BP percentiles and the 95th percentile as the upper limit of normal have been widely accepted for diagnosis and management of hypertension in younger children, adolescents from 16 years of age present a challenge when using BP percentiles for the definition of arterial hypertension and high-normal BP/prehypertension. Some boys aged 16–18 years could not be diagnosed as hypertensive despite having systolic BP values above the adult threshold value of 140 mmHg, because the values of the 95th percentile for systolic BP are much higher than 140 mmHg. On the contrary, in girls aged 16–18 years the 95th percentile values for systolic BP may be in the range of 132–135 mmHg, which means that they would be considered hypertensive by the paediatric definition based on percentiles but they would be normotensive or prehypertensive based on the adult definition of absolute BP values (<140/90). Similar problems have been encountered in children with prehypertensive/high-normal BP, as the 90th percentile increases with age and may reach the threshold of 120 mmHg at 13 years of age in some adolescents. These problems have led to a new classification of BP in children and adolescents as proposed by the ESH in 2016 [8]. In this new classification, adolescents aged 16 years and older have their BP status categorized according to the classification for adults, i.e. based on absolute BP values. Moreover, the definition of BP categories proposed by ESH differs from the original classification by the 4th Task Force Report. ESH defines normal BP as BP below the 90th percentile for children less than 16 years of age and below 130/85 mmHg in adolescents aged 16 years and older. Similarly, in children aged 16 and below, the high-normal BP has been defined as BP equal or higher than the 90th and lower than the 95th percentile, whereas in children 16–18 years of age the definition is based on absolute BP values between 130/85 and 139/89 mmHg. Thus, in contrast to the

US classification, the BP threshold of 120/80 mmHg for a prehypertensive range has not been adopted by the ESH. Importantly, in both US and EU classifications, the diagnosis of high-normal BP/prehypertension may be based on blood pressure values measured on one occasion, which may complicate the assessment of the prevalence of high-normal BP/prehypertension.

In addition to classification based on office BP measurements, prehypertension is also included in the classification of BP based on 24 h ambulatory blood pressure measurements (ABPM). According to paediatric ABPM classification, prehypertension is diagnosed when mean systolic and/or diastolic BP is below 95th percentile but BP load (percentile of BP readings above 95th percentile) is above 25% and below 50% [9].

1.4 Prevalence of High-Normal BP and Hypertension in Children and Adolescents

The real prevalence of high-normal BP/prehypertension in children and adolescents is difficult to assess due to several reasons. First, the definitions of prehypertension/high-normal BP differ between US and Europe as discussed above [6, 8]. Second, the intrinsic variability in repeated BP measurements (even in one clinic setting) and inconsistency in interpretation of the repeated BP measurements (some authors record the first reading only, some prefer the second BP reading, some calculate the average of the second and third readings, etc.) result in a significant heterogeneity within published reports on prehypertension/high-normal BP. Third, the diagnosis of high-normal BP/prehypertension depends on the number of clinic visits. When the definition of prehypertension was based on BP measurements during only one visit (average of three BP readings), the prevalence of prehypertension and hypertension was 9.4% and 9.5%, respectively [10]. However, after three screenings (clinic visits) the prevalence of prehypertension increased to 15.7% and the prevalence of arterial hypertension decreased to 3.2% [10]. These findings indicate that a large amount of adolescents labelled as hypertensive after their first BP screening become prehypertensive on subsequent visits. Similar findings of a decreasing prevalence of elevated BP in high-normal BP/prehypertensive range, was found with repeated measurements [11]. It was found that the prevalence of high-normal BP/prehypertension in 9-year-old children was 12.6% when BP was measured during one visit, but decreased to 9% when BP was measured during three visits. However, the prevalence of high-normal BP/prehypertension increased with age; the prevalence of high-normal BP/prehypertension in 11-year-old children was 14.4% based on one BP measurement and 12.4% when BP was measured over three visits.

In a Polish nationwide study (OLAF) on 21, 414 randomly selected students aged 3–18 years the BP was assessed and documented as the mean of the second and third measurements during one visit. We found that the prevalence of high-normal BP (according to the ESH definition) ranged from 10.8% to 19.7% in boys and from 8.3% to 14.4% in girls aged 11 to 18 years, respectively. The prevalence of high-normal BP did not differ between sexes until 14 years of age, but started to rise during a growth spurt, especially in boys (Figs. 1.1 and 1.2). As shown in Figs. 1.1 and 1.2, the prevalence of high-normal/prehypertension depends on the definition. When the definition based on the 4th Task Force Report guidelines was applied, the prevalence of high-normal blood pressure/prehypertension increased to 49.7% and 25.9%, in boys and girls, respectively. These age- and sex-related differences in the prevalence of prehypertension/high-normal BP have also been reported in other ethnic groups [12]. The prevalence of prehypertension/high-normal BP is

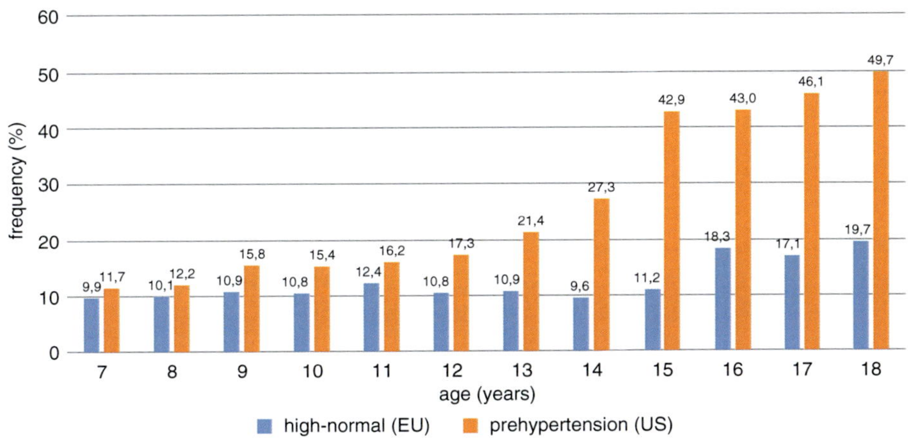

Fig. 1.1 Prevalence of high-normal BP (ESH definition) and prehypertension (4th Task Report definition) in sample of boys ($n = 8321$). OLAF Study, Poland

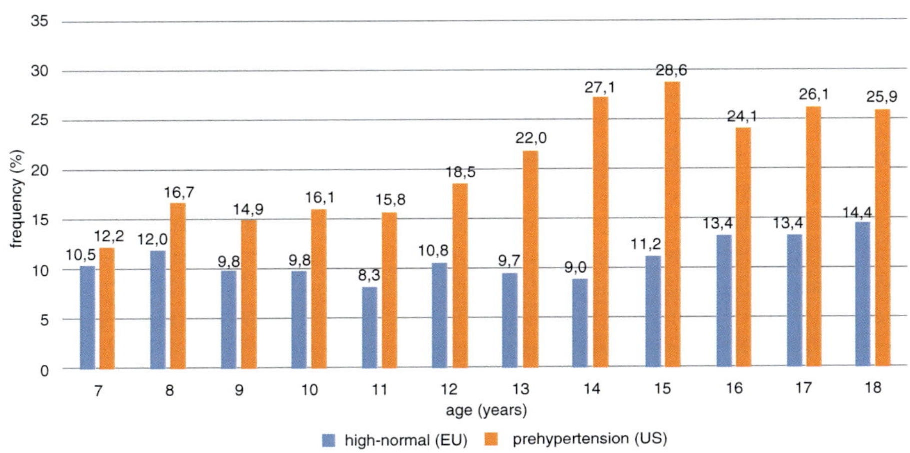

Fig. 1.2 Prevalence of high-normal BP (ESH definition) and prehypertension (4th Task Report definition) in sample of girls ($n = 9107$). OLAF Study, Poland

related to ethnicity and socioeconomic status and these determinants are the same as in arterial hypertension cases. In a study from the USA it was found that prehypertension was more common among African Americans and Hispanic adolescents than among White adolescents [10].

The other potential confounder in the assessment of high-normal BP prevalence is the method of BP measurement used. According to guidelines, the diagnosis of high-normal BP/prehypertension is based on office BP measurements. However, many patients who are referred with office hypertension undergo ABPM and are ultimately diagnosed with ambulatory prehypertension; this may lead to an underestimation of the true prevalence, as reported data on the prevalence of high-normal BP/prehypertension are usually based on office BP measurements only.

All these factors contribute to a significant variation in the prevalence ranging from 2.9% to 31%. However, regardless of the exact point prevalence estimate, it seems that the prevalence of high-normal BP/prehypertension increases over time as suggested by recent publications reporting a higher prevalence compared to earlier reports [13].

1.5 Intermediate Clinical and Laboratory Phenotype of High-Normal BP/Prehypertension in Children

The intermediate phenotype of high-normal BP/prehypertensive children in terms of anthropometrical parameters and metabolic abnormalities is in the middle between normotensive children and children with primary hypertension (PH). The main finding in children and adolescents with high-normal BP/prehypertension is obesity and visceral obesity expressed as increased waist circumference [14, 15]. Children and adolescents with high-normal BP/prehypertension present similar metabolic abnormalities as the children with PH, namely insulin resistance which is otherwise typical of MS. However these abnormalities are of a lower magnitude in comparison with children with PH. Similar to children with PH, children with high-normal BP/prehypertension have higher serum uric acid levels than normotensive children. It was shown that in pre-pubertal children, the risk of high-normal BP/prehypertension increased by 50% for each 1 mg/dL increase of serum uric acid concentration [16]. These metabolic abnormalities are associated with faster biological development, one of the main biological alterations seen across BP strata from normotension to PH in adolescents. In an analysis of data from NHANES II and III, Lauer et al. found that the level at which BP was tracked during childhood was related to growth, obesity and the degree of maturation acquired (expressed as bone age, number of permanent teeth, waist circumference). Children whose BP rose or fell in relation to their peers had body growth and maturation characteristics (bone age, number of permanent teeth, waist circumference) similar to those who maintained their rank order high or low, respectively [17]. In a study of adolescent boys referred to the hypertension clinic due to elevated BP, the difference between bone age and chronological age significantly increased from normotension through prehypertension, through stage 1 and stage 2 hypertension [18]. These findings indicate that an intermediate phenotype of adolescents with high-normal BP/prehypertension is similar to PH and also includes the basic alterations of the processes of biological development indicating a faster biological maturation associated with elevated BP values already in the prehypertensive range.

1.6 Evolution of High-Normal Blood Pressure/Prehypertension in Childhood

High-normal BP/prehypertension exhibits a tracking phenomenon, i.e. children with high-normal BP/prehypertension would more likely continue to have high-normal BP/prehypertension in adulthood [19, 20]. In adults, as many as 26% of patients with prehypertension progressed to hypertension and those patients had a 2.95 times higher risk of CV disease than those who remained at a normal BP or prehypertensive state [21]. It was shown that a significant number of children with high-normal BP/prehypertension progressed to PH later in life and had a worsening in cardiovascular outcome by midlife (i.e. 38 years of age) [22]. The overall incidence of arterial hypertension in the general population of adolescents (10–19 years) is estimated to be 0.5–0.8%. Redwine et al. found that the rate of progression from normotension to hypertension, confirmed by three measurements on three independent visits, was 0.4%/year; yet among adolescents who were prehypertensive it was 1.1%/year [23, 24]. In those who had either a systolic or diastolic BP above the 95th percentile during their first measurement session and who had a BP which later normalized, (<90th percentile or 120/80 mmHg), the incidence rate was 1.4%/year, i.e. the same as among adults with optimal BP.

The recent report from Bogalusa Heart Study on 2732 adults aged 20–51 years who were followed from childhood showed a prevalence of arterial hypertension of 23.5% [25]. However, those who became hypertensive had their BP in the prehypertensive range as children and adolescents. Similar findings were reported in a longitudinal representative birth cohort study from New Zealand, where SBP was reported at ages 7, 11, 18, 26, 32 and 38 years [22]. It was found that at an age of 38 years, adults who became hypertensive had significantly higher SBP trajectory starting already during their 7th year of age and their SBP values were in a prehypertensive range during childhood and adolescence up to mid-adulthood. These subjects also had the steepest rise of systolic BP during adolescence, attaining hypertensive values in early adulthood.

All these studies suggest that high-normal BP/prehypertension detected in childhood will most likely stay high-normal or increase to hypertensive levels later on in life at a much faster rate than among subjects with optimal BP. On the other hand, PH in adulthood develops from high-normal BP/prehypertension in adolescence. In some of these studies, adolescents ultimately labelled as high-normal BP/prehypertensives were originally diagnosed as hypertensive and then lowered their BP to a prehypertensive range. In fact, in aforementioned studies BP classification was not confirmed by ABPM; thus a portion of prehypertensive subjects suffer from white-coat hypertension [26]. Moreover, high-normal BP and prehypertension include a rather wide BP range (19/9 mmHg in US classification and 9/5 mmHg in ESH classification) and there are no data comparing risk of CV disease between those who were labelled as prehypertensive according to the 4th Task Force definition and those who were diagnosed as high-normal BP according to the ESH paediatric guidelines. Nevertheless, the risk of developing PH in adulthood by prehypertensive children concerns all patients in a prehypertensive range, but those who had higher BP values will develop PH faster than those who had a lower range of prehypertensive values [22]. The above-mentioned findings indicate that PH has its origin in childhood; the crucial period determining future BP trajectory and risk of development of PH is puberty and the pubertal growth spurt.

1.7 High-Normal Blood Pressure/Prehypertension in Childhood and Risk of Hypertensive Target Organ Damage

Elevated BP leads to adaptive changes of the CV system which, when elevated BP is sustained and accompanied by immuno-metabolic abnormalities, eventually leads to hypertensive target organ damage (TOD). Although there are only few reports on early subclinical TOD in adolescents with high-normal BP/prehypertension, it is now clear that there is a continuous increase in the risk of hypertensive TOD across all spectrums of BP values. These early subclinical changes include an increase of left ventricular mass index (LVMi), increased carotid intima-media thickness (cIMT), increased stiffness of large arteries expressed as pulse wave velocity (PWV), endothelial dysfunction assessed as flow mediated dilation (FMD) and early remodelling of small capillaries.

It was found that LVMi of prehypertensive adolescents was greater than in normotensive peers and did not differ significantly in comparison with hypertensive adolescents [27] and was of an intermediate nature between normotensive and hypertensive children [28]. Similarly, in a population study including 526 children aged 6–15 years, it was found that increasing BP and the presence of prehypertension (defined as BP in the 90–95th percentile) and arterial hypertension (but not obesity) were associated with concentric cardiac remodelling [15]. Heart rate, a clinical surrogate of the sympathetic drive, also increased within the BP category from normotension through prehypertension to hypertension. There is also evidence that arterial wall remodelling starts in prehypertensive youths. Although it was reported that prehypertensive adolescents had numerically increased cIMT in comparison with normotensive peers, significant differences were found in the carotid bulb and the internal carotid artery [28]. However, these alterations were modified by metabolic abnormalities which accompanied elevated BP.

Increased cIMT in prehypertensive adolescents is accompanied by increased stiffness of the arterial tree. It was reported that carotid-femoral, carotid radial and carotid-dorsal PWV were all significantly increased in prehypertensive adolescents when compared with normotensives [28, 29]. It was also found that PWV of prehypertensive youths was intermediate between normotensive and hypertensive subjects [28]. High-normal BP/prehypertension also exerts its effects on the level of microcirculation. Prehypertensive youths present with early remodelling of retinal arterial vessels which are expressed as central retinal arteriolar equivalents, representing an average arteriolar diameter and are similar to those found in hypertensive adolescents and different from normotensive controls [30]. In summary, high-normal BP/prehypertension is associated with significant adaptive changes in the whole CV system, including the left ventricle, remodelled arterial and arteriolar walls and increased arterial stiffness. These changes are intermediate between those found in normotensive and hypertensive children. The above-described early alterations of CV structure and function were modified by metabolic abnormalities and obesity. This is yet further evidence suggesting that high-normal BP/prehypertension is not an isolated hemodynamic alteration but rather a neuro-immuno-metabolic disease with hemodynamic consequences and signs of early vascular ageing [31, 32].

1.8 Risk of High-Normal BP/Prehypertension in Adolescence and Target Organ Damage and Cardiovascular Disease in Adulthood

At present it is evident from large longitudinal population studies, where elevated BP was defined as higher than the 90th percentile or 120/80 mmHg, that high-normal BP/prehypertension in adolescence is related not only to adaptive changes detected in adolescence but also to the risk of development of hypertensive TOD and CV disease in adulthood. The data was obtained from four studies (The Muscatine Study, Bogalusa Heart Study, Young Finns Study and CDAH Study) in which BP was measured on a minimum of four occasions in adolescent subjects (11.9–14.6 years of age) followed for a mean of 23 years. Individuals with persistently elevated BP (>90th percentile or >120/80 mmHg) had significantly increased cIMT in comparison with those who had optimal BP [33]. However, the risk of increased cIMT in early adulthood was lower if the subjects had elevated BP during adolescence which resolved by adulthood. Liang et al. also showed that the risk of development of PH and hypertensive arterial remodelling (increase of cIMT and carotid-femoral PWV) in early adulthood (mean age 34.5 years) was already increased in those adolescents who had a BP above the 80th percentile and below the 95th percentile, thus below the lower threshold of the prehypertensive range [34].

1.9 How to Manage High-Normal Blood Pressure in Children and Adolescents

According to guidelines, high-normal BP should be treated with non-pharmacological measures [8]. The exception is that in children with diabetes mellitus (DM) or CKD, pharmacological therapy should also be instituted [35]. The basis of non-pharmacological therapy is directed to main risk factors of PH and CV disease, i.e. obesity, associated metabolic abnormalities and physical inactivity. Thus, non-pharmacological treatment is based on lifestyle changes with dietary advice and moderate to intensive physical activity of at least 60–90 min daily. Although the efficacy of physical aerobic exercise in young adults with prehypertension has been questioned recently, detailed analysis shows that it is quite effective when applied and accepted by individuals [36]. Recent meta-analysis of efficacy during physical exercise in young adults (mean age 42.2 years) with prehypertension, defined as BP above 120/80 mmHg and below 140/90 mmHg, revealed that after 3–6 months after starting the intervention, systolic and diastolic BP decreased on average by −4.4 and 4.1 mmHg, respectively, but after 12 months this effect was lost. However, analysis of factors associated with the loss of hypotensive effects of physical exercise revealed that it was due to an increasing rate of patient non-compliance. Thus, the main reason of low efficacy of physical exercise in young adults was the loss of interest and a return to their previous sedentary lifestyle. Interestingly, BP reduction was greater when physical exercise was of vigorous intensity, when it was supervised and when it was associated with significant weight loss. One of the most important factors associated with long-term success of this type of therapy was due to frequency and duration of contact with health care professionals. These findings underscore the fact that similarly to the pharmacological therapy, non-compliance is the main reason for the lack of effect of non-pharmacological therapy. The other conclusion is that young patients with high-normal BP/prehypertension are by definition less physically active and therefore organized/supervised programmes of moderate to vigorous physical activity would be more effective than self-directed low intensity activities. Such conclusions are supported by the results acquired during treatment in adolescents with PH. Twelve months of pharmacological and non-pharmacological treatment, based on angiotensin convertase inhibitors (ACEi) or angiotensin receptor blockers (ARB) and physical exercise in 86 adolescents with PH, caused normalization of BP in 70% of patients, a decrease in the prevalence of metabolic syndrome by 50%, normalization of markers of oxidative stress, along with the regression of left ventricular hypertrophy and subclinical arterial injury. However, the main determinant of TOD regression was not due to a decrease of BP but rather a decrease of waist circumference and amount of visceral fat, assessed by magnetic resonance [37].

There are only a few paediatric studies analysing the effects of non-pharmacological treatment in children with high-normal BP/prehypertension. Most of them have included children with obesity who had elevated BP and who underwent programmes of dietary and physical activity treatment. Fapour-Lambert et al. reported results from a 3-month randomized controlled trial on the effects of physical activity treatment in pre-pubertal obese children with elevated BP (high-normal BP/prehypertension and hypertension) [38]. The study showed that moderate intensity training over a 3-month period (60 min three times weekly) led to significant improvements in endothelial function measured as FMD and nitroglycerin-mediated dilation, along with a decrease in BP and arterial stiffness. These changes were associated with a decrease in body fat and visceral fat. A subgroup of patients was followed for 2 years in whom beneficial effects of physical training on BP were sustained, especially in the children who decreased their body mass index [39]. Importantly, it occurred that the increased physical activity was maintained beyond the end of the 3 month intervention. This observation suggests that lifestyle changes may be implemented with greater success in paediatric patients than in adults.

Although the role of dietary advice and dietary modifications has been well established, it seems that the effects of physical activity on BP and arterial function continue to be more significant. Woo et al. analysed the effects of diet along with diet plus exercise on arterial properties of obese children of a mean age of 10 years (9–12 years) [40]. He found that although both interventions led to a significant decrease of waist-to-hip ratio and the improvement of FMD within 6 weeks, these changes were of a greater magnitude when diet was combined with training. Importantly, these beneficial changes were even more evident after 1 year in the children who continued their dietary and physical activity programmes, yet decreased in those who resigned from the programme.

In conclusion, non-pharmacological interventions based on dietary modifications and physical activity of moderate to vigorous intensity not only lead to normalization of BP but also exert beneficial effects on arterial structure and function by normalizing metabolic abnormalities.

1.10 High-Normal Blood Pressure/Prehypertension in Children with Chronic Kidney Disease and Diabetic Children

In contrast to the general population, children with CKD and those with DM, a BP in the high-normal/prehypertensive range is regarded as an indication for treatment and should be treated pharmacologically. In CKD, the reason for pharmacological treatment of high-normal BP/prehypertension is not only early prevention of CV disease, but also renoprotection based on ACEi or ARBs. The goal of BP lowering therapy depends on proteinuria; in children with proteinuria greater than 0.5 g/day, BP should be lowered below 50 pc of the 24 h mean arterial BP. In the absence of significant proteinuria, the BP should be lowered below 90 pc of the 24 h mean arterial BP and preferably below 75 pc [31, 32, 35].

As in CKD, the aim of antihypertensive treatment in diabetic children is both early prevention of diabetic kidney disease and CV protection. In general, BP in diabetic children should be kept below 90 pc for age, sex and height. In both diabetic children and children with CKD, a more aggressive therapy is indicated along with close monitoring of BP by home BP measurements and repeated ABPM measurements.

1.11 Summary and Perspectives

There is strong evidence that high-normal BP/prehypertension in childhood and adolescence tracks to adulthood, leads to early development of PH and represents a risk factor for CV disease in the fourth decade of life. The adaptive changes of the CV system associated with high-normal BP/prehypertension develop in childhood and are accompanied by neuro-immuno-metabolic abnormalities typical of PH and MS. Normalization of high-normal BP/prehypertension lowers the risk of development of hypertensive TOD and CV disease in adulthood. Interventions based on lifestyle changes with dietary advice and increased physical activity are more efficient when started early and include all family members, but long-term prospective studies are lacking in prehypertensive children. On the contrary, the close association between increased arterial stiffness in adulthood and BP in the range of prehypertensive values in childhood suggests that the threshold of abnormal BP should be lowered to the 90th percentile [41]. Consequently, adolescents with high-normal BP/prehypertension may benefit from a wider diagnostic workup with an assessment of TOD and metabolic CV risk factors, combined with antihypertensive treatment.

References

1. Vasan R, Larson M, Leip E, Evans J, O'Doneel CJ, Kannel WB, Levy D. Impact of high-normal blood pressure on the risk of cardiovascular disease. N Engl J Med. 2001;345:1291–7.
2. Fernandez C, Sander GE, Giles TD. Prehypertension: defining the transitional phenotype. Curr Hypertens Rep. 2016;18:2.
3. Chobanian AV, Bakris GL, Black HR, et al. Seventh report of the joint national committee on prevention, detection, evaluation, and treatment of high blood pressure. Hypertension. 2003;42:1206–52.
4. Feber J, Litwin M. Blood pressure (BP) assessment-from BP level to BP variability. Pediatr Nephrol. 2016;31:1071–9.
5. National Heart, Lung, and Blood Institute. Report of the task force on blood pressure control in children. Pediatrics. 1977;59:797–820.
6. National High Blood Pressure Education Program Working Group on High Blood Pressure in Children and Adolescents. The fourth report on the diagnosis, evaluation, and treatment of high blood pressure in children and adolescents. Pediatrics. 2004;114:555–76.
7. Lurbe E, Cifkova R, Cruickshank JK, Dillon MJ, Ferreira I, Invitti C, Kuznetsova T, Laurent S, Mancia G, Morales-Olivas F, Rascher W, Redon J, Schaefer F, Seeman T, Stergiou G, Wühl E, Zanchetti A, European Society of Hypertension. Management of high blood pressure in children and adolescents: recommendations of the European Society of Hypertension. J Hypertens. 2009;27:1719–42.
8. Lurbe E, Agabiti-Rosei E, Cruickshank JK, Dominiczak A, Erdine S, Hirth A, Invitti C, Litwin M, Mancia G, Pall D, Rascher W, Redon J, Schaefer F, Seeman T, Sinha M, Stabouli S, Webb NJ, Wühl E, Zanchetti A. European Society of Hypertension guidelines for the management of high blood pressure in children and adolescents. J Hypertens. 2016;34:1887–920.
9. Flynn JT, Daniels SR, Hayman LL, Maahs DM, McCrindle BW, Mitsnefes M, Zachariah JP. Urbina EM; American Heart Association Atherosclerosis, Hypertension and Obesity in Youth Committee of the Council on Cardiovascular Disease in the Young: Update: ambulatory blood pressure monitoring in children and adolescents: a scientific statement from the American Heart Association. Hypertension. 2014;63:1116–35.

10. McNiece KL, Poffenbarger TS, Turner JL, Franco K, Sorof J, Portman R. Prevalence of pre-hypertension and hypertension among adolescents. J Pediatr. 2007;150:640–4.
11. Marcovecchio ML, Mohn A, Diddi G, Polidori N, Chiarelli F, Fuiano N. Longitudinal assessment of blood pressure in school-aged children: a 3-year follow-up study. Pediatr Cardiol. 2016;37:255–61.
12. Xu T, Zhu G, Liu J, Han S. Gender-specific prevalence and associated risk factors of high normal blood pressure and hypertension among multi-ethnic Chinese adolescents aged 8–18 years old. Blood Press. 2015;24:189–95.
13. Liang YJ, Xi B, Hu YH, Wang C, Liu JT, Yan YK, et al. Trends in blood pressure and hypertension among Chinese children and adolescents: China health and nutrition surveys 1991–2004. Blood Press. 2011;20:45–53.
14. Acosta AA, Samuels JA, Portman RJ, Redwine KM. Prevalence of persistent prehypertension among adolescents. J Pediatr. 2012;160:757–61.
15. Pieruzzi F, Antolini L, Salerno FR, Giussani M, Brambilla P, Galbiati S, Mastriani S, Rebora P, Stella A, Valsecchi MG, Genovesi S. The role of blood pressure, body weight and fat distribution on left ventricular mass, diastolic function and cardiac geometry in children. J Hypertens. 2015;33:1182–92.
16. Viazzi F, Antolini L, Giussani M, Brambilla P, Galbiati S, Mastriani S, Stella A, Pontremoli R, Valsecchi MG, Genovesi S. Serum uric acid and blood pressure in children at cardiovascular risk. Pediatrics. 2013;132:e93–9.
17. Lauer RM, Anderson AR, Beaglehole R, Burns TL. Factors related to tracking of blood pressure in children. U.S. National Center for Health Statistics Health Examination Surveys Cycles II and III. Hypertension. 1984;6:307–14.
18. Pludowski P, Litwin M, Niemirska A, Jaworski M, Sladowska J, Kryskiewicz E, Karczmarewicz E, Neuhoff-Murawska J, Wierzbicka A, Lorenc RS. Accelarated skeletal maturation in children with primary hypertension. Hypertension. 2009;54:1234–9.
19. Banker A, Bell C, Gupta-Malhotra M, Samuels J. Blood pressure percentile charts to identify high or low blood pressure in children. BMC Pediatr. 2016;16:98.
20. Kagura J, Adair LS, Musa MG, Pettifor JM, Norris SA. Blood pressure tracking in urban black South African children: birth to twenty cohort. BMC Pediatr. 2015;15:78.
21. Ishikawa Y, Ishikawa J, Ishikawa S, Kario K, Kajii E, Jichi Medical School Cohort Investigators Group. Progression from prehypertension to hypertension and risk of cardiovascular disease. J Epidemiol. 2017;27:8–13.
22. Theodore RF, Broadbent J, Nagin D, Ambler A, Hogan S, Ramrakha S, Cutfield W, Williams MJ, Harrington H, Moffitt TE, Caspi A, Milne B, Poulton R. Childhood to early-midlife systolic blood pressure trajectories: early-life predictors, effect modifiers, and adult cardiovascular outcomes. Hypertension. 2015;66:1108–15.
23. Redwine KM, Acosta AA, Poffenbarger T, Portman RJ, Samuels J. Development of hypertension in adolescents with pre-hypertension. J Pediatr. 2012;160:98–103.
24. Redwine KM, Falkner B. Progression of prehypertension to hypertension in adolescents. Curr Hypertens Rep. 2012;14:619–25.
25. Shen W, Zhang T, Li S, Zhang H, Xi B, Shen H, Fernandez C, Bazzano L, He J, Chen W. Race and sex differences of lon-term blood pressure profiles from childhood and adult hypertension. The Bogalusa Heart Study. Hypertension. 2017;70:66–74.
26. Obrycki Ł, Niemirska A, Sarnecki J, Kulaga Z, Litwin M. Central systolic blood pressure and central pulse pressure as predictors of left ventricular hypertrophy in hypertensive children. ESH 2017, Abstract.
27. Stabouli S, Kotsis V, Rizos Z, Toumanidis S, Karagianni C, Constantopoulos A, Zakopoulos N. Left ventricular mass in normotensive, prehypertensive and hypertensive children and adolescents. Pediatr Nephrol. 2009;24:1545–51.
28. Urbina EM, Khoury PR, McCoy C, Daniels SR, Kimball TR, Dolan LM. Cardiac and vascular consequences of pre-hypertension in youth. J Clin Hypertens (Greenwich). 2011;13:332–42.
29. Zhu H, Yan W, Ge D, Treiber FA, Harshfield GA, Kapuku G, Snieder H, Dong Y. Cardiovascular characteristics in American youth with prehypertension. Am J Hypertens. 2007;20:1051–7.

30. Murgan I, Beyer S, Kotliar KE, Weber L, Bechtold-Dalla Pozza S, Dalla Pozza D, Wegner A, Sitnikova D, Stock D, Stock K, Heemann U, Schmaderer C, Baumann M. Arterial and retinal changes in hypertensive and prehypertensive adolescents. Am J Hypertens. 2013;26:400–8.
31. Litwin M, Feber J, Niemirska A, Michałkiewicz J. Primary hypertension is a disease of premature vascular aging associated with neuro-immuno-metabolic abnormalities. Pediatr Nephrol. 2016a;31:185–94.
32. Litwin M, Feber J, Ruzicka M. Vascular Aging: Lessons From Pediatric Hypertension. Can J Cardiol. 2016b;32:642–9.
33. Juhola J, Magnussen CG, Berenson GS, Venn A, Burns TL, Sabin MA, Srinivasan SR, Daniels SR, Davis PH, Chen W, Kähönen M, Taittonen L, Urbina E, Viikari JS, Dwyer T, Raitakari OT, Juonala M. Combined effects of child and adult elevated blood pressure on subclinical atherosclerosis: the International Childhood Cardiovascular Cohort Consortium. Circulation. 2013;128:217–24.
34. Liang Y, Hou D, Shan X, Zhao X, Hu Y, Jiang B, Wang L, Liu J, Cheng H, Yang P, Shan X, Yan Y, Chowienczyk PJ, Mi J. Cardiovascular remodeling relates to elevated childhood blood pressure: Beijing Blood Pressure Cohort Study. Int J Cardiol. 2014;20:836–9.
35. Wühl E, Trivelli A, Picca S, Litwin M, Peco-Antic A, Zurowska A, Testa S, Jankauskiene A, Emre S, Caldas-Afonso A, Anarat A, Niaudet P, Mir S, Bakkaloglu A, Enke B, Montini G, Wingen AM, Sallay P, Jeck N, Berg U, Caliskan S, Wygoda S, Hohbach-Hohenfellner K, Dusek J, Urasinski T, Arbeiter K, Neuhaus T, Gellermann J, Drozdz D, Fischbach M, Möller K, Wigger M, Peruzzi L, Mehls O, Schaefer F, ESCAPE Trial Group. Strict blood-pressure control and progression of renal failure in children. N Engl J Med. 2009;361:1639–50.
36. Williamson W, Foster C, Reid H, Kelly P, Lewandowski AJ, Boardman H, Roberts N, McCartney D, Huckstep O, Newton J, Dawes H, Gerry S, Leeson P. Will exercise advice be sufficient for treatment of young adults with prehypertension and hypertension? A systematic review and meta-analysis. Hypertension. 2016;68:78–87.
37. Litwin M, Niemirska A, Sladowska-Kozlowska J, Wierzbicka A, Janas R, Wawer ZT, Wisniewski A, Feber J. Regression of target organ damage in children and adolescents with primary hypertension. Pediatr Nephrol. 2010;25:2489–99.
38. Farpour-Lambert NJ, Aggoun Y, Marchand LM, Martin XE, Herrmann FR, Beghetti M. Physical activity reduces systemic blood pressure and improves early markers of atherosclerosis in pre-pubertal obese children. J Am Coll Cardiol. 2009;54:2396–406.
39. Maggio AB, Aggoun Y, Martin XE, Marchand LM, Beghetti M, Farpour-Lambert NJ. Long-term follow-up of cardiovascular risk factors after exercise training in obese children. Int J Pediatr Obes. 2011;6:e603–1.
40. Woo KS, Chook P, Yu CW, Sung RY, Qiao M, Leung SS, Lam CW, Metreweli C, Celermajer DS. Effects of diet and exercise on obesity-related vascular dysfunction in children. Circulation. 2004;109:1981–6.
41. Aatola H, Magnussen CG, Koivistoinen T, Hutri-Kähönen N, Juonala M, Viikari JS, Lehtimäki T, Raitakari OT, Kähönen M. Simplified definitions of elevated pediatric blood pressure and high adult arterial stiffness. Pediatrics. 2013;132:e70–6.

History of Prehypertension: Past and Present, a Saga of Misunderstanding and Neglect

2

Reuven Zimlichman, Stevo Julius, and Giuseppe Mancia

The blood pressure measurements became an important clinical tool only a century ago, when Riva Rocci and Korotkoff demonstrated how to use sphygmomanometers to measure the blood pressure in clinical practice. During this relatively short period there was a substantial variation in the definitions of normal and pathologic blood pressure levels [1, 2]. The impact of this variability on the management or treatment of prehypertension and hypertension will be discussed later. At this point it is appropriate to underscore that already in ancient times, by evaluating the pulse, medical practitioners were capable to assess patient's cardiovascular health. Ancient records, as far back as 2600 BC, reported that acupuncture, venesection [3], and bleeding by leeches were the sole means of treating what was called "hard pulse disease." The Ashurbanipal Library at Nineveh (669–626 BC) contains details on the use of the latter two procedures [4]. Remarkable work was done by the Yellow Emperor of China (Chou You-J, 2600 BC), Wang (280 BC), and the Roman Cornelius Celsus [5]. Galen (131–201 AD) [6], Erisitrates, and Hippocrates [5] all recommended venesection. Sorovas of Ephesus in 120 AD recommended cupping the spine to draw out animal spirits [4]. Thanks to two students of medical history [3, 4] we can presently wonder about the wisdom of our ancient colleagues. As early as 2600 BC the Yellow Emperor explained that "In order to examine whether Ying or Yang prevail one must distinguish a gentle pulse from hard and bounding pulse. The

R. Zimlichman (✉)
Sackler Faculty of Medicine, Tel Aviv University, Tel Aviv, Israel
e-mail: zimlich@post.tau.ac.il

S. Julius
Department of Internal Medicine, University of Michigan, Ann Arbor, MI, USA
e-mail: sjulius@umich.edu

G. Mancia
Emeritus Professor of Medicine, University of Milano-Bicocca, Milan, Italy
e-mail: giuseppe.mancia@unimib.it

R. Zimlichman et al. (eds.), *Prehypertension and Cardiometabolic Syndrome*, Updates in Hypertension and Cardiovascular Protection,
https://doi.org/10.1007/978-3-319-75310-2_2

hearth influences the force and fills the pulse with blood." Furthermore, he stated that "If too much salt is used in food, the pulse hardens." He also understood the relationship between hypertension and congestive heart failure by stating that "when the pulse is abundant but tense and hard like a cord, there are dropsical spellings (edema)." Ancient doctors also understood the relationship between excessive food intake and negative health outcomes. Physical exercise as well as decrease in eating were routinely recommended. The Arabic text Al-Azkhora stated that " Nothing is more harmful to an aging person than to have a clever cook and a beautiful concubine."

Since the early nineteens, in the modern era of blood pressure measurement, when the use of sphygmomanometers became ubiquitous, the cutoff levels for normalcy became a moving target and remained such, up till present times. In the late 1950s, when thiazide diuretics were introduced, hypertension was defined as blood pressure levels greater than 180/100 mmHg. However, during the succeeding decades, based on the results of blood pressure lowering trials, the cutoff decreased considerably [7, 8].

In parallel with studies reporting results of antihypertensive treatment, epidemiologic investigations uniformly confirmed that elevation of blood pressure is a strong predictor of cardiovascular morbidity and mortality. However, the interpretation of these findings varied. In fact, the management of hypertension is a classic example of how, facing the same data, people may come to opposing conclusions. All branches of science must develop a nomenclature for the observed data. Unfortunately, in prehypertension and hypertension the semantics of some terms is confusing. A good example is the term "hypertonie essential" coined by Frank in 1925 [9]. It is not quite clear why Frank chose the term "essential" but it can mean two different things. Essential may mean "absolutely necessary, extremely important" but in medicine it also means "disease with not known cause, idiopathic." One would think that such a semantic issue would not cause a problem, but the fact is that a group of physicians believed that the increased blood pressure is an appropriate response to secure the perfusion of tissues in people with increased peripheral resistance. They predicted that lowering the blood pressure would have catastrophic consequences.

In the 1950s, the development of the first ganglionic blockers sharpened the dispute about the benefit of blood pressure reduction. Mainly pioneering and progressive physicians dared to treat their patients with ganglion blockers despite the serious side effects. While discussing the cost-effectiveness of treating severe hypertension, Pickering reported in 1961 that the five-year survival rate in malignant hypertension was zero. But already in 1958, Dustan reported a survival rate of 33% in patients treated with malignant hypertension [10]. The debate regarding the cost-effectiveness of treating hypertension continued. Nonetheless, the publication of the US Veteran study in 1967 reported dramatic improvement in survival in the subgroup of patients with diastolic blood pressure of about 110 mmHg [11]. By this point, treatment of hypertension was fully justified and the focus shifted to populations with milder forms of hypertension. In parallel, since the goal of treatment was to normalize the blood pressure, it was important to define normalcy.

The term "normal" has numerous connotations, ranging from a statistical definition based on variables in healthy people to meanings such as "most common" and "most desirable" [12]. Furthermore, the term "normal" is problematic because it determines that what is not "normal" is "abnormal" [13]. A meta-analysis of epidemiological cohort published in 2002 showed an association of a blood pressure reading of 115/75 mmHg with a minimal risk of cardiovascular mortality, and thus concluded that this constitutes an optimal blood pressure level [14]. However, this mean value did not provide information about the risk in individual subjects. Definitions of normal and abnormal blood pressure are further complicated by the fact that blood pressure, on a population level, is a continuous variable with a Gaussian distribution, i.e., without any clear point that would denote abnormality because the relationship between systolic and diastolic blood pressure and cardiovascular risk is continuous. In a large study that reviewed data of about one million individuals, mortality from cardiovascular disease increased exponentially from blood pressure levels as low as 115/75 mmHg, with an approximate doubling of the risk for every 20/10 mmHg increase above that level [14, 15].

Over time, various terms have been used to classify the degrees of hypertension such as mild, moderate, and severe hypertension; and systolic, diastolic, and systo-diastolic hypertension. On the lower end of classification numerous terms were used to define the group of subjects whose blood pressure was slightly elevated above normal but not yet in the hypertension range. There was substantial research interest in this group but the nomenclature varied. The terms "borderline hypertension," "high-normal blood pressure," and "borderline blood pressure elevation" were most frequently used. In this millennium, in 2003, the American seventh report of the Joint National Committee on Hypertension revitalized the term "prehypertension" [8] and defined it as a blood pressure range of 120–139/80–89 mmHg. Nonetheless, this definition was controversial and many physicians felt that a large number of healthy individuals would be labeled as having as a medical diagnosis. This, in turn, might create anxiety and indicate pharmaceutical treatment in the absence of evidence that lowering blood pressure from this range is beneficial. Previously, in 1984, the Joint National Committee on the Detection, Evaluation and Treatment of High Blood Pressure introduced the concept of high-normal blood pressure (blood pressure in the 130–139/85–89 mmHg range), due to the concern that a moderate blood pressure elevation which was previously considered normal, could increase the risk of premature cardiovascular morbidity and mortality and lead to the development of established hypertension much more frequently than the lower blood pressure range of normal or optimal blood pressure [16]. Nevertheless, the purpose of this action was only to promote awareness in order to stimulate lifestyle modification and the document did not discuss whether and when should pharmacologic blood pressure lowering be considered.

It is well known that if patients are not receiving antihypertensive treatment their blood pressure will increase. The increase is exponential and with passage of time the rise becomes more and more rapid. Just as the size of skeletal muscles grows in response to repetitive increases of exercise, the smooth muscles in the resistance vessels (arterioles) also respond to repetitive bouts of higher blood pressure by decrease of their lumen. This in turn increases the vascular resistance and blood pressure [17].

The fact that untreated blood pressure elevation increases exponentially [14] provided the rationale for the TROPHY (Trial of Preventing Hypertension) study. This trial [18] recruited 772 patients with blood pressure of 130–139 and/or 85–89 mmHg and followed them over a period of 4 years. One group was randomized to 4 years of placebo treatment and the other group was treated with the angiotensin receptor blocker candesartan for 2 years. After 2 years, patients in the candesartan group were switched to placebo. The hypothesis was that 2 years of previous treatment would prevent or postpone the development of stage 1 hypertension during the 2 years of placebo observation. Following are the results of the study: (1) Treatment with candesartan was safe. Rates of adverse events during the 2 years of treatment were similar in both groups. (2) During the 4 years of observation nearly two-thirds of the placebo group developed stage 1 hypertension. Thus, marginal blood pressure elevation at baseline forecasts future hypertension and "prehypertension" is the appropriate term for patients whose baseline blood pressure is in the 130–139 and or 85–89 mmHg range. (3) The risk of new onset hypertension in the previously actively treated group was suppressed. Whereas the difference was statistically significant, the actual difference was modest. The overall conclusion of the study was that pharmacological treatment of prehypertension is feasible but the findings were not sufficiently robust to mandate treatment.

The PHARAO study also showed that blood pressure lowering in prehypertension is safe using the angiotensin-converting enzyme inhibitor ramipril [19].

Whether subjects with a high-normal blood pressure need medical treatment had of course to be ultimately tested by trials in which the goal was prevention of cardiovascular events. Little evidence of this kind has ever been made available, however, for two reasons. First, because in the high-normal blood pressure range cardiovascular risk is lower than in hypertensive patients these trials had to be larger or based on longer follow-up than usual trials, thereby representing a difficult research option. Second, trials showing (mostly by subgroup analysis) that reducing blood pressure from a high-normal range was accompanied by a reduction of cardiovascular events had made use of patients already under antihypertensive treatment, and thus most likely with an original frank blood pressure elevation, this being the case also for the meta-analyses of the available studies. The response in the media to the possibility of expanding treatment to this large subject category was also unsupportive and accusations like "disease mongering" were campaigned in the press.

In the above context, two recent important trials are ACCORD [20] and SPRINT [21] that aimed to determine the optimal target blood pressure to reduce morbidity and mortality, in type 2 diabetic and nondiabetic patients, respectively. Although the interpretation of their results has raised some controversy. These trials have scored in favor of blood pressure targets lower than the traditional ones (<140/90 mmHg) because patients randomized to an on-treatment systolic blood pressure <120 mmHg (achieved value slightly >120 mmHg) showed a reduction of cardiovascular outcomes compared to patients randomized to <140 mmHg (achieved value about

135 mmHg), an incremental benefit that in SPRINT extended to all-cause mortality as well. These findings influenced the guidelines issued in November 2017 by the American College of Cardiology (ACC) and the American Heart Association (AHA) recommend the blood pressure target for treatment to be <130 mmHg systolic value in virtually all hypertensive individuals. The American guidelines recommended to lower the blood pressure range at which physicians should initiate antihypertensive drug treatment because in both trials initial systolic blood pressure was <140 mmHg, thereby falling in the high-normal blood pressure range. This is not immune from criticism, because as for the abovementioned data in both ACCORD and SPRINT patients received antihypertensive treatment at baseline. In the meantime, new data suggested that in untreated subjects with high-normal blood pressure blood pressure lowering does not reduce cardiovascular events. However, the exception is in patients who have a history of cardiovascular events and are therefore at very high risk. Presently the high-normal blood pressure range is considered to be a condition in which active blood pressure lowering treatment is indicated, albeit only when background risk is elevated. This progress along the line formerly traced by the TROPHY study which championed years ago the idea that treatment might benefit subjects even before the state of established hypertension.

Extension of active antihypertensive treatment to the high-normal blood pressure range has prompted the ACC/AHA guidelines to modify the classification of hypertension stages, stage 1 being now the former prehypertension [22]. The implementation of the recently proposed definition for hypertension will classify nearly half (46%) of the adult US population as hypertensive. The new guidelines do not necessarily mean that half the adult population in the USA and in other developed countries should receive medical treatment. Rather, the focus is on individuals with a suboptimal blood pressure, in an effort to convince them to make lifestyle changes and to reduce their cardiovascular risk. Nonetheless, the number of persons that will be treated with pharmacologic agents will increase and this will include patients who were not pharmacologically treated before.

Due to the changing definition of hypertension over the course of decades, it was only natural that the definition of prehypertension would change too. For many years, the notion was widely accepted that "the higher the blood pressure, the higher the morbidity and mortality." Diagnosing and treating persons in the higher blood pressure group has been recognized as the main goal, due to their propensity to faster and more severe end-organ damage. However, the fact that the total number of persons with prehypertension outnumbers those with overt hypertension has been underestimated. Moreover, therapeutic options in the early 1900s were very limited, and entailed severe side effects. Treatment with medications such as ganglion blockers was known not to be simple, due to the multiple side effects that impaired quality of life. Thus, the cost-effectiveness of the treatment was justified mainly for high risk patients.

Surprisingly, during this period, most of the information about blood pressure on the population level, and associated risks of morbidity and mortality, was accumulated by insurance companies and these data were evaluated by physicians and medical statisticians employed by these companies. The insurance viewpoint of an impairment differs from the clinical viewpoint, yet they do not contradict one another. Clinical studies and insurance medicine benefited greatly from each other, and this was true in the early 1900s as it is today. The difference between the approaches is that insurance medicine deals mainly with data of large groups, while clinical medicine focuses on individuals. However, to benefit individuals, clinical medicine needs information about morbidity and mortality in large populations [23]. Life insurance companies mainly study mortality, but also morbidity. Clearly, all people die eventually, but insurance companies determine the longevity of subgroups of populations and correlate them with various medical conditions. Clinical medicine deals more with quality of life, while insurance medicine deals with financial aspects of prognosis. Insurance companies deserve credit for most of the early knowledge that was available to clinicians regarding blood pressure levels and risk. We note that in the past, not all physicians had equipment for blood pressure measurement, nor knowledge of correctly measuring blood pressure.

To fully understand historical attitudes, we will briefly review the development of blood pressure measuring and the difficulties encountered in determining prehypertensive and hypertensive levels.

Sodium restriction was advocated after the role of sodium in hypertension was demonstrated in 1904, and the rice diet of Kempner was popularized in the early 1940s. Sodium thiocyanate was the first chemical substance to be used in the treatment of hypertension, by Treupel and Edinger in 1900, and later by Hines at the Mayo clinic; it was potentially toxic, side effects were many, and it subsequently became unpopular.

In 1978 the WHO defined hypertension as blood pressure levels above 160/95 mmHg, and normotension as levels less than 140/90 mmHg. Blood pressure levels between these two cutoff values were defined as borderline hypertension [23].

Many experts have defined borderline hypertension as intermittent blood pressure levels above 150 mmHg systolic or 90 mmHg diastolic pressure [24]. The Ann Arbor group previously defined borderline hypertension as at least one diastolic measurement below 90 mmHg diastolic among five blood pressure measurements [25]. Since arterial pressure increases with age, these definitions have their limitations. Thus, many investigators have defined target blood pressure ranges according to age groups. Such definition disregards the presence or absence of end-organ damage. In addition, transient elevations in blood pressure have raised debate as to whether these are sufficient to classify a person with borderline hypertension. Moreover, different terminologies have been used, such as the term "labile hypertension," which implies increased blood pressure variability. Furthermore, several studies have demonstrated a lack of correlation between the absolute level of blood pressure and its variability. Blood pressure has been shown to fluctuate in normotensive individuals also. Considering the above, it is not surprising that excessive variability of blood pressure has never been established as a feature of borderline hypertension [25]. The five highest and five lowest blood pressure measurements during a 24 h recording were shown not to correlate to cardiovascular morbidity, while average blood pressure levels carry with them important predictive power [26].

The term prehypertension signifies a condition that most always leads to hypertension. Thus, this diagnosis indicates increased risk of cardiovascular morbidity and mortality. Patients should be informed of their condition, and encouraged to make every effort to change their destiny, by adopting measures that will lower blood pressure and protect them from developing hypertension.

Over the years, the definition of hypertension has changed quite frequently and the definition of prehypertension has changed accordingly. The recent AHA 2017 definition actually added the 130–140/80–90 mmHg range, which was previously classified as prehypertension, to the hypertensive range, with the diagnostic and therapeutic implications of such [22]. Defining the limits of prehypertension and hypertension is problematic since there is no dispute that arterial pressure is a continuous variable and when converted to a logarithmic scale is Gaussian in shape.

The most recent definition of the AHA will likely be disputed by many, and probably by the upcoming guidelines of the European Society of Hypertension, which are currently being finalized. Nonetheless, as mentioned, the courageous definition of the ACC/AHA is not new. In 1930, this was the definition stated by Dr. Lewellys S. Barker of Johns Hopkins University [16]. Dr. Barker stated that "In adults, systolic blood pressure about 140 mm in the male and above 130 in the female, when it is more than transitory from physical exertion or emotional excitement, is looked upon as a pathological increase."

Since blood pressure measuring was deemed compulsory in all insurance policies, huge amounts of data about blood pressure levels and outcomes have accumulated. The average blood pressure of all adults of all ages has been found in life insurance examinations to be 127 mm systolic and 83.5 mm diastolic [16]. From outcome insurance information, the lowest mortality was shown in persons with levels somewhat lower than the average. Sir Thomas Lewis stated in 1933 that in healthy individuals, a blood pressure level below average is an asset, from the standpoint of longevity. Due to the very high relevance of blood pressure level to predicting morbidity and mortality, insurance companies established tables of mean blood pressure measurements according to age groups and their correlation to health and survival outcomes.

The increase in average blood pressure with age is well known, as is the correlation of average blood pressure at various age groups with life expectancy. However, based on insurance company data, if blood pressure remains stable for 20, or even 15 years, then at age 60 years, our prospect for a longer life will be correspondingly increased [16].

Blood pressure reduction was not always considered beneficial. The body build and blood pressure study, performed by the US Society of Actuaries in 1939, showed that among persons with diastolic blood pressure of 88–92 mmHg, mortality was 100% above the average risk for the population. Thus, they concluded that blood pressure lowering may be advantageous [27]. However, during those years (the early 1940s) the prevailing concept of essential hypertension was that blood pressure elevation was essential to perfusion of various organs. An increase in blood pressure was considered a compensatory reflex regulation to preserve tissue perfusion. Thus, interfering with this reflex was considered as impairing tissue perfusion and to be potentially deleterious [28].

The use of ganglion blockers caused several problems. A search was undertaken for patients with stable, severe hypertension for treatment. Treatment of severe hypertension with those "toxic" drugs was limited to patients with "true" hypertension. Patients with labile hypertension were not considered for this treatment because they did not have "established" hypertension [29]. They were assumed to have excessive blood pressure variability, a statement that was never proven. In 1945, Levy et al. showed that transient hypertension predicts future established hypertension with end-organ damage and the development of cardiovascular events [29].

Another problematic matter regarding the treatment of hypertension during the middle of the last century was the idea that patients with labile hypertension were only "nervous" and that tachycardia is a good marker for their nervousness. It is evident today, as it was in the past, that prehypertension and tachycardia are strong predictors of negative outcomes and that they are present in a large proportion of the population.

In recent years three major studies evaluated the benefit of treating patients with blood pressure in the prehypertensive range. The TROPHY trial [18] was designed to investigate whether pharmacologic treatment of prehypertension prevents or postpones stage 1 hypertension. Individuals with systolic blood pressure of 130–159 and diastolic blood pressure of 85–90 mmHg were randomized to 2-year treatment with candesartan or a placebo, followed by 2 years of treatment of a placebo to both groups. When participants reached hypertension, antihypertensive treatment was initiated. After 4 years, hypertension occurred less in the treatment group. Treatment during 2 of the 4 follow-up years resulted in a lower incidence of hypertension [18, 30].

The ACCORD study aimed to determine the target range of blood pressure. A total of 4753 diabetic patients were randomized to two groups. One group was treated with standard therapy that targeted systolic pressure to levels of 140 mmHg and below, while in the second group, blood pressure levels were targeted to less than 120 mmHg. The mean follow-up period in both groups was 4.7 years. The findings of the study showed that for patients with type 2 diabetes at high risk for cardiovascular events, targeting a systolic blood pressure of less than 120 mmHg compared to less than 140 mmHg did not reduce the rate of the composite outcome of fatal and nonfatal cardiovascular events [20].

The SPRINT study [21] also aimed to identify the most appropriate target range of systolic blood pressure to reduce cardiovascular morbidity and mortality, albeit in a larger sample (9361 persons) than the ACCORD study, and among persons without diabetes [21]. The results showed that among persons with systolic blood pressure of 130 mmHg or higher, and with elevated cardiovascular risk but without diabetes, targeting a systolic blood pressure of less than 120 mmHg, compared with less than 140 mmHg, yielded lower rates of fatal and nonfatal major cardiovascular events and death from any cause, although significantly higher rates of some adverse events were observed in the intensive treatment groups [21].

In summary: About 100 years ago, elevated blood pressure was considered a natural compensatory phenomenon that preserved tissue perfusion. However, clinical evidence and research subsequently proved otherwise: elevated blood pressure has become recognized as a cardiovascular risk factor, and treatment of hypertension has been shown to reduce cardiovascular morbidity and mortality.

Several erroneous concepts have hindered the understanding of the development of hypertension and its progression through the stage of prehypertension. Only after many years did physicians finally recognize the importance of tachycardia, which had been interpreted as a sign of "nervousness." The importance of this marker, which implies sympathetic activation that leads to the development of hypertension, was ignored. Another wrong concept was the notion of "labile" versus "established" hypertension, which led to the idea that hypertension is due to overreaction to stress and that repeated episodes of elevated blood pressure are markers of the future development of established hypertension.

Since cardiovascular risk is greater in patients with severe hypertension than prehypertension, during a time period in which only limited therapeutic options were available, and such options were associated with substantial side effects, it was only natural that the main effort of "salvage of end organs" from hypertension focused on patients with severe and established hypertension. However, with the emergence of effective medications with minimal side effects, addressing prehypertension is recognized as important and feasible, for the prevention of future cardiovascular disease.

References

1. Levy RL, White PD, Stroud WD. Transient tachycardia. Prognostic significance alone and in association with transient hypertension. JAMA. 1945;129(9):585–8.
2. Huang Y, Wang S, Cai X, et al. Prehypertension and incidence of cardiovascular disease: a meta-analysis. BMC Med. 2013;11:177.
3. Ruskin A. Classics in arterial hypertension. Springfield, IL: Charles C Thomas; 1956.
4. Freis ED. Origins and development of antihypertensive treatment. In: Laragh JH, Brenner BM, editors. Hypertension: pathophysiology, diagnosis, and management. New York: Raven Press; 1990. p. 2093–4.
5. Hippocrates. Genuine works of Hippocrates, translated by Adams F. London: Sydenham Society; 1949.
6. Galen C. Introduction in Pulsus ad teuthram, interpreted by Gregory M. London: Guliel Rovillius; 1959.
7. Final Report of the Subcommittee on Definition and Prevalence of the 1984 Joint National Committee. Hypertension prevalence and the status of awareness, treatment and control in the United States. Hypertension. 1985;7:457–68.
8. Chobanian AV, Bakris GL, Black HR, et al. For the Joint National Committee. The seventh report of the joint National Committee Report on prehypertension detection, evaluation and treatment of high blood pressure. The JNC VII report. JAMA. 2003;289:2560–72.
9. Esunge PM. From blood pressure to hypertension: the history of research. J R Soc Med. 1991;84:621.
10. Dustan HP, Schneckloth RE, Corcoran AC, Page IH. The effectiveness of long-term treatment of malignant hypertension. Circulation. 1958;18(4 Part 1):644–51.
11. Veterans Administration Cooperative Study Group on Antihypertensive Agents. Effects of treatment on morbidity and mortality in hypertension: I. Results in patients with diastolic blood pressure averaging 115–129 mmHg. JAMA. 1967;202:116–22.

12. Murphy EA. The normal and the perils of sylleptic argument. Perspect Biol Med. 1972;15:566–82.
13. Freitag MH, Vasan RS. What is normal blood pressure? Curr Opin Nephrol Hypertens. 2003;12:285–92.
14. Lewington S, Clarke R, Qizibash N, et al. Age-specific relevance of usual blood pressure to vascular mortality. Lancet. 2002;360:1903–13.
15. Chobanian AV. Guidelines for the management of hypertension. Med Clin N Am. 2017;101:219–27.
16. Livingston JM. Blood pressure, normal and abnormal. Can Med Assoc J. 1934;30(1):54–7.
17. Folkov B. Physiological aspects of primary hypertension. Physiol Rev. 1982;62:347–504.
18. Julius S, Nesbitt SD, Egan BM, et al. For the trial of preventing hypertension (TROPHY) Study Investigators. Feasibility of treating prehypertension with an angiotensin receptor blocker. N Engl J Med. 2006;354:1685–97.
19. Luders S, Schrader J, Berger J, et al. PHARAO Study Group. The PHARAO study: prevention of hypertension with the angiotensin-converting enzyme inhibitor ramipril in patients with high-normal blood pressure: a prospective, randomized controlled prevention trial of the German Hypertension League. J Hypertens. 2008:26:1487–96.
20. The ACCORD Study Group. Effect of intensive blood pressure control in type 2 diabetes mellitus. N Engl J Med. 2010;362:1575–85.
21. The SPRINT Research Group. A randomized trial of intensive versus standard blood pressure control. N Engl J Med. 2015;373:2103–16.
22. Whelton PK, Carey RM, Aronov WS, et al. ACC/AHA/AAPA/ABC/ACPM/AGS/APHA/ASH/ASPC/NMA/PCNA Guidelines for the Prevention, Detection, Evaluation and Management of High blood Pressure in Adults: A Report of the American College of Cardiology/American Heart Association Task Force on Clinical Practice Guidelines. Hypertension, Published online November 13, 2017. http://hyper.Ahajonrnals.Org/early/2017/11/10hgp.0000000000000066.
23. The 1984 report of the Joint National Committee on Detection, Evaluation and Treatment of high blood pressure. Arch Intern Med. 1984;144:1045–57.
24. World Health Organization: Report of a WHO Expert committee. Arterial hypertension. WHO Techn Rep Ser, 628; 1978.
25. Takeshita A, Mark AL. Decreased venous distensibility in borderline hypertension. Hypertension. 1979;1:202.
26. Julius S, Hanson L, Andrew L, Gnbrandsson T, Sivertsson R, Svensson A. Borderline hypertension. Acta Med Scand. 1980;208:481–9.
27. Body build and blood pressure study—US Society of Actuaries 1939.
28. Hay J. The significance of a raised blood pressure. Br Med J. 1931;3679:43–7.
29. Levy RL, White PD, Stroud WD, Hillman CC. Transient tachycardia. JAMA. 1945;129(9):585–60.
30. Julius S, Kacirot N, Egan BM, Nesbitt S, Michelson EL. For the trial of prevention of hypertension (TROPHY) Investigators. TROPHY study: outcomes based on the seventh report of the Joint National Committee on Hypertension definition of hypertension. J Am Soc Hypertens. 2008;2(1):39–43.

3 Parental History of Hypertension as the Determinant of Cardiovascular Function

Katarzyna Stolarz-Skrzypek and Danuta Czarnecka

Parents' health influences the overall, including cardiovascular, health of their offspring, and the effect of a genetic basis and positive family history exists in the development of cardiometabolic risk in children [1]. Offspring usually imitate the unhealthy lifestyle habits of their parents, such as an unbalanced diet, smoking, and physical inactivity, and such shared family habits can also lead to an increased risk for cardiometabolic diseases.

Determination of blood pressure in related and unrelated individuals in a Tecumseh community and calculation of heritability have suggested that genetic components and shared household environment contribute to familial aggregation of blood pressure elevation [2]. Blood pressure correlation between parents and biological offspring ($r = 0.32$ for systolic and $r = 0.37$ for diastolic blood pressure) was significantly closer than that between parents and adopted offspring ($r = 0.09$ and $r = 0.10$, respectively, for systolic and diastolic blood pressure) [3].

In the European Project on Genes in Hypertension (EPOGH) the investigators reported high heritability of various other cardiovascular phenotypes, including left ventricular mass [4], left ventricular diastolic function [5], and vascular properties [6].

In the recent years, the number of evidence has been accumulated that the unfavorable change in the cardiovascular structure and function precede the development of hypertension among the offspring of hypertensive parents.

K. Stolarz-Skrzypek (✉) · D. Czarnecka
First Department of Cardiology, Interventional Electrocardiology and Hypertension, Jagiellonian University Medical College, Krakow, Poland
e-mail: katarzyna.stolarz-skrzypek@uj.edu.pl

R. Zimlichman et al. (eds.), *Prehypertension and Cardiometabolic Syndrome*, Updates in Hypertension and Cardiovascular Protection,
https://doi.org/10.1007/978-3-319-75310-2_3

3.1 Blood Pressure

Associations of parental hypertension with blood pressure elevation in offspring have been indicated by number of cross-sectional studies.

Subjects with a family history of parental hypertension are reported to have a slightly higher office blood pressure in the prehypertensive stage [7].

In an early study by Parati et al., normotensive subjects with both parents hypertensive were characterized by a significant although mild increase in their blood pressure values recorded either at rest and in ambulatory conditions over the 24 h, including night sleep, as compared to normotensive subjects with one parent hypertensive or normotensive subjects with no parental hypertension [8].

In a cross-sectional sample of 217 men and 196 women, selected from the general Caucasian population of Rochester, Minnesota, in the multivariate analyses, paternal but not maternal history of hypertension contributed to the probability of having hypertension in men. Neither paternal nor maternal history of hypertension made a statistically significant contribution to the probability of having hypertension in women [9].

Overwhelming evidence has been recently provided by the longitudinal studies.

In a study by Burke et al., by the time offspring were aged 9 years, systolic blood pressure was significantly higher in sons and daughters of hypertensive fathers than it was in sons and daughters of normotensive fathers. When they were aged 18 years, paternal hypertension predicted blood pressures in men and women independently of their weight at birth, fitness, alcohol consumption and weight for height for age. Systolic blood pressures increased more rapidly (by 0.6 mmHg/year) in men with hypertensive fathers [10].

Van den Elzen et al. examined the relationship between natural history of blood pressure in children aged 5–19 years and level of blood pressure in their parents. Cardiovascular risk factors were measured annually from 1975 through 2002. Repeated blood pressure measurements were studied as a function of tertiles of age-adjusted blood pressure measured in their parents at baseline. They found that systolic blood pressure was consistently higher by 2.7 mmHg from the age of 5 years to the age of 40 years in subjects with parents in the highest tertile of systolic blood pressure, whereas such a parallel shift was not observed for diastolic blood pressure [11].

Wang et al. recruited university students, but they used only data from white men in their analysis. The blood pressure–age relationship within the age range of 20–80 years was shifted upward by ≈2 mmHg in subjects with a parental history of hypertension compared with that in subjects without a parental history [12].

The effects of parental hypertension on longitudinal trends of blood pressure were examined in 2607 subjects (1095 men and 1512 women) who participated in the Tanno-Sobetsu Study from 1977 to 2006. In both men and women with and without parental hypertension, systolic blood pressure increased from the third to eighth decades of life, whereas diastolic blood pressure followed biphasic (inverted U shape) time course during that period. However, the relationships between the parameters and age were significantly shifted upward (by ≈5.3 mm Hg in systolic blood pressure, 2.8 mmHg in diastolic blood pressure) in the group with parental hypertension compared with those in the group without parental hypertension. Both paternal and maternal histories of hypertension were determinants of systolic blood pressure and diastolic blood pressure, and there was no significant interaction between the sides of parental history [13].

3.2 Heart and Vessels

Available evidence is relatively small with regard to morphological and functional changes in the left ventricle in subjects with positive family history of hypertension.

In the Strong Heart Study there was shown a significantly higher thickness of intraventricular septum and left ventricular mass in adolescents and young adults with normal and high normal blood pressure compared to individuals with optimal blood pressure [14].

In the case–control study of normotensive men with positive family history of hypertension and their counterparts without such family history, parental hypertension was independently associated with higher left ventricular relative wall thickness, an early index of concentric remodeling [15].

Furthermore, Grandi et al. showed that normotensive young adults with high genetic risk for hypertension (two parents hypertensive) have higher blood pressure and thicker and overactive left ventricle as compared to subjects with normotensive parents. Handgrip stimulated left ventricular function in offspring of normotensives, but not the already hyperkinetic left ventricle of offspring of hypertensive parents [16].

Moreover, in the Hypertension Genetic Epidemiologic Network (HyperGEN) it was shown that in this large, population-based cohort of nonhypertensive offspring of hypertensive parents, ethnic differences in hemodynamic and echocardiographic profiles exist. Nonhypertensive African American offspring had more abnormalities in left ventricular function than their white counterparts. The authors postulated that these abnormalities may be a precursor of the observed earlier appearance of cardiovascular disease in African Americans compared with whites [17].

In the study by Zizek et al., in normotensive individuals with family history of hypertension, left ventricular morphological and functional changes were found. Offspring of hypertensive families had higher left ventricular mass index and worse left ventricular diastolic function than control subjects (lower E/A ratio, lower E(m) and E(m)/A(m) ratio). Moreover, it was demonstrated that an increase in left ventricular mass and alterations in left ventricular diastolic function are related to endothelial dysfunction [18].

Among individuals recruited for the Bergen Blood Pressure Study, offspring of hypertensive families had lower transmitral early/late peak flow velocities and higher transmitral late peak flow velocities than offspring of normotensive families, but the differences between groups became inconsistent after adjustment for confounding variables (including left ventricular structural parameters). On the other hand, the family history of hypertension was consistently associated with increased transmitral early peak flow velocity and increased transmitral acceleration and deceleration slopes, a pattern suggesting increased left ventricular stiffness [19].

Increased carotid intima-media thickness is considered as an early and valuable cardiovascular risk marker. However, information about the impact of the family burden of hypertension on the remodeling of large vessels in young healthy people are limited.

In the study by Cuomo et al., carried out in 29 participants with parental history of hypertension, higher values of carotid intima-media thickness were found compared to offspring of normotensive parents, also after accounting for blood pressure, body mass index, smoking, lipid levels, apolipoproteins, and lipoprotein (a) [20].

In offspring aged 14–30 years, central augmentation index assessed with SphygmoCor device was significantly higher in subjects with at least one hypertensive parent, after adjusting for sex, age, body mass index, heart rate, smoking cigarettes, total serum cholesterol, and C-reactive protein [21].

Augmentation index, but not brachial pulse wave velocity, was reported as significantly higher in middle-aged offspring of hypertensive parents compared with control subjects [22].

Rajzer et al. in a group of 70 young adults with normal blood pressure after accounting for confounding factors did not find any difference in carotid-femoral pulse wave velocity in relation to family history of hypertension [23].

In a case–control study of 67 normotensive children whose parents had a diagnosis of essential hypertension and 39 normotensive children with no parental history of hypertension, carotid intima-media thickness were significantly different in the study group compared with the control group among all age groups. Aortic systolic and diastolic diameters were larger in normotensive children of hypertensive parents compared with the control group [24].

In the EPOGH cohort, normotensive offspring who had at least one hypertensive parent as compared to normotensive offspring of two normotensive parents had higher central augmentation index and pulse wave velocity. However, complex adjustment including mean arterial pressure and age removed the differences between the offspring in the measures of arterial stiffness [6].

In a sample of 1564 nonhypertensive Framingham Heart Study third-generation cohort participants (mean age: 38 years; 55% women) whose parents were enrolled in the Framingham Offspring Study, parental hypertension was associated with greater offspring mean arterial pressure and with greater forward pressure wave amplitude. Carotid-femoral pulse wave velocity and augmentation index displayed similar dose-dependent relations with parental hypertension in sex-, age-, and height-adjusted models, but associations were attenuated on further adjustment. Offspring with at least one parent in the upper quartile of augmentation index and carotid-femoral pulse wave velocity had significantly higher values themselves. These observations are consistent with higher vascular stiffness at an early stage in the pathogenesis of hypertension [25].

Gopinath et al. showed that a positive parental history of hypertension in healthy prepubertal girls, but not boys, is associated with narrower retinal arteriolar vessels, likely conveying a predisposition to develop hypertension later in life [26].

3.3 Biochemical Disturbances and Life Style

Accumulating epidemiological studies have shown that healthy offspring of hypertensive patients exhibit some metabolic disturbances such as hyperinsulinemia, insulin resistance, lipid disorders, elevated plasma leptin levels, and reduced insulin receptor number, features that may be predictors of future cardiovascular events.

A Japanese study showed that a maternal history of hypertension was significantly associated with the risk of overweight in children [27].

Normotensive adolescent offspring with hypertensive parents were found to have significantly higher serum insulin levels, which indicates that insulin resistance precedes the onset of clinical hypertension in persons genetically predisposed to hypertension [28].

Over 10 years of follow-up of 557 young, nonobese Japanese men who were normotensive at entry, development of hyperinsulinemia was more pronounced in the subjects with a positive family history of hypertension [29].

Furuhashi et al. observed that plasma level of adiponectin, a biomarker correlating with insulin sensitivity, was lower in young men with a parental history of hypertension [30].

Moreover, it was demonstrated that number of insulin receptors is reduced in the erythrocytes of healthy offspring of hypertensive patients in comparison to the offspring of healthy normotensive subjects [31].

Papadopoulos et al. showed that insulin and resistin plasma levels were significantly higher, while adiponectin levels were significantly lower in 18 years old healthy offspring of patients with essential hypertension-positive family history [32].

A recent study in 554 Korean adolescents aged 13–19 years showed that a parental history of hypertension indicates a greater risk for elevated alanine transaminase (ALT) in teenagers, suggestive of nonalcoholic fatty liver disease (NAFLD) [33].

In the long-term observation of the Bogalusa Heart Study, the offspring of hypertensive parents displayed overweight regardless of age, higher levels of blood pressure after age 10 years, and elevations of triglycerides and VLDL cholesterol after age 24 years irrespective of weight [34].

Some groups also reported elevated total serum cholesterol [35] and higher serum glucose [36] in offspring of hypertensive as compared to offspring of normotensive parents.

In the Odense Schoolchild Study, children aged 8–10 years with a parental history of hypertension displayed a significant decrease in physical fitness and a significant increase in obesity and systolic and diastolic blood pressure compared with the rest of the population. After controlling for differences in body size and physical fitness, they also showed significantly higher levels of systolic and diastolic blood pressure [37].

Shook et al. studied fitness and incident hypertension in 6278 participants who were given a preventative medical examination. Thirty-three percent reported a parent with hypertension, and there were 1545 cases of incident hypertension after a mean of 4.7 years. Individuals with both a low level of fitness and a parent with hypertension exhibited a 70% higher risk for developing hypertension compared with high-fit individuals with no parental history. However, individuals with a high level of fitness and a parent with hypertension only experienced a 16% higher risk of developing hypertension compared with fit individuals with no parental history. This significantly lower risk of developing hypertension when progressing from low- to high-fit groups among those with a parental history of hypertension has important clinical implications [38].

3.4 Cardiovascular Regulation

To investigate whether parental hypertension affects children's cardiovascular reactivity over time, a longitudinal study of 315 students was conducted in the public schools of Obion County, Tennessee. The CVR task was a series of video games (taking approximately 10 min to play) given to the same students in their third-, fourth-, fifth-, seventh-, and eighth-grade years. Cardiovascular reactivity was defined as the change in blood pressure or heart rate between before playing and while playing the video game. Increased cardiovascular reactivity was observed in children with parental hypertension compared with children without parental hypertension but was statistically significant only for systolic blood pressure after adjustment for covariates [39].

Among 220 healthy men and women, aged 22–50 years, who completed two 24 h ambulatory blood pressure monitoring sessions, women with two hypertensive parents and elevated norepinephrine levels had higher systolic and diastolic blood pressure during waking and sleep periods. In men the combination of two hypertensive parents and high norepinephrine was related only to diastolic blood pressure during waking [40].

In a case–control study, Pitzalis et al. noticed a shorter resting RR interval and a blunted autonomic modulation of heart rate among offspring of hypertensive parents [41]. In line with this case–control study, in a population-based family study we found among subjects with a positive family history of hypertension a shorter RR interval and a diminished regulation of autonomic balance upon standing [42].

3.5 Impact of Hypertensive Disorders of Pregnancy

An accumulating body of evidence suggests that offspring of mothers with preeclampsia have higher blood pressure during childhood and young adulthood compared with offspring of women without preeclampsia.

In the data for mother-offspring pairs from a United Kingdom prospective birth cohort (the Avon Longitudinal Study of Parents and Children), systolic and diastolic blood pressures were higher in offspring of mothers with gestational hypertension (mean difference, 2.06 mmHg) and preeclampsia (1.12 mmHg) compared with offspring of mothers without hypertensive disorders of pregnancy, adjusting for potential confounders (age, sex, maternal age at delivery, household social class, prepregnancy body mass index, parity, and smoking in pregnancy) [43].

Also in a subsample of 2608 mother-offspring pairs followed for 21 years from an original cohort of 7223 singleton infants whose mothers gave birth in Brisbane, Australia, between 1981 and 1983, unadjusted regression analysis showed that offspring of women who experienced hypertensive disorder of pregnancy have 3.46 mmHg greater systolic and 3.02 mmHg greater diastolic blood pressure at 21 years. This association remained consistent after adjusting for potential confounding and mediating factors including offspring gender, age, percentile birth weight for gestation, placenta weight and body mass index at 21 year, maternal age, education, racial origin, and smoking during pregnancy and their prepregnancy body mass index [44].

Adolescent offspring exposed to maternal preeclampsia have greater relative wall thickness and reduced left ventricular end-diastolic volume, which could be early signs of concentric remodeling and affect future cardiac function as well as risk of cardiovascular disease [45].

According to the recent meta-analysis, maternal hypertensive disorders do appear to be associated with adverse changes in cardiovascular risk in adult offspring, including raised body mass index, overweight and obesity and higher blood pressure. These findings are consistent with those from studies of offspring childhood and early adulthood. This supports the hypothesis that the offspring of women with hypertensive disorders in pregnancy have a risk of clinical cardiometabolic events later in life, including hypertension and stroke [46].

Conclusion

Evaluating the history of parental hypertension could be helpful in predicting offspring with a higher risk of developing cardiometabolic diseases, even in the preclinical stage. The collection of parental history of hypertension should also include the information concerning hypertensive disorders of pregnancy in the mother.

Offspring of hypertensive parents are characterized by elevated blood pressure, alterations in cardiac and arterial structure and function, and biochemical disturbances, even before the development of sustained hypertension. Therefore, preventive measures of and early intervention for cardiometabolic risk in individuals with parental hypertension should be reinforced, with particular attention towards offspring of both hypertensive parents.

References

1. Steinberger J, Daniels SR. American Heart Association Atherosclerosis, Hypertension, and Obesity in the Young Committee (Council on Cardiovascular Disease in the Young); American Heart Association Diabetes Committee (Council on Nutrition, Physical Activity, and Metabolism). Circulation. 2003;107(10):1448–53.
2. Longini IM Jr, Higgins MW, Hinton PC, Moll PP, Keller JB. Environmental and genetic sources of familial aggregation of blood pressure in Tecumseh, Michigan. Am J Epidemiol. 1984;120:131–44.
3. Biron P, Mongeau JG, Bertrand D. Familial aggregation of blood pressure in 558 adopted children. Can Med Assoc J. 1976;115:773–4.

4. Kuznetsova T, Staessen JA, Olszanecka A, Ryabikov A, Stolarz K, Malyutina S, Fagard R, Kawecka-Jaszcz K, Nikitin Y. European Project on Genes in Hypertension (EPOGH) Investigators. Maternal and paternal influences on left ventricular mass of offspring. Hypertension. 2003;41(1):69–74.
5. Kloch-Badelek M, Knez J, Tikhonoff V, Thijs L, Sakiewicz W, Ryabikov A, Stolarz-Skrzypek K, Jin Y, Malyutina S, Casiglia E, Narkiewicz K, Czarnecka D, Kawecka-Jaszcz K, Staessen JA, Kuznetsova T. European Project on Genes in Hypertension (EPOGH) Investigators. Heritability and other determinants of left ventricular diastolic function in the family-based population study. J Hypertens. 2014;32(9):1854–61.
6. Kucerová J, Filipovský J, Staessen JA, Cwynar M, Wojciechowska W, Stolarz K, Kuznetsova T, Gasowski J, Dolejsová M, Grodzicki T, Kawecka-Jaszcz K, Fagard R. Arterial characteristics in normotensive offspring of parents with or without a history of hypertension. Am J Hypertens. 2006;19(3):264–9.
7. Ravogli A, Trazzi S, Villani A, Mutti E, Cuspidi C, Sampieri L, De Ambroggi L, Parati G, Zanchetti A, Mancia G. Early 24-hour blood pressure elevation in normotensive subjects with parental hypertension. Hypertension. 1990;16:491–7.
8. Parati G, Ravogli A, Giannattasio C, et al. Changes in 24 hour blood pressure and in cardiac and vascular structure in normotensive subjects with parental hypertension. Clin Exp Hypertens A. 1992;14:67–83.
9. Rebbeck TR, Turner ST, Sing CF. Probability of having hypertension: effects of sex, history of hypertension in parents, and other risk factors. J Clin Epidemiol. 1996;49:727–34.
10. Burke V, Gracey MP, Beilin LJ, Milligan RA. Family history as a predictor of blood pressure in a longitudinal study of Australian children. J Hypertens. 1998;16:269–76.
11. van den Elzen AP, de Ridder MA, Grobbee DE, Hofman A, Witteman JC, Uiterwaal CS. Families and the natural history of blood pressure: a 27-year follow-up study. Am J Hypertens. 2004;17:936–40.
12. Wang NY, Young JH, Meoni LA, Ford DE, Erlinger TP, Klag MJ. Blood pressure change and risk of hypertension associated with parental hypertension: the Johns Hopkins Precursors Study. Arch Intern Med. 2008;168:643–8.
13. Mitsumata K, Saitoh S, Ohnishi H, Akasaka H, Miura T. Effects of parental hypertension on longitudinal trends in blood pressure and plasma metabolic profile: mixed-effects model analysis. Hypertension. 2012 Nov;60(5):1124–30.
14. Drukteinis JS, Roman MJ, Fabsitz RR, Lee ET, Best LG, Russell M, Devereux RB. Cardiac and systemic hemodynamic characteristics of hypertension and prehypertension in adolescents and young adults: the Strong Heart Study. Circulation. 2007;115:221–7.
15. Pelà G, Pattoneri P, Passera M, Li Calzi M, Goldoni M, Tirabassi G, Montanari A. Normotensive male offspring of essential hypertensive parents show early changes in left ventricular geometry independent of blood pressure. Echocardiography. 2011;28(8):821–8.
16. Grandi AM, Poletti L, Tettamanti F, Finardi G, Venco A. Left ventricular anatomy and function in normotensive young adults with hypertensive parents. Study at rest and during handgrip. Am J Hypertens. 1995;8:154–9.
17. Glasser SP, Lynch AI, Devereux RB, Hopkins P, Arnett DK. Hemodynamic and echocardiographic profiles in African American compared with White offspring of hypertensive parents: the HyperGEN study. Am J Hypertens. 2014;27(1):21–6.
18. Zizek B, Poredos P. Increased left ventricular mass and diastolic dysfunction are associated with endothelial dysfunction in normotensive offspring of subjects with essential hypertension. Blood Press. 2007;16(1):36–44.
19. Mo R, Nordrehaug JE, Omvik P, Lund-Johansen P. The Bergen Blood Pressure Study: prehypertensive changes in cardiac structure and function in offspring of hypertensive families. Blood Press. 1995;4:16–22.
20. Cuomo S, Gaeta G, Guarini P, et al. Increased carotid intima-media thickness in healthy young subjects with a parental history of hypertension (parental hypertension and vascular health). Heart. 2007;93:368–9.

21. Kyvelou SM, Vyssoulis GP, Karpanou EA, Adamopoulos DN, Deligeorgis AD, Cokkinos DV, Stefanadis CI. Arterial stiffness in offspring of hypertensive parents: a pilot study. Int J Cardiol. 2007;129:438–40.
22. Yasmin FR, Brown MJ. Determinants of arterial stiffness in offspring of families with essential hypertension. Am J Hypertens. 2004;17:292–8.
23. Rajzer MW, Klocek M, Kawecka-Jaszcz K, Czarnecka D, Baran W, Dudek K, Petriczek T. Aortic pulse wave velocity in young normotensives with a family history of hypertension. J Hypertens. 1999;17:1821–4.
24. Yildirim A, Kosger P, Ozdemir G, Sahin FM, Ucar B, Kilic Z. Carotid intima-media thickness and elastic properties of aortas in normotensive children of hypertensive parents. Hypertens Res. 2015 Sep;38(9):621–6.
25. Andersson C, Quiroz R, Enserro D, Larson MG, Hamburg NM, Vita JA, Levy D, Benjamin EJ, Mitchell GF, Vasan RS. Association of parental hypertension with arterial stiffness in nonhypertensive offspring: the Framingham Heart Study. Hypertension. 2016;68(3):584–9.
26. Gopinath B, Baur LA, Hardy LL, Wang JJ, Teber E, Wong TY, Mitchell P. Parental history of hypertension is associated with narrower retinal arteriolar caliber in young girls. Hypertension. 2011;58:425–30.
27. Liu J, Sekine M, Tatsuse T, Hamanishi S, Fujimura Y, Zheng X. Family history of hypertension and the risk of overweight in Japanese children: results from the Toyama Birth Cohort Study. J Epidemiol. 2014;24(4):304–11.
28. Grunfeld B, Balzareti M, Romo M, Gimenez M, Gutman R. Hyperinsulinemia in normotensive offspring of hypertensive parents. Hypertension. 1994;23(1 Suppl):I12–5.
29. Masuo K, Mikami H, Ogihara T, Tuck ML. Familial hypertension, insulin, sympathetic activity, and blood pressure elevation. Hypertension. 1998;32:96–100.
30. Furuhashi M, Ura N, Higasiura K, Shimamoto K, Miyazaki Y, Murakami H, Hyakukoku M. Low adiponectin level in young normotensive men with a family history of essential hypertension. Hypertens Res. 2005;28:141–6.
31. Makris TA, Paizis I, Krespi PG, Stavroulakis GA, Papazachou OG, Papadopoulos DP, Hatzizacharias AN, Votteas VV. Insulin receptor number is reduced in healthy offspring of patients with essential hypertension. Am J Hypertens. 2004;17(10):911–4.
32. Papadopoulos DP, Makris TK, Perrea D, Papazachou O, Daskalaki M, Sanidas E, Votteas V. Adiponectin—insulin and resistin plasma levels in young healthy offspring of patients with essential hypertension. Blood Press. 2008;17(1):50–4.
33. Yoo JE, Park HS. Relationship between parental hypertension and cardiometabolic risk factors in adolescents. J Clin Hypertens (Greenwich). 2017;19:678. https://doi.org/10.1111/jch.12991.
34. Bao W, Srinivasan SR, Wattigney WA, Berenson GS. The relation of parental cardiovascular disease to risk factors in children and young adults. The Bogalusa Heart Study. Circulation. 1995;91(2):365–71.
35. Neutel JM, Smith DH, Graettinger WF, Winer RL, Weber MA. Heredity and hypertension: impact on metabolic characteristics. Am Heart J. 1992;124:435–40.
36. Zizek B, Poredos P, Trojar A, Zeljko T. Diastolic dysfunction is associated with insulin resistance, but not with aldosterone level in normotensive offspring of hypertensive families. Cardiology. 2008;111:8–15.
37. Hansen HS, Nielsen JR, Hyldebrandt N, Froberg K. Blood pressure and cardiac structure in children with a parental history of hypertension: the Odense Schoolchild Study. J Hypertens. 1992;10:677–82.
38. Shook RP, Lee DC, Sui X, Prasad V, Hooker SP, Church TS, Blair SN. Cardiorespiratory fitness reduces the risk of incident hypertension associated with a parental history of hypertension. Hypertension. 2012;59(6):1220–4.
39. Li R, Alpert BS, Walker SS, Somes GW. Longitudinal relationship of parental hypertension with body mass index, blood pressure, and cardiovascular reactivity in children. J Pediatr. 2007;150:498–502.

40. Goldstein IB, Shapiro D, Weiss RE. How family history and risk factors for hypertension relate to ambulatory blood pressure in healthy adults. J Hypertens. 2008;26:276–83.
41. Pitzalis MV, Iacoviello M, Massari F, Guida P, Romito R, Forleo C. Influence of gender and family history of hypertension on autonomic control of heart rate, diastolic function and brain natriuretic peptide. J Hypertens. 2001;19:143–8.
42. Stolarz K, Staessen JA, Kuznetsova T, Tikhonoff V, State D, Babeanu S, Casiglia E, Fagard RH, Kawecka-Jaszcz K, Nikitin Y. European Project on Genes in Hypertension (EPOGH) Investigators. Host and environmental determinants of heart rate and heart rate variability in four European populations. J Hypertens. 2003;21(3):525–35.
43. Fraser I, Nelson SM, MacDonald-Wallis C, Sattar N, Lawlor DA. Hypertensive disorders of pregnancy and cardiometabolic health in adolescent offspring. Hypertension. 2013;62(3):614–20.
44. Mamun AA, Kinarivala MK, O'Callaghan M, Williams G, Najman J, Callaway L. Does hypertensive disorder of pregnancy predict offspring blood pressure at 21 years? Evidence from a birth cohort study. J Hum Hypertens. 2012;26(5):288–94.
45. Timpka S, Macdonald-Wallis C, Hughes AD, Chaturvedi N, Franks PW, Lawlor DA, Fraser A. Hypertensive disorders of pregnancy and offspring cardiac structure and function in adolescence. J Am Heart Assoc. 2016;5(11):e003906.
46. Thoulass JC, Robertson L, Denadai L, Black C, Crilly M, Iversen L, Scott NW, Hannaford PC. Hypertensive disorders of pregnancy and adult offspring cardiometabolic outcomes: a systematic review of the literature and meta-analysis. J Epidemiol Community Health. 2016;70(4):414–22.

4 Prehypertension, the Risk of Hypertension and Events

Michael Doumas, Niki Katsiki, and Dimitri P. Mikhailidis

Highlights

- Prehypertension is a precursor of hypertension in a high proportion of individuals.
- Several factors may predispose to the development of prehypertension including uric acid, dietary salt intake, arterial stiffness, autonomic imbalance, obesity, and subclinical inflammation.
- Progression of prehypertension to hypertension has been associated with visceral abdominal fat, sympathetic overactivity, sympathovagal imbalance, endothelial dysfunction, impairment of coronary flow reserve, and metabolic syndrome. Age, gender, ethnicity, and baseline blood pressure may also affect the incidence of hypertension.
- Prehypertension is associated with increased risk for coronary heart disease, stroke, chronic kidney disease, and cardiovascular death, but not all-cause mortality.
- Lifestyle measures and antihypertensive drugs may delay or even prevent the progression of prehypertension to hypertension.

M. Doumas · N. Katsiki
Second Propedeutic Department of Internal Medicine, Medical School, Aristotle University of Thessaloniki, Hippocration Hospital, Thessaloniki, Greece

D. P. Mikhailidis (✉)
Department of Clinical Biochemistry, Royal Free Hospital Campus, University College London Medical School, University College London (UCL), London, UK

R. Zimlichman et al. (eds.), *Prehypertension and Cardiometabolic Syndrome*, Updates in Hypertension and Cardiovascular Protection,
https://doi.org/10.1007/978-3-319-75310-2_4

4.1 Introduction

The concept of "predisease" was first used over a century ago, when a "precancerous" state was described for several tumors, delineating the process from normal tissue morphology to neoplastic development [1–3]. The aim of the "predisease" term was mainly to identify malignancies at an earlier asymptomatic stage in an effort to attenuate the progression to overt disease through specific intervention.

The term "prehypertension" was first used by Robinson and Brucer in 1939 [4]. In a landmark study of 10,883 men and women living in Chicago, they evaluated a range of normal blood pressure (BP) and drew attention to a "danger zone" of BP at 120–139/80–89 mmHg. Participants with BP within this "danger zone" were designated as prehypertensive, stating that: "… there is a difference in the daily changing tensions of the vascular system in the healthy and in the prehypertensive person" and "… about 40% of the adult population is prehypertensive or hypertensive" [4].

The term prehypertension did not gain wide recognition and was almost forgotten for many decades until the Seventh Report of the Joint National Committee on Prevention, Detection, Evaluation and Treatment of High Blood Pressure (JNC-7) re-introduced the term at 2003 [5]. According to the JNC-7 report: "... prehypertension is not a disease category. Rather it is a designation chosen to identify individuals at high risk of developing hypertension, so that both patients and clinicians are alerted to this risk and encouraged to intervene and prevent or delay the disease from developing" [5]. Prehypertension is defined as systolic BP (SBP) values between 120 and 139 mmHg and/or diastolic BP (DBP) values between 80 and 89 mmHg. Prehypertension can be further categorized in stage I and stage II prehypertension (120–129 and/or 80–84 mmHg and 130–139 and/or 85–89 mmHg, respectively).

The relationship between BP and future cardiovascular (CV) events is continuous and graded [6]. Therefore, using a dichotomous approach (hypertension—normotension) or a trichotomous approach (hypertension—prehypertension—normotension) is arbitrary and can only be justified as the effort to draw the line for individuals who will benefit from an intervention. In order to use the "prehypertension" term as a clinically meaningful description of a group of individuals, three major requirements need to be fulfilled: (a) the risk of developing hypertension should be markedly higher in people with prehypertension compared with those without prehypertension, (b) the risk of future CV events should be substantially greater in prehypertensive compared with normotensive individuals, and (c) effective intervention (e.g., lifestyle modification or pharmacological therapy) should substantially reduce the detrimental consequences of prehypertension (the progression from prehypertension to hypertension and future CV events), with the benefits of intervention exceeding its harms.

This review aims to address and critically discuss the first two aspects: the progression from prehypertension to hypertension and the risk for future CV events conferred by prehypertension.

4.2 Progression from Prehypertension to Hypertension

Hypertension is a progressive disease with constant BP elevation over time, mainly due to structural and functional alterations of the vasculature [7]. The Framingham study offered significant information on the residual lifetime risk for developing hypertension in middle-aged individuals. Among 1298 participants aged 55–65 years, the residual lifetime risk for incident hypertension was 90% for both male and female participants, and for both 55- and 65-year-old participants at baseline [8]. In other words, almost all of us will develop hypertension if we live long enough. The real question is whether all individuals with normal BP are at the same risk to develop hypertension or patients with higher BP values (prehypertension) are at increased risk for incident hypertension compared with lower BP (optimal BP). The landmark study by Robinson and Brucer was the first to report the impact of prehypertension on incident hypertension stating that "… men with moderately high systolic pressures (120–140 mmHg) at any age, but especially in the younger group, are probably the ones who will have hypertension years later," and that prehypertension "… is an almost infallible sign of incipient hypertension" [4]. The risk of progression from prehypertension to hypertension has been addressed in several studies. Relevant data comes from large longitudinal cohorts in various populations or the placebo arm of randomized studies.

The first longitudinal study that specifically addressed the progression from prehypertension to hypertension was the Framingham study [9]. A total of 5209 men and women were followed for 26 years. The proportion of males who developed hypertension during the 26-year follow-up period was 70.6% in men with high-normal BP vs. only 33.2% in men with normal BP [relative risk (RR): 2.11; 95% confidence interval (CI): 1.81–2.50]. Similar differences were observed in females: 77.7% of women with high-normal BP developed hypertension compared with only 41.9% of women with normal BP (RR: 1.90; 95% CI: 1.60–2.30). Moreover, the age-adjusted RR for incident hypertension in participants with high-normal BP was 3.36 for males and 3.37 for females. It has to be acknowledged, however, that the definitions of hypertension, prehypertension, and optimal BP were different than the ones currently used. In particular, hypertension diagnosis was based on DBP alone (>90 mmHg), prehypertension was defined as DBP 80–89 mmHg and SBP <140 mmHg, and normotension was defined as BP <140/85 mmHg. Therefore, the findings of the study are representative of stage II prehypertension compared with lower BP (stage I prehypertension and optimal BP).

An updated report of the Framingham study about a decade later overcame the definition problems [10]. Overall, 9845 individuals aged 35–94 years were eligible for analysis of a 4-year follow-up period. In total, progression to hypertension was twice as frequent in older than in younger participants (35 vs. 16%, respectively). In younger participants (35–64 years), progression to hypertension occurred in 37.4% of participants with stage II prehypertension (95% CI: 33.3–41.5%), 17.6% of participants with stage I prehypertension (95% CI: 15.2–20.3%), and 5.3% of participants with optimal BP (95% CI: 4.4–6.3%). The corresponding 4-year rates of progression to hypertension in older participants (65–94 years) were 49.5% (95%

CI: 42.6–56.4%), 25.5% (95% CI: 20.4–31.4%), and 16% (12–20.9%). Compared with optimal BP, the odds ratios for stage II and stage I prehypertension were 11.6 (95% CI: 9.6–14) and 4.1 (95% CI: 3.4–4.9), respectively, in younger participants, and 5.5 (95% CI: 3.4–4.9) and 2.0 (95% CI: 1.4–2.7), respectively, in older participants. The proportions of younger participants with stage II prehypertension who progressed to hypertension at 1, 2, and 3 years were 11.0, 20.8, and 29.6%, while the corresponding rates for participants with stage I prehypertension were 4.7, 9.2, and 13.5%, and for participants with optimal BP were 1.3, 2.7, and 4%. For older participants, the corresponding rates for stage II prehypertension were 15.7, 28.9, and 40.1%, for stage I prehypertension were 7.1, 13.7, and 19.8%, and for optimal BP were 4.3, 8.3, and 12.2%.

Another study included 2048 participants in two British Health and Lifestyle Surveys (HALS 1 and HALS 2) conducted 7 years apart [11]. Compared with participants with optimal BP, participants with stage I prehypertension had a twofold higher risk of developing hypertension (RR: 2.0; 95% CI: 1.6–2.6), while participants with stage II prehypertension had an almost threefold higher risk for incident hypertension (RR: 2.9; 95% CI: 2.3–3.7). Binomial regression analysis revealed that the greater RR for progression to hypertension was observed in younger patients (35–44 years of age at baseline) with stage II prehypertension (RR: 4.4; 95% CI: 3.0–6.3), and the lower RR was observed in older patients (65–74 years of age) with stage I prehypertension (RR: 1.4; 95% CI: 0.7–2.8).

A prospective cohort of 18,865 non-hypertensive individuals (African-Americans: 30.4% and Caucasians 69.6%) aged 18–85 years provides information about the impact of black race on the progression of prehypertension to hypertension [12]. Over a 7-year follow-up period, 63.8% of study participants developed hypertension. Compared with participants with optimal SBP, participants with stage I prehypertension were at an increased risk to develop hypertension [adjusted hazard ratio (HR): 1.50; 95% CI: 1.42–1.58], which was further increased in participants with stage II prehypertension (adjusted HR: 1.75; 95% CI: 1.67–1.84). The corresponding HRs for DBP were 1.18 (95% CI: 1.13–1.24) for stage I and 1.21 (95% CI: 1.15–1.28) for stage II prehypertension, respectively. Compared with Caucasian participants, African-Americans were at an increased risk for incident hypertension (adjusted HR: 1.35; 95% CI: 1.30–1.40). Of note, the median conversion time (when half of participants developed hypertension) was 1 year shorter for African-Americans than Caucasians (626 vs. 991 days; $p < 0.001$).

Two prospective cohorts provide relevant information for Chinese individuals. A population-based sample of 10,525 non-hypertensive Chinese over 40 years of age was followed for a mean of 8.2 years [13]. Overall, 28.9% of male and 26.9% of female participants developed hypertension. The conversion rates were 37.6 and 36.6% for prehypertensive men and women compared with 20.3 and 18.9% for normotensive men and women, respectively. Compared with participants with normal BP, participants with prehypertension were at a significantly higher risk for incident hypertension with a RR of 1.70 for men (95% CI: 1.53–1.88) and 1.64 for women (95% CI: 1.46–1.83) [13]. Another population-based sample of 24,052 rural non-hypertensive Chinese over 35 years of age was followed for a median of 28 months [14]. Overall, hypertension developed in 32.4% of participants with stage II prehypertension, 25.2% with stage I prehypertension, and 21.2% with optimal BP. Compared with participants with optimal BP, participants with stage I prehypertension were at an increased risk for incident hypertension (adjusted HR: 1.16; 95% CI: 1.08–1.24) and the risk was further increased in participants with stage II prehypertension (adjusted HR: 1.28; 95% CI: 1.20–1.36). Further analyses of this cohort identified predictors of progression (age, Mongolian ethnicity, obesity, lifestyle habits) [15] and revealed a higher incidence of conversion in men than in women (12.75 vs. 10.04 for 100 person-years, respectively) [16] and a similarity of progression predictors between prehypertensive and normotensive individuals [17].

In a cohort of more than 12,000 non-hypertensive Japanese workers aged 20–64 years that were followed from 1999 to 2008, hypertension developed in 36.5% of study participants [18]. The rates of incident hypertension increased with age, from 23.1% in participants aged 35–49 years to 50.6% in participants over 50 years of age. Compared with participants with optimal BP, participants with stage I and stage II prehypertension had a significantly increased risk for incident hypertension in all age groups (20–34, 35–49, and 50–64 years). The HRs were from 2.6 to 3.4 for stage I prehypertension and from 5.0 to 9.6 for stage II prehypertension in the 3 age groups in males, and from 2.7 to 3.7 for stage I prehypertension and from 5.1 to 10 for stage II prehypertension in the 3 age groups in females.

Two studies in the USA addressed the progression to hypertension specifically in women and men [19, 20]. The Women's Health Study included 39,322 healthy women older than 45 years of age who were followed for a median of 10.2 years [19]. Overall, 30.1% of study participants developed hypertension. The incidence of conversion to hypertension was substantially higher in participants with stage II prehypertension than in participants with stage I prehypertension or optimal BP (114.7 vs. 41.8 vs. 16.0 age-adjusted incidence per 1000 person-years, respectively). With stage II prehypertension as the reference group, the multivariable-adjusted HRs for stage I prehypertension and optimal BP were 0.42 (95% CI: 0.40–0.44) and 0.17 (95% CI: 0.16–0.18), respectively. Another study evaluated 2303 male Veterans for a median follow-up period of 7.8 years [20]. The incidence rate of progression from prehypertension to hypertension was 34.4 per 1000 person-years. This study provides important information about the impact of prehypertension type on progression risk. The rate of incident hypertension was significantly higher in systolic-diastolic prehypertension (40.7%) than in participants with either isolated systolic prehypertension (32.3%) or isolated diastolic prehypertension (24.3%), and the difference was significant ($p < 0.01$ for all comparisons). Additional important information is the impact of exercise capacity on progression rates. The RR for incident hypertension was progressively higher as exercise capacity decreased, and the association was significant across fitness categories ($p < 0.001$ for high compared with low fit individuals).

The progression rate from prehypertension to hypertension was also assessed in young adulthood. A retrospective analysis of more than 1000 adolescents in Houston revealed a progression rate of 1.1% per year during a mean follow-up period of 21 years in participants with prehypertension compared with a progression rate of 0.3% per year in adolescents with optimal BP [21].

Six prospective, randomized, placebo-controlled trials evaluated the impact of lifestyle modification [22–24] and antihypertensive therapy [25–27] on the risk of incident hypertension in individuals with prehypertension.

The Primary Prevention of Hypertension (PPH) trial randomly assigned 201 individuals with prehypertension in nutritional-hygienic intervention or usual care for 5 years [23]. Progression from prehypertension to hypertension was observed in 19.2% of participants in the control group compared with 8.8% of participants in the intervention group, for an odds ratio of 2.4 (90% CI: 1.2–4.8). Of note, hypertension occurred earlier in participants assigned to the control group than those assigned to the intervention group.

In the Hypertension Prevention Trial (HPT) 841 individuals with prehypertension were randomly assigned to a control treatment group (no dietary counselling) or to 1 of 4 intervention groups (reduced calories, reduced sodium, reduced calories and sodium, or reduced sodium and increased potassium) [24]. Progression from prehypertension to hypertension occurred in 38.7% of participants in the control group during the 3-year follow-up period of the study, while the nutritional intervention was not associated with significant reduction in conversion rates.

The Trial of Hypertension Prevention (TOHP) phase II compared the effects of weight reduction, sodium restriction, and their combination with usual care in 2382 overweight participants with prehypertension [22]. Overall, 44.4% of study participants developed hypertension at the end of the 4-year follow-up period of the study in the usual care group, while the corresponding transition proportions in the 3 intervention groups were 37.6–38.5% and the RRs for incident hypertension were 0.85–0.87 ($p = 0.02$–0.06) in the three intervention groups. The proportions of incident hypertension in the usual care group at 6, 18, and 36 months during the study follow-up were 7.3, 21.1, and 39.2%, respectively.

The Trial of Preventing Hypertension (TROPHY) examined whether early treatment of hypertension with an angiotensin receptor blocker prevents or delays the development of subsequent incident hypertension compared with placebo in individuals with prehypertension [25]. A total of 809 participants were randomized to candesartan or placebo for 2 years, followed by 2 years of placebo for all study participants. Overall, 40.4% developed hypertension at the year-2 visit in the placebo group, and this proportion increased to 63% at the year-4 visit in the same group. The corresponding proportions of incident hypertension in the intervention group were 13.6 and 53.2%, indicating a 66% risk reduction with candesartan at 2 years (RR: 0.34; 95% CI: 0.25–0.44), which was later attenuated to 16% (RR: 0.84; 95% CI: 0.75–0.95) when placebo was administered in the intervention group replacing candesartan. The median time to incident hypertension was 2.2 years in the placebo group and significantly longer (3.3 years) with candesartan. RR reduction with active therapy compared with placebo was evident throughout all prespecified subgroups (by age, gender, body weight, body mass index, and race).

The Prevention of Hypertension with the ACE-inhibitor Ramipril in patients with high-normal blood pressure (PHARAO) study assessed whether treatment of stage II prehypertension with ramipril can prevent or delay the progression to manifest office hypertension compared with placebo [26]. A total of 1008 participants with stage II prehypertension were randomly assigned to ramipril or placebo for 3 years. Overall, 42.9% of participants in the placebo group developed hypertension compared with 30.7% of participants in the ramipril group during the 3-year follow-up period, and the RR reduction was 34.4% (HR: 0.656; 95% CI: 0.533–0.807). A positive correlation of incident hypertension with SBP was identified in multivariate analysis (for each 1 mmHg increment, the risk increased by 5%).

The Prevention of Hypertension in Patients with Prehypertension (PREVER-Prevention) study evaluated the efficacy and safety of a low-dose diuretic for the prevention of hypertension and end-organ damage [27]. A total of 730 individuals with prehypertension were randomly assigned to chlorthalidone/amiloride or placebo for a follow-up period of 18 months. The incidence of hypertension was significantly lower in participants allocated to diuretics compared with participants allocated to placebo (HR: 0.56, 95% CI: 0.38–0.82). The cumulative incidence of progression from prehypertension to hypertension during the 18-month follow-up period of the study was 19.5% with placebo and 11.7% with low-dose diuretics. Moreover, benefits with active therapy were observed for left ventricular mass (assessed by electrocardiography), while new-onset diabetes mellitus was not different between the two groups (5.5% with active therapy vs. 3.3% with placebo, $p = 0.18$).

4.2.1 The Progression Process

Several factors along with baseline demographic characteristics have been associated with the development of prehypertension: uric acid [28–30], dietary salt intake [31], arterial stiffness [32], autonomic imbalance [33, 34], obesity [35], hemoglobin levels [36], and subclinical inflammation [37]. In addition, several factors (along with baseline demographic characteristics) have been associated with the progression of prehypertension to hypertension: visceral abdominal fat [38], sympathetic overactivity [39], sympathovagal imbalance [34], endothelial dysfunction [40], impairment of coronary flow reserve [41, 42], and metabolic syndrome [41].

Target organ damage might contribute to future CV events in addition to elevated BP in individuals with prehypertension compared with individuals with optimal BP. Prehypertension has been associated with several types of target organ damage: metabolic syndrome [28, 43, 44], increased left ventricular mass and left ventricular hypertrophy [44–47], left ventricular diastolic dysfunction [44, 47–50], coronary artery calcification [51, 52], increased minimum coronary resistance [42], arterial stiffness [32], increased arterial intima-media thickness [53, 54], retinal vascular alterations [55], microalbuminuria [56–58], hemorheological abnormalities [59], increased tissue plasminogen activator [60], carotid atherosclerosis [61], poor cognitive performance [62], subclinical inflammation [37, 63], increased low density lipoprotein (LDL) oxidation in vivo [64], increased serum complement [65], excessive sympathetic response [66], and abnormalities in endothelial progenitor cells [67].

In a recent cohort of almost 12,500 Japanese individuals for a median period of 11.8 years, the impact of progression from prehypertension to hypertension on the risk of future CV events was evaluated. Prehypertensive individuals who developed hypertension during the follow-up period had almost a 2-times higher risk of CV disease (adjusted HR: 2.95; 95% CI: 1.05–8.33) compared with individuals who remained prehypertensive during the follow-up period [68].

4.2.2 Attenuation or Delay of Progression

Lifestyle modification has been shown to exert beneficial effects in individuals with prehypertension and is currently recommended for the management of prehypertension [6, 69]. Accumulating data indicate that regular physical exercise and especially aerobic exercise reduces BP, attenuates sympathetic activity, improves arterial stiffness, and should be an essential part of the therapeutic plan for the management of individuals with prehypertension [70–73]. Healthy diet has been also shown to be beneficial in prehypertension [74, 75]. However, long-term maintenance to healthy lifestyle represents the Achilles' heel of lifestyle modification [5, 69]. In a recent meta-analysis, the short-term (3–6 months) benefits of exercise on BP were almost abolished after the first year of initiating an exercise program [76]. Recently, a mobile phone-based intervention was evaluated in 637 individuals with prehypertension in Latin America [77]. However, a small reduction in body weight and an improvement in some dietary habits were not associated with a significant BP reduction with the intervention compared with usual care [77].

The impact of ideal health behaviors was recently evaluated in a cohort of more than 30,000 Chinese individuals with prehypertension [78]. In total, incident hypertension was observed in 47.1% of study participants during a mean follow-up period of 52.2 months. It was found that hypertension was inversely associated with ideal health behaviors and developed in 78.6, 71.1, 63.1, 56.1, and 61.6% of prehypertensive participants carrying ≤1, 2, 3, 4, or ≥5 ideal health behaviors (nonsmoking, regular physical activity, healthy diet, salt restriction) or ideal health factors (total cholesterol <200 mg/dL, blood glucose <100 mg/dL, BP <120/80 mmHg). Compared with participants with one or none ideal health behaviors or factors, the risk ratios for incident hypertension in participants with 2, 3, 4, and ≥5 ideal healthy behaviors or factors were 0.83 (95% CI: 0.79–0.88), 0.71 (95% CI: 0.67–0.75), 0.60 (95% CI: 0.57–0.64), and 0.58 (95% CI: 0.52–0.64), respectively.

Antihypertensive therapy has been evaluated in the aforementioned randomized studies and was shown to delay the progression of prehypertension to hypertension [25–27]. In addition, a meta-analysis of 16 studies with >70,000 participants with prehypertension showed that the stroke risk was significantly reduced (by 22%) with antihypertensive therapy compared with placebo (RR: 0.78; 95% CI: 0.71–0.86) [79]. Moreover, 169 individuals with prehypertension need to be treated with an antihypertensive drug for 4.3 years to prevent one stroke, indicating a relatively high number needed to treat in prehypertension [79]. Collectively, the pharmacological therapy of prehypertension remains a topic of lively discussion and debate [80–83].

4.3 Prehypertension and CV Morbidity

Many longitudinal prospective cohort studies have evaluated the association of prehypertension with CV morbidity and mortality. During the last decade, six meta-analyses sought to report the association of prehypertension with myocardial infarction, stroke, and CV events in total [84–89].

The association of prehypertension with stroke as a separate outcome was assessed in two meta-analyses [84, 85]. The meta-analysis by Lee et al. included data from 12 cohorts with >500,000 participants [84]. Prehypertension was associated with a significantly increased risk for stroke, with a RR of 1.55 (95% CI: 1.35–1.79). A marked heterogeneity of stroke risk was observed within the prehypertension group according to BP. The RR for stroke was not significantly elevated with stage I prehypertension (RR: 1.22; 95% CI: 0.95–1.57), while the respective risk was significantly increased with stage II prehypertension (RR: 1.79; 95% CI: 1.49–2.16). The meta-analysis by Huang et al. was larger and included data from 19 cohorts with >750,000 participants [85]. Compared with individuals with optimal BP, participants with prehypertension had a substantially elevated risk for stroke (RR: 1.66; 95% CI: 1.51–1.81). Similar to the previous meta-analysis, stroke risk was dependent on baseline BP and increased with increasing levels. In particular, the relative stroke risk was 1.44 for participants with stage I prehypertension (95% CI: 1.27–1.63), while the respective risk for stage II prehypertension was 1.95 (95% CI: 1.73–2.21).

The association of prehypertension with coronary heart disease (CHD) as a separate outcome was assessed in two meta-analyses [86, 87]. The meta-analysis by Shen et al. pooled data from 18 prospective cohorts with almost 900,000 participants [86]. Overall, prehypertension was associated with a substantially increased risk for CHD (RR: 1.36; 95% CI: 1.22–1.53). This association was significantly affected by prehypertension staging. Stage I prehypertension was not associated with significantly increased risk for CHD (RR: 1.16; 95% CI: 0.96–1.42). In contrast, stage II prehypertension was associated with a significantly elevated risk for CHD (RR: 1.53; 95% CI: 1.19–1.97). The meta-analysis by Huang et al. pooled data from 17 prospective cohorts with almost 600,000 participants and evaluated whether racial differences exist regarding the association of prehypertension with CHD [87]. Overall, when participants with prehypertension were compared with participants with optimal BP, the risk for CHD was significantly increased (RR: 1.43; 95% CI: 1.26–1.63). Moreover, it was found that significant differences in RR for CHD exist for different races. In particular, Western participants were at significantly higher risk for CHD than Asian participants, and the RRs were 1.70 (95% CI: 1.49–1.94) for Western participants and 1.25 (95% CI: 1.12–1.38) for Asian participants (ratio of RRs: 1.36; 95% CI: 1.15–1.61). This meta-analysis provides another very important piece of information, since the population-attributable risk estimation indicates that 24.1% of CHD in Western participants may be attributed to prehypertension, while only 8.4% of CHD in Asian participants may be attributed to prehypertension [to 73].

Two meta-analyses evaluated the risk for CV events as a whole as well as stroke and myocardial infarction separately [88, 89]. The meta-analysis by Huang et al. included data from 18 prospective cohorts with >450,000 participants [88]. Overall, participants with prehypertension were at significantly higher risk for CV events when compared with participants with optimal BP (RR: 1.55; 95% CI: 1.41–1.71). The respective RRs for CHD and stroke were 1.50 (95% CI: 1.30–1.74) and 1.71 (95% CI: 1.55–1.89). Once again, the RR depended on prehypertension staging. Compared with optimal BP, stage I prehypertension was associated with a significantly increased risk for CV events (RR: 1.46; 95% CI: 1.32–1.62) and the risk was further elevated in stage II prehypertension (RR: 1.80; 95% CI: 1.41–2.31). The meta-analysis by Guo et al. pooled data from 29 cohorts with >1 million participants [89]. Overall, prehypertension was associated with a significantly elevated risk for CV events (RR: 1.44; 95% CI: 1.35–1.53) compared with optimal BP. The respective RRs for stroke and myocardial infarction were 1.73 (95% CI: 1.61–1.85) and 1.79 (95% CI: 1.45–2.22) for participants with prehypertension compared with participants with optimal BP. Similarly to other meta-analyses, the RR was strongly affected by prehypertension staging. Stage I prehypertension was associated with a significantly elevated risk for CV events (RR: 1.24; 95% CI: 1.10–1.39), and the risk was further elevated in stage II prehypertension (RR: 1.56; 95% CI: 1.36–1.78). Likewise, the RRs for stroke and myocardial infarction were 1.35 (95% CI: 1.10–1.66) and 1.43 (95% CI: 1.10–1.86), respectively, in stage I prehypertension and were further elevated to 1.95 (95% CI: 1.69–2.24) and 1.99 (95% CI: 1.59–2.50), respectively, in stage II prehypertension.

4.4 Prehypertension and Chronic Kidney Disease (CKD)

Three recent meta-analyses have addressed the association of prehypertension with end-stage renal disease [90], CKD [91], and decreased estimated glomerular filtration rate (eGFR) in the general population [92].

The first meta-analysis included data from one million individuals who participated in six prospective cohort studies [90]. Individuals with prehypertension were at significantly higher risk for end-stage renal disease (RR: 1.59; 95% CI: 1.39–1.91) when compared with individuals with optimal BP. Moreover, a graded association with end-stage renal disease was observed with increasing BP within the prehypertension range. In particular, stage I prehypertension was associated with significantly increased risk for end-stage renal disease compared with optimal BP (RR: 1.44; 95% CI: 1.19–1.74), and the risk was further increased among individuals with stage II prehypertension (RR:2.02; 95% CI: 1.70–2.40).

The second meta-analysis included >250,000 individuals who participated in seven cohort studies, mainly conducted in the Far East [91]. Prehypertension was associated with an increased risk for CKD compared with optimal BP (pooled RR: 1.28; 95% CI: 1.13–1.44). This association between prehypertension and future development of CKD was gender- and ethnic-dependent. In particular, the association was evident in females (pooled RR: 1.29; 95% CI: 1.01–1.63) but not in males. Similarly, the association was evident in Far East participants (pooled RR: 1.37; 95% CI: 1.18–1.59) but not in European and Middle-East individuals.

In the third meta-analysis data from 16 cohorts with >315,000 participants were pooled and analyzed [92]. Renal function deterioration was observed in 6.6% of participants during a mean follow-up period of 6.5 years. Prehypertension was associated with a significantly increased risk for renal function deterioration defined as a decline in eGFR (RR: 1.19; 95% CI: 1.07–1.33), while the respective RR for hypertensive individuals was 1.76 (95% CI: 1.58–1.97). Moreover, it was found that an increase of SBP and DBP by 10 mmHg was associated with a greater RR for renal function deterioration, which was 1.08 for prehypertension (95% CI: 1.04–1.11) and 1.12 for hypertension (1.04–1.20). Further analysis identified older age as the only significant contributor for renal function deterioration.

A recent very large study from Israel provides further credence on the association between prehypertension and CKD. The study included 2.19 million healthy asymptomatic adolescents 16–19 years old evaluated for military service and followed for a median of 16.8 years [93]. Prehypertension (defined either as BP between the 90th and 95th percentile or BP between 120 and 139 mmHg for SBP and/or 80–89 mmHg for DBP) was associated with a 32% increased risk for future end-stage renal disease (HR: 1.32; 95% CI: 1.11–1.58) compared with adolescents with optimal BP, which was not substantially lower than the respective risk of hypertensive adolescents (HR: 1.44; 95% CI: 1.17–1.79).

A recent study of almost 100,000 individuals aged 80–89 years in Japan unveiled a significant association between prehypertension and glomerular hyperfiltration [94]. The prevalence of glomerular hyperfiltration increased with increasing stages of prehypertension. In particular, when individuals with optimal BP were used as the reference group, those with stage 1 prehypertension had an odds ratio of 1.10 (95% CI: 1.00–1.20), and those with stage 2 prehypertension had an odds ratio of 1.33 (95% CI: 1.21–1.47). Glomerular hyperfiltration is mainly driven by increased intraglomerular pressure in subjects with elevated BP [95] and is considered an early alteration of renal function [96]. Long-term glomerular hyperfiltration contributes to CKD [97, 98] through progressive glomerular sclerosis [99]. Glomerular hyperfiltration is associated with a faster decline of glomerular filtration rate and thus renal function [100], while the prevention of glomerular hyperfiltration is associated with less glomerular injury [101]. Therefore, the timely recognition of prehypertensive individuals with glomerular hyperfiltration can identify those at increased risk for CKD who might benefit from early intervention.

4.5 Prehypertension and CV and All-Cause Mortality

The landmark study by Robinson and Brucer was the first to report the impact of prehypertension on mortality risk: "… the mortality of any random group of 1000 persons with pressures over 120 systolic and 80 diastolic is higher than that of similar group with pressures under these levels" [4]. Several longitudinal studies have evaluated the association of prehypertension with CV and/or all-cause mortality, and three relevant meta-analyses are available [102–104].

The meta-analysis by Wang et al. pooled data from 13 prospective cohort studies involving almost 400,000 participants [102]. Prehypertension was associated with an increased risk for CV mortality (pooled RR: 1.17; 95% CI: 1.07–1.27) when compared with optimal BP. Prehypertension staging significantly affected the association between prehypertension and CV mortality. There was a trend towards increased CV mortality in stage I prehypertension that failed marginally to reach statistical significance (RR: 1.18; 95% CI: 0.98–1.42), while the respective risk was significantly elevated in stage II prehypertension (RR: 1.33; 95% CI: 1.13–1.58). In contrast, no association between prehypertension and all-cause mortality was found. The overall RR conferred by prehypertension was 1.01 (95% CI: 0.95–1.08). Similarly, neither stage I nor stage II prehypertension were associated with elevated all-cause mortality risk (RR: 0.99; 95% CI: 0.88–1.13, and RR: 1.02; 95% CI: 0.97–1,08, respectively).

In the meta-analysis of Guo et al. data from >870,000 individuals participating in 13 prospective cohorts were pooled and analyzed [103]. Prehypertension was associated with an elevated risk for CV mortality (RR: 1.32; 95% CI: 1.16–1.50). The same was evident for stage II prehypertension (RR: 1.26; 95% CI: 1.13–1.41) but not for stage I prehypertension (RR: 1.10; 95% CI: 0.92–1.30). Prehypertension was not associated with all-cause mortality in this meta-analysis as well. The relative all-cause mortality risk was 1.03 (95% CI: 0.91–1.15) for the prehypertension group as a whole, 0.91 (95% CI: 0.81–1.02) for stage I prehypertension, and 1.00 (95% CI: 0.95–1.06) for stage II prehypertension.

The larger meta-analysis was performed by Huang et al. and pooled data from 20 prospective cohorts with >1.1 million participants [104]. Prehypertension significantly increased the risk for CHD and stroke mortality (RR: 1.12; 95% CI: 1.02–1.23, and RR: 1.41; 95% CI: 1.28–1.56, respectively). Likewise, prehypertension was associated with a significantly elevated risk for CV mortality (RR: 1.28; 95% CI: 1.16–1.40). This association was evident for stage II prehypertension (RR: 1.28; 95% CI: 1.16–1.41) but not for stage I prehypertension (RR: 1.08; 95% CI: 0.98–1.18). Finally, prehypertension was not associated with all-cause mortality after adjustments for all covariates (RR: 1.03; 95% CI: 0.97–1.10), and the same applied for both stage I and II prehypertension.

4.6 Critical Evaluation

Collectively, available evidence demonstrates that individuals with prehypertension have a two- to threefold increased risk for incident hypertension compared with individuals with optimal BP. The conversion rates from prehypertension to hypertension vary significantly among the studies, and the variation may be attributed to several factors, such as the duration of the study, baseline BP, age, race, body mass index, physical fitness, and comorbidities. In particular, regarding the duration of follow-up period, it is obvious that the longer the duration of the study, the higher the proportion of participants who will develop hypertension. In addition, the higher the baseline BP, the greater the proportion of participants who will develop hypertension, with >50% increased risk for incident hypertension among individuals with stage II compared with stage I prehypertension. Moreover, African-Americans are more likely to progress from prehypertension to hypertension more rapidly than Caucasians with prehypertension. Furthermore, the higher the body mass index and the older the age, the greater the risk for incident hypertension in prehypertensive individuals. In addition, impaired physical fitness as expressed with limited exercise capacity is associated with increased risk for developing hypertension. Finally, comorbidities such as diabetes mellitus [73] and CKD significantly increase the risk of prehypertensive individuals to develop hypertension.

Overall, available data indicates that prehypertension is associated with a significantly increased risk for CHD, stroke, total CV disease, and CV mortality, but not with all-cause mortality (maybe due to the relatively short follow-up period of several studies). The elevated CV risk strongly depends on prehypertension staging; individuals with stage II prehypertension are at a significantly greater risk for CV morbidity and mortality than individuals with stage I prehypertension. In addition, the impact of prehypertension is greater when fatal and nonfatal CV events are combined compared with the evaluation of fatal CV events alone. In addition, CV events are more likely to occur in prehypertensive individuals who develop hypertension compared with individuals who remain prehypertensive. Moreover, the earlier the progression from prehypertension to hypertension is, the higher the risk for CV events. It has to be acknowledged that all meta-analyses addressing the association of prehypertension with CV outcomes report significantly elevated RRs in prehypertensive compared with normotensive individuals, without reporting (in most cases) however the absolute morbidity and mortality risks, limiting the ability to estimate the number of patients needed to treat over a certain period for the prevention of one event. In general, the absolute risk of prehypertensive individuals is rather low, unless prehypertension is associated with overt CV disease or clustering multiple CV risk factors, or significant target organ damage.

Given, however the high prevalence of prehypertension in the general population (it is estimated that 40 million individuals have stage I and 30 million individuals have stage II prehypertension in the US), and the frequent coexistence of CV risk factors, target organ damage, or overt CV disease, it becomes obvious that prehypertension is a major public health problem that requires immediate attention and management. Pharmacological therapy is a matter of hot debate and is not likely to gain implementation in the near future. In contrast, lifestyle modification is strongly recommended by all guidelines for the management of individuals with prehypertension in the effort to prevent or delay the progression of prehypertension to hypertension. Therefore, primary care physicians should intensity efforts for the widespread implementation and maintenance of healthy measures to limit the detrimental consequences of prehypertension.

Conclusions

Prehypertension is placed between normotension and hypertension. Accumulating evidence proved that prehypertension is a precursor of hypertension in a high proportion of individuals. The progression rates are higher in individuals with stage II prehypertension, obesity, and other comorbidities. Of major clinical importance, prehypertension is associated with increased risk for CHD, stroke, CKD, and CV but not all-cause mortality. The detrimental consequences of prehypertension, especially stage II prehypertension, justify its utility in real life clinical practice and should attract the attention of practicing physicians to appropriately manage prehypertensive individuals.

Declaration of Interest This review was written independently; no company or institution supported the authors financially or by providing a professional writer. M.D. received honoraria from Menarini, WinMedica, Bayer, Boehringer, Merck, and Unipharma. N.K. has given talks, attended conferences, and participated in trials sponsored by Amgen, Angelini, Astra Zeneca, Boehringer Ingelheim, Galenica, MSD, Novartis, Novo Nordisk, Sanofi, and WinMedica. D.P.M. has given talks and attended conferences sponsored by MSD, AstraZeneca, and Libytec.

References

1. Orth J. On the morphology of carcinoma and the parasitic theory of its etiology. Ann Surg. 1904;40:773–81.
2. Levin I. Changes in the tissue surrounding a growing tumor and the significance of the precancerous state. J Exp Med. 1912;16:149–54.
3. Rodman WL. Cancer and precancerous conditions. Ann Surg. 1914;59:47–64.
4. Robinson SC, Brucer M. Range of normal blood pressure: a statistical and clinical study of 11,383 persons. Arch Intern Med. 1939;64:409–44.
5. Chobanian AV, Bakris GL, Black HR, Cushman WC, Green LA, Izzo JL Jr, et al. Seventh report of the Joint National Committee on prevention, evaluation, and treatment of high blood pressure. Hypertension. 2003;42:1206–52.
6. Lewington S, Clarke R, Qizibash N, Peto R, Collins R. Age specific relevance of usual blood pressure to vascular mortality: a meta-analysis of individual data for one million adults in 61 prospective studies. Lancet. 2002;360:1903–13.
7. Laurent S, Boutouyrie P. The structural factor of hypertension: large and small artery alterations. Circ Res. 2015;116:1007–21.
8. Vasan RS, Beiser A, Seshadri S, Larson MG, Kannel WB, D'Agostino RB, et al. Residual lifetime risk for developing hypertension in middle-aged women and men. The Framingham Heart Study. JAMA. 2002;287:1003–10.
9. Leitschuh M, Cupples A, Kannel W, Gagnon D, Chobanian A. High-normal blood pressure progression to hypertension in the Framingham Heart Study. Hypertension. 1991;17:22–7.
10. Vasan RS, Larson MG, Leip EP, Kannel WB, Levy D. Assessment of frequency of progression to hypertension in non-hypertensive participants in the Framingham Heart Study: a cohort study. Lancet. 2001;358:1682–6.
11. Winegarden CR. From prehypertension to hypertension? Additional evidence. Ann Epidemiol. 2005;15:720–5.
12. Selassie A, Wagner S, Laken ML, Ferguson L, Ferdinand K, Egan BM. Progression is accelerated from prehypertension to hypertension in blacks. Hypertension. 2011;58:579–87.
13. Gu D, Wildman RP, Wu X, Reynolds K, Huang J, Chen CS, et al. Incidence and predictors of hypertension over 8 years among Chinese men and women. J Hypertens. 2007;25:517–23.

14. Zheng L, Sun Z, Zhang X, Xu C, Li J, Li M, et al. Risk of progression to hypertension across baseline blood pressure in nonhypertensive participants among rural Chinese adults: a prospective study. J Hypertens. 2010;28:1158–65.
15. Zheng L, Sun Z, Zhang X, Xu C, Li J, Hu D, et al. Predictors of progression from prehypertension to hypertension among rural Chinese adults: results from Liaoning Province. Eur J Cardiovasc Prev Rehabil. 2010;17:217–22.
16. Sun Z, Zheng L, Detrano R, Zhang X, Xu C, Li J, et al. Incidence and predictors of hypertension among rural Chinese adults: results from Liaoning Province. Ann Fam Med. 2010;8:19–24.
17. Sun Z, Zheng L, Detrano R, Zhang X, Xu C, Li J, et al. Risk of progression to hypertension in a rural Chinese women population with prehypertension and normal blood pressure. Am J Hypertens. 2010;23:627–32.
18. Kurioka S, Horie S, Inoue A, Mafune K, Tsuda Y, Otsuji Y. Risk of progression to hypertension in nonhypertensive Japanese workers aged 20–64 years. J Hypertens. 2014;32:236–44.
19. Conen D, Ridker PM, Buring JE, Glynn RJ. Risk of cardiovascular events among women with high normal blood pressure or blood pressure progression: prospective cohort study. BMJ. 2007;335:432.
20. Faselis C, Doumas M, Kokkinos JP, Panagiotakos D, Kheirbek R, Sheriff HM, et al. Exercise capacity and progression from prehypertension to hypertension. Hypertension. 2012;60:333–8.
21. Redwine KM, Acosta AA, Poffenbarger T, Portman RJ, Samuels J. Development of hypertension in adolescents with prehypertension. J Pediatr. 2012;160:98–103.
22. The Trials of Hypertension Prevention Collaborative Group. Effects of weight loss and sodium reduction intervention on blood pressure and hypertension incidence in overweight people with high-normal blood pressure. The Trials of Hypertension Prevention Phase II. Arch Intern Med. 1997;57:657–67.
23. Stamler R, Stamler J, Gosch FC, Civinelli J, Fishman J, McKeever P, et al. Primary prevention of hypertension by nutritional-hygienic means. Final report of a randomized, controlled trial. JAMA. 1989;262:1801–7.
24. Hypertension Prevention Trial Research Group. The Hypertension Prevention Trial: three-year effects of dietary changes on blood pressure. Arch Intern Med. 1990;150:153–62.
25. Julius S, Nesbitt SD, Egan BM, Weber MA, Michelson EL, Kaciroti N, et al. Feasibility of treating prehypertension with an angiotensin receptor blocker. N Engl J Med. 2006;354:1685–97.
26. Lüders S, Schrader J, Berger J, Unger T, Zidek W, Böhm M, et al; PHARAO Study Group. The PHARAO Study: prevention of hypertension with the angiotensin-converting enzyme inhibitor ramipril in patients with high-normal blood pressure—a prospective, randomized, controlled prevention trial of the German Hypertension League. J Hypertens. 2008;26:1487–96.
27. Fuchs SC, Poli-de-Figueiredo CE, Figueiredo Neto JA, Scala LC, Whelton PK, Mosele F, et al. Effectiveness of chlorthalidone plus amiloride for the prevention of hypertension: the PREVER-Prevention randomized clinical trial. J Am Heart Assoc. 2016;5:e004248.
28. Rizzo M, Pbradovic M, Labudovic-Borovic M, Nikolic D, Montalto G, Rizvi AA, et al. Uric acid metabolism in prehypertension and the metabolic syndrome. Curr Vasc Pharmacol. 2014;12:572–85.
29. Jiang M, Gong D, Fan Y. Serum uric acid levels and risk of prehypertension: a meta-analysis. Clin Chem Lab Med. 20171;55:314–21.
30. Liu L, Gu Y, Li C, Zhang Q, Meng G, Wu H, et al. Serum uric acid is an independent predictor for developing prehypertension: a population-based prospective cohort study. J Hum Hypertens. 2017;31:116–20.
31. Zhao X, Yang X, Zhang X, Li Y, Zhao X, Ren L, et al. Dietary salt intake and coronary atherosclerosis in patients with prehypertension. J Clin Hypertens. 2014;16:575–80.
32. Tomiyama H, Yamashina A. Arterial stiffness in prehypertension: a possible vicious cycle. J Cardiovasc Transl Res. 2012;5:280–6.
33. Davis JT, Rao F, Naqshbandi D, Fung MM, Zhang K, Schork AJ, et al. Autonomic and hemodynamic origins of prehypertension. J Am Coll Cardiol. 2012;59:2206–16.
34. Pal GK, Pal P, Nanda N, Amudharaj D, Adithan C. Cardiovascular dysfunctions and sympathovagal imbalance in hypertension and prehypertension: physiological perspectives. Futur Cardiol. 2013;9:53–69.

35. Martín-Espinosa N, Díez-Fernández A, Sánchez-López M, Rivero-Merino I, Lucas-De La Cruz L, Solera-Martínez M, et al. Movi-Kids Group. Prevalence of high blood pressure and association with obesity in Spanish schoolchildren aged 4-6 years old. PLoS One. 2017;12:e0170926.
36. Senthil S, Krishndasa SN. Prehypertension in apparently healthy young adults: incidence and influence of hemoglobin level. J Clin Diagn Res. 2015;9:10–2.
37. Nandeesha H, Bobby Z, Selvaraj N, Rajappa M. Prehypertension: is it an inflammatory state? Clin Chim Acta. 2015;451:338–42.
38. Hwang YC, Fujimoto WY, Kahn SE, Leonetti DL, Boyko EJ. Greater visceral abdominal fat is associated with a lower probability of conversion of prehypertension to normotension. J Hypertens. 2017;35:1213–8.
39. Hering D, Kara T, Kucharska W, Somers VK, Narkiewicz K. Longitudinal tracking of muscle sympathetic nerve activity and its relationship with blood pressure in subjects with prehypertension. Blood Press. 2016;25:184–92.
40. Millgard J, Hägg A, Sarabi M, Lind L. Endothelium-dependent vasodilation in normotensive subjects with a familial history of essential hypertension and in young subjects with borderline hypertension. Blood Press. 2002;11:279–84.
41. Erdogan D, Ozaydin M, Icli A, Gonul E, Yucel H, Arslan A, et al. Echocardiographic predictors of progression from prehypertension to hypertension. J Hypertens. 2012;30:1639–45.
42. Palombo C, Kozakova M, Magagna A, Bigalli G, Morizzo C, Ghiadoni L, et al. Early impairment of coronary flow reserve and increase in minimum coronary resistance in borderline hypertensive patients. J Hypertens. 2010;18:453–9.
43. Katsiki N, Doumas M, Athyros VG, Karagiannis A. Prehypertension and the cardiometabolic syndrome: targeting several risk factors to achieve maximum benefit. Expert Rev Cardiovasc Ther. 2014;12:295–6.
44. Jung MH, Ihm SH, Lee DH, Chung WB, Jung HO, Youn HJ. Prehypertension is associated with early complications of atherosclerosis but not with exercise capacity. Int J Cardiol. 2017;227:387–92.
45. Mousa TM, Akinseye OA, Berekashvili K, Akinboboye OO. Correlation of prehypertension with left ventricular mass assessed by magnetic resonance imaging. Int J Hypertens. 2015;2015, Article no. 742658.
46. Oyama J, Node K. Prevalence of prehypertension and left ventricular hypertrophy. Hypertens Res. 2017;40:544–5.
47. Markus MR, Stritzke J, Lieb W, Mayer B, Luchner A, Döring A, et al. Implications of persistent prehypertension for ageing related changes in left ventricular geometry and function: the MONICA/KORA Augsburg study. J Hypertens. 2008;26:2040–9.
48. Jung JY, Park SK, Oh CM, Kang JG, Choi JM, Ryoo JH, et al. The influence of prehypertension, controlled and uncontrolled hypertension on left ventricular diastolic function and structure in the general Korean population. Hypertens Res. 2017;40:606–12.
49. Jang SY, Kim S, Lee CK, Cho EJ, Cho SJ, Lee SC. Prehypertension and left ventricular diastolic dysfunction in middle-aged Koreans. Korean Circ J. 2016;46:536–41.
50. Santos AB, Gupta DK, Bello NA, Gori M, Claggett B, Fuchs FD, et al. Prehypertension is associated with abnormalities of cardiac structure and function in the Atherosclerosis Risk in Communities Study. Am J Hypertens. 2016;29:568–74.
51. Lehmann N, Erbel R, Mahabadi AA, Kälsch H, Möhlenkamp S, Moebus S, et al. Accelerated progression of coronary artery calcification in hypertension but also prehypertension. J Hypertens. 2016;34:2233–42.
52. Pletcher M, Bibbins-Domingo K, Lewis CE, Wei GS, Sidney S, Carr JJ, et al. Prehypertension during young adulthood and coronary calcium later in life. Ann Intern Med. 2008;149:91–9.
53. Manios E, Michas F, Tsivgoulis G, Stamatelopoulos K, Tsagalis G, Koroboki E, et al. Impact of prehypertension on carotid artery intima-media thickening: actual or masked? Atherosclerosis. 2011;214:215–9.
54. Manios E, Tsivgoulis G, Koroboki E, Stamatelopoulos K, Papamichael C, Toumanidis S, et al. Impact of prehypertension on common carotid artery intima-media thickness and left ventricular mass. Stroke. 2009;40:1515–8.

55. Ikram MK, Witteman JC, Vingerling JR, Breteler MM, Hofman A, de Jong PT. Retinal vessel diameters and risk of hypertension: the Rotterdam study. Hypertension. 2006;47:189–94.
56. Chen J, Muntner P, Hamm LL, Jones DW, Batuman V, Fonseca V, et al. The metabolic syndrome and chronic kidney disease in US adults. Ann Intern Med. 2004;140:167–74.
57. Bianchi S, Bigazzi R, Campese V. Microalbuminuria in essential hypertension: significance, pathophysiology, and therapeutic implications. Am J Kidney Dis. 1999;34:973–95.
58. Lee JE, Kim YG, Choi YH, Huh W, Kim DJ, Oh HY. Serum uric acid is associated with microalbuminuria in prehypertension. Hypertension. 2006;47:962–7.
59. Tripolino C, Gnasso A, Carallo C, Scavelli FB, Irace C. Hemorheological profiles of subjects with prehypertension. Hypertens Res. 2006;39:519–23.
60. Stamler J, Stamler R, Neaton JD. Blood pressure systolic and diastolic, and cardiovascular risks. Arch Intern Med. 1993;153:598–615.
61. Hong H, Wang H, Liao H. Prehypertension is associated with increased carotid atherosclerotic plaque in the community population of Southern China. BMC Cardiovasc Disord. 2013;13:20.
62. Knecht S, Wersching H, Lohmann H, Bruchmann M, Duning T, Dziewas R, et al. High normal blood pressure is associated with poor cognitive performance. Hypertension. 2008;51:663–8.
63. Chrysohoou C, Pitsavos C, Panagiotakos DB, Skoumas J, Stefanadis C. Association between prehypertension status and inflammatory markers related to atherosclerotic disease. Am J Hypertens. 2004;17:568–73.
64. Toikka JO, Laine H, Ahotupa M, Haapanen A, Viikari JS, Hartiala JJ, et al. Increased arterial intima-media thickness and in vivo LDL oxidation in young men with borderline hypertension. Hypertension. 2000;36:929–33.
65. Bao X, Meng G, Zhang Q, Liu L, Wu H, Du H, et al. Elevated serum complement C3 levels are associated with prehypertension in an adult population. Clin Exp Hypertens. 2017;39:42–9.
66. Bond V, Curry BH, Adams RG, Obisesan T, Pemminati S, Gorantla VR, et al. Cardiovascular responses to an isometric handgrip exercise in females with prehypertension. N Am J Med Sci. 2016;8:243–9.
67. Di Stefano R, Barsotti MC, Felice F, Vlachopoulos C, Barbarini A. Endothelial progenitor cells in prehypertension. Curr Pharm Des. 2011;17:3002–19.
68. Ishikawa Y, Ishikawa J, Ishikawa S, Kario K, Kajii E. Progression from prehypertension to hypertension and risk of cardiovascular disease. J Epidemiol. 2017;27:8–13.
69. Mancia G, Fagard R, Narkiewicz K, Redon J, Zanchetti A, Böhm M, et al. ESH/ESC guidelines for the management of arterial hypertension. J Hypertens. 2013;31:1281–357.
70. Saxena Y, Gupta R, Moinuddin A, Narwal R. Blood pressure reduction following accumulated physical activity in prehypertensive. J Family Med Prim Care. 2017;5:349–56.
71. Montero D, Roche E, Martinez-Rodriguez A. The impact of aerobic exercise training on arterial stiffness in pre- and hypertensive subjects: a systematic review and meta-analysis. Int J Cardiol. 2014;173:361–8.
72. Ash GI, Taylor BA, Thompson PD, MacDonald HV, Lamberti L, Chen MH, et al. The antihypertensive effects of aerobic versus isometric handgrip resistance exercise. J Hypertens. 2017;35:291–9.
73. Bushman B. Promoting exercise as medicine for prediabetes and prehypertension. Curr Sports Med Rep. 2014;13:233–9.
74. Slimko ML, Mensah GA. The role of diets, food, and nutrients in the prevention and control of hypertension and prehypertension. Cardiol Clin. 2010;28:665–74.
75. Davinelli S, Scapagnini G. Polyphenols: a promising nutritional approach to prevent or reduce the progression of prehypertension. High Blood Press Cardiovasc Prev. 2016;23:197–202.
76. Williamson W, Foster C, Reid H, Kelly P, Lewandowski AJ, Boardman H, et al. Will exercise advice be sufficient for treatment of young adults with prehypertension and hypertension? A systematic review and meta-analysis. Hypertension. 2016;68:78–87.
77. Rubinstein A, Miranda JJ, Beratarrechea A, Diez-Canseco F, Kanter R, Gutierrez L, et al. Effectiveness of an mHealth intervention to improve the cardiometabolic profile of people with prehypertension in low-resource urban settings in Latin-America: a randomized controlled trial. Lancet Diabetes Endocrinol. 2016;4:52–63.

78. Gao J, Sun H, Liang X, Gao M, Zhao H, Qi Y, et al. Ideal cardiovascular health behaviours and factors prevent the development of hypertension in prehypertensive subjects. Clin Exp Hypertens. 2015;37:650–5.
79. Sipahi I, Swaminathan A, Natesan V, Debanne SM, Simon DI, Fang JC. Effect of antihypertensive therapy on incident stroke in cohorts with prehypertensive blood pressure levels. Stroke. 2012;43:432–40.
80. McInnes G. Prehypertension: how low to go and do drugs have a role? Br J Clin Pharmacol. 2011;73:187–93.
81. Gaddam KK, Ventura H, Lavie CJ. Antihypertensive therapy versus alternative therapeutic options for prehypertension: an evidence-based approach. Futur Cardiol. 2012;8:115–22.
82. Aronow WS. Treating hypertension and prehypertension in older people: when, whom and how. Maturitas. 2015;80:31–6.
83. Collier SR, Landram MJ. Treatment of prehypertension: lifestyle and/or medication. Vasc Health Risk Manag. 2012;8:613–9.
84. Lee M, Saver JL, Chang B, Chang KH, Hao Q, Ovbiagele B. Presence of baseline prehypertension and risk of incident stroke. A meta-analysis. Neurology. 2011;77:1330–7.
85. Huang Y, Cai X, Li Y, Su L, Mai W, Wang S, et al. Prehypertension and the risk of stroke. Neurology. 2014;82:1153–61.
86. Shen L, Ma H, Xiang MX, Wang JA. Meta-analysis of cohort studies of baseline prehypertension and risk of coronary heart disease. Am J Cardiol. 2013;112:266–71.
87. Huang Y, Cai X, Liu C, Zhu D, Hua J, Hu Y, et al. Prehypertension and the risk of coronary heart disease in Asian and Western populations: a meta-analysis. J Am Heart Assoc. 2015;4:e001519.
88. Haung Y, Wang S, Cai X, Mai W, Hu Y, Tang H, et al. Prehypertension and incidence of cardiovascular disease: a meta-analysis. BMC Med. 2013;11:177.
89. Guo X, Zhang X, Guo L, Li Z, Zheng L, Yu S, et al. Association between pre-hypertension and cardiovascular outcomes: a systematic review and meta-analysis of prospective studies. Curr Hypertens Rep. 2013;15:703–16.
90. Huang Y, Cai X, Zhang J, Mai W, Wang S, Hu Y, et al. Prehypertension and incidence of ESRD: a systematic review and meta-analysis. Am J Kidney Dis. 2014;63:76–83.
91. Li Y, Xia P, Xu L, Wang Y, Chen L. A meta-analysis on prehypertension and chronic kidney disease. PLoS One. 2016;11:e0156575.
92. Garofalo C, Borelli S, Pacilio M, Minutolo R, Chiodini P, De Nicola L, et al. Hypertension and prehypertension and prediction of development of decreased estimated GFR in the general population: a meta-analysis of cohort studies. Am J Kidney Dis. 2016;67:89–97.
93. Leiba A, Twig G, Vivante A, Skorecki K, Golan E, Derazne E, et al. Prehypertension among 2.19 million adolescents and future risk for end-stage renal disease. J Hypertens. 2017;35:1290–6.
94. Okada R, Yasuda Y, Tsushita K, Wakai K, Hamajima N, Matsuo S. Glomerular hyperfiltration in prediabetes and prehypertension. Nephrol Dial Transplant. 2012;27:1821–5.
95. Brenner BM, Lawler EV, Mackenzie HS. The hyperfiltration theory: a paradigm shift in nephrology. Kidney Int. 1996;49:1774–7.
96. Losito A, Zampi I, Fortunati I, del Favero A. Glomerular hyperfiltration and albuminuria in essential hypertension. Nephron. 1988;49:84–5.
97. Mogensen CE. Early glomerular hyperfiltration in insulin-dependent diabetics and late nephropathy. Scand J Clin Lab Invest. 1986;46:201–6.
98. Rudberg S, Persson B, Dahlquist G. Increased glomerular filtration rate as a predictor of diabetic nephropathy-an 8-year prospective study. Kidney Int. 1992;41:822–8.
99. Gabbai FB. Renal reserve in patients with high blood pressure. Semin Nephrol. 1995;15:482–7.
100. Sl J, Wiseman MJ, Viberti GC. Glomerular hyperfiltration as a risk factor for diabetic nephropathy: five year report of a prospective study. Diabetologia. 1991;34:59–60.
101. Neuringer JR, Brenner BM. Glomerular hypertension: cause and consequence of renal injury. J Hypertens. 1992;Suppl 10:S91–7.

102. Wang S, Wu H, Zhang Q, Xu J, Fan Y. Impact of baseline prehypertension on cardiovascular events and all-cause mortality in the general population: a meta-analysis of prospective cohort studies. Int J Cardiol. 2013;168:4857–60.
103. Guo X, Zhang Y, Zheng L, Guo L, Li Z, Yu S, et al. Prehypertension is not associated with all-cause mortality: a systematic review and meta-analysis of prospective studies. PLoS One. 2013;8:e61796.
104. Huang Y, Su L, Cai X, Mai W, Wang S, Hu Y, et al. Association of all-cause and cardiovascular mortality with prehypertension: a meta-analysis. Am Heart J. 2014;167:160–8.

5 Prehypertension and the Cardiometabolic Syndrome

Talma Rosenthal

5.1 Definitions of Prehypertension

The USA Joint National Committee Guidelines (JNC7) on hypertension which were published in 2003 [1] combined the two categories: normal blood pressure (BP) and high-normal BP, and thus introduced prehypertension as a new category of BP including individuals with systolic BP 120–139 mmHg or diastolic BP 80–89 mmHg.

However, the European societies ESH/ESC published committee guidelines in 2007 [2] rejected this terminology and the joining of these two BP categories. Their argument was that even in the Framingham study the risk of developing hypertension was higher in subjects with high-normal BP (130–139/85–89 mmHg range) than in patients with normal BP (120–129/80–84 mmHg), therefore there is little reason to combine both groups.

Additionally, considering the ominous significance of the term hypertension, they presumed "prehypertension" may create anxiety and fear in many subjects.

Accordingly, the Framingham study results demonstrated a relatively rapid progression to hypertension in individuals with high-normal BP, in which the incidence of hypertension was 37.3% and 49.5% for the 30- to 64-year and ≥65-year groups, respectively. Whereas a relatively lower risk of developing hypertension was evident among those with normal BP, which progressed over 4 years to hypertensive levels in 17.6% of individuals between 30 and 64 years of age and in 25.5% of those ≥65 years of age [3].

T. Rosenthal
Department of Physiology and Pharmacology,
Tel-Aviv University, Sackler School of Medicine, Tel Aviv, Israel
e-mail: rtalma@post.tau.ac.il

R. Zimlichman et al. (eds.), *Prehypertension and Cardiometabolic Syndrome*, Updates in Hypertension and Cardiovascular Protection,
https://doi.org/10.1007/978-3-319-75310-2_5

Over the years the term prehypertension has been again divided into stage 1 prehypertension which correlates to the previous normal BP while BP in the upper range (130–139/85–89 mmHg) is referred to as stage 2 prehypertension. This division is significant since individuals with BP in the upper-range of prehypertension were shown to be at twice the risk of developing hypertension than individuals with lower BP values [3].

Hypertension is a major modifiable risk factor for cardiovascular morbidity and mortality. Guidelines recommended lowering BP to below 140/90 mmHg in the general population and below 130/80 mmHg in diabetic patients [1, 2]. Thus, even individuals with prehypertension, with BP below the conventional threshold for intervention with antihypertensive drugs, still have an increased risk of cardiovascular disease (CVD). A well-designed meta-analysis showed that particularly those in the upper-range prehypertension (130/80 to 139/89 mmHg) have an increased risk of developing coronary heart disease (CHD) [4]. Moreover, Vasan et al. showed that among the Framingham Heart Study's participants, for individuals with BP in the upper-range of prehypertension, the risk for CVD was 2.5- and 1.6-fold higher among women and men, respectively, than in those with optimal BP (<120/80 mmHg) [5]. Furthermore, a recent meta-analysis of prospective cohort studies indicated that prehypertension was a predictor for cardiovascular events, suggesting subjects in the general population with prehypertension had a 55% and 17% increased risk of CVD and cardiovascular mortality [6]. Nonetheless, the vast majority, especially with stage 1 hypertension have a low absolute risk for CVD, which further questions the benefit of pharmacological treatment [7].

Therefore, all efforts are currently aimed at detection of at-risk individuals with prehypertension and means for preventing their progression to clinical hypertension. Risk scores have been developed for predicting the development of hypertension. The Strong Heart Study, a 12 year longitudinal study, showed baseline systolic BP, diabetes, and increased left ventricular mass were predictive for progression to hypertension in 38% of the 2629 prehypertensive participants [8].

In a recent longitudinal study among 569 healthy individuals, the cumulative 6-year incidence of progression from normotension to prehypertension was 33.5%. The strongest significant predictors of prehypertension were early dysregulation of glucose metabolism and weight gain [9].

Because of these rates of progression, annual or biannual monitoring of BP in prehypertensive individuals has been suggested [9].

5.2 Strategies for Prevention of Hypertension

5.2.1 Nonpharmacological Approaches

To manage or reduce the risk of developing hypertension and to lower cardiovascular risk the established recommendations are termed "Health-promoting Lifestyle Modifications." These include weight loss, dietary recommendations, and increased physical activity.

The final weight loss goal for individuals who are overweight or obese is to maintain a normal body weight (BMI, 18.5–24.9) [1]. The Trials of Hypertension Prevention assessed the efficacy of nonpharmacological interventions (weight loss, sodium restriction, and both interventions together) in a multicenter randomized study including 2383 adults with upper-range prehypertension (130/80 to 139/89 mmHg) and BMI representing 110–165% of desirable body weight. Results showed the interventions were effective already in the short term; at 6-months follow-up BP decreased by 3.7/2.7 mmHg, 2.9/1.6 mmHg, and 4.0/2.8 mmHg in the weight loss, sodium restriction, and combined groups, respectively. Moreover, during the 4-year follow-up, 44% of the usual-care group that was prehypertensive at baseline progressed to hypertension while the three intervention groups showed a significantly reduced relative risk (0.78–0.82) of incident hypertension [10].

The PREMIER 6-month trial assessed the effects of multiple lifestyle interventions based on established recommendations alone and with the addition of the Dietary Approaches to Stop Hypertension (DASH) eating plan, which entails consuming a diet rich in fruits, vegetables, and low-fat dairy products with a reduced content of saturated and total fat. The study included 810 overweight/obese participants average age 50 years, with prehypertension to stage-1 hypertension. Results show that optimal BP control was achieved in 30–35% of the participants in both intervention groups. Further analysis of these results suggests that especially individuals with the metabolic syndrome may benefit in reduced BP levels by adopting the DASH diet [11].

Physical activity recommendations include engaging in a regular routine of aerobic physical activity, such as brisk walking (at least 30 min per day, most days of the week) [1]. An assessment of the benefits of physical activity by a submaximal treadmill exercise test showed the increased aerobic fitness among the PREMIER participants was associated with a reduced prevalence of the metabolic syndrome [12]. Physical fitness has also shown to have a protective effect on progression to hypertension. A graded exercise test conducted in 2303 middle-aged older men with prehypertension showed that within a median of 7.8 years low-fit individuals had a 66% increased risk for developing hypertension compared to high-fit individuals [13]. Another study included 43 prehypertensive young adults who were randomized to 2 exercise training groups (resistance and endurance training) and a control group. The results show both types of exercise training showed effective in reducing BP and peripheral arterial stiffness and in improving resistance artery endothelial function and oxidant/ antioxidant balance in the young prehypertensive participants [14, 15].

Overall studies show engaging in intensive lifestyle interventions can achieve a 20% reduced relative risk of incident hypertension [16].

5.2.2 Pharmacological Approaches

Angiotensin II has been recognized to play a deleterious role in the early course of the atherosclerotic process, thus highlighting the utility in blocking the renin-angiotensin system in patients with hypertension and/or type 2 diabetes with antihypertensive drugs as angiotensin-receptor blockers (ARB) and angiotensin converting enzyme inhibitors (ACEi) [17].

Prevalence rates of prehypertension in adults worldwide are 25–50%. Pharmacological treatment with a single antihypertensive medication can achieve a 34–66% reduced relative risk of progression to incident hypertension [16]. Moreover, early pharmacologic treatment in subjects with high-normal BP with concomitant comorbidities (diabetes, a cluster of cardiovascular risk factors, target organ damage, and metabolic syndrome) has shown beneficial for adequate BP control, which will further contribute to the prevention of cardiovascular complications [18].

The PHARAO trial assessed whether progression to hypertension in prehypertensive individuals can be prevented with pharmacological treatment with ACEi. Participants with BP in the upper range of prehypertension (BP 130–139 and/or 85–89 mmHg) were randomly assigned to 3 years of treatment with Ramipril (505) or placebo (503). The results showed 43% of the group receiving placebo developed hypertension in 3 years. While participants receiving ACEi treatment achieved a 34% reduced relative risk of incident hypertension over 3 years compared with placebo [19].

The TRial Of Preventing HYpertension (TROPHY) aimed at investigating whether pharmacological treatment of prehypertension with ARB prevents or postpones progression to clinical hypertension. Participants with BP in the upper range of prehypertension (BP 130–139 and/or 85–89 mmHg) were randomly assigned to 2 years of treatment with candesartan (409) or placebo (400), followed by 2 years of placebo for all. The TROPHY study results show 63% of prehypertensive individuals aged 30–65 years receiving a placebo developed hypertension within 4 years and >40% after only 2 years [20]. An additional analysis following the new guideline definitions using 2 successive visits showing BP in the upper range of prehypertension, after only 2 years 52% progressed to hypertension in the placebo group [21]. Moreover, participants on ARB medication achieved a 66% reduced risk of incident hypertension at 2 years compared with placebo, and 16% at 4 years (2 years after discontinuation of medication) [20].

The long-term effects of pharmacologic antihypertension therapy, specifically the impact of Health-related quality of life (HRQL—which evaluates the subjective patient experience using both physical and mental components), were assessed among the TROPY participants. The results showed the participants had a relatively high baseline HRQL which was maintained throughout the 2-year treatment period and the 4-year study period [22].

5.3 Early Detection of Prehypertension: Weight, Metabolic Syndrome, and Reduced eGFR

Early detection is aimed at risk stratification of a subset of individuals with prehypertension who are at highest risk of progression to clinical hypertension.

Prehypertension has been associated with the metabolic syndrome. The metabolic syndrome encompasses conditions characterized by various combinations of abnormalities in glucose metabolism, lipid metabolism, and blood pressure [2]. Indeed previous studies have found that not only is the metabolic syndrome associated with prehypertension, it may even precede the elevation in BP. This trend has been established worldwide. For example, a study conducted in China including 1176 urban adults aged 40–70 years found a high prevalence of the metabolic syndrome (evident in lipid metabolism abnormalities) significantly associated with prehypertension detected among these individuals [23].

Accordingly, many studies assessed the utility of early detection of components of the metabolic syndrome, such as weight gain and obesity, lipid metabolism abnormalities as elevated triglycerides, elevated LDL cholesterol, and low levels of HDL cholesterol; dysregulation of glucose metabolism, as insulin resistance and diabetes; and signs of subclinical organ damage as reduced estimated glomerular filtration rate (eGFR) and microalbuminuria and indeed found these associated to prehypertension.

A large study in Japan including 205,382 older adults aged 40–74 years found renal hyperfiltration, the sign of early stage renal damage, detected by reduced eGFR was associated with prehypertension and prediabetes in this large population cohort [24]. A registry study conducted in Spain including 19,041 adults showed prehypertension was associated to markers of insulin resistance assessed by the prevalence of the metabolic syndrome [25]. Similarly, two studies conducted in Taiwan and India found clinical characteristics of insulin resistance syndrome among nondiabetic individuals with prehypertension [26, 27]. While contradictory results regarding the association between prehypertension and insulin resistance were presented in a study conducted in Italy among 1384 healthy adults aged 30–60 years [28].

5.4 The Cardiovascular Metabolic Syndrome

The interplay between a number of risk factors leading to CVD including insulin resistance-diabetes, obesity, endothelial dysfunction, and prehypertension has been termed the cardiovascular metabolic syndrome [29, 30].

The Strong Heart Study included 2629 normotensive participants followed for 12 years. Compared to nondiabetic normotensive participants, the risk for developing incident CVD was 1.8-fold and 2.9-fold higher in participants with prehypertension or diabetes, respectively, with a 3.7-fold increased risk for those with both prehypertension and diabetes [31].

A prospective study included 2376 elderly Koreans, aged >60 years with a median follow-up for 7.6 years. The results showed that hypertensive subjects had a significantly increased risk for CVD mortality. Moreover, compared to normotensive individuals, those with both hypertension and low levels of HDL cholesterol had a twofold higher risk of all-cause mortality [32].

The Coronary Artery Risk Development in Young Adults (CARDIA) Study included 3560 participants age 18–30 followed for 20 years. The results show prehypertension developed in 18% of the cohort before 35 years and was associated with coronary atherosclerosis which is a strong predictor for CHD later in life [33].

Additionally, endothelial dysfunction was found to play a vital role in the progression of atherosclerosis. Diehl et al. employed a unique protocol to assess acute endothelial release of tissue type plasminogen activator (t-PA) in response to bradykinin. Their main finding was a considerably lower (−35%) release of t-PA in prehypertensive men compared with normotensive men [34]. These findings confirm previous work by Hrafnkelsdottir et al. who demonstrated impaired t-PA release in hypertension, by showing that the onset of endothelial fibrinolytic dysfunction with elevated BP manifests in the prehypertensive state [35].

The endothelial consequences of prehypertension are considerable and cannot be overlooked. Along with findings of poor endothelial fibrinolytic capacity, prehypertension is also characterized by reduced nitric oxide-mediated endothelium-dependent vasodilation, increased endothelin-1 vasoconstriction, increased arterial stiffness, and reduced endothelial repair [36].

Evidence has shown that large artery stiffening is one of the most important pathophysiological determinants of isolated systolic hypertension. Moreover, assessments of arterial stiffness have shown to have a predictive value for all-cause mortality and CV morbidity, in patients with essential hypertension [2].

Several prospective studies have identified increased arterial stiffness in prehypertensive subjects as a risk factor for progression to hypertension. While long-term prehypertension may accelerate age-related increase of the arterial stiffness [37]. Suggesting that this vicious cycle towards development of hypertension may be further aggravated by additional CV risk factors as dysregulation of glucose metabolism and aging [38].

Prehypertension and left ventricular dysfunction were found significantly related to vascular inflammation and aortic stiffness, suggesting that an increased inflammatory process is involved in the pathophysiological mechanism of early cardiac and vascular alterations [39].

5.5 Pathophysiological Markers to Detect Risk for Prehypertension

Evidence suggests that inflammation may precede the elevation in BP contributing to the risk for incident hypertension. Using various inflammatory markers, a number of studies have found evidence that insulin resistance is associated with inflammation [29]. The ATTICA study, a cross-sectional population-based survey of 1514 men and 1528 women, revealed an association between prehypertension and inflammatory markers (C-reactive protein (CRP), white blood cells (WBC), tumor necrosis factor-alpha (TNFα), amyloid-a and homocysteine) [40]. Additionally, a new analysis of the WBC counts in participants in the TROPHY trial revealed a significant independent association of WBC counts with baseline BMI and triglycerides showing further evidence that obesity and insulin resistance are associated with inflammation [41].

More recent research has focused on early detection of additional pathophysiological markers as serum complement c3 and serum uric acid that may precede the development of prehypertension and prediabetes. Evidence suggests that circulating serum complement c3 might serve as a signal for an immune process that may lead to the development of impaired glucose tolerance [42]. Two recent studies by the same group of investigators found evidence indicating that elevated serum c3 levels were significantly related to an increased risk of developing prediabetes [43], and prehypertension [44], in an adult population in China, thus suggesting the use of c3 as a biomarker in high-risk individuals to improve primary prevention of these disorders.

A link has been established between highly elevated levels of serum uric acid (hyperuricemia) and CVD. Insight into the pathogenic mechanism of this association has been demonstrated in animal studies. Rat studies have shown that hyperuricemia induced both hypertension as well as endothelial dysfunction which may lead to CVD [45].

Therefore, early detection of elevated SUA levels may provide as a biomarker in individuals at risk of developing prehypertension. A prospective study conducted in Italy included 1156 young to middle-age participants with a median of 11.4 years follow-up. The results showed participants with highly elevated SUA levels had a 31% increased risk of hypertension compared to those with low levels of SUA. Although SUA was an independent predictor of hypertension they also found that physical activity may counteract the pathophysiological mechanisms involved in the association between hyperuricemia and future hypertension [46]. While a study conducted in Brazil among 3412 individuals aged 35–74 years found elevated SUA levels were associated with prehypertension *only* among men [47].

A study among 4817 adults in Singapore found higher SUA levels were associated with prehypertension detected among the study cohort [48]. This association was further confirmed by a meta-analysis including 21,832 prehypertensive individuals which determined a positive association between elevated SUA levels and the risk of prehypertension in the general population [49].

Conclusions

Hypertension is a major modifiable risk factor for cardiovascular morbidity and mortality.

Nonpharmacological treatment interventions with lifestyle modifications (i.e., weight loss, increased physical activity, adopting the DASH diet) are recommended for all patients with prehypertension as these approaches were shown to effectively reduce the risk of CV events. Pharmacological antihypertensive treatment for prehypertensive individuals at increased risk of CV events due to concomitant comorbidities (obesity, diabetes, CV risk factors, target organ damage, and metabolic syndrome) has shown beneficial for adequate BP control, in numerous clinical trials. Risk-stratified, patient-centered approach to the treatment of prehypertension allows an informed, safe, and effective balance of lifestyle and medication interventions to prevent incident hypertension and CVD.

The utility of early detection of various pathophysiological markers (inflammatory markers, endothelial dysfunction, increased arterial stiffness, elevated levels of serum complement c3 and SUA) has shown beneficial for individuals at high risk for developing the cardiovascular metabolic syndrome to improve primary prevention of prehypertension and prediabetes.

References

1. Chobanian AV, Bakris GL, Black HR, Cushman WC, Green LA, Izzo JL Jr, et al. The seventh report of the joint national committee on prevention, detection, evaluation, and treatment of high blood pressure: the JNC 7 report. JAMA. 2003;289(19):2560–71.
2. Mancia G. Guidelines for the management of arterial hypertension: the Task Force for the Management of Arterial Hypertension of the European Society of Hypertension (ESH) and of the European Society of Cardiology (ESC). J Hypertens. 2007;25:1105–87.
3. Vasan RS, Larson MG, Leip EP, Kannel WB, Levy D. Assessment of frequency of progression to hypertension in non-hypertensive participants in the Framingham Heart Study: a cohort study. Lancet. 2001;358(9294):1682–6.
4. Shen L, Ma H, Xiang M-X, Wang J-A. Meta-analysis of cohort studies of baseline prehypertension and risk of coronary heart disease. Am J Cardiol. 2013;112(2):266–71.
5. Vasan RS, Larson MG, Leip EP, Evans JC, O'donnell CJ, Kannel WB, et al. Impact of high-normal blood pressure on the risk of cardiovascular disease. N Engl J Med. 2001;345(18):1291–7.
6. Wang S, Wu H, Zhang Q, Xu J, Fan Y. Impact of baseline prehypertension on cardiovascular events and all-cause mortality in the general population: a meta-analysis of prospective cohort studies. Int J Cardiol. 2013;168(5):4857–60.
7. McInnes G. Pre-hypertension: how low to go and do drugs have a role? Br J Clin Pharmacol. 2012;73(2):187–93.
8. De Marco M, De Simone G, Roman MJ, Chinali M, Lee ET, Russell M, et al. Cardiovascular and metabolic predictors of progression of prehypertension into hypertension. Hypertension. 2009;54(5):974–80.
9. Chobanian AV. Prehypertension revisited. Hypertension. 2006;48:812–4.
10. Effects of weight loss and sodium reduction intervention on blood pressure and hypertension incidence in overweight people with high-normal blood pressure. The Trials of Hypertension Prevention, phase II. The Trials of Hypertension Prevention Collaborative Research Group. Arch Intern Med. 1997;157(6):657–67.
11. Lien LF, Brown AJ, Ard JD, Loria C, Erlinger TP, Feldstein AC, et al. Effects of PREMIER lifestyle modifications on participants with and without the metabolic syndrome. Hypertension. 2007;50(4):609–16.
12. Crist LA, Champagne CM, Corsino L, Lien LF, Zhang G, Young DR. Influence of change in aerobic fitness and weight on prevalence of metabolic syndrome. Prev Chronic Dis. 2012;9:E68.
13. Faselis C, Doumas M, Kokkinos JP, Panagiotakos D, Kheirbek R, Sheriff HM, et al. Exercise capacity and progression from prehypertension to hypertension novelty and significance. Hypertension. 2012;60(2):333–8.
14. Beck DT, Martin JS, Casey DP, Braith RW. Exercise training improves endothelial function in resistance arteries of young prehypertensives. J Hum Hypertens. 2014;28(5):303–9.
15. Beck DT, Martin JS, Casey DP, Braith RW. Exercise training reduces peripheral arterial stiffness and myocardial oxygen demand in young prehypertensive subjects. Am J Hypertens. 2013;26(9):1093–102.

16. Egan BM, Stevens-Fabry S. Prehypertension—prevalence, health risks, and management strategies. Nat Rev Cardiol. 2015;12(5):289–300.
17. Schmieder RE, Hilgers KF, Schlaich MP, Schmidt BMW. Renin-angiotensin system and cardiovascular risk. Lancet. 2007;369(9568):1208–19.
18. Segura J, Ruilope LM. Treatment of prehypertension in diabetes and metabolic syndrome. Diabetes Care. 2009;32(Suppl 2):S284–9.
19. Lüders S, Schrader J, Berger J, Unger T, Zidek W, Böhm M, et al. The PHARAO study: prevention of hypertension with the angiotensin-converting enzyme inhibitor ramipril in patients with high-normal blood pressure—a prospective, randomized, controlled prevention trial of the German Hypertension League. J Hypertens. 2008;26(7):1487–96.
20. Julius S, Nesbitt S, Egan B, Kaciroti N, Schork MA, Grozinski M, et al. Trial of preventing hypertension. Hypertension. 2004;44(2):146–51.
21. Julius S, Kaciroti N, Egan BM, Nesbitt S, Michelson EL, Trial of Preventing Hypertension (TROPHY) Investigators. TROPHY study: outcomes based on the seventh report of the joint National Committee on hypertension definition of hypertension. J Am Soc Hypertens. 2008;2(1):39–43.
22. Williams SA, Michelson EL, Cain VA, Yang M, Nesbitt SD, Egan BM, et al. An evaluation of the effects of an angiotensin receptor blocker on health-related quality of life in patients with high-normal blood pressure (prehypertension) in the trial of preventing hypertension (TROPHY). J Clin Hypertens. 2008;10(6):436–42.
23. Yao W, Sun Y, Wang X, Si Q, Chen H, Wan Z. High prevalence of metabolic syndrome in a middle-aged and elderly population with prehypertension in Tianjin. Clin Exp Hypertens. 2015;37(5):369–74.
24. Okada R, Yasuda Y, Tsushita K, Wakai K, Hamajima N, Matsuo S. The number of metabolic syndrome components is a good risk indicator for both early-and late-stage kidney damage. Nutr Metab Cardiovasc Dis. 2014;24(3):277–85.
25. Cordero A, Laclaustra M, León M, Grima A, Casasnovas JA, Luengo E, et al. Prehypertension is associated with insulin resistance state and not with an initial renal function impairment: a Metabolic Syndrome in Active Subjects in Spain (MESYAS) Registry substudy. Am J Hypertens. 2006;19(2):189–96.
26. Hwu C-M, Liou T-L, Hsiao L-C, Lin M-W. Prehypertension is associated with insulin resistance. QJM. 2009;102(10):705–11.
27. Sathiyapriya V, Nandeesha H, Bobby Z, Pavithran P, Selvaraj N, Rattina DN. Insulin resistance and enhanced protein glycation in men with prehypertension. Clin Chem Lab Med. 2006;44(12):1457–61.
28. Natali A, Muscelli E, Casolaro A, Nilsson P, Melander O, Lalic N, et al. Metabolic characteristics of prehypertension: role of classification criteria and gender. J Hypertens. 2009;27(12):2394–402.
29. Rana JS, Nieuwdorp M, Jukema JW, Kastelein JJP. Cardiovascular metabolic syndrome--an interplay of, obesity, inflammation, diabetes and coronary heart disease. Diabetes Obes Metab. 2007;9(3):218–32.
30. Duprez D, Toleuova A. Prehypertension and the cardiometabolic syndrome: pathological and clinical consequences. Expert Rev Cardiovasc Ther. 2013;11(12):1725–33.
31. Zhang Y, Lee ET, Devereux RB, Yeh J, Best LG, Fabsitz RR, et al. Prehypertension, diabetes, and cardiovascular disease risk in a population-based sample. Hypertension. 2006;47(3):410–4.
32. Kim NH, Cho HJ, Kim YJ, Cho MJ, Choi HY, Eun CR, et al. Combined effect of high-normal blood pressure and low HDL cholesterol on mortality in an elderly Korean population: the South-West Seoul (SWS) study. Am J Hypertens. 2011;24(8):918.
33. Pletcher MJ, Bibbins-Domingo K, Lewis CE, Wei GS, Sidney S, Carr JJ, et al. Prehypertension during young adulthood and coronary calcium later in life. Ann Intern Med. 2008;149(2):91–9.
34. Diehl KJ, Weil BR, Greiner JJ, Wright KP, Stauffer BL, DeSouza CA. Impaired endogenous fibrinolytic capacity in prehypertensive men. J Hum Hypertens. 2015;29(8):468–72.
35. Hrafnkelsdóttir T, Wall U, Jern C, Jern S. Impaired capacity for endogenous fibrinolysis in essential hypertension. Lancet. 1998;352(9140):1597–8.

36. Van Guilder GP. It is time to contend with the endothelial consequences of prehypertension. J Hum Hypertens. 2015;29(8):457.
37. Patil SG, Aithala M, Das KK. Evaluation of arterial stiffness in elderly with prehypertension. Indian J Physiol Pharmacol. 2015;59(1):16–22.
38. Tomiyama H, Yamashina A. Arterial stiffness in prehypertension: a possible vicious cycle. J Cardiovasc Transl Res. 2012;5(3):280–6.
39. Celik T, Yuksel UC, Fici F, Celik M, Yaman H, Kilic S, et al. Vascular inflammation and aortic stiffness relate to early left ventricular diastolic dysfunction in prehypertension. Blood Press. 2013;22(2):94–100.
40. Chrysohoou C, Pitsavos C, Panagiotakos DB, Skoumas J, Stefanadis C. Association between prehypertension status and inflammatory markers related to atherosclerotic disease: The ATTICA Study. Am J Hypertens. 2004;17(7):568–73.
41. Julius S, Egan BM, Kaciroti NA, Nesbitt SD, Chen AK, TROPHY Investigators. In prehypertension leukocytosis is associated with body mass index but not with blood pressure or incident hypertension. J Hypertens. 2014;32(2):251–9.
42. Onat A, Can G, Rezvani R, Cianflone K. Complement C3 and cleavage products in cardiometabolic risk. Clin Chim Acta. 2011;412(13):1171–9.
43. Bao X, Xia Y, Zhang Q, Wu HM, Du HM, Liu L, et al. Elevated serum complement C3 levels are related to the development of prediabetes in an adult population: the Tianjin Chronic Low-Grade Systematic Inflammation and Health Cohort Study. Diabet Med. 2016;33(4):446–53.
44. Bao X, Meng G, Zhang Q, Liu L, Wu H, Du H, et al. Elevated serum complement C3 levels are associated with prehypertension in an adult population. Clin Exp Hypertens. 2017;39(1):42–9.
45. Khosla UM, Zharikov S, Finch JL, Nakagawa T, Roncal C, Mu W, et al. Hyperuricemia induces endothelial dysfunction. Kidney Int. 2005;67(5):1739–42.
46. Saladini F, Mos L, Fania C, Garavelli G, Casiglia E, Palatini P. Regular physical activity prevents development of hypertension in young people with hyperuricemia. J Hypertens. 2017;35(5):994–1001.
47. Lotufo PA, Baena CP, Santos IS, Bensenor IM. Serum uric acid and prehypertension among adults free of cardiovascular diseases and diabetes: baseline of the Brazilian longitudinal study of adult health (ELSA-Brasil). Angiology. 2016;67(2):180–6.
48. Syamala S, Li J, Shankar A. Association between serum uric acid and prehypertension among US adults. J Hypertens. 2007;25(8):1583–9.
49. Jiang M, Gong D, Fan Y. Serum uric acid levels and risk of prehypertension: a meta-analysis. Clin Chem Lab Med. 2017;55(3):314–21.

Prehypertension: Definition and Epidemiology

6

Sadi Gulec and Cetin Erol

6.1 Definition of Prehypertension

Prehypertension is a term used to describe a condition of increased blood pressure (BP) which falls short of a formal definition of hypertension yet confers an increased risk of progression to hypertension and/or cardiovascular disease. The word itself has been first introduced in 2003, when Joint National Committee on Prevention, Detection, Evaluation, and Treatment of High Blood Pressure issued its seventh report (JNC-7) [1]. The report set the threshold for a normal blood pressure reading lower than ever before, at 120/80 millimeters of mercury (mmHg), and it also established a new diagnostic category of "prehypertension" for those with BPs ranging from 120–139 mmHg systolic and/or 80–89 mmHg diastolic. Prehypertension emerged from the fusion of two categories employed by the JNC-6: high-normal BP (130–139/85–89 mmHg) and normal BP (120–129/80–84 mmHg). The decision to establish this new BP category was based on a number of factors. Framingham Heart Study investigators had reported the lifetime risk of hypertension to be approximately 90 percent in individuals whose BP was normal at age 55 years [2]. Furthermore, a meta-analysis of 61 prospective studies had shown that mortality from ischemic heart disease and stroke in individuals aged 40–89 years increases in a log-linear relationship with BP, from levels as low as 115 mmHg systolic and 75 mmHg diastolic [3]. In addition, a WHO report had indicated that about 62% of cerebrovascular disease and 49% of ischemic heart disease were attributable to suboptimal blood pressure (systolic blood pressure >115 mmHg) globally [4]. However, the 2003 European Society of Hypertension-European Society of Cardiology (ESH/ESC) guidelines [5] as well as the 2003 World Health Organization/International

S. Gulec (✉) · C. Erol
Cardiology Department, Medical School of Ankara University, Ankara, Turkey
e-mail: sgulec@ankara.edu.tr

R. Zimlichman et al. (eds.), *Prehypertension and Cardiometabolic Syndrome*, Updates in Hypertension and Cardiovascular Protection,
https://doi.org/10.1007/978-3-319-75310-2_6

Society of Hypertension (WHO/ISH) Statement on management of hypertension [6] did not share JNC-7's view. The point of objection was the inhomogeneity within the prehypertension category in terms of cardiovascular risk. Individuals with BP 130–139/85–89 mmHg were more likely to progress to hypertensive values and to develop cardiovascular disease when compared to those with BP 120–129/80–84 mmHg.

The JNC-7 guidelines made clear that prehypertension was not a disease category and that people labeled prehypertensive should not be treated with drugs. Rather, it was a new designation intended to identify those individuals in whom early intervention by adoption of healthy lifestyle modifications could reduce BP, decrease the rate of progression to clinical hypertension with age, or to prevent hypertension entirely. Although lifestyle modifications have been shown to reduce BP and retard the development of manifest hypertension [7–9], people are reluctant to adopt healthy behaviors [10]. Even a past heart attack does not seem to encourage patients sufficient enough to adopt healthy lifestyle modifications. In PURE study [11], we found that the prevalence of healthy lifestyle behaviors among patients with a CHD or stroke event from countries with varying income levels was less than 5%. Another source of concern for prehypertension was that dealing with large numbers of prehypertensive individuals might place excessive burdens on physicians who already are having difficulty managing hypertensive patients.

Recently, several national and international guidelines for the management of hypertension have been published [12–17]. When these guidelines are reviewed and compared with respect to BP classification, significant discrepancies have been noted in nomenclature (Table 6.1). There appears to be three different approaches for classifying BP when it is in the range of 120–139/80–89 mmHg. First one is to call them all "prehypertensive" as suggested by JNC-7 and ASH/ISH [12] guidelines. Second one is to call them "normal" if it is 120–129/ 80–84 mmHg, and "high-normal" if it is 130–139/85–89 mmHg. European [13], Canadian [14], Australian [15], and Japanese [16] guidelines use this approach. The third and final approach is to ignore them, or call them all "normal" as it is in the British NICE

Table 6.1 Blood pressure classifications in various hypertension guidelines for values of <140/90 mmHg

Guidelines	Classifications	Systolic BP (mmHg)	Diastolic BP (mmHg)
JNC-7, 2003	Prehypertension	120–139	80–89
ASH/ISH, 2013	Normal	<120	<80
ESH/ESC, 2013	Optimal	<120	<80
JSH, 2014	Normal	120–129	80–84
NHFA, 2016	High-normal	130–139	80–84
CHEP, 2017			
NICE, 2011 (Updated in 2016)	Normal	<140	<90

ASH/ISH American Society of Hypertension/International Society of Hypertension, *CHEP* Canadian Hypertension Education Program, *ESH/ESC* European Society of Hypertension/European Society of Cardiology, *JNC-7* Seventh Joint National Committee, *JSH* Japanese Society of Hypertension, *NHFA* National Heart Foundation of Australia, *NICE* National Institute for Clinical Excellence guidelines [17]. Accordingly, if you have a blood pressure of 130/80 mmHg, it will be named as "prehypertension" in USA, "high-normal" in Europe, and "normal" in England. Guidelines like JNC, ESH/ESC, and NICE, are recognized by many physicians from different countries who do not have their own national guidelines. It should be noted that these physicians feel confused and unmotivated because of the disagreements between credible guidelines on major topics [18]. We wish developers of these guidelines would cooperate and make a consensus paper regarding these issues.

Currently, little is known about how often physicians use the prehypertension classification when treating patients, and how patients recall and respond to this information. Researchers from School of Medicine, University of North Carolina, conducted a trial [19] aiming to estimate how often patients with prehypertension are being told about it by their primary care physicians. Participants were asked to indicate whether a doctor or other health care provider had ever told them they had "prehypertension" (Yes/ No); a subsample of patients with measured BP in the prehypertension range was asked the same question. Of 1008 non-hypertensive patients, 1.9% indicated being told they had prehypertension. Among a subsample of 102 patients with measured BP in the prehypertension range, 2.0% indicated being told they had prehypertension. This data may suggest physicians are reluctant to tell patients they have prehypertension and do not talk about lifestyle modification. One other explanation is that, clinicians counsel patients about lifestyle modifications that will reduce their chances of developing hypertension without labeling them with prehypertension. There, actually, is a claim that being labeled prehypertensive may have unintended negative consequences that could limit the potential benefits of early identification of elevated BP. Increases in work absenteeism [20], higher levels of physical symptoms [21], and lower health-related quality of life [22] have been reported among patients who are aware of their hypertension status compared with those who are hypertensive but unaware of the diagnosis. Negative outcomes are not explained by BP elevation itself or by drug treatment, suggesting that psychological effects of being labeled likely play a significant role. Viera et al. [23], examined whether the label of prehypertension exerts a negative effect on patients' perceived health and whether it motivates people to adopt lifestyle recommendations to prevent hypertension. They randomized 97 newly diagnosed prehypertensive adults to either a labeling message or a generic (no label) message. Those in the "label" group received a standardized message delivered by a trained research assistant. The participant was told that he/she had prehypertension; that was followed by a description of various lifestyle recommendations. Within the message the term "prehypertension" was mentioned several times. Those in the "no label" group received a very similar standardized message about lifestyle modifications without any mention of prehypertension. At 3 months there were no differences in reports of changing eating habits, cutting down on salt, reducing alcohol intake, or exercising to try to prevent hypertension. Perception of health parameters was also not different at the end of the follow-up. Being labeled as prehypertensive seems to exert neither harmful nor helpful effects. In a similar study, Spruill et al. [24] evaluated the effects of labeling individuals with prehypertension on BP and health-related quality of life. They randomly assigned 100 patients to either a "Labeled" group in which they were informed of their prehypertension, or an "Unlabeled" group in which they were not informed. Subjects underwent office BP measurement, 24 h ambulatory BP monitoring and completed self-report questionnaires at baseline and 3 months. Their findings suggest that labeling patients with prehypertension does not have negative effects on BP or quality of life, at least in the short term. Thus, few studies with limited number patients suggest that prehypertension labeling may not be harmful to patients. It is also not particularly helpful. Studies are needed to determine approaches to communicate with prehypertensive patients that will increase the likelihood of lifestyle change and lead to improved health outcomes.

6.2 Diagnosis of Prehypertension

Blood pressure screening is sine qua non for the early diagnosis of hypertension. However, the diagnosis process is much more complex than it looks. Consider a patient with an office BP of >140/90 mmHg. Is this patient hypertensive? Indeed, confirmation of the initial BP by subsequent measurement(s) is needed before a patient can be diagnosed as hypertensive. According to the JNC-7, and the ESH/ESC guidelines, BP classification should be based on the average of at least two properly measured, seated BP readings on each of at least two office visits. However, according to the CHEP, five visits with average BPs of >140 and/or >90 mmHg is needed to label a patient as hypertensive. On the other hand, NICE asks physicians to perform ambulatory BP monitoring to confirm the diagnosis of hypertension. If a person is unable to tolerate ambulatory BP monitoring, home BP monitoring of at least 4 days is recommended as a suitable alternative to confirm the diagnosis of hypertension. Indeed, out-of-office BP measurement currently remains the "gold standard" for screening, diagnosis, and management of hypertension. It is crucial for the diagnosis of white-coat effect and masked hypertension. Actual guidelines have proposed that levels of the self-measured BP at home of 135 mmHg systolic or 85 mmHg diastolic or higher and/or 24 h ambulatory BP of 130 mmHg systolic or 80 mmHg diastolic or higher indicate hypertension. However, out-of-office thresholds for prehypertension and/or high-normal BP has not been identified in any of the existing guidelines. This may cause confusion in daily practice. For example, if a patient has an average office BP of 130/80 mmHg, you may call it prehypertension. What if the average home BP of the same patient is 115/75 mmHg? Does he/she really have prehypertension? Or should we call it "white-coat prehypertension" (i.e., prehypertension at office and normotension at home). As another example, what if the office BP is 110/70 mmHg, while the home BP is 130/80 mmHg? Should we call it "masked prehypertension"? (i.e., normotension at office and prehypertension at home). Recently, Niiranen et al. [25] conducted a trial to determine an outcome-driven reference frame for home BP measurement based on individual participant data that includes all existing population cohorts with fatal and nonfatal outcomes available for analysis. They measured home and clinic BP in 6470 participants, and calculated the home BP levels that yielded 10-year absolute risks of cardiovascular, cerebrovascular, or cardiac events similar to those associated with stages 1 (120–129/80–84) and 2 (130–139/85–89) prehypertension on clinic BP measurement. The rounded thresholds amounted to 120/75 and 125/80 mmHg, respectively. Head et al. [26] evaluated 8575 patients to derive ambulatory BP equivalents to clinic BP thresholds for diagnosis of different stages of hypertension. Their analysis has shown that the closer the patient's BP is to normal levels, the closer is the agreement between daytime ambulatory and clinic BP. On the other hand, the higher the BP, the greater the difference between ambulatory and clinic BP. The daytime systolic/diastolic ambulatory BP equivalent to the lower limit of grade 1 or mild hypertension (140/90) was estimated to be 4/3 mmHg lower (136/87) than clinic values; the estimate for grade 2 hypertension (160/100) was 8/4 mmHg lower (152/96) and for grade 3 hypertension (180/100) was 12/6 mmHg lower (168/105). Based on this data, systolic/diastolic ambulatory BP equivalent to the lower limit of prehypertension can be expected to be similar or slightly lower than that of the office value of 120/80 mmHg. More data are needed to identify home and ambulatory BP thresholds for prehypertension.

6.3 Epidemiology of Prehypertension

6.3.1 Prevalence

Numerous epidemiologic studies from different countries have documented the prevalence of prehypertension. Data from the 2011 and 2012 National Health and Nutrition Examination Survey (NHANES III) suggested that the prevalence of prehypertension among adults in the United States was approximately 28% [27]. Reported prevalence of prehypertension for some other countries were as follows: China 36.4% [28], Japan 33% [29], India 33.2% [30], UK 43.9% [31], Canada 27.2% [31], Netherlands 32.8% [32] sub-Saharan Africa 29.8%, [33], Brazil 36.1% [34], Belarus 34.3% [35], and Iran 47.3% [36]. Variations in the BP measurement methodology, age range of study participants, exclusion of individuals with hypertension in some cohorts and the standard population chosen for age adjustment made direct comparisons of the studies difficult. In a systematic review and meta-analysis of 20 cross-sectional and 6 longitudinal studies, the overall prevalence of prehypertension was 36% [37]. In accordance, PURE (Prospective Urban and Rural Epidemiological) study [38], assessing 153,996 individuals in 17 countries, found the prevalence of prehypertension as 36.8% (unpublished data). It turns out that a huge number of people in any given population are actually people with prehypertension.

Recently, data on the temporal changes in the prevalence of prehypertension and hypertension have also been published. A systematic analysis of population-based studies from 90 countries showed that the prevalence of hypertension decreased by 2.6% in high-income countries but increased by 7.7% in low- and middle-income countries from 2000 to 2010 [39]. It has been suggested that aging and urbanization with accompanying unhealthy lifestyle may play a role in the epidemic of hypertension in low- and middle-income countries. Evaluation of two cross-sectional surveys conducted with participants aged >60 years in the same district in Beijing, China, and using the same methods in both 2001 and 2010 showed that the prevalence of prehypertension decreased, whereas the prevalence of hypertension increased with increasing age [40]. This finding was consistent with previous studies [41]. The explanation was that by this age most of the people with prehypertension would have already developed full-blown hypertension. On the other hand, according to the National Health and Nutrition Examination Surveys between 1999 and 2012, the percentage of US adults with prehypertension decreased from 31.2 to 28.2% without any increase in the rate of hypertension [27].

6.3.2 Distribution of Prehypertension by Age, Sex, and Race or Ethnicity

According to the WHO Global Health Observatory reports 2015 (last updated 2017.01.11) [42] the global estimates of age standardized (+18 years old) prevalence of hypertension was 24.1% in men and 20.1% in women while age standardized mean systolic BP was 127.0 and 122.3 mmHg, respectively. Hypertension was more common in males than females in nearly all countries for which data were available, with few exceptions (i.e., Ireland, Tajikistan, and Turkey) where the prevalence was the same in both sexes. Like hypertension, prehypertension has been found to be more prevalent among men than among women [43]. Gender differences in the distribution of prehypertension and hypertension seem to vary from culture to culture, which implies an interaction between social and biological mechanisms. The prevalence of prehypertension increases with age in both genders, except for those >60 years of age because of a higher prevalence of hypertension [44].

In terms of race/ethnic variables, multiethnic comparison studies on prevalence have produced contradictory evidence. Reasons for Geographic and Racial Differences in Stroke (REGARDS) study (n = 5553 individuals with prehypertension) [45] found that the prevalence of prehypertension was higher in African-American participants across all age and gender strata. In line with them, The Bogalusa Heart Study [46] indicated that prehypertension prevalence was higher among black compared to white participants. In the Women's Health Initiative study [47], however, prehypertension was present in 39.5%, 32.1%, 42.6%, 38.7%, and 40.3% of white, black, Hispanic, American Indian, and Asian women, respectively (P = 0.0001 across ethnic groups). The Multi-Ethnic Study of Atherosclerosis (MESA) study [48] investigated the age-specific incidence of hypertension by ethnicity for 3146 participants. After adjustment for age, sex, and study site, the incidence rate ratio for hypertension was increased for blacks age 45–74 years compared with whites. Hispanic participants also had a higher incidence of hypertension compared with whites; however, hypertension incidence did not differ for Chinese and white participants. On the other hand, NHANES III found no difference in the prevalence between Non-Hispanic whites, Non-Hispanic blacks, Mexican Americans, or others [49]. Recent study from China [50], a multi-ethnic country, where minorities have their specific dietary habits and lifestyles, which could influence their blood pressure status, demonstrated that prevalence of prehypertension was statistically different between ethnicities. A study from Europe [32] demonstrated that the prevalence of prehypertension did not differ between the ethnic groups in men African Surinamese and Hindustani Surinamese women, however, had a higher prevalence of prehypertension than White Dutch women.

6.3.3 Incidence

Much less is known about the incidence of newly developed prehypertension than about its prevalence. In a Middle East population-based cohort, during a median follow-up of 9.2 years about half of the individuals who were normotensive at baseline had progressed to prehypertension [51]. Progression was more prominent among men. In a subpopulation of Women's Health Initiative, 3 years incidence of prehypertension was 27.3% among Hispanic women [52]. Very recently, Hardy et al. [53] studied age, racial/ethnic, and sex-specific annual net transition probabilities between categories of BP using three NHANES cross-sectional samples. From ages 8 to 30 years, annual net transition probabilities from normal BP to prehypertension among male individuals were more than two times the net transition probabilities of their female counterparts. The largest net transition probabilities for ages 8–30 years occurred in African American young men, while Mexican American young women aged 8–30 years experienced the lowest normal to prehypertension transition. After age 40 years, normal BP to prehypertension net transition probabilities stabilized or decreased for men, whereas increased rapidly for women. Mexican American women exhibited the largest normal to prehypertension net transition probabilities after age 60 years. Authors suggest that primordial prevention beginning in childhood and into early adulthood is necessary to preempt the development of prehypertension as well as associated racial/ethnic and sex disparities.

6.3.4 Associated Risk Factors

Like hypertension, prehypertension tends to cluster with other cardiovascular risk factors such as dyslipidemia, obesity, and diabetes mellitus [54, 55]. It has been shown that almost 90% of individuals with prehypertension have at least one other traditional cardiovascular risk factor [56]. Association with inflammation [57], microalbuminuria [58], income status, education level, diet [28, 59, 60], and living in an urban or rural area [60] also have been reported with contradictory results. Prehypertension and associated metabolic risk factors will be discussed in detail elsewhere in this book.

References

1. Chobanian AV, Bakris GL, Black HR, et al. The seventh report of the joint national committee on prevention, detection, evaluation, and treatment of high blood pressure: the JNC 7 report. JAMA. 2003;289:2560–71.
2. Vasan RS, Larson MG, Leip EP, et al. Assessment of frequency of progression to hypertension in non- hypertensive participants in the Framingham Heart Study: a cohort study. Lancet. 2001;358:1682–6.
3. Lewington S, Clarke R, Qizilbash N, et al. Age-specific relevance of usual blood pressure to vascular mortality: a meta-analysis of individual data for one million adults in 61 prospective studies. Lancet. 2002;360:1903–13.
4. World Health Report 2002. Reducing risks, promoting healthy life. http://www.who.int/whr/2002/ Accessed 27 June 2017.
5. European Society of Hypertension-European Society of Cardiology Guidelines Committee. European Society of Hypertension-European Society of Cardiology guidelines for the management of arterial hypertension. J Hypertens. 2003;21:1011–53.
6. World Health Organization /International Society of Hypertension Writing group. 2003 World Health Organization (WHO)/International Society of Hypertension (ISH) statement on management of hypertension. J Hypertens. 2003;21:1983–92.
7. Appel LJ, Champagne CM, Harsha DW, et al. Writing Group of the PREMIER Collaborative Research Group. Effects of comprehensive lifestyle modification on blood pressure control: main results of the PREMIER clinical trial. JAMA. 2003;289:2083–93.
8. Prather AA, Blumenthal JA, Hinderliter AL, Sherwood A. Ethnic differences in the effects of the DASH diet on nocturnal blood pressure in individuals with high blood pressure. Am J Hypertens. 2011;24:1338–44.
9. Faselis C, Doumas M, Kokkinos JP, et al. Exercise capacity and progression from prehypertension to hypertension. Hypertension. 2012;60:333–8.
10. Greenlund KJ, Daviglus ML, Croft JB. Differences in healthy lifestyle characteristics between adults with prehypertension and normal blood pressure. J Hypertens. 2009;27:955–62.
11. Teo K, Lear S, Islam S, et al; on behalf of PURE Study Investigators. Prevalence of a healthy lifestyle among individuals with cardiovascular disease in high-, middle- and low-income countries the Prospective Urban Rural Epidemiology (PURE) study. JAMA. 2013;310:959–68.
12. Weber MA, Schiffrin EL, White WB, et al. Clinical practice guidelines for the management of hypertension in the community a statement by the American Society of Hypertension and the International Society of Hypertension. J Hypertens. 2014;32:3–15.
13. Mancia G, Fagard R, Narkiewicz K, et al. The Task Force for the management of arterial hypertension of the European Society of Hypertension (ESH) and of the European Society of Cardiology (ESC). 2013 ESH/ESC guidelines for the management of arterial hypertension. Eur Heart J. 2013;34:2159–219.
14. Leung AA, Daskalopoulou SS, Dasgupta K, et al. Hypertension Canada's 2017 guidelines for diagnosis, risk assessment, prevention and treatment of hypertension in adults. Can J Cardiol. 2017;33:557–76.
15. Gabb GM, Mangoni AA, Anderson CS, et al. Guideline for the diagnosis and management of hypertension in adults, 2016. Med J Aust. 2016;205:85–9.
16. Shimamoto K, Ando K, Fujita T, et al. Japanese Society of Hypertension Committee for Guidelines for the Management of Hypertension: the Japanese Society of Hypertension Guidelines for the Management of Hypertension (JSH 2014). Hypertens Res. 2014;37:253–387.
17. National Institute for Health and Care Excellence. Hypertension: clinical management of primary hypertension in adults (Clinical guideline 127). http://guidance.nice.org.uk/CG127. Accessed 27 June 2017.
18. Gulec S. Early diagnosis saves lives: focus on patients with hypertension. Kidney Int Suppl. 2013;3:332–4.
19. Viera AJ, Bangura F, Mitchell CM, et al. Do clinicians tell patients they have prehypertension? J Am Board Fam Med. 2011;24:117–8.

20. Haynes RB, Sackett DL, Taylor DW, et al. Increased absenteeism from work after detection and labeling of hypertensive patients. N Engl J Med. 1978;299:741–4.
21. Stewart JC, France CR, Sheffield D. Hypertension awareness and pain reports: data from the NHANES III. Ann Behav Med. 2003;26:8–14.
22. Barger SD, Muldoon MF. Hypertension labelling was associated with poorer self-rated health in the Third US National Health and Nutrition Examination Survey. J Hum Hypertens. 2006;20:117–23.
23. Viera AJ, MD MPH, et al. Effects of labeling patients as prehypertensive. J Am Board Fam Med. 2010;23:571–83.
24. Spruill TM, Feltheimer SD, Harlapur M, et al. Are there consequences of labeling patients with prehypertension? An experimental study of effects on blood pressure and quality of life. J Psychosom Res. 2013;74:433–8.
25. Niiranen TJ, Asayama K, Thijs L, et al. for the International Database of HOme blood pressure in relation to Cardiovascular Outcome Investigators. Outcome-driven thresholds for home blood pressure measurement international database of home blood pressure in relation to cardiovascular outcome. Hypertension. 2013;61:27–34.
26. Head GA, Mihailidou AS, Duggan KA, et al. Definition of ambulatory blood pressure targets for diagnosis and treatment of hypertension in relation to clinic blood pressure: prospective cohort study. BMJ. 2010;340:c1104.
27. Booth JN, Li J, Zhang L, et al. Trends in prehypertension and hypertension risk factors in US adults1999–2012. Hypertension. 2017;70(2):275–84.
28. Meng XJ, Dong GH, Wang D, et al. Epidemiology of prehypertension and associated risk factors in urban adults from 33 communities in China—The CHPSNE Study. Circ J. 2012;76:900–6.
29. Ishikawa Y, Ishikawa L, Ishikawa S, et al. for the JMS Cohort Investigators Group. Prevalence and determinants of prehypertension in a Japanese general population: The Jichi Medical School Cohort Study. Hypertens Res. 2008;31:1323–30.
30. Gupta R, Deedwania PC, Achari V, et al. Normotension, prehypertension, and hypertension in urban middle-class subjects in India: prevalence, awareness, treatment, and control. Am J Hypertens. 2013;26:83–94.
31. Joffres M, Falaschetti E, Gillespie C, et al. Hypertension prevalence, awareness, treatment and control in national surveys from England, the USA and Canada, and correlation with stroke and ischaemic heart disease mortality: a cross-sectional study. BMJ Open. 2013;3:e003423. https://doi.org/10.1136/bmjopen-2013-003423.
32. Agyemang C, van Valkengoed I, van den Born BJ, Stronks K. Prevalence and determinants of prehypertension among African Surinamese, Hindustani Surinamese, and White Dutch in Amsterdam, the Netherlands: The SUNSET study. Eur J Cardiovasc Prev Rehabil. 2007;14:775–81.
33. Guwatudde D, Nankya-Mutyoba J, Kalyesubula R, et al. The burden of hypertension in sub-Saharan Africa: a four-country cross sectional study. BMC Public Health. 2015;15:1211. https://doi.org/10.1186/s12889-015-2546-z.
34. Silva DA, Petroski EL, Peres MA, et al. Prehypertension and hypertension among adults in a metropolitan area in southern Brazil: population-based study. Rev Saude Publica. 2012;46:988–98.
35. Podpalov V, Stchastlivenko AI, Zhurova ON, et al. Prevalence of prehypertension, hypertension and cardiovascular risk factors in a Belarus urban population. Eur Heart J. 2013;34(Suppl 1):5960.
36. Tabrizi JS, Bazargani HS, Farahbakhsh M, et al. Prevalence and associated factors of prehypertension and hypertension in Iranian population: Lifestyle Promotion Project (LPP). PLos One. 2016. https://doi.org/10.1371/journal.pone.0165264.
37. Guo X, Zou L, Zhang X, et al. Prehypertension: a meta-analysis of the epidemiology, risk factors, and predictors of progression. Tex Heart Inst J. 2011;38:643–52.
38. Teo K, Chow CK, Vaz M, et al. The Prospective Urban Rural Epidemiology (PURE) study. Am Heart J. 2009;158:1–7.

39. Mills KT, Bundy JD, Kelly TN, et al. Global disparities of hypertension prevalence and control a systematic analysis of population-based studies from 90 countries. Circulation. 2016;134:441–50.
40. Wu L, He Y, Jiang B, et al. Trends in prevalence, awareness, treatment and control of hypertension during 2001–2010 in an urban elderly population of China. PLoS One. 2015;10(8):e0132814. https://doi.org/10.1371/journal.pone.0132814.
41. Chiu YH, Wu SC, Tseng CD, et al. Progression of pre-hypertension, stage 1 and 2 hypertension (JNC 7): a population-based study in Keelung, Taiwan (Keelung Community-based Integrated Screening No. 9). J Hypertens. 2006;24:821–8.
42. WHO Global Observatory data. http://apps.who.int/gho/data/view.main.12467GLOBAL?lang=en. Accessed 22 June 2017.
43. Grotto I, Grossman E, Huerta M, Sharabi Y. Prevalence of prehypertension and associated cardiovascular risk profiles among young Israeli adults. Hypertension. 2006;48:254–9.
44. Wang Y, Wang QJ. The prevalence of prehypertension and hypertension among US adults according to the new Joint National Committee guidelines. Arch Intern Med. 2004;164:2126–34.
45. Glasser SP, Judd S, Basile J, et al. Prehypertension, racial prevalence and association with risk factors: analysis of the REasons for Geographic And Racial Differences in Stroke (REGARDS) Study. Am J Hypertens. 2011;24:194–9.
46. Toprak A, Wang H, Chen W, et al. Prehypertension and black-white contrasts in cardiovascular risk in young adults: Bogalusa heart study. J Hypertens. 2009;27:243–50.
47. Hsia J, Margolis KL, Eaton CB, et al. for the Women's Health Initiative Investigators. Prehypertension and cardiovascular disease risk in the Women's Health Initiative. Circulation. 2007;115:855–60.
48. Carson AP, Howard G, Burke GL. Ethnic differences in hypertension incidence among middle-aged and older adults the multi-ethnic study of atherosclerosis. Hypertension. 2011;57:1101–7.
49. Gu Q, Burt VL, Paulose-Ram R, et al. High blood pressure and cardiovascular disease mortality risk among U.S. adults: the third National Health and Nutrition Examination Survey mortality follow-up study. Ann Epidemiol. 2008;18:302–9.
50. Xu T, Liu J, Zhu G, et al. Prevalence of prehypertension and associated risk factors among Chinese adults from a large-scale multi-ethnic population survey. BMC Public Health. 2016;16:775. https://doi.org/10.1186/s12889-016-3411-4.
51. Hadaegh F, Hasheminia M, Abdi H et al. (2015) Prehypertension Tsunami: a decade follow-up of an Iranian adult population. PLoS One. 10(10):e0139412. https://doi.org/10.1371/journal.pone.0139412.
52. Zambrana RE, López L, Dinwiddie GY, et al. Prevalence and incident prehypertension and hypertension in postmenopausal Hispanic women: results from the Women's Health Initiative. Am J Hypertens. 2014;27:372–81.
53. Hardy ST, Holliday KM, Chakladar S, et al. Heterogeneity in blood pressure transitions over the life course. Age-specific emergence of racial/ethnic and sex disparities in the United States. JAMA Cardiol. 2017;2:653. https://doi.org/10.1001/jamacardio.2017.0652.
54. Gupta AK, McGlone M, Greenway FL, Johnson WD. Prehypertension in disease-free adults: a marker for an adverse cardiometabolic risk profile. Hypertens Res. 2010;33:905–10.
55. Greenlund KJ, Croft JB, Mensah GA. Prevalence of heart disease and stroke risk factors in persons with prehypertension in the United States, 1999–2000. Arch Intern Med. 2004;164:2113–8.
56. Mainous AG 3rd, Everett CJ, Liszka H, et al. Prehypertension and mortality in a nationally representative cohort. Am J Cardiol. 2004;94:1496–500.
57. Chrysohoou C, Pitsavos C, Panagiotakos DB, et al. Association between prehypertension status and inflammatory markers related to atherosclerotic disease: The ATTICA Study. Am J Hypertens. 2004;17:568–73.

58. Navarro-gonzález JF, Mora C, Muros M, et al. Relationship between inflammation and microalbuminuria in prehypertension. J Hum Hypertens. 2013;27:119–25.
59. Yang G, Ma Y, Wang S, et al. Prevalence and correlates of prehypertension and hypertension among adults in Northeastern China: a cross sectional study. Int J Environ Res Public Health. 2016;13:82. https://doi.org/10.3390/ijerph13010082.
60. Hu L, Huang X, You C, et al. Prevalence and risk factors of prehypertension and hypertension in Southern China. PLoS One. 2017;12(1):e0170238. https://doi.org/10.1371/journal.pone.0170238.

7 Prehypertension, Statistics and Health Burden

Andrzej Januszewicz and Aleksander Prejbisz

7.1 Introduction

The decision to establish prehypertension, the new blood pressure category, was based on the number of factors and highlighted the relevance of the observational studies in adults between 40 and 80 years of age. They indicated that the risk of cardiovascular disease [CVD] increased progressively beginning from levels as low as 115/75 mmHg upward with doubling of the incidence of both coronary heart disease [CHD] and stroke for every 20/10 mmHg increment of systolic and diastolic BP [1, 2].

As indicated by several studies since the population continues to age in most countries worldwide and BP increases with age, clinical practice focused on hypertension care becomes more relevant. Therefore designation of prehypertension was established to focus attention on the segment of the population representing higher-than-normal CVD risk and whom therapeutic approaches to prevent or delay the onset of hypertension would be of value [3–5].

Since release of the Seventh Joint National Committee on the Prevention, Detection, Evaluation and Treatment of Hypertension [JNC-7] report in 2003, new data provided a compelling argument for using the concept of prehypertension and focusing attention on the range of systolic blood pressure of 120–139 mmHg and diastolic BP between 80 and 89 mmHg as having clinical and public health significance [6].

Many reports and articles has been published on prehypertension over the past decade and new data have been provided on the prevalence, the rate of progression to hypertension, association with other cardiovascular risk factors and its relationship to the development of cardiovascular disease. It has been clearly documented

A. Januszewicz (✉) · A. Prejbisz
Department of Hypertension, Institute of Cardiology,
Warsaw, Poland

R. Zimlichman et al. (eds.), *Prehypertension and Cardiometabolic Syndrome*,
Updates in Hypertension and Cardiovascular Protection,
https://doi.org/10.1007/978-3-319-75310-2_7

that blood pressure in the prehypertension range is carrying higher rates of incident hypertension and cardiovascular events than optimal BP < 120/<80 mmHg [1–6].

The prehypertensive category has been stratified into stage 1 prehypertension with blood pressure 120–129/80–84 mmHg and stage 2 prehypertension reflecting blood pressure 130–139/85 to 89 mmHg. Of note, most individuals with stage 2 prehypertension have 1 or more concomitant conditions associated with increased cardiovascular risk and this term may better reflect the risk of progression to hypertension and cardiovascular disease than stage 1 prehypertension. However the stage 1 prehypertension with BP in the range of 120 to 129/80 to 84 mmHg is also associated with increased risk but approximately half of that stage 2 prehypertension [6, 7].

Stage 2 prehypertension progresses to hypertension at a rate of about 8–14% annually, which is twofold to threefold higher than blood pressure <120/80 mmHg. Adults with stage 2 prehypertension are also suffering from CVD approximately twice as likely as adults with optimal BP. From 2005 to 2006, approximately 3 of 8 adults in the United States had BP in the stage 1 prehypertensive range of 120 to 139/80 to 89 mmHg and roughly 1 in 8 adults had BP in the range of 130 to 139/85 to 89 mmHg referred as stage 2 prehypertension [1, 6, 7].

Of note, the designation of prehypertension by JNC-7 had raised concerns since this category increased the number of individuals targeted for BP modification by millions in the United States. More importantly, the prehypertensive subgroup represents a heterogenous cohort of individuals with varying risk profiles for cardiovascular disease.

7.2 Prevalence of Prehypertension

7.2.1 Prevalence of Prehypertension in Population-Based Studies

The prevalence of prehypertension and its associated risk factors has been investigated worldwide indicating that prehypertension is a common condition across age, sex, ethnicity, and geographical boundaries in countries with both developed and developing economies. Of note the estimates of prehypertension prevalence are based on office or clinic blood pressure measurements and do not include out-of-office values [6].

Prevalence estimates in population-based samples range from 22 to 38% with only few studies reporting higher prevalence than 50% (Table 7.1). This indicates that data about the prevalence of prehypertension in populations worldwide are not consistent and depend on age, geographical region, and population studied [1–7].

Cross-sectional analysis of national representative data collected from 4805 adults 18 years and older surveyed in the 1999–2000 National Health and Nutrition Examination Survey [NHANES] estimated the prevalence of prehypertension in the United States based on JNC-7 guidelines [8].

Table 7.1 Prevalence of raised blood pressure in representative population samples

Study	Population	Sample size	Age (range or mean; years)	Sex (% female)	BMI (kg/m^2)[a]	Prevalence of prehypertension (%)	Prevalence of hypertension (%)
Prehypertension							
Wu et al. (2002)	China	27,739	35–64	46.3	NA	35.3	NA
Yu et al. (2008)	China, Thailand	10,748	35–74	53.0	23.7	21.0	Excluded
Gu et al. (2009)	China	158,666	55.7	55.8	22.8	34.5	27.7
Erbel et al. (2011)	Germany	4181	59.2	53.0	27.1	26.2	54.2
Janghorbani et al. (2008)	Iran	69,772	44.1	49.7	26.3 (in whole sample)	52.1	23.4
Kokubo et al. (2008)	Japan	5,494	56.0	53.2	22.7	35.2	27.6
Ishikawa et al. (2010)	Japan	11,000	55.1	61.3	23.1	32.3	34.1
Tanaka et al. (2010)	Japan	22,676	62.6	66.2	24.0	25.2	41.1
Fukuhara et al. (2012)	Japan	2634	59.0	57.9	22.9	37.7	37.4
Choi et al. (2006)	Korea	6074	45.9	56.9	23.8	31.6	22.9
Tsai et al. (2005)	Taiwan	2225	49.9	53.3	23.7	34.0	34.7
Onat et al. (2008)	Turkey	3034	48.0	50.5	27.7	32.8	50.3
Liszka et al. (2005)	USA	8986	25–74	54.6	9.4% had BMI >30	33.0	47.0
Kshirsagar et al. (2006)	USA	8960	54.0	53.5	27.7	37.3	Excluded
Hypertension							
Yadav et al. (2008)	Lucknow, North India	1112	49.8	49.0	26.2	32.3	32.2
Ferguson et al. (2008)	Jamaica	1972	36.3	66.5	26.1	30.0	27.5
Tsai et al. (2008)	Taiwan	35,259	51.9	34.2	24.1	33.7	13.6
Vasan et al. (2001)	USA	9845	52.0	57.3	26.7	54.3	Excluded
Asayama et al. (2004)	Omahasa, rural Japan[b]	1702	60.6	61.0	23.5	45.1	29.5
Zhang et al. (2006)	Native Americans, USA	2629	54.8	60.9	30.4	59.4 with DM, 48.2 without DM	Excluded

(continued)

Table 7.1 (continued)

Study	Population	Sample size	Age (range or mean; years)	Sex (% female)	BMI (kg/m^2)[a]		Prevalence of prehypertension (%)	Prevalence of hypertension (%)
Hsia et al. (2007)	Postmenopausal women in USA	60,785	62.8	100	28.9		38.8	34.9
Glasser et al. (2011)	USA	30,150 (9799[c])	≥45.0	55.0	NA		62.9 in black individuals, 54.1 in white individuals	Excluded

Prehypertension defined as 120–139/80–89 mmHg

[a]In individuals with prehypertension

[b]Included patients with comorbidities, including clinical cardiovascular disease

[c]Number without hypertension after excluding adults with blood pressure ≥140 mmHg systolic and/or ≥90 mmHg diastolic and documented or reported use of antihypertensive medication

Abbreviations: *DM* diabetes mellitus, *NA* not available

As evaluated from 1999 to 2000 the prevalence of prehypertension in the United States was approximately 70 million in the age group >20 years and was more common in men [42 million] than in women [28 million], in younger and middle-age than older adults and in Hispanic than African-American individuals [8].

One of the important findings of the NHANES 1999–2000 survey was to show that abdominal obesity is associated with increased risk of prehypertension in American men and women. In this study, abdominal obesity was associated with increased risk of prehypertension in whites, blacks, and Hispanics being independent of age, blood glucose, total cholesterol, exercise, and current smoking [9].

The survey indicated that proportions of risk of prehypertension explained by abdominal obesity were 15.2%, 22%, and 25.8% in white, black, and Hispanic men, respectively. The analogous values in women were 38.8%, 58.6%, and 32.5% clearly demonstrating that prehypertension could have been avoided if abdominal obesity was absent in both men and women of the three ethnic groups [9].

These data further indicated gender differences in the response of abdominal obesity for prehypertension. Approximately 7% of the differences in the risk of developing prehypertension between white and black men and between white and Hispanic men may be attributable to differences in rates of abdominal obesity. The analogous values for women were approximately 39.7% and 16.5%, respectively [9].

In conclusion, despite having lower rates of abdominal obesity than their counterparts, black men, Hispanic men, and Hispanic women had high population attributable risks. This may indicate that other factors than abdominal obesity may have explained power for racial differences in prehypertension in these groups.

Another report from the National Health and Nutrition Examination Survey [NHANES] conducted in 2005 to 2006 showed that approximately 37% of US adults had prehypertension. The number of adults with prehypertension was estimated to be approximately 83 million based on extrapolations from NHANES 2005–2006 [7].

Among this group, roughly 3 of 8 US adults, or approximately 31 million, have stage 2 prehypertension. The NHANES 2005–2006 report showed that prehypertension is associated not only with concomitant cardiovascular risk factors but also with several adverse health outcomes including new-onset diabetes and hypertension, cognitive impairment and increased number of CVD events [7].

Also data on the temporal changes in the prevalence of prehypertension and cardiovascular risk factors were analyzed from 30,958 US adults >20 years of age who participated in the National Health and Nutrition Examination Surveys between [NHANES] 1999 and 2012 [10].

The recent study showed that during this time period, the prevalence of prehypertension has decreased modestly since 1999–2000. However the prevalence of several risk factors for cardiovascular disease and incident hypertension increased among US adults with prehypertension, including prediabetes, diabetes mellitus, overweight, and obesity. There was also nonstatistically decrease in prevalence of adhering to the Dietary Approaches to Stop Hypertension eating pattern [10].

Of note the prospective cohort analysis among 8960 middle-aged adults in the Atherosclerosis Risk in Communities [ARIC] study showed that prehypertension levels of BP were clearly associated with the significant increase in incident cardiovascular disease. The effect of prehypertension was particularly pronounced among blacks, individuals with diabetes mellitus, elevated BMI and relatively low LDL cholesterol levels. These findings may provide compelling evidence for screening and early detection in vulnerable groups [2].

The population-based study included 4272 Mexican adult men and women aged 20–65 years representing northern, middle, and southern parts of Mexico. The results of the study showed the prevalence of prehypertension in 37.5% of Mexican adults [11].

Several studies estimated the prevalence of prehypertension in China in different geographical regions and populations, including urban and urban cohorts.

The prevalence of prehypertension was estimated in a representative sample of 25,196 adults aged 18–74 years in northeast of China. The Control hypertension and Other Risk Factors to Prevent Stroke with Nutrition Education in Urban Area of Northeast China [CHPSNE] Study was a cross-sectional study on hypertension and stroke risk factors among urban residents of northeast China years selected from 2009 to 2010 [12].

Overall, 40.5% of urban Chinese adults had prehypertension with the prevalence of 47.7% and 33.6% in men and women, respectively, and is associated with many risk factors [12].

In another China National Hypertension Survey prospective cohort study including 169,871 Chinese adults aged 40 years and older data on blood pressure were obtained at baseline examination in 1991 and from follow-up examination conducted in 1999–2000. A multistage random cluster sampling design was used to select a representative sample of the general Chinese population from 17 provinces in the mainland China [13].

The results from China National Hypertension Survey Epidemiology Follow-up Study showed that the prevalence of prehypertension was 34.5% and was significantly associated with an increased relative risk of cardiovascular disease [13].

Another population-based, cross-sectional survey of the Chinese Physiological Constant and Health Condition [CPCHC] was conducted between 2008 and 2010 with the aim to estimate the prevalence of prehypertension coexisting with prediabetes. Representative samples of the general population were selected from two urban and two rural areas provinces in mainland China [14].

The study showed that the prevalence of coexisting prehypertension and prediabetes was 11%, was higher in men [14.2%] than in women [8.4%], increased with age and body mass index and was the lowest among Mongolian-Chinese [14].

Three cross-sectional surveys were conducted in Shandong province in the rural population of eastern China. The sample population included 8359, 18,922, and 20,167 subjects included in 1991, 2002, and 2007, respectively [15].

The study documented that among the Chinese rural population, the prevalence of prehypertension increased significantly from 1991 to 2002 and remained high from 2002 until 2007. After adjustment for age and sex the prevalence of prehypertension over the period of 16 years increased from 33.8% in 1991 to 54.6% in 2007. In each survey, the prevalence of prehypertension tended to decline with increasing age in both men and women [15].

In 2007, a cross-sectional population survey of CRF's was carried out among 19,003 adults aged 18–76 years in suburban Beijing indicating that the prevalence of prehypertension was 35.7% [38.2% in men and 31.8% in women]. Overall, 85.3%, 49.8%, and 17.8% of men with prehypertension had one or more, two or more, and three or more CV risk factors, respectively [16].

The prevalence of prehypertension was also evaluated in the other Asian countries. The Jichi Medical School Cohort Study enrolled 11,000 community dwelling persons aged 18–90 years from general Japanese population and then followed for the average of 10.7 years. Participants aged 65 years and older constituted 22.8% of the sample [17].

In this study of a large sample of the Japanese general population the prevalence of prehypertension was 32.3% and was associated with an increased 10-year risk of cardiovascular disease [17].

The Korean National Health and Nutrition Examination Survey [KNHNES], a cross-sectional nationally representative survey conducted in 2001 collected measured blood pressure data and determined the prevalence of prehypertension in association with the risk factors in the Korean population [18].

Data from a comprehensive questionnaire together with a physical examination and blood sample were obtained and analyzed from 6074 Korean adults aged >20 years. The estimated age-adjusted prevalence of prehypertension was 31.6% [41.9% in men and 25.9% in women]. The KNHNES study indicated that male sex, aging, and obesity were predictors of prehypertension. Interestingly, a decreasing prevalence of prehypertension with age was found in this study [18].

The Nutrition and Health Survey in Taiwan [NAHSIT], a cross-sectional survey of 1039 men and 1186 women aged 18–96 years showed the overall prevalence of prehypertension of 34% in Taiwanese adults and was greater in men than in women. Multivariable logistic regression revealed that age and BMI were the determinants of prehypertensive status in men while age, waist circumference, and triglycerides were the determinants in women [19, 20].

Few studies showed a relatively high prevalence of prehypertension in geographically different populations. Between 1991 and 1999, a large population-based sample of 36,424 Israel Defense Forces young healthy employees underwent periodic medical evaluation in Israel. Prehypertension was observed in 48.9% of the subjects and was 50.6% among men and 35.9% among women. The prevalence of prehypertension remained constant across age groups among men but increased with age among women [21].

Multivariate logistic regression analysis showed that male gender was the most powerful predictor of prehypertension and BMI was the strongest modifiable predictor of prehypertension among men and women.

Another study determined the prevalence of prehypertension in Africa in two ethnic groups of 782 individuals representing Sokoto State of northwestern Nigeria. The prevalence rate of prehypertension was 58.7% [men 59.2%, women 58.2%] [22].

The study showed that as compared to hypertension, prehypertension had earlier onset [second versus third decade] and peak [fourth versus fifth decade] of life. Obesity, abnormalities of glucose metabolism, and insulin resistance were the major factors associated with prehypertension.

A nationwide cross-sectional survey of 69,722 adults aged 25–65 years was conducted in Iran from 2004 to 2005 with the objective to estimate the prevalence of prehypertension. It was also found that the estimated prevalence of prehypertension was 59.6% in men and 44.5% in women [23].

Prehypertension tended to increase with age and was more common in overweight and obese men and women and was also associated with the higher prevalence of additional cardiovascular risk factors which result in a high-risk profile [23].

Although the ethnicity most likely plays a role in the pathogenesis of prehypertension, the current studies about the prevalence of prehypertension do not support the hypothesis that difference could be attributable to ethnicity per se.

These results do not indicate an ethnical pattern and for instance the prevalence of prehypertension in selected Chinese populations is similar to the prevalence found in the Mexican population. In addition, the prevalence of prehypertension in the United States [31%] is similar to the prevalence of Korea [31.6%] and Japan [32%]. The variability of prehypertension prevalence emphasizes that in addition to ethnicity, other risk factors play an important role in the development of prehypertension [1–6].

Of note, cross-sectional studies conducted to establish the associated risk factors for developing prehypertension demonstrated that aging, sex, low educational level, smoking, alcohol consumption, BMI, diabetes, elevated plasma glucose, triglycerides, cholesterol levels, and low HDL-c levels were significantly associated with prehypertension [1–8].

7.2.2 Prevalence of Prehypertension in Selected Populations

Prehypertension prevalence in selected population studies is generally similar to the findings in population-based studies, after accounting for differences in age, sex, and inclusion or exclusion of patients with hypertension.

Studies that excluded subjects with hypertension reported a higher prevalence of prehypertension in comparison to those that included individuals with hypertension from the same countries. The prevalence of prehypertension was >30% in all studies including individuals with a mean BMI in the overweight range.

The prevalence of prehypertension in individuals with and without diabetes was estimated in the Strong Heart Study including 2629 participants free from hypertension and cardiovascular disease at baseline examination. They were followed for 12 years to observe the prevalence of incident cardiovascular disease [24].

The results from the Strong Heart Study showed that the prevalence of prehypertension was high in nondiabetic [48.2%] and even higher [59.4%] in diabetic nonhypertensive American Indians. Prehypertension was related to an increased subsequent cardiovascular event rate in both diabetic and nondiabetic participants, but this increase was greater in individuals with diabetes [24].

The prevalence of prehypertension in white and nonwhite postmenopausal women was determined in the Women's Health Initiative [WHI], a large cohort of 60, 785 participants that included black, Hispanic, and Asian women. The prevalence of prehypertension was 39% among WHI study participants at baseline [25].

Prehypertension was identified in 39.9%, 32.1%, 42.6%, 38.7%, and 40.3% of white, black, Hispanic, American Indian, and Asian women, respectively. The distribution of blood pressure categories differed among ethnic groups.

It was found that age, body mass index, and prevalence of diabetes mellitus and hypercholesterolemia increased across the BP categories, whereas current smoking was more prevalent among normotensive women compared with those with prehypertension and hypertension [25].

The differences in cardiovascular event rates between women with prehypertension and hypertension in WHI study were seen and when compared with referent normotensive women, the hazard ratio for the composite cardiovascular outcome was 1.66 for women with prehypertension and 2.89 for those with hypertension [25].

Another study Reasons for Geographic And Racial Differences in Stroke [REGARDS] recruited approximately equal representation of white and black participants of total population of 30,239 aged 45 years and older [26].

The REGARDS study showed that the overall prevalence of prehypertension was 17%—however after excluding subjects with hypertension it was 51%.

It was observed that the prevalence of prehypertension was higher by age and black race and a higher prevalence of prehypertension was observed in obese individuals, self-reported heart disease and those with elevated hsCRP, diabetes and microalbuminuria compared to those without these factors. Heavy alcohol consumption in white participants was associated with increased odds of prehypertension and was even greater in black participants [26].

7.2.3 Prevalence of Prehypertension Based on Meta-Analyses

The prevalence and risk factors for prehypertension were investigated in the meta-analysis which included 20 cross-sectional and 6 longitudinal studies with a total sample of 250,741 individuals of age range from 35 to 60 years. Most of the studies were conducted in East Asia [27].

The results indicated that pooled prevalence of prehypertension was 36% and was higher among males than that among females [40% vs. 33%]. After removing non-East Asian countries it has been found that pooled prevalence of prehypertension in 11 studies from China, Japan, and Korea was 35% and was similar to the overall pooled prevalence [27].

In another meta-analysis of incident cardiovascular disease in 18 prospective studies, estimates of prehypertension prevalence ranged from 25.2 to 46.0% [28].

Of the 18 studies 11 were from Asia [3 from China, 6 from Japan and 2 from Iran], 5 were from the United States and 1 each was from Turkey and Germany. The proportion of Asians was 79.6%. The sample size ranged from 1702 to 158, 666 and the follow-up duration ranged from 2.7 years to 31 years. All studies adjusted adequately for potential confounders—at least five of six factors—including age, sex, diabetes mellitus, BMI cholesterol, and smoking [28].

The results of this meta-analysis showed that the estimates for prehypertension ranged from 32.6 to 41.1% for the five US studies, from 25.2 to 46.0% for the five Japanese studies, and from 30.0 to 35.3% for the three Chinese studies [28].

7.3 Risk of Incident Hypertension

Individuals with prehypertension are carrying a twofold to threefold higher risk of developing hypertension than those who are normotensive. Several factors related to study design may affect annual transition rates from prehypertension to hypertension including the duration of follow-up and whether the population includes the full range of prehypertension [120–139/80–89 mmHg] or only stage 2 prehypertension [1–7].

Several studies indicate that absolute percentages of incident hypertension are generally higher with longer periods of observations when similar baseline blood pressure values are compared, but the annualized rates of incident hypertension are higher for the studies of shorter duration [1–7].

In contrast to annual incident hypertension rates of 8–20% reported in the studies lasting 2–4 years, annualized incident hypertension is 4–9% in studies with the 7–8 follow-up. In one of the studies 57.3% of the original non-hypertensive cohort were hypertensive at 3.5 years, and 60.3% were hypertensive at 7 years [1–8].

Several studies have identified factors which may predict progression from prehypertension to hypertension during the period of observation.

The Framingham Heart Study assessed frequency of progression from prehypertension to hypertension in non-hypertensive participants and showed a stepwise increase in incidence of hypertension across the three non-hypertensive BP categories [29].

It has been demonstrated that 5.3% of participants with optimum BP categories, 17.6% with normal and 37.3% with high-normal BP [stage 2 prehypertension] aged below 65 years progressed to hypertension over 4 years, respectively [29].

The study also documented for patients 65 years and older that corresponding 4-year rates of progression from prehypertension to hypertension were 16%, 25.5%, and 49.5%, respectively. Obesity and weight gain also contributed to the progression and a 5% weight gain on the follow-up was associated with 20–30% increased odds of hypertension [29].

In conclusion, it has been demonstrated that older individuals and those with high-normal BP were more likely to progress to hypertension than younger people and those with normal or optimum BP. Incidence rates of hypertension were similar for men and women and multivariable analyses identified baseline body mass index and weight gain as important determinants of future hypertension. In addition, systolic rather than diastolic BP was the major determinant of progression to hypertension.

In the Trials of Hypertension Prevention, 44% of the usual-care group that was prehypertensive at baseline developed hypertension during the 4-year follow-up. By contrast, the three intervention groups—implementing weight loss, sodium restriction, and both interventions together—had a significantly reduced relative risk [0.78–0.82] of incident hypertension after 4 years [6, 7].

In the TROPHY study, 63% of the placebo treated patients aged 30–65 years with stage 2 prehypertension progressed to hypertension within 4 years, and >40% had progressed after only 2 years. In the PHARAO study, in adults with stage 2 prehypertension, 43% of the group randomly allocated to placebo developed hypertension in 3 years [6, 30].

Of note, the incidence rate in the PHARAO, TROPHY, and Framingham studies are of similar magnitude when the analysis is restricted to individuals with stage 2 prehypertension at baseline.

The ATTICA study showed that increasing age, male sex, low education status, and C-reactive protein were positively associated with the development of hypertension. Also waist circumference was found to be independent predictor [6, 7].

A prospective cohort study of 18,865 non-hypertensive persons [30.4% black, 69.6% white] aged from 18 till 85 years examined electronic health record data from 197 community-based outpatient clinics in the Southeast of the United States. Of note the covariable adjusted median conversion time when 50% became hypertensive was 365 days earlier for blacks than whites [31].

Among covariables, baseline systolic BP 130–139 mmHg and 120–129 mmHg, as well as age >75 and in the range 55–74 years were the strongest predictors for hypertension. Additional predictors included age range 35–54 years, diastolic BP in the range 80–89 mmHg, obesity, and diabetes mellitus. The study showed that conversion from prehypertension to hypertension is accelerated in blacks suggesting that effective interventions in prehypertension could reduce racial disparities in prevalent hypertension [31].

Low levels of physical fitness have also been independently associated with the risk of incident hypertension in men with prehypertension as documented in the study conducted at Veterans Affairs Medical Center, Washington DC, USA. The findings support an increase in the rate of progression to hypertension with decreased exercise capacity [32].

The most pronounced and very similar increase in risk occurred in the two lowest-fit categories, suggesting an S-shaped association. The health benefits are evident at moderate levels of fitness attainable by a brisk walk of 20–40 min most days of the week by most middle-age and older individuals. Fitness attenuated the risk for developing hypertension, regardless of age, BMI, and other traditional risk factors [32].

In another Chinese study it has been demonstrated that older age at baseline, Mongolian race, alcohol-drinking, obesity, high salt intake, low level of physical activity, and family history of hypertension were found to be associated with incident hypertension [14].

7.4 Health Burden

7.4.1 Prehypertension and Cardiovascular Risk

The results of available meta-analyses confirm previous studies and reports indicating that individuals with prehypertension free from cardiovascular disease are carrying increased relative risk of coronary heart disease, stroke, and total cardiovascular disease [33].

Although it is recognized that persons with prehypertension are at higher risk of cardiovascular diseases, the risk may be related to the increased risk of developing hypertension per se. It also remains unresolved whether the mild elevation of BP directly increases the risk of cardiovascular diseases or whether augmented prevalence of other concurrent risk factors may be responsible [33, 34].

Based on the available studies prehypertension increases the risk of myocardial infarction by 3.5 times and coronary artery disease by 1.7 times. When analyzed separately by sex, the risk of myocardial infarction and coronary artery disease was augmented 4.2 and 3.4 times, respectively [6].

Of note, the risk is lower in non-hypertensive individuals as compared to those with hypertension. Among subjects with prehypertension, the risk of coronary artery disease was 2.9 times greater in persons aged 45–64 years and 4.4 times in persons 65 years or older when compared with persons younger than 45 years. It was also higher in subjects with diabetes mellitus [2.1 times] and individuals with hypercholesterolemia [2.5 times] [7].

Among subjects with prehypertension who have at baseline clinical cardiovascular disease, diabetes or both, annualized incidence of cardiovascular disease in the group randomly allocated to placebo averaged approximately 4.3% with an estimated 10-year rate of 43%.

Subject with prehypertension, particularly those in a stage 2 prehypertension, were characterized by multiple cardiovascular risk factors contributing to the augmented risk ratios. In most studies, risk was adjusted for common comorbid factors, such as age, sex, tobacco smoking, and total cholesterol or other lipid fractions, when assessing the risk of prehypertension [6, 7].

7.4.2 Population-Based Studies and Selected Populations

In general, available studies indicate that subjects with prehypertension were characterized by annualized absolute excess risk of cardiovascular disease of approx. 0.39–0.61%, with an average of 0.5% [33].

Of note the studies included in these reports were based on the office BP measurements and also indicate that stage 2 prehypertension was associated with greater risk than stage 1 prehypertension [6, 7].

Given the spectrum of risk factors associated with stage 2 prehypertension, this group has a higher incidence of CVD. Several cohort studies documented a significant contribution of stage 2 prehypertension to CVD risk and the adjusted hazard ratios in these studies ranged from approximately 1.4 to 2.3 [6, 7].

Given an estimated number of 31 million people with stage 2 prehypertension in the United States and the absolute excess CVD risk ranging from 0.39 to 0.61% annually, this population contributes to between 121,000 and 189,000 excess in cardiovascular events annually [6, 7].

On the other hand, the annual incidence of cardiovascular disease among middle-age individuals with stage 2 prehypertension is 1%, with stage 1 prehypertension is 0.8%, and with optimal BP is 0.5%. With an estimated 40 million individuals with stage 1 prehypertension in the United States and an absolute cardiovascular disease risk of 0.8% and an excess of 0.3%, this group would account for approximately 340,000 total and 140,000 excess cardiovascular events annually [6, 7].

Several cohort studies on prehypertension and cardiovascular disease have provided the information on the risk of incident cardiovascular disease in this group (Table 7.2) [6].

Fareed et al. estimated that the population-attributable risk of prehypertension in the United States is 47% for myocardial infarction and 20% for coronary artery disease. This implied that there is a potential for reducing the incidence of myocardial infarction by 47% if prehypertension is treated. Russell et al. found that if prehypertension is eliminated, then hospital admissions would be reduced by 3.4%, nursing home admissions by 6.5%, and mortality by 9.1% [33].

Vasan et al. previously reported that the 10-year cumulative incidence of CVD associated with the high-normal BP [130–139/85–89 mmHg] in the Framingham Heart Study was higher among older participants [>65 years] than younger participants [<65 years]. However the older participants had an elevated incidence of CVD even among those with optimal BP [29].

Liszka et al. reported that in the longitudinal, population-based US cohort, prehypertension was associated with increased risk of major cardiovascular events independently of other cardiovascular risk factors [35].

The authors concluded that low-range prehypertension was associated with increased cardiovascular disease in unadjusted analyses but was not statistically significant in adjusted analyses. High-normal blood pressure remained a predictor of cardiovascular disease in unadjusted and adjusted analyses. It is relevant to consider that the majority of prehypertensive participants had at least one cardiovascular risk factor [35].

The risk for incident cardiovascular disease was also evaluated among 8960 middle-aged adults in the Atherosclerosis Risk in Communities [ARIC] study. The outcome was incident cardiovascular disease defined as fatal/nonfatal coronary heart disease, cardiac procedure, silent myocardial infarction, or ischemic stroke [2].

The study showed that prehypertension levels of BP were clearly associated with significant increase in incident cardiovascular disease. The effect of prehypertension was particularly pronounced among blacks, individuals with diabetes mellitus, elevated BMI, and relatively low LDL cholesterol levels [2].

In the high-normal blood pressure group, the hazard ratio for incident cardiovascular disease compared with optimal blood pressure was 2.49 after adjustment for baseline demographic factors and remained significant after adjustment for traditional risk factors. Both the normal BP and the high-normal BP groups were

Table 7.2 Cardiovascular risk with prehypertension[a]

Study	Sample size	Number with prehypertension	Follow-up (years)	HR (95% CI) for cardiovascular disease	Absolute difference per year (%)	NNT (40%)[b]	NNT (100%)[b]
Morbidity and mortality							
ARIC (2006)	8960	1279	11.6	2.33 (1.85–2.92)	~0.42	60	24
Framingham (2001)	6859	1794	12.0	Men: 1.6 (1.1–2.2)	~0.54 (0.43[c])	48	19
				Women: 2.5 (1.6–4.1)	~0.52 (0.25[c])	50	20
NHANES 1 (2005)	8986	2708[d]	18.0	1.42 (1.09–1.84)	~0.53	48	19
NHEFS 1 (2000)	12,269	1947	7–21	NA	NA	32	13
REGARDS (2013)	27,748	13,407	4.5	1.38 (0.94–2.02)	~0.12[e]	208	83
Strong Heart Study (2006)	2629	1390[d]	12.6	1.80 (1.28–2.54)	~0.61	42	17
Women's Health Initiative (2007)	60,785	23,596[d]	7.7	1.77 (1.52–2.06)	~0.39	65	26
Mortality only							
MRFIT (1994)	347,978	77,248	15.0	CAD: 1.66 (1.56–1.77) CVA: 2.14(95% CI NA)	~0.09	278	111
Taiwan (2008)	35,259	4655	13.0	1.96 (1.5–2.6)	~0.10	250	100

[a]Compared with normal blood pressure levels in individuals without baseline cardiovascular disease

[b]NNT for 10 years to prevent one cardiovascular disease event based on estimated reductions of either 40% or 100% in the absolute excess risk between individuals with prehypertension and those with optimal blood pressure

[c]Age-adjusted

[d]Includes all individuals with prehypertension (120–139/80–89 mmHg), whereas other studies included only those with stage 2 hypertension (130–139/85–89 mmHg)

[e]Stroke was the only cardiovascular outcome reported; for adults aged 45–59 years

Abbreviations: *CAD* coronary artery disease, *CVA* cerebrovascular accident (stroke), *NA* not available, *NNT* number needed to treat

Reprinted with permission from Macmillan Publishers Ltd.: Nature Reviews, Egan B.M., Stevens-Fabry S.: Prehypertension—prevalence, health risks and management strategies. 12, 289–300, copyright 2015 associated with incident coronary heart disease. The majority of cardiovascular events were related to coronary heart disease rather than stroke [2].

The risk for incident cardiovascular disease events was determined in white and nonwhite postmenopausal women determined in the Women's Health Initiative [WHI], a large cohort of 60,785 participants that includes significant numbers of black, Hispanic, and Asian women [25].

Compared with referent normotensive women adjusted hazard ratios for women with prehypertension were 1.58 for cardiovascular death, 1.76 for myocardial infarction, and 1.93 for stroke. Hazards ratios for the composite outcome with prehypertension did not differ between ethnic groups, although the numbers of events among Hispanic and Asian women were small [25].

For every 1000 women with prehypertension, 7 had a first cardiovascular event each year compared to 14 events per year for women with hypertension and 4 events per year for normotensive women. Thus, the population-attributable risk for prehypertension was 3 excess cardiovascular events per year per 1000 women, whereas 8 excess events per year could be attributed for hypertension [25].

The hazard ratios of incident cardiovascular disease associated with prehypertension in individuals with and without diabetes was assessed in the Strong Heart Study in which a total of 2629 participants free from hypertension and cardiovascular disease at baseline examination were followed for 12 years to observe the incident cardiovascular disease. Approximately 42% of the participant had diabetes [24].

The Strong Heart Study findings revealed that in nondiabetic participants, prehypertension increased cardiovascular events 1.8-fold compared with their normotensive counterparts with an absolute increase of 6 cardiovascular events per 1000 persons [24].

Diabetes alone increased the risk of cardiovascular disease by 2.9-fold compared with normotensive nondiabetic participants. Diabetes plus prehypertension increased the cardiovascular disease risk 3.7 times (Fig. 7.1), representing an absolute increase of 19 cardiovascular events per 1000 person-years [24].

When the prehypertensive category was stratified into those with BP 120–129/80–84 mmHg or BP 130–139/85 to 89 mmHg, hazards ratios for those in the higher group were greater, but there was a significant risk even in those in the lower group [24].

The coexistence of impaired glucose tolerance or impaired fasting glucose and prehypertension also increased cardiovascular disease risk significantly when compared with normotensive participants with normal glucose tolerance. The magnitude of the increased cardiovascular disease risk related to the coexistence of prehypertension, glucose intolerance, and diabetes suggest that pharmacological intervention for blood pressure control in these groups may be warranted to prevent cardiovascular disease morbidity and mortality [34].

Qureshi et al. evaluated the association of prehypertension with the incidence atherothrombotic brain infarction and all strokes during follow-up of cohort of 5181 persons who participated in the Framingham Study. It has been demonstrated after adjusting for age, gender, obesity, diabetes mellitus, cigarette smoking

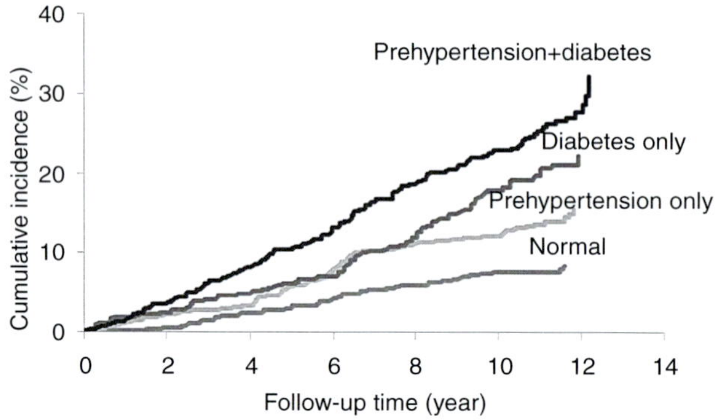

Fig. 7.1 Cumulative cardiovascular disease incidence during 12 years of follow-up by prehypertension and diabetes status in the Strong Heart Study cohort. Reprinted with permission of Wolters Kluwer: Zhang Y., Lee E.T., Devereux R.B. et al.: Prehypertension, diabetes and cardiovascular disease risk in a population-based sample. The Strong Heart Study. Hypertension, 2006, 47, 410–414. http://hyper.ahajournals.org/

hypercholesterolemia and study period that prehypertension is not associated with ischemic or all strokes [34].

An analysis of the nationally representative cohort available in the National Health and Nutrition Examination Survey [NHANES] in 1976–1980 merged with the NHANES II Mortality Study [NHANES2MS] showed that prehypertension was not independently associated with increased all-cause or CVD mortality. Further analysis of subgroups of age >55 years yielded the same lack of association [36].

The Jichi Medical School Cohort Study that included large sample of the Japanese population showed that the risk of CVD for those with prehypertension was 45% greater than those with normal BP [17].

Across the total duration of follow-up the increased CVD hazard risk associated with prehypertension tended to be higher in those under the age of 65 years than those over 65 years. In the separate analysis of the CVD during the first 5 years and second 5 years of the follow-up period, prehypertension was associated with the modest, non-significant increase in the overall hazard risk of CVD during the second 5-year period, but a widening gap between the nonelderly [<65 years] and elderly [>65 years] participants [17].

7.5 Results from Meta-Analyses

In the meta-analysis of incident cardiovascular disease in 18 prospective studies, estimates of prehypertension prevalence ranged from 25.2 to 46.0%, although several reports were not representative [28].

Of the 18 studies 11 were from Asia [3 from China, 6 from Japan, and 2 from Iran], 5 were from the United States, and 1 each was from Turkey and Germany. The

Study or Subgroup	log[Risk Ratio]	SE	Weight	Risk Ratio IV, Random, 95% CI	Year
Mainous 2004	0.077	0.1726	4.9%	1.08 [0.77, 1.51]	2004
Bowman, 2005	0.0198	0.1707	5.0%	1.02 [0.73, 1.43]	2005
Sairenchi 2005	0.1398	0.0868	9.8%	1.15 [0.97, 1.36]	2005
Baldinger 2006	1.1184	0.5128	0.8%	3.06 [1.12, 8.36]	2006
Terry 2007	0.392	0.0211	14.4%	1.48 [1.42, 1.54]	2007
Hsia 2007	0.4574	0.1756	4.8%	1.58 [1.12, 2.23]	2007
Gu 2008	0.207	0.1885	4.3%	1.23 [0.85, 1.78]	2008
Thomas 2008	0.1989	0.117	7.7%	1.22 [0.97, 1.53]	2008
Lee 2009	0.4055	0.3207	1.8%	1.50 [0.80, 2.81]	2009
Pednekar 2009	0.0583	0.0613	11.8%	1.06 [0.94, 1.20]	2009
He 2009	0.3293	0.0461	12.9%	1.39 [1.27, 1.52]	2009
Dorjgochoo 2009	0.239	0.217	3.5%	1.27 [0.83, 1.94]	2009
Lorenzo 2009	0.4383	0.3006	2.1%	1.55 [0.86, 2.79]	2009
Hozawa 2009	0.0953	0.2162	3.5%	1.10 [0.72, 1.68]	2009
Ikeda 2009	0.2469	0.1363	6.5%	1.28 [0.98, 1.67]	2009
Kim 2011	0.1044	0.4721	0.9%	1.11 [0.44, 2.80]	2011
Stojanov 2012	0.5068	0.5365	0.7%	1.66 [0.58, 4.75]	2012
Takashima 2012	0.3365	0.182	4.5%	1.40 [0.98, 2.00]	2012
Total (95% CI)			100.0%	1.28 [1.16, 1.40]	

Heterogeneity: $Tau^2 = 0.01$; $Chi^2 = 45.34$, df = 17 ($P = .0002$); $I^2 = 63\%$
Test for overall effect: Z = 5.22 ($P < .0001$)

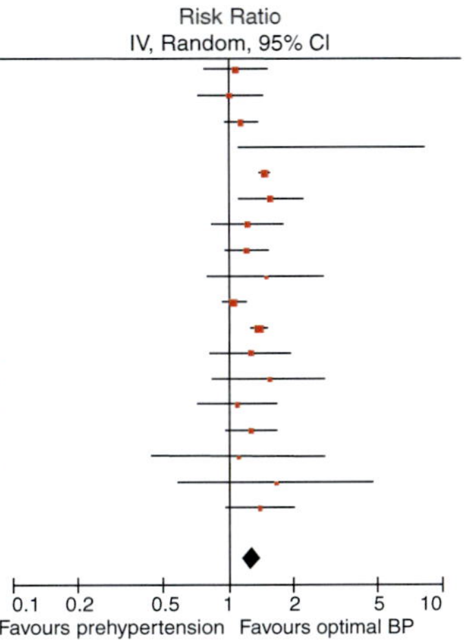

Fig. 7.2 Forest plot of CVD mortality comparison: prehypertension vs. optimal BP. Reprinted from American Heart Journal; 167; Huang Y., Su L., Cai X. et al.; Association of all-cause and cardiovascular mortality with prehypertension: A meta-analysis; 160–168; Copyright (2014), with permission from Elsevier

proportion of Asians was 79.6%. The sample size ranged from 1702 to 158, 666 and the follow-up duration ranged from 2.7 years to 31 years [28].

This meta-analysis found, after controlling for multiple cardiovascular risk factors, significant association between prehypertension and CVD incidence. The results were consistent across age, gender, trial characteristics, ethnicity, and follow-up duration.

More importantly, even low-range prehypertension increased the risk of CVD compared with optimal BP and the risk was higher with high-range prehypertension. The relative risk was significantly higher in the high-range prehypertensive populations than in the low-range populations. It was evaluated that 15.9% of CVD, 14.6% of CHD, and 19.6% of stroke cases could be prevented if prehypertension was eliminated [37].

Also Guo et al. showed in the meta-analysis of prospective studies that the prehypertensive patients have a greater risk of incident stroke, MI, and CVD events in the high prehypertension range.

The meta-analysis of Huang et al. evaluated data from 1,129,098 participants derived from 20 prospective cohort studies. The results showed that after controlling for multiple cardiovascular risk factors, prehypertension is significantly associated with CVD mortality (Fig. 7.2), mostly driven by high-range prehypertension. The risk for stroke mortality was higher than for CHD mortality and it was calculated that 10.5% of CVD, 4.8% of CHD, and 14.6% of stroke death could be prevented if prehypertension was eliminated [38].

It is interesting that in this analysis prehypertension was not associated with all-cause mortality even at high-range prehypertension levels. In the subgroups where participants with CVD at baseline were excluded and the data were adjusted for adequate risk factors, prehypertension was associated with a very slight increase in all-cause mortality. The reason for the discrepancy in the association of prehypertension with cardiovascular and all-cause mortality are unclear. Of note, also Guo et al. showed in their meta-analysis that prehypertension was not associated with all-cause mortality [38, 39].

Lee et al.'s meta-analysis of 12 studies which included total of 518,520 participants showed that prehypertension was associated with the risk of stroke. However among individuals with lower-range prehypertension, stroke risk was not significantly increased. In subjects with higher values within the prehypertensive range, stroke risk was substantially increased indicating that stroke risk is largely driven by the higher values within the prehypertensive range and is particularly relevant in non-elderly individuals [40].

Taken together, the population burden of cardiovascular disease associated with prehypertension is substantial, whereas the absolute excess risk of prehypertension for an individual without previous clinical cardiovascular disease is relatively small.

Taking into consideration the high prevalence of prehypertension, roughly 30% of cardiovascular events in the global population are estimated to occur in those with prehypertension. Of note cardiovascular events are likely to be attributable to elevated blood pressure alone irrespective of other common risk factors.

Consequently, prevention strategies need to be carefully considered to design and implement strategies both to reduce population-attributable risk among the majority of subjects who are at low-to-moderate risk, and to decrease adverse outcomes among individuals with prehypertension who are at high risk.

References

1. Chobanian AV. Prehypertension revisited. Hypertension. 2006;48:812–4.
2. Kshirsgar AV, Carpenter M, Bang H, et al. Blood pressure usually considered normal is associated with an elevated risk of cardiovascular disease. Am J Med. 2006;119:133–41.
3. Assadi F. Prehypertension : a warning sign of future cardiovascular risk. Int J Prev Med. 2014;special issue:S4–9.
4. Whaley-Connell A, Sowers JR. Is it time to target prehypertension. Cardiovasc Ther. 2010;28:337–8.
5. Habib GB, Virani SS, Jneid H. Is 2015 the primetime year for prehypertension ? Prehypertension: a cardiovascular risk factor or simply a risk marker? J Am Heart Assoc. 2015;4:e001792. https://doi.org/10.1161/JAHA/115.00.1792.
6. Egan BM, Stevens-Fabry S. Prehypertension—prevalence, health risks and management strategies. Nat Rev Cardiol. 2015;12:289–300.
7. Egan BM, Lackland DT, Jones DW. Prehypertension: an opportunity for a new public health paradigm. Cardiol Clin. 2010;28:561–9.
8. Wang Y, Wang QJ. The prevalence of prehypertension and hypertension among US adults according to the New Joint National Committee Guidelines. Arch Intern Med. 2004;164:2126–34.
9. Okosun IS, Boltri JM, Anochie LK, et al. Racial / ethnic differences in prehypertension in American adults: population and relative attributable risks of abdominal obesity. J Hum Hypertens. 2004;18:849–55.
10. Booth JN, Li J, Zhang L, et al. Trends in prehypertension and hypertension risk factors in USA adults: 1999–2012. Hypertension. 2017;70:275–84.

11. Rodriguez-Ramirez M, Simental-Mendia L, Gonzalez-Ortiz M, et al. Prevalence of prehypertension in Mexico and its association with hypomagnesemia. Am J Hypertens. 2015;28:1024–30.
12. Meng XJ, Dong GH, Wang D, et al. Epidemiology of prehypertension and associated risk factors in urban adults from 33 communities in China. Circ J. 2012;76:900–6.
13. Gu D, Chen J, Wu X, Duan X, et al. Prehypertension and risk of cardiovascular disease in Chinese adults. J Hypertens. 2009;27:721–9.
14. Wu J, Yan W, Qiu L, et al. High prevalence of coexisting prehypertension and prediabetes among healthy adults in northern and northeastern China. BMC Public Health. 2011;11:794–802.
15. Yang J, Lu F, Zhang C, et al. Prevalence of prehypertension and hypertension in a Chinese rural area from 1991 to 2007. Hypertens Res. 2010;33:331–7.
16. Zhang W-H, Zhang L, An W-F, et al. Prehypertension and clustering of cardiovascular risk factors among adults in suburban Beijing, China. J Epidemiol. 2011;21:440–6.
17. Ishikawa Y, Ishikawa J, Ishikawa S, et al. Prehypertension and the risk for cardiovascular disease in the Japanese general population : the Jichi Medical School Cohort Study. J Hypertens. 2010;28:1630–7.
18. Choi KM, Park HS, Han JH, et al. Prevalence o prehypertension and hypertension in a Korean population : Korean National Health and Nutrition Survey 2001. J Hypertens. 2006;24:1515–21.
19. Tsai P-S, Ke T-L, Huang C-J, et al. Prevalence and determinants of prehypertension status in the Taiwanese general population. J Hypertens. 2005;23:1355–60.
20. Liu L-K, Peng L-N, Chen L-K, et al. Prehypertension among middle-age and elderly people in Taiwan : a five-year follow-up. J Atheroscler Thromb. 2010;17:189–94.
21. Grotto I, Grossman E, Huerta M, et al. Prevalence of prehypertension and associated cardiovascular risk profiles among young Israeli adults. Hypertension. 2006;48:254–9.
22. Isezuo SA, Sabir AA, Ohwovorilole AE, et al. Prevalence, associated factors and relationship between prehypertension and hypertension : a study of two ethnic African populations in Northern Nigeria. J Hum Hypertens. 2011;25:224–30.
23. Janhorbani M, Amini M, Gouya MM, et al. Nationwide survey of prevalence and risk factors of prehypertension and hypertension in Iranian adults. J Hypertens. 2008;26:419–26.
24. Zhang Y, Lee ET, Devereux RB, et al. Prehypertension, diabetes and cardiovascular disease risk in a population-based sample. The Strong Heart Study. Hypertension. 2006;47:410–4.
25. Hsia J, Margolis KL, Eaton CB, et al. Prehypertension and cardiovascular disease risk in the Women's Health Initiative. Circulation. 2007;115:855–60.
26. Glasser SP, Judd S, Basile J, et al. Prehypertension, racial prevalence and its association with risk factors: analysis of the reasons for geographic and racial differences in stroke [REGARDS] study. Am J Hypertens. 2011;24:194–9.
27. Guo X, Zou L, Zhang X, et al. Prehypertension. A meta-analysis of the epidemiology, risk factors, and predictors of progression. Tex Heart Inst J. 2011;38:643–52.
28. Huang Y, Wang S, Cai X, et al. Prehypertension and incidence of cardiovascular disease: a meta-analysis. BMC Med. 2013;11:177–86.
29. Vasan RS, Larson MG, Leip EP, et al. Assessment of frequency of progression to hypertension in non-hypertensive participants in the Framingham Heart Study: a cohort study. Lancet. 2001;358:1682–6.
30. Luders S, Schrader J, Berger J, et al. The PHARAO study: prevention of hypertension with the angiotensin-converting enzyme inhibitor ramipril in patients with high-normal blood pressure—a prospective, randomized, controlled prevention trial of the German Hypertension League. J Hypertens. 2008;26:1487–96.
31. Selassie A, Wagner CS, Laken ML, et al. Progression is accelerated from pre-hypertension to hypertension in African Americans. Hypertension. 2011;58:579–87.
32. Faselis C, Doumas M, Kokkinos JP, et al. Exercise capacity and progression from prehypertension to hypertension. Hypertension. 2012;60:333–8.
33. Suri MFK, Qureshi AI. Prehypertension as a risk factor for cardiovascular diseases. J Cardiovasc Nurs. 2006;21:478–82.

34. Qureshi AI, Suri MFK, Kirmani JF, et al. Is prehypertension a risk factor for cardiovascular disease? Stroke. 2005;36:1859–63.
35. Liszka HA, Mainous AG, King DE, et al. Prehypertension and cardiovascular morbidity. Ann Fam Med. 2005;3:294–9.
36. Mainous AG, Everett CJ, Liszka H, et al. Prehypertension and mortality in a nationally representative cohort. Am J Cardiol. 2004;94:1496–500.
37. Guo X, Zhang X, Guo L, et al. Association between pre-hypertension and cardiovascular outcomes: a systematic review and meta-analysis of prospective studies. Curr Hypertens Res. 2013;15:703–16.
38. Huang Y, Su L, Cai X, et al. Association of all-cause and cardiovascular mortality with prehypertension: a meta-analysis. Am Heart J. 2014;167:160–8.
39. Guo X, Zhang X, Zheng L, et al. Prehypertension is not associated with all-cause mortality: a systematic review and meta-analysis of prospective studies. PLoS One. 2013;8:e61796.
40. Lee M, Saver JL, Chang B, et al. Presence of baseline prehypertension and risk of incident stroke. Neurology. 2011;77:1330–7.

Part II

Organ Damage in Prehypertension

Arterial Stiffness in Early Phases of Prehypertension

8

Stéphane Laurent and Pedro Guimarães Cunha

Children, adolescent, and adults with prehypertension have a high risk for developing hypertension. Modifiable cardiovascular risk factors, such as prediabetes and diabetes mellitus, overweight and obesity, high lipid diet, high salt intake, and lack of regular physical activity play a crucial role in the transition between prehypertension and hypertension. Because these cardiovascular risk factors are key determinants of increased arterial stiffness, and because increased arterial stiffness is a determinant of incident hypertension, the question arises as to whether arterial stiffness plays a crucial role in the transition between early phases of prehypertension and hypertension. In this review, we will analyze the epidemiological and hemodynamic evidences that increased arterial stiffness is a determinant of incident hypertension. We will also address the complexity of this relationship by discussing the hemodynamic and biomechanical pathways involved in the bidirectional influence between arterial stiffness and blood pressure. And then, we will discuss (a) the predictive value of arterial stiffness not only for incident hypertension, but also for cardiovascular events, (b) the influence of low-grade inflammation associated with chronic diseases in the development of arterial stiffness and subsequently

S. Laurent (✉)
Paris-Descartes University, Assistance-Publique Hôpitaux de Paris, Paris, France

Department of Pharmacology and Hôpital Européen Georges Pompidou,
INSERM U970, Paris-Descartes University, Assistance Publique—Hôpitaux de Paris,
Paris, France
e-mail: stephane.laurent@egp.aphp.fr

P. G. Cunha
Center for the Research and Treatment of Arterial Hypertension and Cardiovascular Risk,
Serviço de Medicina Interna do Hospital da Senhora da Oliveira,
University of Minho, Guimarães, Portugal

Life and Health Science Research Institute (ICVS), School of Medicine,
University of Minho, Guimarães, Portugal

R. Zimlichman et al. (eds.), *Prehypertension and Cardiometabolic Syndrome*,
Updates in Hypertension and Cardiovascular Protection,
https://doi.org/10.1007/978-3-319-75310-2_8

hypertension, (c) how the concept of Early Vascular Ageing can help understanding the relationship between arterial stiffness and prehypertension, and (d) the relationships between metabolic syndrome, arterial stiffness, and prehypertension in children.

8.1 Introduction

Children, adolescent, and adults with prehypertension have a high risk for developing hypertension [1–3] and cardiovascular disease [4–6]. Modifiable cardiovascular (CV) risk factors, such as prediabetes and diabetes mellitus, overweight and obesity, high lipid diet, high salt intake, and lack of regular physical activity play a crucial role in the transition between prehypertension and hypertension [1, 7]. Because these CV risk factors are key determinants of increased arterial stiffness, and because increased arterial stiffness is a determinant of incident hypertension, the question arises as to whether arterial stiffness plays a crucial role in the transition between early phases of prehypertension and hypertension.

In this review, we will analyze the epidemiological and hemodynamic evidences that increased arterial stiffness is a determinant of incident hypertension. We will also address the complexity of this relationship by discussing the hemodynamic and biomechanical pathways involved in the bidirectional influence between arterial stiffness and blood pressure. And then, we will discuss (a) the predictive value of arterial stiffness not only for incident hypertension, but also for cardiovascular events, (b) the influence of low-grade inflammation associated with chronic diseases in the development of arterial stiffness and subsequently hypertension, (c) how the concept of Early Vascular Ageing can help understanding the relationship between arterial stiffness and prehypertension, and (d) the relationships between metabolic syndrome, arterial stiffness, and prehypertension in children.

8.2 Arterial Stiffness as a Cause of Incident Hypertension: Epidemiological Evidences

From hemodynamic principles, arterial stiffness is believed to underlie, at least in part, the age-associated changes in SBP. Recent cross-sectional studies have shown a strong association between prehypertension and arterial stiffness. In the Reference Values for Arterial Stiffness' Collaboration study (Reference values 2010), the reference and normal values of arterial stiffness, measured with cfPWV, have been determined in large international cohorts. In this cohort, age and blood pressure were the major determinants of arterial stiffness. Interestingly, cfPWV was higher in subjects with normal (stage 1 prehypertension) and high-normal (stage 2 prehypertension) BP than in age-matched subjects with optimal BP. Thus, prehypertension is associated with arterial stiffening at a given age decade. However, cross-sectional studies are not sufficient and longitudinal studies are needed to demonstrate the temporal relationship between arterial stiffness and BP.

Liao and colleagues [8] prospectively examined the relation between arterial stiffness and the development of hypertension over 6 years of follow-up in a cohort of 6992 normotensive men and women aged 45–64 years at baseline from the biracial, population-based Atherosclerosis Risk in Communities (ARIC) Study. Arterial stiffness was measured at the carotid level, from high-resolution B-mode ultrasound examination of the left common carotid artery, using adjusted stroke change in arterial diameter (in micrometers, simultaneously adjusted for diastolic BP, pulse pressure, pulse pressure squared, diastolic arterial diameter, and height). The incident rates of hypertension from the lowest to the highest quartiles of arterial stiffness were 6.7%, 8.0%, 7.3%, and 9.6%, respectively ($P < 0.01$). One standard deviation increase in arterial stiffness was associated with 15% greater risk of hypertension, independent of established risk factors for hypertension and the level of baseline BP.

Dernellis and coauthors [9] assessed, in a 4 years longitudinal study, the predictive value of aortic stiffness on future hypertension in non-hypertensive subjects with BP < 140/90. Aortic stiffness was determined by echocardiography at a level of 3 cm above the aortic valve, at baseline in 2512 subjects. A stepwise increase in hypertension incidence occurred across the male and older participants: 3.8% of young female individuals, 11.5% of young male, 26.1% of old female, and 58.8% of old male subjects progressed to hypertension over 4 years. In multivariate analysis, aortic stiffness remained significantly associated with the progression to future hypertension after adjustment to classic risk factors in men and women and in young and old populations.

Najjar and colleagues [10] measured carotid-femoral pulse wave velocity (cfPWV) at baseline in 449 normotensive or untreated hypertensive volunteers (age 53 ± 17 years). Repeated measurements of BP were performed during an average follow-up of 4.9 years. After adjusting for covariates including age, body mass index, and mean BP, linear mixed effects regression models showed that cfPWV was a significant and independent determinant of the longitudinal increase in SBP ($P = 0.003$ for the interaction term with time). In a subset of 306 subjects who were normotensive at baseline, hypertension developed in 105 (34%) during a median follow-up of 4.3 years (range 2–12 years). By stepwise Cox proportional hazards models, cfPWV was an independent predictor of incident hypertension (hazard ratio 1.10 per 1 m/s increase in cfPWV, 95% confidence interval 1.00–1.30, $P = 0.03$) in individuals with a follow-up duration greater than the median.

More recently, Kaess and coauthors [11] analyzed the longitudinal community-based Framingham cohort and studied the temporal relationships among BP and 3 measures of arterial stiffness measured through carotid-femoral pulse wave velocity (cfPWV) over a 7-year period. In a multivariable-adjusted regression model, cfPWV at baseline (beta, 1.5 [95% CI, 0.5–2.6] mm Hg per 1 SD; $P = 0.006$) was associated with systolic BP during examination 7 years later. In a model that included systolic and diastolic BP and additional risk factors during examination at baseline, cfPWV was associated with incident hypertension (OR, 1.3 [95% CI, 1.0–1.6] per 1 SD; $P = 0.04$) 7 years later in 1048 participants without hypertension at baseline. Conversely, BP at baseline was not associated with cfPWV 7 years later. Thus, although higher aortic stiffness was associated with higher risk of incident hypertension, the reverse was not observed, i.e., initial BP was not independently associated with risk of progressive aortic stiffening.

In conclusion, longitudinal studies measuring either carotid stiffness (one study) or aortic stiffness (three studies) at baseline and incident hypertension suggest that arterial stiffness measurement could help identify normotensive individuals at risk of incident hypertension. These subjects should be targeted for the implementation of interventions aimed at preventing or delaying the progression of subclinical arterial stiffening, thus preventing or delaying the onset of hypertension. In the following paragraph, we will see how a progressive arterial stiffness can lead to the onset of hypertension.

8.3 Arterial Stiffness as a Cause of Incident Hypertension: Hemodynamic Evidences

The wording "arterial stiffness" is a general term that refers to the loss of arterial compliance and/or changes in arterial wall elastic properties [12]. Compliance of large arteries, including the thoracic aorta that has the major role, represents their ability to dampen the pulsatility of ventricular ejection and to transform a pulsatile pressure (and flow) at the site of the ascending aorta into a continuous pressure (and flow) downstream at the site of arterioles, in order to lower the energy expenditure during organ perfusion and protect small arteries of target organs (mainly the brain and the kidney) from the damaging effects of pressure pulsatility [13]. When arteries stiffen with aging, they lose their ability to dampen the pulsatility of ventricular ejection and small arteries of target organ are damaged.

Another important consequence of arterial stiffening is the increase in systolic BP at the central level. Indeed, the arterial pressure waveform is a composite of the forward pressure wave created by ventricular contraction and a reflected wave. Waves are reflected from the periphery, mainly at branch points or sites of impedance mismatch (i.e., from an elastic to a stiff arterial segment). In elastic vessels, because PWV is low, reflected wave tends to arrive back at the aortic root during diastole. In the case of stiff arteries, because PWV is high, the reflected wave arrives back at the central arteries earlier, adding to the forward wave, and augmenting pressure pulsatility (i.e., SBP *minus* DBP, or pulse pressure—PP) and SBP at the central level (i.e., at the level of the thoracic aorta and carotid arteries).

Importantly, an increase in central SBP and PP can occur without any detectable changes in peripheral SBP and PP, most often measured at the site of the brachial artery. Indeed, as described above, in peripheral arteries, reflection sites are closer than in central arteries, and reflected waves travel faster on peripheral arteries than on central arteries, which are less stiff in young subjects. This has been described as the "amplification phenomenon," which states that the amplitude of the pressure wave is higher in peripheral arteries than in central arteries. Thus, brachial SBP and PP overestimates central SBP and PP in young subjects [13, 14].

A cross-sectional relationship between prehypertension and central pulse pressure and/or amplification has been demonstrated recently. In the Reference Values for Arterial Measurements Collaboration study [14], the reference and normal values of central systolic and pulse pressures, as well as pressure amplification (peripheral SBP *minus* central SBP), have been determined in large international cohorts [14]. In this cohort, age, sex, and blood pressure were the major determinants of central systolic and pulse pressures. Interestingly, central SBP and PP and pressure amplification were higher in subjects with normal (stage 1 prehypertension) and high-normal (stage 2 prehypertension) BP than in those with optimal BP [14]. Thus, prehypertension is associated with increased central SBP, PP, and pressure amplification at a given age decade, and, as described above, the later parameters are the consequence of an increase in arterial stiffness.

Complementary evidence to the increased risk of prehypertension associated with increased central blood pressure values can be extracted from the Anglo Cardiff Collaborative Trial II (ACCT) [15], evaluating central and peripheral blood pressure from 10,613 subjects, to show that: (a) subjects with normal and high-normal peripheral blood pressure had higher central systolic blood pressure than subjects with optimal peripheral BP and (b) 70% of subjects with prehypertension stage 1 and 2 had central systolic pressures values that overlapped with the ones measured for subjects with grade I hypertension. Recently, the mechanical properties of the proximal aorta were studied by cardiovascular resonance imaging in 2001 participants of the Dallas Heart Study [16]. After adjustment on age, mean BP, and a number of clinical characteristics of this multiracial and multiethnic cohort, individuals with prehypertension had lower proximal aorta distensibility and compliance than those with optimal BP, although aortic arch PWV was not significantly different. This evidence is supported by previous findings from Redheuil and coworkers [17], showing that reduced aortic strain and distensibility are early manifestations of stiffness and aging in large vessels. Thus, as discussed in the previous two paragraphs, aortic stiffness is increased in individuals with prehypertension, partly in response to a higher BP and partly independently of mean BP.

Increased arterial stiffening in prehypertension can increase pressure pulsatility and thus damage the heart, kidney, and brain through increased afterload on the heart and increased pulsatility at the site of small brain and kidney arteries. Because target organ damage is a major cause of cardiovascular and renal complications, it is expected that arterial stiffness has a predictive value for cardiovascular events, namely in prehypertensive individuals. Urbina and colleagues [18] and Drukteinis and coworkers in the Strong Heart Study [19] both evaluated populations of very young subjects (children and young adults) showing, after multivariate analysis, that prehypertension was independently associated to target organ damage, namely arterial stiffness (measured by different methods), increased left ventricular mass, and diastolic dysfunction. Manios and coworkers [20] demonstrated the same in a population of 896 adult subjects. Subjects enrolled in the Third National Health and Nutrition Examination Survey (without type 2 Diabetes and normotensive) were examined according to their blood pressure level. Data show that subjects with prehypertension had higher prevalence of microalbuminuria than those with optimal blood pressure [21].

8.4 Hemodynamic and Biomechanical Approach of the Arterial Stiffness–BP Relationship

The bidirectional relationship between arterial stiffness and BP is rendered more complex by two characteristics of hemodynamics and biomechanics (Table 8.1).

First, an insidious positive feedback loop between local mechanobiological responses and global hemodynamics, as suggested by Humphrey and coauthors [25], may explain why central artery stiffening is at the same time a cause of hypertension and one of its consequences. We have seen above that arterial stiffening in early phases of prehypertension may be a major determinant of elevated systolic BP on the long term. Indeed, the longitudinal assessment of the temporal relationship between carotid [8] and aortic stiffness [10, 11] on the one side and incident hypertension on the other side suggests a precursor role of arterial stiffening in future altered systolic hemodynamic load. However, the reverse occurs when hypertension is installed, even at the lower grade of prehypertension. Indeed, arterial stiffening can be a consequence of the rise in mean BP. Early work, in the 1950s–1970s, suggested that sustained increases in BP stimulate matrix synthesis and thus vascular thickness and structural stiffness [26, 27]. In addition, high BP loads the stiff components of the arterial wall and changes the spatial organization between smooth muscle cells and extracellular matrix [28], and eventually increases arterial stiffness.

Table 8.1 The bidirectional relationship of arterial stiffness and prehypertension

	Author/year	Study type	Participants	Result
	Arterial stiffness promotes hypertension			
1.	Liao et al. [8] (ARIC Study)	Longitudinal (6 years follow-up)	6992 Normotensives	1 SD increase in arterial stiffness increased 15% risk of developing HTN
2.	Dernellis et al. [9]	Longitudinal (4 years follow-up)	2571 Normotensives	Increased arterial stiffness was associated with an OR of 1.2 for the development of HTN
3.	Najjar et al. [10] (BLSA)	Longitudinal (4.3 years follow-up)	306 Normotensives	OR of developing HTN increase 1.1 for every 1 m/s increase in PWV
4.	Peralta et al. [22] (mesa)	Longitudinal (4.3 years follow-up)	2512 Normotensives	Higher CIMT and lower aortic distensibility are independent predictors of the development of HTN
5.	Kaess et al. [11] (Framingham)	Longitudinal (7 year follow-up)	1408 Normotensives	OR of developing HTN increased 1.3 per each SD increase in PWV
	Prehypertension promotes increase in arterial stiffness			
6.	Tomyiama et al. [23]	Longitudinal (6 years follow-up)	1503 Normotensives	Subjects with persistent preHTN had higher annual increase in arterial stiffness
7.	AlGhatrif et al. [24] (BLSA)	Longitudinal (9 years follow-up)	775 subjects from general population	Prehypertensives had higher increase in PWV than normotensives

CIMT carotid intima-media thickness, *HTN* hypertension, *preHTN* prehypertension, *PWV* pulse wave velocity, *SD* standard deviation

A good illustration that prehypertension can promote increased arterial stiffness is given by the following two studies. Using brachial-ankle PWV (baPWV) Tomiyama and coworkers [23], evaluated longitudinally 1563 healthy subjects, dividing them by 3 age classes (29–39, 40–59 and >60 years) and evaluating them according to their blood pressure class at the beginning of the study and 6 years later; subjects who persistently maintained BP values of prehypertension were the ones presenting with the most accelerated rate of increase in arterial stiffness (over those who persisted normotensives or who had borderline phenotypes—presenting values of either normo or prehypertension in different evaluations), after adjustment for several other concurrent risk factors. The Baltimore Longitudinal Study of Aging has also contributed to this hypothesis, by showing that in 775 subjects free of cardiovascular disease and followed longitudinally for 9.3 years with several measurements of PWV, it was possible to see that PWV increases with age, but this increase was steeper not only when subjects were hypertensives but also (with a smaller effect) whenever their systolic blood pressure was between 120 and 139 mmHg [24].

Second, arterial stiffening may be paralleled by a remodeling of small resistance arteries. Small and large artery alterations are indeed closely interdependent in sustained grade I hypertension, and likely during the early phases of prehypertension. A temporal relationship is difficult to establish, and we previously suggested that a cross talk, by which small artery alterations influence larger artery phenotype, and conversely large artery alterations influence small artery phenotype, is more likely than a linear sequence [29]. Both small and large artery damages contribute to the rise in central BP, by favoring the generation of wave reflections and their propagation, respectively. This is exemplified by the fact that, in hypertensive patients, media-to-lumen ratio of subcutaneous small resistance arteries and cfPWV are both independent determinants of central SBP [30].

The cross talk between the micro- and the macro-circulation [29] promotes a vicious circle which can be described by starting at the site of small arteries. An increased resistance in small arteries increases mean blood pressure (BP), and then increases arterial stiffness in the large elastic arteries, which in parallel with more pressure wave reflections increases central systolic BP, variability of 24 h ambulatory brachial BP, and ultimately damages target organs [29, 31, 32]. The increased central BP pulsatility in turn is a factor of small resistance artery damage, i.e., increased media-to-lumen ratio of subcutaneous small resistance arteries. This has initially been reported in hypertensive animals [33] and then in hypertensive patients with brachial PP [34] and more recently with central systolic and PPs measured with applanation tonometry [30]. Interestingly, the wall-to-lumen ratio of retinal arteries is significantly correlated with 24 h systolic BP [35], and retinal microcirculation changes can already be found in prehypertensive subjects [36, 37]. Eventually, increased media-to-lumen ratio of subcutaneous small resistance arteries, which is associated with reduced lumen diameter, represents the largest part of the structural part of increased total peripheral resistance, leading to a rise in mean BP, and thus continuing the vicious circle.

8.5 Arterial Stiffness, Prehypertension, and Inflammation

The purpose of this section is not to detail the entire amount of evidence correlating inflammation as a precursor of both increased blood pressure and subclinical arteriosclerosis. It is rather set to pinpoint some key pathophysiologic mechanisms and, most importantly, to report on findings of BP and arterial stiffness in subjects with inflammation-associated pathologies. It is also a call for attention to all clinicians dealing with chronic disease and low-grade inflammation conditions: these are subjects that can have their baseline clinical condition very well controlled with modern available therapies—they will have considerably low morbidity arising from these conditions; on the other hand, they will survive longer and be subjected longer to the inflammatory stimulus and therefore be at higher risk for cardiovascular conditions such as high BP and subclinical arteriosclerosis, eventually progressing to established CVD. It is therefore of paramount importance to survey these subjects more strictly for the development of higher CV risk phenotypes (such as prehypertension and accelerated vascular aging).

A recent review of the molecular and cellular mechanisms involved in the biology of vascular aging has emphasized several aberrations that conduce to an acceleration of the aging process and increase in BP: aberrant signal transduction, oxidative stress, and activation of proinflammatory and pro-fibrotic transcription factors [38]. Several studies have been dedicated to establish a causal role of these biological mechanisms in the development of increased BP and arterial stiffness or to associate inflammatory states with the development of subclinical arteriosclerosis.

Using a randomized sham procedure in 100 healthy individuals, Vlachlopoulos and colleagues [39] compared subjects injected with a vaccine for Salmonella typhi with those receiving placebo, to find that inflammatory markers increased (hs CRP, IL6 and MMP9) in the first group, as did pulse wave velocity.

McEniery and colleagues [15] studied the influence of known polymorphisms of the metalloproteinase-9 (MMP9) gene (a protein with an enzymatic function degrading elastin and other arterial wall proteins) on arterial stiffness, in 865 healthy subjects from a community cohort; MMP-9 is usually released in response to proinflammatory states by neutrophils and monocytes or mechanic stress [15, 40]; the authors described that PWV was in fact increased in subjects carrying such polymorphisms (in the promotor and coding gene of MMP-9) as well as higher levels of MMP-9 in serum.

The Amsterdam Growth and Health Longitudinal Study (AGHLS) investigated if endothelial dysfunction and/or low-grade inflammation could influence the development of arterial stiffness [41], in 293 healthy young adults during a period of 6 years. It showed that higher levels of serum markers of both endothelial dysfunction (soluble intercellular adhesion molecule 1 [sICAM-1], soluble vascular cell adhesion molecule 1, soluble endothelial selectin, and soluble thrombomodulin) and low-grade inflammation (C-reactive protein [CRP], serum amyloid A, interleukin 6, interleukin 8, tumor necrosis factor-α, and sICAM-1) were associated with the development of higher measurements of arterial stiffness at the carotid and femoral levels.

Fifty-three prehypertensive subjects were followed during 3 years by Kim and coworkers [42], and compared to matched normotensives concerning the expression of inflammatory markers and the progression of arterial stiffness measures; the authors report that prehypertensives had higher expression of lysophosphatidylcholines (lysoPCs—with a known effect on vasodilation impairment) and higher circulating Lp-PLA2 activity, oxidized LDL (ox-LDL), interleukin 6 (IL-6), urinary 8-epi-PGF2a, and higher brachial-ankle pulse wave velocity (ba-PWV). They postulated that a proinflammatory state could, through enhanced oxidative stress, lead to higher arteriosclerosis in prehypertensives. The same research team followed 254 prehypertensives for 3.5 years, dividing them in three groups, according to the evolution of BP levels they registered (those who remained prehypertensive, those who became normotensive and those who progressed to hypertension) [43], studying changes in oxidative stress, lipoprotein-associated phospholipase A2 activity, and arterial stiffness. Their results in the group of persistent prehypertensives suggest that increased oxidative stress could enhance arterial stiffness without increase in blood pressure. Tomiyama and coworkers [44] also looked into the chronic influence of inflammation in the development of hypertension and arterial stiffness; evaluating 3274 middle-aged normotensive men during 9 years, they measured annually arterial stiffness, hsCRP, and blood pressure, and showed that higher levels of circulating hsCRP were associated with higher changes in arterial stiffness measurements, which in turn were associated with increases in BP. Similar observations (concerning the influence of low-grade inflammation in the development of arterial stiffness) were also found in the Malmo Diet and Cancer Study [45], following 2338 subjects for 17 years.

This accumulating evidence can be supplemented with findings of increased arterial stiffness and cardiovascular disease in subjects suffering from chronic inflammatory diseases.

Ambrosino and colleagues [46] performed meta-analysis and meta-regression studies to evaluate the impact of Rheumatoid Arthritis (RA) in several arterial stiffness measures (25 articles, 1472 RA patients); they showed that subjects with this condition had higher arterial stiffness, the magnitude of which was influenced by the severity of the inflammatory condition; more importantly, this influence can be seen from the earlier stages of the disease.

Zanolli and coworkers [47] took into consideration the cardiovascular risk paradox evident in patients with inflammatory bowel disease: the feature of malabsorption conditions a reduction in prevalence of obesity, dyslipidemia, and hypertension, but still patients suffer high cardiovascular mortality. They performed a meta-analysis to determine if these subjects have associated increased arteriosclerosis (9 studies included, 342 patients with ulcerative colitis, and 234 patients with Crohn's disease). They reported that these patients have higher arterial stiffness than matched controls, and a meta-regression performed with data from studies including patients treated with anti-TNFα drugs suggested that this later subgroup of patients could have lower arterial stiffness [47].

On this later topic (anti-TNFα treatment and reduction of arteriosclerosis) Tam and colleagues have conducted a systematic review of published information [48], concluding that the existing evidence is leaning to a beneficial effect of these drugs in stopping progression of arteriosclerosis (in these high inflammatory autoimmune pathologies) and even in reversing some of the arterial damage documented before the initiation of the drug.

Much controversy has been surrounding patients with HIV and their association to increased cardiovascular risk, particularly concerning the progression of arteriosclerosis. In spite of conflicting results (mainly derived from heterogeneous study populations, with different treatment strategies, some of which influence themselves the cardiovascular risk of the patient) recent work by Maia Leite and coworkers [49] suggests that HIV-infected patients have higher progression rates of arteriosclerosis and that among main contributors to this effect is the record of a $CD4^+$ T-cell nadir below 200 cells/μL, an expression of previous severe immunosuppression.

A recent meta-analysis and meta-regression of 18 studies including subjects with Obstructive Sleep Apnoea Syndrome (OSAS) has studied the impact of this nosology in the expression of higher levels of inflammatory markers and arterial stiffness [50]; the findings support the increased levels of both inflammatory markers and arterial stiffness measurements in these subjects.

A final word within this section is due to the recent review executed by Liu and coworkers [51], correlating inflammation, autoimmunity, and hypertension. Short of suggesting that hypertension could be an autoimmune disease, the authors did an extensive revision of the role of inflammatory cytokines (some of which induced by Ang II), and especially dwell on the role of tissue transglutaminase in mechanisms promoting hypertension and arterial stiffness through the renin-angiotensin system and cross-linking of extracellular matrix proteins promoting vascular remodeling.

8.6 Measurement of Arterial Stiffness

Details on the measurement of arterial stiffness are given here, in order to better understand the pathophysiological meaning of large artery stiffening, and its consequences on central BP. Arterial stiffness can be evaluated at the systemic, regional, and local levels [12, 31]. In contrast to systemic arterial stiffness, which can only be estimated from models of the circulation, regional and local arterial stiffness can be measured directly, and noninvasively, at various sites along the arterial tree. A major advantage of the regional and local evaluations of arterial stiffness is that they are based on direct measurements of parameters strongly linked to wall stiffness. Reviews have been published on the methodological aspects [12, 31, 52].

The measurement of pulse wave velocity (PWV) is generally accepted as the most simple, noninvasive, robust, and reproducible method with which to determine arterial stiffness. The measurement of PWV between the common carotid artery and the common femoral artery (carotid-femoral PWV) is a direct measurement, and it corresponds to the widely accepted propagative model of the arterial system [13, 31]. Measured along the aortic and aorto-iliac pathway, it is the most clinically relevant, since the aorta and its first branches are what the left ventricle "sees," and are thus responsible for most of the pathophysiological effects of arterial stiffness. Carotid-femoral PWV has been used in most epidemiological studies demonstrating the predictive value of aortic stiffness for CV events, namely in hypertensive patients [53–55]. By contrast, PWV measured outside the aortic track, at the upper (brachial PWV) or lower limb (femoro-tibial PWV), had no predictive value in patients with end-stage renal disease (ESRD) [56].

PWV is usually measured using the foot-to-foot velocity method from various waveforms. These are usually obtained, transcutaneously at the right common carotid artery and the right femoral artery (i.e., "carotid-femoral" PWV—cfPWV), and the time delay (Δt, or transit time) measured between the feet of the two waveforms [12, 57]. The "foot" of the wave is defined at the end of diastole, when the steep rise of the wavefront begins. The transit time is the time of travel of the "foot" of the wave over a known distance. A variety of different waveforms can be used including pressure [57, 58], distension, and Doppler [59]. The distance (D) covered by the waves is usually assimilated to the surface distance between the two recording sites, i.e., the common carotid artery (CCA) and the common femoral artery (CFA). The direct distance ΔD is (CFA to CCA). PWV is calculated as PWV = D (meters)/Δt (seconds). Magnetic resonance imaging allows determining aortic stiffness according to the same methodology [17].

Other methods have been used in pathophysiological and epidemiological studies in prehypertensive subjects. They include, at the regional level, either two-sites methods such as the aortic arch PWV with magnetic resonance imaging [16], brachial-ankle PWV, the heart-ankle PWV, and the finger-toe PWV, or one-site methods such as the QKD, the Arteriograph, and the Mobilograph methods [52]. At the local level, they include high-resolution echotracking methods and magnetic resonance imaging and use the noninvasive determination of arterial distensibility as distensibility = AS/cPP, where AS is arterial strain, defined as relative changes in area (Amax-Amin/Amin) during the systole, and where cPP is the central pulse pressure obtained by tonometry [12, 52].

8.7 Predictive Value of Arterial Stiffness for Cardiovascular Events

Discussing arterial stiffness in the early phases of prehypertension is important, not only because arterial stiffness has predictive value for incident hypertension, but also because arterial stiffness is an independent risk factor for CV events. The largest amount of evidence has been given for aortic stiffness measured through cfPWV. This has been initially reported in the late 1990s-early 2000s [53, 54]. Currently, a meta-analysis [55] of 19 studies showed the predictive value of aortic stiffness for fatal and nonfatal CV events in various populations having different levels of CV risk: general population, hypertensive patients, elderly subjects, type 2 diabetic patients, and patients with end-stage renal disease. In summary, aortic stiffness has demonstrated an independent predictive value for various outcomes (total mortality, CV mortality, coronary events, asymptomatic CAD, stroke, functional outcome after stroke, onset of dialysis) in various population (general population, elderly, hypertensives, diabetics (T2D), CAD, after acute stroke, stroke/TIA, moderate and severe chronic kidney disease—CKD and ESRD, and renal transplant recipients) [31]. Importantly, the predictive value of arterial stiffness for CV events is independent of classical CV risk factors, including risk scores such as the Framingham Risk Score (FRS) and the European risk score (SCORE). Thus, arterial stiffness is able to predict CV events beyond the traditional risk factors. A meta-analysis of 18 longitudinal cohort studies [60] has been performed with another method of determination of arterial stiffness, the measure of the brachial-ankle PWV (baPWV), which significantly predicted the risk of total CV events and all-cause mortality.

Ben Shlomo et al. [61] undertook a systematic review and obtained individual participant data from 16 studies in 17,635 participants, in order to determine the study-specific associations of cfPWV with CV outcomes. Using Cox proportional hazard models and random and after adjusting for conventional risk factors, they showed that cfPWV remained a significant predictor of CV events, namely coronary heart disease events. Moreover, a significant interaction with age was observed, i.e., the younger the subjects the higher the predictive value for CV events.

These data are consistent with previous findings that we obtained 20 years ago, after a biomechanical analysis of the carotid artery wall in normotensives and hypertensives [62]. In order to evaluate the elastic properties of the wall material of the common carotid artery, we determined Young's incremental elastic modulus (Einc) as a function of BP and circumferential wall stress, in 102 patients with never-treated essential hypertension and 40 age- and gender-matched normotensive subjects, using high-resolution echotracking and applanation tonometry. A major finding was that the "intrinsic" stiffness of the arterial wall material, determined through Einc calculated at a common circumferential wall stress, was increased in younger HT patients, but not in middle-aged and older HT patients. Thus, in these later categories, carotid stiffness was mainly due to the increase in BP, loading the stiff components of the arterial wall, whereas in younger subjects arterial stiffness was partly due to some abnormalities in the components of the arterial wall material and partly due to the high BP. The present findings are consistent with the interaction with age observed in the individual meta-analysis by Ben Shlomo et al. [61]. Taken together, they suggest that changes in the complex structure of the arterial wall may occur during the early phases of prehypertension, leading to increased arterial stiffness and ultimately high central and then peripheral systolic BP, whereas adaptive mechanisms occur later, aiming at rendering arterial stiffness only dependent on BP level.

8.8 Early Vascular Aging and Prehypertension

The aging of the large artery wall is characterized by a reduction in the elastin content, as well as an increased content of collagen, associated with changes in cell–matrix interactions, which altogether increase arterial stiffness [28, 63, 64]. In recent years a better understanding of these processes has led to the concept of Early Vascular Ageing (EVA) [65–68] in subjects with higher arterial stiffness than expected for their age and gender. More generally, EVA indicates a pronounced effect of aging on the vascular tree and especially on arterial function. Structurally,

EVA can be seen as an inadequate ability for repairing arterial damage in response to various mechanical, metabolic, and chemical stresses [65]. The arteries in subjects with such accelerated aging, present biological and cardiovascular risk features that would be expected years later, if the aging process would not have been accelerated through the interaction of age with different risk factors (traditional and non-traditional). Here, we use the concept of Early Vascular Ageing (EVA) to better understand the relationship between arterial stiffness and prehypertension.

Vascular aging in general, and EVA more specifically, can be investigated noninvasively through the measurement of a number of parameters, but arterial stiffness has been the most often studied, likely because of the robustness of its measurement. Arterial stiffness, which can be considered as an "imaging" biomarker, may be more predictive than "circulating" biomarkers, like hs-CRP [69], and show a better additional prediction when coupled to classical CV risk scores [70, 71]. Particularly, arterial stiffness can be considered as a measure of the cumulative influence of CV risk factors with aging on the arterial tree. Indeed, arterial stiffness reflects the true arterial wall damage, whereas blood pressure, glycemia, and lipids, which are fluctuating along the follow-up of patients, may not. A temporal dissociation exists between the observed values of classical (i.e., age, blood pressure, total cholesterol) and up-to-date (i.e., hs-CRP, BNP, plasma renin) CV risk factors which can be considered as "snapshots" [29], and arterial stiffness which integrates the long-lasting effects of all identified and non-identified CV risk factors and thus may be considered as relevant "imaging" biomarker [72].

EVA may help understanding the relationship between arterial stiffness and hemodynamic changes in the early phase of prehypertension, leading after years of arterial remodeling and target organ damage to incident hypertension. Interestingly, the Lancet commission on hypertension lead by M. Olsen [73] adopted the EVA concept through a life-course preventive and therapeutic strategy aiming at reducing CV risk factors, target organ damage, and CV events at various periods of life (childhood, young adult, middle-age, advanced age, and elderly). Indeed, a number of modifiable CV risk factors are associated with both EVA, i.e., higher arterial stiffness than expected for age, and prehypertension. These modifiable CV risk factors include classical CV risk factors, such as high BP, hyperglycemia, overweight, impaired glucose tolerance, metabolic syndrome, type 1 and 2 diabetes, chronic kidney disease, high plasma lipid levels, smoking, fat diet, high salt intake, and lack of regular physical activity; they include additional CV risk factors, such as chronic low-grade inflammation, oxidative stress, social deprivation, perceived stress, abnormal sleep pattern, thrombogenic factors, prenatal fetal growth, and hormonal status [1, 2, 12].

Cunha et al. [66] applied the EVA concept in a population from northern Portugal, an area which registers an especially high prevalence of hypertension and stroke incidence by contrast with other southern European people. In this cohort study which enrolled 3038 individuals, individuals were classified with EVA if their cfPWV was at least 97.5th percentile of z-score for mean PWV values adjusted for age, using normal European reference values as comparators (Reference values 2010). The overall prevalence of EVA was higher than expected in this so-called low cardiovascular risk area: 12.5%. Moreover, 26.1% of individuals below 30 years presented with EVA and 40.2% of individuals in that same age strata were placed above the 90th percentile of cfPWV. Thus, high prevalence rates of EVA and noteworthy large artery damage were found in young individuals, a significant percentage of whom had prehypertension. Although not all key factors of EVA in this population have been determined, one must bear in mind the high prevalence of overweight/obesity and adiposity measures, high salt intake, lack of physical activity, and the epidemiological transitions of the population in the last 40 years (Fig. 8.1; [65, 66]).

In fact when developing a logistic regression model for EVA in these subjects, one could see (Table 8.2, adapted from [66]) the expected influence of blood pressure; but it is of particular interest to remark that subjects with High-Normal blood pressure had an OR of 1.7 of developing accelerated vascular aging, when compared with subjects with optimal blood pressure.

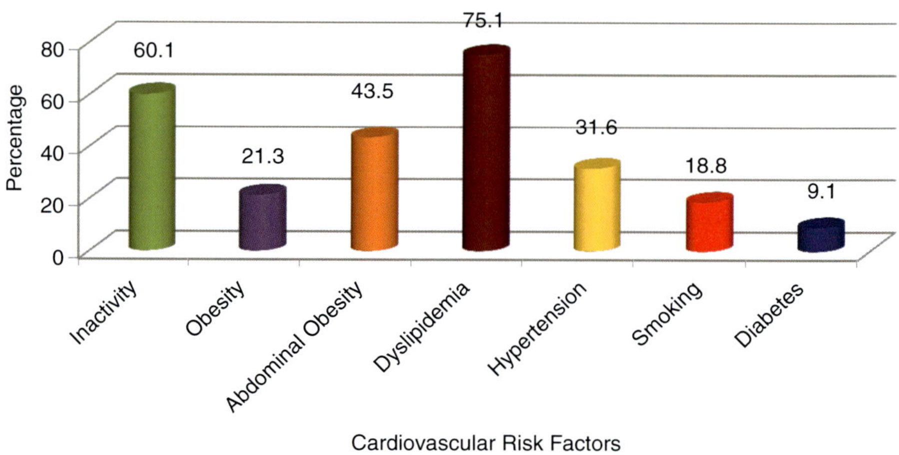

Fig. 8.1 Prevalence of cardiovascular risk factors in the Guimarães/Vizela Study [66]

Table 8.2 Prehypertensives have an increased risk of presenting EVA—Logistic Regression model for Early Vascular Aging (adapted from [66])

	B-Coefficient (SE)	Odds ratio (95% CI)	*p* value
Age < 30 years	1.173 (0.225)	3.232 (2.078–5.026)	<0.001
Age 30–39 years	0.114 (0.228)	1.121 (0.717–1.752)	0.618
Normal BP	0.227 (0.193)	1.255 (0.859–1.834)	0.240
High-normal BP	0.562 (0.220)	1.754 (1.1.40–2.698)	0.011
Grade 1 HT	1.134 (0.260)	3.107 (1.865–5.174)	0.010
Grade 2/3 HT	2.235 (0.630)	9.350 (2.719–32.149)	<0.001
HR > 75 bpm	0.510 (0.187)	1.665 (1.154–2.403)	0.006
Diabetes	1.042 (0.444)	2.832 (1.188–6.789)	0.019
Male sex	0.363(0.165)	1.438 (1.041–1.986)	0.028

EVA early vascular aging, *HR* heart rate, *BP* blood pressure, *HT* hypertension, *bpm* beats per minute, *SE* standard error, *CI* confidence interval using age 40–49 years, Optimal BP, and female sex as reference class

8.9 Metabolic Syndrome, Arterial Stiffness, and Prehypertension in Children

The relationship between arterial stiffness, metabolic syndrome, and BP levels have been discussed in several research articles [74–76] and reviews [66, 68, 77]. Data in adults have been discussed most of the time. We focus here on children and adolescents, since this is at these young ages that most often the early phases of prehypertension occur, and that preventive measures are the most effective [2, 78, 79].

On another perspective, the concept of early vascular aging and the relationship between prehypertension and arterial stiffness are altogether very cohesive with the existing evidence that links the prevalence and progression of cardiovascular risk factors at young ages with premature manifestations of arteriosclerosis and, therefore, earlier excessive cardiovascular risk. The particularly enthusiastic feature of this cohesive link is the notion that, at these stages/ages, cardiovascular risk (and arteriosclerosis, to some extent) can be reversed, as we will demonstrate below.

Blood Pressure and arterial stiffness. In children, diagnostic criteria for elevated BP in general and prehypertension in particular are based on the concept that BP in children increases with age and body size, making it impossible to utilize a single-BP level to define hypertension, as done in adults [78, 79]. Unfortunately, there are no European reference values for BP that incorporate age, sex, and height, throughout the entire pediatric age range. Thus, hypertension definition is based on the normal distribution of BP in healthy children. Hypertension in children is defined as SBP and/or DBP persistently at least 95th percentile for sex, age, and height measured on at least three separate occasions [78, 79]. Children with average SBP and/or DBP at least 90th, but less than 95th are classified as having high-normal BP. Thus, it is expected that about 5% of children have stage 2 prehypertension, according to US Guidelines.

Falkner [2] recently pointed out that, given current estimates, about 10% of adolescents have hypertension or prehypertension, and reported various child and adolescent exposures playing a role in high BP, such as stress [80], dietary salt intake, fructose, lifestyles including food sources (processed and fast foods), sleep patterns, and reductions in physical activity. Particularly, vascular injury may be present in children and adolescent in the early phase of prehypertension and could be considered a risk factor for later hypertension in adulthood [2]. Conversely, elevated BP in childhood has been associated with increased adult arterial stiffness [81–84]. Thus, a vicious feedback loop is exemplified here, through which both arterial stiffness and high BP in childhood increase the occurrence of each other in adulthood. The early publications of the Bogalusa Heart Study [85] described the tracking phenomenon of blood pressure from childhood to adulthood, and showed that children above the 80th percentile of BP (i.e., including prehypertensives) were the most likely to develop hypertension later on. And then, many other studies have devoted to explain the early influence of BP on the development of early damage to the medial wall of large arteries. In the Bogalusa Heart Study, Li et al. [84] demonstrated that SBP in childhood as well as the time of exposure to elevated SBP were the main predictors of increased arterial stiffness in adulthood. The Cardiovascular

Risk in Young Finns Study has followed 2255 subjects from childhood to adulthood (mean follow-up of 21 years), correlating the elevation of several CVRF, including childhood blood pressure to development of decreased distensibility and increased arterial stiffness in early adulthood [83]. More recently, Chu and coworkers [81] have described the influence of several risk factors during childhood on the development of arterial stiffness, 26 years later; 4623 children from the Hanzhong province have been characterized and followed for this time period, showing that those with BP above the 75th percentile (i.e., including children with prehypertension) had higher levels of arterial stiffness revealed in adulthood.

Metabolic syndrome and arterial stiffness. Much evidence has been published concerning the frequent coexistence of prehypertension and several other cardiovascular risk factors in childhood. Srinivasan and coworkers of the Bogalusa Heart Study [86] followed 3255 children until adulthood; analyzing the 721 prehypertensives included, the authors could verify that these subjects, throughout their development had significantly higher adiposity measures, blood pressure levels, and triglycerides beginning in childhood; higher glucose in adolescence; and higher low-density lipoprotein cholesterol, and insulin metabolism abnormalities in adulthood. In a collaborative effort, the Cardiovascular Risk in Young Finns Study, the Bogalusa Heart Study, and the Childhood Determinants of Adult Health (CDAH) Study looked into the influence of childhood dyslipidemia on the development of arterial stiffness during adulthood; 1711 children with mean age between 13 and 15 years at study entrance were followed for 17–21 years; adolescents with dyslipidemia and overweight/obese had markedly higher intima-media thickness at 35 years of age than their counterparts without dyslipidemia, or with dyslipidemia but normal—weight [87]. The Bogalusa Heart Study and the Cardiovascular Risk in Young Finns Study subsequently evaluated 1781 participants aged 9–18 years at baseline with the objective of understanding the influence of childhood Metabolic Syndrome (MS) in the development of subclinical atherosclerosis and type 2 Diabetes Mellitus 14–27 years later; individuals with the MS had 2–3 times higher risk of presenting higher cIMT or T2DM, with prehypertension/hypertension factoring in specifically for higher arterial stiffness. Interestingly higher BMI (overweight/obesity) at study entrance was a variable as discriminative of the risk of both endpoints (cIMT and T2DM) as MS [88], a fact that would be corroborated with more clarity in 1617 participants followed during 31 years in the Cardiovascular Risk in Young Finns Study [89].

Ferreira et al. [82] examined whether the trajectories, from adolescence to young adulthood, of BP, body fatness and fat distribution, blood lipids, cardiorespiratory fitness, and heart rate determined levels of arterial stiffness in young adults. They investigated 373 apparently healthy adults in whom cardiovascular risk factors were repeatedly examined between the ages of 13 and 36 years during the Amsterdam Growth and Health Longitudinal study, and measured carotid stiffness 24 years later, at the age of 36 years. Compared with individuals with less stiff carotid arteries, those with stiffer carotid arteries at the age of 36 years were characterized from ages 13 to 36 years by greater levels of and steeper increases in BP and central fatness, independently of each other and other risk factors. These increases were already present in adolescence, preceded the development of poorer levels of blood lipids, cardiorespiratory fitness, and heart rate, which were evident during adulthood only, and explained to a great extent the deleterious association between these risk factors and carotid stiffness at the age of 36 years.

Finally, at least two large review and collaborative studies have addressed the complex relationships of several cardiovascular risk factors in childhood with the development of arterial stiffness in adulthood. The Cardiovascular Risk in Young Finns Study, the Childhood Determinants of Adult Health Study, the Bogalusa Heart Study, and the Muscatine Study for the International Childhood Cardiovascular Cohort (i3C) Consortium evaluated the capability of a childhood risk score (defined as total cholesterol, triglycerides, BMI, and systolic BP in the highest quintile) to predict adult high levels of carotid intima-media thickness (IMT), showing that exposure to these risk factors between the ages of 9 and 18 years were significantly associated with increased adult carotid IMT [90]. In a large systematic review of 65 observational studies, Lamotte and colleagues [91] confirmed the association between the prevalence of several cardiovascular risk factors (obesity, diabetes mellitus, hypertension, dyslipidemia, and chronic renal disease) and the existence of subclinical arteriosclerosis (increased carotid IMT) during childhood and adolescence, when compared to healthy controls [91].

Early interventions to reduce prehypertension and arterial stiffness. From all of the above described, six particular aspects need to be surveyed and addressed during childhood to prevent the early development of prehypertensiom, adverse cardiometabolic profiles, and early manifestations of arteriosclerosis: (1) The concept of lifetime risk of CVD [92] and the importance of Ideal Cardiovascular Health metrics [93]; (2) The importance of prenatal care and early life surveillance (Low birth weight and small for gestational age children and the influence of the mismatch growth hypothesis on the development of increased blood pressure and early manifestations of arterial stiffness—[94, 95]); (3) Reducing measures of adiposity and insulin resistance; (4) Promotion of Physical activity; (5) Monitor and reduce Blood Pressure; (6) Assume, for each subject, a life course approach to track and control cardiovascular risk factors and promote ideal cardiovascular health, remembering critical points in the human life-course for the development of large artery damage—the race horse hypothesis, discussed by Ferreira and coworkers [82] remembers the clinician that the rate of change of a given risk factor is also important to monitor, as it pinpoints subjects racing faster to increased risk conditions and need of interventional measures.

Several key studies have demonstrated that it is possible to obtain a reduction of the risk of subclinical arteriosclerosis and cardiometabolic disease in adulthood, through early intervention on reducing cardiovascular risk exposure during childhood. A brief review of these meaningful results can be seen in Table 8.3 [96–103].

It is thus of crucial importance to prevent or reduce childhood obesity in order to decrease the prevalence of high BP in childhood. Weight control in overweight and obese children, along with dietary changes [104] and increases in physical activity [105], has benefit on BP levels in childhood, likely through

Table 8.3 Reduction of the risk of subclinical arteriosclerosis and cardiometabolic disease in adulthood

	Author/year	Study type	Participants	Result
1.	Aatola (2010) [96] (CVRYFS)	Longitudinal (27 years follow-up)	1691 subjects (3–18 years old at study entrance)	Decreased number of risk factor and reversal of obesity status from childhood to adulthood are associated with lower PWV in adulthood
2.	Koskinen (2010) [97] (CVRYFS)	Longitudinal (6 years follow-up)	1673 subjects	Subjects who recovered from MetS, presented lower AStiff and better aortic distensibility than those who persisted with or had de novo MetS
3.	Juonala (2011) [98] (ICCCC)	Longitudinal (23 years follow-up)	6328 subjects (from the CVRYFS, BHS, MS and CDAH)	Subjects who reduced adiposity status from childhood to adulthood, eliminated added risk of T2DM, HTN, AStiff, and dyslipidemia in adulthood
4.	Laitinen (2012) [99] (CVRYFS)	Longitudinal (21 years follow-up)	856 subjects (15 years at study entrance)	Higher number of ideal CV health metrics were associated with reduced risk of HTN, T2DM, MS, AStiff, and dyslipidemia in adulthood
5.	Magnussen (2012) [100] (BHS & CVRYFS)	Longitudinal (24.4 years follow-up)	1757 subjects (aged 9–18 at study entrance)	Subjects with MetS at childhood that was reversed by adulthood, had the same risk of developing T2DM and Astiff than those who never had MetS
6.	Oikonen (2013) [101] (ICCCC)	Cross-sectional (young adults from different cohorts)	5785 subjects (from the PFS, MCCS, BHS, CVRYFS and CDAH	The number of ideal CV health metrics were inversely associated with cIMT
7.	Aatola (2014) [102] (CVRYFS)	Longitudinal (21 years follow-up)	1143 subjects	During follow-up, for each point increase in CV health metrics, a reduction of 0.09 m/s in PWV was verified
8.	Kelly (2015) [103] (CDAH)	Longitudinal (20 years follow-up)	798 subjects (9 years at study entrance)	Subjects with elevated BP in childhood who adapted healthy lifestyles had a decreased risk of developing HTN in adulthood

AStiff arterial stiffness, *BHS* Bogalusa Heart Study, *BP* blood pressure, *CDAH* childhood determinants of adult health, *CIMT* carotid intima-media thickness, *CV* cardiovascular, *CVRYFS* cardiovascular risk in Young Finns Study, *HTN* hypertension, *ICCC* International Childhood Cardiovascular Cohort Consortium, *MCCS* Minneapolis Childhood Cohort Studies, *MetS* Metabolic Syndrome, *MS* Muscatine Study, *PFS* Princeton Follow-up Study, *PWV* pulse wave velocity, T2DM Type 2 Diabetes Mellitus

the reduction of the metabolic syndrome. Indeed, Koistoinen and coworkers [106] showed, in 945 subjects participating to the Cardiovascular Risk in Young Finns study and having their baseline data in 1986 (then aged 9–18 years) and adult follow-up in 2007 (then aged 30–39 years), that metabolic syndrome in childhood predicted increased arterial stiffness in adulthood, and recovery from childhood metabolic syndrome was associated with decreased arterial PWV in adulthood. In addition, the favorable BP change from childhood to adulthood reduces the risk of high adult arterial stiffness, as reported by Aatola et al. [107] recently. During the Cardiovascular Risk in Young Finns study, these authors examined the effect of child and adult BP on PWV assessed in adulthood among 1540 white adults followed-up for 27 years since baseline (1980, aged 6–18 years). Individuals with persistently elevated BP and individuals with normal child but elevated adult BP had increased risk of high adult PWV in comparison with individuals with normal (both child and adult) BP. In contrast, individuals with elevated BP in childhood but not in adulthood did not have significantly increased risk of high PWV.

The lack of physical activity participates to epidemics of overweight, obesity and prehypertension in children and adolescent. An increase in physical activity is of crucial importance, not only in children with metabolic syndrome, but also in all children. In this regard, the data obtained in 1417 children (aged 9–15 years) and 999 young adults (aged 18–24 years) from the prospective Cardiovascular Risk in Young Finns study, are of great interest [108]. Participants had questionnaire measures of leisure-time physical activity available from 1986 and ultrasound-derived indices of carotid stiffness measured in 2007. Physical activity at age 18–24 years was directly associated with carotid stiffness 21 years later in males and females, independently of confounding factors. Thus, higher levels of physical activity in youth may benefit future cardiovascular health.

Conclusion

The evidence shown here describes a bidirectional relationship between prehypertension and arterial stiffness, but it also shows that even if they interact to generate higher blood pressure levels or higher large artery damage, they are also not exclusively dependent on each other to progress and increase the cardiovascular risk of an individual per se—this underlines the importance of measuring both, especially in subjects at risk of a faster decline of their vascular health, as described in the previous sections of this chapter.

A number of cohort studies and pathophysiological evidences relating arterial stiffness to cardiovascular risk factors, inflammation and incident hypertension suggest that arterial stiffness measurement could help identify normotensive individuals at risk of incident hypertension. These subjects should be targeted for the implementation of interventions targeting CV risk factors, with the objective of preventing or delaying the progression of subclinical arterial stiffening, thus preventing or delaying the onset of hypertension.

In parallel, we have shown evidence of the association of different cardiovascular risk factors in adulthood, with adverse cardiometabolic profiles promoting subclinical arteriosclerosis and early vascular aging, leaving a positive message concerning the demonstrated possibility of intervening with higher rates of success ate these young ages.

References

1. Egan BM, Stevens-Fabry S. Prehypertension—prevalence, health risks, and management strategies. Nat Rev Cardiol. 2015;12:289–300.
2. Falkner B. Recent clinical and translational advances in pediatric hypertension. Hypertension. 2015;65:926–31.
3. Vasan RS, Larson MG, Leip EP, Evans JC, O'Donnell CJ, Kannel WB, Levy D. Impact of high-normal blood pressure on the risk of cardiovascular disease. N Engl J Med. 2001;345:1291–7.
4. Egan BM, Julius S. Prehypertension: risk stratification and management considerations. Curr Hypertens Rep. 2008;10(5):359–66.
5. Lee M, Saver JL, Chang B, Chang KH, Hao Q, Ovbiagele B. Presence of baseline prehypertension and risk of incident stroke: a meta-analysis. Neurology. 2011;77(14):1330–7.
6. Lorenzo C, Aung K, Stern MP, Haffner SM. Pulse pressure, prehypertension, and mortality: the San Antonio heart study. Am J Hypertens. 2009;22(11):1219–26.
7. Zimlichman R. Treatment of hypertension and metabolic syndrome: lowering blood pressure is not enough for organ protection, new approach-arterial destiffening. Curr Hypertens Rep. 2014;16:479–84.
8. Liao D, Arnett DK, Tyroler HA, Riley WA, Chambless LE, Szklo M, Heiss G. Arterial stiffness and the development of hypertension. The ARIC study. Hypertension. 1999;34:201–6.
9. Dernellis J, Panaretou M. Aortic stiffness is an independent predictor of progression to hypertension in nonhypertensive subjects. Hypertension. 2005;45:426–31.
10. Najjar SS, Scuteri A, Shetty V, Wright JG, Muller DC, Fleg JL, Spurgeon HP, Ferrucci L, Lakatta EG. Pulse wave velocity is an independent predictor of the longitudinal increase in systolic blood pressure and of incident hypertension in the Baltimore Longitudinal Study of Aging. J Am Coll Cardiol. 2008;51:1377–83.
11. Kaess BM, Rong J, Larson MG, Hamburg NM, Vita JA, Levy D, Benjamin EJ, Vasan RS, Mitchell GF. Aortic stiffness, blood pressure progression, and incident hypertension. JAMA. 2012;308:875–81.
12. Laurent S, Cockcroft J, Van Bortel L, Boutouyrie P, Giannattasio C, Hayoz D, Pannier B, Vlachopoulos C, Wilkinson I, Struijker-Boudier H. Expert Consensus Document on arterial stiffnes: methodological aspects and clinical applications. Eur Heart J. 2006;27:2588–605.
13. Nichols WW, O'Rourke MF. McDonald's blood flow in arteries; Theoretical, experimental and clinical principles. 5th ed. Oxford: Oxford University Press; 2005. 624 p.
14. Herbert A, Cruickshank K, Laurent S, Boutouyrie P, on behalf of The Reference Values for Arterial Measurements Collaboration. Establishing reference values for central blood pressure and its amplification in a general healthy population and according to cardiovascular risk-factors. Eur Heart J. 2014;35:3122–33.
15. McEniery CM, Yasmin, McDonnell B, Munnery M, Wallace SM, Rowe CV, Cockcroft JR, Wilkinson IB. Central pressure: variability and impact of cardiovascular risk factors: the Anglo-Cardiff Collaborative Trial II. Hypertension. 2008;51(6):1476–82.
16. Yano Y, Neeland IJ, Ayers C, Peshock R, Berry JD, Lloyd-Jones DM, Greenland P, Mitchell GF, Vongpatanasin W. Hemodynamic and mechanical properties of the proximal aorta in young and middle-aged adults with isolated systolic hypertension: the Dallas Heart Study. Hypertension. 2017;70:158–65.
17. Redheuil A, Yu WC, Wu CO, Mousseaux E, de Cesare A, Yan R, Kachenoura N, Bluemke D, Lima JA. Reduced ascending aortic strain and distensibility: earliest manifestations of vascular aging in humans. Hypertension. 2010;55(2):319–26.
18. Urbina EM, Khoury PR, McCoy C, Daniels SR, Kimball TR, Dolan LM. Cardiac and vascular consequences of pre-hypertension in youth. J Clin Hypertens (Greenwich). 2011;13(5):332–42.
19. Drukteinis JS, Roman MJ, Fabsitz RR, Lee ET, Best LG, Russell M, Devereux RB. Cardiac and systemic hemodynamic characteristics of hypertension and prehypertension in adolescents and young adults: the Strong Heart Study. Circulation. 2007;115(2):221–7.

20. Manios E, Tsivgoulis G, Koroboki E, Stamatelopoulos K, Papamichael C, Toumanidis S, Stamboulis E, Vemmos K, Zakopoulos N. Impact of prehypertension on common carotid artery intima-media thickness and left ventricular mass. Stroke. 2009;40(4):1515–8.
21. Knight EL, Kramer HM, Curhan GC. High-normal blood pressure and microalbuminuria. Am J Kidney Dis. 2003;41(3):588–95.
22. Peralta CA, Adeney KL, Shlipak MG, Jacobs D Jr, Duprez D, Bluemke D, Polak J, Psaty B, Kestenbaum BR. Structural and functional vascular alterations and incident hypertension in normotensive adults: the Multi-Ethnic Study of Atherosclerosis. Am J Epidemiol. 2010;171(1):63–71.
23. Tomiyama H, Hashimoto H, Matsumoto C, Odaira M, Yoshida M, Shiina K, Nagata M, Yamashina A, Doba N, Hinohara S. Effects of aging and persistent prehypertension on arterial stiffening. Atherosclerosis. 2011;217(1):130–4.
24. AlGhatrif M, Strait JB, Morrell CH, Canepa M, Wright J, Elango P, Scuteri A, Najjar SS, Ferrucci L, Lakatta EG. Longitudinal trajectories of arterial stiffness and the role of blood pressure: the Baltimore Longitudinal Study of Aging. Hypertension. 2013;62(5):934–41.
25. Humphrey JD, Dufresne ER, Schwartz MA. Mechanotransduction and extracellular matrix homeostasis. Nat Rev Mol Cell Biol. 2014;15:802–12.
26. Folkow B. "Structural factor" in primary and secondary hypertension. Hypertension. 1990;16:89–101.
27. Wolinsky H. Long-term effects of hypertension on the rat aortic wall and their relation to concurrent aging changes. Morphological and chemical studies. Circ Res. 1972;30:301–9.
28. Lacolley P, Challande P, Osborne-Pellegrin M, Regnault V. Genetics and pathophysiology of arterial stiffness. Cardiovasc Res. 2009;81:637–48.
29. Laurent S, Briet M, Boutouyrie P. Large and small artery cross-talk and recent morbidity-mortality trials in hypertension. Hypertension. 2009;54:388–92.
30. Muiesan ML, Salvetti M, Rizzoni D, Paini A, Agabiti-Rosei C, Aggiusti C, Bertacchini F, Stassaldi D, Gavazzi A, Porteri E, De Ciuceis C, Agabiti-Rosei E. Pulsatile hemodynamics and microcirculation: evidence for a close relationship in hypertensive patients. Hypertension. 2013;61:130–6.
31. Laurent S, Safar M. Large artery damage: measurement and clinical importance in textbook of hypertension. In: Mancia G, Grassi G, Redon J, editors. Informa Healthcare. 2014. p. 191–202.
32. Schillaci G, Bilo G, Pucci G, Laurent S, Macquin-Mavier I, Boutouyrie P, Battista F, Desamericq G, Dolbeau G, Faini A, Salvi P, Mannarino E, Parati G. Relationship between short-term blood pressure variability and large-artery stiffness in human hypertension: findings from 2 large databases. Hypertension. 2012;60:369–77.
33. Christensen KL. Reducing pulse pressure in hypertension may normalize small artery structure. Hypertension. 1991;18:722–7.
34. James MA, Watt PA, Potter JF, Thurston H, Swales JD. Pulse pressure and resistance artery structure in the elderly. Hypertension. 1995;26:301–6.
35. Salvetti M, Agabiti Rosei C, Paini A, Aggiusti C, Cancarini A, Duse S, Semeraro F, Rizzoni D, Agabiti Rosei E, Muiesan ML. Relationship of wall-to-lumen ratio of retinal arterioles with clinic and 24-hour blood pressure. Hypertension. 2014;63:1110–5.
36. Grassi G, Buzzi S, Dell'Oro R, Mineo C, Dimitriadis K, Seravalle G, Lonati L, Cuspidi C. Structural alterations of the retinal microcirculation in the "prehypertensive" high-normal blood pressure state. Curr Pharm Des. 2013;19(13):2375–81.
37. Sharrett AR, Hubbard LD, Cooper LS, Sorlie PD, Brothers RJ, Nieto FJ, Pinsky JL, Klein R. Retinal arteriolar diameters and elevated blood pressure: the Atherosclerosis Risk in Communities Study. Am J Epidemiol. 1999;150(3):263–70.
38. Harvey A, Montezano AC, Touyz RM. Vascular biology of ageing—implications in hypertension. J Mol Cell Cardiol. 2015;83:112–21.
39. Vlachopoulos C, Dima I, Aznaouridis K, Vasiliadou C, Ioakeimidis N, Aggeli C, Toutouza M, Stefanadis C. Acute systemic inflammation increases arterial stiffness and decreases wave reflections in healthy individuals. Circulation. 2005;112(14):2193–200.

40. Blankenberg S, Rupprecht HJ, Poirier O, Bickel C, Smieja M, Hafner G, Meyer J, Cambien F, Tiret L. Plasma concentrations and genetic variation of matrix metalloproteinase 9 and prognosis of patients with cardiovascular disease. Circulation. 2003;107(12):1579–85.
41. van Bussel BC, Schouten F, Henry RM, Schalkwijk CG, de Boer MR, Ferreira I, Smulders YM, Twisk JW, Stehouwer CD. Endothelial dysfunction and low-grade inflammation are associated with greater arterial stiffness over a 6-year period. Hypertension. 2011;58(4):588–95.
42. Kim M, Jung S, Kim SY, Lee SH, Lee JH. Prehypertension-associated elevation in circulating lysophosphatidlycholines, Lp-PLA2 activity, and oxidative stress. PLoS One. 2014;9(5):e96735.
43. Kim M, Yoo HJ, Ahn HY, Park J, Lee SH, Lee JH. Associations among oxidative stress, Lp-PLA2 activity and arterial stiffness according to blood pressure status at a 3.5-year follow-up in subjects with prehypertension. Atherosclerosis. 2017;257:179–85.
44. Tomiyama H, Shiina K, Matsumoto-Nakano C, Ninomiya T, Komatsu S, Kimura K, Chikamori T, Yamashina A. The contribution of inflammation to the development of hypertension mediated by increased arterial stiffness. J Am Heart Assoc. 2017;6(7):e005729.
45. Muhammad IF, Borne Y, Ostling G, Kennback C, Gottsater M, Persson M, Nilsson PM, Engstrom G. Acute phase proteins as prospective risk markers for arterial stiffness: The Malmo Diet and Cancer cohort. PLoS One. 2017;12(7):e0181718.
46. Ambrosino P, Tasso M, Lupoli R, Di Minno A, Baldassarre D, Tremoli E, Di Minno MN. Non-invasive assessment of arterial stiffness in patients with rheumatoid arthritis: a systematic review and meta-analysis of literature studies. Ann Med. 2015;47(6):457–67.
47. Zanoli L, Rastelli S, Granata A, Inserra G, Empana JP, Boutouyrie P, Laurent S, Castellino P. Arterial stiffness in inflammatory bowel disease: a systematic review and meta-analysis. J Hypertens. 2016;34(5):822–9.
48. Tam LS, Kitas GD, Gonzalez-Gay MA. Can suppression of inflammation by anti-TNF prevent progression of subclinical atherosclerosis in inflammatory arthritis? Rheumatology (Oxford). 2014;53(6):1108–19.
49. Maia-Leite LH, Catez E, Boyd A, Haddour N, Curjol A, Lang S, Nuernberg M, Duvivier C, Desvarieux M, Kirstetter M, Girard PM, Cohen A, Boccara F. Aortic stiffness aging is influenced by past profound immunodeficiency in HIV-infected individuals: results from the EVAS-HIV (EValuation of Aortic Stiffness in HIV-infected individuals). J Hypertens. 2016;34(7):1338–46.
50. Wang J, Yu W, Gao M, Zhang F, Gu C, Yu Y, Wei Y. Impact of obstructive sleep apnea syndrome on endothelial function, arterial stiffening, and serum inflammatory markers: an updated meta-analysis and metaregression of 18 studies. J Am Heart Assoc. 2015;4(11):e002454.
51. Liu C, Kellems RE, Xia Y. Inflammation, autoimmunity, and hypertension: the essential role of tissue transglutaminase. Am J Hypertens. 2017;30(8):756–64.
52. Laurent S, Marais L, Boutouyrie P. the non-invasive assessment of vascular ageing. Can J Cardiol. 2016;32:669–79.
53. Boutouyrie P, Tropeano AI, Asmar R, Gautier I, Benetos A, Lacolley P, Laurent S. Aortic stiffness is an independent predictor of primary coronary events in hypertensive patients: a longitudinal study. Hypertension. 2002;39:10–5.
54. Laurent S, Boutouyrie P, Asmar R, Gautier I, Laloux B, Guize L, Ducimetiere P, Benetos A. Aortic stiffness is an independent predictor of all-cause and cardiovascular mortality in hypertensive patients. Hypertension. 2001;37:1236–41.
55. Vlachopoulos C, Aznaouridis K, Stefanadis C. Prediction of cardiovascular events and all-cause mortality with arterial stiffness: a systematic review and meta-analysis. J Am Coll Cardiol. 2010;55:1318–27.
56. Pannier B, Guerin AP, Marchais SJ, et al. Stiffness of capacitive and conduit arteries: prognostic significance for end-stage renal disease patients. Hypertension. 2005;45:592–6.
57. Asmar R, Benetos A, Topouchian J, Laurent P, Pannier B, Brisac AM, Target R, Levy B. Assessment of arterial distensibility by automatic pulse wave velocity measurement. Validation and clinical application studies. Hypertension. 1995;26:485–90.

58. Pauca AL, O'Rourke MF, Kon ND. Prospective evaluation of a method for estimating ascending aortic pressure from the radial artery pressure waveform. Hypertension. 2001;38:932–7.
59. Cruickshank K, Riste L, Anderson SG, Wright JS, Dunn G, Gosling RG. Aortic pulse-wave velocity and its relationship to mortality in diabetes and glucose intolerance: an integrated index of vascular function? Circulation. 2002;106:2085–90.
60. Vlachopoulos C, Aznaouridis K, Terentes-Printzios D, Ioakeimidis N, Stefanadis C. Prediction of cardiovascular events and all-cause mortality with brachial-ankle elasticity index: a systematic review and meta-analysis. Hypertension. 2012;60:556–62.
61. Ben-Shlomo Y, Spears M, Boustred C, May M, Anderson SG, Benjamin EJ, Boutouyrie P, Cameron J, Chen CH, Cruickshank JK, Hwang SJ, Lakatta EG, Laurent S, Maldonado J, Mitchell GF, Najjar SS, Newman AB, Ohishi M, Pannier B, Pereira T, Vasan RS, Shokawa T, Sutton-Tyrell K, Verbeke F, Wang KL, Webb DJ, Hansen TW, Zoungas S, McEniery CM, Cockcroft JR, Wilkinson IB. Aortic pulse wave velocity improves cardiovascular event prediction: an individual participant meta-analysis of prospective observational data from 17,635 subjects. J Am Coll Cardiol. 2014;63(7):636–46.
62. Bussy C, Boutouyrie P, Lacolley P, Challande P, Laurent S. Intrinsic stiffness of the carotid arterial wall material in essential hypertensives. Hypertension. 2000;35:1049–54.
63. Laurent S, Boutouyrie P, Lacolley P. Structural and genetic bases of arterial stiffness. Hypertension. 2005;45:1050–5.
64. Laurent S, Boutouyrie P. The structural factor in hypertension: large and small artery alterations. Circ Res. 2015;116:1007–21.
65. Cunha PG, Boutouyrie P, Nilsson PM, Laurent S. Early Vascular Ageing (EVA): definitions and clinical applicability. Curr Hypertens Rev. 2017;13:8. https://doi.org/10.2174/1573402113666170413094319.
66. Cunha PG, Cotter J, Oliveira P, Vila I, Boutouyrie P, Laurent S, Nilsson P, Scuteri A, Sousa N. Pulse wave velocity distribution in a cohort study–From arterial stiffness to early vascular ageing (EVA). J Hypertens. 2015;33:1438–45.
67. Nilsson P, Boutouyrie P, Cunha P, Kotsis V, Narkiewicz K, Parati G, Rietzschel E, Scuteri A, Laurent S. Early vascular ageing (EVA) in translation—from laboratory investigations to clinical applications in cardiovascular prevention. J Hypertens. 2013;31:1517–26.
68. Nilsson P, Boutouyrie P, Laurent S. Vascular aging: a tale of EVA and ADAM in cardiovascular risk assessment and prevention. Hypertension. 2009;54:3–10.
69. Zethelius B, Berglund L, Sundström J, Ingelsson E, Basu S, Larsson A, Venge P, Arnlöv J. Use of multiple biomarkers to improve the prediction of death from cardiovascular causes. N Engl J Med. 2008;358:2107–716.
70. Sehestedt T, Jeppesen J, Hansen TW, Rasmussen S, Wachtell K, Ibsen H, Torp-Pedersen C, Olsen MH. Thresholds for pulse wave velocity, urine albumin creatinine ratio and left ventricular mass index using SCORE, Framingham and ESH/ESC risk charts. J Hypertens. 2012;30(10):1928–36.
71. Sehestedt T, Jeppesen J, Hansen TW, Wachtell K, Ibsen H, Torp-Pedersen C, Hildebrandt P, Olsen MH. Risk prediction is improved by adding markers of subclinical organ damage to SCORE. Eur Heart J. 2010;31(7):883–91.
72. Wang TJ. Assessing the role of circulating, genetic, and imaging biomarkers in cardiovascular risk prediction. Circulation. 2011;123:551–65.
73. Olsen M, Angell S, Asma S, Boutouyrie P, Burger D, Chirinos J, et al. A call to action and a life-course strategy to address the global burden of raised blood pressure on current and future generations. The Lancet Commission on Hypertension. Lancet. 2016;388:2665–712.
74. Safar ME, Thomas F, Blacher J, Nzietchueng R, Bureau JM, Pannier B, Benetos A. Metabolic syndrome and age-related progression of aortic stiffness. J Am Coll Cardiol. 2006;47(1):72–5.
75. Scuteri A, Cunha PG, Rosei EA, Badariere J, Bekaert S, Cockcroft JR, Cotter J, Cucca F, De Buyzere ML, De Meyer T, Ferrucci L, Franco O, Gale N, Gillebert TC, Hofman A, Langlois M, Laucevicius A, Laurent S, Matta Ceraso FU, Morrell CH, Muiesan ML, Munnery MM, Navickas R, Oliveira P, Orru' M, Pilia MG, Rietzschel ER, Ryliskyte L, Salvetti M, Schlessinger D, Sousa N, Stefanadis C, Strait J, Van daele C, Villa I, Vlachopoulos C, Witteman

J, Xaplanteris P, Nilsson P, Lakatta EG, MARE Consortium. Arterial stiffness and influences of the metabolic syndrome: a cross-countries study. Atherosclerosis. 2014;233:654–60.
76. Scuteri A, Najjar SS, Muller DC, Andres R, Hougaku H, Metter EJ, Lakatta EG. Metabolic syndrome amplifies the age-associated increases in vascular thickness and stiffness. J Am Coll Cardiol. 2004;43:1388–95.
77. Smulyan H, Lieber A, Safar ME. Hypertension, diabetes type II, and their association: role of arterial stiffness. Am J Hypertens. 2016;29:5–13.
78. Lurbe E, Agabiti-Rosei E, Cruickshank JK, Dominiczak A, Erdine S, Hirth A, Invitti C, Litwin M, Mancia G, Pall D, Rascher W, Redon J, Schaefer F, Seeman T, Sinha M, Stabouli S, Webb NJ, Wühl E, Zanchetti A. 2016 European Society of Hypertension guidelines for the management of high blood pressure in children and adolescents. J Hypertens. 2016a;34:1887–920.
79. Lurbe E, Torro MI, Alvarez-Pitti J, Redon P, Redon J. Central blood pressure and pulse wave amplification across the spectrum of peripheral blood pressure in overweight and obese youth. J Hypertens. 2016b;34:1389–95.
80. Su S, Wang X, Kapuku GK, Treiber FA, Pollock DM, Harshfield GA, McCall WV, Pollock JS. Adverse childhood experiences are associated with detrimental hemodynamics and elevated circulating endothelin-1 in adolescents and young adults. Hypertension. 2014;64:201–7.
81. Chu C, Dai Y, Mu J, Yang R, Wang M, Yang J, Ren Y, Xie B, Dong Z, Yang F, Wang D, Yan D, Guo TS, Wang Y. Associations of risk factors in childhood with arterial stiffness 26 years later: the Hanzhong adolescent hypertension cohort. J Hypertens. 2017;35(Suppl 1):S10–S5.
82. Ferreira I, van de Laar RJ, Prins MH, Twisk JW, Stehouwer CD. Carotid stiffness in young adults: a life-course analysis of its early determinants: the Amsterdam Growth and Health Longitudinal Study. Hypertension. 2012;59:54–61.
83. Juonala M, Jarvisalo MJ, Maki-Torkko N, Kahonen M, Viikari JS, Raitakari OT. Risk factors identified in childhood and decreased carotid artery elasticity in adulthood: the Cardiovascular Risk in Young Finns Study. Circulation. 2005;112(10):1486–93.
84. Li S, Chen W, Srinivasan SR, Berenson GS. Childhood blood pressure as a predictor of arterial stiffness in young adults: the Bogalusa heart study. Hypertension. 2004;43(3):541–6.
85. Bao W, Threefoot SA, Srinivasan SR, Berenson GS. Essential hypertension predicted by tracking of elevated blood pressure from childhood to adulthood: the Bogalusa Heart Study. Am J Hypertens. 1995;8(7):657–65.
86. Srinivasan SR, Myers L, Berenson GS. Changes in metabolic syndrome variables since childhood in prehypertensive and hypertensive subjects: the Bogalusa Heart Study. Hypertension. 2006;48(1):33–9.
87. Magnussen CG, Venn A, Thomson R, Juonala M, Srinivasan SR, Viikari JS, Berenson GS, Dwyer T, Raitakari OT. The association of pediatric low- and high-density lipoprotein cholesterol dyslipidemia classifications and change in dyslipidemia status with carotid intima-media thickness in adulthood evidence from the cardiovascular risk in Young Finns study, the Bogalusa Heart study, and the CDAH (Childhood Determinants of Adult Health) study. J Am Coll Cardiol. 2009;53(10):860–9.
88. Magnussen CG, Koskinen J, Chen W, Thomson R, Schmidt MD, Srinivasan SR, Kivimaki M, Mattsson N, Kahonen M, Laitinen T, Taittonen L, Ronnemaa T, Viikari JS, Berenson GS, Juonala M, Raitakari OT. Pediatric metabolic syndrome predicts adulthood metabolic syndrome, subclinical atherosclerosis, and type 2 diabetes mellitus but is no better than body mass index alone: the Bogalusa Heart Study and the Cardiovascular Risk in Young Finns Study. Circulation. 2010;122(16):1604–11.
89. Koskinen J, Magnussen CG, Sabin MA, Kahonen M, Hutri-Kahonen N, Laitinen T, Taittonen L, Jokinen E, Lehtimaki T, Viikari JS, Raitakari OT, Juonala M. Youth overweight and metabolic disturbances in predicting carotid intima-media thickness, type 2 diabetes, and metabolic syndrome in adulthood: the Cardiovascular Risk in Young Finns Study. Diabetes Care. 2014;37(7):1870–7.
90. Juonala M, Magnussen CG, Venn A, Dwyer T, Burns TL, Davis PH, Chen W, Srinivasan SR, Daniels SR, Kahonen M, Laitinen T, Taittonen L, Berenson GS, Viikari JS, Raitakari OT. Influence of age on associations between childhood risk factors and carotid intima-media

thickness in adulthood: the Cardiovascular Risk in Young Finns Study, the Childhood Determinants of Adult Health Study, the Bogalusa Heart Study, and the Muscatine Study for the International Childhood Cardiovascular Cohort (i3C) Consortium. Circulation. 2010;122(24):2514–20.

91. Lamotte C, Iliescu C, Libersa C, Gottrand F. Increased intima-media thickness of the carotid artery in childhood: a systematic review of observational studies. Eur J Pediatr. 2011;170(6):719–29.
92. Berry JD, Dyer A, Cai X, Garside DB, Ning H, Thomas A, Greenland P, Van Horn L, Tracy RP, Lloyd-Jones DM. Lifetime risks of cardiovascular disease. N Engl J Med. 2012;366(4):321–9.
93. Lloyd-Jones DM, Hong Y, Labarthe D, Mozaffarian D, Appel LJ, Van Horn L, Greenlund K, Daniels S, Nichol G, Tomaselli GF, Arnett DK, Fonarow GC, Ho PM, Lauer MS, Masoudi FA, Robertson RM, Roger V, Schwamm LH, Sorlie P, Yancy CW, Rosamond WD. Defining and setting national goals for cardiovascular health promotion and disease reduction: the American Heart Association's strategic impact goal through 2020 and beyond. Circulation. 2010;121(4):586–613.
94. Chen W, Srinivasan SR, Berenson GS. Amplification of the association between birthweight and blood pressure with age: the Bogalusa Heart Study. J Hypertens. 2010;28(10):2046–52.
95. Gamborg M, Byberg L, Rasmussen F, Andersen PK, Baker JL, Bengtsson C, Canoy D, Droyvold W, Eriksson JG, Forsen T, Gunnarsdottir I, Jarvelin MR, Koupil I, Lapidus L, Nilsen TI, Olsen SF, Schack-Nielsen L, Thorsdottir I, Tuomainen TP, Sorensen TI. Birth weight and systolic blood pressure in adolescence and adulthood: meta-regression analysis of sex- and age-specific results from 20 Nordic studies. Am J Epidemiol. 2007;166(6):634–45.
96. Aatola H, Hutri-Kahonen N, Juonala M, Viikari JS, Hulkkonen J, Laitinen T, Taittonen L, Lehtimaki T, Raitakari OT, Kahonen M. Lifetime risk factors and arterial pulse wave velocity in adulthood: the Cardiovascular Risk in Young Finns Study. Hypertension. 2010;55(3):806–11.
97. Koskinen J, Magnussen CG, Taittonen L, Rasanen L, Mikkila V, Laitinen T, Ronnemaa T, Kahonen M, Viikari JS, Raitakari OT, Juonala M. Arterial structure and function after recovery from the metabolic syndrome: the cardiovascular risk in Young Finns Study. Circulation. 2010;121(3):392–400.
98. Juonala M, Magnussen CG, Berenson GS, Venn A, Burns TL, Sabin MA, Srinivasan SR, Daniels SR, Davis PH, Chen W, Sun C, Cheung M, Viikari JS, Dwyer T, Raitakari OT. Childhood adiposity, adult adiposity, and cardiovascular risk factors. N Engl J Med. 2011;365(20):1876–85.
99. Laitinen TT, Pahkala K, Magnussen CG, Viikari JS, Oikonen M, Taittonen L, Mikkila V, Jokinen E, Hutri-Kahonen N, Laitinen T, Kahonen M, Lehtimaki T, Raitakari OT, Juonala M. Ideal cardiovascular health in childhood and cardiometabolic outcomes in adulthood: the Cardiovascular Risk in Young Finns Study. Circulation. 2012;125(16):1971–8.
100. Magnussen CG, Koskinen J, Juonala M, Chen W, Srinivasan SR, Sabin MA, Thomson R, Schmidt MD, Nguyen QM, Xu JH, Skilton MR, Kahonen M, Laitinen T, Taittonen L, Lehtimaki T, Ronnemaa T, Viikari JS, Berenson GS, Raitakari OT. A diagnosis of the metabolic syndrome in youth that resolves by adult life is associated with a normalization of high carotid intima-media thickness and type 2 diabetes mellitus risk: the Bogalusa heart and cardiovascular risk in young Finns studies. J Am Coll Cardiol. 2012;60(17):1631–9.
101. Oikonen M, Laitinen TT, Magnussen CG, Steinberger J, Sinaiko AR, Dwyer T, Venn A, Smith KJ, Hutri-Kahonen N, Pahkala K, Mikkila V, Prineas R, Viikari JS, Morrison JA, Woo JG, Chen W, Nicklas T, Srinivasan SR, Berenson G, Juonala M, Raitakari OT. Ideal cardiovascular health in young adult populations from the United States, Finland, and Australia and its association with cIMT: the International Childhood Cardiovascular Cohort Consortium. J Am Heart Assoc. 2013;2(3):e000244.
102. Aatola H, Hutri-Kahonen N, Juonala M, Laitinen TT, Pahkala K, Mikkila V, Telama R, Koivistoinen T, Lehtimaki T, Viikari JS, Raitakari OT, Kahonen M. Prospective relationship of change in ideal cardiovascular health status and arterial stiffness: the Cardiovascular Risk in Young Finns Study. J Am Heart Assoc. 2014;3(2):e000532.

103. Kelly RK, Thomson R, Smith KJ, Dwyer T, Venn A, Magnussen CG. Factors affecting tracking of blood pressure from childhood to adulthood: the childhood determinants of adult health study. J Pediatr. 2015;167(6):1422–8. e2
104. Couch SC, Saelens BE, Levin L, Dart K, Falciglia G, Daniels SR. The efficacy of a clinic-based behavioral nutrition intervention emphasizing a DASH-type diet for adolescents with elevated blood pressure. J Pediatr. 2008;152:494–501.
105. Leary SDNA, Smith GD, Mattocks C, Deere K, Blair SN, Riddoch C. Physical activity and blood pressure in childhood. Findings from a population-based study. Hypertension. 2008;51:92–8.
106. Koivistoinen T, Hutri-Kähönen N, Juonala M, Aatola H, Kööbi T, Lehtimäki T, Viikari JS, Raitakari OT, Kähönen M. Metabolic syndrome in childhood and increased arterial stiffness in adulthood: the Cardiovascular Risk in Young Finns Study. Ann Med. 2011;43:312–9.
107. Aatola H, Koivistoinen T, Tuominen H, Juonala M, Lehtimäki T, Viikari JSA, Raitakari OT, Kähönen M, Hutri-Kähönen N. Influence of child and adult elevated blood pressure on adult arterial stiffness: the Cardiovascular Risk in Young Finns Study. Hypertension. 2017;70:531–6.
108. Pälve KS, Pahkala K, Magnussen CG, Koivistoinen T, Juonala M, Kähönen M, Lehtimäki T, Rönnemaa T, Viikari JS, Raitakari OT. Association of physical activity in childhood and early adulthood with carotid artery elasticity 21 years later: the cardiovascular risk in Young Finns Study. J Am Heart Assoc. 2014;3:e000594.

9 Central Blood Pressure and Prehypertension

Charalambos Vlachopoulos, Dimitrios Terentes-Printzios, and Dimitrios Tousoulis

9.1 Prehypertension

Measurement of blood pressure (BP) is one of the most important and powerful clinical tools in clinical practice. The classical method that was introduced more than 100 years ago with the emergence of the brachial cuff sphygmomanometer is still in use by physicians [1]. Sphygmomanometry, despite its initial setbacks, stormed throughout the medical community. This was boosted by the early exploitation of insurance companies and was founded on the ease of use, the availability with the wide variety of devices, the good reproducibility and its predictive role [1].

Once peripheral (brachial) BP were established as the gold-standard method of assessing hypertension and optimal BP status, physicians and relevant societies set cutoff points to communicate the risks of hypertension to patients. Prehypertension was firstly defined in the 2003 Joint National Committee on Prevention, Detection, Evaluation, and Treatment of High Blood Pressure Guidelines as a systolic BP of 120–139 mmHg, diastolic BP of 80–89 mmHg, or both [2]. With a different terminology and range, the European guidelines define high-normal BP as a systolic BP between 130 and 139 mmHg [3].

BP is a principal risk factor for morbidity and mortality. This relationship is potent, continuous, and has been established in a range of age groups and populations. On the other hand, BP is a continuous variable and has a normal distribution. Therefore, definition of "hypertension" in terms of risk prediction is rather arbitrary [4]. While hypertension is prevalent in middle-aged and elderly adults there is an increase in prevalence of prehypertension in younger ages in recent years [4]. Overall,

C. Vlachopoulos (✉) · D. Terentes-Printzios · D. Tousoulis
Hypertension and Cardiometabolic Unit, First Department of Cardiology,
Hippokration Hospital, Medical School, National and Kapodistrian University of Athens,
Athens, Greece
e-mail: cvlachop@otenet.gr

R. Zimlichman et al. (eds.), *Prehypertension and Cardiometabolic Syndrome*,
Updates in Hypertension and Cardiovascular Protection,
https://doi.org/10.1007/978-3-319-75310-2_9

prehypertension has an essential deleterious health impact in all ages. Prehypertension is associated with a twofold increased risk of cardiovascular events [4]. In addition, these prehypertensive subjects are more likely to have hypercholesterolemia, increased body-mass index, and/or diabetes compared to individuals with normal blood [5]. Apart from the risks for cardiovascular disease that prehypertension conveys by itself, it should be stressed that prehypertension is precursor of hypertension [4].

Nonetheless, it should be stressed that the ongoing debate for the ideal target of interventional studies [6] has cast shadow on the true value of the concept of prehypertension since there is a tendency to lower the proposed targets to the prehypertension range. For such reasons, in the latest guidelines for Hypertension Management from the American Heart Association the concept of prehypertension has been challenged [7].

9.2 Central Blood Pressures

Peripheral blood pressure may not always be a reliable surrogate of central blood pressure [8]. An indolent dispute between measurements of peripheral (brachial) and central (aortic, carotid) has resurfaced after the introduction of techniques and devises that can easily and accurately estimate noninvasively the central pressure waveform [9]. Analysis of the central waveform can provide clinically useful information, beyond blood pressure measured in the brachial artery [9, 10]. This additional prognostic ability of central pressures stems from the fact that they are more pathophysiologically relevant to end-organ damages on the brain, heart, and kidneys [9–11].

Pathophysiology: Differences between peripheral and aortic pressures vary and are greater at younger ages (Fig. 9.1). In that case, systolic pressure may be up to 40 mmHg higher in the brachial artery than in the aorta, despite the fact that

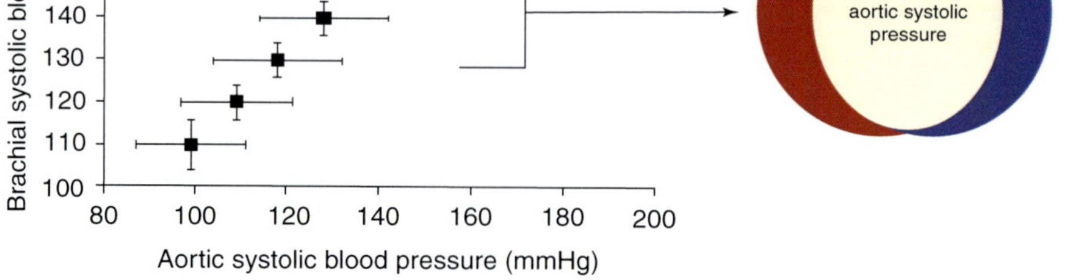

Fig. 9.1 Overlap between categories of aortic (central) and brachial (peripheral) blood pressure categories. Figure adapted from [14]

Table 9.1 Factors determining pressure pulse wave amplification

Factors
Age
Gender
Body size (height)
Heart rate
Blood pressure
Race
Smoking
Dyslipidemia (men only)
Blood glucose

diastolic and mean arterial pressures are rather constant [12]. Among other factors, this is due to the change of the structure of the arterial wall (elastic aorta compared to the stiffer muscular brachial artery) and the resultant increase in arterial stiffness as the pressure wave moves away from the heart. This in turn results in a rapid increase in the systolic pressure, causing an important pulse pressure amplification [12]. Pulse pressure amplification has a large both within- and between-subjects variability that stems from differences in age, gender, race, heart rate, body size and conditions that modify the vascular system and tone (Table 9.1) [13].

Measurement techniques: There are several ways of measurement or estimation of central blood pressure [14]. The most direct classical method is measurement of BP in the ascending aorta using a pressure-sensing catheter during cardiac catheterization. As it is apparent this method is not suitable for screening due to its invasive nature and need for technical expertise and it is used nowadays only for validation of noninvasive devices. In the last two decades numerous noninvasive devices have emerged; pressure waveforms are recorded from sites distal to the aorta, such as the radial, brachial, or carotid arteries, and calibrated to BP measured by cuff sphygmomanometry [9, 14]. Extremely interesting is also the recent development of 24 h measurement of central BP [14]. It remains to be investigated whether the 24 h values have better predictive ability for future events than single measurements of central BPs as already has been shown for 24 h ambulatory peripheral BPs compared to single office blood pressures. As one can expect all these methods have their pros and cons and should be carefully and rigorously validated with a standardized method before entering the market [15].

Prognostic role of central blood pressures: As already mentioned, central pressures are pathophysiologically more relevant than peripheral pressures for the pathogenesis of cardiovascular disease and according to accumulating evidence this results in an essential prognostic role for both cardiovascular and all-cause mortality. A considerable number of studies have examined the ability of central pressures to predict the risk of future fatal and nonfatal cardiovascular events (myocardial infarction, stroke, revascularization, aortic syndromes) and all-cause mortality [10]. Although promising, findings were not consistent in all studies. We meta-analyzed 11 longitudinal studies that estimated central hemodynamics and had followed 5648 subjects for a mean follow-up of 45 months and showed the independent predictive role of central blood pressures and augmentation index to predict future events. When three more recent studies than the respective meta-analysis [13] were included (total 9093 subjects and mean follow-up 54.9 months) the relative risk (RRs) of total cardiovascular events were 1.115 (95% CI 1.029–1.209) for a 10 mmHg-increase of central pulse pressure, and 1.303 (95% CI 1.098–1.546) for a 10%-absolute increase of central augmentation index. Furthermore, a 10%-increase of central augmentation index was associated with a RR of 1.328 (95% CI 1.167–1.511) for all-cause mortality. The important question is whether central pressures have an incremental predictive ability over and beyond peripheral pressures. According to our meta-analysis, central pulse pressure was found to have a marginally better predictive value compared to peripheral pulse pressure ($P = 0.057$). Due to the strong correlation between central and peripheral pressures, large populations are required to provide convincing and meaningful data on the comparison between them. This marginal but existent superiority of central blood pressures was supported by the a recent large individual-data meta-analysis in 22,433 subjects from 15 studies [16], where although the predictive ability for myocardial infarction was similar for central and peripheral systolic BP, there was a statistically significant superiority of central pressure compared to peripheral pressure for the prediction of stroke, especially in subjects below 61 years. However, it must be acknowledged that so far there are no published data of an improved reclassification with the use of central BP with the inclusion of peripheral BP in the model.

In addition to hard-end points, central hemodynamic indices have been shown to be independently associated with end-organ damage and incident cardiovascular disease. The late systolic augmentation of the central pressure waveform is associated with an increase in left ventricular mass index, and carotid systolic blood pressure is an independent predictor of left ventricular wall thickness [17]. Moreover, central pressure is also more closely related to other essential surrogate endpoints, such as vascular hypertrophy, extent of carotid atherosclerosis than brachial pressure [18]. In fact, in a recent meta-analysis, central BP was shown to be slightly, but consistently, superior to the peripheral BP in predicting end-organ damage, such as carotid intima-media thickness, pulse wave velocity, and left ventricular mass index except for albuminuria [19]. The close association of central pressures with intermediate cardiovascular phenotypes is colorfully illustrated in a recent review (Fig. 9.2) [20].

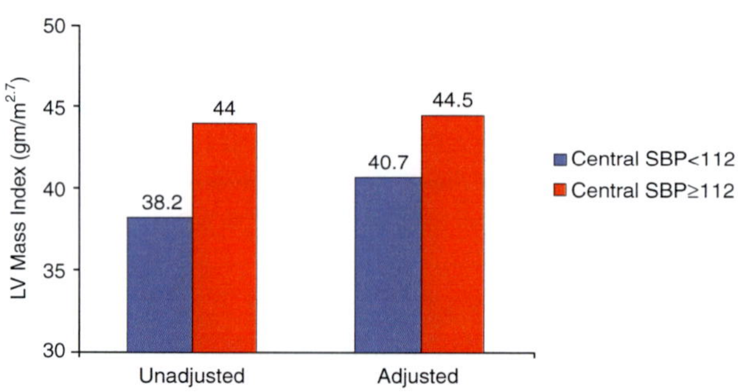

Fig. 9.2 Comparison of left ventricular (LV) mass index in prehypertensives subdivided according to whether central systolic blood pressure (SBP) is <112 or ≥112 mmHg. Figure adapted from [20]

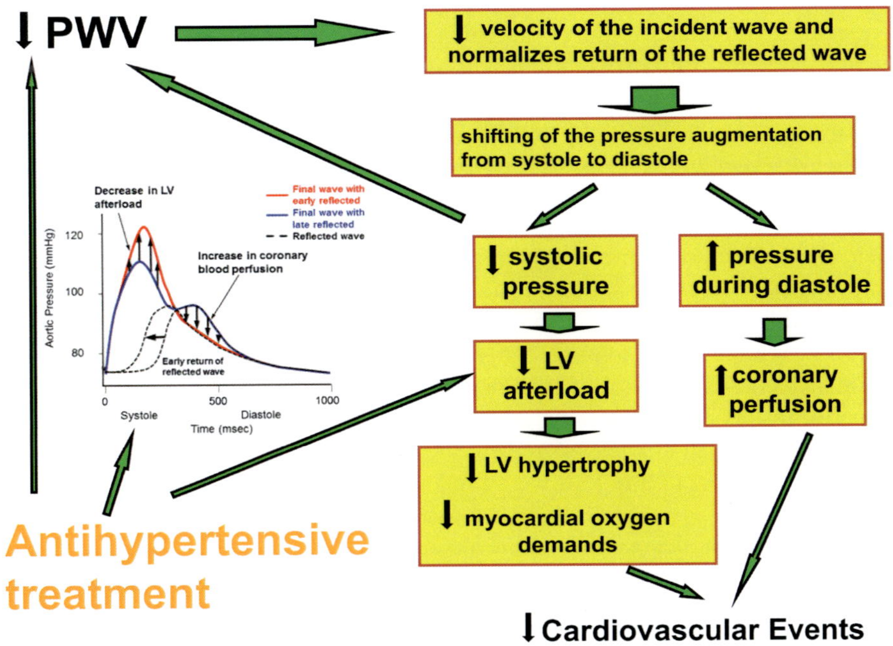

Fig. 9.3 The effects of antihypertensive treatment of wave reflections and aortic stiffness

Modulation of central blood pressures: Despite similar effects on brachial pressure, antihypertensive drugs have differential effects on central pressure and this may explain the advantage of arterial vasodilating drugs in survival studies (Fig. 9.3) [21]. In particular, the relative efficacy of antihypertensive treatment in randomized trials has been principally assessed based on its ability to lower brachial BP. However, due to the essential role of wave reflections, it could be assumed that some classes of antihypertensive regimens with vasodilatory properties could have a greater impact on the reduction of aortic BP that is not apparent in peripheral BP measurements [22]. This discrepancy could translate to different effects both on target-organ damage and future hard endpoints. In the Conduit Artery Function Evaluation (CAFÉ) Study, a substudy of the Anglo-Scandinavian Cardiac Outcomes Trial (ASCOT), a higher treatment-related decrease of central pulse pressure (such a decrease was not evident in brachial pressure measurements) was independently associated with clinical benefit and reduced cardiovascular events [23]. Specifically, central systolic pressure was some 4.3 mmHg lower, and aortic pulse pressure 3.0 mmHg lower in those randomized to the amlodipine–perindopril regimen. Other studies have also shown that endpoints related to organ damage can be predicted by indices of central hemodynamics after therapy. The pREterax in regression of Arterial Stiffness in a contrOlled double-bliNd (REASON) study that compared atenolol against a perindopril–indapamide combination showed that normalization of brachial systolic BP is achieved with a significantly greater reduction of carotid systolic BP after a 12-month treatment with the combination [24]. In this study, compared with atenolol, the perindopril–indapamide combination was associated with a greater fall in left ventricular mass, and this was related to carotid but not brachial blood pressure [25]. Furthermore, the reduction in carotid wall diameter and hypertrophy with antihypertensive treatment is related to carotid pulse pressure but not to mean blood pressure [26]. On the contrary, nebivolol, a beta-blocker with vasodilatory action, apparently reduced central BP compared to placebo in a recent small, randomized, controlled trial with prehypertensive patients [27]. Furthermore, in a randomized study an amlodipine–valsartan combination decreased central (systolic and pulse) pressure and augmentation index more than an amlodipine–atenolol combination, irrespectively of changes in peripheral BP and heart rate [28].

There is a great need to prove the clinical value of central pressures by assigning them as the guiding factor of treatment and testing whether this strategy provides superior results compared to peripheral BP-guided therapy [11]. In this direction, in two recent small studies where central BP in hypertensives [29] and augmentation index in heart failure [30] were used as therapeutic targets there were modest but clinically apparent benefits for the patients. Specifically, in the first case measurement of central pressures led to decrease in the number of antihypertensive medications used, as well as to a marginal improvement in reduction of left ventricular mass; in the second case there was a slight improvement in exercise capacity.

9.3 Prehypertension and Central Pressures

While it has become apparent that prehypertension deserves specific attention, the extrapolation of similar cutoffs to central pressures is neither practical nor documented at this stage. This relates mainly to the variable correspondence between values of peripheral and brachial pressures and to the nonsolid substantiation of the predictive role of central pressures in prehypertensive subjects. More specifically, due to the inherent variability of predictors of pulse pressure amplification, a single model cannot accurately predict this amplification by measurements of pressure in the brachial level. This was elucidated in a large cohort [31] that demonstrated a significant, and highly variable, difference between central and brachial systolic pressure at all ages, as well as a substantial overlap in aortic systolic pressure between different groups of blood pressure. More than 70% of individuals in the "high-normal" brachial systolic pressure had similar central pressures to those with stage 1 hypertension, despite no overlap in brachial pressures (Fig. 9.1). Moreover, approximately 30% of males, and 10% of females, with "normal" brachial BP had similar central pressures to those categorized as having stage 1 hypertension. However, an important clinical assistance was provided by the recent publication of reference values for central BP that will shed more light in the management of hypertension and the stratification of risk [32].

Regarding the second prerequisite, i.e., the predictive role of central blood pressures in prehypertension, this is difficult to substantiate. It should be noted that there are small cross-sectional studies suggesting an early detrimental role of prehypertension on central pressures and markers of arterial function and structure [33–36], as well on other surrogate markers of CVD, such as coronary artery calcification [37]. However, regarding the predictive ability of central pressures in terms of clinical endpoints, there are no such dedicated prospective studies. Nevertheless, such a possible prognostic ability could be extrapolated by relevant studies on the general population and also by the close association of central BPs with other vascular biomarkers that have been shown to be predictive in prehypertensives [11]. Furthermore, scarce data imply an incremental role of central BP over and beyond peripheral BP for the detection of target-organ damage that is stronger in patients with prehypertension [38, 39].

Research on the importance of central pressures in the context of hypertension should be encouraged. The notion that BP targets should be individualized based on assessment of cardiovascular risk [6] has gained significant ground. Central BPs could theoretically be an appealing such tool for individualization of treatment [29, 40].

Conclusions

Assessment of central blood pressures makes its way from the research field to the clinical field. There are still answers that remain to be answered concerning the incremental predictive ability of central blood pressures over peripheral blood pressures, as well as the possible role of the central BP-guided therapy in everyday practice. Prehypertensive subjects lack guidance from randomized studies and their management is based on data from hypertensive patients or from the general population. Therefore, prehypertension could be a breeding ground for central pressures in order to improve our understanding, as well as the management of this population. Although the predictive ability of central pressures for clinical endpoints in the context of hypertension is not currently substantiated, medium-sized studies have shown a small advantage of central pressures compared to peripheral blood pressures at least as far as intermediate endpoints are concerned. Further advancements in central blood pressure technology and acquisition will lead to more widespread use of the new standardized devices for assessment of central blood pressures that will result in lower cost and higher availability. The idea of central pressures at one day replacing peripheral pressures may sound rude and absurd but is not impossible if certain demands are met. As Albert Einstein once said "If at first the idea is not absurd, then there is no hope for it."

References

1. O'Brien E, Fitzgerald D. The history of blood pressure measurement. J Hum Hypertens. 1994;8:73–84.
2. Chobanian AV, Bakris GL, Black HR, Cushman WC, Green LA, Izzo JL Jr, et al. JAMA. 2003;289:2560–72.

3. Mancia G, Fagard R, Narkiewicz K, Redon J, Zanchetti A, Böhm M, et al. 2013 ESH/ESC guidelines for the management of arterial hypertension: the Task Force for the Management of Arterial Hypertension of the European Society of Hypertension (ESH) and of the European Society of Cardiology (ESC). Eur Heart J. 2013;34:2159–219. https://doi.org/10.1093/eurheartj/eht151.
4. Egan BM, Stevens-Fabry S. Prehypertension—prevalence, health risks, and management strategies. Nat Rev Cardiol. 2015;12:289–300. https://doi.org/10.1038/nrcardio.2015.
5. Roger VL, Go AS, Lloyd-Jones DM, Adams RJ, Berry JD, Brown TM, et al. Heart disease and stroke statistics—2011 update: a report from the American Heart Association. Circulation. 2011;123:e18–e209. https://doi.org/10.1161/CIR.0b013e3182009701. Erratum in: Circulation. 2011;124:e426. Circulation 2011;123:e240
6. SPRINT Research Group, Wright JT Jr, Williamson JD, Whelton PK, Snyder JK, Sink KM, et al. A randomized trial of intensive versus standard blood-pressure control. N Engl J Med. 2015;373:2103–16.
7. Whelton PK, Carey RM, Aronow WS, Casey DE Jr, Collins KJ, Dennison Himmelfarb C, et al. ACC/AHA/AAPA/ABC/ACPM/AGS/APhA/ASH/ASPC/NMA/PCNA Guideline for the Prevention, Detection, Evaluation, and Management of High Blood Pressure in Adults: A Report of the American College of Cardiology/American Heart Association Task Force on Clinical Practice Guidelines. J Am Coll Cardiol. 2017. https://doi.org/10.1016/j.jacc.2017.11.006.
8. Picone DS, Schultz MG, Otahal P, Aakhus S, Al-Jumaily AM, Black JA, et al. Accuracy of cuff-measured blood pressure: systematic reviews and meta-analyses. J Am Coll Cardiol. 2017;70:572–86.
9. O'Rourke MF. Central aortic pressure: alive and well at 25 years. J Hypertens. 2015;33:187–8.
10. Vlachopoulos C, Aznaouridis K, O'Rourke MF, Safar ME, Baou K, Stefanadis C. Prediction of cardiovascular events and all-cause mortality with central haemodynamics: a systematic review and meta-analysis. Eur Heart J. 2010;31:1865–71.
11. Vlachopoulos C, Xaplanteris P, Aboyans V, Brodmann M, Cífková R, Cosentino F, et al. The role of vascular biomarkers for primary and secondary prevention. A position paper from the European Society of Cardiology Working Group on peripheral circulation: endorsed by the Association for Research into Arterial Structure and Physiology (ARTERY) Society. Atherosclerosis. 2015;241:507–32.
12. Vlachopoulos C, O'Rourke M. Genesis of the normal and abnormal arterial pulse. Curr Probl Cardiol. 2000;25:303–67.
13. Nichols WW, O'Rourke MF, Vlachopoulos C. McDonald's blood flow in arteries: theoretic, experimental, and clinical principles. 6th ed. London: CRC Press; 2011.
14. McEniery CM, Cockcroft JR, Roman MJ, Franklin SS, Wilkinson IB. Central blood pressure: current evidence and clinical importance. Eur Heart J. 2014;35:1719–25.
15. Sharman JE, Avolio AP, Baulmann J, Benetos A, Blacher J, Blizzard CL, et al. Validation of non-invasive central blood pressure devices: ARTERY Society task force consensus statement on protocol standardization. Eur Heart J. 2017a;38:2805–12. https://doi.org/10.1093/eurheartj/ehw632.
16. McEniery CM. Central blood pressure and cardiovascular risk: an individual participant meta-analysis of prospective observational data from 22,433 subjects. JACC. 2015;65(Suppl 10):A1464.
17. Roman MJ, Ganau A, Saba PS, Pini R, Pickering T, Deveraux R. Impact of arterial stiffening on left ventricular structure. Hypertension. 2000;36:489–94.
18. Roman MJ, Devereux RB, Kizer JR, Lee ET, Galloway JM, Ali T, et al. Central pressure more strongly relates to vascular disease and outcome than does brachial pressure: the Strong Heart Study. Hypertension. 2007;50:197–203.
19. Kollias A, Lagou S, Zeniodi ME, Boubouchairopoulou N, Stergiou GS. Association of central versus brachial blood pressure with target-organ damage: systematic review and meta-analysis. Hypertension. 2016;67:183–90.

20. Roman MJ, Devereux RB. Association of central and peripheral blood pressures with intermediate cardiovascular phenotypes. Hypertension. 2014;63:1148–53.
21. Agabiti-Rosei E, Mancia G, O'Rourke MF, Roman MJ, Safar ME, Smulyan H, et al. Central blood pressure measurements and antihypertensive therapy: a consensus document. Hypertension. 2007;50:154–60.
22. Pucci G, Ranalli MG, Battista F, Schillaci G. Effects of β-blockers with and without vasodilating properties on central blood pressure: systematic review and meta-analysis of randomized trials in hypertension. Hypertension. 2016;67:316–24.
23. Williams B, Lacy PS, Thom SM, Cruickshank K, Stanton A, Collier D, et al. Differential impact of blood pressure-lowering drugs on central aortic pressure and clinical outcomes: principal results of the Conduit Artery Function Evaluation (CAFE) study. Circulation. 2006;113:1213–25.
24. London GM, Asmar RG, O'Rourke MF, Safar ME, on behalf of the REASON Project Investigators. Mechanism(s) of selective systolic blood pressure reduction after a low-dose combination of perindopril/indapamide in hypertensive subjects: comparison with atenolol. J Am Coll Cardiol. 2004;43:92–9.
25. de Luca N, Asmar RG, London GM, O'Rourke MF, Safar ME, REASON Project Investigators. Selective reduction of cardiac mass and central blood pressure on low-dose combination perindopril/indapamide in hypertensive subjects. J Hypertens. 2004;22:1623–30.
26. Boutouyrie P, Bussy C, Hayoz D, Hengstler J, Dartois N, Laloux B, et al. Local pulse pressure and regression of arterial wall hypertrophy during long-term antihypertensive treatment. Circulation. 2000;101:2601–6.
27. Davis JT, Pasha DN, Khandrika S, Fung MM, Milic M, O'Connor DT. Central hemodynamics in prehypertension: effect of the β-adrenergic antagonist nebivolol. J Clin Hypertens (Greenwich). 2013;15:69–74.
28. Boutouyrie P, Achouba A, Trunet P, Laurent S, EXPLOR Trialist Group. Amlodipine-valsartan combination decreases central systolic blood pressure more effectively than the amlodipine-atenolol combination: the EXPLOR study. Hypertension. 2010;55:1314–22.
29. Sharman JE, Marwick TH, Gilroy D, Otahal P, Abhayaratna WP, Stowasser M. Value of Central Blood Pressure for GUIDing ManagEment of Hypertension Study Investigators Randomized trial of guiding hypertension management using central aortic blood pressure compared with best-practice care: principal findings of the BP GUIDE study. Hypertension. 2013;62:1138–45.
30. Borlaug BA, Olson TP, Abdelmoneim Mohamed S, Melenovsky V, Sorrell VL, Noonan K, et al. A randomized pilot study of aortic waveform guided therapy in chronic heart failure. J Am Heart Assoc. 2014;3:e000745.
31. McEniery CM, Yasmin MDB, Munnery M, Wallace SM, Rowe CV, et al. Central pressure: variability and impact of cardiovascular risk factors: the Anglo-Cardiff Collaborative Trial II. Hypertension. 2008;51:1476–82.
32. Herbert A, Cruickshank JK, Laurent S, Boutouyrie P, Reference Values for Arterial Measurements Collaboration. Establishing reference values for central blood pressure and its amplification in a general healthy population and according to cardiovascular risk factors. Eur Heart J. 2014;35:3122–33.
33. Drukteinis JS, Roman MJ, Fabsitz RR, Lee ET, Best LG, Russell M, et al. Cardiac and systemic hemodynamic characteristics of hypertension and prehypertension in adolescents and young adults: the Strong Heart Study. Circulation. 2007;115:221–7.
34. Gedikli O, Kiris A, Ozturk S, Baltaci D, Karaman K, Durmus I, et al. Effects of prehypertension on arterial stiffness and wave reflections. Clin Exp Hypertens. 2010;32:84–9.
35. Tomiyama H, Yamashina A. Arterial stiffness in prehypertension: a possible vicious cycle. J Cardiovasc Transl Res. 2012;5:280–6.
36. Urbina EM, Khoury PR, McCoy C, Daniels SR, Kimball TR, Dolan LM. Cardiac and vascular consequences of pre-hypertension in youth. J Clin Hypertens (Greenwich). 2011;13:332–42.

37. Lehmann N, Erbel R, Mahabadi AA, Kälsch H, Möhlenkamp S, Moebus S, et al. Accelerated progression of coronary artery calcification in hypertension but also prehypertension. J Hypertens. 2016;34:2233–42.
38. Booysen HL, Norton GR, Maseko MJ, Libhaber CD, Majane OH, Sareli P, et al. Aortic, but not brachial blood pressure category enhances the ability to identify target organ changes in normotensives. J Hypertens. 2013;31:1124–30.
39. Hodson B, Norton GR, Ballim I, Libhaber CD, Sareli P, Woodiwiss AJ. Impact of aortic rather than brachial pulsatile haemodynamics on variations in end-organ measures across the full adult blood pressure range. J Hypertens. 2017;35(12):2443–53.
40. Sharman JE, Stanton T, Reid CM, Keech A, Roberts-Thomson P, Stewart S, et al. Targeted LOWering of central blood pressure in patients with hypertension: baseline recruitment, rationale and design of a randomized controlled trial (The LOW CBP study). Contemp Clin Trials. 2017b;62:37–42.

Diurnal and Pulsatile Hemodynamics in Individuals with Prehypertension

10

Thomas Weber, Siegfried Wassertheurer, Bernhard Hametner, Brigitte Kupka, and Kai Mortensen

10.1 Introduction: The Concept of Prehypertension and Out-of-Office Blood Pressure

Prehypertension as a blood pressure (BP) category was introduced in the 7th US Joint National Committee (JNC 7) report on prevention, detection, evaluation, and treatment of high blood pressure [1]. The decision was based on the continuous relationship between BP levels and the risk of cardiovascular events, which starts well below 140/90 mmHg (the usual definition of hypertension). In particular, the incidence of cardiovascular events in individuals with BP levels in the prehypertensive range (120–139/80–89 mmHg) is in between those with optimal BP (<120/80 mmHg) and those with hypertension (>140/90 mmHg) [2]. This categorization is undoubtedly true for population-based studies, and may be useful for early detection of individuals at risk for developing hypertension in order to promote lifestyle changes to reduce this risk. However, a closer look at the JNC 7 report reveals that the BP classification proposed was based on office BP measurements only. It is well known that out-of-office BP monitoring (24 h ambulatory BP monitoring—ABPM and home BP monitoring—HBPM) provides a more reliable assessment of an individual's BP level, as compared to office BP [3]. For instance, BP measured at the doctor's office may be higher than out-of-office BP (white-coat effect), which may lead to different BP classifications for office and

T. Weber (✉)
Cardiology Department, Klinikum Wels-Grieskirchen, Wels, Austria
e-mail: thomas.weber3@liwest.at

S. Wassertheurer · B. Hametner · B. Kupka
Department of Health and Environment, Austrian Institute of Technology, Vienna, Austria

K. Mortensen
University of Lübeck, Lübeck, Germany

R. Zimlichman et al. (eds.), *Prehypertension and Cardiometabolic Syndrome*, Updates in Hypertension and Cardiovascular Protection,
https://doi.org/10.1007/978-3-319-75310-2_10

out-of-office measurements in one single individual ("white-coat hypertension"). On the other hand, office BP may be also lower than out-of-office BP, which could also lead to problems with classification in single individuals. This effect is called "masked hypertension," if office BP is normal and out-of-office BP is elevated. The percentage of individuals with masked hypertension is low with office-based optimal BP, but can be substantial in individuals with office-based prehypertension [4]. As cardiovascular risk is related more closely to out-of-office BP, as compared to office BP [3], a closer look at diurnal BP profiles (i.e., out-of-office BP) in office-based prehypertension is warranted. In a recent study, 83.8% of participants with masked hypertension had prehypertension, and 34.1% of participants with prehypertension had masked hypertension, suggesting substantial overlap between both categories [5].

10.2 Pulsatile Hemodynamics: Basic Principles

Due to the nature of the pump in the human circulation (the heart), pressure and flow is pulsatile, rather than continuous, in large and small arteries. Up to the last decade of the twentieth century, the focus in blood pressure research and treatment was mean and diastolic BP, and hemodynamics of the circulation were described as "cardiac output = mean BP/peripheral resistance." This simplistic approach is valid only for steady-state conditions, and fails to take the mechanical properties of the arteries ("arterial stiffness") into account. To characterize pulsatile phenomena, other measures are needed. The simplest one is **pulse pressure (PP)**, the difference between systolic and diastolic BP. PP is a convenient but crude measurement of pulsatile hemodynamics. PP increases with age and with stiffening of the aorta and the large arteries. PP is more closely related to cardiovascular risk in middle-aged and elderly individuals than other blood pressure components [6], and can be used to identify patients with heart failure with preserved ejection fraction [7]. Brachial pulse pressure > 60 mmHg is a hallmark of asymptomatic organ damage in the elderly, according to the 2013 European Society of Hypertension (ESH)/European Society of Cardiology (ESC) guidelines for the management of arterial hypertension [3]. PP, assessed at the brachial artery, has several limitations: it depends not only on arterial (PP increases with increased arterial stiffness) but also on cardiac function (PP decreases with severely impaired systolic function), which leads to an inverse relationship with outcomes in patients with severely impaired systolic function [8]; PP measured at the brachial artery does not exactly match PP assessed at the ascending aorta (central PP), with brachial PP being higher ("amplified") than aortic PP. The difference or ratio ("pulse pressure amplification—PPA") [9] between central and brachial PP depends among other factors on aortic stiffness, cardiac function, heart rate, and arterial geometry.

In general, measurements of pulsatile hemodynamics can be divided into central (aortic) pressures (central systolic BP—cSBP, central PP—cPP), estimates of wave reflections, and measures of arterial stiffness. **CSBP** and **cPP** are lower than their brachial counterparts, whereas mean BP and diastolic BP decrease by only

1–2 mmHg from the aorta to peripheral arteries. CSBP and cPP are the pressures relevant to vital organs like the heart, brain, and kidney, and have been closer associated with cardiovascular outcomes in some, but not all, studies [10]. Pressure and flow waves are generated with each heartbeat and are propagated towards the periphery where they are reflected backwards (towards the heart) for various reasons (stiffness gradient, presence of bifurcations, abrupt diameter gradient in arterioles). On their return, the reflected waves merge with the antegrade wave and amplify it [11]. With aging, the arrival of reflected waves in the ascending aorta is shifted into systole due to earlier wave return. With vasoconstriction, the amplitude of the reflected pressure waves increases. As a net result of both these processes, cardiac load and oxygen consumption is increased, resulting in an imbalance towards myocardial ischemia and an impairment of (mainly diastolic) left ventricular function [11]. **Wave reflection** can be quantified from pressure waveforms (Pulse Waveform Analysis—PWA), or from simultaneous analysis of pressure and flow waves (Wave Separation Analysis—WSA)—Fig. 10.1. With PWA, an inflection point is identified mathematically on the pressure waveform, which is thought to represent the beginning of the arrival of reflected waves at the ascending aorta. The pressure rise from the inflection point to the systolic peak of the pressure curve is called "**Pressure Augmentation—AP**," and the ratio AP/cPP is called "**Augmentation Index—AIx**"). Using WSA, the amplitudes of the **forward wave** (**Pf**; the pressure wave generated by the heart) and the

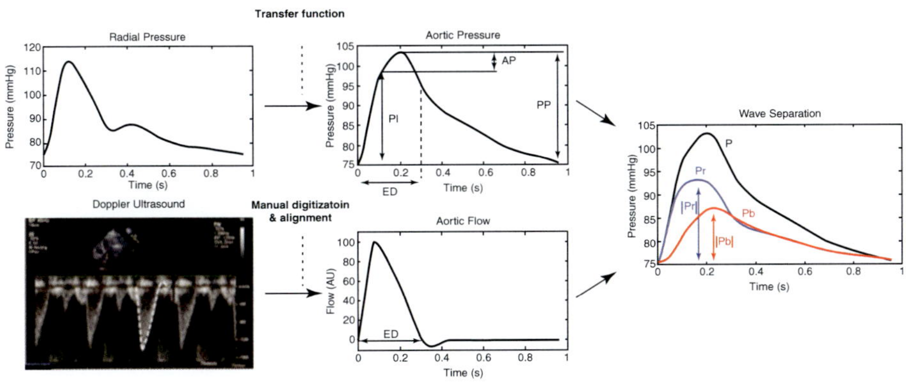

Fig. 10.1 Quantification of wave reflections. Upper panel: A peripheral pressure waveform (here: radial waveform) is obtained. Using a generalized transfer function, the corresponding central pressure waveform is calculated. Pulse waveform analysis (PWA) provides the inflection point; the part of the curve following the inflection point is ascribed to the effects of wave reflection on central pressure and quantified as AP = Augmented Pressure; the ratio AP/PP is called Augmentation Index = AIx); Lower panel: Doppler flow curves are obtained at the left ventricular outflow tract (using the ARCSolver algorithms, they also can be estimated from pressure waves); they are digitized and aligned with the pressure curves; Right figure: Wave Separation Analysis (WSA) using simultaneous analysis of pressure and flow curves yields the amplitudes of the forward (Pf) and the backward (= reflected; Pb) pressure waves. Reproduced with slight modifications with permission of IOP Publishing from Parragh et al., Non-invasive wave reflection quantification in patients with reduced ejection fraction. Physiol Meas 2015;36:179–90

backward wave (**Pb**; the reflected wave) can be calculated, as well as their ratio (**Reflection Magnitude RM**; Pb/Pf). **Arterial stiffness** (particularly **aortic stiffness**) can be measured in vivo, because the speed of propagation of pulse (pressure or flow or distension) waves in an artery is directly related to the mechanical properties of the vessel (the stiffer the vessel, the higher the velocity). Therefore, one has to measure the time delay between the arrival of a pulse wave at two locations (commonly the carotid artery and the femoral artery), and distance between both locations, to calculate the **pulse wave velocity (PWV)** as the most robust measure of arterial stiffness. As the effects of the aging process (i.e., loss of elasticity, increased stiffening) are most pronounced in the human aorta as opposed to the muscular arteries [12], the aortic pathway should be included in the measurement. In addition, the prognostic value is largely limited to pathways including the aorta [13], such as carotid-femoral PWV. Carotid-femoral PWV is a strong independent predictor of cardiovascular events in different groups of high- and low-risk patients and in the general population [14].

10.3 Pulsatile Hemodynamics: Measurement in the Ambulatory Setting

Traditionally, central BP and wave reflections have been estimated, using brachial or radial tonometry to acquire waveforms, which were calibrated with brachial SBP and DBP, further processed with dedicated algorithms (transfer functions) to derive central BP waveforms, and PWA to derive AIx and AP [10]. These techniques have been successfully used in clinical trials. Their value for ambulatory recordings, however, is limited. Therefore, alternatives have been developed, which rely on acquisition of waveforms with a brachial cuff [15, 16] or with a wrist-watch-like tonometer [17]. The device we used in our study (Mobil-O-Graph, I.E.M., Stolberg, Germany) as well as the algorithms used for further processing the brachial waveforms (ARCSolver algorithms [18], AIT Austrian Institute of Technology, Vienna, Austria) have been extensively validated for brachial ABPM [19–21], cSBP [15, 22], and wave reflections [22–24]. In addition, the device with the inbuilt ARCSolver algorithms gives an estimate of aortic PWV, based on an algorithm which incorporates age, SBP, and waveform characteristics. This algorithm has been validated against the gold standard (invasive aortic PWV) in more than 900 patients [25], and against magnetic resonance imaging-based aortic PWV [26]. In office-based recordings, ARCSolver-based estimates of central pressures, wave reflections, and aortic PWV are associated with hypertensive organ damage [7, 24] and clinical endpoints such as all-cause mortality [27, 28] above and beyond brachial BP. Using ABPM-based estimates of pulsatile hemodynamics, 24 h cSBP has a closer relationship with left ventricular mass and left ventricular hypertrophy [29, 30] and to diastolic function [31], as compared to 24 h brachial SBP. In patients with end-stage renal disease undergoing hemodialysis, ambulatory 48 h-based aortic PWV was an independent predictor of cardiovascular events and all-cause mortality [32].

10.4 Aim of Our Study and Characteristics of Study Participants

For the purpose of the recent analysis, we selected individuals free from antihypertensive treatment out of several ongoing studies on 24 h pulsatile hemodynamics. The studies have been approved by regional Ethics committees (D-20-13, EC of Upper Austria, Austria; 1991/2013; EC of Medical University Vienna, Austria). Our aim was twofold: first, to characterize out-of-office BP, based on ABPM, in patients with prehypertension, and to identify patients with masked hypertension among those classified as prehypertensive; and second, to describe 24 h pulsatile hemodynamics in patients with prehypertension and to compare them with normotensives and hypertensives.

10.5 Results: Classification According to 24 h ABPM

Overall, we included 433 individuals (228 men, 205 women). Mean age was 50.6 years (SD 15.8), mean body mass index 26.0 kg/m^2 (SD 4.6).

Based on the JNC 7 classification and office BP, 38 individuals (8.8%) were classified as having optimal BP, 137 (31.6%) as prehypertensives, and 258 (59.6%) as hypertensives (Table 10.1). Age increased from optimal BP (45.7 years, SD 17.2) to prehypertension (49.2 years, SD 17.3) and hypertension (52.2 years, SD 14.5).

When brachial ABPM was taken into account, using a cutoff of 24 h ABPM of 130 mmHg systolic and 80 mmHg diastolic, classification changed substantially—Fig. 10.2: among the 38 individuals with optimal BP, 4 had elevated ABPM values, and accordingly were classified as masked hypertension. Thirty-four individuals with optimal BP had ABPM values in the normal range. Among the 137 participants with prehypertension, 28 (20.4%) had elevated ABPM values, and accordingly were classified as having masked hypertension. One hundred and nine prehypertensives (79.6%) had ABPM values in the normal range. Among the 258 hypertensives, 79 (30.6%) had normal ABPM values, and accordingly were classified as white-coat hypertensives. One hundred and seventy-nine office-based hypertensives (69.4%) had also ABPM values in the hypertensive range.

Table 10.1 Classification of study participants

BP classification	*n*	Office BP (mmHg)	24 h ABPM (mmHg)
Classification based on office BP			
Optimal BP	38	110/71	115/71
Prehypertension	137	126/81	119/75
Hypertension	258	148/96	131/84
Classification based on office BP and ABPM			
True optimal BP	34	109/71	113/70
True prehypertension	109	125/80	116/72
Masked hypertension	32	127/82	132/84
White-coat hypertension	79	143/91	120/74
Sustained hypertension	179	151/99	136/88

BP blood pressure, *ABPM* ambulatory blood pressure monitoring

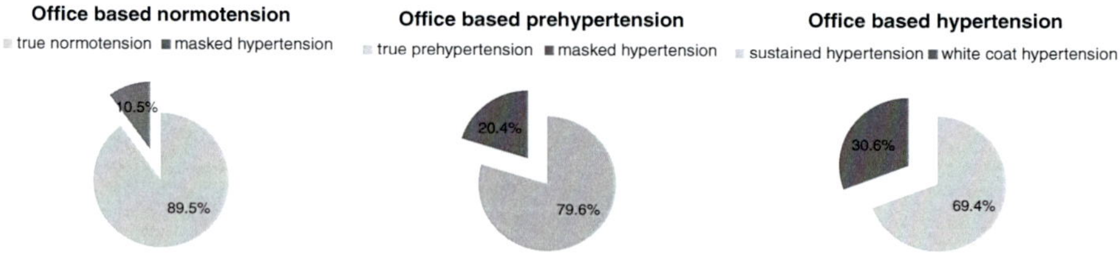

Fig. 10.2 Percentage of individuals with a change of blood pressure category after ambulatory blood pressure monitoring

Table 10.2 24 h pulsatile hemodynamics, according to office-based BP categories

	Optimal BP (n = 38)		Prehypertension (n = 137)		Hypertension (n = 258)		
	Mean	SD	Mean	SD	Mean	SD	p-value
24 h bSBP (mmHg)	114.8	9.0	119.4	9.9	131.0	12.1	<0.01
24 h MAP (mmHg)	91.0	6.8	95.2	7.9	105.4	9.9	<0.01
24 h bDBP (mmHg)	70.9	6.2	74.6	7.3	83.8	9.6	<0.01
24 h bPP (mmHg)	43.9	6.7	44.8	6.8	47.2	8.6	0.01
24 h HR (bpm)	73.1	8.2	71.3	8.8	74.5	8.1	<0.01
24 h cSBP (mmHg)	117.0	9.8	122.3	11.5	132.1	12.2	<0.01
24 h cPP (mmHg)	44.9	7.6	46.5	9.1	47.0	9.8	0.44
24 h AIx75 (%)	23.2	8.5	22.6	8.8	24.0	8.6	0.29
24 h AP (mmHg)	11.7	5.4	12.3	5.9	12.4	6.0	0.86
24 h AIx (%)	24.3	8.4	24.7	8.9	24.4	8.6	0.96
24 h RM (%)	62.9	6.8	64.0	6.6	63.8	5.7	0.64
24 h Pb (mmHg)	18.2	3.6	19.0	4.2	19.1	4.3	0.46
24 h pf (mmHg)	28.5	4.5	29.4	5.7	29.6	6.1	0.65
24 h aPWV (m/s)	7.3	2.0	7.9	2.0	8.4	1.8	<0.01

10.6 Results: Pulsatile Hemodynamics in Office-Based BP Categories

24 h pulsatile hemodynamics, according to office-based BP categories, are shown in Table 10.2. Results for 24 h central pressures in individuals with prehypertension were in between individuals with optimal BP and with hypertension—Fig. 10.3. Roughly the same was true for estimates of 24 h wave reflections, although differences were small and failed to reach statistical significance. 24 h PWV was lowest in individuals with optimal BP, intermediate in prehypertensives, and highest in hypertensives ($p < 0.01$).

10.7 Results: Pulsatile Hemodynamics in Office- and ABPM-Based BP Categories

24 h pulsatile hemodynamics, according to office- and ABPM-based BP categories, are shown in Table 10.3. Individuals with masked hypertension have significantly higher values for 24 h brachial pressures, 24 h central pressures, 24 h wave

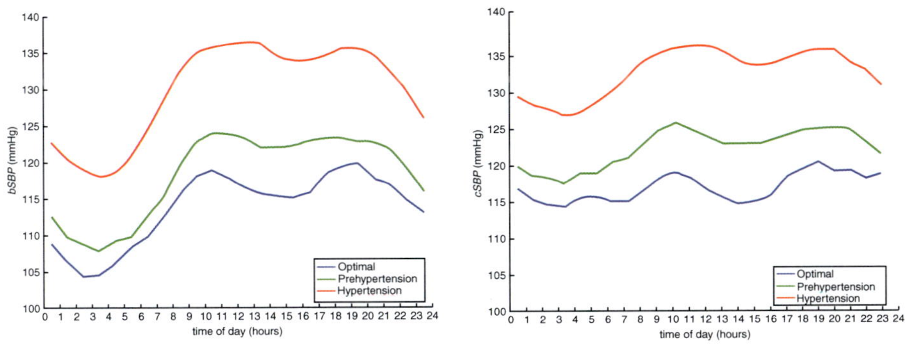

Fig. 10.3 24 h profiles of brachial and central systolic blood pressure, according to office blood pressure-based categories

Table 10.3 24 h pulsatile hemodynamics, according to office- and ABPM-based BP categories

	True optimal BP ($n = 34$)		Masked hypertension ($n = 32$)		True prehypertension ($n = 109$)		White-coat hypertension ($n = 79$)		Sustained hypertension ($n = 179$)		
	Mean	SD	Mean	SD	Mean	SD	Mean	SD	Mean	SD	*p*-value
24 h bSBP (mmHg)	113.1	7.5	131.8	7.3	116.2	7.5	120.4	6.6	135.7	11.0	<0.01
24 h MAP (mmHg)	89.6	5.5	105.8	4.3	92.3	5.8	95.3	4.7	109.9	8.1	<0.01
24 h bDBP (mmHg)	69.6	5.0	83.9	5.0	72.2	5.5	74.0	5.2	88.1	7.7	<0.01
24 h bPP (mmHg)	43.5	6.1	48.0	8.8	44.0	6.0	46.3	7.1	47.5	9.2	<0.01
24 h HR (bpm)	72.9	8.6	70.1	7.7	71.8	8.9	73.4	7.3	75.0	8.4	<0.01
24 h cSBP (mmHg)	115.4	8.7	135.3	10.3	118.9	8.8	122.5	7.3	136.4	11.5	<0.01
24 h cPP (mmHg)	44.7	7.3	50.0	12.0	45.5	7.9	47.3	8.7	46.9	10.3	0.26
24 h AIx75 (%)	22.9	8.7	22.6	9.4	22.8	8.5	23.7	8.6	24.2	8.6	0.63
24 h AP (mmHg)	11.6	5.5	13.7	7.2	11.9	5.4	12.5	6.2	12.3	6.0	0.69
24 h AIx (%)	24.0	8.7	25.4	8.8	24.5	8.8	24.6	9.2	24.4	8.4	0.97
24 h RM	62.8	7.0	64.4	5.8	63.8	6.8	65.0	5.9	63.3	5.6	0.23
24 h Pb (mmHg)	18.1	3.5	20.5	5.5	18.5	3.7	19.4	4.0	18.9	4.5	0.18
24 h pf (mmHg)	28.4	4.2	31.4	7.2	28.8	5.0	29.7	5.3	29.6	6.4	0.28
24 h PWV (m/s)	7.2	1.9	8.9	2.2	7.6	1.8	8.5	2.3	8.4	1.5	<0.01

P-values for comparison across all groups are from ANOVA. Individuals with masked hypertension have significantly higher values for brachial pressures, central pressures, and PWV, as compared to individuals with true prehypertension (all $p < 0.05$, *t*-test or Welch test). For abbreviations see Table 10.2

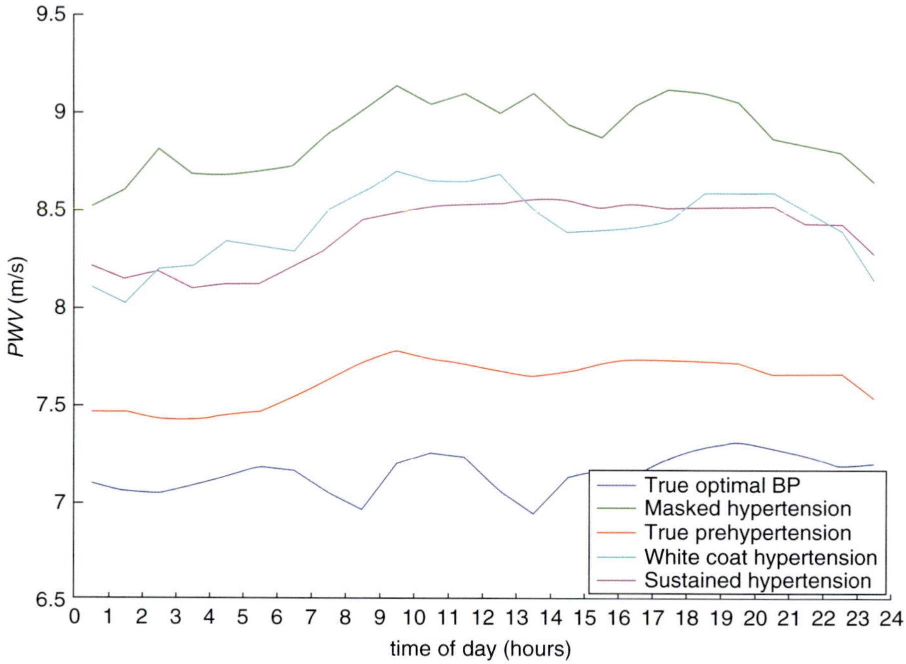

Fig. 10.4 24 h profiles of aortic pulse wave velocity according to office and 24 h ambulatory blood pressure-based categories

reflections, and 24 h PWV, as compared to individuals with true prehypertension. Interestingly, individuals with sustained hypertension have significantly higher values for 24 h bSBP, DBP, and MAP, as well as for 24 h cSBP, but not for most measures of wave reflection and PWV. Individuals with masked hypertension had the highest values for 24 h bPP, 24 h cPP, 24 h wave reflections (AP, AIx, Pb), and 24 h aortic stiffness (PWV)—Fig. 10.4.

10.8 Discussion and Conclusions

Our data clearly show the shortcomings of conventional BP classifications, which are based only on office BP [1]. The prognosis of individuals and patient groups can be easily misclassified, if only office BP is taken into account. In our dataset, 10% of individuals classified as having optimal BP and 20 percent of individuals classified as prehypertensive (both based on office BP), turned out to have actually masked hypertension, a condition with clearly worse prognosis, as compared to true optimal BP [3]. 24 h pulsatile hemodynamics show higher central BP, an increase in wave reflections, and a stiffer aorta (a higher aortic PWV) in the subgroups of individuals with office-based optimal BP or prehypertension, who were finally diagnosed with masked hypertension, as compared to those with true optimal BP or true prehypertension. All of these measures of pulsatile hemodynamics have proven diagnostic value above and beyond brachial BP [7, 10, 13, 24, 27–32]. Therefore, our findings suggest that office-based prehypertension actually comprises individuals with high and low cardiovascular risk. Out-of-office BP measurements, ideally incorporating pulsatile hemodynamics, are a necessity in these individuals.

References

1. Chobanian AV, Bakris GL, Black HR, Cushman WC, Green LA, Izzo JL Jr, Jones DW, Materson BJ, Oparil S, Wright JT Jr, Roccella EJ, Joint National Committee on Prevention, Detection, Evaluation and Treatment of High Blood Pressure. National Heart, Lung, and Blood Institute and National High Blood Pressure Education Program Coordinating Committee. Seventh report of the Joint National Committee on Prevention, Detection, Evaluation, and Treatment of High Blood Pressure. Hypertension. 2003;42:1206–52.
2. Vasan RS, Larson MG, Leip EP, Evans JC, O'Donnell CJ, Kannel WB, Levy D. Impact of high-normal blood pressure on the risk of cardiovascular disease. N Engl J Med. 2001;345:1291–7.
3. Mancia G, Fagard R, Narkiewicz K, Redon J, Zanchetti A, Bohm M, Christiaens T, Cifkova R, De Backer G, Dominiczak A, Galderisi M, Grobbee DE, Jaarsma T, Kirchhof P, Kjeldsen SE, Laurent S, Manolis AJ, Nilsson PM, Ruilope LM, Schmieder RE, Sirnes PA, Sleight P, Viigimaa M, Waeber B, Zannad F. 2013 ESH/ESC guidelines for the management of arterial hypertension: the Task Force for the management of arterial hypertension of the European Society of Hypertension (ESH) and of the European Society of Cardiology (ESC). J Hypertens. 2013;31:1281–357.
4. Schwartz JE, Burg MM, Shimbo D, Broderick JE, Stone AA, Ishikawa J, Sloan R, Yurgel T, Grossman S, Pickering TG. Clinic blood pressure underestimates ambulatory blood pressure in an untreated employer-based US population: results from the masked hypertension study. Circulation. 2016;134:1794–807.
5. Shimbo D, Newman JD, Schwartz JE. Masked hypertension and prehypertension: diagnostic overlap and interrelationships with left ventricular mass: the Masked Hypertension Study. Am J Hypertens. 2012;25:664–71.
6. Franklin SS, Larson MG, Khan SA, Wong ND, Leip EP, Kannel WB, Levy D. Does the relation of blood pressure to coronary heart disease risk change with aging? The Framingham Heart Study. Circulation. 2001;103(9):1245.
7. Weber T, Wassertheurer S, O'Rourke MF, Haiden A, Zweiker R, Rammer M, Hametner B, Eber B. Pulsatile hemodynamics in patients with exertional dyspnea: potentially of value in the diagnostic evaluation of suspected heart failure with preserved ejection fraction. J Am Coll Cardiol. 2013;61:1874–83.
8. Regnault V, Lagrange J, Pizard A, Safar ME, Fay R, Pitt B, Challande P, Rossignol P, Zannad F, Lacolley P. Opposite predictive value of pulse pressure and aortic pulse wave velocity on heart failure with reduced left ventricular ejection fraction: insights from an Eplerenone Post-Acute Myocardial Infarction Heart Failure Efficacy and Survival Study (EPHESUS) substudy. Hypertension. 2014;63:105–11.
9. Avolio AP, Van Bortel LM, Boutouyrie P, Cockcroft JR, McEniery CM, Protogerou AD, Roman MJ, Safar ME, Segers P, Smulyan H. Role of pulse pressure amplification in arterial hypertension: experts' opinion and review of the data. Hypertension. 2009;54:375–83.
10. McEniery CM, Cockcroft JR, Roman MJ, Franklin SS, Wilkinson IB. Central blood pressure: current evidence and clinical importance. Eur Heart J. 2014;35:1719–25.
11. Vlachopoulos C, Xaplanteris P, Aboyans V, Brodmann M, Cifkova R, Cosentino F, De Carlo M, Gallino A, Landmesser U, Laurent S, Lekakis J, Mikhailidis DP, Naka KK, Protogerou AD, Rizzoni D, Schmidt-Trucksass A, Van Bortel L, Weber T, Yamashina A, Zimlichman R,

Boutouyrie P, Cockcroft J, O'Rourke M, Park JB, Schillaci G, Sillesen H, Townsend RR. The role of vascular biomarkers for primary and secondary prevention. A position paper from the European Society of Cardiology Working Group on peripheral circulation: endorsed by the Association for Research into Arterial Structure and Physiology (ARTERY) Society. Atherosclerosis. 2015;241:507–32.

12. O'Rourke MF, Hashimoto J. Mechanical factors in arterial aging: a clinical perspective. J Am Coll Cardiol. 2007;50:1–13.
13. Pannier B, Guerin AP, Marchais SJ, Safar ME, London GM. Stiffness of capacitive and conduit arteries: prognostic significance for end-stage renal disease patients. Hypertension. 2005;45:592–6.
14. Ben-Shlomo Y, Spears M, Boustred C, May M, Anderson SG, Benjamin EJ, Boutouyrie P, Cameron J, Chen CH, Cruickshank JK, Hwang SJ, Lakatta EG, Laurent S, Maldonado J, Mitchell GF, Najjar SS, Newman AB, Ohishi M, Pannier B, Pereira T, Vasan RS, Shokawa T, Sutton-Tyrell K, Verbeke F, Wang KL, Webb DJ, Willum Hansen T, Zoungas S, McEniery CM, Cockcroft JR, Wilkinson IB. Aortic pulse wave velocity improves cardiovascular event prediction: an individual participant meta-analysis of prospective observational data from 17,635 subjects. J Am Coll Cardiol. 2014;63:636–46.
15. Weber T, Wassertheurer S, Rammer M, Maurer E, Hametner B, Mayer CC, Kropf J, Eber B. Validation of a brachial cuff-based method for estimating central systolic blood pressure. Hypertension. 2011;58:825–32.
16. Horvath IG, Nemeth A, Lenkey Z, Alessandri N, Tufano F, Kis P, Gaszner B, Cziraki A. Invasive validation of a new oscillometric device (Arteriograph) for measuring augmentation index, central blood pressure and aortic pulse wave velocity. J Hypertens. 2010;28:2068–75.
17. Williams B, Lacy PS, Yan P, Hwee CN, Liang C, Ting CM. Development and validation of a novel method to derive central aortic systolic pressure from the radial pressure waveform using an n-point moving average method. J Am Coll Cardiol. 2011;57:951–61.
18. Hametner B, Wassertheurer S, Kropf J, Mayer C, Holzinger A, Eber B, Weber T. Wave reflection quantification based on pressure waveforms alone—methods, comparison, and clinical covariates. Comput Methods Prog Biomed. 2013;109:250–9.
19. Jones CR, Taylor K, Chowienczyk P, Poston L, Shennan AH. A validation of the Mobil O Graph (version 12) ambulatory blood pressure monitor. Blood Press Monit. 2000;5:233–8.
20. Franssen PM, Imholz BP. Evaluation of the Mobil-O-Graph new generation ABPM device using the ESH criteria. Blood Press Monit. 2010;15:229–31.
21. Wei W, Tolle M, Zidek W, van der Giet M. Validation of the mobil-O-Graph: 24 h-blood pressure measurement device. Blood Press Monit. 2010;15:225–8.
22. Wassertheurer S, Kropf J, Weber T, van der Giet M, Baulmann J, Ammer M, Hametner B, Mayer CC, Eber B, Magometschnigg D. A new oscillometric method for pulse wave analysis: comparison with a common tonometric method. J Hum Hypertens. 2010;24:498–504.
23. Hametner B, Parragh S, Mayer C, Weber T, Van Bortel L, De Buyzere M, Segers P, Rietzschel E, Wassertheurer S. Assessment of model based (input) impedance, pulse wave velocity, and wave reflection in the Asklepios cohort. PLoS One. 2015;10:e0141656.
24. Weber T, Wassertheurer S, Rammer M, Haiden A, Hametner B, Eber B. Wave reflections, assessed with a novel method for pulse wave separation, are associated with end-organ damage and clinical outcomes. Hypertension. 2012;60:534–41.
25. Weber T, Wassertheurer S, Hametner B, Parragh S, Eber B. Noninvasive methods to assess pulse wave velocity: comparison with the invasive gold standard and relationship with organ damage. J Hypertens. 2015;33:1023–31.
26. Feistritzer HJ, Reinstadler SJ, Klug G, Kremser C, Seidner B, Esterhammer R, Schocke MF, Franz WM, Metzler B. Comparison of an oscillometric method with cardiac magnetic resonance for the analysis of aortic pulse wave velocity. PLoS One. 2015;10:e0116862.
27. Baumann M, Wassertheurer S, Suttmann Y, Burkhardt K, Heemann U. Aortic pulse wave velocity predicts mortality in chronic kidney disease stages 2-4. J Hypertens. 2014;32:899–903.
28. Wassertheurer S, Baumann M. Assessment of systolic aortic pressure and its association to all cause mortality critically depends on waveform calibration. J Hypertens. 2015;33:1884.

29. Protogerou AD, Argyris AA, Papaioannou TG, Kollias GE, Konstantonis GD, Nasothimiou E, Achimastos A, Blacher J, Safar ME, Sfikakis PP. Left-ventricular hypertrophy is associated better with 24-h aortic pressure than 24-h brachial pressure in hypertensive patients: the SAFAR study. J Hypertens. 2014;32:1805–14.
30. Weber T, Wassertheurer S, Sala ER, Ablasser C, Jankowski P, Muisan ML, Giannatasio C, Mang C, Schmidt-Trucksass A, Wilkinson I, McEniery C. Os 13-09 relationship between 24 hour ambulatory central blood pressure and left ventricular mass—a prospective multicenter study. J Hypertens. 2016;34(Suppl 1). —ISH 2016 Abstract Book: e210–e211
31. Zhang Y, Kollias G, Argyris AA, Papaioannou TG, Tountas C, Konstantonis GD, Achimastos A, Blacher J, Safar ME, Sfikakis PP, Protogerou AD. Association of left ventricular diastolic dysfunction with 24-h aortic ambulatory blood pressure: the SAFAR study. J Hum Hypertens. 2015;29:442–8.
32. Sarafidis PA, Loutradis C, Karpetas A, Tzanis G, Piperidou A, Koutroumpas G, Raptis V, Syrgkanis C, Liakopoulos V, Efstratiadis G, London G, Zoccali C. Ambulatory pulse wave velocity is a stronger predictor of cardiovascular events and all-cause mortality than office and ambulatory blood pressure in hemodialysis patients. Hypertension. 2017;70:148–57.

Early Changes in Renal Vasculature in Prehypertension

11

Hermann Haller, Anna Bertram, Klaus Stahl, and Jan Menne

In this chapter the role of the renal vasculature in the pathophysiology of early hypertension or prehypertension will be discussed. Renal vasculature is considered the renal microcirculation, i.e., renal capillaries. We will mostly concentrate on interstitial capillaries and discuss their role in the early changes of the renal interstitium. Figure 11.1 illustrates the underlying mechanisms of this hypothesis. We will in brief describe the role of endothelial cells in this regard and then proceed with the role of the NO system, reactive oxygen species, and microinflammation for the early changes in the renal vasculature. A novel aspect, the importance of the endothelial glycocalyx and its importance for both inflammation and salt sensitivity will also be described and integrated in our model.

Prehypertension is considered to be a condition which precedes and is a precursor of hypertension. It is defined by blood pressure with systolic blood pressure between 120 and 139 mmHg or a diastolic blood pressure between 80 and 89 mmHg, respectively [1]. Prehypertension is a fairly common condition which affects roughly 30% of the population in western countries [2, 3]. The concept of a prehypertensive state which slowly develops into "real" hypertension has been further supported by intervention trials which have demonstrated that exposure of a prehypertensive population to a blood pressure lowering strategy, i.e., angiotensin-receptor blockade prevents and/or postpones the development of hypertension. Interestingly, even 2 years after treatment with ACE-inhibitors or sartans has been stopped, a preventive effect of active treatment is still to be demonstrated [4, 5].

The importance of RAAS in these studies may indicate that the vascular system of the kidney is involved in the pathophysiology of prehypertension. It is important to note that prehypertension is associated with a significantly increased

H. Haller (✉) · A. Bertram · K. Stahl · J. Menne
Department of Nephrology, Hannover Medical School, Hannover, Germany
e-mail: haller.hermann@mh-hannover.de; Bertram.anna@mh-hannover.de; stahl.klaus@mh-hannover.de; menne.jan@mh-hannover.de

R. Zimlichman et al. (eds.), *Prehypertension and Cardiometabolic Syndrome*, Updates in Hypertension and Cardiovascular Protection,
https://doi.org/10.1007/978-3-319-75310-2_11

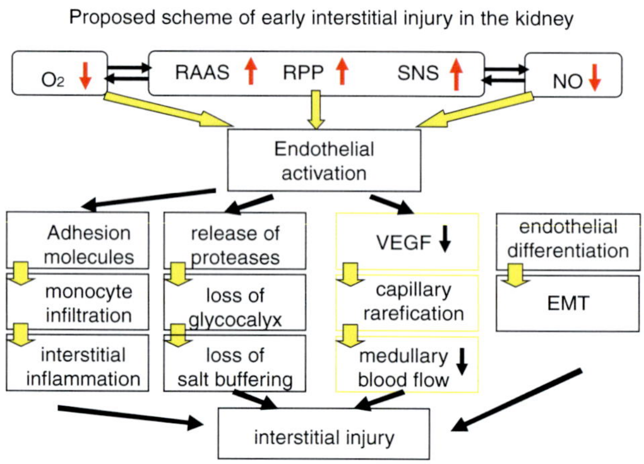

Fig. 11.1 Hypothetical scheme of the putative mechanisms underlying the early vascular and interstitial changes in the hypertensive kidney

cardiovascular risk. An important question is therefore which cardiovascular alterations are associated or may lead to the development of prehypertension and then progress into hypertension. It is obvious that the several pathophysiological systems which are important in the pathophysiology of hypertension could be involved, namely the sympathetic and/or the central nervous system, the heart, the kidney or changes in the vasculature. In this chapter we will discuss the involvement of the renal vasculature in the early stages of hypertension and describe several mechanisms which have been considered to be of importance in the development of prehypertension. We will especially concentrate on the changes of renal vasculature and propose a hypothesis whereby endothelial cell dysfunction in prehypertension may lead to vascular rarefaction and therefore contributing to the development of hypertension in some individuals. Since only few studies exist so far in patients with prehypertension we will also discuss animal models and clinical studies in patients with early forms of hypertension. As in the case of established hypertension it is difficult to define whether the early vascular changes are a result of increased blood pressure or whether the vascular changes are responsible for the development of prehypertension and/or hypertension. In addition, we will limit our discussion on endothelial cells and their functional contribution to the development of hypertension. We will describe the role of the endothelial cell layer (1) in blood pressure regulation and the development of prehypertension and (2) as the structure which is most easily damaged by the small increase in blood pressure [6, 7]. Several investigations have been carried out to define the endothelial cell alterations in prehypertension. Early on Taddei and coworkers have observed that the endothelium-dependent vasodilation is abnormal in the offspring of patients with essential hypertension [8]. Investigations such as these have led to the hypothesis that endothelial dysfunction may promote the development of hypertension. Schlaich and his group have shown that in individuals with a positive family history of hypertension the metabolism of

L-arginine is altered. They could show that the uptake of the essential L-arginine is diminished in these individuals implicating this system in the pathogenesis of early hypertension [9].

The endothelial cell functions which have been analyzed in the early stages of hypertension and/or in prehypertension include the following systems:

- NO and ROS system with an alteration of L-arginine metabolism
- Endothelial cell permeability with increased leakage of albumin and other factors both to the interstitium or in the case of the glomeruli into the urine
- The alterations in endothelial cell progenitor cells in patients with prehypertension
- Inflammatory mechanisms with release of cytokines and enhanced leukocyte adhesion on the endothelial cell surface
- The role of the endothelial glycocalyx

The imbalance between reactive oxygen species (ROS) and nitric oxide (NO) has been named oxidative stress. Oxidative stress indicates a shift and imbalance between the ROS and the NO system. Oxidative stress and NO deficiency have both been implicated in the pathophysiology of hypertension and prehypertension. The NO deficiency can precede the development of hypertension. The imbalance of NO-ROS is therefore important for the pathogenesis of high blood pressure [10, 11]. NO deficiency can be elicited by a decreased activity of the nitric oxide synthase (NOS). Both the expression and the activity of the enzyme have been demonstrated in prehypertension. As mentioned above, a decreased availability of L-arginine can also be the culprit for NO deficiency [12]. Several authors have demonstrated that an inhibitor of the NO system, the asymmetric dimethylargenine (ADMA) as an endogenous and NOS inhibitor, plays a role in the pathogenesis of oxidative stress and NO deficiency. ADMA can reduce the synthesis of NO and in addition induces superoxide reduction by uncoupling NOS [13, 14]. The cellular concentration of ADMA therefore regulates the local NO-ROS balance. We have shown in several studies that ADMA plays an important role in the development of hypertension and can induce high blood pressure in asymptomatic young individuals when it is increased [15, 16]. An increase in ADMA has not only an effect on vasoconstriction in different vascular beds but leads also to functional alterations in the brain, in the heart, and in the kidney [17, 18]. In addition to ADMA, the lack of intracellular antioxidants may play a role in the early stages of hypertension. The glutathione system (GSH) is impaired in an animal model of hypertension prior to the development of hypertension [19]. When these animals are treated with antioxidants such as *N*-acetylcysteine the development of hypertension can be prevented and/or reduced [20]. Another possibility to influence the NO-ROS system is the treatment with L-arginine. The supplementation of prehypertensive animals with L-citrulline prevents the transition from prehypertension to hypertension in this animal model [21, 22]. In summary, the balance of oxidative stress and the NO system may early on influence the reactivity of the vascular wall and lead to high blood pressure [23]. The alterations of the ROS system have been closely associated with alterations of the renin-angiotensin system (RAS). The RAS plays a fundamental role in the regulation of blood pressure in kidney development.

Interestingly, Richard Johnson and his group have early on discovered that angiotensin II induced damage of the kidney, which by itself does only lead to small increases in blood pressure, predisposes the organ to substantial blood pressure rise after exposure to sodium [24, 25]. These findings which have been confirmed by other groups shed an interesting light on the pathophysiological changes in the kidney in the early stages of hypertension [26, 27]. It has been observed that the angiotensin II induced damage leads to endothelial cell injury followed not only by an inflammatory response in the kidney but also to loss of capillaries with a rarefaction of the microvascular system in the kidney. The less perfused kidney which also may show signs of ischemia is extremely sensitive to changes in sodium intake. The following sequence of events is therefore possible: Either via microinflammation or by blood pressure induced damage by the endothelium a cascade is initiated which leads both to microinflammation and to verification of blood vessels. It is of interest that patients with prehypertension have been shown to have reduced nephron number in the kidneys which predisposes them to increases in blood pressure upon exposure to other risk factors [25]. Interestingly, these patients also display an increased sensitivity to salt. Recently, a novel hypothesis has been put forward which links the endothelial cell dysfunction and increased salt sensitivity.

It is well known that an excessive amount of salt in food affects the vascular system, leading to high blood pressure and premature disabilities. Kusche-Vihrog and Oberleithner [26, 27] noted that salt entering the vascular bed is transiently bound to the negatively charged endothelial glycocalyx, thus protecting the endothelium against salt overload. The glycocalyx is a negatively charged, organized mesh of membranous glycoproteins, with core proteoglycans of the syndecan and glypican family carrying highly sulfated, linear glycosaminoglycan attachments (mostly of the heparan, chondroitin, and dermatan sulfate families). Hyaluronic acid and the negatively charged heparan sulfate proteoglycans are its major constituents [28, 29]. This structure of core proteins "decorated" with long glycosaminoglycans provides a sea-grass like surface where components of functional systems such as the coagulation cascade or the complement system can be located and plasma constituents may interact intensely and dynamically (Fig. 11.2). Heparan sulfates displays high affinities for polycationic molecules. In addition, they also provide a significant storage volume which is easily accessible from the fluid phase. Oberleithner et al. suggested that plasma sodium is stored in the glycocalyx partially neutralizing the negative surface charges [26, 27]. A "good" glycocalyx has a high sodium store capacity but still maintains sufficient surface negativity at normal plasma sodium. A "bad" glycocalyx shows the opposite. Thus proteoglycans and glycosaminoglycans (i.e., mainly extracellular polyanions) may provide potential sinks for sodium and may serve as a means of concentrating cations close to the plasma membrane. It was shown that heparan sulfates adsorbed to a surface undergo a conformational change when exposed to flow: Their core proteins unfold from a random coil to an extended filament and their HS chains elongate significantly. This finding was used to illustrate how sodium ions bound to heparan sulfates could not

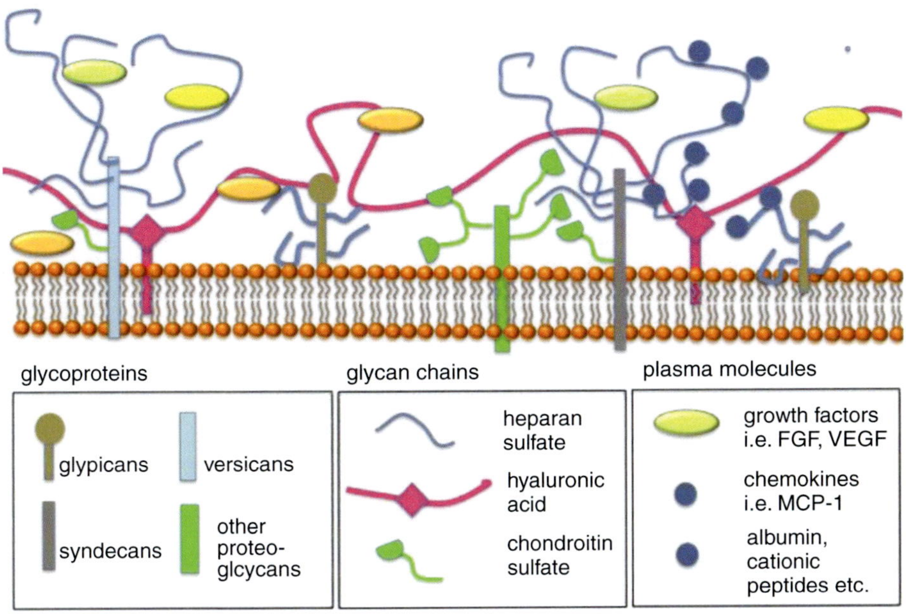

Fig. 11.2 Schematic diagram showing the components and spatial organization of the endothelial glycocalyx

only be stored but be delivered by the stretched glycosaminoglycan to their transporter channels. Such a concept of "storage space" in an intact glycocalyx has important implications for the binding of cations to the heparan sulfates of the glycocalyx, thereby regulating the sodium content in a third space. A degraded glycocalyx (by cardiovascular risk factors) increases the salt permeability of the vascular system resulting in one form of hypertension. In a related study, Pot et al. [30] presented evidence that the SHR rat has an elevated systemic level of proteases, including MMPs, involved in cell membrane receptor cleavage. They showed that RBCs from SHR rats are subject to enhanced glycocalyx cleavage compared to the RBCs of the normotensive WKY rats. These blood-borne MMPs have access to the glycocalyx on cell surfaces, providing a mechanism for the parallel degradation of the glycocalyx. Interestingly, in diabetes and in hypertension the glycocalyx is diminished, further supporting a role of the endothelial cell surface in the early stages of hypertension [31].

The second possibly altered function of the endothelium in the prehypertensive state is microinflammation. In the renal microcirculation the endothelial cells are responsible for release of inflammatory cytokines and adhesion of leukocytes with subsequent transmigration of the inflammatory cells into the surrounding tissue [32–34]. Several studies have shown that there is a link between elevated markers of inflammation and the risk of developing hypertension [35–39]. In recent years a wave study has shown and further investigated the links between inflammation, hypertension, and organ damage (for review [40, 41]). Early on it has been observed that there is a link between the oxidative stress and microinflammation. Inflammatory cells are potent sources of ROS. The interaction between the reactive oxygen species and inflammation is complex. Blood pressure elevations can lead to end-organ damage by driving the generation of ROS in the vasculature, the kidney, and the nervous system. However, other studies have characterized a converse relationship where ROS generated within these cardiovascular organs promote activation of circulating immune cells and thereby results in a dangerous positive feedback system that exaggerates hypertensive response following an initial endothelial cell injury. For the kidney the relationship between inflammation ROS and blood pressure elevation is especially challenging due to the critical role of the kidney in regulating sodium excretion and therefore intravascular volume. Inflammatory responses or oxidative stress localized in the kidney can therefore be the cause of the result of changes in blood pressure. This complicated relationship has not become easier to understand by recent findings that sodium by itself can influence the inflammatory response.

An increase in circulating levels of tumor necrosis factor alpha (TNF-alpha), C-reactive protein (CRP), and leukocytes compared to normotensive controls have been observed [38, 39]. Some studies have shown that higher CRP levels or leukocyte counts may predict the onset of hypertension is associated in prehypertension. Already in the early stages of hypertension elevated levels of endothelial cell adhesion molecules that facilitate the binding of mononuclear cells in the microcirculation of kidney and the heart have been observed [40]. Also released chemokines from the endothelial cells are present in the vasculature of patients in the early stages of hypertension. The major question is whether these patients have an increased immune response which causes an increase in blood pressure or whether the increase in blood pressure induces endothelial cell damage, thereby leading to an inflammatory response.

An important structure which mediates the inflammatory change on the surface of the endothelium is the glycocalyx. The glycocalyx and its glycosaminoglycans play an important role in various aspects of inflammation and in the physiological functioning of a range of inflammatory mediators, including chemokines, growth factors, endothelial adhesion molecules and inflammatory cell emigration. Studies suggest that at least two mechanisms of the glycocalyx, a change in glycosamin composition as well as enzymatic disruption of the proteoglycans, may have a strong effect on inflammatory responses. A change in glycosamin composition of the glycocalyx affects the early inflammatory mechanisms in several ways: van der Vlag and his group have demonstrated that an early response of the glycocalyx to inflammatory stimuli is a change in the N-deacetylase-N-sulfotransferase-mediated composition of the heparan sulfate. They have argued that modulation of heparan sulfates in the endothelial glycocalyx significantly reduces or enhances the inflammatory response in inflammatory kidney disease [42, 43].

In this brief review we have focused on the microvascular changes in patients with prehypertension or in the early stages of hypertension. We have demonstrated that the endothelium is of extreme importance in these early stages. These cells transmit both the injury and the reaction to other stimuli such as hyperlipidemia and hyperglycemia resulting in microinflammation, an increase in reactive oxygen species and decreased NO availability. These early stages may lead to endothelial cell dysfunction and to a cascade of events leading to interstitial injury and rarefaction of the blood vessels in the kidney rendering the organ more susceptible to further damage. In the future it will be important to define which pathophysiology is present in individual patients and design better diagnostic tools to analyze the pathophysiology in our prehypertensive patients. Analysis of the endothelial glycocalyx and its early changes are a promising novel field of diagnosis and, possibly, early treatment strategies.

References

1. Chobanian AV, Bakris GL, Black HR, Cushman WC, Green LA, Izzo JL Jr, Jones DW, Materson BJ, Oparil S, Wright JT Jr, Roccella EJ. Seventh report of the Joint National Committee on Prevention, Detection, Evaluation, and Treatment of High Blood Pressure. Hypertension. 2003;42:1206–52.
2. Wang Y, Wang QJ. The prevalence of prehypertension and hypertension among US adults according to the new joint national committee guide- lines: new challenges of the old problem. Arch Intern Med. 2004;164:2126–34.
3. Julius S, Nesbitt SD, Egan BM, Weber MA, Michelson EL, Kaciroti N, Black HR, Grimm RH Jr, Messerli FH, Oparil S, Schork MA. Feasibility of treating prehypertension with an angiotensin-receptor blocker. N Engl J Med. 2006;354:1685–97.
4. Vasan RS, Larson MG, Leip EP, Evans JC, O'Donnell CJ, Kannel WB, Levy D. Impact of high-normal blood pressure on the risk of cardiovas- cular disease. N Engl J Med. 2001;345:1291–7.
5. Menne J, Ritz E, Ruilope LM, Chatzikyrkou C, Viberti G, Haller H. The Randomized Olmesartan and Diabetes Microalbuminuria Prevention (ROADMAP) observational follow-up study: benefits of RAS blockade with olmesartan treatment are sustained after study discontinuation. J Am Heart Assoc. 2014;3(2):e000810.
6. Deanfield JE, Halcox JP, Rabelink TJ. Endothelial function and dys-function: testing and clinical relevance. Circulation. 2007;115:1285–95.
7. Landmesser U, Hornig B, Drexler H. Endothelial function: a critical determinant in atherosclerosis? Circulation. 2004;109:II27–33.
8. Taddei S, Virdis A, Mattei P, Ghiadoni L, Sudano I, Salvetti A. Defective L-arginine-nitric oxide pathway in offspring of essential hypertensive patients. Circulation. 1996;94:1298–303.
9. Schlaich MP, Parnell MM, Ahlers BA, Finch S, Marshall T, Zhang WZ, Kaye DM. Impaired L-arginine transport and endothelial function in hypertensive and genetically predisposed normotensive subjects. Circulation. 2004;110:3680–6.
10. Baylis C. Nitric oxide synthase derangements and hypertension in kidney disease. Curr Opin Nephrol Hypertens. 2012;21:1–6.
11. Vaziri ND. Roles of oxidative stress and antioxidant therapy in chronic kidney disease and hypertension. Curr Opin Nephrol Hypertens. 2004;13:93–9.
12. Wilcox CS. Oxidative stress and nitric oxide deficiency in the kidney: a critical link to hypertension? Am J Physiol Regul Integr Comp Physiol. 2005;289:R913–35.
13. Teerlink T, Luo Z, Palm F, Wilcox CS. Cellular ADMA: regulation and action. Pharmacol Res. 2009;60:448–60.
14. Schwedhelm E, Böger RH. The role of asymmetric and symmetric dimethylarginines in renal disease. Nat Rev Nephrol. 2011;7:275–85.
15. Kielstein JT, Donnerstag F, Gasper S, Menne J, Kielstein A, Martens-Lobenhoffer J, Scalera F, Cooke JP, Fliser D, Bode-Böger SM. ADMA increases arterial stiffness and decreases cerebral blood flow in humans. Stroke. 2006;37(8):2024–9.

16. Kielstein JT, Simmel S, Bode-Böger SM, Roth HJ, Schmidt-Gayk H, Haller H, Fliser D. Subpressor dose asymmetric dimethylarginine modulates renal function in humans through nitric oxide synthase inhibition. Kidney Blood Press Res. 2004;27(3):143–7.
17. Surdacki A, Nowicki M, Sandmann J, Tsikas D, Boeger RH, Bode-Boeger SM, Kruszelnicka-Kwiatkowska O, Kokot F, Dubiel JS, Froelich JC. Reduced urinary excretion of nitric oxide metabolites and increased plasma levels of asymmetric dimethylarginine in men with essential hypertension. J Cardiovasc Pharmacol. 1999;33:652–8.
18. Tain YL, Baylis C. Determination of dimethylarginine dimethylaminohydrolase activity in the kidney. Kidney Int. 2007;72:886–9.
19. Lee SK, Arunkumar S, Sirajudeen KN, Singh HJ. Glutathione system in young spontaneously hypertensive rats. J Physiol Biochem. 2010;66:321–7.
20. Fan NC, Tsai CM, Hsu CN, Huang LT, Tain YL. *N*-Acetylcysteine prevents hypertension via regulation of the ADMA–DDAH pathway in young spontaneously hypertensive rats. Biomed Res Int. 2013;2013:696317.
21. Chien SJ, Lin KM, Kuo HC, Huang CF, Lin YJ, Huang LT, Tain YL. Two different approaches to restore renal nitric oxide and prevent hypertension in young spontaneously hypertensive rats: L-Citrulline and nitrate. Transl Res. 2014;163:43–52.
22. Carlström M, Persson AE, Larsson E, Hezel M, Scheffer PG, Teerlink T, Weitzberg E, Lundberg JO. Dietary nitrate attenuates oxidative stress, prevents cardiac and renal injuries, and reduces blood pressure in salt-induced hypertension. Cardiovasc Res. 2011;89:574–85.
23. Böger RH, Maas R, Schulze F, Schwedhelm E. Asymmetric dimethylarginine (ADMA) as a prospective marker of cardiovascular disease and mortality—an update on patient populations with a wide range of cardiovascular risk. Pharmacol Res. 2009;60:481–7.
24. Johnson RJ, Gordon KL, Giachelli C, Kurth T, Skelton MM, Cowley AW Jr. Tubulointerstitial injury and loss of nitric oxide synthases parallel the development of hypertension in the Dahl-SS rat. J Hypertens. 2000;18:1497–505.
25. Johnson RJ, Gordon KL, Suga S, Duijvestijn AM, Griffin K, Bidani A. Renal injury and salt-sensitive hypertension after exposure to catecholamines. Hypertension. 1999;34:151–9.
26. Kusche-Vihrog K, Oberleithner H. An emerging concept of vascular salt sensitivity. F1000 Biol Rep. 2012;4:20.
27. Oberleithner H. Vascular endothelium: a vulnerable transit zone for merciless sodium. Nephrol Dial Transplant. 2014;29:240–6.
28. Pries AR, Secomb TW, Gaehtgens P. The endothelial surface layer. Pflugers Arch. 2000;440:653–66.
29. Reitsma S, Slaaf DW, Vink H, van Zandvoort MA, Oude Egbrink MG. The endothelial glycocalyx: composition, functions, and visualization. Pflugers Arch. 2007;454(3):345–59.
30. Pot C, Chen AY, Ha JN, Schmid-Schonbein GW. Proteolytic cleavage of the red blood cell glycocalyx in a genetic form of hypertension. Cell Mol Bioeng. 2011;4:678–92.
31. Kumase F, Morizane Y, Mohri S, Takasu I, Ohtsuka A, Ohtsuki H. Glycocalyx degradation in retinal and choroidal capillary endothelium in rats with diabetes and hypertension. Acta Med Okayama. 2010;64:277–83.
32. Parra G, Quiroz Y, Salazar J, Bravo Y, Pons H, Chavez M, Johnson RJ, Rodriguez-Iturbe B. Experimental induction of salt-sensitive hypertension is associated with lym- phocyte proliferative response to HSP70. Kidney Int Suppl. 2008;74:S55–9.
33. Muller DN, Dechend R, Mervaala EMA, Park J-K, Schmidt F, Fiebeler A, Theuer J, Breu V, Ganten D, Haller H, Luft FC. NF-{kappa}B inhibition ameliorates angiotensin II-induced inflammatory damage in rats. Hypertension. 2000;35:193–201.
34. Muller DN, Shagdarsuren E, Park JK, Dechend R, Mervaala E, Hampich F, Fiebeler A, Ju X, Finckenberg P, Theuer J, Viedt C, Kreuzer J, Heidecke H, Haller H, Zenke M, Luft FC. Immunosuppressive treatment protects against angiotensin II-induced renal damage. Am J Pathol. 2002;161:1679–93.
35. Kim M, Jung S, Yeon Kim S, Lee S-H, Lee JH. Prehypertension-associated elevation in circulating lysophosphatidlycholines, Lp-PLA$_2$ activity, and oxidative stress. PLoS One. 2014;9(5):e96735.

36. Niskanen L, Laaksonen DE, Nyyssonen K, Punnonen K, Valkonen VP, Fuentes R, Tuomainen TP, Salonen R, Salonen JT. Inflammation, abdominal obesity, and smoking as predictors of hypertension. Hypertension. 2004;44:859–65.
37. Gesso HD, Buring JE, Rifai N, Blake GJ, Gaziano JM, Ridker PM. C-reactive protein and the risk of developing hypertension. JAMA. 2003;290:2945–51.
38. Tatsukawa Y, Hsu WL, Yamada M, Cologne JB, Suzuki G, Yamamoto H, Yamane K, Akahoshi M, Fujiwara S, Kohno N. White blood cell count, especially neutrophil count, as a predictor of hypertension in a Japanese popu-lation. Hypertens Res. 2008;31:1391–7.
39. Stumpf C, John S, Jukic J, Yilmaz A, Raaz D, Schmieder RE, Daniel WG, Garlichs CD. Enhanced levels of platelet P- selectin and circulating cytokines in young patients with mild arterial hypertension. J Hypertens. 2005;23:995–1000.
40. McMaster WG, Kirabo A, Madhur MS, Harrison DG. Inflammation, immunity, and hypertensive end-organ damage. Circ Res. 2015;116(6):1022–33.
41. Foss JD, Kirabo A, Harrison DG. Do high-salt microenvironments drive hypertensive inflammation? Am J Physiol Regul Integr Comp Physiol. 2017;312(1):R1–4.
42. Rops AL, Loeven MA, van Gemst JJ, Eversen I, Van Wijk XM, Dijkman HB, van Kuppevelt TH, Berden JH, Rabelink TJ, Esko JD, van der Vlag J. Modulation of heparan sulfate in the glomerular endothelial glycocalyx decreases leukocyte influx during experimental glomerulonephritis. Kidney Int. 2014;86(5):932–42.
43. Rops AL, van den Hoven MJ, Baselmans MM, Lensen JF, Wijnhoven TJ, van den Heuvel LP, van Kuppevelt TH, Berden JH, van der Vlag J. Heparan sulfate domains on cultured activated glomerular endothelial cells mediate leukocyte trafficking. Kidney Int. 2008;73(1):52–62.

12 Heart and Prehypertension

Cesare Cuspidi, Marijana Tadic, and Guido Grassi

12.1 Introduction

Asymptomatic alterations of the cardiovascular system reflect intermediate stages in the disease continuum linking risk factors such as high blood pressure (BP), hypercholesterolemia, diabetes, obesity, and smoking to cardiovascular fatal and nonfatal events. In particular, a variety of manifestations of subclinical target organ damage such as left ventricular hypertrophy (LVH), LV systolic/diastolic dysfunction, abnormalities in small, medium, and large size arteries, and renal impairment have been reported to be associated with systemic hypertension [1, 2].

An increasing and consistent body of evidence supports the view that these markers of cardiac and extra-cardiac organ damage are powerful predictors of cardiovascular disease over and beyond BP levels and traditional risk factors [3–6]. As for the heart, systemic hypertension adversely affects cardiac structure and function by inducing a wide array of morpho-functional changes including myocyte hypertrophy and fibrosis resulting in alterations of both LV contractility and relaxation, left atrial (LA) enlargement and aortic root (AR) dilatation [7, 8]. Hypertensive heart disease, the cardinal marker of subclinical organ damage, is the result of long-term exposure of LV to pressure overload in combination to a variety of unhealthy

C. Cuspidi (✉)
Department of Medicine and Surgery, University of Milano-Bicocca, Milan, Italy

Clinical Research Unit, Istituto Auxologico Italiano, Meda, Italy
e-mail: cesare.cuspidi@unimib.it

M. Tadic
Department of Cardiology, Charité-University-Medicine Campus Virchow Klinikum, Berlin, Germany

G. Grassi
Department of Medicine and Surgery, University of Milano-Bicocca, Milan, Italy

IRCCS Multimedica, Sesto San Giovanni, Milan, Italy

R. Zimlichman et al. (eds.), *Prehypertension and Cardiometabolic Syndrome*, Updates in Hypertension and Cardiovascular Protection,
https://doi.org/10.1007/978-3-319-75310-2_12

non-modifiable and modifiable factors, often associated to elevated BP. In fact, the magnitude of cardiac morpho-functional alterations secondary to hypertension is not only dependent on the severity and time of exposure to BP overload but also to several racial, demographic, and clinical variables, such as black ethnicity, age, gender, type 2 diabetes mellitus, metabolic syndrome, obesity, sleep apnea syndrome, and renal disease.

Prehypertensive status (i.e., BP ranging from 120 to 139 mmHg systolic and/or from 80 to 89 mmHg diastolic in adult subjects not taking any BP lowering drugs) has been consistently shown to be associated with increased risk of incident cardiovascular disease, this is because the linear and continuous relationship between BP levels and cardiovascular events, starting at BP values of 115 and 75 mmHg, has been documented by a historical meta-analysis of 61 prospective studies including approximately one million people [9].

The findings provided by this meta-analysis indicated that mortality from ischemic heart disease and stroke in individuals aged 40–89 years increases in a log-linear relationship with BP, from levels greater or equal to 115/75 mmHg. More recently, subgroup analyses of pooled data from 468,561 participants recruited in 18 prospective cohort studies showed even for low-range prehypertension, the risk of cardiovascular disease was significantly higher than for optimal BP: (RR = 1.46, 95% CI = 1.32–1.62), and further increased with high-range prehypertension (RR = 1.80, 95% CI = 1.41–2.31) [10].

In view of the fact that the prehypertension has been recognized as a risk factor for incident cardiovascular disease, numerous studies, mostly conducted over the past decade, have investigated the relationship between subclinical organ damage and this BP phenotype.

This chapter reviews the literature providing evidence on the association between prehypertension and cardiac abnormalities such as LVH, systolic/diastolic dysfunction, LA and AR dilatation, as assessed by echocardiography. These findings will be discussed in detail in separate subsections.

12.2 Left Ventricular Structure

In early phases of systemic hypertension, LVH can be regarded as a response to pressure overload aimed at reducing ventricular wall stress. At this stage, LVH is an adaptive change facilitating cardiac work primarily via the growth of cardiomyocytes. Two aspects concerning this process need to be considered. First, LVH is associated with expression of fetal isoforms of myocardial proteins such as β-myosin heavy chain, β-troponin, and skeletal α-actin. Thus, LVH is a likely consequence of a re-expression of an early stage of myocardial growth rather than an increased synthesis of normal contractile proteins. Second, the long-term pressure overload may stimulate pro-collagen gene expression and collagen protein synthesis leading to collagen deposition and fibrosis. Myocardial fibrosis, accompanying hypertensive LVH, reflects a very complex process resulting from the imbalance between stimulatory and inhibitory factors that control fibrillar collagen turnover [11].

In the subsequent phases, experimental and clinical studies have proven that persistence/ progression LVH causes several negative effects, such as impaired myocardial relaxation, leading to diastolic dysfunction, LA remodeling, reduced coronary reserve, atrial/ventricular arrhythmias, and ultimately systolic dysfunction, the patho-physiologic substrate carrying a high risk for overt cardiovascular disease.

The first large population-based study aimed to examine specifically the cardiac and systemic hemodynamic status of prehypertension was performed in 1940 adolescent and young adult American Indian participants of the Strong Heart Study (age < 40 years), a population in which obesity, diabetes, and hypertension were highly prevalent [12]. Compared with the non-hypertensive group, prehypertensive participants were more likely to be men (52% vs. 38%), to be obese (65% vs. 53%), and to have type 2 diabetes (9% vs. 6%) and impaired fasting glucose (6% vs. 3%), respectively. Prehypertensive subjects had, on average, thicker interventricular septal and LV posterior walls than normotensive participants. Both LV chamber diameter and relative wall thickness were increased in the prehypertensive groups. As a result, LV mass indexed for body surface area and height to its allometric power of 2.7 was higher in the prehypertensive group. Furthermore, the prevalence of LVH was twofold higher in prehypertensive participants than in their normotensive counterparts. As for classification of LV geometric patterns, according to Ganau et al. [13], eccentric LVH was approximately twofold higher in the cases than in normotensive controls. Of note, in the Strong Heart Study the overall prevalence of concentric LVH was rare (0.4), this was also the case for LV concentric remodeling.

Further important data on the association between prehypertension and LV morphology have obtained in a large, biracial community based cohort of elderly men and women (mean age > 70 years) by the Atherosclerosis Risk in Communities Study Investigators (14). Participants with prehypertension had greater LV mass index (73.6 ± 14.8 g/m^2) and LV wall thickness (0.94 ± 0.11 cm) than those with optimal BP (69.9 ± 16.4 g/m^2 and 0.91 ± 0.12 cm, respectively), but lower than those with hypertension. These differences remained statistically significant after multivariable analysis adjusted by age, sex, race, heart rate, body mass index, diabetes, and estimated glomerular filtration rate. Yet, compared to participants with optimal BP, those with prehypertension had a higher prevalence of abnormal LV geometry (concentric hypertrophy, eccentric hypertrophy, or concentric remodeling) of borderline statistical significance (adjusted P value = 0.05).

Other information comes from studies that have included individuals with a wider range of age and therefore more representative of the impact of prehypertension on cardiac damage in the general population than those restricted to young or elderly population-based samples. Among 10,547 subjects (1651 normotensive, 3616 prehypertensive, and 5280 hypertensive participants) examined in a cross-sectional survey in a northeast rural Chinese area, a gradual and significant increase in absolute LV mass and LV mass index (regardless the type of indexation for body size) was found across the three BP categories [15]. The prevalence LVH resulted to be statistically different among three groups ($P < 0.001$), being the rates of LVH 5.9%, 8.6%, 28.4% by indexing LV mass to height$^{2.7}$ and 4.9%, 5.3%, 19.3% by indexing LV mass to BSA, respectively. Finally, the prevalence rates of abnormal

LV geometric patterns such as eccentric hypertrophy, concentric remodeling, and concentric hypertrophy were 7.3%, 5.3%, and 1.4% in prehypertensive, and 5.1%, 6.4%, and 0.8% in normotensive participants.

The Kangbuk Samsung Cohort Study, which included a very large sample of Korean men and women (55,211, mean age 40 years) undergoing a thorough medical health check-up program, reported a clear dose–response relationship between unfavorable LV structural changes and five BP categories: i.e., normotensive ($n = 35{,}086$), prehypertensive ($n = 9.283$), controlled hypertensive ($n = 4795$), newly recognized hypertensive ($n = 1818$), and uncontrolled hypertensive groups ($n = 1129$) [16]. The proportion of LVH was 0.9% in the normotensive group, 1.6% in the prehypertensive group, 4.9% in controlled hypertensives, 3.4% in newly recognized hypertensives, and 8.1% in uncontrolled hypertensives. The rates of increased relative wall thickness and LV geometry changes also showed similar trends.

Although prehypertension is not a static condition because it can often progress over time to hypertension or less frequently shift to normotension, the clinical significance of such temporal variations to date has been poorly investigated by prospective studies. The Investigators of the MONICA/KORA Augsburg study evaluated whether changes in LV geometry and function that occur with 10 years of ageing differ between individuals who remain normotensive and those who have persistent prehypertension over that period (17). In cross-sectional comparisons of the baseline study, LV mass indexed to height$^{2.7}$ was slightly higher in the prehypertensive group; this was not the case for other echocardiographic parameters such as LV wall thickness, relative wall thickness, LV end-diastolic diameter, and LV mass. At the follow-up examination, the persistent prehypertensive group had significantly higher adjusted mean values for absolute as well as for relative wall thickness, LV mass and LV mass indexed to height$^{2.7}$ as compared with the persistent normotensive group. These findings support the view that long-standing prehypertension appears to be associated with a significantly increased occurrence of LV structural changes.

Emerging evidence indicates that masked hypertension is a BP phenotype associated with increased cardiovascular risk as compared to true normotension. The term masked hypertension, coined for the first time in the early 2000s by Pickering et al. [18], is currently used to define a subgroup hypertensive subjects with normal office and elevated out-of-office BP. Observational studies focusing on demographic and clinical characteristics of masked hypertension reported that prehypertension is a key variable differentiating masked hypertensive individuals from normotensive ones. The Masked Hypertension Study, a worksite-based population, showed that prevalence of masked hypertension was approximately tenfold greater in prehypertensive participants (34.1%) than in those with optimal clinic BP (3.9%) [19]. As for subclinical cardiac damage, compared with subjects with optimal clinic BP, LV mass index was significantly greater in prehypertensive group with masked hypertension, after adjusting for several confounders.

On the whole, consistent findings support the view that even small elevations in BP, as seen with prehypertension, can have detrimental effects on LV structure and geometry across different age ranges and ethnicities [20–22] (Tables 12.1 and 12.2).

Table 12.1 Summary of seven population-based studies reporting data on prevalence of left ventricular hypertrophy, as assessed by echocardiography, in normotensive, prehypertensive, and hypertensive subjects

Author, Reference	Year of publication	Total sample size, *n*	Age, years	Normotensives (%)	Prehypertensives (%)	Hypertensives (%)
Drukteinis et al. [12]	2007	1940	26.8 ± 7.7	6.5	11.4	19.9
Toprak[a]	2009	1204	35.5 ± 5.0	3.6	8.8	n.a.
Kim et al. [36]	2011	1671	52.5 ± 5.3	17.5	22.6	n.a.
Urbina et al. [29]	2011	723	18.0 ± 3.1	7.6	7.7	22.6
Santos et al. [14]	2016	4871	75.0 ± 5.0	36.0	44.0	51.0
Li et al. [15]	2016	10,547	52.0 ± 10.0	459	8.6	28.4
Jung et al. [16]	2017	52,111	40.3 ± 8.1	0.9	1.6	5.0

Data are shown as absolute numbers, percentages, means ± standard deviation. In the study by Santos et al. data regarding prevalence of left ventricular hypertrophy include left ventricular concentric remodeling. Left ventricular mass was indexed by body surface area in the studies by Santos et al. and Jung et al. and by height to allometric power of 2.7 in the other reports

[a]Toprak et al. J Hypertens 2009; 27: 243–250

Table 12.2 Summary of four population-based studies reporting data on prevalence of abnormal left ventricular geometric patterns, as assessed by echocardiography, in normotensive, prehypertensive, and hypertensive subjects

Author, Reference	Year of publication	Total sample size, *n*	Age, years	Normotensives			Prehypertensives			Hypertensives		
				CR (%)	CH (%)	EH (%)	CR (%)	CH (%)	EH (%)	CR (%)	CH (%)	EH (%)
Drukteinis [12]	2007	1940	26.8 ± 7.7	0.7	0.4	6.1	1.4	0.3	11.1	1.8	0	19.9
Urbina [29]	2011	723	18.0 ± 3.1	0.8	3.4	3.4	0	3.1	4.6	5.5	4.7	13.4
Li [15]	2016	10,547	52.0 ± 10.0	6.4	0.8	5.1	5.3	1.4	7.3	8.8	10.6	17.8
Jung [16]	2017	52,111	40.3 ± 8.1	2.2	0.1	0.8	5.0	0.3	1.3	8.7	1.2	3.8

Data are shown as absolute numbers, percentages, means ± standard deviation; *CR* concentric remodeling, *CH* concentric hypertrophy, *EH* eccentric hypertrophy

12.3 Left Ventricular Function

As already mentioned the left ventricular systolic function tends to deteriorate only in advanced stages of the natural history of hypertension. Accordingly, the results concerning conventional and prognostically validated echocardiographic indices of LV systolic function (such as ejection fraction or fractional shortening) obtained in many studies conducted in subjects with hypertension showed no significant changes compared to their counterparts with optimal BP.

However, the development of new imaging modalities and especially the introduction of speckle tracking imaging and strain in clinical research enabled a detailed analysis of cardiac mechanics and detection of subtle subclinical myocardial damage that previously had not been recognized. Only a few studies based on two-dimensional and three-dimensional speckle tracking imaging have addressed this topic in prehypertensive subjects [23, 24].

Our group assessed the presence of subclinical LV myocardial dysfunction in subjects with optimal (n = 49), high-normal BP (n = 50) and untreated arterial hypertension (n = 50), using three-dimensional echocardiography strain analysis [24]. Three-dimensional global longitudinal strain was significantly lower in the high-normal BP group and the hypertensive patients, in comparison with the optimal BP group. Similar results were obtained for three-dimensional global circumferential strain as well for three-dimensional global radial strain, and global area strain.

Therefore, in this section will report in detail data concerning exclusively LV diastolic function, as assessed by conventional Doppler analysis and tissue Doppler imaging.

Echocardiography is the reference method for diagnosing heart failure with preserved ejection fraction and identifying early diastolic alterations in asymptomatic patients at high cardiovascular risk [25].

A large amount of evidence highlights that the assessment of diastolic function by using conventional Doppler and tissue Doppler imaging may provide relevant predictive information about cardiovascular morbidity and mortality independently from LV mass, LV geometry, and traditional risk factors.

Alterations of diastolic properties in the hypertensive heart may be related to a complex interplay of factors including increased BP itself, structural LV changes (i.e., increased collagen matrix, disorganization of collagen fibers, abnormal collagen type I/III ratio), and coronary microcirculation impairment [26]. The association between LVH (and particularly of concentric type) and diastolic dysfunction has been largely reported either in population-based studies as in hypertensive cohorts [27].

The estimation of LV diastolic dysfunction rates in the hypertensive setting is a difficult task due to differences in demographic/clinical characteristics of the subjects examined as well as in diagnostic criteria. Prevalence rates of diastolic dysfunction reported in recent literature indicate that at least one-quarter of asymptomatic hypertensive subjects older than 50 years can have LV diastolic dysfunction [28].

In the prehypertensive setting early LV diastolic alterations have been described cohorts with different demographic and clinical characteristics. In the Strong Heart study, the percentage of young participants with prolonged isovolumic relaxation time was greater in the hypertensive and prehypertensive groups, which also exhibited higher peak mitral late velocity (A) and atrial filling fractions than reference group with optimal BP [14]. Hypertensive and prehypertensive participants had significantly lower mean mitral early diastolic peak flow velocity (E), early to late diastolic peak flow velocity E/A ratios, suggesting slightly impaired LV relaxation counterbalanced by a greater atrial contribution to LV ventricular filling. Similar results have been shown by Urbina et al. [29] in 479 adolescents and young adults in which diastolic function was more completely assessed by both conventional Doppler and tissue Doppler indices. A graded decrease in diastolic function was observed from normotensive, to prehypertensive and to hypertensive subjects.

In keeping with the findings of the aforementioned studies, an independent association between diastolic dysfunction and prehypertension was described by Jang et al. [30] in a large sample of apparently healthy Korean adults aged 40–64 years who underwent routine health examinations.

The proportion of diastolic dysfunction grade 1 or 2 (as defined according to according to the guidelines of the American Society of Echocardiography) was significantly higher in prehypertensive (31.0%) and hypertensive (38.0%) groups compared to the normotensive group (19.1%). Diastolic dysfunction was more frequently found in men than in women and showed a continuous and positive relationship with office BP and body mass index.

In the biracial cohort of elderly men and women examined in the ARIC study, diastolic parameters such as E/A ratio, early (Ei) diastolic annular peak velocity, and the ratio of trans-mitral flow velocity to annular velocity (E/Ei) were impaired in participants with prehypertension which therefore had higher prevalence of mild and moderate-severe diastolic dysfunction compared to those with optimal BP [14]. Of note, these differences in LV diastolic function remained significant after adjusting for important clinical covariates.

12.4 Left Atrium

LA enlargement is currently regarded as a reliable biomarker of LV pressure and volume overload [31]. Consequently, LA size is increased in several cardiac disorders such as mitral, aortic valve disease, myocardial diseases as well as arterial hypertension. In hypertensive heart disease, LA dilatation is an indicator of chronically elevated LV filling pressure and diastolic dysfunction even in the absence of mitral diseases.

A direct correlation between LA size and the circulating levels of brain natriuretic peptide has been reported in patients with chronic heart failure and preserved systolic function as well as in hypertensive patients with LVH and diastolic dysfunction. Although the increase in LA chamber may be a compensatory mechanism counterbalancing early alterations in LV relaxation and filling and the worsening of

LV diastolic performance in the hypertrophied ventricle, LA enlargement can develop well before the onset of a frank LVH.

Some authors have shown that in recently diagnosed essential hypertensive patients without LVH, LA size is directly associated with BP, LV mass index, and brain natriuretic peptide [32].

In general, population-based samples and in hypertensive cohorts LA diameter has been identified as an independent correlate of incident atrial fibrillation and stroke [33, 34]. In addition, a significant association has been reported between LA size and incident CV death or congestive heart failure, after adjusting for major confounders. In the Pressioni Monitorate e Loro Associazioni (PAMELA) study the incidence of new-onset LAE increased significantly from the lowest to the highest tertile of baseline office, home and 24 h BP, body mass index, fasting blood glucose, and LV mass index. In multivariate analysis baseline LA diameter, female gender office systolic BP, body mass index, LV mass index emerged as key predictors of new-onset LA enlargement [35].

Data focusing on the involvement of the LA in prehypertension are really more scant than those addressing the structure and function of the LV. Another limitation that deserves mention refers to different echocardiographic parameters used by various authors to estimate LA size such as anteroposterior diameter, atrial area, non-indexed or indexed for body surface area atrial volume. This heterogeneity of atrial parameters makes it difficult to compare the results of available studies. Prehypertensive subjects enrolled in The Korean Genome Epidemiology Study displayed a significantly higher LA volume (45.3 ± 10.3 mL) than their normotensive counterparts (42.6 ± 10.5 mL), the difference between the two groups persisted to be significant after adjustment for age, gender, body mass index, heart rate, physical activity, smoking, alcohol consumption, fasting glucose, and total cholesterol [36]. A gradual increase in LA size from normotension to hypertension was recently demonstrated by Jung et al. in a general Korean population [16]. Prehypertensive subjects had intermediate LA diameter values (35.4 ± 4.3 mm) between normotensive (33.0 ± 4.3 mm) and hypertensive participants (36.7 ± 4.2 mm).

It is worth of note, however, that other population-based studies failed to demonstrate a more pronounced LA involvement in prehypertension. The largest of these negative reports was the ARIC study [14]. In that elderly population LA volume indexed to body surface area was slightly but not significantly higher in the prehypertensive group (24.0 ± 7.4 mL/m^2) than in those belonging to optimal BP category (23.2 ± 7.4). In line with the aforementioned findings Jang et al. (30) did not find difference in LA volume index between normotensive (26.5 ± 6.5 mL/m^2) and prehypertensive subjects (26.6 ± 6.6 mL/m^2).

12.5 Aortic Root

Growing evidence from studies conducted in the general population and in hypertensive cohorts indicates that AR dilatation may be regarded as a sign of subclinical cardiac organ damage paralleling other markers of established prognostic value such as LVH, LV diastolic dysfunction, and LA dilatation [37]. Indeed, AR dilatation, affecting the most proximal portion of the systemic arterial tree, has been shown to occur more frequently in hypertensive than in normotensives individuals as well as in patients with LVH than in those with normal LV mass [38]. In the PAMELA population office and out-of-office systolic BP and diastolic BP have been shown to have a direct, significant correlation with absolute and indexed AR diameter in univariate analyses; this kind of association persisted significant in multivariate analyses [39]. More importantly, emerging findings, including those recently provided by our group, support the concept that AR dilatation is an independent predictor of cardiovascular morbidity and mortality [39, 40]. Of note, the association between LVH and AR dilatation in the participants of the PAMELA study resulted to be a stronger predictor of long-term cardiovascular outcomes than that entailed by LVH alone.

Literature data addressing the impact of prehypertension on aortic diameter are extremely limited and to the best of our current knowledge no study analyzed specifically this issue. Nevertheless, a couple of studies provided data on AR diameter, as part of the standard echocardiographic examination.

A gender-based analysis focusing on cardiac changes related to prehypertensive status carried out in a relatively small group of apparently healthy Indian subjects ($n = 99$; age range 25–65 years) showed that AR diameter was similar in normotensive and prehypertensive subjects of both sexes [41]. On the contrary, Li et al. [15] assessing echocardiographic variables in large Chinese population-based sample, comprising a total of 10,457 participants, found that AR increased progressively from normotensive (2.16 ± 0.25 cm), to prehypertensive (2.22 ± 0.31 cm) and to hypertensive group (2.28 ± 0.27 cm). From this it is clear that further studies are needed to assess the association between prehypertension and the risk of AR dilatation.

Conclusions

The relevance of systemic hypertension in the pathogenesis of LVH and other markers of subclinical cardiac damage is well established, and a large body of clinical studies has shown strong associations between LV mass and BP in a wide range of values ranging from mild to severe hypertension [42–44]. The present review highlights that cardiac organ damage can occur even in the presence of BP yet within the limits deemed clinically normal. It is worth noting that more robust data on the association between prehypertension and cardiac changes concern subtle but clinically significant increase in LV mass and impairment of diastolic function, whereas less information is available on LA and AR alterations accompanying this BP phenotype. Finally, LV systolic function, as assessed by conventional echocardiographic indexes (i.e., LV ejection fraction) seems to be well preserved in prehypertension, although this conclusion has been recently challenged by the results of studies showing that LV mechanics assessed by three-dimensional echocardiography is significantly impaired in the subjects with high-normal BP. The increased risk of cardiac organ damage in prehypertension is probably related to BP load, due to the continuous relationship between BP and LV mass. However, other factors seem to play a role in this complex relationship. As compared to subjects with optimal BP, higher prevalence rates of masked hypertension, obesity, metabolic syndrome, unhealthy habits such as smoking, drinking, low physical activity have been described in prehypertensive subjects [45]. As widely documented, most of the cited factors may exert an unfavorable effect on cardiac structure and function.

In conclusion, the increased weight of evidence about the clinical and prognostic significance of prehypertension (and this review underlines that subtle cardiac changes can occur before the onset of hypertension) emphasizes the need to intensify current preventive actions by extending them to subjects with prehypertension.

Acknowledgement Disclosure: The authors report no conflicts of interest.

References

1. Martinez MA, Sancho T, Armada E, Rubio JM, Antòn JL, Torre A, Palau J, Seguido P, Gallo J, Saenz I, Polo E, Torres R, Oliver J, Puig JG. Prevalence of left ventricular hypertrophy in patients with mild hypertension in primary care: impact of echocardiography on cardiovascular risk stratification. Am J Hypertens. 2003;16:556–63.
2. de Moraes R, Tibirica E. Early functional and structural microvascular changes in hypertension related to aging. Curr Hypertens Rev. 2017;13:24–32.
3. Vakili BA, Okin PM, Devereux RB. Prognostic implications of left ventricular hypertrophy. Am Heart J. 2001;141:334–41.
4. Cuspidi C, Facchetti R, Bombelli M, Sala C, Tadic M, Grassi G, Mancia G. Prognostic value of left ventricular mass normalized to different body size indexes: findings from the PAMELA population. J Hypertens. 2015;33(5):1082–9.
5. Mathiassen OM, Buus NH, Sihm I, Thybo NK, Morn B, Schroeder AP, Thygesen K, Aalkjaer C, Lederballe O, Mulvany MJ, Christensen KL. Small artery structure is an independent predictor of cardiovascular events in essential hypertension. J Hypertens. 2007;25:1021–6.
6. Ruilope LM, Zanchetti A, Julius S, McInnes GT, Segura J, Stolt P, Hua TA, Weber MA, Jamerson K, VALUE Investigators. Prediction of cardiovascular outcomes by estimated glomerular filtration rate and estimated creatinine clearance in the high-risk hypertension population of the VALUE trial. J Hypertens. 2007;25:1473–9.
7. Ruilope LM, Schmieder RE. Left ventricular hypertrophy and clinical outcomes in hypertensive patients. Am J Hypertens. 2008;21:500–6.
8. Weber KT. Fibrosis and hypertensive heart disease. Curr Opin Cardiol. 2000;15:264–72.
9. Lewington S, Clarke R, Qizilbash N, Peto R, Collins R. Age-specific relevance of usual blood pressure to vascular mortality: a meta-analysis of individual data for one million adults in 61 prospective studies. Lancet. 2002;360:1903–13.
10. Huang Y, Wang S, Cai X, Mai W, Hu Y, Tang H, Xu D. Prehypertension and incidence of cardiovascular disease: a meta-analysis. BMC Med. 2013;11:177.
11. Moreno MU, Eiros R, Gavira JJ, Gallego C, González A, Ravassa S, López B, Beaumont J, San José G, Díez J. The hypertensive myocardium: from microscopic lesions to clinical complications and outcomes. Med Clin North Am. 2017;101:43–52.
12. Drukteinis JS, Roman MJ, Fabsitz RR, Lee ET, Best LG, Russell M, Devereux RB. Cardiac and systemic hemodynamic characteristics of hypertension and prehypertension in adolescents and young adults: the Strong Heart Study. Circulation. 2007;115:221–7.
13. Ganau A, Devereux RB, Roman MJ, de Simone G, Pickering TG, Saba PS, Vargiu P, Simongini I, Laragh JH. Patterns of left ventricular hypertrophy and geometric remodeling in essential hypertension. J Am Coll Cardiol. 1992;19:1550–8.

14. Santos ABS, Gupta DK, Bello NA, Gori M, Claggett B, Fuchs FD, Shah AM, Coresh J, Sharrett AR, Cheng S, Solomon SD. Prehypertension is associated with abnormalities of cardiac structure and function in the atherosclerosis risk in communities study. Am J Hypertens. 2016;29:568–74.
15. Li T, Yang J, Guo X, Chen S, Sun Y. Geometrical and functional changes of left heart in adults with prehypertension and hypertension: a cross-sectional study from China. BMC Cardiovasc Disord. 2016;16:114.
16. Jung JY, Park SK, Oh CM, Kang JG, Choi JM, Ryoo JH, Lee JH. The influence of prehypertension, controlled and uncontrolled hypertension on left ventricular diastolic function and structure in the general Korean population. Hypertens Res. 2017;40:606–12.
17. Markus MR, Stritzke J, Lieb W, Mayer B, Luchner A, Döring A, Keil U, Hense HW, Schunkert H. Implications of persistent prehypertension for ageing-related changes in left ventricular geometry and function: the MONICA/KORA Augsburg study. J Hypertens. 2008;26:2040–9.
18. Pickering TG, Davidson K, Gerin W, Schwartz JE. Masked hypertension. Hypertension. 2002;40:795–6.
19. Shimbo D, Newman JD, Schwartz JE. Masked hypertension and prehypertension: diagnostic overlap and interrelationship with left ventricular mass: the masked hypertension study. Am J Hypertens. 2012;25:664–71.
20. Norton GR, Maseko M, Libhaber E, Libhaber CD, Majane OH, Dessein P, Sareli P, Woodiwiss AJ. Is prehypertension an independent predictor of target organ changes in young-to-middle-aged persons of African descent ? J Hypertens. 2008;26:2279–87.
21. Manios E, Tsivgoulis G, Koroboki E, Stamatelopoulos K, Papamichael C, Toumanidis S, Stamboulis E, Vemmos K, Zakopoulos N. Impact of prehypertension on common carotid artery intima-media thickness and left ventricular mass. Stroke. 2009;40:1515–8.
22. Mousa TM, Akinseye OA, Berekashvili K, Akinboboye OO. Correlation of prehypertension with left ventricular mass assessed by cardiac magnetic resonance imaging. Int J Hypertens. 2015;2015, Article ID 742658.
23. Di Bello V, Talini E, Dell'Omo G, Giannini C, Delle Donne MG, Canale ML, Nardi C, Palagi C, Dini FL, Penno G, Del Prato S, Marzilli M, Pedrinelli R. Early left ventricular mechanics abnormalities in prehypertension: a two-dimensional strain echocardiography study. Am J Hypertens. 2010;23:405–12.
24. Tadic M, Majstorovic A, Pencic B, Ivanovic B, Neskovic A, Badano L, Stanisavljevic D, Scepanovic R, Stevanovic P, Celic V. The impact of high-normal blood pressure on left ventricular mechanics: a three-dimensional and speckle tracking echocardiography study. Int J Cardiovasc Imaging. 2014;30:699–711.
25. Lang RM, Badano LP, Mor-Avi V, Afilalo J, Armstrong A, Ernande L, Flachskampf FA, Foster E, Goldstein SA, Kuznetsova T, Lancellotti P, Muraru D, Picard MH, Rietzschel ER, Rudski L, Spencer KT, Tsang W, Voigt JU. Recommendations for cardiac chamber quantification by echocardiography in adults: an update from the American Society of Echocardiography and the European Association of Cardiovascular Imaging. J Am Soc Echocardiogr. 2015;28:1–39.
26. Frohlich E, Gonzales A, Diez J. Hypertensive left ventricular hypertrophy risk: beyond adaptive cardiomyocytic hypertrophy. J Hypertens. 2011;29:17–26.
27. Chahal NS, Kim TK, Jain P, Chambers JC, Kooner JS, Senior R. New insights into the relationship of left ventricular geometry and left ventricular mass with cardiac function: a population study of hypertensive subjects. Eur Heart J. 2010;31:588–94.
28. Zanchetti A, Cuspidi C, Comarella L, Agabiti-Rosei E, Ambrosioni E, Chiarello M, Leonetti G, Mancia G, Pessina AC, Salvetti A, Trimarco B, Volpe M, Grassivaro N, Vargiu G. Left ventricular diastolic dysfunction in elderly hypertensives: results of the APROS-diadys study. J Hypertens. 2007;25:2158–67.
29. Urbina EM, Khoury PR, McCoy C, Daniels SR, Kimball TR, Dolan LM. Cardiac and vascular consequences of pre-hypertension in youth. J Clin Hypertens. 2011;13:332–42.
30. Jang SY, Kim S, Lee CK, Cho EJ, Cho SJ, Lee SC. Prehypertension and left ventricular diastolic dysfunction in middle-aged Koreans. Korean Circ J. 2016;46:536–41.
31. Douglas P. The left atrium. A biomarker of chronic diastolic dysfunction and cardiovascular disease risk. J Am Coll Cardiol. 2003;42:1206–7.

32. Tsioufis C, Stougiannos P, Taxiarchou E, Skiadas I, Chatzis D, Thomopoulos C, Lalos S, Stefanadis C, Kallikazaros I. The interplay between hemodynamic load, brain natriuretic peptide and left atrial size in the early stages of essential hypertension. J Hypertens. 2006;24:965–72.
33. Benjamin EJ, D'Agostino RB, Belanger AJ, Wolf PA, Levy D. Left atrial size and the risk of stroke and death: the Framingham Heart Study. Circulation. 1995;92:835–41.
34. Bombelli M, Facchetti R, Cuspidi C, Villa P, Dozio D, Brambilla G, Grassi G, Mancia G. Prognostic significance of left atrial enlargement in a general population: results of the PAMELA study. Hypertension. 2014;64:1205–11.
35. Bombelli M, Cuspidi C, Facchetti R, Sala C, Tadic M, Brambilla G, Re A, Villa P, Grassi G, Mancia G. New-onset left atrial enlargement in a general population. J Hypertens. 2016;34:1838–45.
36. Kim SH, Cho GY, Baik I, Lim SY, Choi CU, Lim HE, Kim EJ, Park CG, Park J, Kim J, Shin C. Early abnormalities of cardiovascular structure and function in middle-aged Korean adults with prehypertension: the Korean Genome Epidemiology study. Am J Hypertens. 2011;24:218–24.
37. Cipolli JA, Souza FAS, Ferreira-Sae MCS, Magalhaes JAP, Figueiredo ES, Vidotti VG, Matos-Souza JR, Franchini KG, Nadruz W. Sex-specific hemodynamic and non-hemodynamic determinants of aortic root size in hypertensive subjects with left ventricular hypertrophy. Hypertens Res. 2009;32:956–61.
38. Covella M, Milan A, Totaro S, Cuspidi C, Re A, Rabbia F, Veglio F. Echocardiographic aortic root dilatation in hypertensive patients: a systematic review and meta-analysis. J Hypertens. 2014;32:1928–35.
39. Gardin JM, Arnold AM, Polak J, Jackson S, Smith V, Gottdiener J. Usefulness of aortic root dimension in persons >65 years of age in predicting heart failure, stroke, cardiovascular mortality, all-cause mortality and acute myocardial infarction (from the Cardiovascular Health Study). Am J Cardiol. 2006;97:270–5.
40. Cuspidi C, Facchetti R, Bombelli M, Re A, Cairo M, Sala C, Tadic M, Grassi G, Mancia G. Aortic root diameter and risk of cardiovascular events in a general population: data from the PAMELA study. J Hypertens. 2014;32:1879–8.
41. Bajpai JK, Sahay AP, Agarwal AK, De AK, Garg B, Goel A. Impact of prehypertension on left ventricular structure, function and geometry. J Clin Diagn Res. 2014;8:BC07–10.
42. Mancia G, Carugo S, Grassi G, Lanzarotti A, Schiavina R, Cesana GC, Sega R. Prevalence of left ventricular hypertrophy in hypertensive patients without and with blood pressure control: data from the PAMELA population. Hypertension. 2002;39:744–9.
43. Abdalla M, Booth JN, Diaz KM, Sims M, Muntner P, Shimbo D. Hypertension and alterations in left ventricular structure and geometry in African Americans: the Jackson Heart Study. J Am Soc Hypertens. 2016;10:550–8.
44. Nakanishi K, Jin Z, Homma S, Elkind MSV, Rundek T Tugcu A, Sacco RL, Di Tullio MR. Association of blood pressure control level with left ventricular morphology and function and with subclinical cerebrovascular disease. J Am Heart Assoc. 2017;6(8):e006246.
45. Guo X, Zou L, Zhang X, Li J, Zheng L, Sun Z, Hu J, Wong ND, Sun Y. Prehypertension : a meta-analysis of the epidemiology, risk factors, and predictors of progression. Tex Heart Inst J. 2011;38:643–52.

Hemodynamics of Prehypertension

13

Peter W. de Leeuw, Barry van Varik, Daan J. L. van Twist, and Abraham A. Kroon

13.1 Introduction

Despite decades of intensive research, the etiology of essential hypertension remains unknown. Once this disorder has reached its established phase, it is characterized hemodynamically by an elevated peripheral vascular resistance and a normal or slightly reduced cardiac output [1]. In addition, vascular stiffness is increased which over time will result in a further rise in systolic pressure and vascular resistance. This creates a vicious cycle with, if left untreated, an ever-increasing blood pressure. Other pathophysiological features that characterize the phase of established hypertension are reduced renal blood flow, increased filtration fraction, and a tendency towards a lower plasma volume. Both the sympathetic nervous system (SNS) and the renin-angiotensin-aldosterone system (RAAS) have been implicated in these abnormalities but their precise role in the initiation and development of the hypertensive process has still not been fully clarified.

The elucidation of the pathogenetic processes leading to established hypertension requires that the factors responsible for the initiation of the disease be known. The ideal way of investigating these factors would be to follow-up normotensive individuals up to the point where they become hypertensive. For obvious reasons, such studies are not feasible, not the least because one would not know who will become hypertensive and who not. In fact, many if not most of them may never

P. W. de Leeuw (✉)
Department of Medicine, Maastricht University Medical Centre, Maastricht, The Netherlands

Department of Medicine, Zuyderland Medical Center, Geleen/Heerlen, The Netherlands
e-mail: p.deleeuw@maastrichtuniversity.nl

B. van Varik · D. J. L. van Twist
Department of Medicine, Zuyderland Medical Center, Geleen/Heerlen, The Netherlands

A. A. Kroon
Department of Medicine, Maastricht University Medical Centre, Maastricht, The Netherlands

R. Zimlichman et al. (eds.), *Prehypertension and Cardiometabolic Syndrome*,
Updates in Hypertension and Cardiovascular Protection,
https://doi.org/10.1007/978-3-319-75310-2_13

develop hypertension at all. Alternatively, one could study the offspring of hypertensive patients and compare this offspring to that of normotensive parents. In doing so, one enriches the population with people who are likely to develop hypertension at some point in their life. This type of approach has been repeatedly applied, but again it is uncertain whether children from hypertensive parents will, indeed, ever become hypertensive. In addition, one runs the risk of mixing up true genetic influences with familial ones such as environment and diet.

Finally, one could attempt to investigate individuals who are already somewhere on their way from the normotensive to the hypertensive state. Again, this is not an easy category to study but it comprises the people who could be labeled as being prehypertensive. It seems that this group of patients is not too dissimilar from that which was designated in the past with such terms as "labile hypertension" or "borderline hypertension." The term "labile hypertension" has been largely abandoned because, in fact, nearly all patients with hypertension have some degree of lability of their blood pressure. Borderline hypertensives are people who sometimes cross the line of normality in terms of blood pressure but who at other times are completely normotensive. According to a much-used definition it is a condition in which blood pressure is sometimes below but more often above the arbitrary 140/90 mmHg cutoff point that separates normotension from hypertension. One would think, therefore, that this is a transitory state in which an individual gradually moves from being truly normotensive to being truly hypertensive. As such, one could label this state also as prehypertension although it is not entirely the same. Prehypertension was defined in the Seventh Report of the Joint National Committee (JNC-7) as a blood pressure, based on the average of two or more properly measured, seated, readings on each of two or more office visits from 120 to 139 mmHg systolic or from 80 to 89 mmHg diastolic [2]. Thus, an evolutionary scheme could be: true normotension-prehypertension-borderline hypertension-true hypertension. Admittedly, we do not know with certainty whether people go, indeed, through these stages of prehypertension and borderline hypertension and in the past borderline hypertension has often been considered as an "illness" in its own right. Still, data from the Framingham study suggest that a normal or high-normal blood pressure frequently progresses to full hypertension [3] and that this is associated with an increased cardiovascular risk [4]. So, until there is firm evidence to the contrary, we do best to consider prehypertension and borderline hypertension as, presumably transient, phases in the hypertensive process.

13.2 Systemic Hemodynamics in Borderline Hypertension

Blood pressure (BP), in hemodynamic terms, is determined by cardiac output (CO) and total peripheral resistance (TPR) according to the formula: BP = CO × TPR. Whether the very early phases of hypertension are related to a rise in vascular resistance or in cardiac output or both has for years been a matter of vigorous debate. Initially, the hemodynamic studies focused primarily on young, borderline hypertensives. Most of these studies found that cardiac output, when corrected for body size and expressed as cardiac index (L/m^2), as well as heart rate is increased by about 15% in borderline hypertensives as compared to matched normotensives [5, 6]. Since cardiac output is the product of heart rate and stroke volume, in theory both components could be involved. However, it turns out that the rise in cardiac output in borderline hypertensives is mainly due to an elevated heart rate and far less to alterations in stroke volume. In a series of elegant experiments, Julius and coworkers have shown that both enhanced sympathetic and reduced parasympathetic activity can be held accountable for the "hyperkinetic" heart [7]. These investigators found that heart rate became normal after total autonomic blockade with propranolol and atropine combined (but not after any one of these alone) which suggests that the pacemaker by itself acts normally but that it is rendered overactive by neurogenic influences. The same researchers also found stroke volume index to be slightly increased but several other studies failed to find a difference in this variable between normotensives and borderline hypertensives. Overall, therefore, the case for a hyperkinetic heart in borderline hypertension seems to be stronger with respect to frequency than to stroke volume. It must be emphasized, though, that in virtually all publications only mean values are presented for the hemodynamic data. Nevertheless, interindividual variations were substantial and true increases are apparent in only about one-third of the patients [6]. Finally, total peripheral resistance was, on average, increased in the group with borderline hypertension. Even though resistance was numerically normal in those with a hyperkinetic heart, it was inappropriately high for the degree of systemic flow. Therefore, it is safe to conclude that borderline hypertension, if we consider this to be an early phase of hypertension, is characterized by an augmented vascular resistance either with or without a hyperkinetic heart.

13.3 Systemic Hemodynamics in Prehypertension

If we want to try to catch potential hemodynamic abnormalities in even earlier phases of the hypertensive process, it is worthwhile to explore systemic hemodynamics in individuals with prehypertension. This has been done, for instance, in the Strong Heart Study which is a population-based survey of cardiovascular risk factors and cardiovascular disease in several American Indian communities [8]. At the fourth follow-up examination of this study, Drukteinis and coworkers recruited 1940 participants below 40 years of age (average age 27 years) of whom 971 were normotensive, 294 were hypertensive, and 675 fulfilled the criteria of prehypertension (35%). In all these participants, echocardiographic measurements were obtained to estimate cardiac mass and performance. Compared to normotensives, heart rate and cardiac output were significantly higher in the prehypertensives. However, cardiac index did not differ between groups and averaged 2.67 and 2.73 mL/min m^2, respectively, in the normotensives and prehypertensives (Fig. 13.1). These numbers are notably lower than those registered in earlier studies in borderline hypertension [6]. Of note, in the prehypertension group more people were obese and/or had diabetes or impaired glucose tolerance. However, adjustment for

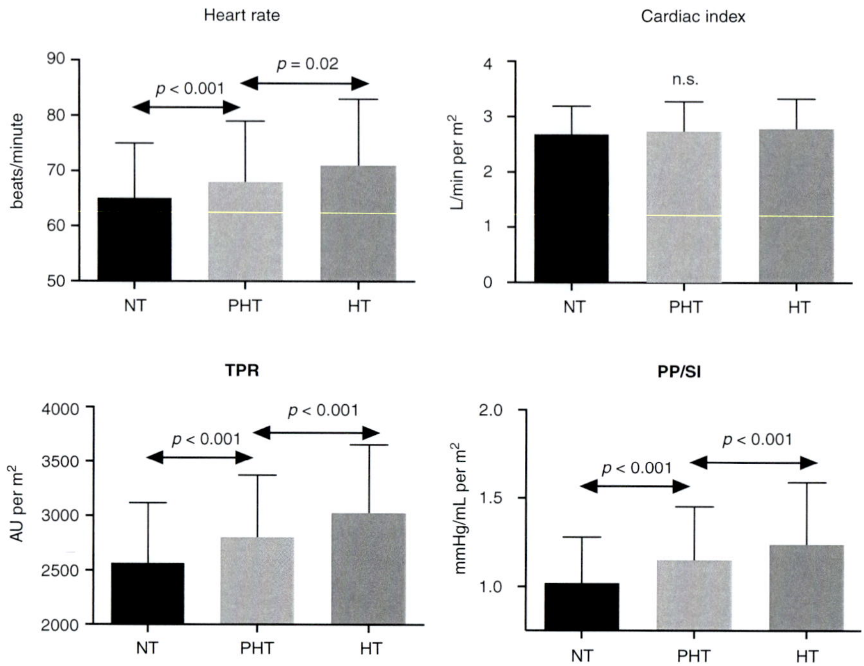

Fig. 13.1 Systemic hemodynamics in normotension (NT), prehypertension (PHT), and hypertension (HT). Adapted from the Strong Heart Study [8]

these confounders did not change the results. Total peripheral resistance index was higher in prehypertension and so was the pulse pressure/stroke index quotient. The latter can be considered as a proxy for arterial stiffness, which apparently is already increased in prehypertension as well. In addition, the prehypertensive group showed a greater left ventricular mass and more often frank left ventricular hypertrophy. Incidentally, besides a higher systolic pressure, the presence of left ventricular hypertrophy also appeared to be a predictor of further progression from prehypertension to hypertension [9].

Almost at the same time, Zhu and coworkers reported on their findings in an even younger group (average age 17 years) with prehypertension [10]. In white prehypertensives, these investigators also found a higher heart rate and total peripheral resistance together with a normal cardiac index (measured with impedance cardiography), which is in line with the data from the Strong Heart Study. However, in blacks they found the opposite hemodynamic pattern, i.e., a higher cardiac index but a normal heart rate and total peripheral resistance. Again, the latter still is inappropriately high in relation to the prevailing level of cardiac output because resistance should have fallen in the face of the high systemic flow (Fig. 13.2). Another race-related feature was arterial stiffness which was greater in white prehypertensives compared to white normotensives but not different between the two blood pressure groups in blacks.

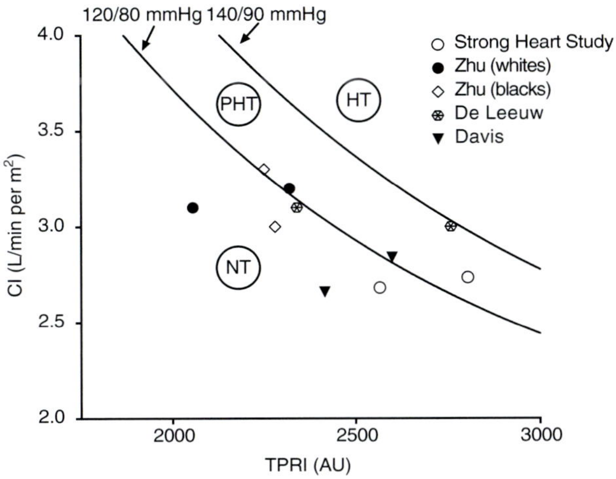

Fig. 13.2 Balance between cardiac index (CI = cardiac output normalized for body surface area) and total peripheral resistance index (TPRI = resistance indexed for body surface area) in normotensives (NT), prehypertensives (PHT), and hypertensives (HT). The "isobars" indicating the lines for a pressure of 120/80 mmHg and 140/90 mmHg mark the boundaries between prehypertension and normotension and between prehypertension and hypertension, respectively. Note that in prehypertensives even a high cardiac output is already associated with an inappropriately elevated vascular resistance. Data derived from Drukteinis et al. [8], Zhu et al. [10], Davis et al. [11], and De Leeuw et al. [13]

A little later, Davis and associates published their results with respect to the autonomic and hemodynamic origins of prehypertension [11]. They obtained their data from the UCSD twin/family study and compared 340 prehypertensives with 337 normotensives of comparable age. For the hemodynamic measurements, an oscillometric device was used which collects several cardiac and vascular functional data. Also in this study, mean heart rate and cardiac output were significantly higher in the prehypertensive group and so was stroke volume. Remarkably, when normalized for body surface area the differences persisted. Total peripheral resistance was numerically similar in the two groups but one could argue that this was still inappropriately elevated for the height of cardiac output in the prehypertensives (Fig. 13.2). Other striking findings in the prehypertensives included enhanced cardiac contractility, a wider pulse pressure and reduced brachial artery distensibility and systemic vascular compliance, which is indicative for an increased vascular stiffness.

Finally, Pal and colleagues studied a group of 118 normotensives and 58 prehypertensives of approximately 20 years of age and found both cardiac output and total peripheral vascular resistance to be significantly higher in the latter [12]. Although body mass index was substantially higher in the prehypertensives, the authors failed to normalize their hemodynamic data. Thus, we do not know whether the increase in cardiac output was also elevated in relation to body surface area or not. But regardless of cardiac index, their data also point to at least an increase in vascular resistance.

In our own laboratory, we have studied a small group of young, male medical students who at one time had proven to be hypertensive, but later had blood pressures in the prehypertensive range [13]. They were compared to another group of young individuals, who were normotensive all the time. In each one of them we recorded blood pressure and noninvasively determined cardiac output and left ventricular ejection time by means of impedance cardiography. Importantly, all participants were put on a mildly sodium-restricted diet to avoid salt-dependent interindividual variations. In our hands, there were no differences in heart rate, stroke volume, cardiac output, and left ventricular ejection time between the two groups. Total peripheral vascular resistance, however, was significantly higher in the prehypertensives. Moreover, the pulse pressure over stroke index ratio as a proxy for systemic arterial stiffness was increased as well in these prehypertensives.

Taken together, the results of the various studies using different populations and different methodology are rather consistent in the sense that they suggest that even in prehypertension the peripheral vasculature is the main source of the elevated pressure. Moreover, an increase in vascular stiffness is a uniform finding [8, 10–15]. Undoubtedly, abnormalities in the microcirculation contribute to enhanced vascular stiffness on the one hand and an increased burden to the heart on the other.

13.4 Comparison with Established Hypertension

As little information there is concerning hemodynamics in prehypertension, as much is there about hemodynamic patterns in patients with established hypertension [6]. There is general agreement that in those in whom hypertension is still uncomplicated, the elevated pressure is maintained by an increased total peripheral resistance. By and large, heart rate remains higher in the hypertensives as well, but cardiac output is either normal or only slightly reduced.

In the Strong Heart Study, prehypertensives were not only compared to normotensives but also to hypertensives with respect to their hemodynamic indices [8]. These data also show that heart rate was significantly higher in the hypertensives while cardiac index was similar. Total peripheral vascular resistance, when indexed for body surface area, was significantly greater in the hypertensives as well. The pulse pressure to stroke index ratio, as proxy for vascular stiffness, was clearly greater in the hypertensives compared to the normotensives with the prehypertensives taking an intermediate position.

In their twin study, Davis and coworkers found significant trends across their groups of normotensives, prehypertensives, and hypertensives with respect to heart rate, cardiac index, pulse pressure, and vascular stiffness [11]. These were all lowest in the normotensives and highest in the hypertensives. The opposite trend was seen for brachial artery distensibility which was lowest in the hypertensives. Except for pulse pressure, however, post hoc analysis failed to find statistical differences in any of these variables between the prehypertensives and the hypertensives. Total peripheral vascular resistance was not different across or between the three groups.

Even though conventional significance levels were not reached in most of the post hoc analyses, the trends are clearly in agreement with the data from the Strong Heart Study in that the "transition" from prehypertension to frank hypertension is associated with an invariably increased heart rate, no or only small changes in cardiac output, and a further rise in arterial stiffness. In numerical terms, vascular resistance may remain unaltered but even then, it signifies an inability to vasodilate properly in response to a normal or enhanced systemic flow.

In our own study on the medical students, we also compared the prehypertensives to a group of matched hypertensives (unpublished data). The latter had a lower cardiac index and a higher vascular resistance and stiffness, without any difference in heart rate. Regarding the vascular abnormalities, therefore, these data also tally well with the previous ones.

13.5 Regional Hemodynamics

Total peripheral resistance is the sum of the resistances (calculated as for parallel circuits) in the various organs of the body. The magnitude of resistance to blood flow in any single organ determines which fraction of the cardiac output will be directed to it. Thus, if we would be able to simultaneously measure cardiac output and regional flows we could explore whether the rise in total resistance is a generalized phenomenon or preferentially occurs in specific organs. A rise in resistance occurs in all vascular beds that have been studied in hypertensives but it is particularly striking in that of the kidney [16]. Renal fraction, which is the proportion of cardiac output that flows through the kidneys, falls with age in hypertensives, indicating that the degree of vasoconstriction in the kidney becomes progressively greater than the rise in resistance elsewhere in the body. However, it is impossible to tell whether this preferential renal vasoconstriction is the cause or the consequence of a higher blood pressure.

Even in this established phase of the hypertensive process glomerular filtration rate is well maintained for a long time so that filtration fraction which is defined as glomerular filtration rate as a percentage of the renal plasma flow gradually rises with the increase in renal vascular resistance. This suggests that the postglomerular resistance increases faster or more than preglomerular resistance. Only when the delivery of blood to the kidneys becomes severely compromised, filtration will fall. Although these pathophysiological features have been well described for established hypertension, only limited information is available with respect to the early phases of hypertension. If we turn again to borderline hypertension, the data from Messerli and coworkers on the renal and the splanchnic vascular beds are of relevance. These investigators studied 41 patients with borderline hypertension who were subdivided in groups with low, normal, or high cardiac output [17]. Except for cardiac output they also measured renal and splanchnic blood flow by means of radio-iodinated PAH and indocyanine green clearance, respectively. Both renal and splanchnic blood flow correlated significantly with cardiac output indicating that, at least in this patient population, the fractional distribution of systemic flow to the kidneys and the splanchnic organs remains unaltered. In other words, the observed increase in vascular resistance at this stage is generalized and not preferential in, for instance, the kidneys. In a later study, Messerli's group explored the relationship of renal blood flow and cardiac output with age in normotensives and in borderline hypertensives [18]. In both groups, they found a parallel decline in systemic and renal flow with ageing. In other words, at any age the distribution of cardiac output over the kidneys and probably other organs is comparable in normotensives and borderline hypertensives. Thus, if there is no sustained hypertension, there is no preferential vasoconstriction in the renal vasculature.

Although a few studies have addressed regional flow patterns in prehypertension, no such data exist in combination with estimations of cardiac output except those from our own study in the medical students. In those, renal fraction was not different either between the normotensives and the prehypertensives and, if anything, even slightly higher in the latter (22 vs. 20%). Renal vascular resistance in the prehypertensives was numerically comparable to that in normotensives, but given the slightly higher blood pressure in the former, one could still consider this as being too high.

Despite the increase in renal vascular resistance, perfusion of the kidneys was even somewhat greater in the prehypertensive students than in their normotensive counterparts. Such a pattern of relative "overperfusion" has been seen in other studies as well and seems to "affect" about one-third of young people in their early stages of hypertension [19, 20]. The reason for the increased flow rate is not clear but may involve a mechanism to protect the glomeruli. Indeed, when glomerular filtration rate remains intact for a very long time despite a progressive decline in renal plasma flow, this will lead to an increased filtration fraction just as in patients with established hypertension. It is thought that a rise in postglomerular resistance is necessary to maintain filtration in the face of an enhanced preglomerular resistance but this may also expose some glomeruli to the detrimental effect of an augmented intraglomerular pressure. If the kidney now recruits dormant nephrons and increases total flow in order to perfuse these recruited nephrons, the filtration process can be divided over a greater surface area without the necessity to raise pressure in these glomeruli. This hypothetical sequence of events, however, needs to be confirmed in proper experiments.

As for other organs, there is a study from Turkey in 40 individuals with prehypertension and 50 healthy volunteers who underwent transthoracic Doppler echocardiography to assess cardiac dimensions and coronary flow reserve (CFR) [21]. The two groups did not differ with respect to left ventricular mass and heart rate but CFR was significantly lower in the prehypertension group. Although these data point towards an increased resistance in the coronary vascular bed of prehypertensives, it is impossible to know whether this increase is proportional to that of systemic vascular resistance.

Finally, Italian investigators have shown that in people with prehypertension frequently abnormalities of the retinal circulation are found, including arteriolar narrowing and, consequently, a reduced arteriolar-to-venular ratio [22].

13.6 Follow-up Studies

All of the data described above have been obtained in cross-sectional studies which have only limited value for our understanding of the natural evolution of the hypertensive process. Thus, longitudinal studies are indispensable to explore how hemodynamics change over time. By far the most informative (and only) long-term study in this regard is that of Lund-Johansson [6]. This investigator has followed a group of young hypertensive individuals and age-matched normotensive controls for a period of 20 years with similar invasive hemodynamic measurements after 10 and 20 years. Although the hypertensives had slightly elevated blood pressures which precluded a diagnosis of borderline hypertension, they could be considered to be in a very early phase of hypertension that still did not require treatment. At the start of the study, heart rate and cardiac index were about 15% higher in the hypertensives who were then 17–29 years of age. After 10 years, blood pressure had changed remarkably little. Nevertheless, total peripheral resistance had increased significantly, while cardiac index and stroke volume index had fallen. Compared to the normotensives, heart rate remained elevated. During the following 10 years, all these changes progressed so that at the 20-year follow-up evaluation cardiac performance was even lower and vascular resistance higher with only minor changes in heart rate.

In our laboratory, we performed repeat examinations of systemic and renal hemodynamics in the prehypertensive group of medical students as well as in the matched hypertensives after 2 years of follow-up [13]. During this time only the hypertensive participants received antihypertensive medication which was discontinued prior to the measurements. Although cardiac output and stroke volume showed a tendency to fall over the two-year period in the prehypertensives, the differences were not statistically significant. The same was true for total peripheral resistance which tended to rise slightly. Heart rate did not change and arterial stiffness remained invariably increased. In the hypertensives, cardiac output fell to a greater extent, together with a rise in resistance and arterial stiffness. Renal blood flow fell slightly in both the prehypertensives and the hypertensives with a rise in renal vascular resistance that was proportional to that in systemic resistance in both groups.

13.7 Pathophysiological Considerations

According to the classical concept of whole-body autoregulation an increased cardiac output will elicit a vasoconstrictor response to prevent overperfusion of tissues and a disturbance of homeostasis [23]. This, in turn, will bring back cardiac output to its original level but at the expense of a raised vascular resistance and, hence, an increased blood pressure. It has long been thought that this sequence of events, which was based on observations in experimental animals, would be applicable to hypertensive humans as well. Many of the hemodynamic observations that have been obtained in patients in different stages of their hypertension do, indeed, suggest that also in man hypertension evolves from a high-output, normal resistance state into a low-output, high-resistance state. The high-output state at the early phase of hypertension or during the period of prehypertension is often explained by enhanced sympathetic activity or altered volume homeostasis. The increase in resistance over time is then seen as the equivalent of the whole-body autoregulation mechanism. There are, however, several arguments against the hypothesis of this hemodynamic transition. First, a high-output state does not necessarily lead to an increased resistance or to hypertension. Clinical examples include severe anemia, hyperthyroidism, arteriovenous anastomoses as in Paget's disease, beri-beri, and Gorlin's syndrome. These are all conditions in which cardiac output may sometimes be extremely high, yet is not followed by a (progressive) rise in vascular resistance. Secondly, an autoregulatory vasoconstrictor response occurs only when tissue perfusion exceeds metabolic demands (so-called luxury perfusion) but this does not occur in humans [6]. Indeed, the rise in cardiac output is entirely proportional to oxygen consumption. Thirdly, not all patients with borderline hypertension or prehypertension have an increased cardiac output. Thus, a hyperkinetic circulation is not at all a prerequisite to develop sustained hypertension. Finally, there are patients with high-output borderline hypertension or prehypertension who will never progress to the state of hypertension and sometimes may even "regress" again to normotension.

As a matter of fact, there is no need to invoke a cardiac driver of hypertension if we focus more on vascular resistance itself. As already outlined above, even a numerically normal vascular resistance is still elevated in the face of the prevailing level of cardiac output, regardless of whether output is increased or not. With a high systemic flow that is appropriate in relation to tissue demands, the normal response would be peripheral vasodilation to prevent a rise in blood pressure. Thus, effectively all hemodynamic studies point to a disturbance of vasoregulation, even in the very early stages of hypertension or prehypertension. If we accept the fact that hypertension always starts as an abnormal vasoconstrictor state (from whatever cause), we could see an increased variability of blood pressure and cardiac output just as secondary phenomena. Whether cardiac output will be normal or high will then depend on what "force" is needed for adequate tissue perfusion.

Collectively, the available data strongly suggest that in prehypertension and borderline hypertension or, for that matter, the early stages of hypertension there is no preferential increase in vascular resistance in any specific organ and certainly not in the kidney. This renders an initiating role of (relative) renal ischemia as the cause of hypertension less likely. It is beyond the scope of this chapter to elaborate on the possible causes of the abnormal resistance but likely genetic, endothelial, and neurohumoral factors will play an important role. Whatever mechanisms are involved, any theory on the pathogenesis of hypertension must account for this generalized, hence non-localized, increase in resistance.

Conclusions

If we try to reconcile the findings described above in a hypothetical scheme concerning the development of hypertension, it is likely that the transition from normotension to established hypertension may first go through a phase of prehypertension and then borderline hypertension. Likely, the duration of these phases is variable and unpredictable with some people progressing very fast and others staying in one of these phases for a long time with perhaps even a return to normal pressures. The general increase in resistance as seen in prehypertension causes only a minor rise in blood pressure which is maintained because cardiac output cannot fall because of the metabolic demands. In principle, this phase can last for a long time. On the long run, systemic resistance probably further increases due to (inappropriate) vascular remodeling, i.e., increased vascular stiffness, resulting in propagation to borderline and established hypertension. Perhaps it is only when the renal fraction falls and the kidney gets jeopardized that the transition to full-blown hypertension is set in motion with the kidney now probably taking on a culprit role. While these are hypothetical thoughts, they may form a good starting point for future hemodynamic studies in prehypertension and hypertension.

References

1. Birkenhäger WH, De Leeuw PW, Schalekamp MADH. Control mechanisms in essential hypertension. Amsterdam: Elsevier Biomedical Press; 1982.
2. Chobanian AV, Bakris GL, Black HR, Cushman WC, Green LA, Izzo JL Jr, et al. The seventh report of the joint National Committee on prevention, detection, evaluation, and treatment of high blood pressure: the JNC 7 report. JAMA. 2003;289(19):2560–72.
3. Vasan RS, Larson MG, Leip EP, Kannel WB, Levy D. Assessment of frequency of progression to hypertension in non-hypertensive participants in the Framingham Heart Study: a cohort study. Lancet. 2001;358(9294):1682–6.
4. Vasan RS, Larson MG, Leip EP, Evans JC, O'Donnell CJ, Kannel WB, et al. Impact of high-normal blood pressure on the risk of cardiovascular disease. N Engl J Med. 2001;345(18):1291–7.
5. Birkenhager WH. A critical interpretation of juvenile borderline hypertension. J Hypertens. 1991;9(Suppl 6):S2–9.
6. Omvik P, Lund-Johansen P. Hemodynamics of hypertension. In: Mancia G, Grassi G, Redon J, editors. Manual of hypertension of the European Society of Hypertension. 2nd ed. Boca Raton, FL: CRC Press; 2014. p. 101–14.
7. Julius S, Esler M. Autonomic nervous cardiovascular regulation in borderline hypertension. Am J Cardiol. 1975;36(5):685–96.
8. Drukteinis JS, Roman MJ, Fabsitz RR, Lee ET, Best LG, Russell M, et al. Cardiac and systemic hemodynamic characteristics of hypertension and prehypertension in adolescents and young adults: the Strong Heart Study. Circulation. 2007;115(2):221–7.
9. De Marco M, de Simone G, Roman MJ, Chinali M, Lee ET, Russell M, et al. Cardiovascular and metabolic predictors of progression of prehypertension into hypertension: the Strong Heart Study. Hypertension. 2009;54(5):974–80.
10. Zhu H, Yan W, Ge D, Treiber FA, Harshfield GA, Kapuku G, et al. Cardiovascular characteristics in American youth with prehypertension. Am J Hypertens. 2007;20(10):1051–7.
11. Davis JT, Rao F, Naqshbandi D, Fung MM, Zhang K, Schork AJ, et al. Autonomic and hemodynamic origins of pre-hypertension: central role of heredity. J Am Coll Cardiol. 2012;59(24):2206–16.
12. Pal GK, Adithan C, Ananthanarayanan PH, Pal P, Nanda N, Thiyagarajan D, et al. Association of sympathovagal imbalance with cardiovascular risks in young prehypertensives. Am J Cardiol. 2013;112(11):1757–62.

13. De Leeuw PW, Kho TL, Birkenhäger WH. Pathophysiologic features of hypertension in young men. Chest. 1983;83(2 Suppl):312–4.
14. Gedikli O, Kiris A, Ozturk S, Baltaci D, Karaman K, Durmus I, et al. Effects of prehypertension on arterial stiffness and wave reflections. Clin Exp Hypertens. 2010;32(2):84–9.
15. Davis JT, Pasha DN, Khandrika S, Fung MM, Milic M, O'Connor DT. Central hemodynamics in prehypertension: effect of the beta-adrenergic antagonist nebivolol. J Clin Hypertens (Greenwich). 2013;15(1):69–74.
16. Birkenhäger WH, De Leeuw PW, Derkx FHM. The kidney in hypertension-background and practical implications. Hypertens Res. 1993;16(1):3–15.
17. Messerli FH, De Carvalho JG, Christie B, Frohlich ED. Systemic and regional hemodynamics in low, normal and high cardiac output borderline hypertension. Circulation. 1978;58(3 Pt 1):441–8.
18. Schmieder RE, Schachinger H, Messerli FH. Accelerated decline in renal perfusion with aging in essential hypertension. Hypertension. 1994;23(3):351–7.
19. Bianchi G, Cusi D, Gatti M, Lupi GP, Ferrari P, Barlassina C, et al. A renal abnormality as a possible cause of "essential" hypertension. Lancet. 1979;1(8109):173–7.
20. Hollenberg NK, Borucki LJ, Adams DF. The renal vasculature in early essential hypertension: evidence for a pathogenetic role. Medicine (Baltimore). 1978;57(2):167–78.
21. Erdogan D, Yildirim I, Ciftci O, Ozer I, Caliskan M, Gullu H, et al. Effects of normal blood pressure, prehypertension, and hypertension on coronary microvascular function. Circulation. 2007;115(5):593–9.
22. Grassi G, Buzzi S, Dell'Oro R, Mineo C, Dimitriadis K, Seravalle G, et al. Structural alterations of the retinal microcirculation in the "prehypertensive" high-normal blood pressure state. Curr Pharm Des. 2013;19(13):2375–81.
23. Guyton A. Arterial pressure and hypertension. Philadelphia: WB Saunders Company; 1980.

Microvascular Structural Alterations and Tissue Perfusion in Hypertension/Diabetes

14

Damiano Rizzoni, Carolina De Ciuceis, Enzo Porteri, Enrico Agabiti-Rosei, and Claudia Agabiti-Rosei

14.1 Microvascular Structure in Hypertension

Resistance arteries are key elements in the control of blood pressure. The main drop in hydrostatic pressure occurs at the level of the resistance vasculature: i.e. small resistance arteries (<350 μm of lumen diameter), arterioles (<100 μm of lumen diameter) and capillaries (about 7 μm of lumen diameter) [1, 2]. Total peripheral resistance in terminal arteries and arterioles amounts to 45–50%, in capillaries to 23–30%, in venules to 3–4%, and to 3% in veins [2]. Thus, structural changes in the microcirculation may directly and strongly affect blood pressure values. In fact, it is now widely accepted that structural abnormalities of microvessels are common alterations associated with chronic hypertension [1, 3–5]. A thickened arterial wall together with a reduced lumen (a process known as remodelling) may play an important role in the increase of vascular resistance, and may also be an adaptive response to the increased haemodynamic load. As described by Poiseuille's law, resistance is inversely proportional to the radius to the forth power; therefore, slight alterations in arterial lumen result in significant effects on vascular resistance. In addition, hypertension seems to be associated with a reduction (rarefaction) in the number of capillaries [6–8].

In the last few years, several evidences have suggested that hypertensive injury of small arteries may participate also in the pathophysiology of its complications.

D. Rizzoni (✉)
Clinica Medica, Department of Clinical and Experimental Sciences, University of Brescia, Brescia, Italy

Division of Medicine, Istituto Clinico Città di Brescia, Brescia, Italy
e-mail: damiano.rizzoni@unibs.it

C. De Ciuceis · E. Porteri · E. Agabiti-Rosei · C. Agabiti-Rosei
Clinica Medica, Department of Clinical and Experimental Sciences, University of Brescia, Brescia, Italy

R. Zimlichman et al. (eds.), *Prehypertension and Cardiometabolic Syndrome*, Updates in Hypertension and Cardiovascular Protection,
https://doi.org/10.1007/978-3-319-75310-2_14

Hence, the study of structural alterations of resistance vessels in essential hypertension, the possibility of their regression with antihypertensive treatment as well as their contribution to the prognosis of patients with essential hypertension should be considered of great clinical and scientific interest.

14.2 Microvascular Structure in Diabetes Mellitus

Microvascular complications are major contributors to morbidity, mortality and costs of both non-insulin-dependent (NIDDM) and insulin-dependent diabetes mellitus (IDDM) [9]. Damage of the small vessels in the kidney can lead to end-stage renal disease, structural alterations of the smaller vessels that supply nutrients and oxygen to peripheral nerves contribute to neuropathy while damage of the microvasculature of the eye is the leading cause of loss of vision in working-age adults. The clinical manifestations of microvascular disease are so characteristic of the disease that diabetes itself is defined primarily by the level of hyperglycaemia which causes microvascular complications.

Alterations in the microcirculation involve small resistance arteries, arterioles, capillaries and post capillary venules. A relevant role in the impairment of vascular distensibility may be played by advanced glycosylation end products (AGE), which may be involved in the formation of collagen cross-links [10]. While there is a huge number of data about microangiopathy (capillary and arterioles), quite few data about morphology of small resistance arteries (diameter ranging from 100 to 350 μm) in diabetes mellitus are presently available. In one study [11], no difference in subcutaneous small artery structure was observed between control subjects and patients with insulin-dependent diabetes mellitus (IDDM). On the contrary, it has been demonstrated that, in both hypertensive and normotensive patients with NIDDM, marked alterations in small artery structure are present [12], and that these alterations are more pronounced in hypertensive patients with NIDDM than in patients with essential hypertension or in normotensive diabetics (Fig. 14.1) [12]. In addition, in diabetic patients a clear increase in the media cross-sectional area of the vessels was observed, thus suggesting the presence of hypertrophic remodelling (vascular smooth muscle cells hypertrophy or hyperplasia) [12, 13] (Fig. 14.1). This was not the case of patients with essential hypertension. A weak, but significant correlation between circulating levels of insulin and media-to-lumen ratio of subcutaneous small arteries was observed in diabetic patients, thus suggesting a possible role of insulin or insulin-like growth factor-1 in the genesis of hypertrophic remodelling in these patients [12] However, an alternative explanation for the presence of hypertrophic remodelling in these vessels has been proposed [13]. In fact, a possible stimulus for hypertrophic remodelling could be the increased wall stress, as a consequence of the impaired myogenic response. Myogenic response is a pressure-induced vasoconstriction, which is the key component of blood flow autoregulation and stabilization of capillary pressure. The observation by Schofield et al. [13] of the lack of such a myogenic response in diabetic patients may therefore be responsible for the development of hypertrophic

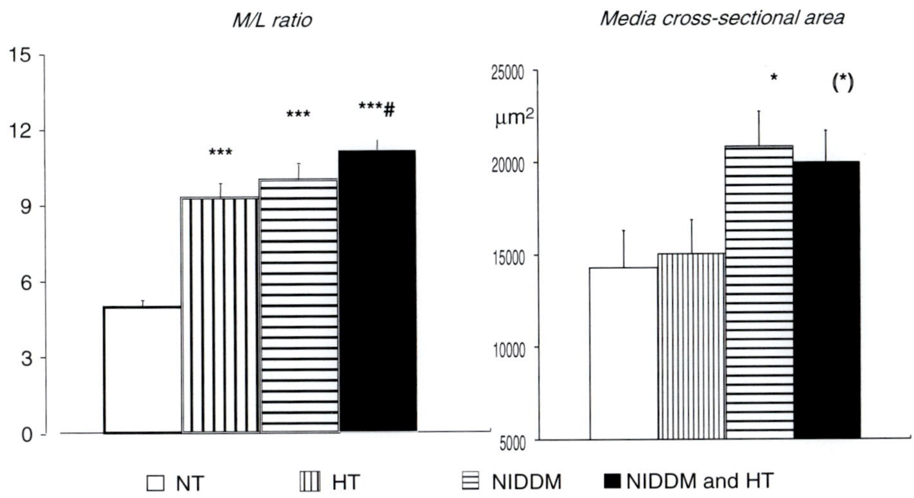

Fig. 14.1 Subcutaneous small resistance arteries structure in hypertensive and diabetic patients. Left: Media-to-lumen ratio in subcutaneous small resistance arteries from normotensive subjects (NT), essential hypertensive patients (HT), normotensive patients with non-insulin-dependent diabetes mellitus (NIDDM) and hypertensive patients with NIDDM (NIDDM and HT). A clear increase may be observed in all the three pathologic groups, which is more evident in hypertensive patients with NIDDM. Right: Medial cross-sectional area in subcutaneous small resistance arteries from normotensive subjects (NT), essential hypertensive patients (HT), normotensive patients with NIDDM and hypertensive patients with NIDDM (NIDDM and HT). An increase may be observed in the diabetic patients, which is more evident in normotensive patients with NIDDM. (*)$p = 0.06$, *$p < 0.05$ vs. Normotensives. Mean ± SEM. (re-drawn, data from [12])

remodelling of small arteries (Fig. 14.2) [13]. As mentioned, while small resistance arteries and arterioles may undergo a remodelling process and fibrosis in pathological conditions, capillaries may undergo a functional or structural rarefaction, with consequent reduction in the density per area units of tissue. This process of vascular rarefaction was previously observed in patients with hypertension [7, 8] but also in patients with NIDDM [14, 15].

On the contrary, in other vascular districts such as the retina, microvascular proliferation may also be observed. In fact, diabetic retinopathy results either from capillary leakage or from new vessel formation (neovascularization, angiogenesis), caused by capillary closure and retinal ischaemia. The capillaries leak lipid products and fluid in the area around the fovea and thicken the retina, which may lead to macular oedema. Angiogenesis is the result of retinal ischaemia, and retinal haemorrhages are the consequence of the fragility of neovessels. The haemorrhage can enter the vitreous and cause sudden loss of vision. Several mechanisms and metabolic abnormalities, acting alone or in concert with each other, may lead to capillary death, leakage and occlusion and to the release of growth factors, finally resulting in new vessel formation and increase vascular permeability. A relevant role is played by vascular endothelial growth factor (VEGF). Whereas VEGF is involved in

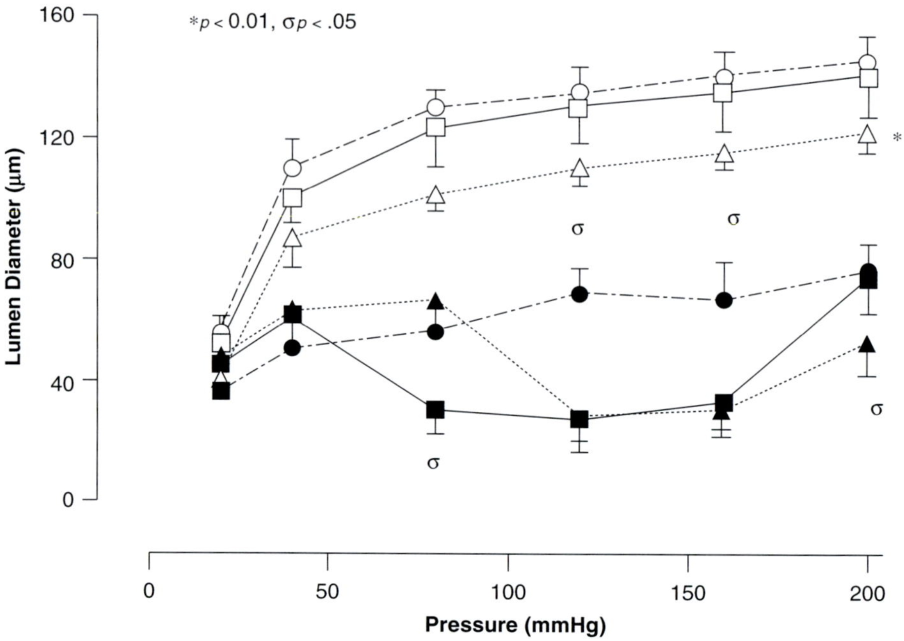

Fig. 14.2 Myogenic response in subcutaneous small resistance arteries in patients with NIDDM. Passive pressure–lumen diameter relations for arteries from control subjects (square), patients with EH (triangle), and hypertensive patients with NIDDM (circle). * = $p < 0.05$, ANOVA, vs. control. Active pressure–lumen diameter relations for arteries from control subjects (filled square), patients with essential hypertension (filled triangle), and hypertensive patients with NIDDM (filled circle). σ = $p < 0.05$ vs. control vessels (from [13])

vascular leakage and angiogenesis, growth hormones and the insulin-like growth factor-1 (IGF-1) are involved, as mediators, in angiogenesis.

14.3 Microvascular Structural Alterations and Organ Perfusion

As previously mentioned, the extent of structural alterations in small resistance vessels is more pronounced in patients with both diabetes mellitus and hypertension, thus suggesting that clustering of risk factors may have synergistic deleterious effects on the vasculature [12, 13]. An important pathophysiological and clinical consequence of the presence of structural alterations in small resistance arteries and arterioles may be an impairment of vasodilator reserve [16]. In fact, as previously reported, remodelling of small resistance arteries is characterized by a narrowing of the lumen, which leads to an increase of flow resistance even at full dilatation, i.e. in the absence of vascular tone. A significant correlation between coronary flow reserve and subcutaneous small resistance artery remodelling has been observed in hypertensive patients, suggesting that structural alterations in small resistance arteries may be present at the same time in different vascular districts, including those of paramount clinical importance, such as the coronary circulation [17]. Recently, we have observed a correlation between media-to-lumen ratio of cerebral small resistance arteries and cerebral blood flow in the cortical grey matter, basal ganglia, thalami and subcortical white matter (Fig. 14.3), thus, again, suggesting that more pronounced alterations of small vessels may be associated to an impaired tissue perfusion [18]. Cerebral autoregulation, a mechanism aimed at maintaining constant brain flow in the presence of changes in mean blood pressure is shifted rightward in hypertension [19], and this may have a consequence in terms of excessive reduction in cerebral perfusion during abrupt reductions in blood pressure [19, 20].

It was observed also that a relatively close correlation exists between structure of subcutaneous small resistance arteries of normotensive subjects and hypertensive patients and microvessel density in the derma, as evaluated by an immunohistochemical approach (immunostaining for CD 31), thus suggesting that structural changes in the microcirculation may be present simultaneously at different levels [21] (Fig. 14.4).

An impaired microvascular hyperaemic response (which may reflect an altered flow reserve) has been observed in children with diabetes mellitus [22] as well as in adult patients with NIDDM [23]. Thus, alterations in the microcirculation may play an important role in the development of organ damage not only in hypertension but also in diabetes mellitus. In fact, a relevant prognostic role of an increased media-to-lumen ratio of subcutaneous small resistance arteries in a high-risk population (including normotensive and hypertensive diabetic patients) has been previously demonstrated [24]. Also the characteristics of the vascular remodelling, i.e. eutrophic vs. hypertrophic remodelling was taken into account. For the same values of internal diameter, those subjects who suffered cardiovascular events had a greater

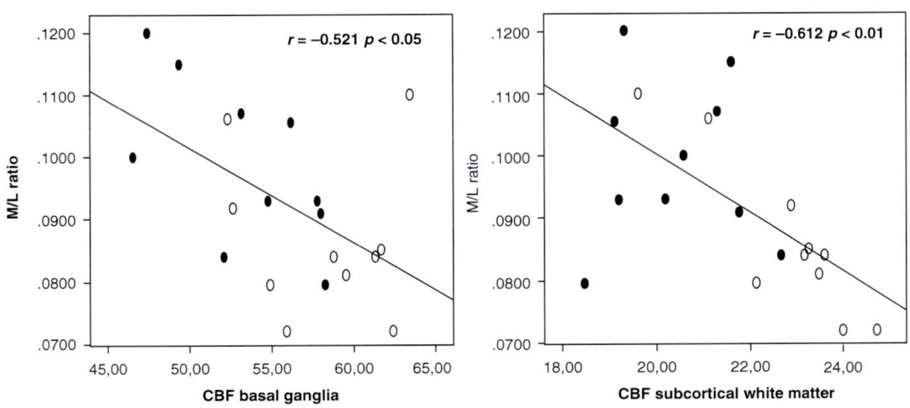

Fig. 14.3 Left graph: correlation between cerebral blood flow (CBF) in the basal ganglia and media-to-lumen (M/L) ratio of cerebral arteries. Right graph: correlation between CBF in the subcortical white matter and M/L ratio of cerebral arteries. Empty circles normotensive subjects, full circles hypertensive patients (from [18])

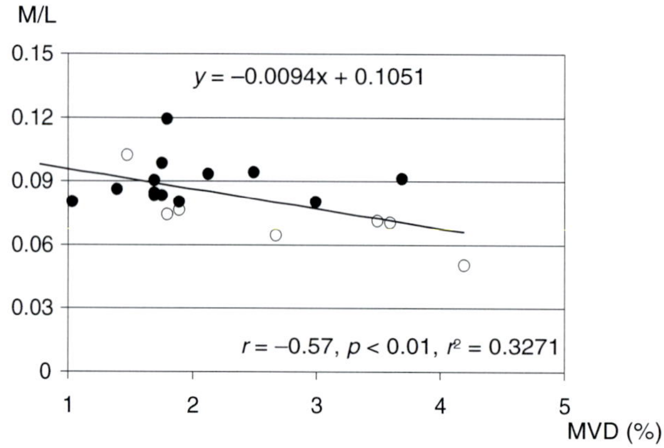

Fig. 14.4 Correlation between media-to-lumen ratio (M/L) of subcutaneous small resistance artery and microvessels density (MVD) in the derma of normotensive subjects (empty circles) and hypertensive patients (full circles). Reprinted from [21], with permission from IOS Press

media-cross-sectional area, in comparison with those without cardiovascular events [25]. Therefore, it seems that, for the same size of the vessels explored, a more consistent cell growth (hypertrophic remodelling, such as that observed in diabetic patients) means an even worse prognosis. It has been also suggested, as previously reported, that an impairment of myogenic response may have a relevant role in the development of hypertrophic remodelling in patients at high cardiovascular risk. In addition, an impaired myogenic response in small vessels may also induce an increase of high blood pressure flow to target organs and downstream increase in capillary pressure, with consequent increased permeability and capillary leakage. Fluid extravasation may induce organ damage. Some data support the presence of an increased capillary pressure in patients with diabetes mellitus [26], especially if they have increased blood pressure values [27], although at present time there is no general agreement about this issue.

The increase in capillary pressure seems to be related to the extent of clinical complications as well as to metabolic control [28]. Also vascular rarefaction per se may have important consequences in terms of tissue perfusion. In fact, it has been demonstrated that in patients with NIDDM, the mechanisms through which insulin is able to increase total limb flow or achieve optimal microvascular perfusion is impaired [14].

As mentioned, hypertension seems to be also associated with a reduction (rarefaction) in the number of parallel-connected arterioles and capillaries [6, 29], with possibly important consequences in terms of tissue perfusion [6]. Microvascular density may be evaluated non-invasively by videomicroscopy/capillaroscopy in specific cutaneous regions or in the nailfold [7, 8, 29]. In general, a functional rarefaction (reduction of capillaries perfused in basal condition) or a structural rarefaction (reduction of capillaries that may be recruited, i.e. after venous congestion) may be observed in essential hypertension [6, 29]. Therefore, capillary rarefaction observed in hypertension is very likely a permanent anatomical change rather than a functional one. Whether it is pathologically important in terms of worsening the disease or generating complications is still a matter of debate, although it is probable that it might be associated to increased peripheral resistance and impaired tissue perfusion, thus, consequently, to organ damage [30]. At present, however, we do not have convincing evidence of a prognostic value of a decreased capillary density in hypertension [29], at difference to what demonstrated for small resistance artery remodelling [24].

Tissue perfusion might be altered, especially in diabetes mellitus, also due to impaired myogenic properties of small vessels [13] (Fig. 14.2). In normal controls and in essential hypertension, an increase in intraluminal or transmural pressure is associated with vasoconstriction, in order to protect tissues from an overperfusion. This autoregulatory function is also vital to ensure stabilization of distal capillary pressures and, hence, to prevent, or limit, organ damage. Indeed in any animal model studied, when myogenic autoregulation is affected, target organ damage ensues [31]. Myogenic autoregulation is damaged in diabetes mellitus [13] (Fig. 14.2), and an excessive transmission of flow and energy to the periphery might be involved in the development of hypertrophic remodelling, usually seen in the vasculature of diabetic patients [31]. An impaired myogenic tone was also observed to be present in the cerebral or cardiac vasculature [32, 33], at least in animal models.

In any case, it is well accepted that cerebral lacunar infarctions [34], or large white matter hyperintensities [35], are usually expression of cerebral microvascular disease. Pulsatility index was associated with lower memory scores and worse performance on tests assessing executive function. When magnetic resonance imaging measures (grey and white matter volumes, white matter hyperintensity volumes and prevalent subcortical infarcts) were included in cognitive models, haemodynamic associations were attenuated or no longer significant, consistent with the hypothesis that increased aortic stiffness and excessive flow pulsatility damage the microcirculation, leading to quantifiable tissue damage and reduced cognitive performance. Marked stiffening of the aorta is associated with reduced wave reflection at the interface between carotid and aorta, transmission of excessive flow pulsatility into the brain, microvascular structural brain damage and lower scores in various cognitive domains [36]. Middle cerebral artery pulsatility was also demonstrated to be the strongest physiological correlate of leukoaraiosis, independent of age, and it resulted dependent on aortic diastolic blood pressure and pulse pressure and on aortic and middle cerebral artery stiffness, supporting the hypothesis that large artery stiffening results in increased arterial pulsatility with transmission to the cerebral small vessels resulting in leukoaraiosis [36].

Therefore, it seems that a close relationship has been established between brain microvascular damage and indices of age and large artery stiffness (pulse pressure, aortic pulse wave velocity, and augmentation index) [36]. A possible pathophysiological explanation of this link can be offered on the basis of differential input impedance in the brain and kidney, compared with other systemic vascular beds: torrential flow and low resistance to flow in these organs exposes small arterial vessels to the high-pressure fluctuations that exist in the carotid, vertebral, and renal arteries. Such fluctuations, measurable as central pulse pressure, increase three- to fourfold with age. Exposure of small vessels to highly pulsatile pressure and flow explains microvascular damage, renal insufficiency and intellectual deterioration [36].

Finally, another issue possible relevant in respect with impaired tissue perfusion in pathological conditions is represented by the loss of anticontractile activity of perivascular fat.

A large body of evidence has accumulated suggesting that adipose tissue is probably highly metabolically active [37, 38]. This has important implications for the vasculature where the perivascular adipose tissue (PVAT) exerts an anticontractile effect through the paracrine actions of vasodilator adipokines. These adipose-derived vasodilators act independently of the endothelium and include adiponectin, nitric oxide, hydrogen sulphide and palmitic acid methyl ester [36]. In patients with metabolic syndrome there is clear evidence that this anticontractile function is lost [39]: the perivascular environment becomes inflamed with increased oxidative stress, macrophage activation [40] and the release of a number of cytokines that can influence the bioavailability of key vasodilator molecules such as adiponectin [39]. The lack of a vasodilator effect mediated by perivascular fat might expose peripheral tissue to hypoperfusion [36].

14.4 Effect of Treatment on Microvascular Structural Alterations

Since changes in microvascular structure have a profound and direct effect on the development of hypertension complications and cardio-cerebrovascular events [24], it is expected that prevention/regression by appropriated treatment of these alterations may be associated with a better prognosis [41, 42].

In hypertension, some intervention studies with specific drugs have demonstrated an improvement or even an almost complete normalization of the structure of subcutaneous small resistance arteries with angiotensin converting enzyme (ACE) inhibitors (cilazapril, perindopril, lisinopril), calcium channel blockers (nifedipine, amlodipine, isradipine), angiotensin II receptor blockers (losartan, irbesartan, candesartan, olmesartan and valsartan) [3, 29, 43]. On the contrary, the β-blocker atenolol and the diuretic hydrochlorothiazide had limited effects on resistance vessels, despite a similar blood pressure reduction [3, 29, 43]. ACE inhibitors proved to be significantly more effective than the β-blocker atenolol in terms of changes in media-to-lumen ratio [43]. The same result was obtained comparing dihydropyridinic calcium channel blockers and atenolol, or angiotensin receptor blockers and atenolol [43]. It should also be noted that, during antihypertensive treatment, the regression of microvascular structural alterations in the subcutaneous small arteries of hypertensive patients is paralleled by an improvement of coronary flow reserve [42, 44].

Basal and total capillary density is increased in effectively treated antihypertensives [45–47]. Hypertensive patients with their blood pressure well controlled with the combination perindopril/indapamide [45, 46] or lercadipine/enalapril [47] showed an improvement/normalization of capillary density, whereas other antihypertensive treatments, including the combination lercanidipine/hydrochlorothiazide, had less effect despite similar blood pressure control [45, 47]. An improvement in retinal capillary rarefaction was observed recently after valsartan treatment in hypertensive patients [48].

Inhibitors of angiogenesis, extensively used in oncology, may induce an increase in blood pressure values also through a reduction in capillary density [49]. This effect might have a clinical relevance in terms of cardiovascular risk and/or management of these patients [49].

Few data are presently available about the possibility to improve or restore the anticontractile effect of PVAT in humans. Blockade of the renin-angiotensin system [50] or antioxidants such as melatonin [51] seem to be effective, while also bariatric surgery seems to reverse the obesity-induced alteration to PVAT anticontractile function [52]. This reversal is attributable to reductions in local adipose inflammation and oxidative stress with improved adiponectin and nitric oxide bioavailability [52].

Similarly, there are not many data about the effect of treatment on structural and functional alterations in the microcirculation of patients with diabetes mellitus. In the United Kingdom Prospective Diabetes Study (UKPDS), a large randomized controlled trial that included almost 5000 patients, it has been demonstrated that a tight haemodynamic and metabolic control is associated with a lower incidence of microvascular disease [53], and, in general, of clinical endpoints related to microvascular disease [54].

Even fewer data are presently available about the effects of antihypertensive drugs on small artery structure in hypertensive diabetic patients. Despite effective antihypertensive treatment, resistance arteries from hypertensive diabetic patients showed marked remodelling, greater than that of vessels from untreated, nondiabetic, hypertensive subjects, in agreement with the high cardiovascular risk of subjects suffering from both diabetes and hypertension [55]. A study has compared the effects of 1 year treatment with the ACE inhibitor (enalapril) or the angiotensin II receptor blocker (candesartan), on subcutaneous small artery structure in hypertensive patients with NIDDM [56]. The two drugs were equally effective in reducing media-to-lumen ratio of small arteries (Fig. 14.5), however, candesartan was more effective than enalapril in normalizing vascular collagen content, probably through a more pronounced stimulation of the local production of metalloproteinase 9 (a collagen-degrading enzyme). At variance to what is observed in the majority of studies in normoglycaemic hypertensive patients, media-to-lumen ratio of small arteries in treated diabetic patients did not reach the values observed in normotensive controls, therefore suggesting that a complete regression of vascular hypertrophic remodelling is probably more difficult to obtain [56]. Angiotensin II receptor blockers seem to be effective in diabetic hypertensive patients also when given on top of an ACE inhibitor treatment [57].

It has been recently proposed that drugs that may stimulate PPARα or PPAR γ receptors (such as fibrates of glitazones) may be useful in terms of vascular protection and regression of structural alterations in the microcirculation although no convincing data is presently available. The sodium-glucose cotransporter 2 inhibitor, dapagliflozin was demonstrated to be able to favourably affect microvascular and macrovascular circulation [58].

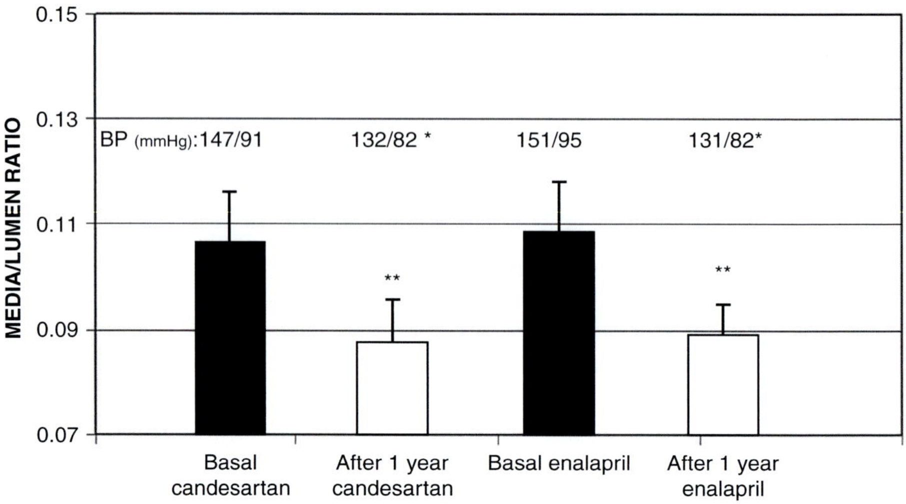

Fig. 14.5 Media-to-lumen ratio in subcutaneous small resistance arteries from hypertensive patients with NIDDM, before and after 1-year treatment with the ACE inhibitor enalapril or the angiotensin II receptor blocker candesartan. A significant and similar reduction was observed with both drugs. *BP* blood pressure. ** = $p < 0.01$ vs. Basal. (re-drawn, data from [56]

Few data about patients with type 1 diabetes mellitus are presently available. A study from Greenstein et al. [59] suggests that, with poor metabolic control, small arteries from patients with type 1 diabetes mellitus show hypertrophic growth in response to elevated blood pressure, similar to that seen in type 2 diabetes mellitus. However, metabolic improvements enable eutrophic remodelling to occur in response to an increase in blood pressure [59].

Conclusion

Probably, more than affecting resistance, microvascular rarefaction has the potential to disturb the cellular delivery of nutrients and oxygen, thus contributing to hypertensive end-organ damage [60]. Circumstantial evidence along this line comes from measurements of tissue partial pressure of oxygen in rat models of hypertension, where relative hypoxia occurred in the cremaster, a muscle in which rarefaction was consistently demonstrated, but not the spinotrapezius, a muscle in which no rarefaction was found [60]. The theoretical impact of rarefaction on tissue oxygenation was also investigated by modelling the spatial distribution of partial pressure of oxygen with a finite element method; in that simulation, suppression of 25% of microvessels generated extended areas of profound hypoxia, especially in the presence of high cellular demand for oxygen [60].

Alterations in the microcirculation represent a common finding, and microangiopathy is one of the most important mechanisms involved in the development of organ damage as well as of clinical events in patients with diabetes mellitus [61, 62]. Both patients with essential hypertension and those with NIDDM are characterized by alterations in the resistance vasculature, i.e. an increased media-to-lumen ratio, that in diabetics is the consequence of the so-called hypertrophic remodelling [61, 62]. Structural alterations of small arteries are associated with an increased cardiovascular risk in hypertensive and diabetic patients, perhaps as a consequence of an impaired organ flow reserve in several vascular districts, including the coronary vascular bed [61, 62]. In fact, it has been observed that the presence of an increased wall-to-lumen ratio in the subcutaneous resistance arteries is associated with a worse prognosis in high-risk patients [61]. Hypertrophic remodelling, such as that observed in diabetic patients, seems to be associated with an even worse prognosis [25]. Data about the effect of therapy on microvascular structure in diabetic patients are scarce; however, renin-angiotensin system blockade seems to be effective in regressing, at least in part, the microvascular structure [61]. Blockers of the angiotensin-aldosterone system and calcium antagonists are effective in regressing small resistance artery remodelling in hypertension [43], and this regression seems to be clinically advantageous [41]; the same drug classes together with the diuretic indapamide were also able to improve microvascular density [45–47], however, in this case we do not know whether this improvement is associated with a better clinical prognosis.

References

1. Mulvany MJ, Aalkjaer C. Structure and function of small arteries. Physiol Rev. 1990;70:921–71.
2. Christensen KL, Mulvany MJ. Location of resistance arteries. J Vasc Res. 2001;38:1–12.
3. Schiffrin EL. Remodeling of resistance arteries in essential hypertension and effects of antihypertensive treatment. Am J Hypertens. 2004;17:1192–200.
4. Mulvany MJ. Structural abnormalities of the resistance vasculature in hypertension. J Vasc Res. 2003;40:558–60.
5. Bund SJ, Lee RMKW. Arterial structural changes in hypertension: a consideration of methodology, terminology and functional consequences. J Vasc Res. 2003;40:547–57.
6. Levy BI, Ambrosio G, Pries AR, Struijker-Boudier HAJ. Microcirculation in hypertension. A new target for treatment? Circulation. 2001;104:735–40.
7. Antonios TF, Singer DR, Markandu ND, Mortimer PS, MacGregor GA. Rarefaction of skin capillaries in borderline essential hypertension suggests an early structural abnormality. Hypertension. 1999;34:655–8.
8. Antonios TF, Singer DR, Markandu ND, Mortimer PS, MacGregor GA. Structural skin capillary rarefaction in essential hypertension. Hypertension. 1999;33:998–1001.
9. Blonde L. State of diabetes care in the United States. Am J Manag Care. 2007;13(Suppl 2):S36–40.
10. Aronson D. Cross-linking of glycated collagen in the pathogenesis of arterial and myocardial stiffening of aging and diabetes. J Hypertens. 2003;21:3–12.
11. McNally PG, Watt PAC, Rimmer T, Burden AC, Hearnshaw JR, Thurston H. Impaired contraction and endothelium-dependent relaxation in isolated resistance vessels from patients with insulin-dependent diabetes mellitus. Clin Sci. 1994;87:31–6.
12. Rizzoni D, Porteri E, Guelfi D, Muiesan ML, Valentini U, Cimino A, Girelli A, Rodella L, Bianchi R, Sleiman I, Agabiti Rosei E. Structural alterations in subcutaneous small arteries of normotensive and hypertensive patients with non insulin dependent diabetes mellitus. Circulation. 2001;103:1238–44.

13. Schofield I, Malik R, Izzard A, Austin C, Heagerty AM. Vascular structural and functional changes in type 2 diabetes mellitus. Evidence for the role of abnormal myogenic responsiveness and dyslipidemia. Circulation. 2002;106:3037–43.
14. Clark MG, Barrett EJ, Wallis MG, Vincent MA, Rattigan S. The microvasculature in insulin resistance and type 2 diabetes. Semin Vasc Med. 2002;2:21–31.
15. Jumar A, Harazny JM, Ott C, Friedrich S, Kistner I, Striepe K, Schmieder RE. Retinal capillary rarefaction in patients with type 2 diabetes mellitus. PLoS One. 2016;11(12):e0162608.
16. Folkow B. Physiological aspects of primary hypertension. Physiol Rev. 1982;62:347–504.
17. Rizzoni D, Palombo C, Porteri E, Muiesan ML, Kozàkovà M, La Canna G, Nardi M, Guelfi D, Salvetti M, Morizzo C, Vittone F, Agabiti Rosei E. Relationships between coronary vasodilator capacity and small artery remodeling in hypertensive patients. J Hypertens. 2003;21:625–32.
18. De Ciuceis C, Cornali C, Porteri E, Mardighian D, Pinardi C, Fontanella MM, Rodella LF, Rezzani R, Rizzoni D, Boari GE, Agabiti Rosei E, Gasparotti R. Cerebral small-resistance artery structure and cerebral blood flow in normotensive subjects and hypertensive patients. Neuroradiology. 2014;56:1103–11.
19. Agabiti Rosei E, Rizzoni D. In:Coca A, editor. Pathophysiology of brain damage in hypertension: small vessels disease. In: Hypertension and brain damage. Cham: Springer International Publishing AG Switzerland; 2016. p. 47–60.
20. Vaughan CJ, Delanty N. Hypertensive emergencies. Lancet. 2000;356(9227):411–7.
21. Paiardi S, Rodella LF, De Ciuceis C, Porteri E, Boari GE, Rezzani R, Rizzardi N, Platto C, Tiberio GA, Giulini SM, Rizzoni D, Agabiti-Rosei E. Immunohistochemical evaluation of microvascular rarefaction in hypertensive humans and in spontaneously hypertensive rats. Clin Hemorheol Microcirc. 2009;42(4):259–68.
22. Shore AC, Price KJ, Sandeman DD, Greeen EM, Tripp JH, Tooke JE. Impaired microvascular hyperhaemic response in children with diabetes mellitus. Diabet Med. 1991;8:619–23.
23. Strain WD, Chaturvedi N, Nihoyannopoulos P, Bulpitt CJ, Rajkumar C, Shore AC. Differences in the association between type 2 diabetes and impaired microvascular function among Europeans and African Caribbeans. Diabetologia. 2005;48:2269–77.
24. Rizzoni D, Porteri E, Boari GEM, De Ciuceis C, Sleiman I, Muiesan ML, Castellano M, Miclini M, Agabiti-Rosei E. Prognostic significance of small artery structure in hypertension. Circulation. 2003;108:2230–5.
25. Izzard AS, Rizzoni D, Agabiti-Rosei E, Heagerty AM. Small artery structure and hypertension: adaptive changes and target organ damage. J Hypertens. 2005;23:247–50.
26. Parving HH, Viberti GC, Keen H, Christensen JS, Lassen NA. Hemodynamic factors in the genesis of diabetic microangiopathy. Metabolism. 1983;32:943–9.
27. Fegan PG, Tooke JE, Gooding KM, Tullet JM, MacLeod KM, Shore AC. Capillary pressure in subjects with type 2 diabetes and hypertension and the effect of antihypertensive therapy. Hypertension. 2003;41:1111–7.
28. Sandeman DD, Shore AC, Tooke JE. Relation of skin capillary pressure in patients with insulin-dependent diabetes mellitus to complications and metabolic control. N Engl J Med. 1992;327:760–4.
29. Agabiti Rosei E, Rizzoni D. The effects of hypertension on the structure of human resistance arteries. In: Lip GYH, Hall JE, editors. Comprehensive hypertension, vol. 207, chapter 47. Amsterdam: Mosby Elsevier; 2007. p. 579–90.
30. Levy BI, Schiffrin EL, Mourad JJ, Agostini D, Vicaut E, Safar ME, Struijker- Boudier HA. Impaired tissue perfusion: a pathology common to hypertension, obesity, and diabetes mellitus. Circulation. 2008;118:968–76.
31. Sonoyama K, Greenstein A, Price A, Khavandi K, Heagerty T. Vascular remodeling: implications for small artery function and target organ damage. Ther Adv Cardiovasc Dis. 2007;1:129–37.
32. Delaney PJ, Burnham MP, Heagerty AM, Izzard AS. Impaired myogenic properties of cerebral arteries from the Brown Norway rat. J Hypertens. 2012;30:926–31.
33. Izzard AS, Heagerty AM. Myogenic properties of brain and cardiac vessels and their relation to disease. Curr Vasc Pharmacol. 2014;12:829–35.

34. Hashimoto J, Aikawa T, Imai Y. Large artery stiffening as a link between cerebral lacunar infarction and renal albuminuria. Am J Hypertens. 2008;21(12):1304–9.
35. Brisset M, Boutouyrie P, Pico F, Zhu Y, Zureik M, Schilling S, Dufouil C, Mazoyer B, Laurent S, Tzourio C, Debette S. Large-vessel correlates of cerebral small-vessel disease. Neurology. 2013;80:662–9.
36. Rizzoni D, Agabiti-Rosei C, Agabiti-Rosei E. Hemodynamic consequences of changes in microvascular structure. Am J Hypertens. 2017;30:939. https://doi.org/10.1093/ajh/hpx032.
37. Ahima RS. Adipose tissue as an endocrine organ. Obesity. 2006;14(Suppl 5):242S–9S.
38. Guerre-Millo M. Adipose tissue hormones. J Endocrinol Investig. 2002;25:855–61.
39. Greenstein AS, Khavandi K, Withers SB, Sonoyama K, Clancy O, Jeziorska M, Laing I, Yates AP, Pemberton PW, Malik RA, Heagerty AM. Local inflammation and hypoxia abolish the protective anticontractile properties of perivascular fat in obese patients. Circulation. 2009;119:1661–70.
40. Withers SB, Agabiti Rosei C, Livingstone DM, Little MC, Aslam R, Malik RA, Heagerty AM. Studies in CD11b-DTR macrophage deficient mice prove that macrophage activation is responsible for the loss of anticontractile function in inflamed perivascular adipose tissue. Arterioscler Thromb Vasc Biol. 2011;31:908–13.
41. Buus NH, Mathiassen ON, Fenger-Grøn M, Præstholm MN, Sihm I, Thybo NK, Schroeder AP, Thygesen K, Aalkjær C, Pedersen OL, Mulvany MJ, Christensen KL. Small artery structure during antihypertensive therapy is an independent predictor of cardiovascular events in essential hypertension. J Hypertens. 2013;31:791–7.
42. Agabiti-Rosei E, Rizzoni D. Microvascular structure as a prognostically relevant endpoint. J Hypertens. 2017;35:914–21.
43. Agabiti-Rosei E, Heagerty AM, Rizzoni D. Effects of antihypertensive treatment on small artery remodelling. J Hypertens. 2009;27:1107–14.
44. Buus NH, Bøttcher M, Jørgensen CG, Christensen KL, Thygesen K, Nielsen TT, Mulvany MJ. Myocardial perfusion during long-term angiotensin-converting enzyme inhibition or beta-blockade in patients with essential hypertension. Hypertension. 2004;44:465–70.
45. Rizzoni D. Impact of different antihypertensive treatments on the microcirculation. Microcirc Cardiovasc Dis. 2012;7:3–7.
46. Debbabi H, Bonnin P, Levy BI. Effects of blood pressure control with perindopril/indapamide on the microcirculation in hypertensive patients. Am J Hypertens. 2010;23:1136–43.
47. De Ciuceis C, Salvetti M, Rossini C, Muiesan ML, Paini A, Duse S, La Boria E, Semeraro F, Cancarini A, Agabiti Rosei C, Sarkar A, Ruggeri G, Caimi L, Ricotta D, Rizzoni D, Agabiti Rosei E. Effect of antihypertensive treatment on microvascular structure, central blood pressure and oxidative stress in patients with mild essential hypertension. J Hypertens. 2014;32:565–74.
48. Jumar A, Harazny JM, Ott C, Kistner I, Friedrich S, Schmieder RE. Improvement in retinal capillary rarefaction after valsartan treatment in hypertensive patients. J Clin Hypertens (Greenwich). 2016;18:1112–8.
49. Rizzoni D, Paini A, Salvetti M, Rossini C, De Ciuceis C, Agabiti-Rosei C, Muiesan ML. Inhibitors of angiogenesis and blood pressure. Curr Cardiovasc Risk Rep. 2013;7(3):244–7.
50. Agabiti Rosei C, Withers SB, Belcaid L, De Ciuceis C, Rizzoni D, Heagerty AM. Blockade of the renin-angiotensin system in small arteries and anticontractile function of perivascular adipose tissue. J Hypertens. 2015;33:1039–45.
51. Agabiti-Rosei C, De Ciuceis C, Rossini C, Porteri E, Rodella LF, Withers SB, Heagerty AM, Favero G, Agabiti-Rosei E, Rizzoni D, Rezzani R. Anticontractile activity of perivascular fat in obese mice and the effect of long-term treatment with melatonin. J Hypertens. 2014;32:1264–74.
52. Aghamohammadzadeh R, Greenstein AS, Yadav R, Jeziorska M, Hama S, Soltani F, Pemberton PW, Ammori B, Malik RA, Soran H, Heagerty AM. Effects of bariatric surgery on human small artery function: evidence for reduction in perivascular adipocyte inflammation, and the restoration of normal anticontractile activity despite persistent obesity. J Am Coll Cardiol. 2013;62:128–1235.

53. Adler AI, Stratton IM, Neil HA, Yudkin JS, Matthews DR, Cull CA, Wright AD, Turner RC, Holman RR. Association of systolic blood pressure with macrovascular and microvascular complications of type 2 diabetes (UKPDS 36): prospective observational study. BMJ. 2000;321:412–9.
54. Tight blood pressure control and risk of macrovascular and microvascular complications in type 2 diabetes: UKPDS 38. UK Prospective Diabetes Study Group. BMJ 1998;317:703–13.
55. Endemann DH, Pu Q, De Ciuceis C, Savoia C, Virdis A, Neves MF, Touyz RM, Schiffrin EL. Persistent remodeling of resistance arteries in type 2 diabetic patients on antihypertensive treatment. Hypertension. 2004;43:399–404.
56. Rizzoni D, Porteri E, De Ciuceis C, Sleiman I, Rodella L, Rezzani R, Paiardi S, Bianchi R, Ruggeri G, Boari GE, Muiesan ML, Salvetti M, Zani F, Miclini M, Rosei A. Effect of treatment with candesartan or enalapril on subcutaneous small artery structure in hypertensive patients with non insulin-dependent diabetes mellitus. Hypertension. 2005;45:659–65.
57. Savoia C, Touyz RM, Endemann DH, Pu Q, Ko EA, De Ciuceis C, Schiffrin EL. Angiotensin receptor blocker added to previous antihypertensive agents on arteries of diabetic hypertensive patients. Hypertension. 2006;48:271–7.
58. Ott C, Jumar A, Striepe K, Friedrich S, Karg MV, Bramlage P, Schmieder RE. A randomised study of the impact of the SGLT2 inhibitor dapagliflozin on microvascular and macrovascular circulation. Cardiovasc Diabetol. 2017;16(1):26.
59. Greenstein AS, Price A, Sonoyama K, Paisley A, Khavandi K, Withers S, Shaw L, Paniagua O, Malik RA, Heagerty AM. Eutrophic remodeling of small arteries in type 1 diabetes mellitus is enabled by metabolic control: a 10-year follow-up study. Hypertension. 2009;54(1):134–41.
60. Feih F, Liaudet L, Waeber B, Levy BI. Hypertension: a disease of the microcirculation? Hypertension. 2006;48:1012–7.
61. Agabiti Rosei E, Rizzoni D. Small artery remodelling in diabetes. J Cell Mol Med. 2010;14:1030–6.
62. Rizzoni D, Agabiti Rosei E. Small artery remodeling in diabetes mellitus. Nutr Metab Cardiovasc Dis. 2009;19:587–92.

Obesity-Hypertension Physiopathology and Treatment: A Forty-Year Retrospect

15

Jonathan Owen, Stephen Morse, Angela McLean, and Efrain Reisin

15.1 Introduction

During the past 40 years of research into obesity, hypertension, and chronic kidney disease, we have gained considerable knowledge on the effects of excess weight gain to alter numerous metabolic and hormonal processes, which can ultimately result in type 2 diabetes, cardiovascular disease, and chronic kidney failure. Over this span of time, we have witnessed the naming of these metabolic and hormonal alterations as a new condition, the Metabolic Syndrome. Additionally, we have noted that hypertension in obesity appears to have some unique differences to essential hypertension in the normal weight population, and have preferred the term Obesity-Hypertension in our description of this process. Unfortunately, also during this timeframe, the obesity epidemic worldwide has continued to surge unabated, and research into this topic is now more poignant than ever. This review will focus on an overview of this condition from insights gained over the preceding 40 plus years of research experience in this field, with an emphasis on Obesity-Hypertension.

Obesity and excess body weight result from the increase in the size and amount of fat cells. Obesity as a disorder is defined as excess body fat, and the most typical screening tool for the measurement of obesity in the general population is the Body

J. Owen
Division of Nephrology, Department of Internal Medicine, University of New Mexico Health Sciences Center, Albuquerque, NM, USA

S. Morse · E. Reisin (✉)
Section of Nephrology and Hypertension, Department of Medicine, Louisiana State University Health Sciences Center, New Orleans, LA, USA
e-mail: ereisi@lsuhsc.edu

A. McLean
Section of Internal Medicine, Department of Medicine, Louisiana State University Health Sciences Center, New Orleans, LA, USA

R. Zimlichman et al. (eds.), *Prehypertension and Cardiometabolic Syndrome*, Updates in Hypertension and Cardiovascular Protection,
https://doi.org/10.1007/978-3-319-75310-2_15

Mass Index (BMI). This measure is calculated by dividing a person's weight in kilograms by the square of a person's height in meters. The World Health Organization has developed the following definitions using BMI for normal weight (BMI 18.5 kg/m^2 to <25 kg/m^2), overweight (BMI 25 kg/m^2 to <30 kg/m^2), and obesity (BMI 30 kg/m^2 or greater) [1]. The definition of obesity has likewise been further subcategorized into three categories: class 1 (BMI 30 kg/m^2 to <35 kg/m^2), class 2 (BMI 35 kg/m^2 to <40 kg/m^2), and class 3 (BMI 40 kg/m^2 or greater) [2]. The term "morbid obesity" has also frequently been used to describe patients with BMI > 40 kg/m^2, although some have proposed this definition should include obesity at any stage with an obesity-related illness such as type 2 diabetes or obesity-hypertension [3]. Though BMI has been a useful tool for describing obesity in the general population, it should be noted that it is not a direct measure of adiposity in the individual, and substantial variations can occur individually based upon adiposity and muscle mass [4]. Additionally, BMI also has limitations in that it does not allow for differentiation of visceral adiposity versus ectopic adiposity, which appears to have important consequences in regard to metabolic disease, as we will discuss later. Nonetheless, given its widespread adoption and ease of calculation, and the general correlation with adiposity in most patients, it has been the most widely used of the definitions for obesity in the general population, and unless specified will be the definition used for the purposes of this review [5].

Regardless of definition, obesity has become a worldwide epidemic, with a doubling of rates across the globe since the 1980s, and increases have been seen in all regions during this timeframe, including Sub-Saharan Africa, an area previously low risk to this condition [6, 7]. In other analyses, body weight has been previously recognized as the sixth most important risk factor contributing to the overall burden of disease worldwide, and was felt to overtake smoking as the main preventable cause of death in the United States as of 2005 [8]. Though a multitude of genetic and environmental factors likely play a role in the surging rates of obesity worldwide, the most commonly implicated cause is an increasingly sedentary lifestyle seen with advancing technologies, coupled with the increased availability of energy dense, highly processed foods containing an excess of added fats, sugars, or both.

Obesity has long been recognized as a substantial contributor to the development of hypertension, with early data from the Community Hypertension Evaluation Clinic (CHEC) trial demonstrating the prevalence of hypertension up to two times higher in those who were overweight compared to individuals of normal weight, and three times higher for those individuals with low weight [9]. Similarly, it has been estimated that three-fourths of the overall prevalence of hypertension in the general population is felt to be attributable to obesity [10]. It has been recognized as early as the 1940s and 1950s that upper body obesity carries a higher risk of metabolic and cardiovascular complications, and over time this has been redefined to describe the variations as visceral fat accumulation versus ectopic fat accumulation, with a substantial body of evidence demonstrating a much more dangerous metabolic profile with visceral fat deposits [11–15]. In addition to the risk of hypertension, visceral adiposity is strongly associated with the development of the Metabolic Syndrome, a strong predictor of future cardiovascular events and the development of type 2 diabetes mellitus. Though various definitions exist, the metabolic syndrome is generally recognized by the following: increased waist circumference (>40 inches for men and >35 inches for women); increased serum triglyceride levels (>150 mg/dL); elevated blood pressure

(>130/85 mmHg); increased fasting glucose levels (>100 mg/dL); and decreased high-density lipoprotein cholesterol (<40 mg/dL for men and <50 mg/dL for women) [6].

Hypertension remains one of the strongest risk factors for cardiovascular disease, including the development of stroke, congestive heart failure, and peripheral vascular disease. The risk for coronary heart disease death doubles for each increase of 20 mmHg in systolic blood pressure over a baseline of 115 mmHg and for each 10 mmHg increase in diastolic blood pressure beginning at 75 mmHg [16]. In addition, long-standing hypertension can result in cardiac myocyte cell growth, resulting in both concentric (increased thickness and mass of the left ventricle) and eccentric (increased septal thickness) hypertrophy; and obesity coupled with hypertension nearly doubles the risk of both forms of cardiac hypertrophy compared to patients with hypertension and normal weight [17]. Beyond cardiovascular disease, hypertension remains the second leading cause of end-stage kidney disease, and it appears obesity may have additive effects, in addition to contribution from associated hypertension, in the development of this condition [18, 19].

We will focus the remainder of this review on the pathophysiology of obesity-hypertension, the treatment of this condition and relative impacts of weight loss via lifestyle modification, medications and bariatric surgery, and the role of pharmacotherapy for the treatment of hypertension in obesity.

15.2 Pathophysiology of Obesity-Hypertension

The physiology of hypertension in obesity and the metabolic syndrome is complex, with an increasingly recognized number of potential mechanisms contributing to this condition. Traditionally, the development of this condition was explained as a result of increasing plasma volume expansion and cardiac output in the setting of increased body mass, with impaired urinary sodium excretion. Vasodilation in the setting of increasing cardiac output subsequently results in glomerular hyperfiltration and increased distal tubular sodium delivery. Hyperinsulinemia, upregulation of the renin-angiotensin-aldosterone system, and the increase in sympathetic tone in obesity causes increased distal sodium reabsorption and impaired natriuresis, thus resulting in hypertension [20–33].

Although this explanation remains pivotal in the understanding of this condition, the precise mechanism underlying these changes appear increasingly complex, and a variety of newly discovered neuro-hormonal peptides, cytokines and adipokines likely additionally contribute to this condition, including leptin, ghrelin, glucagon-like peptide 1 (GLP-1), and adiponectin.

We will explore the potential contribution of these components, as well as other physiological derangements in obesity in further detail.

15.2.1 Hemodynamic Alterations

The increase in cardiac output and plasma volume are long observed effects of obesity, and it was long ago described by Guyton that impaired natriuresis in this condition must account for the development of hypertension [30]. The elevated stroke volume and the increased intravascular volume cause eccentric cardiac hypertrophy and the elevated blood pressure in the same patients is followed by a concentric ventricular hypertrophy. Consequently the cardiac remodeling of the obese hypertensive patients is characterized by a concentric-eccentric ventricular hypertrophy that may be the cause for the increased prevalence of congestive heart failure, arrhythmia, and sudden death in the obese population [20]. The elevated sympathetic activity in obese subjects may cause more arrhythmia and coronary artery disease but the effect of hyperleptinemia and hyperinsulinemia in cardiac remodeling remain controversial [21]. Reisin et al. reported in 1987 that both normotensive and hypertensive obese patients have increases in renal blood flow, cardiac output and blood volume, in the setting of decreased overall peripheral vascular resistance in comparison to patients of normal weight [31]. Thus, in this setting of increased renal blood flow and glomerular hyperfiltration, mechanisms must exist to account for impaired natriuresis, and to account for the difference observed between obese hypertensive patients and obese normotensive patients. The higher increase in glomerular filtration ratio compared with the renal flow will increase the filtration fraction and all these hemodynamic changes are the cause for glomerulosclerosis [24].

In an early model of obesity, Reisin et al. described the changes that are associated with obesity and hypertension in rats with ventromedial hypothalamic electrolytic lesions compared with sham controls. These animals developed both obesity and hypertension. The cardiac output increased slightly but the peripheral resistance remained unchanged [32] (Fig. 15.1).

Hall et al. were able to demonstrate in 1993 the physiologic changes of obesity in an elegant model where dogs fed to obese states on a high-fat diet were compared to normal weight matched controls. The obese dogs developed hypertension during the 5 week study, and were demonstrated to have a marked increase in heart rate and cardiac output, though cardiac index remained unchanged, suggesting the increase was solely a product of increasing body mass. Increases in blood flow to the kidneys and glomerular filtration rate (GFR) were confirmed to develop in these animals. Through daily measurement of urinary electrolytes, the obese animals were demonstrated to have a cumulative net sodium gain of 507 ± 107 mmol compared to the normal weight animals. Further corroborating existing models of obesity-hypertension is that the obese fed animals had a net fluid gain of 15.7 L compared to the normal weight dogs. These animals were further found to have elevated plasma insulin and renin activity levels, consistent with the insulin resistant state of the metabolic syndrome observed in humans [23].

In a separate animal model using rabbits fed to an obese state and compared to normal weight controls, Carrol et al. demonstrated similar findings with respect to cardiac output, heart rate, cardiac index, and peripheral vascular resistance. In this model, however, the group was able to demonstrate significant differences with respect to regional organ blood flow rates. The obese rabbits in this example showed significant increases in blood flow to the kidneys, ovaries, ventricles, and lungs. Regional flow to adipose tissue, however, was decreased. Thus, it is hypothesized that as cardiac output increases with adiposity and increased body size, the relative avascularity of adipose tissue leads to an increase in flow to vital organs in

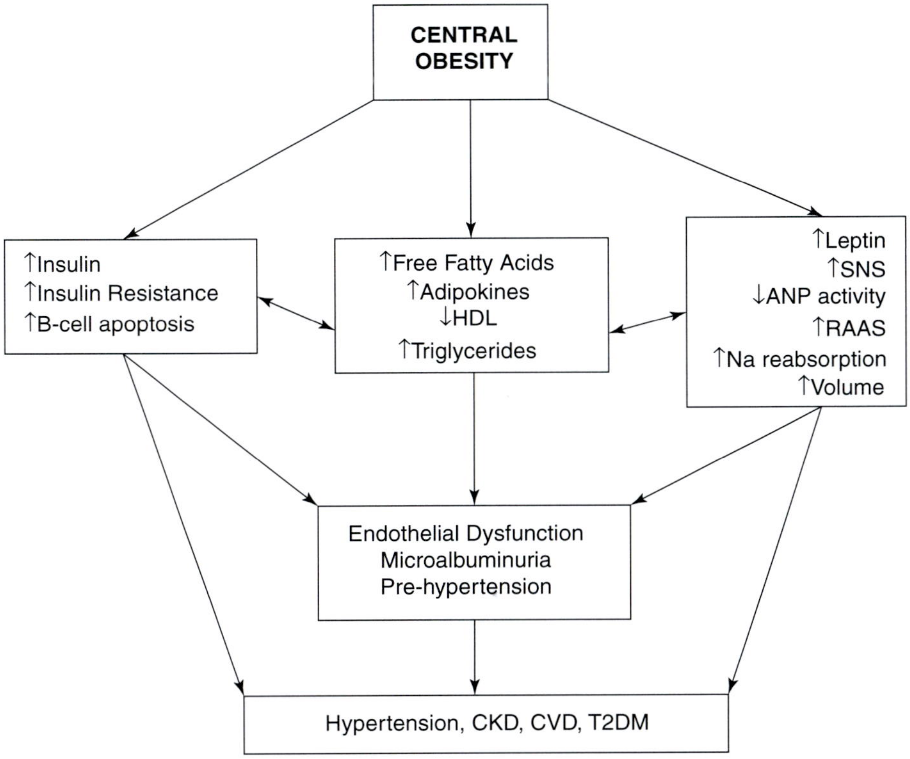

Fig. 15.1 Components and pathways of the metabolic syndrome. *HDL* High-density lipoprotein, *SNS* Sympathetic nervous system, *ANP* Atrial natriuretic peptide, *RAAS* Renin-angiotensin aldosterone system, *Na* Sodium, *CKD* Chronic kidney disease, *CVD* Cardiovascular disease, *T2DM* Type 2 diabetes mellitus. (Figure reprinted with permission from Morse S, Zhang R, Thakur V, Reisin E. Hypertension and the Metabolic Syndrome. Am J Med Sci. 2005;330(6):303–10)

comparison to adipose tissue, accounting for difference seen within renal blood flow and glomerular hyperfiltration. It should be noted that in this study the weights of vital organs increased in the obese subjects as well, and this was mostly attributed to lean mass. Therefore, increased metabolic demand in obesity may also account for differences in regional blood flow rates [33].

Though animal models have limitations when compared to human subjects, these findings correlate well to observations seen in human subjects and provide a vital framework in our understanding of obesity-hypertension. As these changes in cardiac output and renal blood flow are seen in both "obese normotensive" individuals and obese hypertensive subjects in the metabolic syndrome, other important features must exist within the metabolic syndrome to account for impaired natriuresis encountered in obesity-hypertension.

When the renal and systemic hemodynamic findings in obese and lean normotensive and hypertensive subjects were studied, the obese patients had an increased renal blood flow, increased total blood volume and increased cardiac output, as compared to the lean normotensive and hypertensive patients. The total peripheral and renal vascular resistance was decreased. These investigators have shown that elevated cardiac output and volume expansion in obese patients also increased renal perfusion and decreased renal vascular resistance [32]. The higher increase in glomerular filtration ratio compared with the renal flow will increase the filtration fraction and these hemodynamic changes are the likely mechanism for glomerulosclerosis [24].

In summary, the pathological lesion that characterizes the pathology of the human kidney in obesity-hypertension subjects is the development of glomerulomegaly with focal and segmental glomerulosclerosis [19].

15.2.2 Renin-Angiotensin-Aldosterone System Dynamics in Obesity-Hypertension

Upregulation of the Renin-Angiotensin-Aldosterone System (RAAS) is perhaps the best described mechanism accounting for impaired natriuresis in this condition. Upregulation of the RAAS system occurs despite a volume expanded state, which in normal physiology would downregulate RAAS expression. Multiple likely mechanisms for RAAS upregulation exist and include: (1) direct renin secretion via β-adrenergic stimulation by the sympathetic nervous system, (2) increased expression of RAAS components by the adipocyte itself and particularly inflamed adipocytes as seen in visceral obesity, (3) extrinsic renal parenchymal compression via intra-abdominal fat, and (4) extra-adrenal secretion of aldosterone from adipocytes [30, 34].

In the normal state, renin is produced by the juxtaglomerular (JG) apparatus in response to renal hypoperfusion in the setting of hypotension, and by catecholamine induced activation of β-1 adrenergic receptors located on the JG apparatus. Renin then converts free circulating angiotensinogen into angiotensin I, which is subsequently converted to angiotensin II in the lungs by the angiotensin-converting enzyme type 1 (ACE-1). Angiotensin II then binds to angiotensin receptor 1 (ATR1) on vascular smooth muscle cells, resulting in vasoconstriction. Additionally, angiotensin II directly stimulates the ATR1 in the proximal tubule to increase sodium reabsorption, and it stimulates the ATR1 in the zona glomerulosa of the adrenal gland to produce aldosterone, which results in increased sodium and water reabsorption in the distal tubule. In addition to this, ACE-1 also inactivates bradykinin and kallidin, which are potent vasodilators. In the setting of hypotension or shock, the RAAS system provides a useful mechanism to raise arterial blood pressure and minimize sodium and water wasting. However, in chronically activated states, such as in catecholamine excess seen in obesity, this results in excess sodium and volume retention and the development of hypertension [35].

The increase in baseline sympathetic tone in obesity is well documented and is likely a major component of chronic RAAS activation in obesity hypertension [36–38]. Both increases in muscle sympathetic nerve activity and baseline catecholamine levels have been observed in obese human subjects [38–40]. One potential mechanism for this increase in sympathetic tone is via the hyperinsulinemic state seen in the insulin resistant metabolic syndrome. Insulin has been shown to directly stimulate the sympathetic nervous system in human normotensive and pre-hypertensive patients, however concomitant vasodilation in response to insulin infusion limits rise in arterial pressure in response to insulin in the normal state [41, 42]. It is not clear, however, if the vasodilatory properties of acute insulin release persist in the chronic hyperinsulinemic state, with some suggestion that in the setting of insulin resistance, the sympathetic effects of insulin may persist but without the vasodilatory properties. It has been well documented that chronic hyperinsulinemia is a strong predictor of hypertension, and hyperinsulinemia has been associated with hypertension independent of body mass index [43, 44].

Further, patients with normotension but hyperinsulinemia in the fasting state have been shown to have a twofold higher risk of developing hypertension in a four-year follow-up compared to normal controls [45].

In addition to hyperinsulinemia due to insulin resistance in obesity, obese human subjects have also been found to have leptin resistance and hyperleptinemia [46, 47]. In the normal state, leptin, a peptide hormone produced by adipocytes, stimulates receptors within the hypothalamus that signals overfeeding and induces a feeling of satiety, and via activation of the proopiomelanocortin pathway stimulates the sympathetic nervous system resulting in sympathetic activation [48–50]. Leptin infusion in the rare cases of leptin deficiency results in thermogenesis, anorexia, and weight loss [51–54]. However, in the hyper-leptin obese scenario, it no longer appears to have an influence on food intake or weight regulation, though it continues to exert an effect on sympathetic upregulation [55].

Further corroboration of the potential role of leptin in the development of blood pressure and SNS activation is the observation that mutations of melanocortin pathway and inactivation of the leptin receptor delete hypertension despite hyperleptinemia, and that animals undergoing chronic leptin infusion developed hypertension [56–59]. Furthermore, the hypertensive effect of leptin appears to be abolished with α- and β-adrenergic blockade, reinforcing the hypothesis that leptin's hypertensive effects are potentiated via sympathetic activation [60].

Finally, sympathetic overactivation is also felt to occur because of sleep disordered breathing and obstructive sleep apnea, which has been consistently shown to occur with greater frequency in obesity. Frequent nocturnal arousals in this condition have been shown to result in sympathetic bursts and result in increased baseline sympathetic tone in individuals with this condition [61–64]. More recently, it has been shown that volume expansion in obesity and rostral fluid shifts leading to palatial and neck edema at night when patients are supine may be the underlying mechanism accounting for sleep apnea in obese individuals [65, 66]. Therefore, though OSA is a consequence of volume expansion, its occurrence appears to result in a vicious cycle of further sympathetic activation and sodium retention, worsening the condition as well as the development of hypertension.

Beyond the sympathetic induced activation of RAAS in obese subjects, it appears that the adipocyte itself may have an important influence in increasing RAAS expression in obesity. All components of the RAAS system have been found within adipose tissue, and the renin receptor has been isolated to the adipocyte cell wall

[35, 67, 68]. Intriguingly, the renin receptor concentration was found to be much greater on visceral adipocytes than in ectopic adipocytes, suggesting adipocyte derived RAAS expression may account for some of the metabolic and hypertensive differences observed between visceral and ectopic obesity [69]. RAAS expression within the adipocyte appears to have an important role in visceral fat differentiation and growth, and interestingly, mice with angiotensin receptor inactivation and angiotensinogen knockout mice were both found to be immune to the development of diet induced obesity and hypertension despite a high-fat diet [70–74]. Increased expression of RAAS components is felt to influence systemic RAAS expression either from direct systemic secretion of these products from the adipocyte, or from "spillage" from the adipocyte, particularly in the setting of adipocyte hypoxia commonly seen in visceral obesity [35, 75–77]. It has been demonstrated in mice that as much as 30% of circulating angiotensinogen can be derived from the adipocyte [78]. Additionally, increased adipocyte derived angiotensinogen gene expression has been demonstrated in obese humans [77, 79].

A theorized but unconfirmed potential mechanism for increased RAAS expression in obesity-hypertension is from external compression of the kidneys from visceral fat deposits seen in severely advanced stages of obesity [35]. Retroperitoneal fat in humans tightly encases the renal capsule and can invade the renal sinuses. This compression, in theory, could result in reduced effective renal blood flow and distal tubule sodium delivery, which would then be sensed by the macula densa, and RAAS expression would be increased via the tubuloglomerular feedback mechanism. Strong correlations between retroperitoneal fat and hypertension risk were reported from both the Framingham Heart Study cohort and the Dallas Heart study to support this hypothesis [80, 81].

Finally, in addition to increased adrenal production of aldosterone in response to elevated angiotensin II levels with RAAS upregulation, the adipocyte itself has more recently been shown to be a source of extra-adrenal aldosterone [82]. The extra-adrenal production of aldosterone by the adipocyte may account for the findings of increased circulating aldosterone levels in visceral adiposity [83–87]. The degree to which extra-adrenal aldosterone contributes to obesity hypertension is less clear at this time, though numerous studies have linked hyperaldosteronism with inflammation and fibrosis of the vasculature and major organs, and this appears to be an important target for future investigation [88–90]. Further supporting this finding is the observation that aldosterone antagonists appear to have a greater effect at reducing systemic blood pressure in patients with central adiposity as compared to other patients with resistant hypertension [91].

15.2.3 Sympathetic Nervous System in Obesity-Hypertension

Beyond RAAS stimulation, the increase in sympathetic tone in obesity additionally may result in alpha mediated vasoconstriction, beta mediated increased cardiac output, and direct increase in urinary sodium reabsorption via the proximal tubule and loop of Henle, resulting in elevated mean arterial pressure. The potential impact of the sympathetic system influencing impaired natriuresis was well demonstrated in a follow-up study using the dog model described earlier in the chapter. In this follow-up study, the obesity induced hypertensive dogs were shown to have resolution of hypertension after undergoing renal sympathetic nerve denervation, a powerful demonstration of the influence of sympathetic system on natriuresis [92].

Increase in efferent renal sympathetic nerve activity has been shown to increase sodium retention, and this has been a suspected target for the impairment of natriuresis seen in obesity hypertension [39]. Unfortunately, despite numerous animal models and several early human trials demonstrating dramatic improvements in blood pressure with renal denervation, its use in human patients is currently inconclusive, with disappointing results for denervation when compared to sham renal artery catheter placement in the simplicity-3 trial [93]. Therapeutic application with this technique is therefore uncertain for now and will require further investigation [94].

Nonetheless, the likely prominence of the role of the sympathetic nervous system as a major mechanism in the development of obesity hypertension is reinforced by the finding that systolic blood pressure and mean arterial pressure is reduced by a greater amount by combined α-, β-blockade in hypertensive subjects with obesity versus lean hypertensive patients [95]. These findings suggest a more significant role of the sympathetic system in obesity hypertension when compared to other forms of hypertension.

15.2.4 Ghrelin, GLP-1, and Other Hormones

A multitude of relatively newly discovered gut peptide hormones, cytokines and adipokines may additionally contribute to the development of obesity hypertension. One intriguing possibility is the potential role of Ghrelin, a peptide hormone derived from gastric cells in response to caloric restriction. Ghrelin typically stimulates appetite in response to diminished food intake [96]. In human patients, Ghrelin infusion was shown to have a hypotensive effect, resulting in a drop in both systolic and diastolic blood pressure in both obese and lean subjects. Despite this hypotensive effect, Ghrelin infusion resulted in increased muscle sympathetic nerve activity and a rise in serum cortisol levels. Though the study was small, the obese subjects were noted to have a more pronounced reduction in systolic blood pressure compared to the normal weight subjects (−11 mmHg vs. −6 mmHg) [97]. Ghrelin overexpression has not been found to be associated with most forms of human obesity, and in fact obese subjects have been associated with low serum Ghrelin levels, raising the possibility that the absence of this hormone and its antihypertensive effects may influence the development of hypertension in obesity [98].

The role of ghrelin is further complicated, however, from observations from bariatric surgery. Gastric reduction surgeries, such as laparoscopic gastric banding, result in increased levels of circulating ghrelin in the postoperative state; whereas gastric resection type surgeries, such as the sleeve gastrectomy or the Roux-en-Y gastric bypass results in a further decrease in circulating ghrelin levels [99–101].

Paradoxically though, the resection type surgeries are associated with a far superior improvement in hypertension compared to reduction surgeries, though other factors may complicate this such as the degree of weight loss [102]. Nonetheless, the potential impact of ghrelin on obesity hypertension is incompletely understood and requires more investigation.

Glucagon-like peptide-1 has more recently gained notice as a potential contributor to both the development of the metabolic syndrome and possibly as well to obesity hypertension. GLP-1 affects gastric emptying and influences insulin sensitivity [103]. The GLP-1 agonists liraglutide and exenatide have been shown to have modest effects at lowering weight and blood pressure in patients with type II diabetes mellitus, and the blood pressure reduction with these medications appears to be greater than would be expected to a corresponding weight reduction alone [104–107]. In contrast to these findings, however, Krisai et al. demonstrated a linear correlation between fasting plasma GLP-1 levels and ambulatory blood pressure in human subjects [108]. Additionally, studies on infusions of GLP-1 have been mixed, with some findings demonstrating acute infusions raising blood pressure, while others have showed a chronic infusion resulting in natriuresis via release of atrial natriuretic peptide [109–111].

Finally, adiponectin, an adipokine secreted by healthy adipose tissue, appears to have numerous positive effects on the cardiovascular system, with higher levels associated with lower blood pressure, improved insulin sensitivity, and reduced basal sympathetic tone [112–114]. Levels of adiponectin are reduced however in visceral obesity, and it is felt that this may additionally contribute to the development of obesity hypertension, though the mechanism is unclear at this time.

Beyond ghrelin, GLP-1, and adiponectin, a myriad of additional gut peptides, adipokines and inflammatory cytokines appear to be altered in obesity and the metabolic syndrome. The potential of these other agents to affect blood pressure in obesity hypertension is incompletely understood. Certainly, the complexity of this condition will continue to widen with future investigations into this interesting pathology (Fig. 15.2).

15.3 Treatment of Obesity-Hypertension

15.3.1 Weight Loss: Lifestyle Modification

It has long been proven by Reisin et al. that weight loss, regardless of sodium restriction, results in significant improvement in arterial blood pressure [115]. In addition to effects on blood pressure, weight loss in obese subjects has been shown to result in significant improvement in other cardiometabolic risk factors of the metabolic syndrome including hyperglycemia and dyslipidemia [116–121]. As a result of these findings, it has been universally recommended that all patients with obesity and metabolic syndrome undergo lifestyle modification with a focus on weight loss through diet and exercise. Unfortunately, sustained weight loss with lifestyle modification alone is difficult to achieve in practice, and poor overall

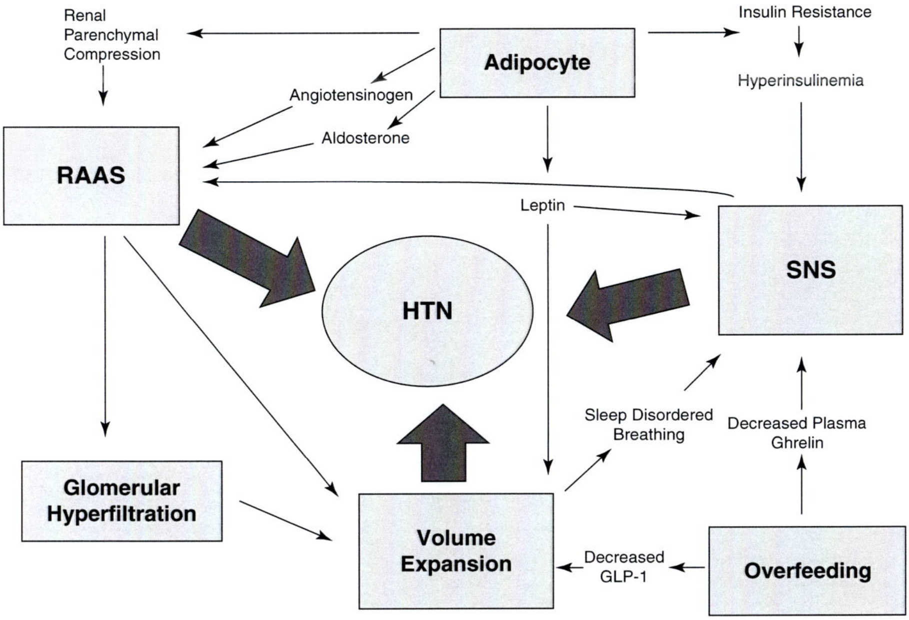

Fig. 15.2 Mechanisms of Obesity-Hypertension. (Figure reprinted with permission from Owen JG, Yazdi F, Reisin E. American Journal of Hypertension 2017;31(1):11–17)

weight loss has been observed in long-term studies [122–124]. Further complicating matters, an ever-increasing number of weight-reducing diet plans now exist and the metabolic impact of each style of diet is uncertain [125]. Likewise, the potential impact of diet versus exercise or both, as well as the type of exercise performed and its impact on hypertension and other metabolic components, is also a matter of debate [126–129].

In terms of the magnitude of blood pressure improvement to be expected with weight loss, several meta-analyses have now been conducted regarding the available studies. In 2003, Neter et al. conducted a review of 25 randomized controlled trials of the effect of weight loss on hypertension [130]. A total of 4874 patients were included in the analysis. In this analysis, an average weight reduction of 5.1kg, or 5.8% of initial body weight, resulted in a decrease in systolic blood pressure (SBP) of 4.44 mmHg, and a decrease in diastolic blood pressure of 3.57 mmHg. In sub-analysis, greater weight loss resulted in larger decreases in both systolic and diastolic blood pressure, with weight loss of greater than 5.0 kg resulting in a reduction in SDP of 6.24 mmHg, and DBP to 4.97 mmHg, compared to 2.44 mmHg SBP and 1.97 mmHg DBP in those with weight loss of less than 5.0 kg. The reduction in this study corresponded to a reduction of 1.1/0.9 mmHg SBP/DBP per kilogram of body weight lost, which corresponded well to an earlier smaller analysis of randomized controlled trials by Stassen et al. demonstrating a decrease of 1.2/1.0 mmHg SBP/DBP per kilogram body weight lost [131].

A later review by Aucott et al. in 2005 sought to determine the durability of blood pressure reduction with weight loss over time [132]. This analysis examined a total of 14 studies, with a total of 4952 patients, and ranging in follow-up from 2 to 11 years. The study was confounded by inclusion of trials with surgical weight loss as well as medication induced weight loss. Though a rough correlation of a 1:1 ratio of blood pressure decrease mmHg per kilogram body weight was observed in the short term; when examining results greater than 2 years after weight loss this dissipated to a predicted drop in blood pressure of 6.0/4.6 mmHg per 10 kg of body weight lost. Thus, it was concluded that long-term reduction in blood pressure with weight loss might be roughly half that estimated from shorter term trials. A separate, later review of eight clinical trials by the same group in 2009, predicted a drop of SBP by 5.6 mmHg for 5 kg weight loss, confirming the earlier estimates, however the reduction could not be predicted from the data for diastolic blood pressure and appeared to become less reliable for follow-up of greater than 3 years, again calling into question the long-term durability of blood pressure reduction after weight loss [133].

Most recently, a Cochrane review by Semlitsch et al. has again reexamined this issue [134]. In this review, a total of eight randomized controlled trials met criteria for review, with a total of 2100 patients. Overall, a reduction of 4.5/3.2 mmHg was observed with an average weight reduction of 4 kg, consistent with the roughly 1:1 mmHg/kg weight loss from baseline reduction in blood pressure as noted from previous reports. Therefore, though these results are overall modest, the consistent finding of an improvement in blood pressure with weight loss, coupled with observed improvements in other cardiometabolic risk factors with weight loss, reinforce the importance of the recommending weight loss for all patients with obesity-hypertension.

The ideal type of diet, which should induce weight reduction and improvement in cardiometabolic risk factors, remains controversial. The so-called DASH diet, adopted from the Dietary Approaches to Stop Hypertension (DASH) trial, is perhaps the most well studied of the available popular diet plans. In the original trial, 459 patients with blood pressures less than 160/95 mmHg were recruited [135]. In the first 3 weeks, all patients were given the control diet, which was felt typical of the average diet in the United States at the time of the study. After the 3-week run in period, the patients were then stratified into one of three dietary pattern groups for the next 8 weeks. In the first group, the patients continued to receive the control diet. In the second group, the patients were given a diet rich in fruits and vegetables compared to the control group. Finally, in the third group, the patients were given a "combination" diet rich in fruits and vegetables, as well as low-fat dairy and with an emphasis on reduction of saturated fat compared to the control group and group two. All meals and snacks for the participants were prepared by the study sites and participants were not allowed outside food. Importantly, all participants in all three groups were restricted to 3 gm daily of sodium. In both intervention arms, the potassium target was 4700 mg per day, compared to 1700 mg per day in the control arm. Both intervention arms in the DASH trial produced significant reductions in blood pressure, with the most improvement in the third "combination group." The fruit and vegetable only group saw a decrease overall of 2.8/1.1 mmHg in blood pressure versus the control group, and the combination group saw an improvement of 5.5/3.0 mmHg in blood pressure versus the controls. More impressively, when the patients with hypertension at study inclusion were sub-analyzed, the hypertensive patients in the combination group saw a reduction of blood pressure of 11.4/5.5 mmHg compared to the control group. Likewise, the hypertension patients in the fruit and vegetable group saw an improvement in blood pressure of 7.2/2.8 mmHg compared to the control group. The combination group diet from DASH emphasizing increased fruits and vegetables, increased low-fat dairy, and decreased saturated fat intake has since become known as the DASH diet. It should be noted, however, that in popular culture the DASH diet is often referred to as a low sodium diet, and while naturally low in sodium, the original study had no differences in sodium intake between the intervention arms and the control group. Therefore, the differences in blood pressure reduction could not be explained from sodium restriction with this diet, but must occur via alternate mechanisms such as increased intake of potassium, intake of antioxidants and other micronutrients from fruits/vegetables, from decreased saturated fat intake and improvement in omega-3 fatty acid consumption, or possibly via increased intake of milk proteins [136, 137].

The ENCORE study was a subsequent evaluation of the DASH diet alone or in combination with a weight loss and exercise plan compared to controls, and demonstrated that the DASH diet combined with weight loss was far superior to DASH diet alone in reducing blood pressure [138]. This study demonstrated an impressive reduction of blood pressure of 16.1/9.9 mmHg when the DASH diet was combined with exercise and weight loss versus a reduction in pressure of 11.2/7.5 mmHg via the DASH diet alone. In a secondary analysis of the ENCORE study, the same group sought to examine the effects of the DASH diet on other parameters of the metabolic syndrome; notably insulin sensitivity, fasting lipid profile, and exercise capacity [139]. Interestingly, this analysis demonstrated improvement in these features only in the group weight loss and exercise combined with DASH diet. The DASH diet alone had no changes in these features compared with the control diet. Thus, it was concluded that although DASH diet is helpful in improving blood pressure alone; weight loss is essential to improve other cardiovascular risk factors of the metabolic syndrome. Furthermore, a meta-analysis of nine studies on the DASH diet published by Shirani et al. in 2013 failed to demonstrate improvements in fasting blood glucose or insulin resistance with the DASH diet, though improvement in fasting insulin concentration was seen, though this appeared to be strongly influenced by one study calling in to question this conclusion [140].

The Mediterranean diet has been more recently popularized, and shares many features of the DASH diet including high consumption of fruits and vegetables but emphasizes increased consumption of monounsaturated and polyunsaturated fats via nuts, fish, legumes and olive oil; and the regular but moderate consumption of wine with meals. Enthusiasm for this diet was bolstered by an observational study involving 22,043 patients in Greece that demonstrated a lower risk of all-cause mortality, death from coronary artery disease, and death from cancer in patients with the highest dietary compliance to the traditional components of this diet [141]. The PREDIMED study was a later, randomized controlled trial of 7447 patients who were randomized to receive either instruction on a low-fat diet, instruction on the Mediterranean diet with supplementation of 1 L of olive oil to be ingested per week, or instruction on the Mediterranean diet with supplementation of 30gm of mixed nuts per week (walnuts, hazelnuts, and almonds) [142]. In this trial, there was a significant reduction in cardiovascular events in both the olive oil group (HR 0.7; 95% CI 0.54–0.92) and the nut groups (HR 0.72; 95% CI 0.54–0.96). However, a subsequent criticism is that the control arm, despite instruction in low-fat diet, failed to achieve adequate fat intake reduction in practice and thus comparison of Mediterranean diet to a low-fat diet was limited in this model. In regard to blood pressure reduction with the Mediterranean diet, two sites in Spain who recruited into the PREDIMED trial also randomized patients into a prospective arm evaluating ambulatory blood pressure response to the Mediterranean diet versus control at one year following randomization [143]. In this sub-study, the patients receiving the Mediterranean diet supplemented with olive oil saw a reduction in ambulatory blood pressure of 2.3/1.2 mmHg; and those patients receiving the Mediterranean diet supplemented with nuts saw a reduction in ambulatory blood pressure of 2.6/1.2 compared to an increase of ambulatory blood pressure of 1.7/0.7 mmHg in the patients on the control diet. This study was small in overall size, however. A later sub-analysis of the PREDIMED data group revealed a modest improvement in diastolic, but not systolic blood pressure with both Mediterranean diet groups when compared to the control diet [144]. Finally, in a meta-analysis by Gay et al., examining different dietary approaches and impact on hypertension, the authors examined four trials on the Mediterranean diet and noted a small but significant reduction in diastolic but not systolic blood pressure [145]. Diastolic pressure was reduced by 1.44 mmHg in this analysis with the Mediterranean diet. However, this compared poorly to the DASH diet, which had the greatest blood pressure reduction of all diets compared in this systematic review with an average reduction of 7.62/4.22 mmHg.

More recently, low carbohydrate and very low carbohydrate diets have gained in popularity. Concerns have persisted since the introduction of these diets as carbohydrates are generally replaced with either fat or protein. Given the earlier studies on low-fat diets and improvement in metabolic parameters, several have questioned whether these diets may confer increased cardiovascular risks over time, particularly if the fat substituted is in the form of saturated fats [146]. Additionally, as high protein intake has been associated with accelerated renal function decline in animal models, concern has also been expressed regarding the long-term effects on the kidney with high protein diets [147, 148]. Somewhat surprisingly, however, early data on low carbohydrate diets suggest they may be superior to low-fat diets for weight loss as well as in improving cardiometabolic risk factors for many patients. In 2003, two initial and groundbreaking trials were published in the New England Journal of Medicine supporting the potential benefit of low carbohydrate over low-fat diets. In the first study by Samaha et al., 132 patients with high prevalence of metabolic syndrome or diabetes were randomized into a low carbohydrate diet versus a low-fat diet. The low carbohydrate group lost 3.9 kg more than the low-fat group, had a greater reduction in their serum triglycerides (−20% vs. −4%), and had greater improvement in insulin sensitivity [149]. In the second study by Foster et al., 63 patients were randomized to a low carbohydrate versus a low protein diet. Similarly, in the short term, patients on the low carbohydrate diet lost more weight than in the low-fat group, though effect was less at 1 year. The low carbohydrate group also saw greater improvements in triglycerides and HDL cholesterol, though LDL and blood pressure was similar between the two groups [150]. Since that time, numerous reports have continued to demonstrate favorability of low carbohydrate diets in regard to weight loss and improvement in cardiometabolic risk factors [151–154].

In terms of blood pressure improvement with carbohydrate restriction, an analysis of the DiOGenes study demonstrated an approximately 2.2 mmHg lower systolic blood pressure in the high protein group versus the control diet [155]. Similarly, in the OmniHeart study, replacement of carbohydrate with protein resulted in mean improvement in systolic blood pressure of 1.4 mmHg in normotensive patients, and by 3.5 mmHg in hypertensive subjects. In this same trial, replacement of carbohydrate with monounsaturated fat also lowered mean systolic blood pressure by 1.3 mmHg in normotensive patients and 2.9 mmHg in hypertensives, thus arguing for benefit of carbohydrate restriction in obesity-hypertension [156]. Longer term cardiovascular outcomes with these diets, however, are still lacking, and very little information exists regarding long-term renal outcomes, though early data on short term renal effects is reassuring [147, 157].

15.3.2 Weight Loss: Pharmacotherapy

Several weight-loss inducing drugs are now available and are being increasingly used as adjunct therapy with lifestyle medication to promote weight loss. The currently available drugs include phentermine, phentermine in combination with topiramate, orlistat, lorcaserin, bupropion, and liraglutide. These drugs exert effects through a variety of mechanisms: sympathetic activation, serotonin agonism, antidepression, and via GLP-1 agonism. The precise impact of each medication on patients with hypertension is less clear at this time, though a cause of concern given their mechanisms of action. Previously, sibutramine was withdrawn from the market as a weight loss agent due to effects of increasing blood pressure and concern for exacerbating cardiovascular events. A recent, large systematic review was conducted on the available pharmacologic agents and their effect on patients with hypertension. Orlistat, an intestinal fat absorption blocker, was found to have a benefit in lowering blood pressure, with an average reduction of 2.5/1.9 mmHg. There was insufficient data, however, on the remaining weight loss inducing drugs for the authors to make conclusions regarding these drugs and blood pressure [158].

15.3.3 Weight Loss: Bariatric Surgery

Intentional weight loss through lifestyle modification with diet and exercise is recommended in all cases of obesity-hypertension. As noted, however, sustained weight loss through lifestyle modification alone is difficult in practice, and most patients meet with long-term or failure or unsatisfactory magnitude of weight loss in their efforts. Increasingly, patients are opting for surgical weight loss via bariatric procedures. Bariatric surgery has been proven to be the most reliable and durable method for sustained weight loss in patients with obesity, with substantial improvements and in many cases resolution of features of the metabolic syndrome [102, 159]. Control of diabetes mellitus type II has been proven to have superior results following bariatric surgery versus intensive lifestyle modification alone, and these results appear to persist long term [160–162]. Though a significant improvement is seen in hypertension as well in the short term following bariatric surgery, significant concern has existed about the long-term durability of hypertension control after an initial report from the Swedish Obese Subjects (SOS) trial [163]. In this trial, approximately 2000 patients were randomized to intensive lifestyle modification or bariatric surgery involving either traditional Roux-en-Y gastric bypass, vertical banded gastroplasty, or adjustable gastric banding. The incidence of hypertension at 2 and 10 years was not found to be different between the surgical group and the control group in the initial report; though the resolution of pre-existing hypertension in the study did favor surgery, suggesting an effect.

In 2012, however, the SOS data was reexamined by the authors due to an increased number of available 10 year follow-up data and to evaluate for a difference in the rates of hypertension control in patients who had a malabsorptive procedure (byass) versus a gastric restrictive procedure (banding) [164]. The re-analysis was more favorable to surgery for long-term control of hypertension in patients undergoing gastric bypass, with an average reduction of 12.1/7.3 mmHg at 2 years, and 5.1/5.6 mmHg at 10 years. Gastric banding was found to have roughly half the reduction in blood pressure of gastric bypass at 2 years, but at 10 years there was no difference in hypertension compared to controls. Similar to other studies, gastric bypass in this analysis demonstrated superior weight loss to gastric banding.

Reassuringly, several large meta-analyses have been conducted demonstrating consistent benefits of bariatric surgery in regard to hypertension (Table 15.1). Though the range of follow-up in the available studies examined varies, the results of these analyses suggest that approximately 60–80% of patients will have some degree of improvement or resolution of hypertension following bariatric surgery [159, 165–169]. These analyses also suggest a lessened effect with restrictive surgeries, such as the laparoscopic adjustable band, when compared to the malabsorptive surgeries or those involving gastric resection such as the Roux-en-Y gastric bypass, the duodenal switch, and the sleeve gastrectomy. In the first major meta-analysis by Buchwald et al., the resolution of hypertension following gastric banding was 38.4% versus 75.4% with traditional Roux-en-Y and 81.3% after biliopancreatic diversion [159]. Likewise, Courcoulus et al. reported remission of hypertension after three years in 38.2% of patients undergoing Roux-en-Y gastric bypass versus 17.4% of patients who had a laparoscopic adjustable gastric band placed [170]. As evidenced by these studies, it can be safely assumed that bariatric surgery does result in reduction of blood pressure, though this effect may lessen over time, and that procedures involving resection of the stomach or malabsorption produce roughly twice the effect of gastric banding procedures.

Table 15.1 Summary of findings from major meta-analysis examining hypertension outcomes following bariatric surgery

Meta-analysis and date	# of studies evaluated	# of patients included in analysis	Type of surgery performed and impact on hypertension	Length of follow up
Sarkhosh et al.—2015	33	3997	LSG	12–48 months
			– 58% resolution at 1 year	
			– 75% resolution or improvement	
Ricci et al.—2014	22	4160	RYGB, BPD, DS, LSG, LAGB, GB, VBG	24–65 months
			– 48% reduction in risk of hypertension[a]	
Wilhelm, Young Kale-Pradhan—2014	57	52,151	RYGB, BPD, DS, LSG, LAGB, GB, VBG	1 week–7 years
			– 50% overall resolution	
			– Improvement in 63.7%[a]	
Vest et al.—2012	73	19,543	RYGB, BPD, DS, LSG, LAGB, VBG	3–176 months
			– 62.5% resolved or improved[a]	
Heneghan et al.—2011	52	16,867	RYGB, BPD, LAGB, LAGB, VBG	3–155 months
			– 68% overall with resolution or improvement (all surgeries)	
			– RYGB—60% resolution or improvement	
			– BPD—79% resolution or improvement	
			– VBG—81% resolution or improvement	
			– LAGB—58% resolution or improvement	
Buchwald et al.—2004	136	22,094	RYGB, BPD, DS, LAGB, VBG	Follow-up length of studies unavailable
			– 61.7% overall resolution; 78.5% improved (all surgeries)	
			– RYGB—67.5% resolved; 87.2% improved	
			– BPD-DS—83.4% resolved; 75.1% improved	
			– LAGB—43.2% resolved; 70.8% improved	

Study definitions vary for resolution and improvement. Abbreviations: *BPD* biliopancreatic diversion, *DS* duodenal switch, *GB* gastric banding, *LAGB* laparoscopic gastric banding, *LSG* laparoscopic sleeve gastrectomy, *RYGB* Roux-en-Y gastric bypass, *VBG* vertical banded gastroplasty

Table reprinted with permission from Owen JG, Yazdi F, Reisin E. American Journal of Hypertension 2017 [102]

[a]Studies did not breakdown outcomes by type of surgery performed

As a result of the robust data on the ability of bariatric surgery to improve the cardiometabolic risk factors of obesity and improve weight loss, a joint clinical guidelines recommendation was made by the American Association of Clinical Endocrinologists, the Obesity Society, and the American Society for Metabolic and Bariatric surgery recommending a weight loss surgery for all patients with a Body Mass Index (BMI) greater than 40 kg/m^2 regardless of comorbidities, for patients with a BMI of greater than 35 kg/m^2 for patients with one or more obesity-related comorbidities, and for patients with a BMI of greater than 30 kg/m^2 with diabetes mellitus type II [171].

15.3.4 Pharmacotherapy for Hypertension in Obesity

Pharmacotherapy for hypertension in obesity should be selected to achieve a blood pressure goal of at least less than 140/90 mmHg while targeting the underlying physiology of this condition and minimizing adverse side effects. The ideal drug or combination of drugs for this condition, however, has been a matter of some debate [34]. Thiazide type diuretics were recommended as first-line blood pressure agents in 2003 in the 7th Report of the Joint National Committee on Prevention, Detection, Evaluation and Management of high blood pressure (JNC 7) [172], and the use of these drugs has been considerable since that time. Significant concern, however, was expressed over this recommendation due to the known effect of thiazide type diuretics to worsen insulin resistance and fasting glucose levels, raise serum uric acid and triglyceride levels, and the potential for these agents to convert metabolic syndrome to overt diabetes [173–177]. The original JNC 7 recommendation was based on the land-mark Antihypertensive and Lipid Lowering to Treatment to Prevent Heart Attack Trial (ALLHAT), which demonstrated a reduced rate of congestive heart failure with chlorthalidone as compared to Lisinopril or amlodipine for blood pressure, and a non-inferiority of chlorthalidone compared to these two drugs in regard to other cardiovascular events [178]. Earlier evidence from the multicenter TROPHY study, however, demonstrated superiority of Lisinopril to hydrochlorothiazide specifically in patients with obesity and hypertension in regard to both achievement of blood pressure targets as well as more favorable cardiometabolic profiles [179].

Since the initial JNC 7 report, numerous post hoc analyses of the ALLHAT data have shed some additional light on this controversy. In the first of these analyses, Barzilay et al. evaluated the development of diabetes in patients in the ALLHAT trial, and demonstrated a reduced odds ratio of the development of type 2 diabetes in patients taking Lisinopril or amlodipine when compared to chlorthalidone (0.55 and 0.73, respectively) [180]. Similarly, Black et al. examined the development of diabetes in patients in ALLHAT sub-grouped to those with and without metabolic syndrome at study inception [181]. In this analysis, it was found that in patients with metabolic syndrome, the percent of patients who develop overt diabetes was increased with chlorthalidone when compared to Lisinopril, but not amlodipine (17.1% vs. 12.6% vs. 16%). In those patients without pre-existing metabolic syndrome, however, diabetes developed in a greater number of patients taking chlorthalidone than either Lisinopril or amlodipine (7.7% vs. 4.7 vs. 4.2%, respectively). However, despite the worrisome increased risks of diabetes with chlorthalidone in these analyses, it is important to note that neither analysis found an increase of cardiovascular events, total mortality, or ESRD in the chlorthalidone group; and the study by Black et al. confirmed the previously noted decrease in congestive heart failure with chlorthalidone when compared to amlodipine in these patients.

Though the lack of cardiovascular events in these analyses is reassuring, consideration has been given as to whether the follow-up period was sufficiently long to see an effect of the worsening glycemic control with chlorthalidone. In an intriguing analysis from the ALLHAT Diabetes Extension Study, a 4 year post study follow-up of 22,418 patients found that though patients with diabetes had a greater risk of developing coronary artery disease compared with nondiabetics, the risk was less in those patients assigned to chlorthalidone versus lisinopril (HR 1.18 vs. 2.54; $p = 0.04$) [182]. This study seemed to suggest that patients who had chlorthalidone induced diabetes carried less risk than the other patients in the amlodipine and lisinopril groups, and thus it was suggested that diabetes that developed in the amlodipine and lisinopril groups might represent a true worsening of insulin resistance and the metabolic syndrome, whereas some of the chlorthalidone induced diabetes may have simply been a result of decreased insulin secretion in response to hypokalemia induced by chlorthalidone, a finding that has been suggested in other studies [183, 184].

In a slightly different concept, Reisin et al. sought to examine if there were differences in blood pressure control between the antihypertensive regimens of ALLHAT when the patients were stratified into normal weight (BMI <25 kg/m^2), overweight (BMI 25–29.9 kg/m^2), or obese (BMI >30 kg/m^2) [185]. The results of this analysis showed that there were no significant differences in blood pressure control between the amlodipine, chlorthalidone, and lisinopril groups when patients were stratified per weight. Secondly, the choice of medication did not seem to have a major influence on the rate of cardiovascular events when patients were stratified by weight, and thus it was concluded that in obese subjects with hypertension, overall blood pressure control appears more important for risk reduction than use of any one single class of antihypertensive. Despite these above assurances, concerns still exist, especially in younger patients, in regard to worsening glycemic control with the use of chlorthalidone.

Given the significant role of the RAAS in the development of obesity-hypertension as outlined in the pathophysiology section, angiotensin-converting enzyme inhibitors (ACE) and angiotensin receptor blockers (ARB) would seem to be the ideal antihypertensive agent for this condition.

Supporting a significant impact on the underlying pathophysiology of this disease, a sub-analysis of the Target to Treat study found significant improvements in HDL cholesterol levels, fasting blood glucose, serum triglycerides and waist circumference in patients treated with irbesartan or irbesartan in combination with hydrochlorothiazide [186]. These effects, and the diminishment of the negative effects of hydrochlorothiazide, were hypothesized to be the result of peroxisome proliferator-receptor gamma (PPARγ) agonist activity of this drug. Both irbesartan and telmisartan have been found to have PPARγ agonist activity, arguing for a potential role of these two agents in obesity and the metabolic syndrome [187, 188]. Likewise, a separate study showed that valsartan in combination with hydrochlorothiazide also ameliorated the negative effects of the thiazide diuretic compared to hydrochlorothiazide alone [189].

A sub-analysis of diabetic patients enrolled in the Captopril Prevention Project found that patients treated with captopril versus a traditional approach using diuretics and/or with the addition of beta-blockers found that the captopril group experienced significantly lower risk of myocardial infarctions (RR = 0.34; $P = 0.002$) as well as total mortality (RR = 0.54; $P = 0.034$) [190]. This was notable as in the larger parent study no difference was found between the two groups, arguing that in subset of patients with diabetes and metabolic syndrome RAAS blockade may be superior to other drugs. However, it should be noted that beta-blockers, as we will discuss below, also have been implicated in worsening glycemic control and weight gain, and thus these results could argue that the additive negative metabolic effects of diuretics with beta-blockers account for the findings, rather than positive effects of ACE inhibition.

Traditional beta-blockers have been associated with exacerbating weight gain and worsening glycemic control, with an unacceptable rate of development of diabetes ranging from 15% to 28% in several major antihypertensive trials [191–193]. For this reason, beta-blockers have been eliminated as first-tier medications for hypertension in most antihypertensive guidelines unless a cardiac indication exits. We feel practitioners should be especially mindful of these effects in the obese population. A small amount of literature exists that suggests the "vasodilating beta-blockers" carvedilol, labetalol, and nebivolol may have a more favorable or even positive metabolic effects, though this needs confirmation with larger trials [194–200], and virtually no comparative outcome trials between vasodilating and traditional beta-blockers have been conducted. Nonetheless, if a beta-blocker is required as an add on antihypertensive in the case of resistant hypertension, we favor use of one from the vasodilating class for this reason.

Calcium channel blockers are generally well tolerated drugs and are metabolically neutral with regard to insulin resistance and lipid abnormalities [201]. For this reason, these drugs are favored over thiazide diuretics by many as a first-line agent for the treatment of obesity-hypertension, despite the previously mentioned ALLHAT trial failing to demonstrate superiority and suggesting lower heart failure risks with chlorthalidone.

The subsequent large, multicenter Avoiding Cardiovascular Events through Combination Therapy in Patients Living with Systolic Hypertension (ACCOMPLISH) trial, which compared a combination treatment of benazepril/amlodipine to benazepril/hydrochlorothiazide, initially seemed to support this approach when the trial was stopped early due to the benazepril/amlodipine group showing a reduced rate of the primary endpoint of combined cardiovascular morbidity or mortality [202]. However, this result has received some criticism as the trial used hydrochlorothiazide, rather than the more potent and longer acting chlorthalidone, which was used in ALLHAT [203]. Furthermore, the overall differences between the groups, though statistically significant, were small and it was suggested this difference may not have been present with chlorthalidone due to its longer duration of action, more like that of amlodipine. Intriguingly, when a sub-analysis was performed of the ACCOMPLISH data stratifying the patients into normal weight, overweight, and obese categories, the amlodipine and hydrochlorothiazide groups no longer had significant differences, whereas the lower weight groups continued to favor amlodipine [204]. This was a surprising discovery as it contradicted a major hypothesis that the negative metabolic effects of thiazides would result in more negative cardiovascular outcomes in obese subjects.

Nonetheless, given the easy tolerability of calcium channel blockers and their noted neutral metabolic effects, most of the recent hypertension guidelines recommend initial therapy to consist of either a calcium channel blocker and/or an ACEi or ARB for the treatment of hypertension in patients with obesity and metabolic syndrome, with the choice of a thiazide diuretic as an alternative to calcium channel blocker if there is difficulty in tolerating that medication, or if a third agent as required [205–207]. Generally, we agree with this approach.

In conclusion, as patients with stage II hypertension (BP >160/100) will almost inevitably require at least two drugs to achieve hypertension control, we favor an ACEi or ARB plus calcium channel blocker combination as initial therapy, and agree the third medication added should be a thiazide diuretic, preferably chlorthalidone. We also feel that based upon existing available data, excessive fear of thiazide diuretics in this population is not necessary, and these drugs are a good alternative to use in combination with ACEi/ARBs in the rare setting of calcium channel blocker intolerance. Additionally, in cases of obesity-hypertension with stage 1 hypertension where monotherapy is adequate, we prefer to initiate treatment with an ACEi or ARB given its effects on the underlying pathophysiology, though likewise this can be substituted for a calcium channel blocker or as a second choice a thiazide diuretic if the patient is intolerant to the either of these medications.

We feel strongly that the beta-blockers should be reserved for fourth tier purposes, unless specific cardiac indications exit, and prefer to use a vasodilating beta-blocker when required for the purposes of hypertension. All other drug classes should be considered only after these choices have been exhausted.

Conclusion

During the last 40 years of research into Obesity-Hypertension and its impact on the cardiovascular and renal systems, we have witnessed an explosion of knowledge in the field, which has paralleled the rise of the obesity epidemic. The pathophysiology of this condition is complex, and involves an ever increasingly recognized number of hormones, cytokines, gut-peptides and adipokines, which result in large systemic hemodynamic alterations. These alterations, if untreated, lead to cardiovascular disease, congestive heart failure, and progression of chronic kidney disease.

Weight loss should be the cornerstone in management of this condition, with lifestyle modification the first approach in all cases. If patients are unsuccessful in this approach, as often occurs in practice, the underutilized option of bariatric surgery should be considered.

It is imperative, however, that antihypertensive therapy not be delayed while patients are attempting weight loss. We favor and agree with most current guidelines recommendations that first-line therapy should consist of an angiotensin receptor blocker or an angiotensin-converting enzyme inhibitor in combination with a calcium channel blocker for patients with stage 2 hypertension. Though either drug can be used alone in stage 1 hypertension, we favor the use of ACE inhibitors or ARBs due to the ability of these drugs to target the underlying physiology. Likewise, thiazide diuretics appear safe in this condition, and can be substituted if the patient is intolerant to either of the other agents, and these agents make an ideal third drug addition if one is required.

We look forward to the next 40 years of research in the field of obesity and hypertension. Though the impact of this disease is growing, we are confident that new, targeted therapies that will improve outcomes are just around the corner.

References

1. World Health Organization. Obesity: preventing and managing the global epidemic. In: World Health Organization; 2000.
2. Centers for Disease Control and Prevention. Defining overweight and obesity. https://www.cdc.gov/obesity/adult/defining.html.
3. Sturm R. Increases in morbid obesity in the USA: 2000–2005. Public Health. 2007;121(7):492–6.
4. Kyle UG, Schutz Y, Dupertuis YM, Pichard C. Body composition interpretation: contributions of the fat-free mass index and the body fat mass index. Nutrition. 2003;19(7–8):597–604.
5. Garrow JS, Webster J. Quetelet's Index (W/H2) as a measure of fatness. Int J Obes (Lond). 1985;9(2):147–53.
6. Owen J, Reisin E. Non-communicable disease: a welcome and long needed addition to the WHO's 2012 World Health Statistics. Curr Hypertens Rep. 2012;14(6):475–7.
7. World Health Organizataion. World Health Statistics 2012. http://www.who.int/gho/publications/world_health_statistics/EN_WHS2012_Full.pdf.
8. Haslam DW, James WP. Obesity. Lancet. 2005;366(9492):1197–209.
9. Stamler R, Stamler J, Riedlinger WF, Algera G, Roberts RH. Weight and blood pressure: findings in hypertension screening of 1 million Americans. JAMA. 1978;240(15):1607–10.
10. Krauss RM, Winston M, Fletcher BJ, Grundy SM. Obesity: impact on cardiovascular disease. Circulation. 1998;98(14):1472–6.
11. Vague J. La differenciation sexuelle; facteur determinant des formes de l'obesite. La Presse Medicale. 1947;55(30):339.
12. Kannel WB, Brand N, Skinner JJ Jr, Dawber TR, McNamara PM. The relation of adiposity to blood pressure and the development of hypertension: the Framingham study. Ann Intern Med. 1967;67(1):48–59.
13. Matsuzawa Y, Shimomura I, Nakamura T, Keno Y, Kotani K, Tokunaga K. Pathophysiology and pathogenesis of visceral fat obesity. Obes Res. 1995;3(Suppl 2):S187–94.

14. Hayashi T, Boyko EJ, Leonetti DL, McNeely MJ, Newell-Morris L, Kahn SE, Fujimoto WY. Visceral adiposity is an independent predictor of hypertension in Japanese Americans. Ann Intern Med. 2004;140(12):992–1000.
15. Peiris AN, Sothmann MS, Hoffmann RG, Hennes MI, Wilson CR, Gustafson AB, Kissebah AH. Adiposity, fat distribution, and cardiovascular risk. Ann Intern Med. 1989;110(11):867–72.
16. Lewington S, Clarke R, Qizilbash N, Peto R, Collins R, Prospective Studies Collaboration. Age-specific relevance of usual blood pressure to vascular mortality: a meta-analysis of individual data for one million adults in 61 prospective studies. Lancet. 2002;360(9349):1903–13.
17. de Simone G, Devereux RB, Roman MJ, Alderman MH, Laragh JH. Relation of obesity and gender to left ventricular hypertrophy in normotensive and hypertensive adults. Hypertension. 1994;23(5):600–6.
18. Griffen KA. Hypertensive kidney injury and the progression of chronic kidney disease. Hypertension. 2017;70:687–94.
19. Kambham N, Markowitz GS, Valeri AM, Lin J, D'Agati VD. Obesity-related glomerulopathy: an emerging epidemic. Kidney Int. 2001;59(4):1498–509.
20. Good D, Morse SA, Ventura HO, Reisin E. Obesity, hypertension, and the heart. J Cardiometab Syndr. 2008;3:168–72.
21. Morse S, Zhang R, Thakur V, Reisin E. Hypertension and the metabolic syndrome. Am J Med Sci. 2005;330(6):303–10.
22. Hall JE. The kidney, hypertension, and obesity. Hypertension. 2003;41:625–33.
23. Hall JE, Brands MW, Dixon WN, Smith MJ. Obesity induced hypertension: renal function and systemic hemodynamics. Hypertension. 1993;22(3):292–9.
24. Thakur V, Morse S and Reisin E. "Functional and structural renal changes in the early stages of obesity" Wolf G 9ed Obesity and the Kidney Contrib. Nephrol. Basel, Karger; 2006, vol 151, pp 135-150.
25. Kotchen T. Obesity-related hypertension: epidemiology, pathophysiology, and clinical management. Am J Hypertens. 2010;23(11):1170–8.
26. Segal-Lieberman G, Rosenthal T. Animal models in obesity and hypertension. Curr Hypertens Rep. 2013;15:190–5.
27. DeMarco VG, Aroor AR, Sowers JR. The pathophysiology of hypertension in patients with obesity. Nat Rev Endocrinol. 2014;10:364–76.
28. Singer GM, Setaro JF. Secondary hypertension—obesity and the metabolic syndrome. J Clin Hypertens. 2008;10(7):567–74.
29. Rahmouni K, Correia MLG, Haynes WG, Mark AL. Obesity-associated hypertension: new insights into mechanisms. Hypertension. 2005;45:9–14.
30. Guyton AC, Coleman TG, Cowley AV Jr, Scheel KW, Manning RD Jr, Norman RA Jr. Arterial pressure regulation: overriding dominance of the kidneys in long-term regulation and in hypertension. Am J Med. 1972;52(5):584–94.
31. Reisin E, Messerli FG, Ventura HO, Frohich ED. Renal haemodynamic studies in obesity hypertension. J Hypertens. 1987;5:397–400.
32. Reisin E, Suarez DH, Frolich ED. Haemodynamic changes associated with obesity and high blood pressure in rats with ventromedial hypothalamic lesions. Clin Sci. 1980;59:397s–9s.
33. Carroll JF, Huang M, Hester RL, Cockrell KH, Mizelle L. Hemodynamic alterations in hypertensive obese rabbits. Hypertension. 1995;26:465–70.
34. Owen JG, Reisin E. Anti-hypertensive drug treatment of patients with the metabolic syndrome and obesity: a review of evidence, meta-analysis, post hoc and guidelines publications. Curr Hypertens Rep. 2015;17:46.
35. Marcus Y, Shefer G, Stern N. Adipose tissue renin-angiotensin-aldosterone system (RAAS) and progression of insulin resistance. Mol Cell Endocrinol. 2013;378:1–14.
36. Grassi G. Sympathetic overdrive and cardiovascular risk in the metabolic syndrome. Hypertens Res. 2006;29:839–47.

37. Trossi RJ, Weiss ST, Parker DR, Sparrow D, Young JB, Landsberg L. Relation of obesity and diet to sympathetic nervous system activity. Hypertension. 1991;17:669–77.
38. Grassi G, Seravalle G, Cattaneo BM, Bolla GB, Lanfanchi A, Colombo M, Giannattasio C, Brunani A, Cavagnini F, Mancia G. Sympathetic activation in obese normotensive subjects. Hypertension. 1995;25:560–3.
39. DiBona GF. Sympathetic nervous system and hypertension. Hypertension. 2013;61:556–60.
40. Kalil GZ, Haynes WG. Sympathetic nervous system in obesity-related hypertension—mechanisms and clinical implications. Hypertens Res. 2012;35(1):4–16.
41. Anderson EA, Hoffman RP, Balon TW, Sinkey CA, Mark AL. Hyperinsulinemia produces both sympathetic neural activation and vasodilation in normal humans. J Clin Investig. 1991;87:2246–52.
42. Anderson EA, Balon TW, Hoffman RP, Sinkey CA, Mark AL. Insulin increases sympathetic activity but not blood pressure in borderline hypertensive humans. Hypertension. 1992;19(6):621–67.
43. Reaven GM, Lithell H, Landsberg L. Hypertension and associated metabolic abnormalities—the role of insulin resistance and the sympathoadrenal system. N Engl J Med. 1996;334(6):374–81.
44. Kazumi T, Kawaquchi A, Katoh J, Iwahashi M, Yoshino G. Fasting insulin and leptin serum levels are associated with systolic blood pressure independent of percentage body fat and body mass index. J Hypertens. 1999;17(10):1451–5.
45. Park SE, Rhee EJ, Park CY, Oh KY, Park SW, Kim SW, Lee WY. Impact of hyperinsulinemia in the development of normotensive, nondiabetic adults: a 4 year follow up study. Metabolism. 2013;62(4):532–8.
46. Considine RV, Sinha MK, Heiman ML, Kriauciunas A, Stephens TW, Nyce MR, Ohannesian JP, Marco CC, Mckee LJ, Bauer TL, Caro JF. Serum immunoreactive-leptin concentrations in normal-weight and obese humans. N Engl J Med. 1996;334(5):292–5.
47. Bravo PE, Morse S, Borne DM, Aguilar EA, Reisin E. Leptin and hypertension in obesity. Vasc Health Risk Manag. 2006;2(2):163–9.
48. Collins S, Kuhn CM, Petro AE, Swick AG, Chrunyk BA, Surwit RS. Role of leptin in fat regulation. Nature. 1996;380(6576):677.
49. da Silva AA, do Carmo JM, Wang Z, Hall JE. The brain melanocortin system, sympathetic control, and obesity hypertension. Physiology. 2014;29:196–202.
50. Hall JE, da Silva AA, do Carmo JM, Dubinion J, Hamza S, Munusamy S, Smith G, Stec DE. Obesity-induced hypertension: role of sympathetic nervous system, leptin, and melanocortins. J Biol Chem. 2010;285(23):17,271–6.
51. Oral EA, Simha V, Ruiz E, Andewelt A, Premkumar A, Snell P, Wanger AJ, DePaoli AM Reitman ML, Taylor SI, Gorden P, Garg A. Leptin-replacement therapy for lipodystrophy. N Engl J Med. 2002;346(8):570–80.
52. Farooqi IS, Matarese G, Lord GM, Keogh JM, Lawrence E, Agwu C, Sanna V, Jebb SA, Perna F, Fontana S, Lechler RI, DePaoli AM, O'Rahily S. Beneficial effects of leptin on obesity, T cell hyporesponsiveness, and neuroendocrine/metabolic dysfunction of human congenital leptin deficiency. J Clin Investig. 2002;110(8):1093–103.
53. Paz-Filho G, Mastronardi CA, Licinio J. Leptin treatment: facts and expectations. Metabolism. 2015;64(1):146–56.
54. Vatier C, Fetita S, Boudou P, Tchankou C, Deville L, Riveline J, Young J, Mathivon L, Travert F, Morin D, Cahen J, Lascols O, Andreeli F, Reznik Y, Mongeois E, Madeline I, Vantyghem M, Gautier J, Vigouroux C. One-year metreleptin improves insulin secretion in patients with diabetes linked to genetic lipodystrophic syndromes. Diabetes Obes Metab. 2016;18(7):693–7.
55. Belin de Chanteme'le EJ, Mintz JD, Rainey WE, Stepp DW. Impact of leptin-mediated sympatho-activation on cardiovascular function in obese mice. Hypertension. 2011;58:271–9.
56. da Silva AA, Kuo JJ, Hall JE. Role of hypothalamic melanocortin ¾-receptors in mediating chronic cardiovascular, renal, and metabolic actions of leptin. Hypertension. 2004;43(6):1312–7.

57. Tallam LS, da Silva AA, Hall JE. Melanocortin-4 receptor mediates chronic cardiovascular and metabolic actions of leptin. Hypertension. 2006;48(1):58–64.
58. do Carmo JM, da Silva AA, Cai Z, Lin S, Dubinion JH, Hall JE. Control of blood pressure, appetite, and glucose in mice lacking leptin receptors in proopiomelanocortin neurons. Hypertension. 2011;57(5):918–26.
59. Shek EW, Brands MW, Hall JE. Chronic leptin infusion increases arterial pressure. Hypertension. 1998;31:409–14.
60. Aizawa-Abe M, Ogawa Y, Masuzaki H, Ebihara K, Satoh N, Iwai H, Matsuoka N, Hayashi T, Hosoda K, Inoue G, Yoshimasa Y, Nakao K. Pathophysiological role of leptin in obesity-related hypertension. J Clin Investig. 2000;105:1243–52.
61. Somers VK, Dyken ME, Clary MP, Abboud FM. Sympathetic neural mechanisms in obstructive sleep apnea. J Clin Invest. 1995;96:1897–904.
62. Calhoun DA. Obstructive sleep apnea and hypertension. Curr Hypertens Rep. 2010;12:189–95.
63. Borgel J, Sanner BM, Keskin F, Bittlinsky A, Bartels NK, Buchner N, Huesing A, Rump LC, Mugge A. Obstructive sleep apnea and blood pressure: Interaction between the blood pressure-lowering effects of positive airway pressure therapy and antihypertensive drugs. Am J Hypertens. 2004;17:1081–7.
64. Dudenbostel T, Calhoun DA. Resistant hypertension, obstructive sleep apnoea, and aldosterone. J Hum Hypertens. 2012;26(5):281–7.
65. Abdel-Kader K, Dohar S, Shah N, Jhamb M, Reis SE, Strollo P, Buysse D, Unruh ML. Resistant hypertension and obstructive sleep apnea in the setting of kidney disease. J Hypertens. 2012;30(5):960–6.
66. Owen J, Reisin E. Obstructive sleep apnea and hypertension: is the primary link simply volume overload. Curr Hypertens Rep. 2013;15:131–3.
67. Karlsson C, Lindell K, Ottosson M, Sjostrom L, Carlsson B, Carlsson LM. Human adipose tissue expresses angiotensinogen and enzymes required for its conversion to angiotensin II. J Clin Endocrinol Metabol. 1998;83(11):3925–9.
68. Engeli S, Gorzelniak K, Kreutz R, Runkel N, Distler A, Sharma AM. Co-expression of renin-angiotensin system genes in human adipose tissue. J Hypertens. 1999;17(4):555–60.
69. Achard V, Boullu-Ciocca S, Desbriere R, Nguyen G, Grino M. Renin receptor expression in human adipose tissue. Am J Physiol Regul Integr Comp Physiol. 2007;292(1):R274–82.
70. Kouyama R, Suganami T, Nishida J, Tanaka M, Toyoda T, Kiso M, Chiwata T, Miyamoto Y, Yoshimasa Y, Fukamizu A, Horiuchi M, Hirata Y, Ogawa Y. Attenuation of diet-induced weight gain and adiposity through increased energy expenditure in mice lacking angiotensin II type 1a receptor. Endocrinology. 2005;146(8):3481–9.
71. Yvan-Charvet L, Even P, Bloch-Faure M, Guerre-Millo M, Moustaid-Moussa N, Ferre P, Quignard-Boulange A. Deletion of the angiotensin type 2 receptor (AT2R) reduces adipose cell size and protects from diet-induced obesity and insulin resistance. Diabetes. 2005;54:991–9.
72. Massiera F, Seydoux J, Geloen A, Quignard-Boulange A, Turban S, Saint-Marc P, Fukamizu A, Negrel R, Ailhaud G, Teboul M. Angiotensinogen-deficient mice exhibit impairment of diet-induced weight gain with alteration in adipose tissue development and increased locomotor activity. Endocrinology. 2001;142(12):5220–5.
73. Massiera F, Bloch-Faure M, Ceiler D, Murakami K, Fukamizu A, Gasc JM, Quignard-Boulange A, Negrel R, Ailhaud G, Seydoux J, Meneton P, Teboul M. Adipose angiotensinogen is involved in adipose tissue growth and blood pressure regulation. FASEB J. 2001;15(14):2727–9.
74. Yiannikouris F, Gupte M, Putnam K, Thatcher S, Charnigo R, Rateri DL, Daugherty A, Cassis LA. Adipocyte deficiency of angiotensinogen prevents obesity-induced hypertension in male mice. Hypertension. 2012;60:1524–30.
75. Hosogai N, Fukuhara A, Oshima K, Miyata Y, Tanaka S, Segawa K, Furukawa S, Tochino Y, Komuro R, Matsuda M, Shimomura I. Adipose tissue hypoxia and its impact on adipocytokine dysregulation. Diabetes. 2007;56:901–11.

76. Wree A, Mayer A, Westphal S, Beilfuss A, Canbay A, Schick RR, Gerken G, Vaupel P. Adipokine expression in brown and white adipocytes in response to hypoxia. J Endocrinol Invest. 2012;35(5):522–7.
77. Yasue S, Masuzaki H, Okada S, Ishii T, Kozuka C, Tanaka T, Fujikura J, Ebihara K, Hosoda K, Katsurada A, Ohashi N, Urushihara M, Kobori H, Morimoto N, Kawazoe T, Naitoh M, Okada M, Sakaue H, Suzuki S, Nakao K. Adipose tissue-specific regulation of angiotensinogen in obese humans and mice: impact of nutritional status and adipocyte hypertrophy. Am J Hypertens. 2010;23(4):425–31.
78. Yvan-Charvet L, Quignard-Boulange A. Role of adipose tissue renin-angiotensin system in metabolic and inflammatory diseases associated with obesity. Kidney Int. 2011;79:162–8.
79. Van Harmelen V, Ariapart P, Hoffstedt J, Lundkvist I, Bringman S, Arner P. Increased adipose angiotensinogen gene expression in human obesity. Obes Res. 2000;8(4):337–41.
80. Foster MC, Hwang SJ, Porter SA, Massaro JM, Hoffmann U, Fox CS. Fatty kidney, hypertension, and chronic kidney disease: the Framingham Heart Study. Hypertension. 2011;58:784–90.
81. Chandra A, Neeland IJ, Berry JD, Ayers CR, Rohatgi A, Das SR, Khera A, McGuire DK, de Lemos JA, Turer AT. The relationship of body mass and fat distribution with incident hypertension: observations from the Dallas Heart Study. J Am Coll Cardiol. 2014;64:997–1002.
82. Briones AM, Nguyen Dinh Cat A, Callera GE, Yogi A, Burger D, He Y, Correa JW, Gagnon AM, Gomez-Sanchez CE, Gomez-Sanchez EP, Sorisky A, Ooi TC, Ruzicka M, Burns KD, Touyz RM. Adipocytes produce aldosterone through calcineurin-dependent signaling pathways: implications in diabetes mellitus-associated obesity and vascular dysfunction. Hypertension. 2012;59:1069–78.
83. Engeli S, Bohnke J, Gorzelniak K, Janke J, Schling P, Bader M, Luft FC, Sharma AM. Weight loss and the renin-angiotensin-aldosterone system. Hypertension. 2005;45(3):356–62.
84. Dubenostel T, Ghazi L, Liu M, Li P, Oparil S, Calhoun DA. Body mass index predicts 24-hour urinary aldosterone levels in patients with resistant hypertension. Hypertension. 2015;68(4):995–1003.
85. Laffin LJ, Majewski C, Liao C, Bakris G. Relationship between obesity, hypertension, and aldosterone production in postmenopausal Africa American Women: a pilot study. J Clin Hypertens. 2016;18(12):1216–21.
86. Goodfriend TL, Egan BM, Kelley DE. Aldosterone in obesity. Endocr Res. 1998;24(3):789–96.
87. Rossi GP, Belfiore A, Bernini G, Fabris B, Caridi G, Ferri C, Giacchetti G, Letizia C, Maccario M, Mannelli M, Palumbo G, Patalano A, Rizzoni D, Rossi E, Pessina AC, Mantero F, Primary Aldosteronism Prevalence in Hypertension Study Investigators. Body mass index predicts plasma aldosterone concentrations in overweight-obese primary hypertensive patients. J Clin Endocrinol Metabol. 2008;93(7):2566–71.
88. Brown NJ. Contribution of aldosterone to cardiovascular and renal inflammation and fibrosis. Nat Rev Nephrol. 2013;9(8):459–69.
89. Huby AC, Antonova G, Groenendyk J, Gomez-Sanchez CE, Bollaq WB, Filosa JA, Belin de Chanemele EJ. Adipocyte-derived hormone leptin is a direct regulator of aldosterone secretion, which promotes endothelial dysfunction and cardiac fibrosis. Circulation. 2015;132(22):2134–45.
90. Buglioni A, Cannone V, Sangaralingham SJ, Heublein DM, Scott CG, Bailey KR, Rodeheffer RJ, Sarzani R, Burnett JC. Aldosterone predicts cardiovascular, renal and metabolic disease in the general community: a 4-year follow up. J Am Heart Assoc. 2015;4(12):pii: e002505.
91. de Souza F, Muxfeldt E, Fiszman R, Salles G. Efficacy of spironolactone therapy in patients with true resistant hypertension. Hypertension. 2010;55:147–52.
92. Henegar JR, Zhang Y, De Rama R, Hata C, Hall ME, Hall JE. Catheter based radiofrequency renal denervation lowers blood pressure in obese hypertensive dogs. Am J Hypertens. 2014;27(10):1285–92.
93. Bhatt DL, Kandzari DE, O'Neill WW, D'Agostino R, Flack JM, Katzen BT, Leon MB, Liu M, Mauri L, Negoita M, Coehn SA, Oparil S, Rocha-Singh K, Townsend RR, Bakris GL,

Symplicity HTN-3 Investigators. A controlled trial of renal denervation for resistant hypertension. N Engl J Med. 2014;370(15):1393–401.

94. Coppolino G, Pisano A, Rivoli L, Bolignano D. Renal denervation for resistant hypertension. Cochrane Database Syst Rev. 2017;2:CD011499.
95. Wofford MR, Anerson DC Jr, Brown CA, Jones DW, Miller ME, Hall JE. Antihypertensive effect of alpha- and beta- adrenergic blockade in obese and lean hypertensive subjects. Am J Hypertens. 2001;14(7):694–8.
96. Lilleness BM, Frishman WH. Ghrelin and the cardiovascular system. Cardiol Rev. 2016;24:288–97.
97. Lambert E, Lamber G, Ika-Sari C, Dawood T, Lee K, Chopra R, Straznicky N, Eikelis N, Drew S, Tilbrook A, Dixon J, Esler M, Schlaich MP. Ghrelin modulates sympathetic nervous system activity and stress response in lean and overweight men. Hypertension. 2011;58(1):43–50.
98. Tschop M, Weyer C, Tataranni PA, Devanarayan V, Rayussin E, Heiman ML. Circulating ghrelin levels are decreased in human obesity. Diabetes. 2001;50:707–9.
99. Wang Y, Liu J. Plasma ghrelin modulation in gastric band operation and sleeve gastrectomy. Obes Surg. 2009;19:357–62.
100. Hady HR, Golaszewski P, Zbucki RL, Dadan J. The influence of laparoscopic adjustable gastric banding and laparoscopic sleeve gastrectomy on weight loss, plasma ghrelin, insulin, glucose and lipis. Folia Histochem Cytobiol. 2012;50:292–303.
101. Sista F, Abruzzese V, Clementi M, Carandina S, Amicucci G. Effect of resected gastric volume of ghrelin and GLP-1 plasma levels: a prospective study. J Gastrointest Surg. 2016;20:1931–41.
102. Owen JG, Yazdi F, Reisin E. Bariatric surgery and hypertension. Am J Hypertens. 2017;31:11–7. Epub ahead of print. https://doi.org/10.1093/ajh/hpx112.
103. Baggio LL, Drucker DJ. Biology of incretins: GLP-1 and GIP. Gastroenterology. 2007;132(6):2137–57.
104. Wang B, Zhong J, Lin H, Zhao Z, Yan Z, He H, Ni Y, Liu D, Zhu Z. Blood pressure- lowering effects of GLP-1 receptor agonists exenatide and liraglutide: a meta-analysis of clinical trials. Diabetes Obes Metab. 2013;15(8):737–49.
105. Goud A, Zhong J, Peters M, Brook RD, Rajagopalan S. GLP-1 agonists and blood pressure: a review of the evidence. Curr Hypertens Rep. 2016;18(2):16.
106. Okerson T, Yan P, Stonehouse A, Brodows R. Effects of exenatide on systolic blood pressure in subjects with type 2 diabetes. Am J Hypertens. 2010;23(3):334–9.
107. Robinson LE, Holt TA, Rees K, Randeva HS, O'Hare JP. Effects of exenatide and liraglutide on heart rate, blood pressure and body weight: systematic review and meta-analysis. BMJ Open. 2013;3(1):e001986.
108. Krisai P, Aeschbacher S, Schoen T, Bossard M, van der Stouwe JG, Dorig L, Todd J, Estis J, Risch M, Risch L, Conen D. Glucgon-like peptide-1 and blood pressure in young and healthy adults from the general population. Hypertension. 2015;65:306–12.
109. Yamamoto H, Lee CH, Marcus JN, Williams TD, Overton JM, Lopez ME, Hollenberg AN, Baggio L, Saper CB, Drucker DJ, Elmquist JK. Glucagon-like peptide-1 receptor stimulation increases blood pressure and heart rate and activates autonomic regulatory neurons. J Clin Investig. 2002;110(1):43–52.
110. Barragan JM, Rodriguez RE, Blazquez E. Changes in arterial blood pressure and heart rate induced by glucagon-like peptide-1-(7-36) amide in rats. Am J Physiol. 1994;266(3):459–66.
111. Kim M, Platt MJ, Shibasaki T, Quaggin SE, Backx PH, Seino S, Simpson JA, Drucker DJ. GLP-1 receptor activation and Epac2 link atrial natriuretic peptide secretion to control of blood pressure. Nat Med. 2013;19(5):567–75.
112. Takahashi N, Anan F, Nakagawa M, Yufu K, Shinohara T, Tsubone T, Goto K, Masaki T, Katsuragi I, Tanaka K, Kakuma T, Hara M, Saikawa T, Yoshimatus H. Hypoadiponectinemia in type 2 diabetes mellitus in men is associated with sympathetic overactivity as evaluated by cardiac 123I-metaiodobenzylguanidine scintigraphy. Metabolism. 2007;56(7):919–24.

113. Vasunta RL, Kesaniemi YA, Ukkola O. Plasma adiponectin concentration is associated with ambulatory daytime systolic blood pressure but not with the dipping status. J Hum Hypertens. 2010;24(8):545–51.
114. Kim DH, Kim C, Ding EL, Townsend MK, Lipsitz LA. Adiponectin levels and the risk of hypertension: a systematic review and meta-analysis. Hypertension. 2013;62(1):27–32.
115. Reisin E, Abel R, Modan M, Silverberg DS, Eliahou HE, Modan B. Effect of weight loss without salt restriction on the reduction of blood pressure in overweight hypertensive patients. N Engl J Med. 1978;298(1):1–6.
116. Dansigner ML, Gleason JA, Giffith JL, Selker HP, Schaefer EJ. Comparison of the Atkins, Ornish, Weight Watchers, and Zone diets for weight loss and heart disease risk reduction: a randomized trial. JAMA. 2005;293(1):43–5.
117. Straznicky NE, Lambert EA, Lambert GW, Masu K, Esler MD, Nestel PJ. Effects of dietary weight loss on sympathetic activity and cardiac risk factors associated with the metabolic syndrome. J Clin Endocrinol Metabol. 2005;90(11):5998–6005.
118. Busetto L, Sergi G, Enzi G, Segato G, De Marchi F, Foletto M, De Luca M, Pigozzo S, Favretti F. Short-term effects of weight loss on the cardiovascular risk factors in morbidly obese patients. Obes Res. 2004;12(8):1256–63.
119. McTigue KM, Harris R, Hemphill B, Lux L, Sutton S, Bunton AJ, Lohr KN. Screening and interventions for obesity in adults: summary of the evidence for the U.S. Preventative Services Task Force. Ann Intern Med. 2003;139(11):933–49.
120. Esposito K, Pontillo A, Di Palo C, Giugliano G, Masella M, Marfella R, Giugliano D. Effect of weight loss and lifestyle changes on vascular inflammatory markers in obese women: a randomized trial. JAMA. 2003;289(14):1799–804.
121. Miller ER 3rd, Erlinger TP, Young DR, Jehn M, Charleston J, Rhodes D, Wasan SK, Appel LJ. Results of the diet, exercise and weight loss intervention trial (DEW-It). Hypertension. 2002;40(5):612–8.
122. Dalle Grave R, Melchionda N, Calugi S, Centis E, Tufano A, Fatati G, Fusco MA, Marchesini G. Countinues care in the treatment of obesity: an observational multicenter study. J Intern Med. 2005;258(3):265–73.
123. Sundstrom J, Bruze G, Ottosson J, Marcus C, Naslund I, Neovius M. Weight loss and heart failure: a nationwide study of gastric bypass surgery versus intensive lifestyle treatment. Circulation. 2017;135(17):1577–85.
124. Motesi L, El Goch M, Brodosi L, Calugi S, Marchesini G, Dalle Grave R. Long-term weight loss maintenance for obesity: a multidisciplinary approach. Diabetes Metab Syndr Obes. 2017;9:37–46.
125. Bloch AS. Low carbohydrate diets, pro: time to rethink our current strategies. Nutr Clin Pract. 2005;20(1):3–12.
126. Verheggen RJHM, Maessen MFH, Green DJ, Hermus ARMM, Hopman MTE, Thijssen DHT. A systematic review and meta-analysis on the effects of exercise training versus hypocaloric diet: distinct effects on body weight and visceral adipose tissue. Obes Rev. 2016;17(8):664–90.
127. Ismail I, Keating SE, Baker MK, Johnson NA. A systematic review and meta-analysis of the effect of aerobic vs. resistance exercise training on visceral fat. Obes Rev. 2011;13:68–91.
128. Goodpaster BH, Delany JP, Otto AD, Kuller L, Vockley J, South-Paul JE, Thomas SB, Brown J, McTigue K, Hames KC, Lang W, Jakicic JM. Effects of diet and physical activity interventions on weight loss and cardiometabolic risk factors in severely obese adults: a randomized trial. JAMA. 2010;304(16):1795–802.
129. Slentz CA, Bateman LA, Willis LH, Granville EO, Pinner LW, Samsa GP, Setji TL, Muehlbauer MJ, Huffman KM, Bales CW, Kraus WE. Effects of exercise training alone vs a combined exercise and nutritional lifestyle intervention on glucose homeostasis in prediabetic individuals: a randomized controlled trial. Diabetologia. 2016;59:2088–98.

130. Neter JE, Stam BE, Kok FJ, Grobbee DE, Geleijnse JM. Influence of weight reduction on blood pressure: a meta-analysis of randomized controlled trials. Hypertension. 2003;42:878–84.
131. Staessen J, Fagard R, Amery A. The relationship between body weight and blood pressure. J Hum Hypertens. 1988;2(4):207–17.
132. Aucott L, Poobalan A, Smith WCS, Avenell A, Jung R, Broom J. Effects of weight loss in overweight/obese individuals and long-term hypertension outcomes: a systematic review. Hypertension. 2005;45:1035–41.
133. Aucott L, Rothnie H, McIntyre L, Thapa M, Waweru C, Gray D. Long-term weight loss from lifestyle intervention benefits blood pressure: a systemtatic review. Hypertension. 2009;54:756–62.
134. Semlitsch T, Jeitler K, Berghold A, Horvath K, Posch N, Poggenburg S, Siebenhofer A. Long-term effects of weight-reducing diets in people with hypertension. Cochrane Database Syst Rev. 2016;3:CD008274.
135. Appel LJ, Moore TJ, Obarzanek E, Vollmer WM, Svetkey LP, Sacks FM, Bray GA, Vogt TM, Cutler JA, Windhauser MM, Lin PH, Karanja N, For the DASH Collaborative Research Group. A clinical trial of the effects of dietary patterns on blood pressure. N Engl J Med. 1997;336(16):1117–24.
136. Lin PH, Allen JD, Li YJ, Yu M, Lien L, Svetky LP. Blood pressure-lowering mechanisms of the DASH dietary pattern. J Nutr Metab. 2012;2012:472396.
137. McGregor RA, Poppitt SD. Milk protein for improved metabolic health: a review of the evidence. Nutr Metab. 2013;10:46.
138. Blumenthal JA, Babyak MA, Hinderliter A, Watkins LL, Craighead L, Lin PH, Caccia C, Johnson J, Waugh R, Sherwood A. Effects of the DASH diet alone and in combination with exercise and weight loss on blood pressure and cardiovascular biomarkers in men and women: the ENCORE study. Arch Intern Med. 2010;170(2):126–35.
139. Blumenthal JA, Babyak MA, Sherwood A, Craighead L, Lin PH, Johnson J, Watkins LL, Wang JT, Kuhn C, Feinglos M, Hinderliter A. Effects of the dietary approaches to stop hypertension diet alone and in combination with exercise and caloric restriction on insulin sensitivity and lipids. Hypertension. 2010;55:1199–205.
140. Shirani F, Salehi-Abargouei A, Azadbakht L. Effects of dietary approaches to stop hypertension (DASH) diet on some risk for developing type 2 diabetes: a systematic review and meta-analysis on controlled clinical trials. Nutrition. 2013;29:939–47.
141. Trichopoulou A, Costacou T, Bamia C, Trichopoulos D. Adherence to a Mediterranean diet and survival in a Greek population. N Engl J Med. 2003;348(26):2599–608.
142. Estruch R, Ros E, Salas-Salvado J, Covas MI, Corella D, Aros F, Gomez-Gracia E, Ruiz-Gutierrez V, Fiol M, Lapetra J, Lamuela-Raventos RM, Serra-Majem L, Pinto X, Basora J, Munoz MA, Soril JV, Martinez JA, Martinez-Gonzalez MA, PREDIMED Study Investigators. Primary prevention of cardiovascular disease with a Mediterranean diet. N Engl J Med. 2013;368(14):1279–90.
143. Domenech M, Roman P, Lapetra J, de la Corte FJ G, Sala-Vila A, de la Torre R, Corella D, Salas-Salvado J, Ruiz-Gutierrez V, Lamuela-Raventos RM, Toledo E, Estruch R, Coca A, Ros E. Mediterranean diet reduces 24-hour ambulatory blood pressure, blood glucose, and lipids: one-year randomized, clinical trial. Hypertension. 2014;64:69–76.
144. Toledo E, Hu FB, Estruch R, Buil-Cosiales P, Corella D, Salas-Salvado J, Covas MI, Aros F, Gomez-Gracia E, Fiol M, Lapetra J, Serra-Majem L, Pinto X, Lamuela-Raventos RM, Saez G, Bullo M, Ruiz-Gutierrez V, Ros E, Sorli JV, Martinez-Gonzalez MA. Effect of the Mediterranean diet on blood pressure in the PREDIMED trial: results from a randomized controlled trial. BMC Med. 2013;11:207.
145. Gay HC, Rao SG, Vaccarino V, Ali MK. Effects of different dietary interventions on blood pressure: systematic review and meta-analysis of randomized controlled trials. Hypertension. 2016;67:733–9.
146. St Jeor ST, Howard BV, Prewitt TE, Boyee V, Bazzare T, Eckel RH, Nutrition Committee of the Council on Nutrition, Physical Activity, and Metabolism of the American Heart Association. Dietary protein and weight reduction: a statement for healthcare professionals

from the Nutrition Committee of the Council on Nutrition, Physical Activity, and Metabolism of the American Heart Association. Circulation. 2001;104(15):1869–74.

147. Friedman AN, Ogden LG, Foster GD, Klein S, Stein R, Miller B, Hill JO, Brill C, Bailer B, Rosenbaum DR, Wyatt HR. Comparative effects of low-carbohydrate high protein versus low-fat diets on the kidney. Clin J Am Soc Nephrol. 2012;7(7):1103–11.
148. Brinkworth GD, Buckley JD, Noakes M, Clifton PM. Renal function following long-term weight loss in individuals with abdominal obesity on a very-low-carbohydrte diet vs high carbohydrate diet. J Am Diet Assoc. 2010;110(4):633–8.
149. Samaha FF, Iqbal N, Seshadri P, Chicano KL, Daily DA, McGrory J, Williams T, Williams M, Gracely EJ, Stern L. A low-carbohydrate as compared with a low-fat diet in severe obesity. N Engl J Med. 2003;348:2074–81.
150. Foster GD, Wyatt HR, Hill JO, McGuckin BG, Brill C, Mohammed S, Szapary PO, Rader DJ, Edman JS, Klein S. A randomized trial of a low-carbohydrate diet for obesity. N Engl J Med. 2003;348:2082–90.
151. Stern L, Iqbal N, Seshadri P, Chicano KL, Daily DA, McGrory J, Williams M, Gracely EJ, Samaha FF. The effects of low-carbohydrate versus conventional weight loss diets in severely obese adults—one year follow-up of a randomized trial. Ann Intern Med. 2004;140:778–85.
152. Yancy WS Jr, Olsen MK, Guyton JR, Bakst RP, Westman EC. A low-carbohydrate, ketogenic diet versus a low-fat diet to treat obesity and hyperlipidemia. Ann Intern Med. 2004;140:769–77.
153. Farnsworth E, Luscombe ND, Noakes M, Wittert G, Argyiou E, Clifton PM. Effect of a high-protein, energy-restricted diet on body composition, glycemic control, and lipid concentrations in overweight and obese hyperinsulinemic men and women. Am J Clin Nutr. 2003;78:31–9.
154. Brehm BJ, Seely RJ, Daniels SR, D'Alessio DA. A randomized trial comparing a very low carbohydrate diet and a calorie-restricted low fat diet on body weight and cardiovascular risk factors in healthy women. J Clin Endocrinol Metab. 2003;88:1617–23.
155. Engberink MF, Geleijnse JM, Bakker SJL, Larsen TM, Handjieva-Darlesnka T, Kafatos A, Martinez JA, Pfeiffer AFH. Effect of a high-protein diet on maintenance of blood pressure levels achieved after initial weight loss: the DiOGenes randomized study. J Hum Hypertens. 2015;29:58–63.
156. Appel LJ, Sacks FM, Carey VJ, Obarzanek E, Swain JF, Miller ER 3rd, Conlin PR, Erlinger TP, Rosner BA, Laranio NM, Charleston J, McCarron P, Bihop LM, OmniHeart Collaborative Research Group. Effects of protein, monounsaturated fat, and carbohydrate intake on blood pressure and serum lipids. JAMA. 2005;294(19):2455–64.
157. Oyabu C, Hashimoto Y, Fukuda T, Tanaka M, Asano M, Yamazaki M, Fukui M. Impact of low-carbohydrate diet on renal function: a meta-analysis of over 1000 individuals from nine randomized controlled trials. Br J Nutr. 2016;116:632–8.
158. Siebenhofer A, Jeitler K, Horvath K, Berghold A, Posch N, Meschik J, Semlitsch T. Long-term effects of weight-reducing drugs in people with hypertension. Cochrane Database Syst Rev. 2016;3:CD007654.
159. Buchwald H, Avidor Y, Braunwald E, Jensen MD, Pories W, Fahrbach K, Schoelles K. Bariatric surgery: a systematic review and meta-analysis. JAMA. 2004;292(14):1724–37.
160. Mingrone G, Panunzi S, De Gaetano A, Guidone C, Iaconelli A, Leccessi L, Nanni G, Pomp A, Castagneto M, Ghirlanda G, Rubino F. Bariatric surgery versus conventional medical therapy for type 2 diabetes. N Engl J Med. 2012;366(17):1577–85.
161. Schauer PR, Bhatt DL, Kirwan JP, Wolski K, Brethauer SA, Navaneethan SD, Aminian A, Pothier CE, Kim ES, Nissen SE, Kashyap SR, Investigators STAMPEDE. Bariatric surgery versus intensive medical therapy for diabetes—3 year outcomes. N Engl J Med. 2014;370(21):2002–13.
162. Schauer PR, Bhatt DL, Kirwan JP, Wolski K, Aminian A, Brethauer SA, Navaneethan SD, Singh RP, Pothier CE, Nissen SE, Kashyap SR, STAMPEDE Investigators. Bariatric surgery versus intensive medical therapy for diabetes—5-year outcomes. N Engl J Med. 2017;376(7):641–51.

163. Sjöström L, Lindroos AK, Peltonen M, Torgerson J, Bouchard C, Carlsson B, Dahlgren S, Larsson B, Narbro K, Sjöström CD, Sullivan M, Wedel H, Swedish Obese Subjects Study Scientific Group. Lifestyle, diabetes, and cardiovascular risk factors 10 years after bariatric surgery. N Engl J Med. 2004;351:2683–93.
164. Hallersund P, Sjöström L, Olbers T, Lönroth H, Jacobson P, Wallenius V, Näslund I, Carlsson LM, Fändriks L. Gastric bypass surgery is followed by lowered blood pressure and increased diuresis - long term results from the Swedish Obese Subjects (SOS) study. PLoS One. 2012;7:e49696.
165. Sarkhosh K, Birch DW, Shi X, Gill RS, Karmali S. The impact of sleeve gastrectomy on hypertension: a systematic review. Obes Surg. 2012;22:832–7.
166. Ricci C, Gaeta M, Rausa E, Asti E, Bandera F, Bonavina L. Long-term effects of bariatric surgery on type II diabetes, hypertension and hyperlipidemia: a meta-analysis and meta-regression study with 5-year follow-up. Obes Surg. 2015;25:397–405.
167. Wilhelm SM, Young J, Kale-Pradhan PB. Effect of bariatric surgery onhypertension: a meta-analysis. Ann Pharmacother. 2014;48:674–82.
168. Vest AR, Heneghan HM, Agarwal S, Schauer PR, Young JB. Bariatric surgery and cardiovascular outcomes: a systematic review. Heart. 2012;98:1763–77.
169. Heneghan HM, Meron-Eldar S, Brethauer SA, Schauer PR, Young JB. Effect of bariatric surgery on cardiovascular risk profile. Am J Cardiol. 2011;108:1499–507.
170. Courcoulas AP, Christian NJ, Belle SH, Berk PD, Flum DR, Garcia L, Horlick M, Kalarchian MA, King WC, Mitchell JE, Patterson EJ, Pendler JR, Pomp A, Pories WJ, Thirlby RC, Yanovski SZ, Wolfe BM, Longitudinal Assessment of Bariatric Surgery (LABS) Consortium. Weight change and health outcomes at 3 years after bariatric surgery among individuals with severe obesity. JAMA. 2013;310:2416–25.
171. Mechanick JI, Youdim A, Jones DB, Garvey WT, Hurley DL, McMahon MM, Heinberg LJ, Kushner R, Adams TD, Shikora S, Dixon JB, Brethauer S. Clinical practice guidelines for the perioperative nutritional, metabolic, and nonsurgical support of the bariatric surgery patient—2013 update: cosponsored by American Association of Clinical Endocrinologists, the Obesity Society, and American Society for Metabolic and Bariatric Surgery. Obesity. 2013;21(Supplement 1):S1–27.
172. Chobanian AV, Bakris GL, Black HR, Cushman WC, Green LA, Izzo JL Jr, Jones DW, Materson BJ, Oparil S, Wright JT Jr, Roccella EJ, National Heart, Lung, and Blood Institute Joint National Committee on Prevention, Detection, Evaluation, and Treatment of High Blood Pressure, National High Blood Pressure Education Program Coordinating Committee. The seventh report of the joint national committee on prevention, detection, evaluation and treatment of high blood pressure: the JNC 7 report. JAMA. 2003;289(19):2560–72.
173. Amery A, Berthaux P, Bulpitt C, Deruyttere M, de Schaepdryver A, Dollery C, Fagard R, Forette F, Hellemans J, Lund-Johansen P, Mutsers A, Tuomilehto J. Glucose intolerance during diuretic therapy: results of trial by the European working party on hypertension in the elderly. Lancet. 1978;1(8066):681–3.
174. Plavinik FL, Rodrigues C, Zanella MT, Ribeiro AB. Hypokalemia, glucose intolerance, and hyperinsulinemia during diuretic therapy. Hypertension. 1992;19(2 suppl):26–9.
175. Harper R, Ennis CN, Heaney AP, Sheridan B, Gormley M, Atkinson AB, Johnston GD, Bell PM. A comparison of the effects of low and conventional dose thiazide diuretic on insulin action in hypertensive patients with NIDDM. Diabetologia. 1995;38(7):853–9.
176. Punzi HA, Punzi CF. Antihypertensive and lipid-lowering heart attack trial study; trinity hypertension research institute. Metabolic issues in the antihypertensive and lipid-lowering heart attack trial study. Curr Hypertens Rep. 2004;6(2):106–10.
177. Harper R, Ennis CN, Sheridan B, Atkinson AB, Johnston GD, Bell PM. Effects of low dose versus conventional dose thiazide diuretic on insulin action in essential hypertension. Br Med J. 1994;309(6949):226–30.
178. ALLHAT Officers and Coordinators for the ALLHAT Collaborative Research Group, The Antihypertensive and Lipid-Lowering Treatment to Prevent Heart Attack Trial. Major outcomes in high-risk hypertensive patients randomized to angiotensin-converting enzyme

inhibitor or calcium channel blocker vs diuretic: the Antihypertensive and Lipid-Lowering Treatment to Prevent Heart Attack Trial (ALLHAT). JAMA. 288(23):2002, 2981.

179. Reisin E, Weir MR, Falkner B, Hutchinson HG, Anzalone DA, Tuck ML. Lisinopril versus hydrochlorothiazide in obese hypertensive patients: a multicenter placebo-controlled trial. For the Treatment in Obese Patients with Hypertension (TROPHY) study group. Hypertension. 1997;30(1):140–5.
180. Barzilay JI, Davis BR, Cutler JA, Pressel SL, Whelton PK, Basile J, Margolis KL, Ong ST, Sadler LS, Summerson J, ALLHAT Collaborative Research Group. Fasting glucose levels and incident diabetes mellitus in older nondiabetic adults randomized to receive 3 different classes of antihypertensive treatment: a report from the Antihypertensive and Lipid-Lowering Treatment to Prevent Heart Attack Trial (ALLHAT). Arch Intern Med. 2006;166(2):2191–201.
181. Black HR, Davis B, Barzilay J, Nwachuku C, Baimbridge C, Marginean H, Wright JT Jr, Basile J, Wong ND, Whelton P, Dart RA, Thadani U, Antihypertensive and Lipid-Lowering Treatment to Prevent Heart Attack Trial. Metabolic and clinical outcomes in nondiabetic individuals with the metabolic syndrome assigned to chlorthalidone, amlodipine, or Lisinopril as initial treatment for hypertension: a report from the Antihypertensive and Lipid-Lowering treatment to prevent Heart Attack Trial (ALLHAT). Diabetes Care. 2008;31(2):353–60.
182. Barzilay JI, Davis BR, Pressel SL, Cutler JA, Einhorn PT, Black HR, Cushman WC, Ford CE, Margolis KL, Moloo J, Oparil S, Piller LB, Simmons DL, Sweeney ME, Whelton PK, Wong ND, Wright JT Jr, ALLHAT Collaborative Research Group. Long-term effects of incident diabetes mellitus on cardiovascular outcomes in people treated for hypertension: the ALLHAT diabetes extension study. Circ Cardiovasc Qual Outcomes. 2012;5(2):153–62.
183. Rapoport MI, Hurd HF. Thiazide-induced glucose intolerance treated with potassium. Arch Intern Med. 1964;113:405–8.
184. Helderman JH, Elahi D, Andersen DK, Raizes GS, Tobin JD, Shocken D, Andres R. Prevention of the glucose intolerance of thiazide diuretics by maintenance of body potassium. Diabetes. 1983;32(2):106–11.
185. Reisin E, Graves JW, Yamal JM, Barzilay JI, Pressel SL, Einhorn PT, Dart RA, Retta TM, Saklayen MG, Davis BR, ALLHAT Collaborative Research Group. Blood pressure control and cardiovascular outcomes in normal-weight, overweight, and obese hypertensive patients treated with three different antihypertensives in ALLHAT. J Hypertens. 2014;32(7):1503–13.
186. Kintscher U, Bramlage P, Paar WD, Thoenes M, Unger T. Irbesartan for the treatment of hypertension in patients with the metabolic syndrome: a sub analysis of the treat to target post authorization survey. Prospective, observational two armed study in 14,200 patients. Cardiovasc Diabetol. 2007;6:12.
187. Benson SC, Pershadsingh HA, Ho CI, Chittiboyina A, Desai P, Prevenec M, Qi N, Wang J, Avery MA, Kurtz TW. Identification of telmisartan as a unique angiotensin II receptor antagonist with selective PPAR gamma modulating activities. Hypertension. 2004;43(5):993–1002.
188. Schupp M, Janke J, Clasen R, Unger T, Kintsher U. Angiotensin type I receptor blockers induce peroxisome proliferator-activated receptor-gamma activity. Circulation. 2004;109(17):2054–7.
189. Zappe DH, Sowers JR, Hsueh WA, Haffner SM, Deedwania PC, Fonseca VA, Keeling L, Sica DA. Metabolic and antihypertensive effects of combined angiotensin receptor blocker and diuretic therapy in Prediabetic hypertensive patients with the cardiometabolic syndrome. J Clin Hypertens. 2008;10(12):894–903.
190. Niskanen L, Hedner T, Hanson L, Lanke J, Niklason A, CAPPP Study Group. Reduced cardiovascular morbidity and mortality in hypertensive diabetic patients on first-line therapy with an ACE inhibitor compared with a diuretic/β-blocker-based Treatment Regimen: a subanalysis of the captopril prevention project. Diabetes Care. 2001;24:2091–6.
191. Gress TW, Nieto FJ, Shahar E, Wofford MR, Brancati FL. Hypertension and antihypertensive therapy as risk factors for type 2 diabetes mellitus. Atherosclerosis risk in communities study. N Engl J Med. 2000;342:905–12.
192. Dahlof B, Devereux RB, Kjeldsen SE, Julius S, Beevers G, de Faire U, Fyhrquist F, Ibsen H, Kristiansson K, Lederballe-Pedersen O, Lindholm LH, Nieminen MS, Omvik P, Oparil

S, Wedel H, LIFE Study Group. Cardiovascular morbidity and mortality in the Losartan Intervention for Endpoint reduction in hypertension study (LIFE): a randomized trial against atenolol. Lancet. 2002;359:995–1003.

193. Pepine CJ, Handberg EM, Cooper-DeHoff RM, Marks RG, Kowey P, Messerli FH, Mancia G, Cangiano JL, Garcia-Barreto D, Keltaj M, Erdine S, Bristol HA, Kolb HR, Bakris GL, Cohen JD, Parmley WW, INVEST Investigators. A calcium antagonist versus a non-calcium antagonist hypertension treatment strategy for patients with coronary artery disease. The International Verapamil-Trandolapril Study (INVEST): a randomized controlled trial. JAMA. 2003;290:2805–16.
194. Jacob S, Balletshofer B, Henriksen EJ, Volk A, Mehnert B, Loblein K, Haring HU, Rett K. Beta-blocking agents in patients with insulin resistance: effects of vasodilating beta-blockers. Blood Press. 1999;8(5-6):261–8.
195. Jacob S, Henriksen EJ. Metabolic properties of vasodilating beta blockers: management considerations for hypertensive diabetic patients and patients with the metabolic syndrome. J Clin Hypertens. 2004;6(12):690–6.
196. Fonseca VA. Effects of beta-blockers on glucose and lipid metabolism. Curr Med Res Opin. 2010;26(3):615–29.
197. Taylor AA, Bakris GL. The role of vasodilating beta-blockers in patients with hypertension and the cardiometabolic syndrome. Am J Med. 2010;123(7 Supplement 1):S21–6.
198. Deedwania P. Hypertension, dyslipidemia, and insulin resistance in patients with diabetes mellitus or the cardiometabolic syndrome: benefits of vasodilating beta-blockers. J Clin Hypertens. 2011;13(1):52–9.
199. Fares H, Lavie CJ, Ventura HO. Vasodilating versus first-generation beta-blockers for cardiovascular protection. Postgrad Med. 2012;124(2):7–15.
200. Fergus IV, Connell KL, Ferdinand KC. A comparison of vasodilating and non-vasodilating beta-blockers and their effects on cardiometabolic risk. Curr Cardiol Rep. 2015;17:38.
201. Reisin E, Owen J. Treatment: special conditions. Metabolic syndrome: obesity and the hypertension connection. J Am Soc Hypertens. 2015;9(2):156–9.
202. Jamerson K, Weber MA, Bakris GL, Dahlof B, Pitt B, Shi V, Hester A, Gupte J, Gatlin M, Velazquez EJ, ACCOMPLISH Trial Investigators. N Engl J Med. 2008;359(23):2417–28.
203. Ernst ME, Carter BL, Basile JN. All thiazide-like diuretics are not chlorthalidone: putting the ACCOMPLISH study into perspective. J Clin Hypertens. 2009;11(1):5–10.
204. Weber MA, Jamerson K, Bakris GL, Weir MR, Zappe D, Zhang Y, Dahlof B, Velazquez EJ, Pitt B. Effects of body size and hypertension treatments on cardiovascular event rates: subanalysis of the ACCOMPLISH randomized controlled trial. Lancet. 2013;381:537–45.
205. National Clinical Guideline Centre. Hypertension: the clinical management of primary hypertension in adults: update of clinical guidelines 18 to 34. Royal College of Physicians (UK) 2011.
206. The Task Force for the management of arterial hypertension of the European Society of Hypertension (ESH) and the European Society of Cardiology (ESC). 2013 ESH/ESC guidelines for the management of arterial hypertension. J Hypertens. 2013;31:1281–357.
207. Dasqupta K, Quinn RR, Zarnke KB, Rabi DM, Ravani P, Daskalopoulou SS, Rabkin SW, Trudeau L, Feldman RD, Cloutier L, Prebtani A, Herman RJ, Bacon SL, Gilbert RE, Ruzicka M, McKay DW, Campbell TS, Grover S, Honos G, Schiffrin EL, Bolli P, Wilson TW, Lindsay P, Hill MD, Coutts SB, Gubitz G, Gelfer M, Vallee M, Prasad GV, Lebel M, McLean D, Arnold JM, Moe GW, Howlett JG, Boulanger JM, Larochelle P, Leiter LA, Jones C, Ogilvie RI, Woo V, Kaczorowski J, Burns KD, Petrella RJ, Hiremath S, Milot A, Stone JA, Drouin D, Lavoie KL, Lamarre-Cliché M, Tremblay G, Hamet P, Fordor G, Carruthers SG, Pylypchuk GB, Burgess E, Lewanczuk R, Dresser GK, Penner SB, Hegele RA, McFarlane PA, Khara M, Pipe A, Oh P, Selby P, Sharma M, Reid DJ, Tobe SW, Padwal RS, Poirer L, Canadian Hypertension Education Program. The 2014 Canadian hypertension education program recommendations for blood pressure measurement, diagnosis, assessment of risk, prevention, and treatment of hypertension. Can J Cardiol. 2014;30(5):485–501.

Pre-chronic Kidney Disease (CKD)? Is It Time for a New Staging?

16

Alexander H. Kirsch and Alexander R. Rosenkranz

16.1 There is Prehypertension and Prediabetes: Do We Need Pre-CKD?

The worldwide prevalence of chronic kidney disease (CKD) is about 12% in the general population [1], and the cardiovascular morbidity and mortality increases dramatically with reduced renal function [2]. It is well known that, at least in Europe, 50% of patients reaching the advanced stage 5 of CKD (CKD G5) suffer from diabetes and/or hypertension [3]. Such patients usually have a long history of disease before they progress to end-stage renal disease. Hypertension as well as diabetes, both have pre-stages of the disease, which are called "prehypertension" or "prediabetes" [4]. In particular, previous definitions of hypertension were revised on the basis of the recognition that values below the defining thresholds for arterial hypertension were associated with higher risk for adverse outcomes [5].

Prediabetes is defined as impaired glucose tolerance or impaired fasting plasma glucose ≥100 and <126 mg/dL) [4], while prehypertension is defined as arterial blood pressure ranging between 130 and 139 mmHg systolic or 80–89 mmHg diastolic [6]. Although these terms are somehow artificial because the risk associated with higher blood glucose levels and blood pressure increases continuously rather than at a certain stage, the questions remains: is it time for a comparable stage in nephrology for CKD, and what could be the possible definition and/or markers [7].

The risk for stroke or coronary artery disease increases continuously starting with a systolic blood pressure of more than 120 mmHg [8]. Even mildly elevated "pre-hypertonic" systolic blood pressure levels higher than 120 mmHg or diastolic levels of 85 mmHg in the adolescent phase are associated with higher

A. H. Kirsch (✉) · A. R. Rosenkranz
Clinical Division of Nephrology, Department of Internal Medicine, Medical University of Graz, Graz, Austria
e-mail: alexander.kirsch@medunigraz.at; alexander.rosenkranz@medunigraz.at

R. Zimlichman et al. (eds.), *Prehypertension and Cardiometabolic Syndrome*, Updates in Hypertension and Cardiovascular Protection,
https://doi.org/10.1007/978-3-319-75310-2_16

cardiovascular mortality later in life [9]. In addition, high-normal blood pressure is associated with increased risk of cardiovascular disease [5]. These findings emphasize the need to determine whether lowering high-normal blood pressure can reduce the risk of cardiovascular disease. Indeed, recent evidence points in the direction that untreated prehypertension leads to stage 1 hypertension, as shown in the TROPHY study, where the intervention could significantly reduce this transition [10].

Individuals with prediabetes are at high risk for the development of diabetes and, of course, for increased risk of cardiovascular disease [4]. Therefore, screening for prediabetes does make sense to flag patients for earlier intervention, which may slow or even prevent the progression to overt diabetes. Guidelines for diabetes screening already exist and have been updated recently [11]. For the general population, screening should start at age 45, while high-risk individuals should be screened regardless of age. Interestingly, the American Diabetes Association recommends screening for albuminuria as well as measurement of serum creatinine including the calculation of an estimated glomerular filtration rate (eGFR) upon diagnosis of prediabetes or diabetes and annually thereafter [12]. Before we introduce the term "pre-CKD", we have to define the standards of screening for CKD, which are not absolutely clear. Also, when and how frequently to screen is unfortunately not strongly supported by evidence.

16.2 What Could Pre-CKD Be?

In 2009, Kidney Disease Improving Global Outcome (KDIGO) published clinical practice guidelines for the diagnosis, evaluation, prevention, and treatment of CKD-MBD (mineral and bone disorders) [13]. In this publication CKD is defined as an abnormality in renal structure or function which persists for more than three months and has implications for the affected individual's health. One would have to define pre-CKD as abnormalities which are not detected by the currently employed classification system and screening tools employed in today's clinical practice and which would predispose an individual to progression to CKD (which is without doubt of consequence to the subject's health). The current staging system considers eGFR, albuminuria, and other evidence of structural or functional abnormality, and in addition has nicely put the albuminuria in the center as an important risk factor for cardiovascular disease. In addition, a landmark study by Hemmelgarn and coworkers examined several adverse outcomes and demonstrated the independent contribution and importance of distinguishing GFR from albuminuria [14]. More importantly, screening for CKD, especially in the general population, has not been accepted as a cost-effective tool as stated by the United States Prevention Services Task Force in 2012 [15]. A Dutch study by Van der Velde recently put the screening for albuminuria in the center of attention by showing that an urine albumin ratio >20 mg/g creatinine leads to the lowest numbers needed to screen to detect cardiovascular high-risk patients with decreasing eGFR [16]. And finally, the National Institute for Health and Care Excellence (NICE) suggest screening for eGFR and albumin/creatinine ratio only in risk patients with diabetes, hypertension, cardiovascular disease, or a positive family history of end-stage renal disease [17].

Based on the abovementioned staging for CKD, there would be no space for a stage called pre-CKD, or is pre-CKD somehow subsumed in the term CKD G1? On the other hand, we also have to be aware that renal function deteriorates with age to a certain degree in some patients [18]. Therefore, assessing pre-CKD solely based on a decreased eGFR would put large numbers of elderly people in a pre-CKD state, and would not take into account the "normal" ageing process. Although there are some patients with normal eGFR (or at least higher than 60 mL/min/1.73 m^2) and albuminuria (it is well established that albuminuria is a cardiovascular risk factor), this definition would not be an exact one. There is good evidence that even lower levels than 30 mg/g creatinine (stage A1 of the CKD staging system) are associated with the development of adverse outcomes such as hypertension, cardiovascular disease, and death. Also, the universal cutoff of >30 mg/g creatinine may not be appropriate as some authors have suggested that ethnicity- and more importantly gender-specific cutoffs and reference ranges may be more appropriate [19]. Indeed, in the abovementioned study from Groeningen which evaluated more than 3300 patients, a cutoff of >20 mg/g creatinine was used as definition of albuminuria showing higher GFR loss and higher cardiovascular risk in this cohort [16]. On the other hand, eGFR levels higher than normal GFR could be a possible indicator of a pre-state for developing CKD. It is well known that a possible precursor of developing albuminuria is the mechanism of hyperfiltration seen in patients with diabetes as well as obesity (reviewed in [20]). Still, both options (low albuminuria as well as hyperfiltration) do not fit in the current definition of CKD. In addition, we have the problem of measuring or estimating renal function. Especially when looking for hyperfiltration, we would need urine collections or direct clearance measurements (inulin, iothalamate, EDTA, or iohexol) which are considered the "gold standard" for measuring GFR. However, they are impractical, expensive, time-consuming, and invasive in the clinical setting. For this reason, eGFR-formulas have been introduced that take into account endogenous filtration markers such as serum creatinine and demographic factors. Creatinine generation is affected by age, sex, race, muscle mass, and body weight independently from GFR [21]. eGFR appears to be a more accurate estimate of GFR than serum creatinine alone [22]. However, these equations cannot account for individual differences in muscle mass for a given age, sex, or race, which may be considerable. Muscle wasting is especially common in CKD and the elderly and it is associated with lower creatinine generation therefore, providing a bias toward falsely high eGFR.

16.3 Biomarkers for Pre-CKD

Looking for a clear definition of pre-CKD, one would expect a biomarker to be the best option. In recent years, a number of biomarkers have been evaluated in CKD (the most promising ones listed in Table 16.1[23]), but so far they have not been

Table 16.1 Based on a review by Wasung et al. [20]

	Legend	Source	Physiological action
Plasma asymmetric dimethylarginine	ADMA	Endothelial cells	Impaired clearance or increased production
Fibroblast growth factor 23	FGF23	osteocytes	
Monocyte chemoattractant protein -1	MCP-1	All nucleated cells, renal cells	
Neutrophil gelatinase-associated lipocalin	NGAL	Leukocytes, loop of Henle and collecting ducts	Released from lysosomes, brush-border and cytoplasm of proximal tubular epithelial cells
Urinary cystatin-C	Cystatin C	All nucleated cells	
Liver-type fatty acid-binding protein	L-FABP	Hepatocytes, kidney: proximal tubular cells	
Connective tissue growth factor	CTGF	All tissues	Excessive production of profibrotic growth factors and extracellular matrix
Transforming growth factor—β1	TGF-β1	All tissues	
Collagen IV	COLIV	Kidney, eye, skin	
Plasma cystatin C	Cystatin C	All nucleated cells	Impaired GFR
Podocalyxin	PCX	Podocytes	Podocyte structure defect
Nephrin	Nep	Podocytes	Integral component of the podocyte slit diaphragm; released by podocytes when damaged

evaluated as a marker for pre-CKD. Monitoring those markers which could provide rapid, noninvasive, and specific detection of renal tissue pathologies could be used as a marker for pre-CKD. This could be similar to "supranormal" blood pressure or slightly elevated blood sugar levels as markers of prehypertension or prediabetes. Early identification of patients with pre-CKD would be important in order to perform early interventions and reduce progression to kidney failure or cardiovascular events.

In recent years, several researchers have promoted the use of cystatin C (CyC) for measuring renal function more accurately. CyC is a 13 kDa protein synthesized at a constant rate in all nucleated cells, and is freely filtered in the glomerulus and reabsorbed and catabolized completely in the proximal tubule with a lack of tubular secretion [24]. CyC is less affected by muscle mass than serum creatinine, and is considered to be a better marker of early kidney dysfunction and a more reliable marker of renal function [25]. Investigators from CKD-EPI developed a set of three eGFR equations for CyC and compared these equations to measured GFR: using CyC alone, CyC with demographic factors, and CyC with creatinine and demographic factors. The equation that included CyC, creatinine, and demographic coefficients provided the most accurate eGFR [26]. Still, the problem remains that pre-CKD would not fit into a categorization based on the eGFR levels. Therefore, GFR-independent biomarkers, which still show renal damage or starting disturbances of renal function would be preferable.

The role of neutrophil gelatinase-associated lipocalin (NGAL) has been evaluated especially in the field of acute kidney injury. Unfortunately, despite high expectations in the beginning, NGAL has failed to fulfil most and recent evidence showed that NGAL is not a good biomarker to predict AKI [27]. NGAL is expressed by tubular epithelial cells in response to injury and tubulointerstitial damage that is a common pathway in progression of most forms of kidney disease [28]. NGAL has performed well as a biomarker in CKD (mostly concerning renal function) in small cohorts. In children, NGAL levels were inversely associated with the GFR; and as renal function was lower than 30 mL/min/1.73 m^2, NGAL outperformed CyC as a biomarker for kidney function [29]. In adults urinary NGAL to creatinine ratio (uNCR) was associated with a higher risk for death and initiation of dialysis independent from renal and cardiovascular risk factors [30]. The authors concluded that measuring uNCR improves the prediction of renal disease progression in this population. In addition, plasma NGAL levels also predicted the progression of CKD in adults, even after adjustment for eGFR [31]. However, in this study the small sample size has to be taken into consideration. Still, a possible role in predicting early renal changes or CKD progression has not been sufficiently evaluated in those studies leaving us without a possible hint for defining a pre-CKD-stage.

To date, nephrologists are focusing on mineral and bone disorders associated with reduced renal function as extensively evaluated in the new KDIGO 2017 Clinical Practice Guideline Update for the Diagnosis, Evaluation, Prevention, and Treatment of CKD-MBD [32]. As renal function declines due to a decrease in the number of functioning nephrons, single nephron phosphate excretion has to increase to maintain serum phosphate levels within normal ranges. Ultimately, this compensatory mechanism falls short and serum phosphate levels begin to rise. Also, renal calcitriol production declines and as a result calcium tends to decrease. Fibroblast growth factor 23 (FGF23) is a 32-kDa protein secreted primarily by osteocytes that plays an important role in controlling serum phosphate concentration. It acts as an endocrine hormone by inhibiting parathyroid hormone secretion, decreasing levels of calcitriol, and by inducing phosphaturia [33]. Circulating levels of FGF23 increase progressively as renal function declines below 60 mL/min/1.73 m^2 [34]. A considerable amount of evidence has shown that an elevated level of FGF23 is an independent risk factor for adverse outcomes in CKD such as faster progression, higher incidence of cardiovascular disease, and increased mortality [35, 36].

Here we have to consider the possible interaction of phosphate levels as well as increased FGF23 in patients with normal renal function. Many studies show a significant association between elevated serum phosphorus levels, poor clinical outcome and vascular calcification. The Framingham Offspring study showed a steadily increasing association between phosphate levels and incidence of cardiovascular disease [37]. First of all, this study showed that even within normal serum phosphate ranges, there is an increasing risk for cardiovascular disease [37]. Secondly, this has been observed in adults with normal renal function [37]! This has been supported by the Atherosclerosis Risk in Community (ARIC) study including more than 15,000 persons, where the authors could show an association between serum phosphate levels and stroke as well as serum phosphate levels and death [38]. Although the presented studies imply that phosphate even in normal range is a therapeutic target, it is not clear how to manage phosphate metabolism in real life. And, most of all, it will be difficult to interpret the effect of phosphate lowering within the normal range of the lab value. Therefore, it would be of utmost importance to have a biomarker with a better "discrimination." Could FGF23 be such a useful biomarker?

The landmark study of Gutierrez et al. in 2008 showed for the first time in dialysis patients that FGF23 is a much better predictor of mortality at the initiation of dialysis than phosphorus [39]. For years, we nephrologists have followed the path set out by Block et al., who showed an association between phosphate levels and mortality—the higher the phosphate levels the higher the mortality [40]. The relative increase in risk was only 30%, still statistically significant, but compared to the newer data of FGF23 in the Gutierrez study nearly negligible. In addition, even lower serum phosphate levels (within the normal range and below), showed an association with mortality [40]. Going into the data of the Gutierrez study, we see an association between serum phosphorus levels and mortality as well, but this pales in comparison to the association between FGF23 and the mortality. The authors concluded that FGF23 is a much better predictor for mortality, at least in the dialysis population at that time [39]. Those data have been supported by a post hoc analysis of the EVOLVE study. The EVOLVE study was planned to show a reduction of mortality in dialysis patients receiving the calcimimetic cinacalcet compared to standard care (in most cases active vitamin D), and the study failed to show its primary objective [41]. This came surprising, since earlier the ADVANCE study had shown that dialysis patients on cinacalcet had a significant reduction in cardiovascular calcification [42]. And it is well known by the work of Gerard London that vascular calcification is the driving force behind mortality in the dialysis population [43]. A post hoc analysis of the EVOLVE study by Sharon Moe nicely revealed an important role of FGF23 as a marker of treatment success. Those patients who had a reduction in FGF23 by cinacalcet also showed a significant decrease of mortality [44]. So, one could conclude that FGF23 is on the one hand a good marker for cardiovascular risk, and on the other hand a good marker to follow the treatment success. Still, one has to admit that the studies described here have been undertaken in the dialysis population with terminal end-stage renal disease.

Even a study on the association between FGF23 levels and progression of kidney disease, meaning loss of kidney function, showing that levels of FGF23 higher than 35 pg/mL were associated with a higher rate of decline in renal function, has been performed in advanced stages of kidney disease [45]. Still, we are not sure what to think about the use of this biomarker in patients (or more accurate "individuals") with normal renal function. Eventually, FGF23 could be a link to higher cardiovascular mortality without reduction in renal function on the one hand, and on the other FGF23 could be an early marker of renal dysfunction and then set the stage for "Pre-CKD".

Once again the group of Gutierrez has set the stage for such speculations: The group showed an association between FGF23 levels and cardiac hypertrophy in patients with reduced renal function, a finding which was surprising at that time [46]. Recently, this was clarified by the findings of Grabner et al. [47]. They revealed that the fibroblast growth factor receptor 4 (FGFR4) on myocardial cells mediates the pro-hypertrophic cardiac effects of FGF23 (mostly elevated in patients with CKD, but probably also in early renal dysfunction). Activation of FGFR4/calcineurin/NFAT signaling is sufficient to induce cardiac hypertrophy in mice, while FGFR4 blockade attenuates cardiac hypertrophy in a rat model of CKD [47]. Still, these are only data in CKD patients. But several recent studies extend the findings in those patients to individuals with a renal function that would not be diagnosed as CKD in today's clinical practice. A community-based study in elderly persons (Prospective Investigation of the Vasculature in Uppsala Seniors (PIVUS) study) with normal renal function (mean eGFR approximately 80 mL/min/1.73 m^2) showed an association between serum FGF23 and total body atherosclerosis [48]. This comes hand in hand with findings from a cohort of patients with mild renal disease, showing that patients with stage CKD G1 (eGFR >90 mL/min/1.73 m^2) have elevated levels of FGF23 [49]. This allows for speculation that these could be patients with early renal injury. FGF23, therefore, could not only be a marker for individuals with renal dysfunction, but also for those with elevated risk for cardiovascular complications. This has been nicely shown in a recent study of patients with eGFR between 70 and 80 mL/min/1.73 m^2 [50]: the incidence of mortality as well as cardiovascular events correlated with higher levels of FGF23 [50].

Conclusion

Taken together, the field has been opened and prepared to further evaluate the role of FGF23 as a biomarker of pre-CKD. Current evidence supports further evaluation in larger cohorts or community-based studies to be initiated. We could have a strong tool in our hands not only to identify persons at risk for cardiovascular events as well as renal dysfunction, but also to more accurately direct therapeutic interventions. Our increasing understanding of the role of FGF23, not only as a phosphatonin, but also as a mediator of cardiovascular risk should stimulate further research on the role of FGF23 as well as the potential therapeutic implications of this hormone.

References

1. Coresh J, et al. Prevalence of chronic kidney disease in the United States. JAMA. 2007;298:2038–47.
2. Go AS, Chertow GM, Fan D, McCulloch CE, Hsu C-Y. Chronic kidney disease and the risks of death, cardiovascular events, and hospitalization. N Engl J Med. 2004;351:1296–305.
3. Prischl FC, et al. Diabetes-related end-stage renal disease in Austria 1965–2013. Nephrol Dial Transplant. 2015;30:1920–7.
4. Nathan DM, et al. Impaired fasting glucose and impaired glucose tolerance: implications for care. Diabetes Care. 2007;30:753–9.
5. Vasan RS, et al. Impact of high-normal blood pressure on the risk of cardiovascular disease. N Engl J Med. 2001;345:1291–7.

6. Chobanian AV, et al. The Seventh Report of the Joint National Committee on Prevention, Detection, Evaluation, and Treatment of High Blood Pressure: the JNC 7 report. JAMA. 2003;289:2560–72.
7. Curhan GC. Prediabetes, prehypertension … is it time for pre-CKD? Clin J Am Soc Nephrol. 2010;5:557–9.
8. Lewington S, et al. Age-specific relevance of usual blood pressure to vascular mortality: a meta-analysis of individual data for one million adults in 61 prospective studies. Lancet. 2002;360:1903–13.
9. Sundstrom J, Neovius M, Tynelius P, Rasmussen F. Association of blood pressure in late adolescence with subsequent mortality: cohort study of Swedish male conscripts. BMJ. 2011;342:d643.
10. Julius S, et al. Feasibility of treating prehypertension with an angiotensin-receptor blocker. N Engl J Med. 2006;354:1685–97.
11. Chamberlain JJ, et al. Pharmacologic therapy for type 2 diabetes: synopsis of the 2017 American Diabetes Association Standards of Medical Care in Diabetes. Ann Intern Med. 2017;166:572–8.
12. American Diabetes Association. Classification and diagnosis of diabetes mellitus. Diabetes Care. 2017;40:S11–24.
13. Kidney Disease: Improving Global Outcomes (KDIGO) CKD-MBD Work Group. KDIGO clinical practice guideline for the diagnosis, evaluation, prevention, and treatment of Chronic Kidney Disease-Mineral and Bone Disorder (CKD-MBD). Kidney Int Suppl. 2009;76:S1–130.
14. Hemmelgarn BR, et al. Relation between kidney function, proteinuria, and adverse outcomes. JAMA. 2010;303:423–9.
15. Moyer VA, U.S. Preventive Services Task Force. Screening for chronic kidney disease: U.S. Preventive Services Task Force recommendation statement. Ann Intern Med. 2012;157:567–70.
16. van der Velde M, de Jong PE, Gansevoort RT. Comparison of the yield of different screening approaches to detect chronic kidney disease. Nephrol Dial Transplant. 2010;25:3222–30.
17. Carville S, Wonderling D, Stevens P, Guideline Development G. Early identification and management of chronic kidney disease in adults: summary of updated NICE guidance. BMJ. 2014;349:g4507.
18. Wetzels JF, Kiemeney LA, Swinkels DW, Willems HL, den Heijer M. Age- and gender-specific reference values of estimated GFR in Caucasians: the Nijmegen Biomedical Study. Kidney Int. 2007;72:632–7.
19. Mattix HJ, Hsu C-Y, Shaykevich S, Curhan G. Use of the albumin/creatinine ratio to detect microalbuminuria: implications of sex and race. J Am Soc Nephrol. 2002;13:1034–9.
20. Tonneijck L, et al. Glomerular hyperfiltration in diabetes: mechanisms, clinical significance, and treatment. J Am Soc Nephrol. 2017;28:1023–39.
21. Stevens LA, Coresh J, Greene T, Levey AS. Assessing kidney function—measured and estimated glomerular filtration rate. N Engl J Med. 2006;354:2473–83.
22. Levey AS, Stevens LA. Estimating GFR using the CKD Epidemiology Collaboration (CKD-EPI) creatinine equation: more accurate GFR estimates, lower CKD prevalence estimates, and better risk predictions. Am J Kidney Dis. 2010;55:622–7.
23. Wasung ME, Chawla LS, Madero M. Biomarkers of renal function, which and when? Clinica chimica acta. Int J Clin Chem. 2015;438:350–7.
24. Abrahamson M, Dalboge H, Olafsson I, Carlsen S, Grubb A. Efficient production of native, biologically active human cystatin C by Escherichia coli. FEBS Lett. 1988;236:14–8.
25. Hojs R, Bevc S, Ekart R, Gorenjak M, Puklavec L. Serum cystatin C as an endogenous marker of renal function in patients with mild to moderate impairment of kidney function. Nephrol Dial Transplant. 2006;21:1855–62.
26. Stevens LA, et al. Estimating GFR using serum cystatin C alone and in combination with serum creatinine: a pooled analysis of 3,418 individuals with CKD. Am J Kidney Dis. 2008;51:395–406.

27. Ribitsch W, et al. Neutrophil gelatinase-associated lipocalin (NGAL) fails as an early predictor of contrast induced nephropathy in chronic kidney disease (ANTI-CI-AKI study). Sci Rep. 2017;7:41300.
28. Kuncio GS, Neilson EG, Haverty T. Mechanisms of tubulointerstitial fibrosis. Kidney Int. 1991;39:550–6.
29. Mitsnefes MM, et al. Serum neutrophil gelatinase-associated lipocalin as a marker of renal function in children with chronic kidney disease. Pediatr Nephrol. 2007;22:101–8.
30. Smith ER, et al. Urinary neutrophil gelatinase-associated lipocalin may aid prediction of renal decline in patients with non-proteinuric stages 3 and 4 chronic kidney disease (CKD). Nephrol Dial Transplant. 2013;28:1569–79.
31. Bolignano D, et al. Neutrophil gelatinase-associated lipocalin (NGAL) and progression of chronic kidney disease. Clin J Am Soc Nephrol. 2009;4:337–44.
32. Ketteler M, et al. Executive summary of the 2017 KDIGO Chronic Kidney Disease-Mineral and Bone Disorder (CKD-MBD) Guideline update: what's changed and why it matters. Kidney Int. 2017;92:26–36.
33. Isakova T, Wolf MS. FGF23 or PTH: which comes first in CKD ? Kidney Int. 2010;78: 947–9.
34. Gutierrez O, et al. Fibroblast growth factor-23 mitigates hyperphosphatemia but accentuates calcitriol deficiency in chronic kidney disease. J Am Soc Nephrol. 2005;16:2205–15.
35. Isakova T, et al. Fibroblast growth factor 23 is elevated before parathyroid hormone and phosphate in chronic kidney disease. Kidney Int. 2011;79:1370–8.
36. Isakova T, et al. Fibroblast growth factor 23 and risks of mortality and end-stage renal disease in patients with chronic kidney disease. JAMA. 2011;305:2432–9.
37. Dhingra R, et al. Relations of serum phosphorus and calcium levels to the incidence of cardiovascular disease in the community. Arch Intern Med. 2007;167:879–85.
38. Foley RN, Collins AJ, Ishani A, Kalra PA. Calcium-phosphate levels and cardiovascular disease in community-dwelling adults: the Atherosclerosis Risk in Communities (ARIC) Study. Am Heart J. 2008;156:556–63.
39. Gutiérrez OM, et al. Fibroblast growth factor 23 and mortality among patients undergoing hemodialysis. N Engl J Med. 2008;359:584–92.
40. Block GA, Hulbert-Shearon TE, Levin NW, Port FK. Association of serum phosphorus and calcium × phosphate product with mortality risk in chronic hemodialysis patients: a national study. Am J Kidney Dis. 1998;31:607–17.
41. The EVOLVE Trial Investigators. Effect of cinacalcet on cardiovascular disease in patients undergoing dialysis. N Engl J Med. 2012;367:2482–94. https://doi.org/10.1056/NEJMoa1205624.
42. Raggi P, et al. The ADVANCE study: a randomized study to evaluate the effects of cinacalcet plus low-dose vitamin D on vascular calcification in patients on hemodialysis. Nephrol Dial Transplant. 2011;26:1327–39.
43. Blacher J, Guerin AP, Pannier B, Marchais SJ, London GM. Arterial calcifications, arterial stiffness, and cardiovascular risk in end-stage renal disease. Hypertension. 2001;38:938–42.
44. Moe SM, et al. Cinacalcet, fibroblast growth factor-23, and cardiovascular disease in hemodialysis: the Evaluation of Cinacalcet HCl Therapy to Lower Cardiovascular Events (EVOLVE) trial. Circulation. 2015;132:27–39.
45. Fliser D, et al. Fibroblast growth factor 23 (FGF23) predicts progression of chronic kidney disease: the Mild to Moderate Kidney Disease (MMKD) study. J Am Soc Nephrol. 2007;18:2600–8.
46. Gutiérrez OM, et al. Fibroblast growth factor 23 and left ventricular hypertrophy in chronic kidney disease. Circulation. 2009;119:2545–52.
47. Grabner A, et al. Activation of cardiac fibroblast growth factor receptor 4 causes left ventricular hypertrophy. Cell Metab. 2015;22:1020–32.
48. Mirza MA, et al. Relationship between circulating FGF23 and total body atherosclerosis in the community. Nephrol Dial Transplant. 2009;24:3125–31.

49. Evenepoel P, et al. Fibroblast growth factor-23 in early chronic kidney disease: additional support in favor of a phosphate-centric paradigm for the pathogenesis of secondary hyperparathyroidism. Clin J Am Soc Nephrol. 2010;5:1268–76.
50. Parker BD, et al. The associations of fibroblast growth factor 23 and uncarboxylated matrix Gla protein with mortality in coronary artery disease: the Heart and Soul Study. Ann Intern Med. 2010;152:640–8.

Prehypertension and Vascular-Renal Impairment

17

Celine Dreyfuss-Tubiana, Michel E. Safar, and Jacques Blacher

17.1 Introduction

The concept of prehypertension has been developed in late 1930s following a series of studies showing a progressive increase of premature death from cardiovascular disease (CVD) in persons with blood pressure (BP) between 120 and 140 mmHg [1].

More than 60 years later, in 2003, prehypertension, been defined as 120–139 mmHg for systolic blood pressure (SBP) and/or 80–89 mmHg for diastolic blood pressure (DBP), entered the American hypertension guidelines, because of longitudinal data obtained from Framingham Heart Study, that indicated that this range of values was associated with a more than twofold increase in relative risk for CVD compared with those with BP levels below 120/80 mmHg [2]. This designation was intended to identify those individuals in whom early intervention by adoption of healthy lifestyle could reduce BP, decrease the rate of progression of BP to hypertensive levels with age and finally prevent hypertension [3].

In this context, it remained essential to understand and study prehypertension. Over 60% of incident CVD events occurred in participants with SBP/DBP <140/90 mmHg. This represented a fundamental shift from previous decades when the majority of incident CVD events occurred among US adults with SBP/DBP >140/90 mmHg [4]. The finding that the majority of incident CVD events in the modern era occurred in participants with SBP/DBP <140/90 mmHg represented a change from studies conducted in prior eras. These data highlighted the need for primordial prevention of hypertension, earlier detection and treatment of hypertension, and additional CVD risk reduction strategies for adults with hypertension once BP control has been achieved [3, 4].

C. Dreyfuss-Tubiana · M. E. Safar · J. Blacher (✉)
AP-HP, Diagnosis and Therapeutic Center, Paris-Descartes University, Hôtel Dieu University Hospital, Paris, France
e-mail: jacques.blacher@aphp.fr

R. Zimlichman et al. (eds.), *Prehypertension and Cardiometabolic Syndrome*, Updates in Hypertension and Cardiovascular Protection,
https://doi.org/10.1007/978-3-319-75310-2_17

Since then, many authors studied the physiopathology of prehypertension, investigated its etiology, and designed protocols to highlight the need of treatments for prehypertensive patients. In this chapter, we will focus on vascular and/or renal impairment in prehypertension: its physiopathology, its role in prehypertension, the method of its diagnosis, treatment, and the importance of prevention.

17.2 Physiopathology-Role of Salt

It has been shown that hereditary and environmental factors were related to the development of hypertension. Among all environmental factors, salt intake has attracted great attention. The character of reversibility has also been discussed. In the Diabetes Control and Complications Trial of type 1 diabetes mellitus, the group that originally received intensive therapy had lower incidence of cardiovascular disease compared with conventional control, although the hemoglobin A1c levels in the two groups had converged. The authors proposed the concept of metabolic memory to illustrate this phenomenon [5]. Some authors have suggested that transient high-salt diet on weanling Dahl salt-sensitive rats (DS rats) for 6 weeks was capable of inducing permanent hypertension [6]. Therefore, the effects of temporary exposure to a high-salt diet on the development of hypertension and whether or not salt memory exists was examined in a complete study [7]. In this article, Oguchi and colleagues experimented law-salt, normal-salt, high-sodium/normal-chloride diet in DS rats on blood pressure and urine protein excretion. Moreover, they transplanted kidneys from DS rats to spontaneously hypertensive rats (SHR) fed with high-sodium diet and conversely for the kidneys and the diet. In this study, they showed that transient high-salt intake during early phases in the development of hypertension induced sustained elevation of BP in hypertensive model rats. This phenomenon was named salt memory. Jax [5] proposed that microvascular changes mediated by hyperglycemia could play an important role in the development of metabolic memory observed in the Diabetes Control and Complications Trials in diabetes mellitus, so that the change in renal microvasculature through increase in BP at a certain important period could play a major role, resulting in the occurrence of the salt memory. No major differences were found in other arterioles of similar size than the renal arterioles, which underscored the importance of the kidney arterioles in the vascular response to high-salt treatments. One potential mechanism by which a high-salt diet in the presence of high Angiotensin II levels caused renal vascular injury could involve an increase in oxidative stress [8]. It was reported that intrarenal angiotensinogen was enhanced in DS rats on high-salt diet [9] and that an augmented intrarenal renin–angiotensin system (RAS) during high-salt diet might contribute to the development of renal injury in SHR [10]. Another report demonstrated that renal angiotensin II played an important role in causing renal cortical damage and decreased in renal hemodynamics independent of BP elevation [11]. It meant that renal RAS activation induced by a high-salt diet could cause renal vascular injury independently of BP elevation. Finally, Oguchi also tested whether the location of salt memory was in the kidneys by performing cross transplantation. It allowed to establish that salt memory was mainly localized in the kidney [7].

17.3 Diagnosis and Interactions

To track prehypertension, measuring blood pressure could be enough. But, it's still not recommended to treat. Nevertheless, some authors proposed to specify other comorbidities when prehypertension is discovered. Indeed, in prehypertension, SBP was associated with microalbuminuria. In the evaluation of increased blood pressures, microalbuminuria should be investigated even in prehypertensive stages. According to some authors, subjects with increased blood pressures should get medical treatment to prevent the effects on vascular structure even in prehypertensive stage [12]. Wang et al. studied the association of glycemic status with MA in prehypertensive and ideal BP subjects and to evaluate the interaction between glycemic and blood pressure status as risk factors for MA prevalence [13]. More than 1000 subjects aged 40–70 without hypertension who were recruited from six districts of Tianjin were divided into prehypertensive group (622 cases) and optimal BP (437 cases). Subjects of prehypertensive group and optimal BP group were divided respectively into three subgroups: normoglycemia subgroup, prediabetes subgroup, and diabetes subgroup. The prevalence of MA in the above three subgroups of subjects with prehypertension and optimal BP were assessed. The differences in prehypertensive group were statistically significant. There was no interaction between prediabetes and BP status regarding microalbuminuria. In prehypertensive group, multivariate logistic regression models showed that the diabetes subgroup had a significant association with microalbuminuria. However, there was no significant association of glycemic status with MA in optimal BP group. Those findings suggested that there was a statistically significant association between diabetes and microalbuminuria only in prehypertensive subjects. In addition, this study highlighted the interaction between prehypertension and diabetes as a risk factor for MA.

Other parameters could help to evaluate the level of cardiovascular risk in prehypertensive patients. Jia and colleagues highlighted that coronary computed tomography could provide multiple aortic elasticity related indices for prehypertensive patients, without additional contrast media consumption and radiation dose. It was hypothesized that the early detection of ascending aortic elasticity index changes, especially for aortic distensibility, were essential for identifying the high-risk individuals in the prehypertensive populations [14].

17.4 Pathophysiologic Changes Associated with Prehypertension

Many studies confirm the considerable vascular and renal risks in the prehypertensive blood pressure range, namely a significant increase in the risks of cardiovascular mortality and all-cause mortality [15]. It is clear that prehypertension is characterized by greater thrombotic tendency, namely increased plasma levels of fibrinogen, thrombomodulin, and plasminogen activator inhibitor-1 antigen [16]. Chronic elevations in blood pressure in the prehypertensive range are atherogenic, contributing to widespread vascular and structural damage to all organs and tissues, particularly the heart, brain, and kidneys. Increased carotid intima-media thickness, coronary artery calcification, abnormal left ventricular morphology and diastolic dysfunction, reduced large-artery elasticity, aortic stiffening and vascular endothelial dysfunction are some of the major abnormalities that commence and progress in the prehypertensive stage [17].

At the renal level, several studies and large meta-analysis have demonstrated that prehypertension is associated with a statistically significant increased risk of chronic kidney disease, namely end-stage renal disease, after controlling for several cardiovascular risk factors. The association is independent of age, sex, and other risk factors, such as diabetes, body mass index, and smoking [18–20].

17.5 Interventional Studies

17.5.1 Animal Models

Some studies have shown in animals that the transient treatment of stroke-prone spontaneously hypertensive rats or Dahl salt-sensitive rats (DS rats) during an early phase in the development of hypertension with angiotensin receptor blocker (ARB) resulted in attenuation of hypertension [21, 22] and found that development of renal arteriolar injury was also suppressed in these models. It was also shown that transient administration of angiotensin II (Ang II) caused renal vascular injury and renin–angiotensin system (RAS) activation, resulting in sustained hypertension after cessation of Ang II treatment in spontaneously hypertensive rat (SHR) [21, 22].

17.5.2 Human Studies

Abnormalities in cardiovascular structure and function and in neuroendocrine control occurred in young adults with a predisposition to hypertension. In rats with spontaneous hypertension, brief treatment of young animals with a renin–angiotensin antagonist has lifelong effects in reducing blood pressure. Therefore, one can hypothesize that an intervention in humans with prehypertension might alter the natural history and prevent or delay the onset of established hypertension [3].

Non-pharmacological interventions have been experimented in prehypertensive patients with favorable results, in term of delaying a future diagnosis of hypertension. Then, since the JNC VI, in 1997 [23], current guidelines recommend that prehypertension be managed with changes in the participant's lifestyle, weight loss, salt restriction, exercise, and dietary modifications [24–28]. Despite intensive community efforts to promote healthful lifestyles, however, the prevalence of prehypertension continues to increase, stressing the opportunity of a pharmacological treatment in patients with prehypertension. Indeed, several points are in favor of an earlier pharmacological treatment in prehypertension : (i) blood pressure remains a strong predictor of cardiovascular events after adjustment for other risk factors, suggesting that lowering blood pressure might be beneficial ; (ii) hypertension is a self-accelerating condition. The transition from prehypertension to established hypertension reflects, in part, ongoing changes such as arteriolar hypertrophy [29] and endothelial dysfunction [30]. Third, increased vasoconstriction and diminished vasodilatation, consistent with these structural and functional findings, have been described in prehypertension [31].

The first trial came from the TROPHY study [32]. The Trial of Preventing Hypertension (TROPHY) was an investigator-initiated study to examine whether early treatment of prehypertension, defined for this study as systolic pressure of 130–139 mmHg and diastolic pressure of 89 mmHg or lower and systolic pressure of 139 mmHg or lower and diastolic pressure of 85–89 mmHg, might prevent or delay the development of subsequent incident hypertension. The TROPHY study seeks only the proof of principle that early pharmacological treatment of prehypertension might delay or prevent development of clinical (stage 1) hypertension [32]. The TROPHY study assessed the safety, tolerability, and efficacy of two years of treatment in participants with prehypertension. This four-year, multicenter, randomized study involved untreated participants 30–65 years of age with blood pressure on study entry in the high-normal range. Participants were eligible for the trial if they were not being treated for hypertension, if at the first clinic visit the blood pressure was lower than 160/100 mmHg, and if the average of the three blood pressure readings at the three visits was a systolic pressure of 130–139 mmHg and a diastolic pressure of 89 mmHg or lower or a systolic pressure of 139 mmHg or lower and a diastolic pressure of 85–89 mmHg. The study consisted of a two-year, double-blind, placebo-controlled phase that was followed by a two-year phase in which all study patients received placebo. The main study end point was the development of clinical hypertension. Eight hundred and nine participants (409 assigned to candesartan and 400 assigned to placebo) were eligible for enrollment. Data on 772 participants (391 in the candesartan group and 381 in the placebo group) were available for further analysis. New onset of hypertension was significantly reduced in the candesartan group at 2 years ($P < 0.001$) and 4 years ($P < 0.001$). The absolute reduction in the incidence of new-onset hypertension at 2 years with candesartan was 26.8%, as compared with 8% with the most successful lifestyle intervention in the Trials of Hypertension Prevention [33]. Indeed, authors were clear about untreated prehypertension. It was a self-accelerating condition. Evolving arteriolar hypertrophy and endothelial dysfunction facilitated the later increase of blood pressure and contributed to the transition from prehypertension to established hypertension. Treatment of prehypertension with candesartan monotherapy decreased incident hypertension in participants in this study. This therapy decreased the development of hypertension and the proportion of patients who became hypertensive.

Another trial, the PHARAO study, demonstrated that ramipril, an ACE inhibitor, given to prehypertensives, reduced the risk of hypertension by 34%, compared to those not taking an antihypertensive drug. However, there was no difference in CV events (stroke or myocardial infarction) [34].

Moreover, the role of therapy in persons at intermediate risk (defined as an annual risk of major cardiovascular events of approximately 1%) who do not have vascular disease and who have a systolic blood pressure of less than 160 mmHg (who represent the majority of middle-aged and older persons) remains less clear. This was evaluated in the Heart Outcomes Prevention Evaluation (HOPE)-3 trial

[35]. The trial evaluated blood-pressure-lowering therapy with a fixed-dose combination of an angiotensin receptor blocker (ARB) and a thiazide diuretic, cholesterol-lowering therapy with a statin, and the combination of both interventions in persons at intermediate cardiovascular risk. The trial included men 55 years of age or older and women 65 years of age or older who had at least one of the following cardiovascular risk factors: elevated waist-to-hip ratio, history of low concentration of high-density lipoprotein cholesterol, current or recent tobacco use, dysglycemia, family history of premature coronary disease, and mild renal dysfunction and women 60 years of age or older who had at least two such risk factors. Participants were randomly assigned to the daily administration of either a fixed-dose combination of candesartan at a dose of 16 mg and hydrochlorothiazide at a dose of 12.5 mg or placebo; participants were also randomly assigned to receive either rosuvastatin at a dose of 10 mg or placebo. The prespecified primary efficacy outcome was the composite of death from cardiovascular causes, nonfatal myocardial infarction, or nonfatal stroke. From April 2007 through November 2010, 12,705 participants (86.5%) underwent randomization; 6356 participants were randomly assigned to candesartan plus hydrochlorothiazide, and 6349 to placebo. At baseline, the mean blood pressure decreases from baseline during the trial were 10.0 ± 13.1 mmHg in the active-treatment group and 4.0 ± 12.9 mmHg in the placebo group, and the average difference between the groups was 6.0 ± 13.0 mmHg. Concerning diastolic BP, the mean decreases from baseline during the trial were 5.7 ± 8.2 mmHg in the active-treatment group and 2.7 ± 7.9mmHg in the placebo group and the average difference between the groups was 3.0 ± 8.0 mmHg. There were no significant differences between the active-treatment group and the placebo group in the incidence of the primary outcome. Then, they divided the participants who received the treatment in three groups, according to the baseline BP value. Only participants in the subgroup for the upper third of systolic blood pressure (>143.5 mmHg; mean, 154.1 ± 8.9 mmHg) who were in the active-treatment group had nominally significantly lower rates than those in the placebo group with respect to the primary outcome (hazard ratio, 0.73; 95% CI: 0.56–0.94) showing that this trial did not show any cardiovascular benefit of treating normotensive and prehypertensive subjects with a combination of two antihypertensive drugs. Only patients with hypertension at inclusion decreased their cardiovascular risk.

Finally, it seems reasonable to conclude that data coming from therapeutic trials are not convincing enough to largely propose a pharmacological treatment in patients with prehypertension.

17.6 Prehypertension at the Population Level

The problem of prehypertension, such as the problem of hypertension, is quite heterogeneous in different countries according to their economic status. In this respect, it is interesting to analyze the results of the PURE study. The overall Prospective Urban Rural Epidemiology (PURE) study was a prospective, standardized collaborative study in which they reported a cross-sectional analysis of baseline data to assess the prevalence, awareness, treatment, and control of hypertension by the economic status of countries and by sex, age group, location (urban vs. rural), and education of the participants. In the PURE study, the overall aim was to examine the relationship of societal influences on lifestyle behaviors, cardiovascular risk factors, and incidence and mortality of chronic diseases [36].The PURE study enumerated 382,341 individuals from 107,599 households in 628 communities (348 urban and 280 rural) in 17 countries on 5 continents from January 2003 to December 2009. This study found a large gap between both detection and control of hypertension across all countries studied. It showed that while initial therapy was started in the large majority of individuals who were detected to have hypertension, control in participants receiving treatment was very poor. Awareness, treatment, and control were lower in participants with primary or no education, most likely reflecting a combination of low socioeconomic status, which might influence access to care, lack of knowledge of the sequelae of uncontrolled hypertension, and differing values with respect to the importance of the future. This important fact, recorded in a very large panel of population could urge us to develop strategies and treatment before having sustained hypertension. So, we understood the role of salt intake, and salt memory so that we indicated the importance of avoiding excess salt intake and undergoing an appropriate antihypertensive treatment intervention at the early stage of the development of hypertension [4–6].

Conclusion

Prehypertension, a frequent condition at the population level, is undoubtedly atherogenic, contributing to widespread vascular and structural damage to all organs and tissues, particularly the blood vessels, heart, brain and kidneys. Increased carotid intima-media thickness, coronary artery calcification, abnormal left ventricular morphology and diastolic dysfunction, reduced large-artery elasticity, aortic stiffening and vascular endothelial dysfunction are some of the major abnormalities that commence and progress in the prehypertensive stage. Prehypertensive patients have a significant increase in the risks of cardiovascular mortality and all-cause mortality.

In thsis respect, prehypertension is a major health challenge that requires more attention. The first-line treatment for prehypertensives should be based on adaption of a healthy lifestyle, especially if there are other associated CV or renal risk factors, with special emphasis on salt restriction. More research is needed to clarify the place of pharmacological treatments in patients with prehypertension.

References

1. Robinson SC, Brucer M. Range of normal blood pressure: a statistical and clinical study of 11,383 persons. Arch Intern Med. 1939;64:409–44.
2. Chobanian AV, Bakris GL, Black HR, Cushman WC, Green LA, Izzo JL Jr, Jones DW, Materson BJ, Oparil S, Wright JT Jr, Roccella EJ, The Seventh Report of the Joint National Committee on Prevention, Detection, Evaluation, and Treatment of High Blood Pressure, National Heart, Lung, and Blood Institute, National High Blood Pressure Education Program

Coordinating Committee. Seventh report of the Joint National Committee on Prevention, Detection, Evaluation, and Treatment of High Blood Pressure. JAMA. 2003;289:2560–72.

3. Albarwani S, Al-Siyabi S, Tanira MO. Prehypertension: underlying pathology and therapeutic options. World J Cardiol. 2014;6:728–43.
4. Tajeu GS, Booth JN, Colantonio LD, Gottesman RF, Howard G, Lackland DT, O'Brien E, Oparil S, Ravenell JE, Safford MM, Seals SR, Shimbo D, Shea S, Spruill TM, Tanner RM, Muntner P. Incident cardiovascular disease among adults with blood pressure <140/90 mmHg. Circulation. 2017;136:798–812. https://doi.org/10.1161/CIRCULATIONAHA.117.027362.
5. Jax TW. Metabolic memory: a vascular perspective. Cardiovasc Diabetol. 2010 Sep;9:51.
6. Dahl LK, Knudsen KD, Heine MA, Leitl GJ. Effects of chronic excess salt ingestion. Modification of experimental hypertension in the rat by variations in the diet. Circ Res. 1968;22:11–8.
7. Oguchi H, Sasamura H, Shinoda K, Morita S, Kono H, Nakagawa K, Ishiguro K, Hayashi K, Nakamura M, Azegami T, Oya M, Itoh H. Renal arteriolar injury by salt intake contributes to salt memory for the development of hypertension. Hypertension. 2014;64:784–91.
8. Lara LS, McCormack M, Semprum-Prieto LC, Shenouda S, Majid DS, Kobori H, Navar LG, Prieto MC. AT1 receptor-mediated augmentation of angiotensinogen, oxidative stress, and inflammation in ANG II-salt hypertension. Am J Physiol Renal Physiol. 2012;302:F85–94.
9. Kobori H, Nishiyama A, Abe Y, Navar LG. Enhancement of intrarenal angiotensinogen in Dahl salt-sensitive rats on high salt diet. Hypertension. 2003;41:592–7.
10. Susic D, Frohlich ED, Kobori H, Shao W, Seth D, Navar LG. Salt-induced renal injury in SHRs is mediated by AT1 receptor activation. J Hypertens. 2011;29:716–23.
11. Lin L, Phillips WE, Manning RD. Intrarenal Angiotensin II is associated with inflammation, renal damage and dysfunction in Dahl salt-sensitive hypertension. J Am Soc Hypertens. 2009;3:306–14.
12. Tenekecioglu E, Yilmaz M, Yontar OC, Karaagac K, Agca FV, Tutuncu A, Kuzeytemiz M, Bekler A, Senturk M, Aydin U, Demir S. Microalbuminuria in untreated prehypertension and hypertension without diabetes. Int J Clin Exp Med. 2014;7(10):3420–9.
13. Wang Q, Huang J, Sun Y, Zhang W, Gao Y, Yao W, Bian B, Li Y, Wu X, Niu K. Association of microalbuminuria with diabetes is stronger in people with prehypertension compared to those with ideal blood pressure. Nephrology (Carlton). 2017. [Epub ahead of print]. https://doi.org/10.1111/nep.13082.
14. Jia CF, Jiang YN, Yang ZQ, Sun XX, Yu Y, Wang H, Lu Y, Chen AJ, Wang ZQ. Ascending aortic elasticity and related risk factors study on prehypertension patients. Am J Hypertens. 2017;30(1):61–6.
15. Huang Y, Su L, Cai X, Mai W, Wang S, Hu Y, Wu Y, Tang H, Xu D. Association of all-cause and cardiovascular mortality with prehypertension: a meta-analysis. Am Heart J. 2014;167:160–8.
16. Papadopoulos D, Mourouzis I, Kotrotsou A, Papazachou U, Sanidas E, Tsioufis K, Makris T. Hemostasis parameters disturbances in healthy individuals with prehypertension. Clin Exp Hypertens. 2012;34:385–8.
17. Van Guilder GP. It is time to contend with the endothelial consequences of prehypertension. J Hum Hypertens. 2015;29(8):457.
18. Garofalo C, Borrelli S, Pacilio M, Minutolo R, Chiodini P, De Nicola L, Conte G. Hypertension and prehypertension and prediction of development of decreased estimated GFR in the general population: a meta-analysis of cohort studies. Am J Kidney Dis. 2016;67:89–97.
19. Huang Y, Cai X, Zhang J, Mai W, Wang S, Hu Y, Ren H, Xu D. Prehypertension and Incidence of ESRD: a systematic review and meta-analysis. Am J Kidney Dis. 2014;63:76–83.
20. Li Y, Xia P, Xu L, Wang Y, Chen L. A meta-analysis on prehypertension and chronic kidney disease. PLoS One. 2016;11:e0156575.
21. Nakaya H, Sasamura H, Hayashi M, Saruta T. Temporary treatment of prepubescent rats with angiotensin inhibitors suppresses the development of hypertensive nephrosclerosis. J Am Soc Nephrol. 2001;12:659–66.

22. Nakaya H, Sasamura H, Mifune M, Shimizu-Hirota R, Kuroda M, Hayashi M, Saruta T. Prepubertal treatment with angiotensin receptor blocker causes partial attenuation of hypertension and renal damage in adult Dahl salt-sensitive rats. Nephron. 2002;91:710–8.
23. The Sixth Report of the Joint National Committee on Prevention, Detection, Evaluation, and Treatment of High Blood Pressure (JNC VI). Bethesda, MD: National Heart, Lung, and Blood Institute; 1997. (NIH publication no. 98-4080).
24. The Trials of Hypertension Prevention Collaborative Research Group. Effects of weight loss and sodium reduction intervention on blood pressure and hypertension incidence in overweight people with high-normal blood pressure: the Trials of Hypertension Prevention, phase II. Arch Intern Med. 1997;157:657–67.
25. Hypertension Prevention Trial Research Group. The Hypertension Prevention Trial: three-year effects of dietary changes on blood pressure. Arch Intern Med. 1990;150:153–62.
26. Jennings G, Nelson L, Nestel P, Esler M, Korner P, Burton D, Bazelmans J. The effects of changes in physical activity on major cardiovascular risk factors, hemodynamics, sympathetic function, and glucose utilization in man: a controlled study of four levels of activity. Circulation. 1986;73:30–40.
27. Neaton JD, Grimm RH Jr, Prineas RJ, Stamler J, Grandits GA, Elmer PJ, Cutler JA, Flack JM, Schoenberger JA, McDonald R, et al. Treatment of mild hypertension: final results. JAMA. 1993;270:713–24.
28. Appel LJ, Moore TJ, Obarzanek E, Vollmer WM, Svetkey LP, Sacks FM, Bray GA, Vogt TM, Cutler JA, Windhauser MM, Lin PH, Karanja N. A clinical trial of the effects of dietary patterns on blood pressure. N Engl J Med. 1997;336:1117–24.
29. Folkow B. Physiological aspects of primary hypertension. Physiol Rev. 1982;62:347–504.
30. Panza JA, Casino PR, Kilcoyne CM, Quyyumi AA. Role of endothelium-derived nitric oxide in the abnormal endothelium-dependent vascular relaxation of patients with essential hypertension. Circulation. 1993;87:1468–74.
31. Egan B, Panis R, Hinderliter A, Schork N, Julius S. Mechanism of increased alpha adrenergic vasoconstriction in human essential hypertension. J Clin Invest. 1987;80:812–7.
32. Julius S, Nesbitt S, Egan B, Kaciroti N, Schork MA, Grozinski M, Michelson E, TROPHY Study Group. Trial of preventing hypertension: design and 2-year progress report. Hypertension. 2004;44:146–51.
33. Julius S, Nesbitt SD, Egan BM, Weber MA, Michelson EL, Kaciroti N, Black HR, Grimm RH Jr, Messerli FH, Oparil S, Schork MA. Feasibility of treating prehypertension with an angiotensin-receptor blocker. Trial of Preventing Hypertension (TROPHY) Study Investigators. N Engl J Med. 2006;354:1685–97.
34. Lüders S, Schrader J, Berger J, Unger T, Zidek W, Böhm M, Middeke M, Motz W, Lübcke C, Gansz A, Brokamp L, Schmieder RE, Trenkwalder P, Haller H, Dominiak P, PHARAO Study Group. The PHARAO study: prevention of hypertension with the angiotensin-converting enzyme inhibitor ramipril in patients with high-normal blood pressure: a prospective, randomized, controlled prevention trial of the German Hypertension League. J Hypertens. 2008;26:1487–96.
35. Lonn EM, Bosch J, Lopez-Jaramillo P, Zhu J, Liu L, Pais P, Diaz R, Xavier D, Sliwa K, Dans A, Avezum A, Piegas LS, Keltai K, Keltai M, Chazova I, Peters RJ, Held C, Yusoff K, Lewis BS, Jansky P, Parkhomenko A, Khunti K, Toff WD, Reid CM, Varigos J, Leiter LA, Molina DI, McKelvie R, Pogue J, Wilkinson J, Jung H, Dagenais G, Yusuf S. Blood-pressure lowering in intermediate-risk persons without cardiovascular disease. HOPE-3 Investigators. N Engl J Med. 2016;374:2009–20.
36. Chow CK, Teo KK, Rangarajan S, Islam S, Gupta R, Avezum A, Bahonar A, Chifamba J, Dagenais G, Diaz R, Kazmi K, Lanas F, Wei L, Lopez-Jaramillo P, Fanghong L, Hassim Ismail N, Puoane T, Rosengren A, Szuba A, Temizhan A, Wielgosz A, Yusuf R, Yusufali A, McKee M, Liu L, Mony P, Yusuf S, PURE (Prospective Urban Rural Epidemiology) Study Investigators. Prevalence, awareness, treatment, and control of hypertension in rural and urban communities in high-, middle-, and low-income countries. JAMA. 2013;310:959–68.

Subclinical Vascular Damage in Prehypertension

18

Enrico Agabiti-Rosei, Anna Paini, and Massimo Salvetti

18.1 Introduction

Epidemiological data clearly indicate that the association between blood pressure (BP) and cardiovascular events is continuous [1], with a relation that is consistent in both men and women, among different racial groups, in young and elderly people and therefore the distinction between normotension and hypertension is arbitrary. However in everyday practice, cut-off BP values are universally used [2]. The term prehypertension was proposed in 1939 on the basis of early studies that had demonstrated a relationship between blood pressure values recorded during physical examination for life insurance purposes and subsequent fatal and nonfatal events. In 2003, the JNC7 (Seventh Report of the Joint National Committee on Prevention, Detection, Evaluation, and Treatment of High Blood Pressure) [3] classified subjects with systolic blood pressure (SBP) between 120 and 139 mmHg with diastolic blood pressure (DBP) <90 mmHg or DBP between 80 and 89 mmHg with SBP <140 mmHg not taking antihypertensive drugs as having prehypertension. Similarly, European Hypertension Guidelines define "high-normal BP" (HN BP), as a SBP between 130 and 139 and/or a DBP between 85 and 89 mmHg. Despite the differences in cut-off values, studies have shown that both conditions are associated with a greater risk of developing hypertension, with a greater prevalence of organ damage, and with an increased risk of developing end stage renal disease and cardiovascular events [4, 5].

Because little is known on the progression of organ damage during follow-up in patients with high-normal BP we considered it to be worthwhile to assess the prevalence of HN BP and of associated cardiovascular target organ damage (TOD) in 420 subjects (age 50 ± 8 years, 46% males) from a general population sample living in

E. Agabiti-Rosei (✉) · A. Paini · M. Salvetti
Department of Medical and Surgical Sciences, University of Brescia, Brescia, Italy
e-mail: enrico.agabitirosei@unibs.it

R. Zimlichman et al. (eds.), *Prehypertension and Cardiometabolic Syndrome*, Updates in Hypertension and Cardiovascular Protection,
https://doi.org/10.1007/978-3-319-75310-2_18

a small town in Northern Italy and who were participating in a prospective epidemiological study aimed at measuring the association between CV risk factors and TOD (Vobarno study). Normotension was defined as a SBP/DBP <130/85 mmHg, HN BP was defined as SBP/DBP ≥130/85 and <140/90 mmHg and hypertension (HT) as SBP/DBP ≥140/90 mmHg. A follow-up (FU) visit, laboratory examinations, echocardiography and carotid intima-media thickness (IMT) measurement were performed after 9 years.

18.2 Baseline

At baseline 34% of subjects were normotensives, 36% were hypertensives and 30% ($n = 126$) of subjects were classified as HN. As compared to NT, subjects with HN BP were older, were more often male, and had a greater body mass index. Furthermore, as compared to NT subjects, those with HN BP had greater plasma glucose values, creatinine and uric acid levels (all $p < 0.05$). The prevalence of metabolic syndrome was 3.5% in NT, 29.4% in HN and 34% in HT ($p < 0.05$ vs. NT for both HT and HN; p = ns for the comparison between HN and HT) (Fig. 18.1). Left ventricular mass index (LVMI, expressed in gm/m^2 [7]) and relative wall thickness (RWT) progressively increased form NT to HN to HT and, in particular, LVMI and RWT were significantly greater in HN as compared to NT (ANOVA p, with Bonferroni correction, <0.05) (Fig. 18.2). Carotid IMT (both meanmax and CBMMax) were greater in HT as compared to NT and HN (all $p < 0.05$). No significant difference in IMT was observed between HN and NT.

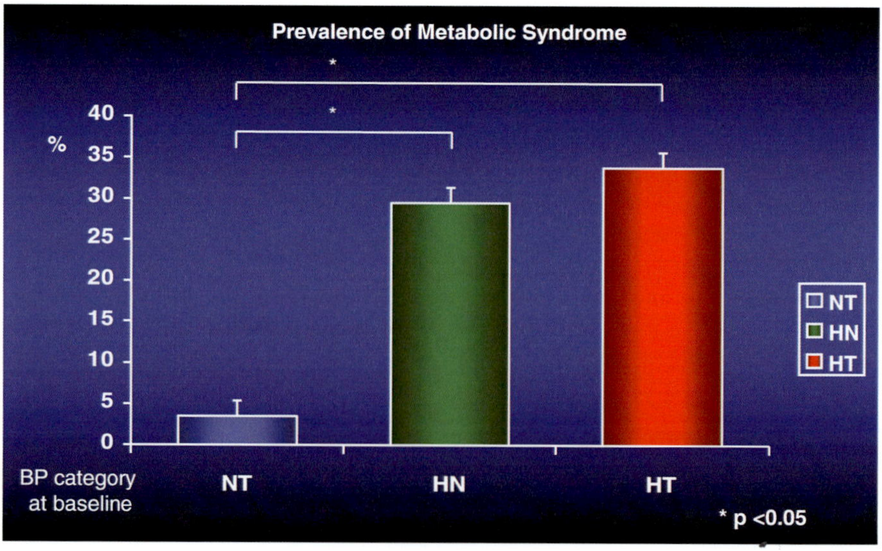

Fig. 18.1 Prevalence of metabolic syndrome at baseline according to BP categories

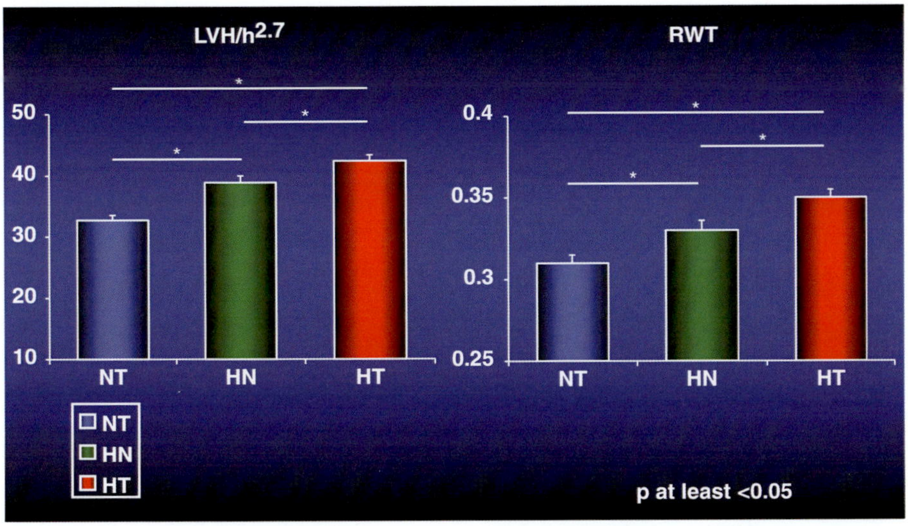

Fig. 18.2 Left ventricular mass and relative wall thickness at baseline according to BP category

18.3 Follow-Up

A second visit was performed after a FU of 8.6 ± 2.2 years. Among subjects classified as NT at baseline, 34% had progressed to HT, 23% had HN BP, while 43% had normal BP (Fig. 18.3). Among those classified as HT at baseline, most (84%) were classified as hypertensive at FU visit, 11% had HN BP and 5% were NT. Interestingly, among the 126 subjects classified as HN at baseline, at follow-up visit 71% had progressed to HT, 18% had HN BP and only 11% had BP values within the normal range.

When cardiac organ damage was analysed at FU, subjects classified as having HN BP at baseline had a LVMI that was significantly greater than those classified as NT at baseline (Fig. 18.4). Similarly, in patients classified as HN at baseline, relative wall thickness at FU was greater than in NT ($p < 0.05$), indicating the development of a more concentric geometry in these subjects. The E/A ratio of transmitral flow was lower and the isovolumic relaxation time was significantly greater in patients classified at baseline as HN BP as compared to NT; also left atrial dimensions were greater in these patients than in NT, thus indicating a tendency to an earlier development of diastolic dysfunction in this group.

Also vascular damage was more prominent in subjects classified as having HN BP at baseline. In particular, both Meanmax and CBMMax IMT were significantly greater in subjects who had HN BP at baseline as compared to those classified as NT. The greatest values were observed in patients classified as hypertensives at baseline (p at least <0.05 for all comparisons) (Fig. 18.5).

When changes over time in measures of TOD during the nine-year follow-up period were analysed, in subjects classified as HN BP at the baseline visit the progression of IMT was progressively greater from patients classified as NT, as HN BP

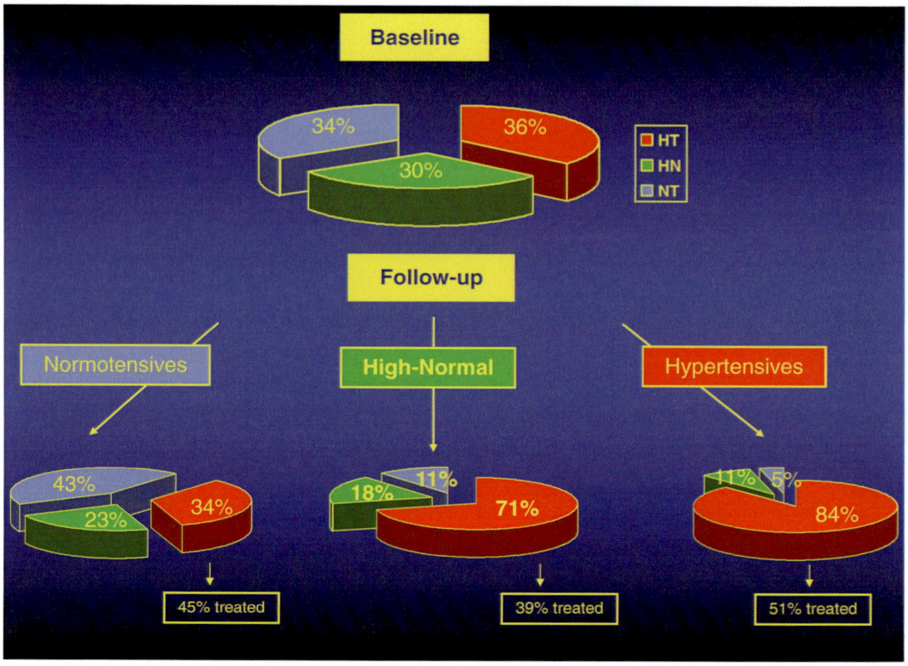

Fig. 18.3 Percentage of patients with normal BP, with high-normal BP, and with arterial hypertension, at baseline and at follow-up

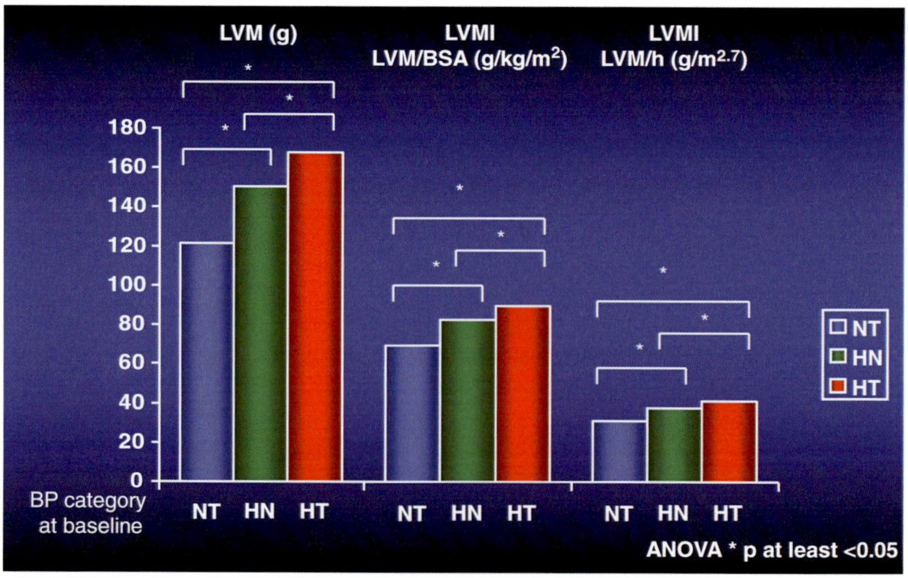

Fig. 18.4 Left ventricular mass at FU according to baseline BP category

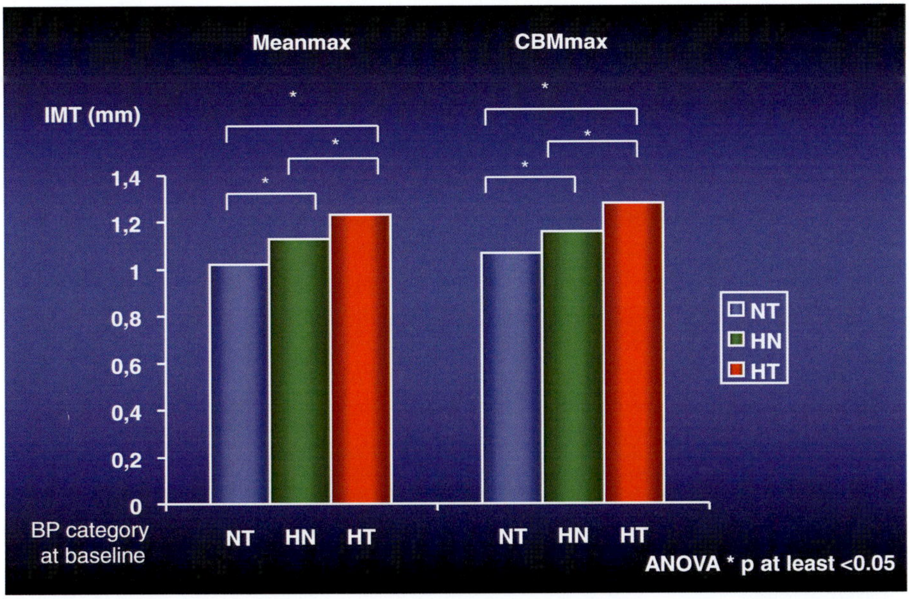

Fig. 18.5 Carotid artery intima-media thickness at FU according to baseline BP category

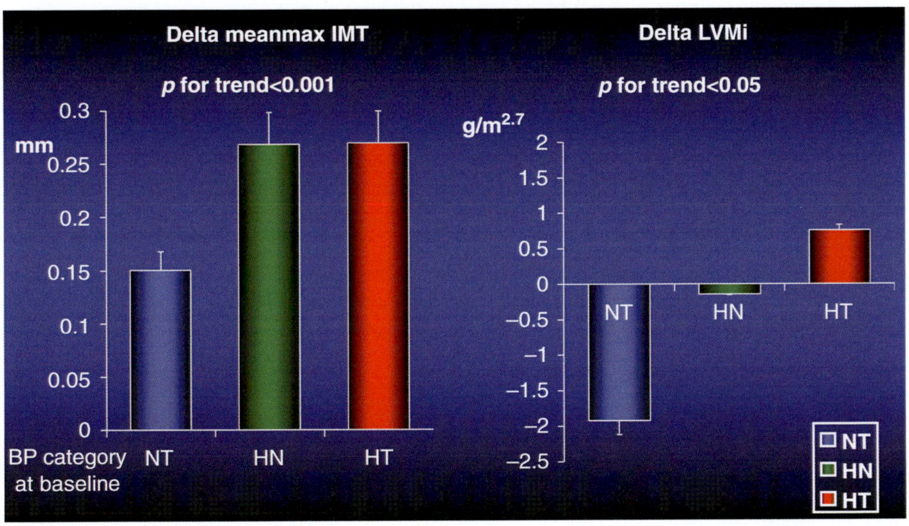

Fig. 18.6 Intima-media thickness and left ventricular mass index changes over time in subjects untreated at follow-up

and as HT at baseline (p for trend <0.01). A similar trend was also observed for left ventricular mass index, but the finding did not reach statistical difference. When limiting the analysis to untreated patients ($n = 295$), the results remained substantially unchanged for IMT, and were statistically significant ($p < 0.05$) also for the change of LVMI over time (Fig. 18.6).

Conclusion

Our findings indicate that a significant proportion (30%) of apparently healthy subjects from an unselected sample of a general population in Northern Italy have HN BP, and that this group of subjects have higher BMI, and a worst cardiovascular risk profile as compared to normotensives (higher plasma glucose, creatinine and uric acid) and that about one third of them have metabolic syndrome. Furthermore, our results confirm that these subjects frequently progress to hypertension: in fact, among the 126 subjects classified as HN at baseline, 71% had progressed to HT after about 9 years, and only 11% had BP values within the normal range. Finally, our results indicate that progression of organ damage is more rapid in patients with high-normal blood pressure, with an increase in carotid intima-media thickness and in left ventricular mass index which is intermediate between that observed in normotensives and in hypertensives. Our findings may contribute to explain [6–8] the increase in the risk of cardiovascular events observed in subjects with high-normal blood pressure and prehypertension.

References

1. Lewington S, Clarke R, Qizilbash N, Peto R, Collins R, Prospective Studies Collaboration. Age-specific relevance of usual blood pressure to vascular mortality: a meta-analysis of individual data for one million adults in 61 prospective studies. Lancet. 2002;360:1903–13.
2. Mancia G, Fagard R, Narkiewicz K, Redon J, Zanchetti A, Bohm M, et al. 2013 ESH/ESC Guidelines for the management of arterial hypertension: the task force for the management of arterial hypertension of the European Society of Hypertension (ESH) and of the European Society of Cardiology (ESC). J Hypertens. 2013;31(7):1281–357.
3. Chobanian AV, Bakris GL, Black HR, Cushman WC, Green LA, Izzo JL Jr, Jones DW, Materson BJ, Oparil S, Wright JT Jr, Roccella EJ, National Heart, Lung, and Blood Institute Joint National Committee on Prevention, Detection, Evaluation, and Treatment of High Blood Pressure, National High Blood Pressure Education Program Coordinating Committee. The Seventh Report of the Joint National Committee on Prevention, Detection, Evaluation, and Treatment of High Blood Pressure: the JNC 7 report. JAMA. 2003;289(19):2560–72.
4. Vasan RS, Larson MG, Leip EP, Evans JC, O'Donnell CJ, Kannel WB, Levy D. Impact of high-normal blood pressure on the risk of cardiovascular disease. N Engl J Med. 2001;345(18):1291–7.
5. Kokubo Y, Kamide K, Okamura T, Watanabe M, Higashiyama A, Kawanishi K, et al. Impact of high-normal blood pressure on the risk of cardiovascular disease in a Japanese urban cohort: the Suita Study. Hypertension. 2008;52:652–9.
6. Muiesan ML, Salvetti M, Rizzoni D, Castellano M, Donato F, Agabiti-Rosei E. Association of change in left ventricular mass with prognosis during long-term antihypertensive treatment. J Hypertens. 1995;13:1091–7.
7. Devereux RB, Wachtell K, Gerdts E, Boman K, Nieminen MS, Papademetriou V, Rokkedal J, Harris K, Aurup P, Dahlöf B. Prognostic significance of left ventricular mass change during treatment of hypertension. JAMA. 2004;292:2350–6.
8. Muiesan ML, Salvetti M, Monteduro C, Bonzi B, Paini A, Viola S, Poisa P, Rizzoni D, Castellano M, Agabiti-Rosei E. Left ventricular concentric geometry during treatment adversely affects cardiovascular prognosis in hypertensive patients. Hypertension. 2004;43:731–8.

Systolic Hypertension in Youth

19

James D. H. Goodman, Ian B. Wilkinson,
and Carmel M. McEniery

19.1 Introduction

Isolated systolic hypertension (ISH) represents one of several different sub-forms of hypertension. It is the most common form of hypertension in the elderly and associated with increased large artery stiffness. However, ISH is also frequently found in young adults, especially males. According to the European Society of Hypertension (ESH) guidelines, ISH in youth [1] (0–15 years) is defined as SBP ≥95th and DBP <90th percentile for age, sex and height. In those aged 16 and over, ISH is defined as SBP ≥140 mmHg and DBP <90 mmHg [2].

The cardiovascular risks associated with hypertension in adulthood are widely recognised and accepted. This contrasts with the ongoing debate concerning the importance of ISH in young individuals, where questions remain over whether ISH represents artefactual or 'spurious' hypertension, a precursor to hypertension or a true hypertensive state with increased cardiovascular risk [3–6]. In addition, prospective longitudinal trials of ISH in youth are lacking, which has caused uncertainty regarding the clinical significance of the condition and whether pharmacological treatment is necessary. In part, the obesity epidemic in young adults and changes in nutrition and lifestyle habits have further contributed to the increased prevalence of ISH in youth, and hence there is added importance regarding stratifying risk for these patients and their subsequent management.

This chapter provides an overview of the current understanding of ISH in youth, concentrating on the epidemiology, pathophysiological mechanisms, association with outcomes and treatment considerations.

J. D. H. Goodman (✉) · I. B. Wilkinson · C. M. McEniery
Experimental Medicine and Immunotherapeutics, University of Cambridge, Cambridge, UK
e-mail: jdhg3@medschl.cam.ac.uk

R. Zimlichman et al. (eds.), *Prehypertension and Cardiometabolic Syndrome*,
Updates in Hypertension and Cardiovascular Protection,
https://doi.org/10.1007/978-3-319-75310-2_19

19.2 Prevalence of ISH in Youth

Many observational studies now demonstrate that ISH is the most common form of hypertension in adolescents and young adults, especially in males. Staessen et al. [7] was one of the first investigators to identify the U-shaped association between ISH prevalence and age, with a 2–8% frequency of ISH in those aged around 30 years, 0.1–0.8% in those aged 40–50, and over 12.6% in those aged over 70. In another study, Sorof [8] examined 2460 school children aged 12–16 years and found 17% of these to be hypertensive, of whom 88% (363/413) were found to have ISH. Mahmud and Feely [9] subsequently examined 174 medical students, confirming ISH in 11, although the authors referred to these individuals as having 'spurious' systolic hypertension (see section below). Along with Sorof, they reported that the number of BP measurements at the time of establishing the formal diagnosis of ISH affects its frequency. Mahmud and Feely stated that repeat BP measurements at intervals of 1 min after 5 min of rest reduced the ISH rate in young adults from 12.6% to 8.5% [8, 9]. In addition, recent data has shown that young adults (18–39 years) with ISH had the slowest rates of receiving an initial diagnosis (of ISH), or starting antihypertensive medication, compared to those with isolated diastolic hypertension (IDH) or systolic diastolic hypertension (SDH) [10]. However, this could also reflect previously published data showing coronary heart disease is more related to diastolic, rather than systolic blood pressure (SBP), although this topic is controversial [11, 12].

In 2003, Mallion [13] reported findings in 27783 untreated individuals in France, finding a 6.8% prevalence of ISH in males aged 25–29 years and a 0.3% prevalence in females of the same age. Then in 2005, the ENIGMA study recruited 1008 young adults in the UK (mean age 20 years of which 43% were male) observing a high prevalence of ISH in males and also noting these individuals to be taller, heavier and with a higher BMI compared to their normotensive controls [14]. In a further study of 750 young adults (aged 26–31) from the Atherosclerosis Risk in Young Adults study [15], ISH was identified in 57 men and 3 women, further confirming the predominance of ISH in men.

The HARVEST study [16], a prospective observational trial, enrolled Italian subjects aged 18–45 years with hypertension, but excluded those with secondary forms of hypertension, diabetes and cardiovascular or renal disease. Out of 1141 subjects, the prevalence of ISH was 13.8%, IDH was 24.8%, and SDH was 61.4%. In agreement with other studies, they confirmed a high prevalence of ISH in those who were young and male—48% in men aged 18–21. Other clinical characteristics of ISH in youth include smoking history [17], more active in sport [18] and those with a higher resting heart rate [19].

Data from the National Health and Nutrition Examination Survey (NHANES) suggests that not only is ISH in youth common but that the frequency is on the rise. For US adults aged 18–39, the prevalence of untreated ISH increased from 0.7% between 1988 and 1994 to 1.6% between 1999 and 2004 [17]. This further increased to 1.9% between 2005 and 2010, and overall, there was a 3.3% prevalence among males aged 18–39 compared to 0.5% for females of the same age [20]. Apart from male sex, smoking, African-American race and obesity were all associated with ISH in the latter NHANES study [17, 20, 21].

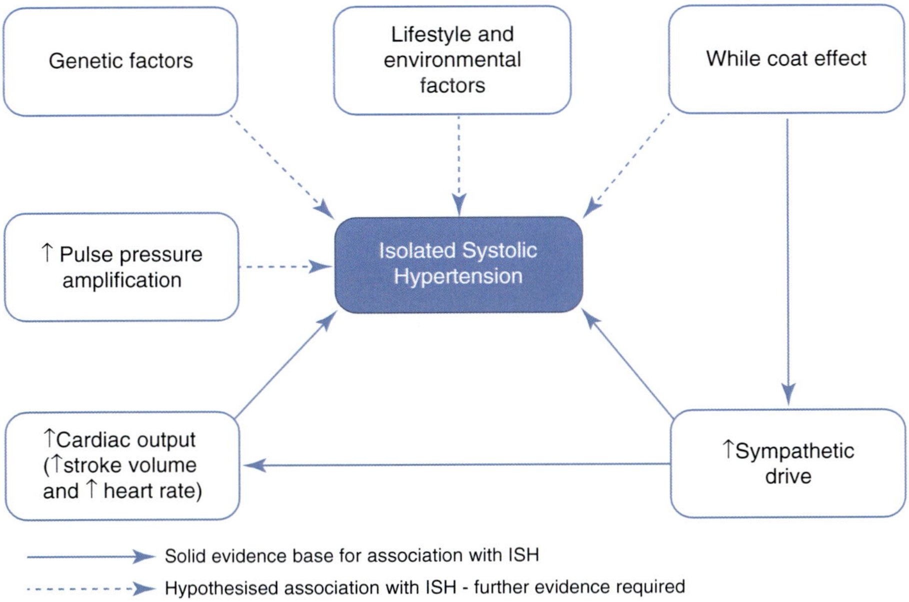

Fig. 19.1 Diagram showing proposed mechanisms of ISH in young adults

19.3 Pathophysiology of ISH in Youth

A number of pathophysiological mechanisms (as illustrated in Fig. 19.1) have been proposed as contributing to ISH in youth including enhanced pulse pressure amplification and increased sympathetic drive with increased cardiac output, stroke volume and heart rate. The following sections review the evidence base for these potential mechanisms in further detail.

19.4 'Spurious' ISH in Youth, Pulse Pressure Amplification and Central (Aortic) Blood Pressure

The term spurious (or pseudo) hypertension has traditionally been applied to elderly individuals where blood vessel calcification causes incompressibility of the artery [22, 23]. This subsequently leads to falsely elevated, or 'spurious' non-invasive brachial cuff blood pressures, but normal intraarterial measurements when measured invasively. Spurious hypertension has also been applied to ISH in young individuals. O'Rourke et al. [18] were the first investigators to describe pseudo-hypertension in an observational study with six healthy young men aged 14–23 with ISH. Using the SphygmoCor system, the authors described these young individuals as having a 'normal' aortic SBP (119 mmHg) but exaggerated central aortic-to-peripheral pressure wave amplification and labelled the condition as pseudo-systolic hypertension. This was further examined by Mahmud and Feely [9] in 174 medical students, again using the SphygmoCor system to estimate the central blood pressure (CBP). Eleven of these were identified as having spurious systolic hypertension with a mean brachial SBP of 147 mmHg, a normal DBP (70 mmHg) and normal aortic pressure waveform and CBP of 116/70. In view of this 'normal' CBP, they suggested that spurious systolic hypertension of youth is unlikely to carry increase cardiovascular risk and does not require antihypertensive treatment.

The physiological mechanism underlying 'spurious' systolic hypertension has been proposed as being due to highly elastic arteries with a low peripheral vascular resistance, a high pulse pressure amplification and low wave reflection [24]. Alternative mechanisms which may explain increased amplification include differences in the transmission properties of the brachiocephalic system itself such as arterial stiffening [25]. It most commonly occurs in those who are male, younger, taller and obese and have a higher resting heart rate (partly because of higher heart rate) [24–27]. This contrasts with the elderly where increased aortic stiffness and early return of reflected waves result in smaller pulse pressure amplification [24].

Both O'Rourke et al. [18] and Mahmud and Feely [9] based their definition of spurious systolic hypertension on a 'normal' systolic pressure in the aorta (i.e. 119 mmHg and 116 mmHg, respectively). Central aortic pressure reflects the pressure experienced by the major organs (heart, kidneys and brain). It should, therefore, better correlate with target organ damage, left ventricular hypertrophy/mass and cardiovascular disease when compared to brachial pressure. Ideally, invasive measurement with cardiac catheterisation is necessary to accurately record central BP. However, this is impractical, particularly in younger individuals, and, therefore, non-invasive estimation of CBP is performed using waveform analysis of distal arterial sites (e.g. carotid, brachial and radial). Analysis of these distal waveforms is performed automatically, with calibration using BP measurements obtained at the brachial artery. One problem with these non-invasive analyses is that the brachial systolic and diastolic cuff pressures required for calibration tend to underestimate the 'true' (invasive) brachial artery pressure, in turn leading to falsely low estimates of central pressure [28].

Leaving these technical points aside, using waveform analysis, McEniery et al. [14] showed that central SBP <110 mmHg corresponded to an optimal BP at the brachial artery (i.e. SBP <120 mmHg). The authors also observed that central SBP was ~22 mmHg higher in young subjects with ISH (121 mmHg) versus normotensives (99 mmHg). Reference values for CBP and pulse pressure amplification have recently been published [29]. 45,426 subjects (from 77 studies) were grouped according to their brachial blood pressure—normotensives, with no cardiovascular risk factors (termed 'normal population'), or hypertensives/normotensives with cardiovascular risk factors (termed 'reference population'). Males aged 20–29 years in the 'normal population' had a central SBP of 103 mmHg, similar to that shown by McEniery et al., and this compared to a central SBP of 110 mmHg in the 'reference population'. Therefore it is apparent that the subjects with spurious ISH described

Table 19.1 Mean central and peripheral systolic blood pressures, in those with isolated systolic hypertension and normotension

ISH studies	Central SBP (mmHg)		Brachial SBP (mmHg)	
	ISH	NT	ISH	NT
O'Rouke et al. (2000) [18]	119	–	153 (radial BP)	–
Mahmud and Feely (2003) [9]	116 (males)	97 (males)	147 (males)	121 (males)
McEniery et al. (2005) [31]	121	99	147	116
Hulsen et al. (2006) [32]	117	106	145	126
Saladini et al. (2011) [33]	130 (ISH—high)[a] 114 (ISH—low)[a]	113	152(ISH—high)[a] 146 (ISH—low)[a]	124
Lurbe et al. (2016) [1]	104	90	132	105

ISH isolated systolic hypertension, *NT* normotension

[a]Saladini divided participants according to whether their central SBP, measured with applanation tonometry, was above (ISH—high) or below (ISH—low) the median (120.5 mmHg). The values here represent the mean of each group

in the studies by O'Rourke et al. or Mahmud and Feely had significantly higher central SBP values than the 'normal' values identified by either McEniery et al. or Herbert et al. [30] (Table 19.1).

It is worth noting that calibration of distal waveforms using brachial BP is highly variable within individuals [27], and as such, caution is required when analysing CBP and pulse pressure amplification results for young adults with ISH. Notwithstanding this, the above data supports the fact that individuals with ISH are actually amplifying an already elevated central SBP rather than amplifying a 'normal' central SBP as previously suggested by O'Rourke et al. and Mahmud and Feely.

19.5 Sympathetic Nervous System Over-Activation in ISH

Stevo Julius was one of the first researchers to link a hyperkinetic state [34] to hypertension in the Tecumseh study, performed in 691 healthy subjects (mean age 32.6 years). A hyperkinetic state (characterised by increased heart rate, increased cardiac index and higher plasma noradrenaline level) was found to be more common in those with borderline hypertension (37.4%) compared to normotensives (10%), thus suggesting a higher degree of sympathetic activity in borderline hypertension. Further studies have supported this view demonstrating that cardiac output and heart rate are also elevated in borderline hypertension, with ISH being a predominant phenotype [35, 36]. However, other European studies have failed to show a positive association between ISH and a hyperkinetic state [32, 33].

Several studies [37, 38] support the hypothesis that in the early stages of hypertension, sympathetic nervous system over-activation, or adrenergic overdrive, is present, particularly in young subjects, although not all studies support an association [39, 40]. What is harder to know is whether this sympathetic activation precedes and subsequently drives an elevated blood pressure. Data from the Framingham Heart Study supports this, demonstrating that young adults with a resting tachycardia were more likely to develop hypertension over the following years compared to age-matched controls with a normal heart rate [41]. Furthermore, Lund-Johansen [42] demonstrated in men that those with borderline hypertension and a high cardiac output transformed over time to sustained essential hypertension via a cascade of haemodynamic adaptations including increased peripheral vascular resistance. If correct, cardiac output could potentially be a valuable biomarker and possible risk stratifier for future hypertension in youth, although further longitudinal data in young adults who are in the early phases of BP elevation will be required [6].

The HARVEST study [43] also explored the role of the autonomic system in the development of sustained hypertension in 163 subjects with stage 1 hypertension and 28 normotensive controls. Those with reduced heart rate variability and signs of sympathetic predominance were more likely to develop sustained hypertension during the 6-year follow-up period. Therefore, interventions aimed at modifying these systems may be beneficial, although it is likely that targeting other risk factors such as obesity, increased salt intake and a lack of physical exercise will also contribute.

19.6 White Coat Effect and ISH

The white coat effect may further contribute to the hyperkinetic state experienced by young adults with ISH. Young adults with hyperkinetic hypertension have significantly higher office BPs compared to home BPs, whereas those with normokinetic hypertension and normotensive individuals show little difference between office and home BP [5]. The white coat effect was examined in 593 overweight children (mean age 12.2 years) [1]. The largest difference between office and central SBP corresponded to the ISH group where only 25% of participants had high central SBP (compared to 50% in IDH group). The highest pulse pressure amplitude was in the ISH group. Furthermore, 75% of the ISH patients were in fact 'white coat' compared to just 10% with IDH. The association between 'white coat' hypertension and ISH is not surprising given that stress results in sympathetic activation, leading to increased stroke volume and cardiac output. This results in a widened pulse pressure as SBP is elevated disproportionately to DBP [44]. The elevation in SBP thus results in an increased frequency of ISH in those with reported 'white-coat' hypertension.

19.7 Other Pathophysiology in ISH in Youth

The ENIGMA study describes the largest group of young adults in whom ISH and its underlying physiological mechanisms have been studied [14]. McEniery et al. measured peripheral and central BP, aortic pulse wave velocity, cardiac output, stroke volume and peripheral vascular resistance in 1008 young adults aged 17–27 years. Compared to normotensive subjects, those with ISH showed higher peripheral and central BPs, aortic pulse wave velocity, cardiac output and stroke volume. However, there were no differences in pulse pressure amplification, heart rate and peripheral vascular resistance between the groups. Compared to hypertensive subjects, those with ISH had higher pulse pressure amplification, aortic pulse wave velocity, cardiac output and stroke volume, while mean blood pressure, heart rate and peripheral vascular resistance were all lower. The authors thus concluded that ISH results from an increased stroke volume and/or aortic stiffness. This contrasts with SDH, in which the major haemodynamic abnormality is an elevated peripheral vascular resistance.

Echocardiography studies in adolescents and children add weight to the above studies by showing an increase in cardiac output and stroke volume in those with persistently elevated SBP [45, 46]. Of note, those of African-American descent were not included in the ENIGMA study. Importantly, African-Americans [47] and blacks [48] tend to have higher peripheral vascular resistance from a younger age. This suggests that different haemodynamic mechanisms contribute to the development of hypertension in different ethnicities, and therefore, the ENIGMA study results may not be generalizable to all ethnic groups.

In a follow-up analysis of the ENIGMA study cohort [49] in 2502 individuals, elevated cardiac output was the haemodynamic factor most strongly associated with increased SBP in lean individuals, but cardiac output was elevated in overweight individuals, irrespective of the level of BP. Instead, peripheral vascular resistance is distinguished between levels of SBP in overweight individuals, suggesting that different haemodynamic mechanisms are likely to drive increased SBP and ISH in young subjects, depending on body size. This may hold important implications for the treatment of ISH in the young, particularly in light of the growing obesity epidemic in the developed world and increasing prevalence of ISH—associated with obesity.

19.8 Association Between SBP and ISH in Youth and Sustained Hypertension

SBP tracks from childhood into adulthood [50], and into later life [51], in almost all societies worldwide. A birth cohort study involving 975 individuals, with multiple BP measurements taken from 7 to 38 years, showed it was possible to identify four discrete trajectories based on SBP and retrospectively identify these from 7 years of age [52]. Those individuals in the two higher SBP trajectories were considered prehypertensive and hypertensive, respectively, by the age of 38 and, in addition, had a worse metabolic profile. Smoking and elevated BMI were associated with increased SBP across all four groups. It is thus possible to predict, with a good degree of accuracy, which children will go on to develop hypertension in adulthood.

Specifically with regard to ISH, The HARVEST study [16] followed 1141 young adults (mean age 33.7 years) for a median of 72.9 months. Subjects were grouped according to their entry BP (ISH, IDH and SDH). When compared to normotensive subjects, the risk of developing hypertension according to their office BP was 5.2 (95% CI 2.9–9.2) for SDH subjects, 2.6 (95% CI 1.5–4.5) among IDH subjects and

2.2 (95% CI 1.2–4.5) for ISH subjects. When sustained hypertension was measured with ambulatory BP (mean daytime BP ≥135/85), the odds ratios were 5.1 (95% CI 3.1–8.2), 5.6 (95% CI 3.2–9.8) and 3.3 (95/% CI 1.7–6.3), respectively. The results thus indicate that young adults with ISH are at increased risk of developing sustained hypertension in later life, although the risk is smaller compared to those with SDH or IDH [3].

A further analysis of the HARVEST trial [33] after 9.5 years of follow-up demonstrated that ISH subjects with high central BP had a risk of developing sustained hypertension and requiring treatment which was similar to those with SDH (OR 6.2; 95% CI 1.8–21.1, $p = 0.003$). In contrast, those with ISH with a low central BP had a risk of developing sustained hypertension which was similar to that of normotensives (OR 1.10, 95% CI 0.2–5.3, $p = 0.90$), indicating that there is potential value in using CBP as a risk stratifier in young adults. Indeed, Hulsen et al. [32] also observed that those younger subjects with ISH and a high central BP (≥121 mmHg vs. <121 mmHg) were at higher risk of developing hypertension that required treatment over a 10-year follow-up period (50% vs. 15.2%) [33]. However, it is worth noting the mean age in the HARVEST trial was 38.9 years, and prospective longitudinal data involving adolescents and young adults is required to confirm the true value of central BP as a stratifier of risk in young subjects.

19.9 Association Between SBP and ISH in Youth and Cardiovascular Risk

The evidence outlined above establishes a strong association between ISH in youth and sustained hypertension in later life. It is not unexpected, therefore, that elevated SBP in youth increases cardiovascular risk in later life. Sundstrom et al. [53] followed 1.2 million Swedish male military conscripts (mean age 18.4 years) over 24 years finding a U-shaped relationship between total mortality and SBP (lowest risk at 130 mmHg) which was primarily driven by non-cardiovascular mortality, whereas there was a monotonic and positive association between cardiovascular mortality and SBP. However, the relationship with DBP and total mortality was stronger compared to that of SBP indicating that DBP should not be ignored. In a study involving 8354 Glasgow University students (mean age 20.5 years) followed over a median of 41.3 years, both SBP and DBP were associated with increasing risk of CHD and CVD mortality, although this did not reach significance for DBP. However, regarding stroke mortality specifically, there was a strong positive association with DBP, but little correlation with SBP. A further study involving 10327 Harvard University former students (under age 30) showed that SBP >130 mmHg, elevated BMI, short body stature and smoking status predicted nonfatal stroke during the follow-up period of 26–50 years [54].

While a number of studies, including those described, assess SBP and DBP individually, there is a distinct lack of prospective studies in young people assessing hypertension by subtype, such as ISH. Two studies by Rutan [55] and Strandberg [56] prospectively assess ISH, although, in both of these studies, ISH was defined as SBP ≥160 mmHg and DBP <90 mmHg. Rutan assessed 317871 white men aged 35–57 years, showing those with ISH had the highest all-cause and cardiovascular mortality over a 6-year follow-up period. Strandberg examined 3267 Finnish men aged 30–45 years. The presence of ISH failed to predict either all-cause or cardiovascular mortality—although only 17 participants were actually classified as having ISH.

The best current evidence for the long-term risk associated with ISH in young subjects is provided by the Chicago Heart Association Detection in Industry Programme [19], which examined 15868 men and 11213 women aged 18–49 (mean age 34) during a 31-year follow-up. Participants were categorised into one of five groups (optimal BP, high-normal BP, IDH, SDH and ISH defined by SBP ≥140 mmHg and DBP <90 mmHg) depending upon their seated brachial blood pressure and according to the Joint National Committee on Prevention, Detection, Evaluation and Treatment of High Blood Pressure (7th report) [57]. In total, there were 1728 deaths from cardiovascular disease, 1168 from coronary heart disease and 223 deaths from stroke. Overall, men with ISH had an increased risk of cardiovascular disease and coronary heart disease mortality when compared to optimal BP. The risk was similar to those with high-normal BP but lower compared to those with IDH and SDH. However, females with ISH showed a higher cardiovascular mortality risk when compared to all other BP categories apart from those with SDH. While it remains unclear how the pathophysiology of hypertension differs between sexes, it is known that at any given age from adolescence, females operate at a lower BP than males [58]. However, females tend to have a relatively higher CBP (due to greater central arterial wave augmentation and smaller pressure amplification) [4, 59], which may render females at greater cardiovascular risk for any given peripheral BP than males.

The results of the Chicago Heart Association study demonstrate for the first time that ISH in younger to middle-aged adults is associated with increased future risk and should not be considered an innocuous condition. Importantly, the study began before the onset of the current obesity epidemic and, therefore, has not captured the impact of ISH associated with obesity, which is increasing in prevalence [17], and may well drive even greater risk. By establishing an association between ISH in youth and increased cardiovascular risk, one can conclude that ISH is unlikely to be artefactual and, instead, necessitates active management and treatment.

19.10 Treatment of ISH in Youth

Modifying diet (reducing salt intake), increasing physical activity, reducing weight and stopping smoking are recommended first-line options in young individuals with hypertension and are advocated, even if pharmacological therapy is necessary. Formal guidelines are otherwise lacking, and while the management of ISH is alluded to, there is no mention on the management or treatment of ISH relating to youth in either the UK National Institute for Health and Clinical Excellence (NICE) guidelines [60], the JNC guidelines [61] or the National Heart Foundation of

Australia guidelines [62]. The 2016 ESH guidelines for children and adolescents [2] do acknowledge the lack of understanding regarding prognosis and treatment in young adults with ISH. Lifestyle modifications and close monitoring are suggested, whereas pharmacological therapy is not, unless there are hypertensive symptoms or target organ damage. Instead, the ESH guidelines suggest that aortic BP measurements may be useful in the assessment of those with ISH (without target organ damage) but do not provide further guidance regarding management. Stratifying risk according to CBP is promising but lacks universally agreed reference ranges and widespread uptake, particularly in primary care settings, and suffers from a lack of evidence in the area.

The underlying pathophysiology in ISH would suggest that reducing cardiac output and/or aortic stiffness would be reasonable therapeutic options. Indeed, beta blockers would seem sensible, and propranolol, labetalol and nebivolol all reduce SBP, DBP and cardiac output in healthy, normotensive individuals (average age 32) [63]. However, non-vasodilating beta blockers (such as atenolol) show less benefit in reducing central aortic pressure when compared to newer beta blockers that either simultaneously block alpha receptors (carvedilol) or cause vasodilation via nitric oxide stimulation (nebivolol) [64–66]. The results of two comprehensive meta-analyses [67, 68], along with comparison studies including the ASCOT trial [69], demonstrate that atenolol is inferior to other major antihypertensive drug classes in preventing cardiovascular events. In addition, haemodynamic and physiological effects of selective B1 antagonists in young adults are poorly understood, and there may be long-term risks associated with lowering cardiac output in children although, as yet, data are very sparse and this area of research is poorly understood.

Once established, hypertension is irreversible, and therefore strategies aimed at preventing or delaying the condition from an early stage are of primary importance. Targeting key mechanisms underlying ISH in the young may well lead to more effective BP control and reduce cardiovascular risk. The lack of treatment guidance reflects underlying uncertainty, both in terms of the optimum treatment strategy and future prognosis, due to a lack of long-term prospective studies.

Conclusion

Evidence increasingly points towards ISH in youth being associated with sustained hypertension in adulthood and thus carries an increased cardiovascular risk. Standardised screening investigations for underlying causes and target organ damage, plus ambulatory blood pressure monitoring to confirm ISH, remain first-line investigations. Measurement of CBP should help to provide additional evidence regarding underlying risk and target organ damage and to confirm or refute true ISH (rather than white coat); however its reproducibility and relevance as a marker of risk remain questionable.

Once confirmed then ISH should be actively managed with lifestyle advice. While the long-term risks and benefits of pharmacological treatment associated with ISH in the elderly are undisputed, the evidence of antihypertensive drugs in ISH in youth remains poorly supported by both the literature and current international hypertension guidelines and has been the subject of continued debate.

Nevertheless, pharmacological therapy should be initiated in this group of patients to achieve a target BP within the designated range.

Studies in this chapter draw their data from a wide range of ages from children to middle-aged adults. Drawing direct comparisons and comparing outcome data between these studies are challenging, as SBP naturally increases into and throughout adult life, and therefore assessing future cardiovascular risk for an otherwise identical individual, aged either 18 or 35 years with the same SBP of 145 mmHg, is markedly different. Furthermore, the use of risk calculators in deciding whether to initiate treatment is not suitable in adolescents or young adults, due to their very low absolute risks (e.g. over 10–20 years).

Elevated cardiac output (with increased stroke volume and heart rate) and increased sympathetic activation, rather than pulse pressure amplification, are the dominant haemodynamic traits in children, adolescents and young adults with ISH. These may serve as useful biomarkers of future risk. Further, long-term prospective studies with ISH subjects, involving different ethnic groups, and with hard end points, are required to better understand the pathophysiology, natural history and clinical consequences of ISH in youth.

References

1. Lurbe E, et al. Central blood pressure and pulse wave amplification across the spectrum of peripheral blood pressure in overweight and obese youth. J Hypertens. 2016;**34**(7):1389–95.
2. Lurbe E, et al. European Society of Hypertension guidelines for the management of high blood pressure in children and adolescents. J Hypertens. 2016;34(10):1887–920.
3. Saladini F, Palatini P. Isolated systolic hypertension in young individuals: pathophysiological mechanisms, prognostic significance, and clinical implications. High Blood Press Cardiovasc Prev. 2017;24(2):133–9.
4. Yano Y, Lloyd-Jones DM. Isolated systolic hypertension in young and middle-aged adults. Curr Hypertens Rep. 2016;18(11):78.
5. Lurbe E, Redon J. Isolated systolic hypertension in young people is not spurious and should be treated: con side of the argument. Hypertension. 2016;68(2):276–80.
6. McEniery CM, et al. Isolated systolic hypertension in young people is not spurious and should be treated: pro side of the argument. Hypertension. 2016;68(2):269–75.
7. Staessen J, Amery A, Fagard R. Isolated systolic hypertension in the elderly. J Hypertens. 1990;8(5):393–405.
8. Sorof JM, et al. Isolated systolic hypertension, obesity, and hyperkinetic hemodynamic states in children. J Pediatr. 2002;140(6):660–6.
9. Mahmud A, Feely J. Spurious systolic hypertension of youth: fit young men with elastic arteries. Am J Hypertens. 2003;16(3):229–32.
10. Johnson HM, et al. Differential diagnosis and treatment rates between systolic and diastolic hypertension in young adults: a multidisciplinary observational study. J Clin Hypertens (Greenwich). 2015;17(11):885–94.
11. Bulpitt CJ. Is systolic pressure more important than diastolic pressure? J Hum Hypertens. 1990;4(5):471–6.
12. Pickering TG, et al. Recommendations for blood pressure measurement in humans and experimental animals: part 1: blood pressure measurement in humans: a statement for professionals from the Subcommittee of Professional and Public Education of the American Heart Association Council on High Blood Pressure Research. Hypertension. 2005;45(1):142–61.

13. Mallion JM, et al. Isolated systolic hypertension: data on a cohort of young subjects from a French working population (IHPAF). J Hum Hypertens. 2003;17(2):93–100.
14. McEniery CM, et al. Increased stroke volume and aortic stiffness contribute to isolated systolic hypertension in young adults. Hypertension. 2005;46(1):221–6.
15. Oren A, et al. The Atherosclerosis Risk in Young Adults (ARYA) study: rationale and design. Eur J Epidemiol. 2003;18(7):715–27.
16. Saladini F, et al. Natural history of hypertension subtypes in young and middle-age adults. Am J Hypertens. 2009;22(5):531–7.
17. Grebla RC, et al. Prevalence and determinants of isolated systolic hypertension among young adults: the 1999–2004 US National Health And Nutrition Examination Survey. J Hypertens. 2010;28(1):15–23.
18. O'Rourke MF, Vlachopoulos C, Graham RM. Spurious systolic hypertension in youth. Vasc Med. 2000;5(3):141–5.
19. Yano Y, et al. Isolated systolic hypertension in young and middle-aged adults and 31-year risk for cardiovascular mortality: the Chicago Heart Association Detection Project in Industry study. J Am Coll Cardiol. 2015;65(4):327–35.
20. Liu X, Rodriguez CJ, Wang K. Prevalence and trends of isolated systolic hypertension among untreated adults in the United States. J Am Soc Hypertens. 2015;9(3):197–205.
21. Franklin SS, et al. Blood pressure categories, hypertensive subtypes, and the metabolic syndrome. J Hypertens. 2006;24(10):2009–16.
22. Sutton-Tyrrell K, et al. Relationship of ankle blood pressures to cardiovascular events in older adults. Stroke. 2008;39(3):863–9.
23. Taguchi JT, Suwangool P. "Pipe-stem" brachial arteries. A cause of pseudohypertension. JAMA. 1974;228(6):733.
24. Avolio AP, et al. Role of pulse pressure amplification in arterial hypertension: experts' opinion and review of the data. Hypertension. 2009;54(2):375–83.
25. Cockcroft JR, McEniery CM, Wilkinson IB. Pseudo hypertension of youth: too much of a good thing? Am J Hypertens. 2003;16(3):262–4.
26. Protogerou AD, et al. Increased pulse pressure amplification in treated hypertensive subjects with metabolic syndrome. Am J Hypertens. 2007;20(2):127–33.
27. McEniery CM, et al. Central pressure: variability and impact of cardiovascular risk factors: the Anglo-Cardiff Collaborative Trial II. Hypertension. 2008;51(6):1476–82.
28. McEniery CM, et al. Central blood pressure: current evidence and clinical importance. Eur Heart J. 2014;35(26):1719–25.
29. Herbert A, et al. Establishing reference values for central blood pressure and its amplification in a general healthy population and according to cardiovascular risk factors. Eur Heart J. 2014;35(44):3122–33.
30. McEniery CM, Wilkinson IB, Cockcroft JR. Systolic hypertension in young adults: spurious definition of a genuine condition. J Hypertens. 2006;24(11):2316–7. author reply 2317-9.
31. McEniery CM, et al. Normal vascular aging: differential effects on wave reflection and aortic pulse wave velocity: the Anglo-Cardiff Collaborative Trial (ACCT). J Am Coll Cardiol. 2005;46(9):1753–60.
32. Hulsen HT, et al. Spurious systolic hypertension in young adults; prevalence of high brachial systolic blood pressure and low central pressure and its determinants. J Hypertens. 2006;24(6):1027–32.
33. Saladini F, et al. Isolated systolic hypertension of young-to-middle-age individuals implies a relatively low risk of developing hypertension needing treatment when central blood pressure is low. J Hypertens. 2011;29(7):1311–9.
34. Julius S, et al. Hyperkinetic borderline hypertension in Tecumseh, Michigan. J Hypertens. 1991;9(1):77–84.
35. Messerli FH, et al. Borderline hypertension: relationship between age, hemodynamics and circulating catecholamines. Circulation. 1981;64(4):760–4.
36. Messerli FH, et al. Borderline hypertension and obesity: two prehypertensive states with elevated cardiac output. Circulation. 1982;66(1):55–60.

37. Esler M, et al. Assessment of human sympathetic nervous system activity from measurements of norepinephrine turnover. Hypertension. 1988;11(1):3–20.
38. Grassi G, Mark A, Esler M. The sympathetic nervous system alterations in human hypertension. Circ Res. 2015;116(6):976–90.
39. Rea RF, Hamdan M. Baroreflex control of muscle sympathetic nerve activity in borderline hypertension. Circulation. 1990;82(3):856–62.
40. Schobel HP, et al. Evidence against elevated sympathetic vasoconstrictor activity in borderline hypertension. J Am Soc Nephrol. 1998;9(9):1581–7.
41. Gudmundsdottir H, et al. Do screening blood pressure and plasma catecholamines predict development of hypertension? Twenty-year follow-up of middle-aged men. Blood Press. 2008;17(2):94–103.
42. Lund-Johansen P. Haemodynamics in essential hypertension. Clin Sci (Lond). 1980;59(Suppl 6):343s–54s.
43. Palatini P, et al. Evolution of blood pressure and cholesterol in stage 1 hypertension: role of autonomic nervous system activity. J Hypertens. 2006;24(7):1375–81.
44. Yoon HJ, et al. Can pulse pressure predict the white-coat effect in treated hypertensive patients? Clin Exp Hypertens. 2012;34(8):555–60.
45. Sinaiko AR, et al. Cardiac status of adolescents tracking with high and low blood pressure since early childhood. J Hypertens Suppl. 1986;4(5):S378–80.
46. Schieken RM, Clarke WR, Lauer RM. The cardiovascular responses to exercise in children across the blood pressure distribution. The Muscatine study. Hypertension. 1983;5(1):71–8.
47. Dysart JM, et al. Ethnic differences in the myocardial and vascular reactivity to stress in normotensive girls. Am J Hypertens. 1994;7(1):15–22.
48. Soto LF, et al. Echocardiographic functions and blood pressure levels in children and young adults from a biracial population: the Bogalusa Heart Study. Am J Med Sci. 1989;297(5):271–9.
49. Middlemiss JE, et al. Mechanisms underlying elevated SBP differ with adiposity in young adults: the Enigma study. J Hypertens. 2016;34(2):290–7.
50. Chen X, Wang Y. Tracking of blood pressure from childhood to adulthood: a systematic review and meta-regression analysis. Circulation. 2008;117(25):3171–80.
51. Wills AK, et al. Population heterogeneity in trajectories of midlife blood pressure. Epidemiology. 2012;23(2):203–11.
52. Theodore RF, et al. Childhood to early-midlife systolic blood pressure trajectories: early-life predictors, effect modifiers, and adult cardiovascular outcomes. Hypertension. 2015;66(6):1108–15.
53. Sundstrom J, et al. Association of blood pressure in late adolescence with subsequent mortality: cohort study of Swedish male conscripts. BMJ. 2011;342:d643.
54. Paffenbarger RS Jr, Wing AL. Chronic disease in former college students. XI. Early precursors of nonfatal stroke. Am J Epidemiol. 1971;94(6):524–30.
55. Rutan GH, et al. Mortality associated with diastolic hypertension and isolated systolic hypertension among men screened for the Multiple Risk Factor Intervention Trial. Circulation. 1988;77(3):504–14.
56. Strandberg TE, et al. Isolated diastolic hypertension, pulse pressure, and mean arterial pressure as predictors of mortality during a follow-up of up to 32 years. J Hypertens. 2002;20(3):399–404.
57. Chobanian AV, et al. Seventh report of the Joint National Committee on Prevention, Detection, Evaluation, and Treatment of High Blood Pressure. Hypertension. 2003;42(6):1206–52.
58. Wiinberg N, et al. 24-h ambulatory blood pressure in 352 normal Danish subjects, related to age and gender. Am J Hypertens. 1995;8(10 Pt 1):978–86.
59. Shim CY, et al. Sex differences in central hemodynamics and their relationship to left ventricular diastolic function. J Am Coll Cardiol. 2011;57(10):1226–33.
60. Ritchie LD, Campbell NC, Murchie P. New NICE guidelines for hypertension. BMJ. 2011;343:d5644.

61. James PA, et al. 2014 evidence-based guideline for the management of high blood pressure in adults: report from the panel members appointed to the Eighth Joint National Committee (JNC 8). JAMA. 2014;311(5):507–20.
62. Gabb GM, Mangoni AA, Arnolda L. Guideline for the diagnosis and management of hypertension in adults—2016. Med J Aust. 2017;206(3):141.
63. Cheymol G, et al. Pharmacokinetics of beta-adrenoceptor blockers in obese and normal volunteers. Br J Clin Pharmacol. 1997;43(6):563–70.
64. Sabovic M, Safar ME, Blacher J. Is there any additional prognostic value of central blood pressure wave forms beyond peripheral blood pressure? Curr Pharm Des. 2009;15(3):254–66.
65. McEniery CM. Antihypertensive drugs and central blood pressure. Curr Hypertens Rep. 2009;11(4):253–9.
66. Soanker R, et al. Effect of beta-1-blocker, nebivolol, on central aortic pressure and arterial stiffness in patients with essential hypertension. Indian J Pharm. 2012;44(3):407–11.
67. Carlberg B, Samuelsson O, Lindholm LH. Atenolol in hypertension: is it a wise choice? Lancet. 2004;364(9446):1684–9.
68. Lindholm LH, Carlberg B, Samuelsson O. Should beta blockers remain first choice in the treatment of primary hypertension? A meta-analysis. Lancet. 2005;366(9496):1545–53.
69. Dahlof B, et al. Prevention of cardiovascular events with an antihypertensive regimen of amlodipine adding perindopril as required versus atenolol adding bendroflumethiazide as required, in the Anglo-Scandinavian Cardiac Outcomes Trial-Blood Pressure Lowering Arm (ASCOT-BPLA): a multicentre randomised controlled trial. Lancet. 2005;366(9489):895–906.

The Role of Perivascular Fat in Raising Blood Pressure in Obesity and Diabetes

20

Reza Aghamohammadzadeh and Anthony M. Heagerty

Abbreviations

ACE	Angiotensin converting enzyme
ADRF	Adipose-derived relaxing factor
AMPK	5′ Adenosine monophosphate-activated protein kinase
BMI	Body mass index
BP	Blood pressure
CNS	Central nervous system
eNOS	Endothelial nitric oxide synthase
G6PD	Glucose-6-phosphate dehydrogenase
MCP-1	Monocyte chemotactic protein-1
MetS	Metabolic syndrome
MR	Mineralocorticoid receptor
NADPH	Nicotinamide adenine dinucleotide phosphate
NO	Nitric oxide
NOS	Nitric oxide synthase
OSA	Obstructive sleep apnoea
PAME	Palmitic acid methyl ester
PVAT	Perivascular adipose tissue
RAAS	Renin-angiotensin-aldosterone system
ROS	Reactive oxygen species
SHR	Spontaneously hypertensive rat
SNS	Sympathetic nervous system
WC	Waist circumference

R. Aghamohammadzadeh (✉) · A. M. Heagerty
Division of Cardiovascular Sciences, The University of Manchester, Manchester, UK
e-mail: reza.zadeh@manchester.ac.uk

R. Zimlichman et al. (eds.), *Prehypertension and Cardiometabolic Syndrome*, Updates in Hypertension and Cardiovascular Protection,
https://doi.org/10.1007/978-3-319-75310-2_20

20.1 The Clinical Problem

Obesity has more than doubled since 1980, with nearly 2 billion overweight (39%) and 600 million obese (13%) adults worldwide [1]. In England nearly a quarter and in the USA close to a third of all adults are obese [2, 3].

Our contemporary understanding of obesity focuses on our ancestors and the fact that fat was the energy store developed in times of plenty which could then be utilised during times of famine. This theory suggests that genes predisposing to obesity would confer survival benefits and such individuals would live long enough to reproduce which is often seen as nature's ultimate aim. Whilst adaptive variations in weight in the animal kingdom continue to serve their pro-survival purpose, we are observing a worrying trend in weight gain often associated with diseases that shorten the lifespan of the affected individual or at the very least don't confer any survival benefits. Susceptible individuals are no longer exposed to periods of famine and are instead able to access easily high energy foods without expending much energy [4, 5]. Hunting and gathering food has been replaced by as little effort as a simple click of a button on the computer or a short drive to the nearest supermarket. In the hibernating mammal, short-term obesity and insulin resistance help direct glucose to the brain to keep the animal alive; however obesity has inflicted the modern man with chronic illnesses with significant associated cardiovascular morbidity and mortality, often requiring treatments such as polypharmacy or surgery in the extreme cases [6].

A clue to the complexity of obesity-related disorders is that whilst the presence of obesity is thought to be detrimental to health, simple and intuitive measurements such as BMI, waist circumference and waist-to-hip ratio do not improve cardiovascular disease risk prediction substantially when information such as blood pressure, lipid profile and a history of diabetes are available [7]. This highlights the fact that there is more to obesity than the shape or size of the individual and there may well be obese individuals whose cardiovascular risk profile is not particularly adverse. This cohort of individuals has been labelled as the 'metabolically healthy obese'. A better understanding of the physiology of these individuals will no doubt help guide future therapies to potentially transform those with MetS into 'metabolically healthy' individuals without resorting to drastic measure to achieve significant weight loss. Nonetheless, obesity and metabolic syndrome remain strong predictors of future cardiovascular events. In those with disproportionately high WC for a given BMI, assessment of further cardiometabolic risk factors is encouraged [8], thus highlighting the specific properties of individual fat depots and providing clues that certain depots convey a worse risk profile.

Hypertension affects nearly one third of the US population [9], and in England it was reported in over 45% of those in the obese group, compared with around 30% of the overweight and 15% of those in the normal weight category [2]. Globally over a billion people have raised blood pressure, that is, 24% of the adult male and 20% of adult female population in 2015 [10]. The Framingham Heart Study identifies obesity as a contributory factor in 60–70% of essential hypertension [11], and obese individuals have a 3.5-fold increase in the likelihood of developing hypertension [12].

The co-occurrence of obesity and hypertension has prompted the scientific community to further investigate the pathophysiology of obesity-related hypertension as well as its links to diabetes. Contemporary hypotheses have described prediabetes as a disease of the microvasculature under the influence of its surrounding perivascular adipose tissue (PVAT).

There are many mechanisms via which obesity can lead to hypertension. In the acute phase, both bolus oral ingestion and the intravenous infusion of fat by normotensive obese individuals result in a significant rise in systolic blood pressure, attenuated endothelial function, increased oxidative stress markers and activation of the sympathetic nervous system [13].

Genetic causes of obesity are rare, and the majority of cases are a consequence of indulgence in readily available and calorie-rich foods which provide significant proportion of the recommended daily allowance of salt and fat. High-salt diets accelerate the development of hypertension in diet-induced obese rats without raising the ceiling of the systolic blood pressure beyond that observed in diet-induced obese rats fed a low-salt diet [14]. This effect may be a consequence of the increase in oxidative stress levels in the vasculature as evidenced by significantly higher superoxide levels within aortic rings of high-fat and high-salt diet fed animals.

There are numerous facilitators of obesity-related hypertension. These include the renin-angiotensin-aldosterone system (RAAS), the overactive sympathetic nervous system, metabolic dysregulation including hyperinsulinaemia, adipokine imbalance, and PVAT damage. There is currently no direct evidence to suggest that a loss of PVAT vasorelaxant function leads to systemic hypertension in man, but we have reported a correlation between the loss of PVAT vasorelaxant effect and a rise in BP in a murine model of obesity [15] and believe that such a correlation might also exist in man.

20.2 Fat Depots

This chapter reviews the role of perivascular adipose tissue in MetS, but it is vital to point out that the distribution of fat around the body determines not only the obese phenotype but also its consequences. Intra-abdominal and visceral fat depots have been linked with an adverse cardiometabolic profile and mortality associated with obesity [16, 17]. The total amount of internal fat rises with increasing subcutaneous adiposity, but even individuals classed as thin may have more visceral fat than some obese individuals. Fat accumulation in some fat depots seems to be more favourable. Increased gluteofemoral fat mass negatively correlates with levels of inflammatory cytokines and is positively linked to raised concentrations of adipokines resulting in decreased metabolic and cardiovascular risk [18]. In human experiments, this is the fat depot that is most easily accessible and studied in ex vivo protocols.

Adipose tissue depots have unique inflammatory profiles. Perivascular adipose tissue from murine aortic arch expresses lower levels of adipocyte-associated genes compared with subcutaneous and visceral fat [19]. Visceral adipose tissue exhibits a more inflammatory profile with a higher macrophage content than subcutaneous fat [20]. This may somewhat explain the stronger link between central obesity and hypertension than between BMI and raised blood pressure [21].

Epicardial adipose tissue thickness correlates well with waist circumference, visceral adipose tissue mass, fasting insulin and diastolic blood pressure [22, 23] and has been shown to be significantly greater in patients with MetS than those without [24].

PVAT surrounding human coronary vessels is made up of smaller, more irregularly shaped adipocytes as compared with visceral and subcutaneous fat depots. Coronary PVAT secretes lower levels of adiponectin and higher levels of cytokines such as IL-8 and IL-6 as compared with subcutaneous and visceral adipocytes [19]. Exposure to IL-6 has been linked with a reduction in adiponectin production by human adipocytes [25]. Interestingly, there is a high level of macrophage infiltration and lower adiponectin mRNA levels in the epicardial fat tissue of patients with coronary artery disease [26]. Coronary PVAT contains higher levels of monocyte chemotactic protein-1 (MCP-1) as compared with visceral and subcutaneous tissue [19, 27–29]. Lower levels of adiponectin in epicardial tissue have also been associated with hypertension [30, 31] and increased risk of myocardial infarction [32].

In this chapter we will focus mainly on PVAT as the fat depot of interest.

20.3 Perivascular Adipose Tissue

Adipocytes surround almost every blood vessel in the body. They are biological active cells that produce and secrete a number of molecules called adipokines with metabolic and vasoactive properties. In the adult man, these are predominantly white adipocytes and form the perivascular adipose tissue or PVAT. In 2005, Yudkin et al. proposed that PVAT might be the link between obesity and the development of diabetes and MetS as a consequence of an adverse effect on the microvasculature [33]. In health, PVAT could produce adipokines that influence metabolism and the control of local microvessel tone. They suggested that the loss of these adipokines would result in a change in vessel function and development of insulin resistance. The effect of circulating insulin on NO-mediated vasodilatation is of paramount importance in modulating the postprandial increase in nutritive flow, and the authors postulated that this could be challenged by the paracrine action of adipokines released from local fat stores in obesity. They further highlighted the role inflammation may play and that higher concentrations of TNF-α in obesity could disrupt the crosstalk between fat and blood vessels. Only recently we have been able to provide the evidence in support of the Yudkin hypothesis, but we are far from identifying definitive therapeutic strategies to treat prediabetes and pre-hypertension before the onset of MetS.

The effect of PVAT on its surrounding vasculature is not only dependent on the properties of the adipocytes but also the presence of a variety of cells coexisting within PVAT. In chronic inflammatory conditions such as obesity, there is an increase in numbers of inflammatory cells including macrophages and eosinophils within PVAT which distorts the properties of 'healthy PVAT' and leads to a less favourable profile.

At first glance, a simple review of the vast literature on the properties of PVAT can appear somewhat confusing or contradictory. There are reports of both vasorelaxant and pro-contractile properties which can bemuse the casual reader. We know now that PVAT can behave differently, depending on the specific species and vascular beds being studied. The distinctive properties of PVAT also depend on the agents used to the tissue. In health, PVAT from both human and murine mesenteric vessel beds exerts a vasorelaxant effect. That is to say that in a simple organ bath or myography experiment, in the presence of PVAT, the adjacent small vessel constricts significantly less than a skeletonised vessel when stimulated with a vasoconstrictor agent. In obesity this effect is not observed.

There is evidence to suggest that the vasorelaxant property is due to a number of molecules being secreted from PVAT as well as a degree of contribution from the 'sponging effect' of PVAT forming a physical barrier and obstructing the flow of the provocative agents from reaching the vessel. We have shown previously that damage to the PVAT vasorelaxant property directly correlates with BP elevation in a murine model of obesity [15]. This is a significant finding as it is the first evidence of a correlation between PVAT function and blood pressure. Quantifying PVAT vasorelaxant effect is a novel endeavour. In brief, animals were fed a high-fat diet to establish an environmental model of obesity. Vessel segments from their mesenteric beds were assessed, and the degree of contraction of their adjacent skeletonised vessel was quantified as a ratio of the degree of contraction of the PVAT-intact segment of the same vessel to KPSS (potassium-rich physiological saline solution). We reported a correlation between this derived figure and systemic BP. This means that as the animals gained weight and lost their PVAT vasorelaxant effect, there was an attendant elevation in blood pressure. This remains the most convincing evidence of a link between weight gain and PVAT function correlating with a rise in BP.

20.4 PVAT as a Vasorelaxant Organ

We have already discussed that healthy PVAT exerts a vasorelaxant effect on adjacent microvasculature when subject to vasoconstrictors [34]. This is true in the majority of vascular beds. A number of mechanisms have been proposed to describe this phenomenon with just as many outstanding questions requiring further investigation.

Experimental protocols have identified both endothelium-dependent and endothelium-independent [35] mechanisms, and a number of molecules have been implicated which will be discussed briefly in this chapter.

White and brown adipocytes have similar yet distinguishably different secretion profiles [36], but the vasorelaxant property of PVAT has been documented in both white and brown tissues [37, 38].

Adiponectin is the most abundant adipokine with a significant vasorelaxant effect on small arteries and is able to reverse endothelial dysfunction in diet-induced obese rats via the AMPK-eNOS pathway [39]. Adiponectin levels are low in hypertension and improve with antihypertensive treatment [40]. Adiponectin secreted from murine PVAT modulates the tone of the adjoining microvessel segment by functioning as an adipose-derived relaxant factor or ADRF [41]. Further data from our group demonstrated that adiponectin receptor type 1 blockade abolishes PVAT vasorelaxant effect on adjacent small arteries obtained from healthy biopsies [42], thus clearly demonstrating that adiponectin is an ADRF in man. Recently we have reviewed in detail the properties of this adipokine and its role as an ADRF [43].

Adiponectin directly stimulates the production of nitric oxide in endothelial cells using the phosphatidylinositol 3-kinase-dependent pathways involving phosphorylation of eNOS at Ser1179 by AMPK. This vasodilator action of adiponectin may in part explain the effects of adiponectin in augmenting the metabolic actions of insulin in vivo [44].

Serum levels of the adipocyte-derived proteins adiponectin and leptin correlate with insulin resistance (HOMA-IR) and BMI. Levels of expression of MCP-1 and TNF-alpha in visceral adipose tissue are also higher in those with BMI $\geq$25. Inflammation plays a major role in diabetes, and a growing body of evidence is pointing to obesity-induced PVAT damage as a precursor to the development of diabetes in obesity. In obesity, adipocytes outgrow their blood supply and exist in a state of chronic low-grade hypoxia. We have shown previously that there is increased staining for TNF-alpha receptor in obese compared with lean PVAT [42] and that following bariatric surgery, there is a significant reduction in staining for the TNF-alpha cytokine in the PVAT which correlates with a reduction in adipocyte size following weight loss [45]. It has been shown that TNF-alpha in visceral adipose tissue correlates with HOMA-IR [46] and those with type 2 diabetes have higher circulating levels of TNF-alpha [47].

Treatment with TNF-alpha leads to a reduction in adiponectin mRNA levels in 3T3-L1 adipocytes, and this can be partially recovered by treatment with a c-Jun N-terminal kinase (JNK) inhibitor or the PPAR-gamma agonist rosiglitazone [48].

Decreased total and HMW adiponectin and increased IL-6 and TNF-alpha levels are characteristic of patients with metabolic syndrome and type 2 diabetes [47, 49]. Adiponectin itself can reduce inflammation. The mRNA expression of TNF-alpha, IL-6 and ICAM-1 is elevated in db/db mice, and adiponectin treatment decreases these expressions in the aorta. Adiponectin may contribute to an increase in nitric oxide bioavailability by decreasing superoxide production as well as by inhibiting inflammation and adhesion molecules in the aorta in type 2 diabetic mice [50].

Nacci et al. have used streptozotocin (STZ)-induced diabetic mice and investigated whether treatment with the TNF-alpha blocking antibody infliximab can normalise the expression of adiponectin and adiponectin receptors in different fat depots and if this effect correlates with improved endothelial activity and vasodilator function. The STZ mice were studied at 1 and 2 weeks after diabetes onset and compared to age-matched infliximab-treated diabetic (I-STZ) and control animals (CTRL). In STZ mice, activation of pro-inflammatory JNK signalling was faster in PVAT than in visceral (VAT), epididymal (EAT) and subcutaneous (SAT) adipose depots and associated with reduced adiponectin synthesis and dysregulated AdipoR1/R2 levels. Compared with controls, activation of JNK in aortic endothelial cells and mesenteric arteries was associated with reduced expression/phosphorylation of eNOS and impaired ACh-mediated vasodilation. Infliximab treatment abrogated JNK activation, ameliorated adiponectin protein expression and normalised expression of both AdipoR1 and AdipoR2 in PVAT, concomitantly improving eNOS expression and vessel relaxation in mesenteric arteries. These data highlight the early susceptibility of PVAT to activation of pro-inflammatory JNK signalling and its potential importance in early vascular changes of T1DM [51].

PVAT secretes a number of other adipokines with vasorelaxant properties in addition to adiponectin; these include angiotensin 1–7 (Ang 1–7), nitric oxide (NO), leptin, hydrogen sulphide and palmitic acid methyl ester (PAME).

Angiotensin 1–7 stimulates the release of endothelial NO, activating Ca-dependent potassium channels in arteries [37] and voltage-dependent potassium channels in veins [52]. In keeping with this, Angiotensin 1–7 receptor antagonists attenuate PVAT vasorelaxant function [53]. Ang 1–7 is also able to function via AT2 and Mas receptors to reduce the nerve-stimulated overflow of noradrenaline [54]. This may prove to be of paramount importance as sympathetic nerve over-activity contributes to pathophysiology of obesity-related hypertension, and we shall discuss this further in this chapter. An oral preparation of Ang 1–7 has been produced [55], and assessment of its in vivo effect on vessel tone may provide another therapeutic opportunity in treating obesity-related hypertension.

Healthy white adipose tissue [56] and PVAT [57] produce nitric oxide (NO). Insulin [58] and leptin [59] stimulate NO production in adipocytes, and it follows that the increased levels of insulin and leptin in obesity should enhance NO concentrations in PVAT. In early diet-induced obesity, there is enhanced NO bioavailability in mesenteric PVAT of rats [57], but factors such as elevated superoxide levels in chronic obesity lead to a diminution of NO bioavailability in obese PVAT [15].

Leptin is another molecule secreted from white adipocytes, and its plasma levels are elevated in obesity. Its central actions include its effects on the hypothalamus resulting in appetite suppression as well as an increase in the activity of the sympathetic nervous system [60]. Leptin also has a direct endothelial NO-dependent vasorelaxant effect in health. Leptin-deficient ob/ob mice are severely obese, but remain normotensive [61]. Leptin stimulates endothelial NO release in the vasculature; thus an acute rise in leptin concentrations does not significantly affect blood pressure despite elevated SNS activity. In obesity, leptin levels are chronically elevated and confounded by endothelial dysfunction and a reduction in NO bioavailability [62]; therefore its vasopressor effects become more prominent.

Hydrogen sulphide functions via KCNQ [63], whilst palmitic acid methyl ester (PAME) functions via K_v channels, independent of nitric oxide and endothelium [64], and its release is Ca-dependent. These two molecules have been more recent additions to the list of ADRFs. There is a reduction in the release of PAME from PVAT of 20-week-old SHR as compared with pre-hypertensive SHR and normotensive Wistar-Kyoto rats. Exogenously applied PAME has a reduced vasorelaxant effect on de-endothelialised aortic rings of SHR as compared with its significant vasorelaxant effect on pre-constricted vessels from pre-hypertensive SHR and normotensive rats [64]. Clearly PAME plays a role in pre-hypertension and is worthy of further clinical investigation in this context.

It has become apparent that there is more than one PVAT-derived molecule that satisfies the criteria for ADRF. We have shown that adiponectin is the ADRF from human subcutaneous PVAT [42], but other ADRFs may well play a significant role in human PVAT.

20.5 PVAT as a Pro-contractile Tissue

In obesity, the vasorelaxant function of PVAT is attenuated or lost completely.

A number of explanations and theories exist as to the cause of this loss of function. Amongst the most likely are the effects of oxidative stress and inflammation, as well as adipokine dysregulation and increased sympathetic nervous system action.

We have shown previously that incubation of healthy PVAT with the inflammatory cytokines TNF-alpha and IL-6 leads to a significant attenuation of PVAT vasorelaxant properties similar to that observed in obesity [42]. In keeping with the complexity of PVAT studies, we have reported that there is no homogenous effect from the presence of different white blood cells within the PVAT. In particular, we have studied both macrophages and eosinophils within PVAT. Macrophages secrete a number of inflammatory cytokines including TNF-α and free radicals such as the superoxide anion. We used experimental hypoxia in tissue baths to approximate obesity-induced PVAT damage and observed that macrophage recruitment and activation in adipose tissue is an essential step resulting in the loss of PVAT vasorelaxant function [65]. On the contrary, mice deficient of eosinophils lack the PVAT vasorelaxant effect, and eosinophil reconstitution did lead to enhanced adiponectin and PVAT-derived NO bioavailability leading to the restoration of PVAT vasorelaxant function [66]. As previously mentioned, fat depots seem to have specific characteristics, and the PVAT surrounding rat thoracic aorta expresses brown adipose tissue genes and appears to resist inflammation and macrophage infiltration in diet-induced obesity [67], so it is possible that in obesity, not all fat depots are affected equally.

The paramount role of macrophages in PVAT damage cannot be overstated; thus macrophage recruitment into PVAT tissue has been studied in some detail. Monocyte chemotactic protein-1 (MCP-1) levels are increased in adipose tissue and in plasma of genetically obese and diet-induced obese mice [68], as well in obese humans [69]. Moreover, insulin increases the secretion of MCP-1 from insulin-resistant 3T3-L1 adipocytes and in ob/ob mice [70]; in this way the hyperinsulinaemic state in obesity leads to PVAT macrophage recruitment and subsequent release of cytokines which attenuate its vasorelaxant function. Fractalkine or CX3CL1 is a protein secreted from adipocytes that promotes monocyte adhesion to human adipocytes [71]. Fractalkine levels are increased in diabetes as well as in obesity [72]. There is also direct evidence for involvement of fractalkine in hypertension. The expression of CX3CL1 receptor gene in blood leukocytes from patients with arterial hypertension has been shown to be significantly increased [73]. This protein may well play a significant facilitator role in the process of initiation of the macrophage-induced loss of PVAT vasorelaxant function and is worthy of further consideration from a therapeutic target viewpoint.

Chemerin is another adipokine that plays a potentially significant role in the loss of PVAT vasorelaxant function by behaving as a possible link between obesity, BMI [74], PVAT, diabetes [75] and hypertension both in adults and children [76, 77].

Adipose tissue explants from obese patients exhibit significantly higher chemerin secretion compared with lean controls, and higher chemerin release is associated with insulin resistance and insulin-induced antilipolysis. Chemerin stimulates vascular smooth muscle cell proliferation and migration via a ROS-dependent signalling pathway, and at least in theory, this vascular remodelling can contribute to raising blood pressure [78]. Moreover, chemerin evokes direct vasoconstriction, as well as enhancing agonist-induced contractions in human and rat vessels through G_i proteins, resulting in the activation of L-type Ca^{2+} channels, as well as Src, and Rho kinase [79]. Levels of chemerin correlate well with clinical parameters too. Its plasma concentration is raised in obesity, insulin resistance and inflammatory conditions, and levels positively correlate with increases in BMI and abdominal visceral fat accumulation [80]. It has been linked with increasing BP in mice, and importantly, its levels fall with loss of adipocyte mass following exercise or bariatric surgery [81].

We have discussed chemerin's role in the vasculature, but it also plays a role in disrupting glucose homeostasis. Chemerin induces insulin resistance in human skeletal muscle cells at the level of insulin receptor substrate 1, Akt and glycogen synthase kinase 3 phosphorylation and glucose uptake, and ERK inhibition prevents chemerin-induced insulin resistance [74]. Following weight loss, the significant decrease in chemerin levels in 3 months after bariatric surgery is associated with a decrease in HOMA-IR and blood glucose [82].

From an inflammatory perspective, chemerin induces ICAM-1 and E-selectin expression in endothelial cells [83]. Given that it plays a role in monocytes recruitment, insulin resistance and vasoconstriction and its levels correlate with weight gain and drop following weight loss, chemerin is one of the major adipokines that could be targeted in therapeutic strategies to treat MetS.

No doubt further PVAT-derived pro-contractile entities will be described much the same way as there is now a list of candidates for PVAT-derived vasorelaxant factors.

20.6 The RAAS Within PVAT

In obesity, there are raised circulating levels of the components of the renin-angiotensin-aldosterone system (RAAS). Adipocytes have an intrinsic RAAS system including ACE and angiotensin type 1 and type 2 receptors, and they secrete angiotensinogen, the levels of which are raised in obesity [84]. The source of the adipocyte renin activity remains controversial and unclear [85].The raised circulating aldosterone levels in obesity correlate with the degree of visceral adiposity and waist-to-hip ratio [86–88]. In the context of obesity-related hypertension, the raised aldosterone concentrations have a twofold effect: they contribute to increased blood volume by increasing sodium reabsorption and lead to the generation of reactive oxygen species (ROS). Aldosterone activates NADPH oxidase, thus increasing ROS levels leading to oxidative posttranslational changes to guanylyl cyclase rendering it NO-insensitive [89]. ROS can also reduce NO bioavailability by forming molecules such as peroxynitrite, thus contributing to endothelial dysfunction. ROS can also stimulate the mineralocorticoid receptor (MR) [90], thereby theoretically contributing to further elevations in ROS levels, forming a vicious circle. At the endothelial level, aldosterone decreases glucose-6-phosphate dehydrogenase (G6PD) activity. G6PD is a cytosolic enzyme and the main source of intracellular NADPH which functions to limit ROS activity [91]. There are two aldosterone receptor antagonists in clinical use: spironolactone is a nonselective aldosterone receptor antagonist, whereas eplerenone is a selective aldosterone receptor antagonist which has a lower degree of cross-reactivity with sex-steroid hormones and a longer half-life than spironolactone [92]. Spironolactone increases the expression of G6PD and its activity, as well as raising NADPH levels leading to a reduction in ROS generation in aortas of aldosterone-treated mice [91]. Aldosterone increases the expression of TNF-α from macrophages within PVAT, and we have reviewed the role of macrophages and TNF-alpha in PVAT damage. Eplerenone leads to a reduction of ROS generation and increased levels of adiponectin in obese and diabetic mice [93].

It is not clear to what extent the blood pressure reduction is a result of blood volume and cardiac output reduction secondary to reduced sodium reabsorption, or due to a reduction in sympathetic activity through the direct CNS effect of aldosterone [94, 95]. Certainly, a reduction in ROS generation within PVAT would partly restore the favourable vasorelaxant profile lost, in part, following hypoxia-induced inflammatory damage in obesity.

The ROS-induced PVAT damage in obesity would suggest that antioxidants and free radical scavengers could be therapeutic agents to reverse this damage and possibly lower blood pressure in obesity. We've shown in ex vivo experiments that SOD and catalase can restore the PVAT vasorelaxant property in both human and murine models of obesity [15, 45]. A 3-week administration of desmethyltirilazad (lazaroid), a potent antioxidant, significantly ameliorates blood pressure in SHR rats [96].

We have shown also that MR blockade using eplerenone is able to reduce macrophage activation and rescue aldosterone-induced and hypoxia-induced PVAT damage [65]. Intuitively, it has been proposed that prevention of ROS generation using NADPH oxidase inhibitors may be a better way of tackling oxidative stress than scavenging the free radicals once they have been generated, although clinical studies need to assess the feasibility of this theory [97].

Vessel stiffness is another important contributing factor in the pathophysiology of obesity-related hypertension. The association of vessel stiffness is strongest for waist circumference and visceral adiposity, rather than global obesity as measured by BMI [98]. Obesity is a complex multifaceted disorder, and dysregulation of any number of factors can affect vascular stiffness. The adipokine leptin has been linked with impairment of arterial distensibility, and its raised levels in obesity may well be a contributing factor in arterial stiffness [99].

Inflammation, oxidative stress and monocyte recruitment all play their part in initiating endothelial dysfunction in obesity. There is also disruption to the fine balance between the vasoconstrictor action of endothelin-1 and the vasodilator effect of NO in endothelial cells. In health, insulin activates phosphoinositide 3-kinase leading to increased NO production secondary to eNOS phosphorylation [100]. Postprandial physiological surge in insulin concentrations leads to dilatation of precapillary arterioles, thus improving blood flow and delivery of nutrients to tissues, a process known as nutritive flow [33]. In obesity, NO-mediated vasorelaxation is impaired, leading to vasoconstriction via unopposed endothelin-1 action [33, 100]. Reduced endothelial nitric oxide bioavailability in obesity is a significant consequence of the reactions between free radicals and NO. Reactive oxygen species such as the superoxide anion react with nitric oxide to produce peroxynitrite and deplete endothelial NO levels. The role of nitric oxide in vessel tone modulation and its fate in inflammatory diseases have been extensively reviewed by Jin and Loscalzo [101]. We now know that PVAT is a source of NO which contributes to the PVAT vasorelaxant function, but in obesity, the generation of ROS depletes this vital source of NO; the microvessel is faced with reduced NO bioavailability from both outside the vessel, the PVAT, and inside, the endothelium.

There is a close correlation between obesity, obstructive sleep apnoea (OSA) and hypertension. There is a dose-response relationship between sleep-disordered breathing and hypertension, independent of confounding factors [102]. Almost half of all hypertensive patients suffer from sleep apnoea, and half of all sleep apnoea patients are hypertensive [86]. Whilst fat deposition around the upper airway in obesity is thought to be the most significant contributor to the development of OSA in obesity, there are a number of potential mechanisms linking OSA with hypertension, including endothelial dysfunction, CNS stimulation, oxidative stress and inflammation [103]. The most significant factor is thought to be the elevated oxidative stress levels initiated by intermittent hypoxia, coupled with hyperleptinaemia [104] with its direct stimulatory effects on the sympathetic nervous system. The elevated levels of aldosterone in OSA also correlate with severity of OSA. Once again, this highlights the significance of ROS and aldosterone generation, both of which are generated by hypoxic and inflamed adipocytes.

20.7 Sympathetic Nerves Within PVAT

PVAT is innervated by nerves from the sympathetic nervous system. Obesity has a differential effect on local SNS activity. Hypertensive obese individuals show an increased sympathetic activity in both cardiac and renal nerves [105].There is also evidence of central stimulation of the SNS by reactive oxygen species, the levels of which are raised in obesity. Animal studies suggest that NADPH oxidase-dependent oxidative stress in the brain may be a cause of increased sympathetic tone leading to hypertension in high-fat fed animals [106].

The heightened sympathetic state in obesity and presence of nerve endings within PVAT have led to further evaluation of the effects of SNS on PVAT using electric field stimulation (EFS) protocols. Work by Gao et al. has shown that superoxide generated by NADPH oxidase in response to electric field stimulation enhances the contractile response of adjacent small arteries [107]. It has been shown that candesartan (angiotensin II type 1 receptor antagonist) reduces this PVAT-mediated potentiation of EFS-induced contractile response, thus providing another potential explanation for the increased vascular resistance in obesity where there are both increased sympathetic nerve activity and increased angiotensin II levels [108].

Circulating adiponectin levels also increase by nearly 70% post gastric bypass and by around 36% post gastric banding procedures. The greatest increase is after the loss of 35% of the original body weight, with a strong correlation between percentage increase in adiponectin levels and percentage decrease in BMI [109]. This is not true of weight loss by other surgical means. After liposuction, despite a 10% weight reduction, no improvements in adiponectin or insulin resistance have been noted [110]. This is likely due to the differing qualities of adipose tissue depots with visceral fat exhibiting a more inflammatory profile as compared with subcutaneous adipose tissue [111].

Weight loss or bariatric surgery remains the most reliable means to achieve and maintain significant weight loss. Bariatric surgery has also been shown to improve the inflammatory profile of obese individuals [112]. In subcutaneous adipose tissue, the expression of IL-6 and TNF-α mRNA decreases significantly, and expression of adiponectin and its receptors increases after dramatic weight loss post surgery [113]. The significant degree of weight loss, together with improvements in adipokine and inflammatory cytokine profile, as well as resolution or improvement in diabetes status [114] makes this an invaluable procedure in those suffering from morbid obesity and its sequelae. We have reported that 6 months following significant weight loss post bariatric surgery, PVAT regains its vasorelaxant function, despite the individuals still weighing in the obese category. This shows that there is more to weight loss than purely loss of mass, and other factors such as the reduced adipocyte size and a reduction in PVAT inflammation as a consequence of a more balanced oxygen supply may be the fundamental trigger leading to our observation [45].

Vitamin D is a perfect example to highlight the need for tissue-specific or tissue-targeted therapies, given that it can suppress renin transcription, and transgenic animals devoid of vitamin D receptor develop hypertension, but they remain lean with smaller adipocytes on a high-fat diet. Overexpression of the receptors on adipocytes leads to a suppression of lipolysis, thermogenesis and resultant obesity [115, 116]. This is a perfect example of the challenges facing researchers trying to identify a molecule that can treat one condition without causing detrimental off-target effects. The (re)search continues.

Conclusion

Perivascular adipose tissue plays a crucial role in modulating vessel tone and blood glucose homeostasis. In obesity, PVAT is damaged and dysfunctional. Rescuing the damaged PVAT and restoring the healthy PVAT phenotype before the onset of hypertension and diabetes should be the focus of future studies.

Acknowledgments *Sources of Funding*: Dr. Aghamohammadzadeh is an NIHR Academic Clinical Lecturer in Cardiology at the University of Manchester.

References

1. WHO. Obesity and overweight (Factsheet 311). 2016 [updated 2016; cited 04 July 2017]. http://www.who.int/mediacentre/factsheets/fs311/en/index.html.

2. The NHS Information Centre LS. Statistics on Obesity, Physical Activity and Diet: England, 2011. 24 Feb 2011.
3. CDC. U.S. Obesity Trends. 2011 [updated 2011; cited 2011 18 Aug 2011]. http://www.cdc.gov/obesity/data/trends.html#State.
4. Neel JV. Diabetes mellitus: a "thrifty" genotype rendered detrimental by "progress"? Am J Hum Genet. 1962;14:353–62.
5. Diamond J. The double puzzle of diabetes. Nature. 2003;423(6940):599–602.
6. Scott EM, Grant PJ. Neel revisited: the adipocyte, seasonality and type 2 diabetes. Diabetologia. 2006;49(7):1462–6.
7. Emerging Risk Factors Collaboration, Wormser D, Kaptoge S, Di Angelantonio E, Wood AM, Pennells L, et al. Separate and combined associations of body-mass index and abdominal adiposity with cardiovascular disease: collaborative analysis of 58 prospective studies. Lancet. 2011;377(9771):1085–95.
8. Cornier MA, Despres JP, Davis N, Grossniklaus DA, Klein S, Lamarche B, et al. Assessing adiposity: a scientific statement from the American Heart Association. Circulation. 2011;124:1996–2019.
9. CDC. Hypertension. 2011 [updated 2011; cited 2011 18 Aug 2011]. http://www.cdc.gov/nchs/fastats/hyprtens.htm.
10. WHO. Blood pressure. 2017 [updated 2017; cited 2017 04 July 2017]. http://apps.who.int/gho/data/view.main.2464GLOBALSTANDARD?lang=en.
11. Henry SL, Barzel B, Wood-Bradley RJ, Burke SL, Head GA, Armitage JA. The developmental origins of obesity-related hypertension. Clin Exp Pharmacol Physiol. 2012;39:799–806.
12. Kotchen TA. Obesity-related hypertension: epidemiology, pathophysiology, and clinical management. Am J Hypertens. 2010;23(11):1170–8.
13. Gosmanov AR, Smiley DD, Robalino G, Siquiera J, Khan B, Le NA, et al. Effects of oral and intravenous fat load on blood pressure, endothelial function, sympathetic activity, and oxidative stress in obese healthy subjects. Am J Physiol Endocrinol Metab. 2010;299(6):E953–8.
14. Dobrian AD, Schriver SD, Lynch T, Prewitt RL. Effect of salt on hypertension and oxidative stress in a rat model of diet-induced obesity. Am J Physiol Ren Physiol. 2003;285(4):F619–28.
15. Aghamohammadzadeh R, Unwin RD, Greenstein AS, Heagerty AM. Effects of obesity on perivascular adipose tissue vasorelaxant function: nitric oxide, inflammation and elevated systemic blood pressure. J Vasc Res. 2015;52(5):299–305.
16. Fox CS, Massaro JM, Hoffmann U, Pou KM, Maurovich-Horvat P, Liu CY, et al. Abdominal visceral and subcutaneous adipose tissue compartments: association with metabolic risk factors in the Framingham Heart Study. Circulation. 2007;116(1):39–48.
17. Gesta S, Tseng YH, Kahn CR. Developmental origin of fat: tracking obesity to its source. Cell. 2007;131(2):242–56.
18. Manolopoulos KN, Karpe F, Frayn KN. Gluteofemoral body fat as a determinant of metabolic health. Int J Obes. 2010;34(6):949–59.
19. Chatterjee TK, Stoll LL, Denning GM, Harrelson A, Blomkalns AL, Idelman G, et al. Proinflammatory phenotype of perivascular adipocytes: influence of high-fat feeding. Circ Res. 2009;104(4):541–9.
20. Dorresteijn JA, Visseren FL, Spiering W. Mechanisms linking obesity to hypertension. Obes Rev. 2011;13:17–26.
21. Lee CM, Huxley RR, Wildman RP, Woodward M. Indices of abdominal obesity are better discriminators of cardiovascular risk factors than BMI: a meta-analysis. J Clin Epidemiol. 2008;61(7):646–53.
22. Iacobellis G, Assael F, Ribaudo MC, Zappaterreno A, Alessi G, Di Mario U, et al. Epicardial fat from echocardiography: a new method for visceral adipose tissue prediction. Obes Res. 2003;11(2):304–10.
23. Iacobellis G, Ribaudo MC, Assael F, Vecci E, Tiberti C, Zappaterreno A, et al. Echocardiographic epicardial adipose tissue is related to anthropometric and clinical parameters of metabolic syndrome: a new indicator of cardiovascular risk. J Clin Endocrinol Metab. 2003;88(11):5163–8.

24. Iacobellis G, Willens HJ, Barbaro G, Sharma AM. Threshold values of high-risk echocardiographic epicardial fat thickness. Obesity (Silver Spring). 2008;16(4):887–92.
25. Simons PJ, van den Pangaart PS, Aerts JM, Boon L. Pro-inflammatory delipidizing cytokines reduce adiponectin secretion from human adipocytes without affecting adiponectin oligomerization. J Endocrinol. 2007;192(2):289–99.
26. Baker AR, Silva NF, Quinn DW, Harte AL, Pagano D, Bonser RS, et al. Human epicardial adipose tissue expresses a pathogenic profile of adipocytokines in patients with cardiovascular disease. Cardiovasc Diabetol. 2006;5:1.
27. Eiras S, Teijeira-Fernandez E, Shamagian LG, Fernandez AL, Vazquez-Boquete A, Gonzalez-Juanatey JR. Extension of coronary artery disease is associated with increased IL-6 and decreased adiponectin gene expression in epicardial adipose tissue. Cytokine. 2008;43(2):174–80.
28. Iacobellis G, Pistilli D, Gucciardo M, Leonetti F, Miraldi F, Brancaccio G, et al. Adiponectin expression in human epicardial adipose tissue in vivo is lower in patients with coronary artery disease. Cytokine. 2005;29(6):251–5.
29. Iacobellis G, di Gioia CR, Cotesta D, Petramala L, Travaglini C, De Santis V, et al. Epicardial adipose tissue adiponectin expression is related to intracoronary adiponectin levels. Horm Metab Res. 2009;41(3):227–31.
30. Teijeira-Fernandez E, Eiras S, Grigorian-Shamagian L, Fernandez A, Adrio B, Gonzalez-Juanatey JR. Epicardial adipose tissue expression of adiponectin is lower in patients with hypertension. J Hum Hypertens. 2008;22(12):856–63.
31. Ohashi K, Kihara S, Ouchi N, Kumada M, Fujita K, Hiuge A, et al. Adiponectin replenishment ameliorates obesity-related hypertension. Hypertension. 2006;47(6):1108–16.
32. Pischon T, Girman CJ, Hotamisligil GS, Rifai N, Hu FB, Rimm EB. Plasma adiponectin levels and risk of myocardial infarction in men. JAMA. 2004;291(14):1730–7.
33. Yudkin JS, Eringa E, Stehouwer CD. "Vasocrine" signalling from perivascular fat: a mechanism linking insulin resistance to vascular disease. Lancet. 2005;365(9473):1817–20.
34. Soltis EE, Cassis LA. Influence of perivascular adipose tissue on rat aortic smooth muscle responsiveness. Clin Exp Hypertens A. 1991;13(2):277–96.
35. Gao YJ, Lu C, Su LY, Sharma AM, Lee RM. Modulation of vascular function by perivascular adipose tissue: the role of endothelium and hydrogen peroxide. Br J Pharmacol. 2007;151(3):323–31.
36. Galvez-Prieto B, Bolbrinker J, Stucchi P, de Las Heras AI, Merino B, Arribas S, et al. Comparative expression analysis of the renin-angiotensin system components between white and brown perivascular adipose tissue. J Endocrinol. 2008;197(1):55–64.
37. Lu C, Su LY, Lee RM, Gao YJ. Alterations in perivascular adipose tissue structure and function in hypertension. Eur J Pharmacol. 2011;656(1-3):68–73.
38. Dubrovska G, Verlohren S, Luft FC, Gollasch M. Mechanisms of ADRF release from rat aortic adventitial adipose tissue. Am J Physiol Heart Circ Physiol. 2004;286(3):H1107–13.
39. Deng G, Long Y, Yu YR, Li MR. Adiponectin directly improves endothelial dysfunction in obese rats through the AMPK-eNOS Pathway. Int J Obes. 2010;34(1):165–71.
40. Yilmaz MI, Sonmez A, Caglar K, Celik T, Yenicesu M, Eyileten T, et al. Effect of antihypertensive agents on plasma adiponectin levels in hypertensive patients with metabolic syndrome. Nephrology (Carlton). 2007;12(2):147–53.
41. Fesus G, Dubrovska G, Gorzelniak K, Kluge R, Huang Y, Luft FC, et al. Adiponectin is a novel humoral vasodilator. Cardiovasc Res. 2007;75(4):719–27.
42. Greenstein AS, Khavandi K, Withers SB, Sonoyama K, Clancy O, Jeziorska M, et al. Local inflammation and hypoxia abolish the protective anticontractile properties of perivascular fat in obese patients. Circulation. 2009;119(12):1661–70.
43. Aghamohammadzadeh R, Withers SB, Lynch FM, Greenstein AS, Malik R, Heagerty AM. Perivascular adipose tissue from human systemic and coronary vessels: the emergence of a new pharmacotherapeutic target. Br J Pharmacol. 2012;165:670–82.
44. Chen H, Montagnani M, Funahashi T, Shimomura I, Quon MJ. Adiponectin stimulates production of nitric oxide in vascular endothelial cells. J Biol Chem. 2003;278(45):45021–6.

45. Aghamohammadzadeh R, Greenstein AS, Yadav R, Jeziorska M, Hama S, Soltani F, et al. The effects of bariatric surgery on human small artery function: evidence for reduction in perivascular adipocyte inflammation, and the restoration of normal anticontractile activity despite persistent obesity. J Am Coll Cardiol. 2013;62:128–35.
46. Kang YE, Kim JM, Joung KH, Lee JH, You BR, Choi MJ, et al. The roles of adipokines, proinflammatory cytokines, and adipose tissue macrophages in obesity-associated insulin resistance in modest obesity and early metabolic dysfunction. PLoS One. 2016;11(4):e0154003.
47. Qiao YC, Shen J, He L, Hong XZ, Tian F, Pan YH, et al. Changes of regulatory T cells and of proinflammatory and immunosuppressive cytokines in patients with type 2 diabetes mellitus: a systematic review and meta-analysis. J Diabetes Res. 2016;2016:3694957.
48. Kim KY, Kim JK, Jeon JH, Yoon SR, Choi I, Yang Y. c-Jun N-terminal kinase is involved in the suppression of adiponectin expression by TNF-alpha in 3T3-L1 adipocytes. Biochem Biophys Res Commun. 2005;327(2):460–7.
49. Lee JM, Kim SR, Yoo SJ, Hong OK, Son HS, Chang SA. The relationship between adipokines, metabolic parameters and insulin resistance in patients with metabolic syndrome and type 2 diabetes. J Int Med Res. 2009;37(6):1803–12.
50. Lee S, Zhang H, Chen J, Dellsperger KC, Hill MA, Zhang C. Adiponectin abates diabetes-induced endothelial dysfunction by suppressing oxidative stress, adhesion molecules, and inflammation in type 2 diabetic mice. Am J Physiol Heart Circ Physiol. 2012;303(1):H106–15.
51. Nacci C, Leo V, De Benedictis L, Potenza MA, Sgarra L, De Salvia MA, et al. Infliximab therapy restores adiponectin expression in perivascular adipose tissue and improves endothelial nitric oxide-mediated vasodilation in mice with type 1 diabetes. Vasc Pharmacol. 2016;87:83–91.
52. Lu C, Zhao AX, Gao YJ, Lee RM. Modulation of vein function by perivascular adipose tissue. Eur J Pharmacol. 2011;657(1-3):111–6.
53. Lee RM, Bader M, Alenina N, Santos RA, Gao YJ, Lu C. Mas receptors in modulating relaxation induced by perivascular adipose tissue. Life Sci. 2011;89:467–72.
54. Byku M, Macarthur H, Westfall TC. Inhibitory effects of angiotensin (1-7) on the nerve stimulation-induced release of norepinephrine and neuropeptide y from the mesenteric arterial bed. Am J Physiol Heart Circ Physiol. 2009;289:H457–65.
55. Marques FD, Ferreira AJ, Sinisterra RD, Jacoby BA, Sousa FB, Caliari MV, et al. An oral formulation of angiotensin-(1-7) produces cardioprotective effects in infarcted and isoproterenol-treated rats. Hypertension. 2011;57(3):477–83.
56. Ribiere C, Jaubert AM, Gaudiot N, Sabourault D, Marcus ML, Boucher JL, et al. White adipose tissue nitric oxide synthase: a potential source for NO production. Biochem Biophys Res Commun. 1996;222(3):706–12.
57. Gil-Ortega M, Stucchi P, Guzman-Ruiz R, Cano V, Arribas S, Gonzalez MC, et al. Adaptative nitric oxide overproduction in perivascular adipose tissue during early diet-induced obesity. Endocrinology. 2010;151:3299–306.
58. Ribiere C, Jaubert AM, Sabourault D, Lacasa D, Giudicelli Y. Insulin stimulates nitric oxide production in rat adipocytes. Biochem Biophys Res Commun. 2002;291(2):394–9.
59. Mehebik N, Jaubert AM, Sabourault D, Giudicelli Y, Ribiere C. Leptin-induced nitric oxide production in white adipocytes is mediated through PKA and MAP kinase activation. Am J Phys Cell Physiol. 2005;289(2):C379–87.
60. Rahmouni K, Correia ML, Haynes WG, Mark AL. Obesity-associated hypertension: new insights into mechanisms. Hypertension. 2005;45(1):9–14.
61. Mark AL, Shaffer RA, Correia ML, Morgan DA, Sigmund CD, Haynes WG. Contrasting blood pressure effects of obesity in leptin-deficient ob/ob mice and agouti yellow obese mice. J Hypertens. 1999;17(12 Pt 2):1949–53.
62. da Silva AA, do Carmo J, Dubinion J, Hall JE. The role of the sympathetic nervous system in obesity-related hypertension. Curr Hypertens Rep. 2009;11(3):206–11.
63. Schleifenbaum J, Kohn C, Voblova N, Dubrovska G, Zavarirskaya O, Gloe T, et al. Systemic peripheral artery relaxation by KCNQ channel openers and hydrogen sulfide. J Hypertens. 2010;28(9):1875–82.

64. Lee YC, Chang HH, Chiang CL, Liu CH, Yeh JI, Chen MF, et al. Role of perivascular adipose tissue-derived methyl palmitate in vascular tone regulation and pathogenesis of hypertension. Circulation. 2011;124:1160–71.
65. Withers BS, Agabiti-Rosei C, Linvingstone DM, Little MC, Aslam R, Malik RA, et al. Macrophage activation is responsible for loss of anticontractile function in inflamed perivascular fat. Arterioscler Thromb Vasc Biol. 2011;31:908–13.
66. Withers SB, Forman R, Meza-Perez S, Sorobetea D, Sitnik K, Hopwood T, et al. Eosinophils are key regulators of perivascular adipose tissue and vascular functionality. Sci Rep. 2017 Mar 17;7:44571.
67. Fitzgibbons TP, Kogan S, Aouadi M, Hendricks GM, Straubhaar J, Czech MP. Similarity of mouse perivascular and brown adipose tissues and their resistance to diet-induced inflammation. Am J Physiol Heart Circ Physiol. 2011;301(4):H1425–37.
68. Kanda H, Tateya S, Tamori Y, Kotani K, Hiasa K, Kitazawa R, et al. MCP-1 contributes to macrophage infiltration into adipose tissue, insulin resistance, and hepatic steatosis in obesity. J Clin Invest. 2006;116(6):1494–505.
69. Kim CS, Park HS, Kawada T, Kim JH, Lim D, Hubbard NE, et al. Circulating levels of MCP-1 and IL-8 are elevated in human obese subjects and associated with obesity-related parameters. Int J Obes. 2006;30(9):1347–55.
70. Sartipy P, Loskutoff DJ. Monocyte chemoattractant protein 1 in obesity and insulin resistance. Proc Natl Acad Sci U S A. 2003;100(12):7265–70.
71. Shah R, Hinkle CC, Ferguson JF, Mehta NN, Li M, Qu L, et al. Fractalkine is a novel human adipochemokine associated with type 2 diabetes. Diabetes. 2011;60(5):1512–8.
72. Sirois-Gagnon D, Chamberland A, Perron S, Brisson D, Gaudet D, Laprise C. Association of common polymorphisms in the fractalkine receptor (CX3CR1) with obesity. Obesity (Silver Spring). 2010;19(1):222–7.
73. Timofeeva AV, Goryunova LE, Khaspekov GL, Kovalevskii DA, Scamrov AV, Bulkina OS, et al. Altered gene expression pattern in peripheral blood leukocytes from patients with arterial hypertension. Ann N Y Acad Sci. 2006;1091:319–35.
74. Sell H, Laurencikiene J, Taube A, Eckardt K, Cramer A, Horrighs A, et al. Chemerin is a novel adipocyte-derived factor inducing insulin resistance in primary human skeletal muscle cells. Diabetes. 2009;58(12):2731–40.
75. Ouwens DM, Bekaert M, Lapauw B, Van Nieuwenhove Y, Lehr S, Hartwig S, et al. Chemerin as biomarker for insulin sensitivity in males without typical characteristics of metabolic syndrome. Arch Physiol Biochem. 2012;118(3):135–8.
76. Schipper HS, Nuboer R, Prop S, van den Ham HJ, de Boer FK, Kesmir C, et al. Systemic inflammation in childhood obesity: circulating inflammatory mediators and activated CD14++ monocytes. Diabetologia. 2012;55(10):2800–10.
77. Verrijn Stuart AA, Schipper HS, Tasdelen I, Egan DA, Prakken BJ, Kalkhoven E, et al. Altered plasma adipokine levels and in vitro adipocyte differentiation in pediatric type 1 diabetes. J Clin Endocrinol Metab. 2011;97(2):463–72.
78. Kunimoto H, Kazama K, Takai M, Oda M, Okada M, Yamawaki H. Chemerin promotes the proliferation and migration of vascular smooth muscle and increases mouse blood pressure. Am J Physiol Heart Circ Physiol. 2015;309(5):H1017–28.
79. Ferland DJ, Darios ES, Neubig RR, Sjogren B, Truong N, Torres R, et al. Chemerin-induced arterial contraction is Gi- and calcium-dependent. Vasc Pharmacol. 2017;88:30–41.
80. Shin H-Y, Lee DC, Chu SH, Jeon JY, Lee MK, Im JA, et al. Chemerin levels are positively correlated with abdominal visceral fat accumulation. Clin Endocrinol. 2012;77(1):47–50.
81. Chakaroun R, Raschpichler M, Kloting N, Oberbach A, Flehmig G, Kern M, et al. Effects of weight loss and exercise on chemerin serum concentrations and adipose tissue expression in human obesity. Metabolism. 2011;61(5):706–14.
82. Sell H, Divoux A, Poitou C, Basdevant A, Bouillot JL, Bedossa P, et al. Chemerin correlates with markers for fatty liver in morbidly obese patients and strongly decreases after weight loss induced by bariatric surgery. J Clin Endocrinol Metab. 2010;95(6):2892–6.

83. Landgraf K, Friebe D, Ullrich T, Kratzsch J, Dittrich K, Herberth G, et al. Chemerin as a mediator between obesity and vascular inflammation in children. J Clin Endocrinol Metab. 2012;97(4):E556–64.
84. Van Harmelen V, Ariapart P, Hoffstedt J, Lundkvist I, Bringman S, Arner P. Increased adipose angiotensinogen gene expression in human obesity. Obesity. 2000;8(4):337–41.
85. Engeli S, Negrel R, Sharma AM. Physiology and pathophysiology of the adipose tissue renin-angiotensin system. Hypertension. 2000;35(6):1270–7.
86. Goodfriend TL, Calhoun DA. Resistant hypertension, obesity, sleep apnea, and aldosterone: theory and therapy. Hypertension. 2004;43(3):518–24.
87. Goodfriend TL, Egan BM, Kelley DE. Aldosterone in obesity. Endocr Res. 1998;24(3-4):789–96.
88. Goodfriend TL, Kelley DE, Goodpaster BH, Winters SJ. Visceral obesity and insulin resistance are associated with plasma aldosterone levels in women. Obes Res. 1999;7(4):355–62.
89. Maron BA, Zhang YY, Handy DE, Beuve A, Tang SS, Loscalzo J, et al. Aldosterone increases oxidant stress to impair guanylyl cyclase activity by cysteinyl thiol oxidation in vascular smooth muscle cells. J Biol Chem. 2009;284(12):7665–72.
90. Wang H, Shimosawa T, Matsui H, Kaneko T, Ogura S, Uetake Y, et al. Paradoxical mineralocorticoid receptor activation and left ventricular diastolic dysfunction under high oxidative stress conditions. J Hypertens. 2008;26(7):1453–62.
91. Leopold JA, Dam A, Maron BA, Scribner AW, Liao R, Handy DE, et al. Aldosterone impairs vascular reactivity by decreasing glucose-6-phosphate dehydrogenase activity. Nat Med. 2007;13(2):189–97.
92. Maron BA, Leopold JA. Aldosterone receptor antagonists: effective but often forgotten. Circulation. 2010;121(7):934–9.
93. Guo C, Ricchiuti V, Lian BQ, Yao TM, Coutinho P, Romero JR, et al. Mineralocorticoid receptor blockade reverses obesity-related changes in expression of adiponectin, peroxisome proliferator-activated receptor-gamma, and proinflammatory adipokines. Circulation. 2008;117(17):2253–61.
94. de Paula RB, da Silva AA, Hall JE. Aldosterone antagonism attenuates obesity-induced hypertension and glomerular hyperfiltration. Hypertension. 2004;43(1):41–7.
95. Rahmouni K, Barthelmebs M, Grima M, Imbs JL, De Jong W. Involvement of brain mineralocorticoid receptor in salt-enhanced hypertension in spontaneously hypertensive rats. Hypertension. 2001;38(4):902–6.
96. Vaziri ND, Ni Z, Oveisi F, Trnavsky-Hobbs DL. Effect of antioxidant therapy on blood pressure and NO synthase expression in hypertensive rats. Hypertension. 2000;36(6):957–64.
97. Drummond GR, Selemidis S, Griendling KK, Sobey CG. Combating oxidative stress in vascular disease: NADPH oxidases as therapeutic targets. Nat Rev Drug Discov. 2011;10(6):453–71.
98. Safar ME, Czernichow S, Blacher J. Obesity, arterial stiffness, and cardiovascular risk. J Am Soc Nephrol. 2006;17(4 Suppl 2):S109–11.
99. Singhal A, Farooqi IS, Cole TJ, O'Rahilly S, Fewtrell M, Kattenhorn M, et al. Influence of leptin on arterial distensibility: a novel link between obesity and cardiovascular disease? Circulation. 2002;106(15):1919–24.
100. Kotsis V, Stabouli S, Papakatsika S, Rizos Z, Parati G. Mechanisms of obesity-induced hypertension. Hypertens Res. 2010;33(5):386–93.
101. Jin RC, Loscalzo J. Vascular nitric oxide: formation and function. J Blood Med. 2010;2010(1):147–62.
102. Peppard PE, Young T, Palta M, Skatrud J. Prospective study of the association between sleep-disordered breathing and hypertension. N Engl J Med. 2000;342(19):1378–84.
103. Wolk R, Shamsuzzaman AS, Somers VK. Obesity, sleep apnea, and hypertension. Hypertension. 2003;42(6):1067–74.
104. Yang R, Sikka G, Larson J, Watts VL, Niu X, Ellis CL, et al. Restoring leptin signaling reduces hyperlipidemia and improves vascular stiffness induced by chronic intermittent hypoxia. Am J Physiol Heart Circ Physiol. 2011;300(4):H1467–76.

105. Rumantir MS, Vaz M, Jennings GL, Collier G, Kaye DM, Seals DR, et al. Neural mechanisms in human obesity-related hypertension. J Hypertens. 1999;17(8):1125–33.
106. Nagae A, Fujita M, Kawarazaki H, Matsui H, Ando K, Fujita T. Sympathoexcitation by oxidative stress in the brain mediates arterial pressure elevation in obesity-induced hypertension. Circulation. 2009;119(7):978–86.
107. Gao YJ, Takemori K, Su LY, An WS, Lu C, Sharma AM, et al. Perivascular adipose tissue promotes vasoconstriction: the role of superoxide anion. Cardiovasc Res. 2006;71(2):363–73.
108. Lu C, Su LY, Lee RM, Gao YJ. Mechanisms for perivascular adipose tissue-mediated potentiation of vascular contraction to perivascular neuronal stimulation: the role of adipocyte-derived angiotensin II. Eur J Pharmacol. 2011;634(1-3):107–12.
109. Butner KL, Nickols-Richardson SM, Clark SF, Ramp WK, Herbert WG. A review of weight loss following Roux-en-Y gastric bypass vs restrictive bariatric surgery: impact on adiponectin and insulin. Obes Surg. 2010;20(5):559–68.
110. Compher C, Badellino KO. Obesity and inflammation: lessons from bariatric surgery. JPEN J Parenter Enteral Nutr. 2008;32(6):645–7.
111. Ibrahim MM. Subcutaneous and visceral adipose tissue: structural and functional differences. Obes Rev. 2009;11(1):11–8.
112. Forsythe LK, Wallace JM, Livingstone MB. Obesity and inflammation: the effects of weight loss. Nutr Res Rev. 2008;21(2):117–33.
113. Moschen AR, Molnar C, Geiger S, Graziadei I, Ebenbichler CF, Weiss H, et al. Anti-inflammatory effects of excessive weight loss: potent suppression of adipose interleukin 6 and tumour necrosis factor {alpha} expression. Gut. 2010;59:1259–64.
114. Blackburn GL, Wollner SB, Jones DB. Bariatric surgery as treatment for type 2 diabetes. Curr Diab Rep. 2010;10(4):261–3.
115. Wong KE, Szeto FL, Zhang W, Ye H, Kong J, Zhang Z, et al. Involvement of the vitamin D receptor in energy metabolism: regulation of uncoupling proteins. Am J Physiol Endocrinol Metab. 2009;296(4):E820–8.
116. Wong KE, Kong J, Zhang W, Szeto FL, Ye H, Deb DK, et al. Targeted expression of human vitamin D receptor in adipocytes decreases energy expenditure and induces obesity in mice. J Biol Chem. 2011;286:33804–10.

Part III

Alteration of Cardiovascular Control Systems

Endothelial Dysfunction in Early Phases of Hypertension

21

Stefano Taddei, Rosa Maria Bruno, and Stefano Masi

21.1 Introduction

Nitric oxide (NO) is produced from the amino acid L-arginine by an enzyme called NO synthase (NOS) and represents a key molecule regulating vascular homeostasis [1]. Cofactors, such as nicotinamide adenine dinucleotide phosphate, flavin mononucleotide, flavin adenine dinucleotide, tetrabiopterin and heme, are necessary for NOS activity. NOS is present in three isoforms in different tissues: neuronal NOS, inducible NOS and endothelial NOS (eNOS). The latter is a constitutive enzyme isoform, first discovered in endothelial cells. The activity of eNOS, as well as NO release from the endothelium, is stimulated by receptor-mediated mechanisms (acetylcholine, bradykinin, serotonin, substance P, adenosine diphosphate) but also by mechanical stimuli (Fig. 21.1). In particular shear stress, namely, tangential cyclic stress generated on vascular walls by blood flow, is the most powerful mechanism of stimulated NO release. In turn, main stimuli with a negative influence on eNOS expression are hypoxia, tumour necrosis factor-α and inflammatory cytokines. False eNOS substrates, such as *N*-monomethyl-L-arginine (L-NMMA), can also reduce NO bioavailability and are commonly used to test the degree of endothelium-dependent vasodilation [2].

Endothelial dysfunction is detected in several pathological conditions and is characterised by an imbalance between substances with vasodilating, antimitogenic and anti-thrombogenic properties and substances with vasoconstricting, prothrombotic and proliferative characteristics (also known with the generic term endothelium-derived contracting factors, EDCFs) (Fig. 21.1). Thus, given that NO exerts vasodilatory action on vascular smooth muscle cells but also inhibits platelet adhesion and aggregation, leukocyte adhesion and migration as well as smooth

S. Taddei (✉) · R. M. Bruno · S. Masi
Department of Internal Medicine, University of Pisa, Pisa, Italy
e-mail: stefano.taddei@med.unipi.it

R. Zimlichman et al. (eds.), *Prehypertension and Cardiometabolic Syndrome*, Updates in Hypertension and Cardiovascular Protection,
https://doi.org/10.1007/978-3-319-75310-2_21

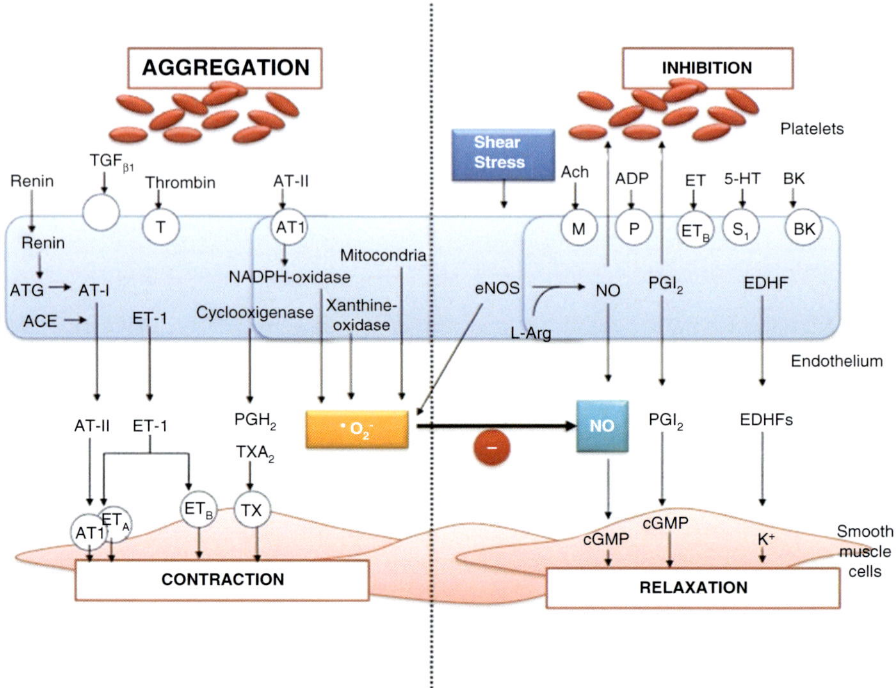

Fig. 21.1 Nitric oxide (NO) and other endothelium-derived factors and their role in vascular homeostasis. *TGF* transforming growth factor, *AT* angiotensin, *ATG* angiotensinogen, *ET* endothelin, *ACE* angiotensin converting enzyme, *TX* thromboxane, *PG* prostaglandin, *NADPH* nicotinamide dinucleotide phosphate, *eNOS* endothelial NO synthase, *L-Arg* L-Arginine, *Ach* acetylcholine, *ADP* adenosine diphosphate, *cGMP* cyclic guanosine monophosphate, *EDHF* endothelium-derived hyperpolarizing factors, *5-HT* serotonin, *BK* Bradykinin. From [2], with permission

muscle cell proliferation [3], it appears evident that reduced NO bioavailability in the vasculature is the main pathophysiological alteration encountered in endothelial dysfunction.

21.2 How to Assess Endothelial Function

Different techniques have been developed to assess vascular properties in humans, including biochemical and genetic markers, as well as vascular reactivity tests [4].

The first demonstration of endothelial dysfunction in atherosclerotic coronary arteries dates back to 1986 [5]. Later, peripheral vascular beds that were easily accessible, such as the upper limbs, were interrogated to assess the presence and severity of endothelial dysfunction in humans, using minimally invasive or non-invasive techniques [4]. While each approach has its advantages and disadvantages, as well as its peculiar characteristics (Table 21.1), all these vascular tests are based on the same principle. In healthy conditions, arteries dilate in response to non-pharmacological (i.e. reactive hyperemia) or pharmacological stimuli

Table 21.1 Advantages and disadvantages of the most commonly used techniques to assess endothelial function

Technique	Vascular bed	Advantages	Disadvantages	Stimulus (examples)
Coronary epicardial vasoreactivity (quantitative coronary angiography)	Epicardial macrovascular Conduit arteries	Assessment directly in the coronary vascular bed Gold standard	Invasive Expensive Time consuming Limited to those undergoing coronary angiography	Ach Exercise Pacing Cold Pressor Test
Coronary microvascular function (Doppler wire)	Coronary microvascular Resistance arteries	Assessment directly in the coronary microvasculature	Invasive Expensive Time consuming Limited to those undergoing coronary angiography	Ach Adenosine Papaverine
Coronary microvascular function (PET)	Coronary microvascular	Coronary district assessment Non-invasive	Less endothelium-specific	Adenosine/dipyridamole Cold pressor test Mental stress
Venous occlusion plethysmography	Forearm vasculature Microvasculature	Easy access Vasoactive substances infused to generate a dose-response relationship Contralateral arm as a control Accurate and reproducible	Invasive (cannulation of the brachial artery) Time consuming Challenging for serial measurements	Ach and other vasoactive substances
Flow-mediated dilation	Brachial artery Conduit artery	Easy access Correlation with invasive epicardial vascular function Many outcome studies Inexpensive Possibility to assess other important parameters (flow, baseline arterial diameter, flow-mediated constriction)	Challenging to perform well Disparate protocols for performance and standardisations Need for standardisation	Reactive Hyperemia
Peripheral arterial tonometry	Peripheral arteries	Non-invasive, easy to use, not user-dependent, automatic analysis, reliable and reproducible	Expense of disposable finger probes Less endothelium-specific	Reactive Hyperemia

Ach Acetylcholine. Adapted from Flammer AJ et al., and [71], with permission (acetylcholine, bradykinin or serotonin) (Fig. 21.1). In disease states the vasodilation induced by these stimuli is reduced or absent, as a result of a reduced NO availability. Endothelium-dependent responses should always be compared to endothelium-independent responses (obtained by exogenous NO donors or other vasodilators), to exclude structural vascular alterations and alterations in smooth muscles cells.

21.2.1 Invasive Techniques

21.2.1.1 Coronary Epicardial Function and Microvascular Function

Endothelial function can be measured in epicardial as well as resistance coronary vessels using several methods. Although these methods are limited by the invasive nature, their advantage is to measure endothelial function directly in this clinically important vascular bed.

The epicardial endothelial function is evaluated by quantitative coronary angiography or intravascular ultrasound, measuring changes in vessel diameter and cross-sectional area in response to endothelium-dependent stimuli. After acetylcholine infusion, vessels and segments with an intact endothelium vasodilate, whereas vessels and segments with dysfunctional or disrupted endothelium, will respond with vasoconstriction due to a direct activation of muscarinic receptors on vascular smooth muscle cells [5].

Changes in coronary or myocardial blood flow in response to endothelium-dependent vasodilators can be used as a surrogate parameter for microvascular function [6]. Other methods to estimate microvascular function have been introduced, such as the measurement of the number of cineangiographic frames that it takes to fill a distal vessel with a proximal injection of contrast (the so-called corrected TIMI frame count) [7]. Recently, non-invasive functional tests have been developed, among them positron emission tomography, myocardial perfusion imaging, blood oxygen level-dependent (BOLD) MRI and echocardiography [8].

21.2.1.2 Peripheral Microcirculation

Venous plethysmography is a semi-invasive technique providing information on the changes in forearm blood volume before and after infusion of vasoactive substances into a cannulated brachial artery, with virtually no systemic effects. Thus, this technique allows the accurate exploration of microvascular pathophysiological mechanisms in health and disease [9]. Furthermore, endothelial function in the forearm microcirculation correlated well with that of the cardiac district [10].

Subcutaneous microcirculation can be studied using the Halpern-Mulvany myograph system, an in vitro ex vivo technique [11]. This technique allows to assess functional characteristics of isolated resistance arterioles (lumen diameter 150–300 μm), taken from subcutaneous tissue obtained by skin biopsies. Once cleaned of adherent connective tissue, vessels are investigated with the "wire myograph" or the "pressure myograph". The first technique implies that two wires are threaded through the vessel, while in the pressurised system, the artery is slipped into two glass microcannula and exposed to a constant pressure. Both techniques have documented a reduced endothelial function in small subcutaneous arteries of hypertensive patients [12]. As an in vitro technique, such methodology allows exploration of several pathways and testing of many compounds not applicable in vivo, although the prognostic value of endothelial dysfunction in isolated small vessels from hypertensive patients is still under debate.

21.2.2 Non-invasive Techniques

Non-invasive techniques to assess macrovascular as well as microvascular endothelial function in peripheral arteries have been developed. These measurements have been shown to correlate reasonably with coronary vascular function, confirming that endothelial dysfunction is a systemic condition [13, 14].

21.2.2.1 Flow-Mediated Vasodilation of Brachial Artery

Among different techniques measuring endothelial function, brachial artery flow-mediated dilation (FMD) is one of the most used for its non-invasiveness. This technique is based on the physiological response of endothelial cells to shear stress that stimulates production of NO and other endothelium-derived relaxing factors, ultimately leading to vasodilation [15]. FMD involves measurement, by means of high-resolution ultrasound, of the change in diameter of a conduit artery (the brachial or radial artery) in response to increased flow, typically induced by a period of ischaemia in the distal circulatory bed [4]. Accordingly, FMD is a tool for examining the pathophysiology of CVD, identifying subjects at increased risk for future CV events, but also has merit in examining the impact of physiological and pharmacological interventions in humans. In recent years, a large number of studies demonstrated the prognostic value of brachial artery FMD for prediction of CV events, as summarised in several meta-analyses [16].

Despite concerns about its reproducibility, strong evidence shows that highly reliable FMD measurements are achieved when specialised laboratories follow strict standardised protocols [12].

21.2.2.2 Finger Plethysmography

Another technique which can be used to assess endothelial function is peripheral arterial tonometry, which is based on the finger arterial pulse wave amplitude (EndoPAT, Itamar Medical) [17]. Augmentation of the pulse amplitude after reactive hyperemia relies on the complex vascular response that also involves NO. As such, the EndoPAT has been suggested as a reliable measure of endothelial function [18].

Similar to the assessment of endothelial function with FMD, a pressure cuff is placed on one arm, and after obtaining baseline blood volume changes, the blood pressure cuff is inflated above systolic pressure and deflated after 5 min to induce reactive hyperemia on the same arm. The main advantages of the system are the use of the contralateral arm as an internal control and the nonoperator dependency.

However, to date a number of methodological, pathophysiological and clinical aspects still need to be clarified before the future and possible application of this user-friendly technique will be defined [19].

21.3 Endothelial Dysfunction: Clinical Aspects

21.3.1 Endothelial Function and Cardiovascular Risk Factors

Endothelial dysfunction, involving both micro- and macrocirculation of cardiac and peripheral districts, is a common trait of essentially all cardiovascular risk factors [20]. Impaired endothelial homeostasis (commonly detected in the form of an abnormal vasomotor response) is observed with ageing, after chronic or acute smoking, in hypercholesterolemia or hypertriglyceridemia, in type I and II diabetes mellitus and in hypertension and metabolic syndrome [20]. A meta-analysis of 211 cross-sectional studies, including almost 12,000 patients, found a significant relationship between FMD and Framingham risk score, which is more evident in low-risk subjects [21]. Thus, endothelial dysfunction may represent the sum of the detrimental effect of these risk factors on vascular health.

Endothelial dysfunction is an early step in the pathogenesis of atherosclerosis. In a cross-sectional study in middle-aged healthy men, there is no evident correlation between brachial FMD and the carotid intima-media thickness (IMT) [22], whereas FMD predicted IMT progression both in healthy subjects [23] and in hypertensive, postmenopausal women [24]. Similarly, endothelial function is not related to arterial stiffness, measured as pulse wave velocity, in healthy individuals [25], while the relationship is significant in patients with cardiovascular risk factors such as diabetes [26].

21.3.2 Endothelial Function and Cardiovascular Events

The presence of endothelial dysfunction is an independent predictor of all different type of clinical events. Its prognostic role has been demonstrated peripheral arterial diseases as well as coronary heart disease, independently from the endothelial stimulus used to test vascular reactivity [27, 28]. Several studies have assessed whether endothelial function provides additional prognostic information to estimate the risk of cardiovascular disease compared to traditional risk factors and risk score algorithms. In recent years, a large number of studies demonstrated the prognostic value of brachial artery FMD for prediction of CV events, as summarised in several meta-analyses [16, 28–30]. These meta-analyses showed a significant pooled relative risk reduction of 8–13% in CV events per percent point increase in brachial FMD, despite the heterogeneity of study selection criteria populations included. This reduction was either similar in high- and low-risk populations [28, 30] or greater in patients with established CVD [16, 29].

Several [31–35], but not all [36], population studies recognised the added value of the endothelial function in primary prevention. In the Multi-Ethnic Study of Atherosclerosis, FMD predicted future cardiovascular events, even after adjusting for the Framingham risk score [37]. Though the addition of FMD to the Framingham risk score did not improve c-statistics, it led to a significant reclassification improvement of patients at low, intermediate or high cardiovascular risk for cardiovascular disease when compared to the Framingham risk score alone [37].

Taken together, these studies indicate that the measure of endothelial function adds additional information to the patient cardiovascular risk stratification, going beyond the detrimental effects of classical cardiovascular risk factors on endothelium. New variables reflecting different aspects of vascular function might also have predictive value. Both hyperemia-induced shear stress and velocity changes showed even stronger correlations with the presence of cardiovascular risk factors than FMD [38]. In the FATE study, which included 1574 middle-aged, apparently healthy men at low cardiovascular risk, hyperemic velocity in the brachial artery, but not FMD, was associated with future clinical events, independently from Framingham risk score [39]. In another community-based cohort study, forearm microvascular endothelial function, assessed with Ach infusion, but not FMD, was associated with cardiovascular events in elderly patients, improving cardiovascular risk stratification compared to the Framingham risk score alone [40]. Similarly, microvascular endothelial dysfunction, measured by peripheral arterial tonometry, predicted adverse cardiac events in 270 outpatients, independently from cardiovascular risk factors [41]. Despite endothelial function measurements are not yet recommended by guidelines for cardiovascular prevention [42, 43], these studies, together with advances in the standardisation of non-invasive approaches, might make the assessment of endothelial function an important tool to refine cardiovascular risk stratification in clinical practice in the future.

21.4 Endothelial Function in Essential Hypertension

Several studies have demonstrated that endothelial dysfunction is a hallmark of arterial hypertension [44], but it is not a consequence of high blood pressure values [45]. Indeed, impaired endothelium-dependent vasodilation is observed in young offspring of hypertensive subjects despite the presence of normal blood pressure values [46]. In addition, there is no relationship between endothelium-dependent relaxation and blood pressure values; such a relationship is instead observed with levels of LDL-cholesterol [47, 48]. Finally, the simple reduction of blood pressure does not restore or improve endothelium-dependent vasodilation [49, 50]. The beneficial effect on endothelial function observed for different classes of antihypertensive medications is independent on blood pressure normalisation and likely related to specific pleiotropic effects of a drug or classes of drugs. Collectively, this evidence suggests that endothelial dysfunction may precede the onset of hypertension, does not reflect the severity of the disease and should not be used to monitor the efficacy of blood pressure lowering treatment.

An increased production of reactive oxygen species (ROS) and elevated vascular wall oxidative stress are important determinants of endothelial dysfunction in hypertension [9]. ROS, mainly superoxide anions, consist of radical and non-radical oxygen species formed by the partial reduction of oxygen. They rapidly react with NO producing peroxynitrites, thus reducing NO availability (Fig. 21.1) [2]. In addition, peroxynitrites have several negative effects on vascular function and structure. The importance of ROS in mediating endothelial dysfunction is confirmed by the evidence that infusion of ROS scavengers, such as vitamin C, can acutely restore NO bioavailability and improve endothelium-dependent vasodilation in hypertensive patients [9]. Several enzymatic and nonenzymatic sources of ROS have been described within the arterial wall, including NAD(P)H-oxidase, xanthine oxidase, cyclooxygenase and uncoupled endothelial NO synthase [51] (Fig. 21.1). In clinical conditions characterised by reduced NO-dependent vasodilation, such as essential hypertension, the endothelium produces another relaxing factor, known as an endothelium-derived hyperpolarising factor (EDHF). This controls vasomotor tone inducing the opening of the smooth muscle large-conductance K_{Ca} channels, therefore promoting potassium efflux and hyperpolarisation of vascular smooth muscle cells [52] (Fig. 21.1).

21.4.1 Endothelium-Derived Contracting Factors: Human Evidence

The endothelium controls the vasomotor tone also by production of several vasoconstricting agents, collectively identified as endothelium-derived contracting factors (EDCFs). These EDCFs might play an important role in controlling vasomotor tone in several pathological conditions, including essential hypertension [53].

The principal EDCF is endothelin-1 (ET-1), generated by the vascular endothelium, which acts through specific ETA and ETB receptors. ETA receptors are located on smooth muscle cells and promote growth and contraction. ETB receptors are located on both endothelial and smooth muscle cells, with opposite effects. Activation of smooth muscle cell ETB evokes contraction, whereas activation of endothelial ETB induces relaxation [54]. The overall biological effect of these activated receptors on the vasculature results from the balance between their protective and deleterious effects. By utilising the isolated forearm technique, an increased vasoconstrictor activity of endogenous ET-1 was demonstrated in essential hypertensive patients in comparison to normotensive individuals [54].

Endoperoxides derived from the metabolism of arachidonic acid by COX activity represent other important EDCFs [55]. Human and animal experiments confirm the role of COX in mediating endothelial dysfunction in hypertension. For example, the production of ROS following acetylcholine infusion in spontaneously hypertensive rat aorta is prevented by indomethacin, suggesting COX as a main source of ROS in such conditions. In turn, ROS can amplify the EDCF-mediated effect, either by triggering EDCF-mediated responses or indirectly by reducing the availability of NO, thus favouring the occurrence of EDCF response [55, 56].

21.4.2 The Source of EDCFs

Several animal experiments confirm that the metabolism of arachidonic acid via endothelial COX generates molecules which contribute to endothelium-dependent vasoconstriction. These COX-derived EDCFs diffuse to the underlying vascular smooth muscle cells and, through the activation of specific receptors (TP receptors), induce smooth muscle cell contraction [57]. Accordingly, most COX-mediated EDCFs effects are inhibited by TP-receptor antagonists [58, 59].

Most of the available data on EDCFs in humans have been obtained in essential hypertensive patients. As already mentioned, human hypertension is associated with a reduced NO availability [44]. The first experiments assessing the role of EDCFs on endothelial dysfunction in the forearm microcirculation of essential hypertensive patients demonstrated that intraarterial administration of the COX inhibitor indomethacin improved the vasodilation to acetylcholine and restored the inhibitory effect of L-NMMA on that response, indicating that COX generates substances that reduce the availability of NO [60]. Moreover, intraarterial infusion of the ROS scavenger ascorbic acid evoked similar effect as indomethacin in these patients, with no further potentiation of the vasodilatory response when the two compounds were confused [9]. These findings demonstrate that the COX pathway is a source of ROS in essential hypertension. Of note, COX-inhibition failed to affect the acetylcholine-induced relaxation in the forearm microcirculation of patients with secondary forms of hypertension [61], thus suggesting that EDCFs production is not a consequence of a mere blood pressure increase, but might be genetically related to essential hypertension.

21.4.3 Vascular COX-2 Isoform

There are two different isoforms of COX: COX-1 and COX-2 [62]. In most tissues, COX-1 is constitutively expressed, accounting for a baseline production of physiological prostanoids, while COX-2 is often induced by a number of stimuli, including inflammation or growth factors [63]. Nevertheless, endothelial and vascular smooth muscle cells constitutively express both isoforms, with COX-1 being usually expressed to a greater extent than COX-2 [63]. Recently, we investigated which COX isoform contributes to ROS generation in human hypertension. Using small resistance arteries from hypertensive patients, we showed that the blunted vascular response to acetylcholine was not improved by the COX-1 inhibitor SC-560, while it was significantly enhanced by the selective COX-2 inhibitor Dup-697, which also partially restored the inhibitory effect of L-NAME on acetylcholine [40]. In addition, we documented an augmented COX-2 protein expression in vessels from these patients, with a marked upregulation of COX-2 mainly in the vascular media layer [55]. These alterations in COX-2 expression were accompanied by an increased concentration of vascular superoxide anions, which was dramatically reduced after incubation with the selective COX-2 inhibitor and moderately blunted by the antioxidant apocynin. These data provided the first evidence that in small arteries isolated from essential hypertensive

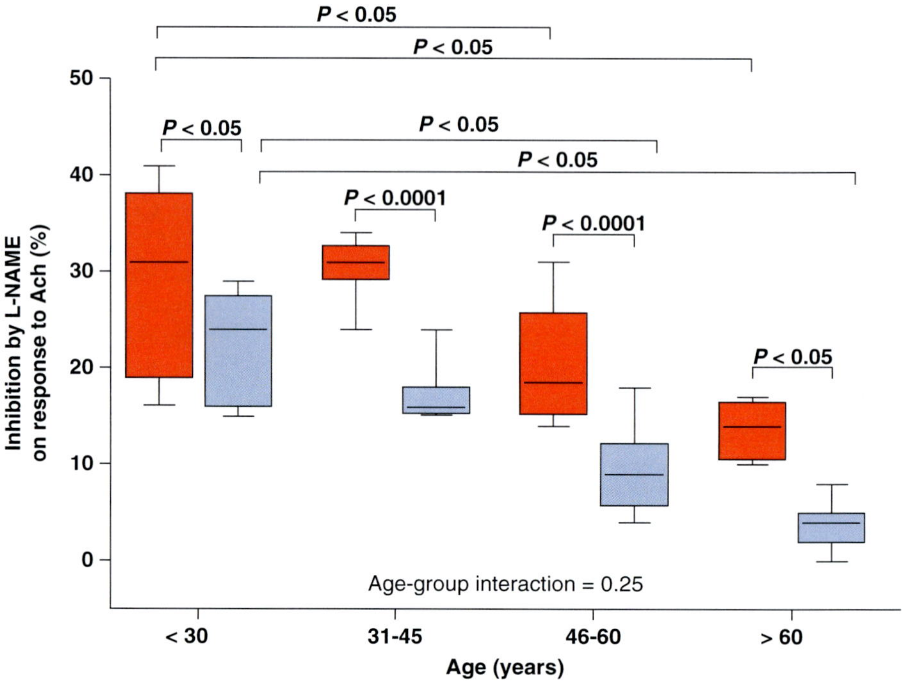

Fig. 21.2 Hypertension causes premature ageing of endothelial function in isolated small arteries from humans. *L-NAME*, N(G)-Nitro-L-arginine methyl ester; Ach, acetylcholine. Red box-plots, normotensive individuals; light blue box-plots, hypertensive individuals. Adapted from [12], with permission

patients, COX-2 is overexpressed and hyperactivated, playing a major role in reducing NO availability by increasing vascular levels of superoxide anions. In addition, as apocynin is a selective inhibitor of the NAD(P)H-oxidase, our data suggested that this enzyme is likely to account for most of the increased superoxide anion production observed in small arteries of hypertensive patients as a result of COX-2 hyperactivation. Other evidence has since confirmed the role of COX-2 as a major source of ROS generation in essential hypertension (Fig. 21.2).

21.4.4 Endothelial Dysfunction and Ageing

Ageing per se is the most powerful determinant of endothelial dysfunction and is accompanied by a progressive worsening of NO availability in resistance vessels [12, 64, 65] (Fig. 21.2). The earliest alteration of vascular homeostasis accounting for the endothelial dysfunction observed with ageing is a reduced availability of L-arginine, the substrate necessary for NO production by the eNOS. Indeed, L-arginine supplementation improves endothelial dysfunction in young adults (<30 years) [64]. With advancing age, however, along with the impaired L-arginine-NO pathway,

COX-dependent EDCF production becomes the prominent pathway accounting for age-related endothelial dysfunction. Indeed, in middle-aged adults (31–45 years), indomethacin or vitamin C begins to show some effect on endothelial-dependent vasodilation. This effect becomes highly significant in late adult and elderly patients (46–60 and >60 years) [64]. Such age-related transition in the pathways accounting for endothelial dysfunction is anticipated by hypertension, as confirmed by the evidence of an increased production of COX-dependent EDCFs and ROS in the vascular wall of hypertensive compared to normotensive subjects.

In conclusion, ageing is an important factor altering endothelium-dependent vasodilation. The most important mechanisms accounting for age-related endothelial dysfunction include a defect in the L-arginine-NO pathway and an upregulated production of COX-dependent EDCFs. Whereas in normotensive subjects the age-related alteration of both NO and EDCF production is detected only in old age, in patients with hypertension, these pathways seem to be altered early and to anticipate the age-related increase of blood pressure values through accelerated vascular remodelling.

21.5 Endothelial Dysfunction in Prehypertension

Considering the evidence that endothelial dysfunction can precede the onset of hypertension, it is conceivable that prehypertension might be characterised by a generalised endothelial alteration.

In line with this possibility, a study from Weil et al. [66] confirms the presence of impaired endothelium-dependent vasodilation in patients with prehypertension and that this alteration is characterised by a reduced NO availability. Using the perfused forearm technique, the authors demonstrated that the vasodilation to acetylcholine is significantly lower (around 30%) in prehypertensive patients as compared to matched normotensive subjects. Because the response to sodium nitroprusside was similar in the two study subgroups, the altered response to acetylcholine must be considered specific for an altered endothelial cell function, resulting in a compromised microvascular reactivity. Remarkably, infusion of L-NMMA, an eNOS antagonist, significantly blunted the vasodilating effect of acetylcholine in healthy controls but did not cause changes prehypertensive patients. These results demonstrate that prehypertension is characterised by impaired endothelium-dependent vasodilation caused by impaired NO availability, an alteration which is commonly observed in patients with established essential hypertension.

Over and above the role of intracellular pathways, an altered repair capacity by the endothelial progenitor cells (EPCs) is also associated with the endothelial dysfunction observed in prehypertension. Giannotti G et al. [67] demonstrated that in vivo endothelial repair capacity of early EPCs is reduced in patients with prehypertension, due to early cellular senescence, and is related to impaired endothelial function, assessed by brachial artery FMD. Importantly, the authors showed that similar alterations were detectable in a matched group of patients with hypertension, although they were more severe compared to prehypertensive subjects.

Whether endothelial dysfunction is cause or consequence of an altered EPCs repair capacity in prehypertension remains unknown. Indeed, a reduced NO availability typically observed in endothelial dysfunction compromises EPCs mobilisation from the bone marrow as well as their maturation. This is confirmed by studies conducted in premenopausal women, in whom EPCs function and mobilisation in prehypertension remain unchanged due to a preserved NO availability [68]. We confirmed the ability of endogenous oestrogen to protect endothelium-dependent relaxation from the age-related endothelial dysfunction which characterises hypertensive women [69].

Some study has also documented a contribution of ET system to the endothelial dysfunction observed in prehypertensive patients. Infusion of BQ-123, a selective ETA receptor antagonist, causes a greater increase in the forearm blood flow of prehypertensive patients as compared to healthy controls [70], demonstrating an increase of the ETA-mediated vasoconstrictor tone in prehypertension.

Conclusions

There is increasing evidence that endothelial dysfunction (1) is associated with almost all cardiovascular risk factors; (2) precedes the development of atherosclerosis; (3) predicts cardiovascular events independently of classical risk scores; (4) might identify a subset of patients in which conventional treatment is not sufficient; and (5) accompanies prehypertension. After three decades of research, non-invasive techniques for endothelial function assessment are finally reaching solid standardisation and good reproducibility. Thus, although by now endothelial function assessment is not recommended by current guidelines, it might have promising clinical applications in several settings.

Acknowledgments *Disclosures*: ST received research grants from Novartis, Servier, Recordati, Menarini and Boehringer and is on the speaker's bureau for Servier, Recordati, Novartis and Boehringer.

References

1. Furchgott RF, Zawadzki JV. The obligatory role of endothelial cells in the relaxation of arterial smooth muscle by acetylcholine. Nature. 1980;288:373–6.
2. Bruno RM, Taddei S. Nitric Oxide. In: Mooren FC, Skinner JS, editors. Encyclopedia of exercise medicine in health and disease. Berlin Heidelberg: Springer-Verlag; 2011.
3. Ross R. Atherosclerosis—an inflammatory disease. N Engl J Med. 1999;340:115–26.
4. Deanfield J, Donald A, Ferri C, Giannattasio C, Halcox J, Halligan S, Lerman A, Mancia G, Oliver JJ, Pessina AC, Rizzoni D, Rossi GP, Salvetti A, Schiffrin EL, Taddei S, Webb DJ. Endothelial function and dysfunction. Part I: methodological issues for assessment in the different vascular beds: a statement by the Working Group on Endothelin and Endothelial Factors of the European Society of Hypertension. J Hypertens. 2005;23:7–17.
5. Ludmer PL, Selwyn AP, Shook TL, Wayne RR, Mudge GH, Alexander RW, Ganz P. Paradoxical vasoconstriction induced by acetylcholine in atherosclerotic coronary arteries. N Engl J Med. 1986;315:1046–51.
6. Camici PG, Crea F. Coronary microvascular dysfunction. N Engl J Med. 2007;356:830–40.

7. Gibson CM, Cannon CP, Daley WL, Dodge JT Jr, Alexander B Jr, Marble SJ, McCabe CH, Raymond L, Fortin T, Poole WK, Braunwald E. TIMI frame count: a quantitative method of assessing coronary artery flow. Circulation. 1996;93:879–88.
8. Leung DY, Leung M. Non-invasive/invasive imaging: significance and assessment of coronary microvascular dysfunction. Heart. 2011;97:587–95.
9. Taddei S, Virdis A, Ghiadoni L, Magagna A, Salvetti A. Vitamin C improves endothelium-dependent vasodilation by restoring nitric oxide activity in essential hypertension. Circulation. 1998;97:2222–9.
10. Anderson TJ, Uehata A, Gerhard MD, Meredith IT, Knab S, Delagrange D, Lieberman EH, Ganz P, Creager MA, Yeung AC, et al. Close relation of endothelial function in the human coronary and peripheral circulations. J Am Coll Cardiol. 1995;26:1235–41.
11. Virdis A, Savoia C, Grassi G, Lembo G, Vecchione C, Seravalle G, Taddei S, Volpe M, Rosei EA, Rizzoni D. Evaluation of microvascular structure in humans: a 'state-of-the-art' document of the Working Group on Macrovascular and Microvascular Alterations of the Italian Society of Arterial Hypertension. J Hypertens. 2014;32:2120–9. discussion 2129
12. Bruno RM, Duranti E, Ippolito C, Segnani C, Bernardini N, Di Candio G, Chiarugi M, Taddei S, Virdis A. Different impact of essential hypertension on structural and functional age-related vascular changes. Hypertension. 2017;69:71–8.
13. Bonetti PO, Pumper GM, Higano ST, Holmes DR Jr, Kuvin JT, Lerman A. Noninvasive identification of patients with early coronary atherosclerosis by assessment of digital reactive hyperemia. J Am Coll Cardiol. 2004;44:2137–41.
14. Takase B, Uehata A, Akima T, Nagai T, Nishioka T, Hamabe A, Satomura K, Ohsuzu F, Kurita A. Endothelium-dependent flow-mediated vasodilation in coronary and brachial arteries in suspected coronary artery disease. Am J Cardiol. 1998;82:1535–9. A7-8
15. Celermajer DS, Sorensen KE, Gooch VM, Spiegelhalter DJ, Miller OI, Sullivan ID, Lloyd JK, Deanfield JE. Non-invasive detection of endothelial dysfunction in children and adults at risk of atherosclerosis. Lancet. 1992;340:1111–5.
16. Matsuzawa Y, Kwon TG, Lennon RJ, Lerman LO, Lerman A. Prognostic value of flow-mediated vasodilation in brachial artery and fingertip artery for cardiovascular events: a systematic review and meta-analysis. J Am Heart Assoc. 2015;4:e002270.
17. Reriani MK, Lerman LO, Lerman A. Endothelial function as a functional expression of cardiovascular risk factors. Biomark Med. 2010;4:351–60.
18. Nohria A, Gerhard-Herman M, Creager MA, Hurley S, Mitra D, Ganz P. Role of nitric oxide in the regulation of digital pulse volume amplitude in humans. J Appl Physiol. 2006;101:545–8.
19. Bruno RM, Gori T, Ghiadoni L. Endothelial function testing and cardiovascular disease: focus on peripheral arterial tonometry. Vasc Health Risk Manag. 2014;10:577–84.
20. Brunner H, Cockcroft JR, Deanfield J, Donald A, Ferrannini E, Halcox J, Kiowski W, Luscher TF, Mancia G, Natali A, Oliver JJ, Pessina AC, Rizzoni D, Rossi GP, Salvetti A, Spieker LE, Taddei S, Webb DJ. Endothelial function and dysfunction. Part II: association with cardiovascular risk factors and diseases. A statement by the Working Group on Endothelins and Endothelial Factors of the European Society of Hypertension. J Hypertens. 2005;23:233–46.
21. Witte DR, Westerink J, de Koning EJ, van der Graaf Y, Grobbee DE, Bots ML. Is the association between flow-mediated dilation and cardiovascular risk limited to low-risk populations? J Am Coll Cardiol. 2005;45:1987–93.
22. Yan RT, Anderson TJ, Charbonneau F, Title L, Verma S, Lonn E. Relationship between carotid artery intima-media thickness and brachial artery flow-mediated dilation in middle-aged healthy men. J Am Coll Cardiol. 2005;45:1980–6.
23. Halcox JP, Donald AE, Ellins E, Witte DR, Shipley MJ, Brunner EJ, Marmot MG, Deanfield JE. Endothelial function predicts progression of carotid intima-media thickness. Circulation. 2009;119:1005–12.
24. Rossi R, Nuzzo A, Olaru AI, Origliani G, Modena MG. Endothelial function affects early carotid atherosclerosis progression in hypertensive postmenopausal women. J Hypertens. 2011;29:1136–44.

25. Koivistoinen T, Virtanen M, Hutri-Kahonen N, Lehtimaki T, Jula A, Juonala M, Moilanen L, Aatola H, Hyttinen J, Viikari JS, Raitakari OT, Kahonen M. Arterial pulse wave velocity in relation to carotid intima-media thickness, brachial flow-mediated dilation and carotid artery distensibility: The Cardiovascular Risk in Young Finns Study and the Health 2000 Survey. Atherosclerosis. 2012;220:387–93.
26. Bruno RM, Penno G, Daniele G, Pucci L, Lucchesi D, Stea F, Landini L, Cartoni G, Taddei S, Ghiadoni L, Del Prato S. Type 2 diabetes mellitus worsens arterial stiffness in hypertensive patients through endothelial dysfunction. Diabetologia. 2012;56:1847–55.
27. Lerman A, Zeiher AM. Endothelial function: cardiac events. Circulation. 2005;111:363–8.
28. Inaba Y, Chen JA, Bergmann SR. Prediction of future cardiovascular outcomes by flow-mediated vasodilatation of brachial artery: a meta-analysis. Int J Card Imaging. 2010;26:631–40.
29. Ras RT, Streppel MT, Draijer R, Zock PL. Flow-mediated dilation and cardiovascular risk prediction: a systematic review with meta-analysis. Int J Cardiol. 2013;168:344–51.
30. Xu Y, Arora RC, Hiebert BM, Lerner B, Szwajcer A, McDonald K, Rigatto C, Komenda P, Sood MM, Tangri N. Non-invasive endothelial function testing and the risk of adverse outcomes: a systematic review and meta-analysis. Eur Heart J Cardiovasc Imaging. 2014;15:736–46.
31. Rossi R, Nuzzo A, Origliani G, Modena MG. Prognostic role of flow-mediated dilation and cardiac risk factors in post-menopausal women. J Am Coll Cardiol. 2008;51:997–1002.
32. Yeboah J, Crouse JR, Hsu FC, Burke GL, Herrington DM. Brachial flow-mediated dilation predicts incident cardiovascular events in older adults: the Cardiovascular Health Study. Circulation. 2007;115:2390–7.
33. Shechter M, Issachar A, Marai I, Koren-Morag N, Freinark D, Shahar Y, Shechter A, Feinberg MS. Long-term association of brachial artery flow-mediated vasodilation and cardiovascular events in middle-aged subjects with no apparent heart disease. Int J Cardiol. 2009;134:52–8.
34. Neunteufl T, Heher S, Katzenschlager R, Wolfl G, Kostner K, Maurer G, Weidinger F. Late prognostic value of flow-mediated dilation in the brachial artery of patients with chest pain. Am J Cardiol. 2000;86:207–10.
35. Hirsch L, Shechter A, Feinberg MS, Koren-Morag N, Shechter M. The impact of early compared to late morning hours on brachial endothelial function and long-term cardiovascular events in healthy subjects with no apparent coronary heart disease. Int J Cardiol. 2011;151:342–7.
36. Shimbo D, Grahame-Clarke C, Miyake Y, Rodriguez C, Sciacca R, Di Tullio M, Boden-Albala B, Sacco R, Homma S. The association between endothelial dysfunction and cardiovascular outcomes in a population-based multi-ethnic cohort. Atherosclerosis. 2007;192:197–203.
37. Yeboah J, Folsom AR, Burke GL, Johnson C, Polak JF, Post W, Lima JA, Crouse JR, Herrington DM. Predictive value of brachial flow-mediated dilation for incident cardiovascular events in a population-based study: the multi-ethnic study of atherosclerosis. Circulation. 2009;120:502–9.
38. Philpott AC, Lonn E, Title LM, Verma S, Buithieu J, Charbonneau F, Anderson TJ. Comparison of new measures of vascular function to flow mediated dilatation as a measure of cardiovascular risk factors. Am J Cardiol. 2009;103:1610–5.
39. Anderson TJ, Charbonneau F, Title LM, Buithieu J, Rose MS, Conradson H, Hildebrand K, Fung M, Verma S, Lonn EM. Microvascular function predicts cardiovascular events in primary prevention: long-term results from the Firefighters and Their Endothelium (FATE) study. Circulation. 2011;123:163–9.
40. Lind L, Berglund L, Larsson A, Sundstrom J. Endothelial function in resistance and conduit arteries and 5-year risk of cardiovascular disease. Circulation. 2011;123:1545–51.
41. Rubinshtein R, Kuvin JT, Soffler M, Lennon RJ, Lavi S, Nelson RE, Pumper GM, Lerman LO, Lerman A. Assessment of endothelial function by non-invasive peripheral arterial tonometry predicts late cardiovascular adverse events. Eur Heart J. 2010;31:1142–8.
42. Graham I, Atar D, Borch-Johnsen K, Boysen G, Burell G, Cifkova R, Dallongeville J, De Backer G, Ebrahim S, Gjelsvik B, Herrmann-Lingen C, Hoes A, Humphries S, Knapton M, Perk J, Priori SG, Pyorala K, Reiner Z, Ruilope L, Sans-Menendez S, Op Reimer WS,

Weissberg P, Wood D, Yarnell J, Zamorano JL, Walma E, Fitzgerald T, Cooney MT, Dudina A, Vahanian A, Camm J, De Caterina R, Dean V, Dickstein K, Funck-Brentano C, Filippatos G, Hellemans I, Kristensen SD, McGregor K, Sechtem U, Silber S, Tendera M, Widimsky P, Altiner A, Bonora E, Durrington PN, Fagard R, Giampaoli S, Hemingway H, Hakansson J, Kjeldsen SE, Larsen L, Mancia G, Manolis AJ, Orth-Gomer K, Pedersen T, Rayner M, Ryden L, Sammut M, Schneiderman N, Stalenhoef AF, Tokgozoglu L, Wiklund O, Zampelas A. European guidelines on cardiovascular disease prevention in clinical practice: full text. Fourth Joint Task Force of the European Society of Cardiology and other societies on cardiovascular disease prevention in clinical practice (constituted by representatives of nine societies and by invited experts). Eur J Cardiovasc Prev Rehabil. 2007;14(Suppl 2):S1–113.

43. Greenland P, Alpert JS, Beller GA, Benjamin EJ, Budoff MJ, Fayad ZA, Foster E, Hlatky MA, Hodgson JM, Kushner FG, Lauer MS, Shaw LJ, Smith SC Jr, Taylor AJ, Weintraub WS, Wenger NK, Jacobs AK, Anderson JL, Albert N, Buller CE, Creager MA, Ettinger SM, Guyton RA, Halperin JL, Hochman JS, Nishimura R, Ohman EM, Page RL, Stevenson WG, Tarkington LG, Yancy CW. 2010 ACCF/AHA guideline for assessment of cardiovascular risk in asymptomatic adults: a report of the American College of Cardiology Foundation/American Heart Association Task Force on Practice Guidelines. J Am Coll Cardiol. 2010;56:e50–103.
44. Mordi I, Mordi N, Delles C, Tzemos N. Endothelial dysfunction in human essential hypertension. J Hypertens. 2016;34:1464–72.
45. Taddei S, Bruno RM. Endothelial dysfunction in hypertension: achievements and open questions. J Hypertens. 2016;34:1492–3.
46. Taddei S, Virdis A, Mattei P, Ghiadoni L, Sudano I, Salvetti A. Defective L-arginine-nitric oxide pathway in offspring of essential hypertensive patients. Circulation. 1996;94:1298–303.
47. John S, Schmieder RE. Impaired endothelial function in arterial hypertension and hypercholesterolemia: potential mechanisms and differences. J Hypertens. 2000;18:363–74.
48. Benjamin EJ, Larson MG, Keyes MJ, Mitchell GF, Vasan RS, Keaney JF Jr, Lehman BT, Fan S, Osypiuk E, Vita JA. Clinical correlates and heritability of flow-mediated dilation in the community: the Framingham Heart Study. Circulation. 2004;109:613–9.
49. Ghiadoni L, Magagna A, Versari D, Kardasz I, Huang Y, Taddei S, Salvetti A. Different effect of antihypertensive drugs on conduit artery endothelial function. Hypertension. 2003;41(6):1281.
50. Ried K, Sullivan TR, Fakler P, Frank OR, Stocks NP. Effect of cocoa on blood pressure. Cochrane Database Syst Rev. 2012;8:CD008893.
51. Munzel T, Gori T, Bruno RM, Taddei S. Is oxidative stress a therapeutic target in cardiovascular disease? Eur Heart J. 2010;31:2741–8.
52. Taddei S, Versari D, Cipriano A, Ghiadoni L, Galetta F, Franzoni F, Magagna A, Virdis A, Salvetti A. Identification of a cytochrome P450 2C9-derived endothelium-derived hyperpolarizing factor in essential hypertensive patients. J Am Coll Cardiol. 2006;48:508–15.
53. Luscher TF. Imbalance of endothelium-derived relaxing and contracting factors. A new concept in hypertension? Am J Hypertens. 1990;3:317–30.
54. Taddei S, Virdis A, Ghiadoni L, Sudano I, Magagna A, Salvetti A. Role of endothelin in the control of peripheral vascular tone in human hypertension. Heart Fail Rev. 2001;6:277–85.
55. Virdis A, Bacca A, Colucci R, Duranti E, Fornai M, Materazzi G, Ippolito C, Bernardini N, Blandizzi C, Bernini G, Taddei S. Endothelial dysfunction in small arteries of essential hypertensive patients: role of cyclooxygenase-2 in oxidative stress generation. Hypertension. 2013;62:337–44.
56. Taddei S, Virdis A, Ghiadoni L, Salvetti A. Vascular effects of endothelin-1 in essential hypertension: relationship with cyclooxygenase-derived endothelium-dependent contracting factors and nitric oxide. J Cardiovasc Pharmacol. 2000;35:S37–40.
57. Vanhoutte PM, Feletou M, Taddei S. Endothelium-dependent contractions in hypertension. Br J Pharmacol. 2005;144:449–58.
58. Yang D, Feletou M, Boulanger CM, Wu HF, Levens N, Zhang JN, Vanhoutte PM. Oxygen-derived free radicals mediate endothelium-dependent contractions to acetylcholine in aortas from spontaneously hypertensive rats. Br J Pharmacol. 2002;136:104–10.

59. Virdis A, Colucci R, Fornai M, Duranti E, Giannarelli C, Bernardini N, Segnani C, Ippolito C, Antonioli L, Blandizzi C, Taddei S, Salvetti A, Del Tacca M. Cyclooxygenase-1 is involved in endothelial dysfunction of mesenteric small arteries from angiotensin II-infused mice. Hypertension. 2007;49:679–86.
60. Taddei S, Virdis A, Ghiadoni L, Magagna A, Salvetti A. Cyclooxygenase inhibition restores nitric oxide activity in essential hypertension. Hypertension. 1997;29:274–9.
61. Taddei S, Virdis A, Mattei P, Salvetti A. Vasodilation to acetylcholine in primary and secondary forms of human hypertension. Hypertension. 1993;21:929–33.
62. Simmons DL, Botting RM, Hla T. Cyclooxygenase isozymes: the biology of prostaglandin synthesis and inhibition. Pharmacol Rev. 2004;56:387–437.
63. Feletou M, Huang Y, Vanhoutte PM. Endothelium-mediated control of vascular tone: COX-1 and COX-2 products. Br J Pharmacol. 2011;164:894–912.
64. Taddei S, Virdis A, Ghiadoni L, Salvetti G, Bernini G, Magagna A, Salvetti A. Age-related reduction of NO availability and oxidative stress in humans. Hypertension. 2001;38:274–9.
65. Taddei S, Virdis A, Mattei P, Ghiadoni L, Gennari A, Fasolo CB, Sudano I, Salvetti A. Aging and endothelial function in normotensive subjects and patients with essential hypertension. Circulation. 1995;91(7):1981.
66. Weil BR, Stauffer BL, Greiner JJ, DeSouza CA. Prehypertension is associated with impaired nitric oxide-mediated endothelium-dependent vasodilation in sedentary adults. Am J Hypertens. 2011;24:976–81.
67. Giannotti G, Doerries C, Mocharla PS, Mueller MF, Bahlmann FH, Horvath T, Jiang H, Sorrentino SA, Steenken N, Manes C, Marzilli M, Rudolph KL, Luscher TF, Drexler H, Landmesser U. Impaired endothelial repair capacity of early endothelial progenitor cells in prehypertension: relation to endothelial dysfunction. Hypertension. 2010;55:1389–97.
68. Zhen Y, Xiao S, Ren Z, Shen HW, Su H, Tang YB, Zeng H. Increased endothelial progenitor cells and nitric oxide in young prehypertensive women. J Clin Hypertens (Greenwich). 2015;17:298–305.
69. Virdis A, Ghiadoni L, Sudano I, Buralli S, Salvetti G, Taddei S, Salvetti A. Endothelial function in hypertension: role of gender. J Hypertens Suppl. 2002;20:S11–6.
70. Weil BR, Westby CM, Greiner JJ, Stauffer BL, DeSouza CA. Elevated endothelin-1 vasoconstrictor tone in prehypertensive adults. Can J Cardiol. 2012;28:347–53.
71. Flammer AJ, Anderson T, Celermajer DS, Creager MA, Deanfield J, Ganz P, Hamburg NM, Luscher TF, Shechter M, Taddei S, Vita JA, Lerman A. The assessment of endothelial function: from research into clinical practice. Circulation. 2012;126:753–67.

Prehypertension and the Renin-Angiotensin-Aldosterone System

22

Elena Kaschina and Thomas Unger

22.1 Introduction

The renin-angiotensin system (RAS) plays a central role in blood pressure regulation. The main effector peptides of this system, the octapeptide angiotensin II (Ang II; Ang 1–8) and the heptapeptide angiotensin III (Ang III; Ang 2–8), act at least on four different receptor subtypes (ATR 1–4). Most of the classical angiotensin actions are mediated by the AT1 receptor (AT1R). They include generalized vasoconstriction, increased release of noradrenaline, stimulation of proximal tubular reabsorption of sodium ions, secretion of aldosterone from the adrenal cortex, and cell growth in the arterial wall and in the heart [1]. Ang II induces endothelial dysfunction, activates prooxidant and proinflammatory processes, and promotes cardiovascular remodeling, thus contributing to vascular tone regulation as well as to the development and progression of hypertension [2, 3].

In the past two decades, novel RAS peptides and receptors have been identified, including the angiotensin AT2 receptor (AT2R), angiotensin-converting enzyme 2 (ACE2), and Ang (1–7) with its G-protein-coupled receptor Mas. The AT2R and the MasR form heterodimers and are functionally closely related [4]. These components are considered as the "protective arm" of RAS because they mainly activate opposing actions compared to those mediated by the AT1R.

E. Kaschina
Center for Cardiovascular Research (CCR), Charité—Universitätsmedizin Berlin, Freie Universität Berlin, Humboldt-Universität zu Berlin, and Berlin Institute of Health, Institute of Pharmacology, Berlin, Germany

T. Unger (✉)
CARIM—School for Cardiovascular Diseases, Maastricht University, Maastricht, The Netherlands
e-mail: t.unger@maastrichtuniversity.nl

R. Zimlichman et al. (eds.), *Prehypertension and Cardiometabolic Syndrome*, Updates in Hypertension and Cardiovascular Protection,
https://doi.org/10.1007/978-3-319-75310-2_22

Prehypertension is characterized by functional and structural changes in the microcirculation. A reduction of small arterial elasticity, the earliest predictor for hypertension development [5], along with endothelial dysfunction, nitric oxide deficiency, accumulation of extracellular matrix, and inflammation, contributes to early vascular remodeling. Increased circulating and local expression of RAS components in the vasculature and subsequently enhanced Ang II production are involved in these pathological processes [6]. Experimental studies in "prehypertensive" rats provided first evidence for the unique effect of RAS interaction on vasculature and blood pressure: Inhibiting the RAS by ACE inhibitors or angiotensin AT1 receptor antagonists (ARBs) prevented the progression of hypertension and vascular remodeling in young "prehypertensive" spontaneously hypertensive rats (SHR) [7–12]. Later on, investigations in humans [13–15] provided evidence that interfering with the RAS not only lowered blood pressure but also improved vascular factors determining vascular tone.

The present overview deals with the role of "harmful" and "protective" arms of RAS in prehypertension particularly in the context of early vascular remodeling. Furthermore, studies on pharmacological blockade of the RAS in prehypertensive humans are discussed.

22.2 Classical Renin-Angiotensin System

22.2.1 AT1 Receptor

Ang II constricts precapillary arterioles by activating AT1 receptors of vascular smooth muscle cells (VSMC). Direct *vasoconstriction* in the kidney leads to reduced renal flow and subsequent efferent arteriole constriction resulting in increased filtration pressure. Blood pressure-driven diuresis and sodium excretion generate a feedback loop on renin release. Furthermore, Ang II facilitates peripheral noradrenergic neurotransmission by augmenting norepinephrine release from sympathetic nerve terminals and by enhancing the vascular response to norepinephrine. This facilitating effect is mediated by presynaptically localized AT1 receptors [16]. Expression of endothelin-1 in response to Ang II also contributes to vasoconstriction [17] (Fig. 22.1).

The pathophysiological mechanisms of *vascular remodeling* are attributed to an Ang II-dependent increase of NAD(P)H oxidase activity via the AT1R in endothelial and VSMCs [18, 19], thereby stimulating reactive oxygen species (ROS) and nitrogen (RNS) formation in the vessel wall [20]. ROS products such as superoxide and H_2O_2 may activate mitogen-activated protein kinases, tyrosine kinases, phosphatases, calcium channels, and redox-sensitive transcription factors [20]. Activation of these signaling pathways results in cell growth and expression of proinflammatory genes.

Above hypertrophic effects on the vascular wall, actions of Ang II mediated by ROS include vasoconstriction and decreased vasodilatation. The ROS, which is generated especially by NAD(P)H oxidase, causes lipid peroxidation and generation

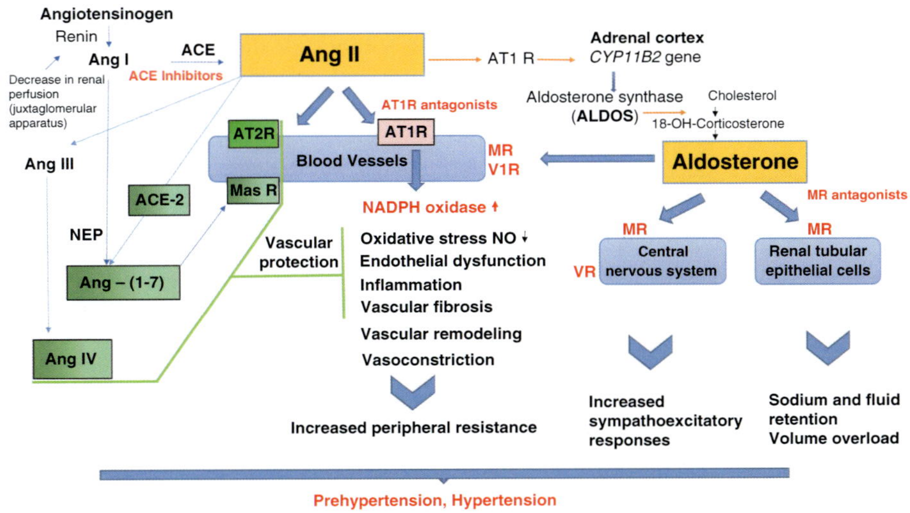

Fig. 22.1 Mechanisms of RAS—mediated prehypertension. *Ang* angiotensin, *AT1R* angiotensin AT1 receptor, *AT2R* angiotensin AT2 receptor, *ACE* angiotensin converting enzyme, *ALDOS* aldosterone synthase, *MR* mineralocorticoid receptor, *NADPH* Nicotinamidadenindinucleotidphosphat, *NO* nitric oxide, *NEP* neprilysin, *VR* vasopressin receptor, *V1R* type 1 vasopressin receptor, *Mas R* Mas receptor

of various vasoconstricting molecules such as F2 isoprostanes. On the other hand, ROS/RNS reduce the availability of the major vasodilator NO by reacting with superoxide [21].

Furthermore, via AT1R activation, Ang II controls cellular growth, migration, and intercellular matrix deposition and hence influences chronic adaptive changes in vascular growth and remodeling. Ang II stimulates the accumulation of extracellular matrix proteins, like collagen, elastin, fibrillin, fibronectin, and proteoglycans, which induce a phenotype switch in VSMC from contractile to proliferative/synthetic [22].

22.2.2 Vasopressin

Acting on AT1 receptors in hypothalamus and brainstem, Ang II or Ang III influence drinking behavior, sodium intake, natriuresis, and vasopressin release [23]. Vasopressin, an antidiuretic hormone, induces volume expansion followed by elevation of blood pressure. The pressor and antidiuretic actions are mediated by different vasopressin receptor subtypes, V1a, V1b, and the V2 receptors (V1aR, V1bR, V2R). The V1aR are expressed abundantly in the vascular smooth muscle cells, and their stimulation is responsible for the vasopressor effect. Blockade of the V1aR for 4 weeks in prehypertensive SHR could attenuate the development of hypertension in adult SHR [24]. This was recently supported by an increase of plasma vasopressin and of renal V1aR gene and protein expressions parallel to hypertension development in SHR [25]. However, in well-hydrated volunteers and in patients with a mild form of essential hypertension, V1R blockade did not alter blood pressure [26, 27]. Thus, the potential contribution of vasopressin to the development of hypertension from prehypertension requires further investigations.

22.2.3 Aldosterone

In 1958, Franz Gross postulated a physiological link between the RAS and aldosterone secretion in the zona glomerulosa of the adrenal gland [28]. Later on, several groups of investigators confirmed that Ang II stimulates aldosterone secretion [29]. Aldosterone, the primary mineralocorticoid, acts via the mineralocorticoid receptors (MR) in the kidneys and plays a central role in the regulation of blood pressure, blood volume, and salt household. Importantly, aldosterone contributes to the pathogenesis of hypertension beyond primary aldosteronism via several pathogenetic pathways, e.g., renal sodium and water retention, increased peripheral resistance, and stimulation of the sympathetic nervous system [30]. Since aldosterone levels within the upper part of the physiological range predispose normotensive subjects to the development of hypertension [31], it can be assumed that aldosterone also contributes to prehypertension.

The effects of aldosterone on blood pressure regulation extend beyond increased intravascular fluid retention and volume overload. Aldosterone modulates vascular tone by upregulation of the AT1R, by limiting bioavailability of endothelial NO, by increasing pressor responses to catecholamines, and by impairing the vasodilatory response to acetylcholine [32]. In addition, aldosterone excess activates inflammation and oxidative stress alters fibrinolysis by increasing plasminogen activator inhibitor-1 expression [33] and promotes vascular hypertrophy followed by increased arterial stiffness [34]. All these cellular pathways, regulated by aldosterone via the MR and by Ang II via its AT1R, can reinforce each other [35].

In an experimental model of prehypertension in young SHR, treatment with the MR antagonist, spironolactone resulted in prolonged blood pressure reduction and decreased collagen deposition [36]. Nevertheless, compared to the AT1R antagonist, losartan, the transient effect of spironolactone treatment was less impressive.

22.3 "Protective" Arm of the RAS

Recently, attention has been paid to the "protective" arm of RAS [37] that consists of several angiotensin peptides and their fragments and receptors with actions at least partly opposing the classical RAS concept. Some of these angiotensin peptides, related enzymes, and receptors are of particular interest because they play a protective role in the cardiovascular system.

Angiotensin-converting enzyme 2 *(ACE2)* has been described to be a potent negative regulator of the RAS, counterbalancing the multiple functions of ACE [38].

ACE2 converts the decapeptide, angiotensin I, to angiotensin Ang (1–9), which can be further converted by ACE to a shorter peptide, *Ang (1–7)*. Alternatively, Ang (1–7) can also be formed directly from Ang I via neutral endopeptidase (NEP, neprilysin). Interestingly, in prehypertensive SHR, the ACE2 levels are reduced [39].

Ang (1–7) evokes a range of acute central and peripheral effects such as vasodilatation, inhibition of VSMC proliferation, and inhibition of vasopressin release [40]. Although some of these effects depend on the acute activation of eNOS or inhibition of NADPH oxidase [41, 42], others may point to a potential role of Ang (1–7) in endothelial regeneration [43].

Furthermore, Ang (1–7) is known to be the endogenous ligand for the *Mas receptor*, a seven-transmembrane domain G-protein-coupled receptor sharing a 31% sequence identity with the AT2R [38, 44]. Other studies have suggested that the Mas receptor can heterodimerize with AT1R to inhibit the effects of Ang II [45]. A recent study shows heterodimerization and close functional relationship of the Mas R and the AT2R [4]. Mas receptor activation promotes often opposing effects to those of the AT1R such as anti-inflammation, antiproliferation [46], and blood pressure reduction as shown in DOCA-salt-induced hypertension in rats [47].

Ang IV (3–8) is formed via the cleavage of Ang III (Ang 2–8) by aminopeptidase B or N. Ang IV was reported to activate anti-inflammation and antiproliferation through a poorly defined AT4R and to induce vasodilatation and vascular protection via eNOS activation and subsequent NO release [48]. In addition, chronic treatment with Ang IV improved endothelial dysfunction in ApoE-deficient mice. This vasoprotective effect most likely resulted from increased NO bioavailability [49].

The angiotensin AT2 receptor (AT2R) is much less expressed under basal conditions compared to the AT1R. However, in cardiovascular diseases, such as hypertension or left ventricular hypertrophy, the AT2R expression is upregulated [3, 50]. The AT2R is a seven-transmembrane domain G-coupled receptor [51] that acts via several intracellular signaling pathways such as NO/cGMP activation [52], inhibition of mitogen-activated protein kinases (MAPKs) by protein phosphatases [53], phospholipase A2 stimulation [54], or disruption of AT1R signaling by AT_1R-AT_2R heterodimerization [55]. Similar to the MasR, AT2R activation promotes often opposing effects to those of the AT1R such as anti-inflammation, vasodilatation, and cell proliferation [1]. Activated AT2R also inhibits sympathetic activity [56] and through the phosphorylation of MAP kinase counteracts AT1R-mediated actions [57]. Notably, the AT2R mediates activation of bradykinin/NO/cGMP system in endothelial cells [58], in the heart [59] and in the aorta of prehypertensive stroke-prone spontaneously hypertensive rats (SHR-SP) [52]. In SHR-SP, the AT2-mediated increase in aortic cGMP is mediated by bradykinin B2 receptors, which activate NO synthase, followed by NO production and formation of the cGMP. cGMP, in turn, exerts antihypertensive and tissue protective effects such as vasodilatation, natriuresis, and antigrowth [60]. In addition, AT2 knockout mice have slightly elevated blood pressure, low basal levels of renal bradykinin and cGMP, as well as low NO production [61]. Conversely, AT2 receptor overexpression activated the vascular kinin system and caused vasodilatation [62]. In humans, the AT2-mediated vasorelaxation has been directly demonstrated in isolated coronary artery [63] and gluteal vasculatures [64]. Whereas acute vasodilator role of AT2R is well described, chronic decrease of blood pressure seems to be minimal after AT2R stimulation [65, 66].

Nevertheless, the AT2R has consistently been shown to be important in the prevention of vascular remodeling. In experimental studies performed in prehypertensive rats, AT2R stimulation with a selective AT2R agonist, compound 21 [67], reduced vascular fibrosis [68] and improved endothelial function and vascular composition by reducing oxidative stress, collagen content, fibronectin, and inflammatory cell infiltration [69]. AT2R stimulation also protected against nephropathy in doxorubicin-treated rats [70] and in 2K1C hypertension [71]. Furthermore, in a mouse model of type 1 diabetes, AT2R showed microvascular vasodilator properties [72].

In addition, AT2R exerts an anti-remodeling effect with regard to atherosclerotic lesions [73] and neointimal formation [74]. Iwai and colleague [75] demonstrated that AT2R/ApoE-double knockout mice fed a high-cholesterol diet display exaggerated atherosclerotic lesion development parallel with increased NADPH oxidase activity and superoxide production when compared to ApoE knockout mice. In humans, AT2Rs are expressed in the atherosclerotic and aneurysmatic lesions being mainly localized in the endothelium of *vasa vasorum* [76].

Taken collectively, an AT2 receptor-mediated increase in production of vasodilators (nitric oxide, cGMP), as well as the antigrowth and antifibrotic and anti-inflammatory features of this receptor, might contribute to blood pressure lowering and prevent remodeling in prehypertension.

22.4 Pharmacological Blockade of the RAS in Prehypertension

In view of the above-described contribution of the RAS to pathological changes in the vasculature and other target organs, given the availability of pharmacological inhibitors of this system and stimulated by experimental data in spontaneous hypertensive rats [7, 11, 12], the idea was borne to delay or even prevent the development of hypertension in prehypertensive individuals via pharmacological blockade of the RAS.

These considerations led to the conception of the so-called TROPHY (Trial of Preventing Hypertension) study "Feasibility of treating prehypertension with an angiotensin-receptor blocker" by Stevo Julius and colleagues [14]. The aim of this clinical trial was to investigate "… whether pharmacological treatment of prehypertension prevents or postpones stage 1 hypertension."

Participants with systolic blood pressure, between 130 and 139 mmHg and diastolic blood pressures of 89 mmHg or lower, were treated for 2 years with the angiotensin AT1 receptor blocker, candesartan, or with placebo followed by placebo for 2 years for both groups. When a participant became hypertensive (stage 1), he or she was continued on candesartan. Advice for "healthy living" to reduce blood pressure was given to both groups throughout the study.

Data from 772 participants could be analyzed, roughly half and with respect to groups. During the first 2 years, 154 participants reached the endpoint in the placebo group, compared to only 53 participants in the candesartan group, corresponding to a risk reduction of more than 66%. After 4 years, 240 individuals had developed hypertension in the placebo group, compared to 208 in the candesartan group. Thus, there was still a significant risk reduction of 16% in the group that had been started on candesartan.

The results of this trial demonstrate, first, that prehypertension can indeed be considered a precursor of hypertension in a substantial number of individuals (nearly two thirds) and, second, that a period of early intervention with an inhibitor of the RAS can delay the appearance of hypertension.

While the design of this study appeared relatively straightforward and the results on first glance quite clear, TROPHY fueled a lot of discussion and received positive as well as negative critiques.

On the negative side, the authors were criticized for using an "odd clinical endpoint" [77]. Without going into too much detail here, this point was answered by the authors in a reappraisal of their outcome data using the criteria of the "Joint National Committee on Hypertension (JNC)" [78]. There were only very minor differences between this analysis and that of the original report.

Even more serious was the criticism that TROPHY did, according to scenarios developed by its authors in an interim report [79], not prevent or delay the development of hypertension but instead caused a "slow unmasking" of hypertension [77]. Indeed, although the endpoints in both groups were still significantly different with less incidence of hypertension in the candesartan group, the slope of the cumulative incidence curve rose promptly after 2 years when candesartan treatment was replaced by placebo. Continuing on their respective slopes, the curves of both groups would have probably met after another 2 years or so. Thus, the study did indeed not show that hypertension can be prevented by a transient pharmacological intervention but that it can be delayed. The authors, although playing with the thought of prevention on several occasions, did not make this claim in the abstract of their original paper but just mention that "treatment with candesartan reduced the risk of incident hypertension during the study period" which is certainly not over-interpreting the data.

The authors further conclude cautiously that "treatment of prehypertension is feasible." This statement, too, is justified by the data of their study, but does it make sense, clinically? Would it imply that, if taken seriously, 25 million prehypertensive US Americans would have to be treated pharmacologically with an inhibitor of the RAS notwithstanding the "rest of the world"? Would the usual lifestyle adaptations (weight loss, salt restriction, exercise and dietary modifications) as more or less authoritatively advocated around the world not have the same effect without "chemistry"?

Kjeldsen et al. [80] argue against this by alluding to the fact that the prevalence of prehypertension has increased despite intensive efforts to promote such healthy lifestyles [81]. They argue further that, just taking the US American population, of the 25 million US Americans with TROPHY-like blood pressures, almost 16 million will become hypertensive over the next 4 years according to the experience from the TROPHY placebo group. Should one not intervene as early as possible in these individuals given the fact that prehypertension already carries pathological abnormalities in cardiovascular structure and function? If one follows this argument, the question is not any more whether or not it is possible to delay the onset of hypertension by transient pharmacological intervention, but to prevent hypertension altogether by early-onset, continuous treatment in prehypertensive individuals. Kjeldsen et al. [80] deliver a strong argument in favor of such early intervention: If one uses the absolute difference in risk reduction between groups in TROPHY, one can calculate that four individuals with prehypertension need to be treated to prevent one case of hypertension in 2 years.

Two years after TROPHY, another clinical study, named PHARAO (*P*revention of *H*ypertension with the *A*ngiotensin-converting enzyme inhibitor *RA*mipril in patients with high-n*O*rmal blood pressure), was published [15].

The objective was quite similar to the one in TROPHY, namely, to address "whether the progression to manifest hypertension in patients with high-normal blood pressure can be prevented with treatment." The study included 505 individuals in the ramipril and 503 individuals in the placebo group, lasted 3 years and, in addition, used ambulatory blood pressure monitoring to confirm the diagnosis of hypertension. After 3 years of treatment, 153 individuals in the ramipril group (30.7%) and 216 (42.9%) in the placebo group reached the primary endpoint (relative risk reduction 34.4%; $p < 0.0001$). Ramipril also reduced the incidence of office hypertension in participants with high-normal blood pressure established by ambulatory blood pressure monitoring (ABPM). The authors concluded that "treatment of patients with high-normal office blood pressure with the angiotensin-converting enzyme inhibitor was well tolerated, and significantly reduced the risk of progression to manifest hypertension." Analysis of the data further revealed that ramipril not only shifted the incidence of manifest hypertension downward in a parallel manner to the placebo group but, in addition, diminished the slope of the graph during the treatment period. This was interpreted to mean that the ACE inhibitor not only lowered blood pressure per se but also interfered with the vascular or neurohumoral factors determining vascular tone.

As with the angiotensin AT1 receptor blocker, candesartan, in TROPHY, it is now a member of another class of RAS inhibitors, the ACE inhibitor ramipril, which yielded such a preventive antihypertensive effect suggesting that a specific interference with the harmful arm of the RAS would reduce the risk toward manifest hypertension. However, in the absence of comparable studies with other classes of antihypertensive drugs, this idea, despite its theoretical plausibility, remains speculative.

References

1. Unger T. The angiotensin type 2 receptor: variations on an enigmatic theme. J Hypertens. 1999;17(12 Pt 2):1775–86.
2. Kaschina E, Unger T. Angiotensin AT1/AT2 receptors: regulation, signalling and function. Blood Press. 2003;12:70–88.

3. Namsolleck P, Recarti C, Foulquier S, Steckelings UM, Unger T. AT(2) receptor and tissue injury: therapeutic implications. Curr Hypertens Rep. 2014;16:416.
4. Leonhardt J, Villela DC, Teichmann A, Münter LM, Mayer MC, Mardahl M, et al. Evidence for heterodimerization and functional interaction of the angiotensin type 2 receptor and the receptor MAS. Hypertension. 2017;69(6):1128–35.
5. Peralta CA, Adeney KL, Shlipak MG, Jacobs D Jr, Duprez D, Bluemke D, et al. Structural and functional vascular alterations and incident hypertension in normotensive adults: the Multi-Ethnic Study of Atherosclerosis. Am J Epidemiol. 2010;171:63–71.
6. Paul M, Poyan Mehr A, Kreutz R. Physiology of local renin-angiotensin systems. Physiol Rev. 2006;86(3):747–803.
7. Harrap SB, Van der Merwe WM, Griffin SA, Macpherson F, Lever AF. Brief angiotensin converting enzyme inhibitor treatment in young spontaneously hypertensive rats reduces blood pressure long-term. Hypertension. 1990;16:603–14.
8. Lundie MJ, Friberg P, Kline RL, Adams MA. Long-term inhibition of the renin-angiotensin system in genetic hypertension: analysis of the impact on blood pressure and cardiovascular structural changes. J Hypertens. 1997;15:339–48.
9. Lee RM, Berecek KH, Tsoporis J, McKenzie R, Triggle CR. Prevention of hypertension and vascular changes by captopril treatment. Hypertension. 1991;17:141–50.
10. Unger T, Mattfeldt T, Lamberty V, Bock P, Mall G, Linz W, Schölkens BA, Gohlke P. Effect of early onset angiotensin converting enzyme inhibition on myocardial capillaries. Hypertension. 1992;20:478–82.
11. Wu JN, Berecek KH. Prevention of genetic hypertension by early treatment of spontaneously hypertensive rats with the angiotensin converting enzyme inhibitor captopril. Hypertension. 1993;22:139–46.
12. Unger T, Rettig R. Development of genetic hypertension. Is there a "critical phase"? Hypertension. 1990;16(6):615.
13. Schiffrin EL, Deng LY, Larochelle P. Effects of a beta-blocker or a converting enzyme inhibitor on resistance arteries in essential hypertension. Hypertension. 1994;23:83–91.
14. Julius S, Nesbitt SD, Egan BM, Weber MA, Michelson EL, Kaciroti N, et al. Trial of Preventing Hypertension (TROPHY) Study Investigators. Feasibility of treating prehypertension with an angiotensin-receptor blocker. N Engl J Med. 2006;20(354):1685–97.
15. Lüders S, Schrader J, Berger J, Unger T, Zidek W, Böhm M, et al. The PHARAO study: prevention of hypertension with the angiotensin-converting enzyme inhibitor ramipril in patients with high-normal blood pressure: a prospective, randomized, controlled prevention trial of the German Hypertension League. J Hypertens. 2008;26:1487–96.
16. Balt JC, Mathy MJ, Pfaffendorf M, van Zwieten PA. Sympatho-inhibitory properties of various AT1 receptor antagonists. J Hypertens Suppl. 2002;20:S3–11.
17. Hahn AW, Regenass S, Kern F, Bühler FR, Resink TJ. Expression of soluble and insoluble fibronectin in rat aorta: effects of angiotensin II and endothelin-1. Biochem Biophys Res Commun. 1993;192:189–97.
18. Griendling KK, Minieri CA, Ollerenshaw JD, Alexander RW. Angiotensin II stimulates NADH and NADPH oxidase activity in cultured vascular smooth muscle cells. Circ Res. 1994;74:1141–8.
19. Zafari AM, Ushio-Fukai M, Akers M, Yin Q, Shah A, Harrison DG, Taylor WR, Griendling KK. Novel role of NADH/NADPH oxidase-derived hydrogen peroxide in angiotensin 11-induced hypertrophy of rat smooth muscle cells. Hypertension. 1998;32:488–95.
20. Montezano AC, Touyz RM. Reactive oxygen species, vascular Noxs, and hypertension: focus on translational and clinical research. Antioxid Redox Signal. 2014;20:164–82.
21. Robert Li Y. Free radical biomedicine: principles, clinical correlations, and methodologies: Bentham eBooks; 2012. https://doi.org/10.2174/97816080532231120101.
22. Lacolley P, Regnault V, Nicoletti A, Li Z, Michel JB. The vascular smooth muscle cell in arterial pathology: a cell that can take on multiple roles. Cardiovasc Res. 2012;15(95):194–204.
23. Culman J, Baulmann J, Blume A, Unger T. The renin-angiotensin system in the brain: an update. J Renin Angiotensin Aldosterone Syst. 2001;2:96–102.

24. Burrell LM, Phillips PA, Risvanis J, Aldred KL, Hutchins AM, Johnston CI. Attenuation of genetic hypertension after short-term vasopressin V1A receptor antagonism. Hypertension. 1995;26:828–34.
25. Burrell LM, Risvanis J, Dean RG, Patel SK, Velkoska E, Johnston CI. Age-dependent regulation of renal vasopressin V(1A) and V_2 receptors in rats with genetic hypertension: implications for the treatment of hypertension. J Am Soc Hypertens. 2013;7:3–13.
26. Bussien JP, Waeber B, Nussberger J, Schaller MD, Gavras H, Hofbauer K, et al. Does vasopressin sustain blood pressure of normally hydrated healthy volunteers? Am J Physiol. 1984;246(1 Pt 2):H143–7.
27. Waeber B, Nussberger J, Hofbauer KG, Nicod P, Brunner HR. Clinical studies with a vascular vasopressin antagonist. J Cardiovasc Pharmacol. 1986;8(Suppl 7):S111–6.
28. Gross F. Renin and hypertension, physiological or pathological agents? Klin Wochenschr. 1958;36:693–706.
29. Weir MR, Dzau VJ. The renin-angiotensin-aldosterone system: a specific target for hypertension management. Am J Hypertens. 1999;12(12 Pt 3):205–13.
30. Tomaschitz A, Pilz S, Ritz E, Obermayer-Pietsch B, Pieber TR. Aldosterone and arterial hypertension. Nat Rev Endocrinol. 2010;6:83–93.
31. Vasan RS, Evans JC, Larson MG, Wilson PWF, Meigs JB, Rifai N, et al. Serum aldosterone and the incidence of hypertension in nonhypertensive persons. N Engl J Med. 2004;351: 33–41.
32. Connell JMC, Davies E. The new biology of aldosterone. J Endocrinol. 2005;186(1):1–20.
33. Schrier RW, Masoumi A, Elhassan E. Aldosterone: role in edematous disorders, hypertension, chronic renal failure, and metabolic syndrome. Clin J Am Soc Nephrol. 2010;5:1132–40.
34. Briet M, Schiffrin EL. Treatment of arterial remodeling in essential hypertension. Curr Hypertens Rep. 2013;15:3–9.
35. Lemarié CA, Paradis P, Schiffrin EL. New insights on signaling cascades induced by cross talk between angiotensin II and aldosterone. J Mol Med. 2008;86:673–8.
36. Baumann M, Megens R, Bartholome R, Dolff S, van Zandvoort M, Smits J, Sruijker-Boudier HA, De Mey J. Prehypertensive renin-angiotensin-aldosterone system blockade in spontaneously hypertensive rats ameliorates the loss of long-term vascular function. Hypertens Res. 2007;30:853–61.
37. Unger T, Steckelings UM, dos Santos RAS, editors. The protective arm of the renin angiotensin system—functional aspects and therapeutic implications. 1st ed. London: Academic Press, Elsevier; 2015.
38. Iwai M, Horiuchi M. Devil and angel in the renin-angiotensin system: ACE-angiotensin II AT1 receptor axis vs. ACE2 angiotensin-(1-7)-Mas receptor axis. Hypertens Res. 2009;32:533–6.
39. Rentzsch B, Todiras M, Iliescu R, Popova E, Campos LA, Oliveira ML, et al. Transgenic angiotensin-converting enzyme 2 overexpression in vessels of SHRSP rats reduces blood pressure and improves endothelial function. Hypertension. 2008;52:967–73.
40. Santos RA, Ferreira AJ, Verano-Braga T, Bader M. Angiotensin-converting enzyme 2, angiotensin-(1–7) and Mas: new players of the renin-angiotensin system. J Endocrinol. 2013;216:R1–R17.
41. Sampaio WO, Souza dos Santos RA, Faria-Silva R, da Mata Machado LT, Schiffrin EL, Touyz RM. Angiotensin-(1-7) through receptor Mas mediates endothelial nitric oxide synthase activation via Akt-dependent pathways. Hypertension. 2007;49:185–92.
42. Bodiga S, Zhong JC, Wang W, Basu R, Lo J, Liu GC, et al. Enhanced susceptibility to biomechanical stress in ACE2 null mice is prevented by loss of the p47(phox) NADPH oxidase subunit. Cardiovasc Res. 2011;91:151–61.
43. Durik M, Sevá Pessôa B, Roks AJ. The renin-angiotensin system, bone marrow and progenitor cells. Clin Sci (Lond). 2012;123:205–23.
44. Santos RA, Simoes e Silva AC, Maric C, Silva DM, Machado RP, de Buhr I, et al. Angiotensin-(1–7) is an endogenous ligand for the G protein-coupled receptor Mas. Proc Natl Acad Sci U S A. 2003;100:8258–63.

45. Kostenis E, Milligan G, Christopoulos A, Sanchez-Ferrer CF, Heringer-Walther S, Sexton PM, et al. G-protein-coupled receptor Mas is a physiological antagonist of the angiotensin II type 1 receptor. Circulation. 2005;111:1806–13.
46. Villela D, Leonhardt J, Patel N, Joseph J, Kirsch S, Hallberg A, et al. Angiotensin type 2 receptor (AT2R) and receptor Mas: a complex liaison. Clin Sci. 2015;128:227–34.
47. Singh Y, Singh K, Sharma PL. Effect of combination of renin inhibitor and Mas-receptor agonist in DOCA-salt-induced hypertension in rats. Mol Cell Biochem. 2013;373:189–94.
48. Patel JM, Martens JR, Li YD, Gelband CH, Raizada MK, Block ER. Angiotensin IV receptor-mediated activation of lung endothelial NOS is associated with vasorelaxation. Am J Physiol. 1998;275(6 Pt 1):L1061–8.
49. Vinh A, Widdop RE, Drummond GR, Gaspari TA. Chronic angiotensin IV treatment reverses endothelial dysfunction in ApoE-deficient mice. Cardiovasc Res. 2008;77:178–87.
50. De Gasparo M, Catt KJ, Inagami T, Wright JW, Unger T. International union of pharmacology. XXIII. The angiotensin II receptors. Pharmacol Rev. 2000;52:415–72.
51. Zhang H, Han GW, Batyuk A, Ishchenko A, White KL, Patel N, et al. Structural basis for selectivity and diversity in angiotensin II receptors. Nature. 2017;544:327–32.
52. Gohlke P, Pees C, Unger T. AT2 receptor stimulation increases aortic cyclic GMP in SHRSP by a kinin-dependent mechanism. Hypertension. 1998;31:349–55.
53. Fischer TA, Singh K, O'Hara DS, Kaye DM, Kelly RA. Role of AT1 and AT2 receptors in regulation of MAPKs and MKP-1 by ANG II in adult cardiac myocytes. Am J Physiol. 1998;275:H906–16.
54. Nouet S, Nahmias C. Signal transduction from the angiotensin II AT2 receptor. Trends Endocrinol Metab. 2000;11:1–6.
55. AbdAlla S, Lother H, Abdel-tawab AM, Quitterer U. The angiotensin II AT2 receptor is an AT1 receptor antagonist. J Biol Chem. 2001;276:39721–6.
56. Gao J, Zhang H, Le KD, Chao J, Gao L. Activation of central angiotensin type 2 receptors suppresses norepinephrine excretion and blood pressure in conscious rats. Am J Hypertens. 2011;24:724–30.
57. Inagami T, Eguchi S, Numaguchi K, Motley ED, Tang H, Matsumoto T, Yamakawa T. Cross-talk between angiotensin II receptors and the tyrosine kinases and phosphatases. J Am Soc Nephrol. 1999;10(Suppl 11):S57–61.
58. Wiemer G, Schölkens BA, Wagner A, Heitsch H, Linz W. The possible role of angiotensin II subtype AT2 receptors in endothelial cells and isolated ischemic rat hearts. J Hypertens Suppl. 1993;11:S234–5.
59. Liu YH, Yang XP, Sharov VG, Nass O, Sabbah HN, Peterson E, Carretero OA. Effects of angiotensin-converting enzyme inhibitors and angiotensin II type 1 receptor antagonists in rats with heart failure. Role of kinins and angiotensin II type 2 receptors. J Clin Invest. 1997;99:1926–35.
60. Kraehling JR, Sessa WC. Contemporary approaches to modulating the nitric oxide-cGMP pathway in cardiovascular disease. Circ Res. 2017;120:1174–82.
61. Siragy HM, Inagami T, Ichiki T, Carey RM. Sustained hypersensitivity to angiotensin II and its mechanism in mice lacking the subtype-2 (AT2) angiotensin receptor. Proc Natl Acad Sci U S A. 1999;96:6506–10.
62. Tsutsumi Y, Matsubara H, Masaki H, Kurihara H, Murasawa S, Takai S, et al. Angiotensin II type 2 receptor overexpression activates the vascular kinin system and causes vasodilation. J Clin Invest. 1999;104:925–93.
63. Batenburg WW, Garrelds IM, Bernasconi CC, Juillerat-Jeanneret L, van Kats JP, Saxena PR, Danser AH. Angiotensin II type 2 receptor-mediated vasodilation in human coronary microarteries. Circulation. 2004;109:2296–301.
64. Savoia C, Touyz RM, Volpe M, Schiffrin EL. Angiotensin type 2 receptor in resistance arteries of type 2 diabetic hypertensive patients. Hypertension. 2007;49:341–6.
65. Widdop RE, Jones ES, Hannan RE, Gaspari TA. Angiotensin AT2 receptors: cardiovascular hope or hype? Br J Pharmacol. 2003;140:809–24.

66. Steckelings UM, Paulis L, Namsolleck P, Unger T. AT2 receptor agonists: hypertension and beyond. Curr Opin Nephrol Hypertens. 2012;21:142–6.
67. Wan Y, Wallinder C, Plouffe B, Beaudry H, Mahalingam AK, Wu X, et al. Design, synthesis, and biological evaluation of the first selective nonpeptide AT2 receptor agonist. J Med Chem. 2004;47:5995–6008.
68. Paulis L, Becker STR, Lucht K, Schwengel K, Slavic S, Kaschina E, et al. Direct angiotensin II type 2 receptor stimulation in Nω-nitro-L-arginine-methyl ester-induced hypertension: the effect on pulse wave velocity and aortic remodeling. Hypertension. 2012;59:485–92.
69. Rehman A, Leibowitz A, Yamamoto N, Rautureau Y, Paradis P, Schiffrin EL. Angiotensin type 2 receptor agonist compound 21 reduces vascular injury and myocardial fibrosis in stroke-prone spontaneously hypertensive rats. Hypertension. 2012;59(2):291–9.
70. Hrenák J, Arendášová K, Rajkovičová R, Aziriová S, Repová K, Krajčírovičová K, et al. Protective effect of captopril, olmesartan, melatonin and compound 21 on doxorubicin-induced nephrotoxicity in rats. Physiol Res. 2013;62(Suppl 1):S181–9.
71. Matavelli LC, Huang J, Siragy HM. Angiotensin AT_2 receptor stimulation inhibits early renal inflammation in renovascular hypertension. Hypertension. 2011;57:308–13.
72. Begorre MA, Dib A, Habchi K, Guihot AL, Bourreau J, Vessieres E, et al. Microvascular vasodilator properties of the angiotensin 2 receptor in a mouse model of type 1 diabetes. Sci Rep. 2017;7:45625.
73. Sales VL, Sukhova GK, Lopez-Ilasaca MA, Libby P, Dzau VJ, Pratt RE. Angiotensin type 2 receptor is expressed in murine atherosclerotic lesions and modulates lesion evolution. Circulation. 2005;112:3328–36.
74. Nakajima M, Hutchinson HG, Fujinaga M, Hayashida W, Morishita R, Zhang L, et al. The angiotensin II type 2 (AT2) receptor antagonizes the growth effects of the AT1 receptor: gain-of-function study using gene transfer. Proc Natl Acad Sci U S A. 1995;92:10663–7.
75. Iwai M, Chen R, Li Z, Shiuchi T, Suzuki J, Ide A, et al. Deletion of angiotensin II type 2 receptor exaggerated atherosclerosis in apolipoprotein E-null mice. Circulation. 2005;112:1636–43.
76. Kaschina E, Scholz H, Steckelings UM, Sommerfeld M, Kemnitz UR, Artuc M, Schmidt S, Unger T. Transition from atherosclerosis to aortic aneurysm in humans coincides with an increased expression of RAS components. Atherosclerosis. 2009;205:396–403.
77. Meltzer JI. A specialist in clinical hypertension critiques the TROPHY trial. Am J Hypertens. 2006;19:1098–100.
78. Julius S, Kaciroti N, Egan BM, Nesbitt S, Michelson EL. Trial of Preventing Hypertension (TROPHY) Investigators. TROPHY study: outcomes based on the Seventh Report of the Joint National Committee on Hypertension definition of hypertension. J Am Soc Hypertens. 2008;2:39–43.
79. Julius S, Kjeldsen SE, Weber M, Brunner HR, Ekman S, Hansson L, et al. Outcomes in hypertensive patients at high cardiovascular risk treated with regimens based on valsartan or amlodipine: the VALUE randomised trial. Lancet. 2004;363(9426):2022–31.
80. Kjeldsen SE, Narkiewicz K, Hedner T. An American TROPHY in the prevention of hypertension. Blood Press. 2006;15:132–4.
81. Qureshi AI, Suri MF, Kirmani JF, Divani AA. Prevalence and trends of prehypertension and hypertension in United States: National Health and Nutrition Examination Surveys 1976 to 2000. Mred Sci Monit. 2005;11:CR403–9.

Tachycardia in Prehypertension

23

Paolo Palatini

23.1 Introduction

Measurement of resting heart rate is a medical maneuver that dates back to the old times when doctors relied on this clinical parameter to assess the health status of their patients. However, high heart rate emerged as a cardiovascular risk factor only in the modern era when some epidemiologists realized that this clinical variable remained included in survival models together with major cardiovascular risk factors and was a strong independent predictor of cardiovascular events and mortality. The first leading study to observe a link between elevated heart rate and development of myocardial infarction was the Chicago People Gas Co. study [1] followed by the Framingham study [2, 3] and the NHANES study [4]. The association appeared particularly strong for sudden death, as shown by the Framingham [2, 3], the Paris Prospective Study I [5], and the CASTEL study [6]. In most studies the relationship between heart rate and cardiovascular mortality was stronger among males than females and was maintained even after excluding individuals who died in the first years after baseline evaluation [2, 3, 6]. In the last 20 years, numerous new data confirmed those previous findings, and two recent meta-analyses unequivocally showed that high heart rate is an independent predictor of adverse outcomes [7, 8]. Zhang et al. in a meta-analysis of general populations encompassing over 1 million people showed that for each 10 bpm increase in resting heart rate, there was a 9% increase in risk of all-cause mortality [7]. For people with heart rate equal to or higher than 80 bpm, there was a 45% increase in risk compared to people with heart rate lower than 60 bpm. Similar results were observed for cardiovascular mortality with an 8% increase in risk for each 10 bpm increment in heart rate. More recently, in a new meta-analysis on the association between heart rate and risk of

P. Palatini
Department of Medicine, University of Padova, Padua, Italy
e-mail: palatini@unipd.it

R. Zimlichman et al. (eds.), *Prehypertension and Cardiometabolic Syndrome*, Updates in Hypertension and Cardiovascular Protection,
https://doi.org/10.1007/978-3-319-75310-2_23

cardiovascular events, the same group of investigators confirmed the predictive capacity of high heart rate for adverse outcome [8]. Using data from 45 prospective cohort studies, these authors found that an increment of 10 bpm in resting heart rate implied a 12% (95% confidence interval [CI] 9%–14%) increase in risk for coronary artery disease, a 5% increase (95% CI 1%–8%) for stroke, a 12% increase (2%–24%) for sudden death, and a 16% increase (95% CI 12%–21%) in risk for non-cardiovascular diseases. All of these relations were linear for either fatal or nonfatal events. After excluding studies involving patients with hypertension or diabetes, similar results were obtained for coronary artery disease, stroke, and non-cardiovascular diseases, while no association was found for sudden death.

23.2 Prehypertension

Prehypertension, e.g., a blood pressure between 120/80 and 139/89 mmHg, affects a large number of people in western as well as underdeveloped societies. However, this condition is very heterogeneous, and the cardiovascular risk differs in relation to many clinical variables, such as age, blood pressure level, and associated risk factors. Among these, heart rate emerged as a novel cardiovascular risk factor in prehypertension. A large number of general population studies have shown that individuals with elevated heart rates also have high blood pressure readings [9]. In addition, heart rate has been found to be associated with a variety of other risk factors including body mass index, metabolic variables, and hematocrit [9]. A number of studies performed in hypertensive populations have shown that the heart rate-mortality association remained significant also when all the above risk factors and other possible confounders were included in the survival analyses [7, 9]. A large Chinese study has shown that resting heart rate plays an important role on the progression to hypertension in subjects with prehypertension [10]. In the Kailuan study, participants diagnosed as prehypertensive were selected as the observation cohort, and the rate of the progression to hypertension was compared among five groups with increasing level of resting heart rate using Cox proportional hazard analysis [10]. A total of 25,392 patients were involved in the final statistics after excluding patients who died or were lost to follow-up. Of these, 13,228 (52.1%) patients developed hypertension during follow-up. The rate of the progression to hypertension increased with the resting heart rate being 50.1% in the subjects with 70–74 bpm and 57.5% in those with ≥85 bpm. Patients in the latter group carried 1.25 times higher risk for developing hypertension than patients in the former group after adjustment for age, gender, systolic blood pressure, diastolic blood pressure, waist circumference, body mass index, triglyceride, total cholesterol, low-density lipoprotein cholesterol, high-density lipoprotein cholesterol, fasting blood glucose, serum uric acid, C-reactive protein, smoking, drinking, physical exercise, and family history of hypertension at baseline. This longitudinal association has been demonstrated not only for baseline heart rate but also for the change in heart rate over time. In the HARVEST study, both baseline and follow-up heart rates were potent predictors of subsequent development of hypertension needing drug therapy [11]. Similarly, in a recent study from China [12] over a period of 3.5 years, fast heart rate (>90 bpm) was associated with a significantly higher hazard ratio of hypertension.

23.3 Tachycardia and the Cardiovascular Risk in Prehypertension and Hypertension

High heart rate is a common feature in patients with hypertension. A large number of studies have shown that heart rate is higher in hypertensive than normotensive people and that tachycardia is more common in the former. Among the stage 1 hypertensive subjects participating in the HARVEST study, over 15% had a baseline resting heart rate ≥85 bpm, and 27% had a heart rate ≥80 bpm (Fig. 23.1) [13]. In a large Italian study performed in general practices, over 30% of the hypertensive patients had a resting heart rate ≥80 bpm [14].

A positive association between heart rate and adverse outcome has been found also in subjects with prehypertension [15]. The Atherosclerosis Risk in Communities (ARIC) study examined 3275, 45–64-year-old prehypertensive subjects, during a mean follow-up of 10.1 years [15]. The primary outcomes were coronary artery disease and all-cause mortality. Participants with elevated resting heart rate had 50% higher all-cause mortality than people with lower resting heart rate (hazard ratio [HR] 1.50, 95% confidence interval [CI] 1.0–2.15), also after controlling for age, ethnicity, gender, diabetes, smoking status, LDL cholesterol, exercise, and use of antilipemic agents. In unadjusted analyses, the risk of coronary artery disease was 49% higher for people with increased heart rate than in those with normal heart rate (HR 1.49, 95% CI 1.03–2.14). In adjusted analyses, elevated resting heart rate remained an independent risk of coronary artery disease in women but not in men. The authors concluded that resting heart rate is an easily accessible tool that may be helpful for stratifying coronary artery disease and mortality risk in people with prehypertension.

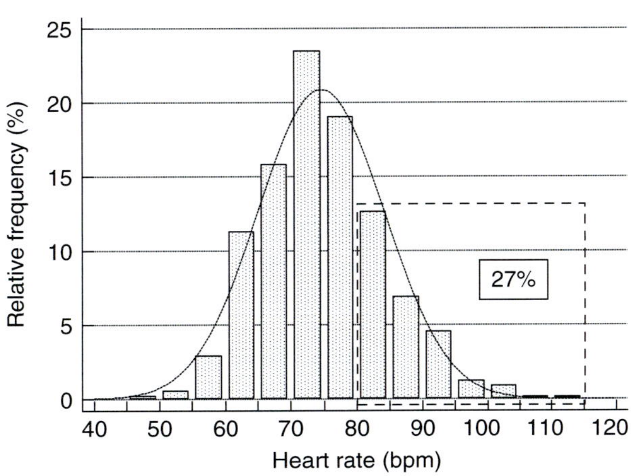

Fig. 23.1 Distribution of resting heart rate measured in the lying posture in 1204, 18–45-year-old subjects screened for stage 1 hypertension from the HARVEST study. Data are related to baseline assessment and are the average of six readings taken during two consecutive visits. Heart rate was ≥80 bpm in 27% of the participants and was ≥85 bpm in 15%

In a cohort of 6100 residents (2600 males and 3500 females) of Kangwha County, Korea, 55–99-year-old, the risk of all-cause and cardiovascular mortality was evaluated by resting heart rate and hypertension during a 21-year follow-up [16]. The hazard ratios associated with resting heart rate >80 bpm were higher in hypertensives, with hazard ratios of 1.43 (95% CI 1.00–1.92) on all-cause mortality for prehypertension, 3.01 (95% CI 1.07–8.28) on cardiovascular mortality for prehypertension, and 8.34 (95% CI 2.52–28.19) for stage 2 hypertension. Increased risk (HR 3.54, 95% CI 1.16–9.21) was observed among those with both a resting heart rate ≥80 bpm and prehypertension on cardiovascular mortality. Thus, these data showed that individuals with coexisting elevated resting heart rate and high blood pressure, even in prehypertensive range, have a greater risk for all-cause and cardiovascular mortality compared to those with elevated resting heart rate or hypertension alone.

Similar heart rate-risk relationships were found in cohort studies which recruited subjects with hypertension [17–21]. In a cohort of over 5000 patients from the Framingham study followed for 36 years, Gillman et al. found that the relative risk of cardiovascular death adjusted for age and blood pressure was 1.68 among men and 1.70 among women for an increase in heart rate of 40 bpm [18]. The risks were even greater for all-cause mortality: 2.18 and 2.14, respectively, and for sudden death they were 1.93 and 1.37, respectively. These associations remained significant also after adjusting for smoking, serum cholesterol, and left ventricular hypertrophy. In addition, serial analyses taking account of events that occurred within the past 6 years, those which took place in the past 4 years, and those which occurred in the past 2 years, confirmed the predictive value of heart rate for mortality, making it unlikely that this relationship was due to an underlying illness producing tachycardia. Similar results were obtained by Benetos et al. in a cohort of 12,123 men from a French population between the ages of 40 and 69 [17]. All-cause and cardiovascular mortality steadily increased with higher heart rates in both normotensive and hypertensive men. For death from ischemic heart disease, the increase in risk was present only among the hypertensive men, while the trend, though present, was not significant among the normotensive men. In contrast, relationships were weaker and nonsignificant among the women. The Glasgow Blood Pressure Clinic study [21] was the first to investigate the effect of a combination of baseline and follow-up heart rates on outcomes. Hypertensive patients with a heart rate persistently >80 bpm had an increased risk of all-cause and cardiovascular mortality. The highest risk of all-cause mortality was found for a final heart rate of 81–90 bpm and the lowest risk for a final heart rate of 61–70 bpm. Within the cohort of the Cooper Clinic study [19], hypertensive individuals with resting heart rate ≥80 bpm were found to be at greater risk for cardiovascular and all-cause mortality compared with those with hypertension and heart rate <60 bpm.

High heart rate proved to be associated with adverse outcomes also in clinical trials of hypertensive patients. In the Systolic Hypertension in Europe (Syst-Eur) trial [22], elderly patients with HR >79 bpm (top quintile) had a 1.89 greater risk of all-cause mortality and a 1.60 greater risk of cardiovascular mortality than subjects with heart rate below that level. In the hypertensive patients with electrocardiographic left ventricular hypertrophy from the LIFE study, a 10 bpm increment in heart rate was associated with a 25% increased risk of cardiovascular mortality and a 27% greater risk of all-cause death [23]. Follow-up heart rate contributed additional prognostic information because persistence or development of a heart rate ≥84 bpm was associated with an 89% greater risk of cardiovascular death and a 97% increased risk of all-cause mortality. In addition, a significant interaction was found between baseline and follow-up heart rate. Even more important are the results obtained in the patients with hypertension and coronary artery disease from the INternational VErapamil-SR/Trandolapril (INVEST) study [24], in which both baseline and follow-up heart rates after treatment with cardiac slowing drugs were tested in survival analyses. In that study, a 5 bpm increment in baseline resting heart rate was associated with a 6% excess risk in the primary composite outcome (all-cause death, nonfatal myocardial infarction, or nonfatal stroke). However, follow-up heart rate after treatment with atenolol or verapamil showed a stronger association with outcome and excluded baseline heart rate from the final multivariable model. An interesting finding of the INVEST was that the heart rate-risk relationship was not linear, as a tendency to an upturn in risk was observed for the lowest heart rates with a nadir at 59 bpm. The heart rate nadir was 64 bpm for people with prior myocardial infarction. Thus, this study indicated that in coronary patients optimal heart rate target should be around 60 bpm. New information on the clinical importance of high heart rate in hypertension was provided by an analysis of the VALUE study [25], in high-risk hypertensive patients treated with either valsartan- or amlodipine-based therapy. In the VALUE study, patients were stratified according to whether they had high heart rate (top quintile) or lower heart rate and whether their blood pressure was controlled or uncontrolled by antihypertensive treatment. As expected, the highest risk was found in the patients with elevated heart rate and blood pressure uncontrolled by treatment. However, the risk remained high also in the patients whose blood pressure was well controlled but heart rate was elevated. A much lower risk was found in the patients with blood pressure uncontrolled and a low heart rate and the lowest risk in the group with blood pressure well controlled and low heart rate. Thus, this study highlighted the important role of tachycardia in hypertension showing that the risk of hypertensive patients can be lowered only marginally by antihypertensive treatment if their heart rate remains elevated. Also in the ASCOT-BPLA study [26], heart rate measured after 6 weeks was a better predictor of cardiovascular events than baseline heart rate. Heart rate predicted all-cause, non-cardiovascular, and cardiovascular mortality that occurred during the follow-up, but not nonfatal cardiovascular events. Finally, an analysis of the ONTARGET and TRANSCEND studies showed that the risk of cardiovascular mortality increased by 41%–58% among the patients with a heart rate >70 bpm and by 77% in those with heart rate >78 bpm [27]. In recent years, the prognostic significance of heart rate has also been evaluated in patients with resistant hypertension [28]. In multivariable Cox regression, both slow heart rate (<60 bpm for clinic or <55 bpm for nighttime heart rate) and fast heart rate (>75 bpm or >70 bpm, respectively) were associated with worse cardiovascular outcomes in comparison with the reference group (60–75 bpm), indicating that in resistant hypertension there is a U-shaped relationship between heart rate and prognosis [28].

23.4 Ambulatory Versus Clinic Heart Rate

In the abovementioned study by Salles et al., ambulatory heart rates were more significant risk markers than office heart rate [28]. Recent research by others confirms the results of that study. In the ABP-International study, the authors investigated whether heart rate measured with intermittent ambulatory recording was a better predictor of cardiovascular events than office heart rate in 7600 untreated hypertensive patients aged 52 ± 16 years [29]. Data were adjusted for several clinical variables including age, gender, blood pressure, smoking, diabetes, serum total cholesterol, and serum creatinine. In a multivariable Cox model, nighttime heart rate emerged as the strongest predictor of fatal combined with nonfatal events with a hazard ratio of 1.13 (95% CI, 1.04–1.22) for a 10 bpm increment of the nighttime heart rate. When subjects taking beta-blockers during the follow-up (hazard ratio 1.15; 95% CI, 1.05–1.25) or subjects who had an event within 5 years after enrollment (hazard ratio 1.23; 95% CI, 1.05–1.45) were excluded from analysis, the association was even stronger. In the ABP-International study, office heart rate was a weaker predictor of outcome than was ambulatory heart rate, and after inclusion of systolic and diastolic blood pressures as covariates in the model, it was no longer a significant predictor of cardiovascular events. When participants were classified according to the level of office and nighttime heart rate, people with masked tachycardia had a higher risk of cardiovascular events and mortality than people with normal office and nighttime heart rate (Fig. 23.2) [30]. In contrast, participants with white-coat tachycardia did not show an increase in risk. Results from smaller studies confirm that heart rate recorded during sleep is the most accurate predictor of adverse outcome. In a Japanese general population followed for 12 years, both daytime and nighttime heart rates predicted non-cardiovascular disease mortality but not cardiovascular mortality [31]. However, when nighttime heart rate and day-to-night heart rate fall were simultaneously included in the Cox model, only nighttime heart rate independently predicted all-cause mortality with a hazard ratio of 1.29 (95% CI, 1.07–1.54) for a 10 bpm increase in heart rate. In the Syst-Eur study, the positive relationship between clinic heart rate and the incidence of fatal endpoints found in the main study was confirmed in the ambulatory monitoring subgroup, although ambulatory heart rate did not provide prognostic information over and above clinic heart rate [22]. In the IDACO study, daytime heart rate did not predict mortality, but nighttime heart rate predicted all of the mortality outcomes (hazard ratios ≥1.15). In a study of 457 Japanese hypertensive patients followed for 72 months, increased nighttime heart rate and nondipping of heart rate were associated with increased risk of cardiovascular and all-cause

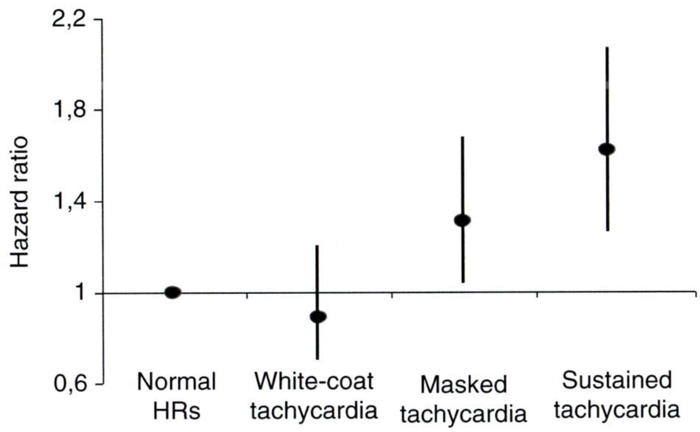

Fig. 23.2 Risk of cardiovascular events in 7602 hypertensive participants from the ABP-International study. Subjects were stratified according to their office and nighttime heart rate (HR). For office heart rate, the cutoff between normal and high heart rate was set at 85 bpm. For nighttime heart rate, the cutoff was set at 73 bpm. Using these cutoffs four different groups were identified: (1) people with normal office and nighttime HRs ($N = 5238$), (2) white-coat tachycardia (high office HR and normal nighttime HR, $N = 998$), (3) masked tachycardia (normal office HR and high nighttime HR, $N = 796$), and (4) sustained tachycardia (high office and nighttime HRs, $N = 570$). The hazard ratios and corresponding two-sided 95% confidence intervals were derived from the regression coefficients in Cox models and were adjusted for age, body mass index, blood pressure, serum glucose, and total serum cholesterol and creatinine concentrations, which were fitted as continuous variables, and for gender, smoking, alcohol intake, and diabetes, which were fitted as categorical variables. Adapted from P. Palatini et al. [30]

mortality, whereas awake heart rate was not [32]. Results obtained with beat-to-beat Holter recordings are in keeping with the above data. In the Copenhagen Holter study [33], average 24 h heart rate, nighttime heart rate, and office heart rate were all associated with all-cause mortality. However, after adjusting for cardiovascular risk factors, the association with resting heart rate and 24 h heart rate disappeared, and only nighttime heart rate remained in the model (hazard ratio, 1.17 (95% CI, 1.05–1.30)). In a comparative analysis of differing heart rate measurement modalities, resting heart rate measured with 24 h Holter recording was found to be marginally superior as a predictor of cardiovascular morbidity and mortality during a 17-year follow-up [33]. In multivariate Cox regression analyses, hazard ratios were 1.02 ($p = 0.079$) for office heart rate, 1.04 ($p = 0.036$) for average of the lowest 3 hourly heart rates, and 1.03 ($p = 0.093$) for mean Holter heart rate for each 10 bpm increment [34]. In conclusion, the majority of the published studies show that ambulatory heart rate, and nighttime heart rate in particular, has a greater prognostic accuracy for cardiovascular and total mortality than office heart rate. A possible explanation is that heart rate during sleep is more representative of the overall hemodynamic load on the arteries and the heart than daytime heart rate and can, thus, better reflect cumulative arterial injury from mechanical stress on the arterial wall. In addition, persistent increased sympathetic activity may be better represented by a high heart rate during sleep than by heart rate measured in the office.

23.5 Pathogenetic Mechanisms

23.5.1 Heart Rate and Physical Fitness

The data from the literature consistently demonstrated that heart rate is a potent predictor of mortality and/or cardiovascular disease in prehypertension and hypertension. However, according to some authors, the relationship between high heart rate and cardiovascular outcomes might be explained by tachycardia merely reflecting poor physical fitness [35–37]. This issue was investigated in several studies which showed that this is unlikely to occur. In the FINRISK Study [38], the effect of resting heart rate toward cardiovascular mortality was determined after excluding people with preexisting coronary heart disease, angina, and heart failure or on antihypertensive therapy. In women, a positive association was observed with a 32% increment in mortality for a 15 bpm increment in heart rate (hazard ratio 1.32, 95% CI, 1.08–1.60). In men, each 15 bpm increase in heart rate was associated with an adjusted hazard ratio of 1.24 (95% CI, 1.11–1.40). It should be pointed out that in this study data were also adjusted for physical activity. Results obtained within the frame of the Cooper Clinic study [19] are in keeping with the above data, showing a protective role of low resting heart rate on all-cause and cardiovascular disease mortality. Patients with a heart rate ≥80 bpm were at greater risk for cardiovascular and all-cause mortality compared with those with heart rate <60 bpm irrespective of physical fitness. Among the unfit individuals, those with high heart rate had the greatest risk of cardiovascular and all-cause mortality, whereas those with low heart rate had a similar risk for cardiovascular and all-cause mortality as the fit with high heart rate. In the Copenhagen Male Study [39], heart rate was inversely related to physical fitness and was associated with mortality in a graded manner also after adjusting for physical fitness, leisure-time physical activity, and other cardiovascular risk factors. In this study, the risk of mortality increased by 16% (95% CI, 10–22%) per 10 bpm increment in heart rate. In conclusion, the above studies showed that elevated heart rate is a risk factor for mortality independent of physical fitness or leisure-time physical activity and that heart rate and cardiorespiratory fitness independently contribute to the risk of mortality. The heart rate-adverse outcome association remained significant after exclusion of people with comorbidities and events occurring within the first years of observation, indicating that the temporal sequence would be compatible with a causal relationship.

23.5.2 Heart Rate and Metabolic Abnormalities

A large number of epidemiologic studies have shown that high heart rate is associated with obesity and metabolic disturbances such as increased glycemia, total cholesterol, triglycerides, and body mass index [34, 40–42]. Longitudinal studies suggest that increased sympathetic tone may be the reason for these associations. Results from the HARVEST study have shown that subjects with sympathetic predominance at heart rate variability developed hypertension, obesity, and metabolic disturbances later in life [43, 44]. In a multivariable Cox regression, baseline clinic heart rate ($P = 0.02$) and follow-up changes in clinic heart rate ($P < 0.001$) were independent predictors of overweight or obesity at the end of a 7-year follow-up. Several cohort studies in Japanese individuals also showed that high heart rate is a precursor of obesity and metabolic abnormalities [45, 46]. Shigetoh et al. [46] found that individuals with baseline heart rate ≥80 bpm had an increased risk of developing obesity, abdominal obesity, metabolic syndrome, and diabetes 20 years later compared to people with heart rate <60 bpm. The adjusted risk was 2.34 (95% CI, 1.09–5.90) for obesity and 5.39 (95% CI, 1.34–21.8) for diabetes. A recent analysis in healthy subjects from the Netherlands Study of Depression and Anxiety (NESDA) showed that several measures of sympathetic activity were predictors of the metabolic syndrome during a 2-year follow-up [47]. In the Chicago Heart Association Detection Project in Industry [48], the adjusted odds of having diabetes after 65 years of age was 1.10 (95% CI, 1.05–1.16) per 12 bpm higher baseline heart rate. In this study, higher heart rate was also associated with diabetes mortality (odds ratio 1.21; 95% CI, 1.03–1.41). A large Japanese study in apparently healthy men and women aged 30–59 years confirmed those findings [49]. In this study, the adverse effects of fast heart rate and high blood pressure were independent of each other as well as of the influences of major risk factors. In the Australian Diabetes, Obesity, and Lifestyle study [50], participants with a heart rate ≥80 bpm were more likely to develop diabetes (odds ratio 1.89; 95% CI, 1.07–3.35) compared with participants with a heart rate <60 bpm. The association between baseline heart rate and future diabetes was also found in a prospective cohort study of patients with clinically manifest vascular diseases from the SMART study [51]. Every 10 bpm increase in heart rate increased the risk for type 2 diabetes (hazard ratio 1.10; 95% CI, 1.00–1.21). The risk was independent of the type of vascular disease or beta-blocker use. The relationship between resting heart rate and metabolic syndrome was also investigated in a large Chinese cohort from Kailuan/Tangshan in a 4-year follow-up [52]. The metabolic syndrome was cross-sectionally associated to resting heart rate with an odds ratio of 1.49 (95% CI, 1.32–1.69) in subjects with heart rate at 95–104 bpm compared with those at 55–64 bpm, after adjusting for confounders and risk factors. In addition, the longitudinal analysis in the participants without metabolic syndrome at baseline showed that heart rate was predictive of the risk of developing the metabolic syndrome 4 years later with a hazard ratio of 1.42 (1.23–1.62) for the top heart rate group compared to the bottom group. Whether a dose-response relationship exists between heart rate and the metabolic syndrome is unclear. This issue was addressed by a recent meta-analysis which used restricted cubic spline function to assess the dose-response relationship [53]. Seven prospective cohort studies and 10 cross-sectional studies with a total of 169,786 participants were included. The pooled relative risk was 2.10 (95% CI 1.80–2.46) for the highest versus reference heart rate category and 1.28 (95% CI 1.23–1.34) for each 10 bpm increment in heart rate. In this study, no evidence was found for a nonlinear dose-response association between heart rate and metabolic syndrome ($P = 0.20$). In conclusion, the above studies demonstrate that high heart rate is a precursor of obesity and metabolic abnormalities and suggest that resting heart rate has a potential for screening subjects at high risk of undiagnosed diabetes.

23.5.3 Role of Autonomic Nervous System in Prehypertension

Why some individuals have a faster resting heart rate than others still remains poorly understood. This is unlikely to be due to an inherently faster cardiac pacemaker, as demonstrated in leading pharmacological studies by Julius et al. [54, 55]. Using intravenous injections of propranolol to block β receptors and atropine to block parasympathetic receptors in a group of healthy volunteers, these authors showed that intrinsic heart rate after blockade was 110 bpm in younger and gradually decreased to about 85 in older individuals [54]. Intrinsic heart rate was measured also in patients with hyperkinetic prehypertension and a group of normotensive subjects of control. In the prehypertensive group, the heart rate remained higher than in the normotensive controls after the β blockade, and addition of parasympathetic blockade with atropine increased heart rate to the same level in the two groups. This experiment showed that tachycardia in prehypertension was due to a different autonomic nervous control of a normal pacemaker. In prehypertensive subjects there was a larger decrease of heart rate after β-blocker administration, and the parasympathetic blockade elicited a smaller increase of heart rate. This indicates that patients with prehypertension have an increased sympathetic and a decreased vagal tone. Tachycardia and sympathetic overactivity are closely intertwined in prehypertension, and both components play an important role in the development of hypertension and cardiovascular disease. Indeed, a body of evidence suggests that fast heart rate is a reliable marker of increased sympathetic activity both in the general population and in hypertensive patients. In the HARVEST study, people with clinical signs of sympathetic predominance at spectral analysis of heart rate variability had a much higher heart rate than people with normal autonomic nervous system tone (Fig. 23.3) [43]. This association was confirmed by Grassi et al., who measured heart rate, plasma catecholamines, and muscle sympathetic nerve activity in four groups of subjects with different clinical characteristics: (1) healthy volunteers (controls), (2) hypertensive patients, (3) obese individuals, and (4) patients with heart failure [56]. In the overall population, a significant correlation of heart rate was found with both markers of sympathetic activity indicating that high heart rate reflects increased sympathetic tone. Hypertension is accompanied not only by increased sympathetic tone but also by reduced parasympathetic activity. In the HARVEST study, young subjects with sympathetic predominance had both an increase in the low-frequency component (mainly marker of sympathetic activity) and the high-frequency component (mainly marker of vagal activity) at spectral analysis of heart rate variability (Fig. 23.3) [43]. A reduced vagal tone in hypertension has also been shown by pharmacological studies [57].

23.5.4 Effect of High Heart Rate on Vascular Wall and Target Organs

Hypertension if left untreated is a self-accelerating condition. In prehypertensive subjects the acceleration is usually slow and nearly linear, but when hypertension

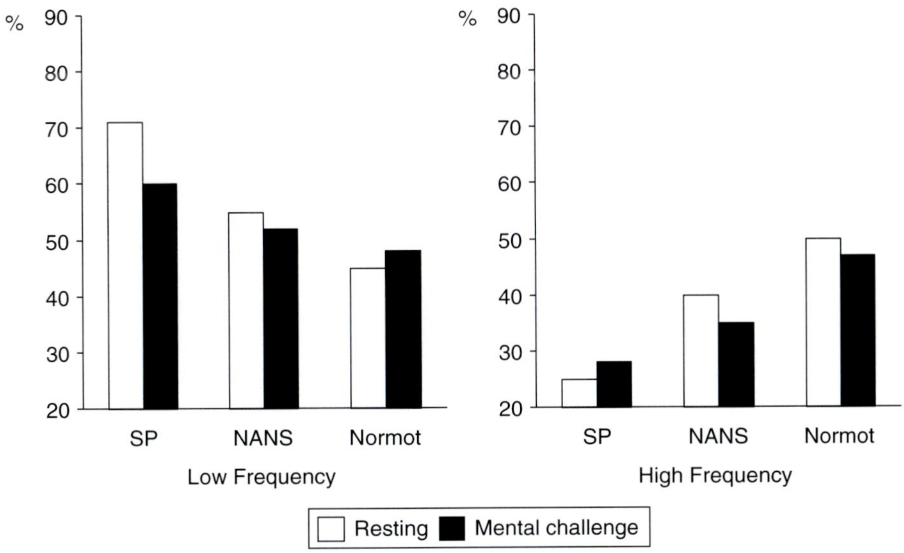

Fig. 23.3 Frequency-domain indexes of heart rate variability in two groups of young-to-middle-age stage 1 hypertensive subjects and a group of normotensive controls (Normot). Group 1, subjects with sympathetic predominance (SP). Group 2, subjects with normal autonomic nervous system activity (NANS). Power spectral densities were computed from 512-s periods by the maximum entropy method using an autoregressive model. Low-frequency power (LF, 0.04–0.15 Hz) and high-frequency power (HF, 0.15–0.40 Hz) are expressed as percent of total power (0.04–0.40 Hz). Parameters of heart rate variability were recorded in resting conditions and during Stroop's color mental test, a computerized conflict-evoking test. For both data obtained at rest and during the mental challenge, there was a progressive decrease of the low-frequency component from the hypertensive subjects with SP to the normotensive subjects of control and a progressive increase in the high-frequency component. Mean ± SEM resting heart rate was 79.1 ± 1.7 bpm in Group 1 and was 67.8 ± 0.9 in Group 2, $p < 0.001$. Adapted from P. Palatini et al. [43]

develops the increase of blood pressure is faster and even becomes exponential due to the blood pressure-induced restructuring of the arterioles. Arteriolar wall thickens because of smooth muscle hypertrophy and arteriolar remodeling with consequent increase of vascular resistance. In addition, high heart rate exposes the arteries to turbulent blood flow chiefly at points where vessels bifurcate [34, 58]. The low shear stress and the increased tensile stress generated by tachycardia favor the development of atherosclerotic plaques and increase the stiffness of large blood vessels [40–42].

The effect of tachycardia on coronary arteries was examined in several studies of cynomolgus monkeys consuming an atherogenic diet [59–63]. Evidence that heart rate lowering might retard coronary atherogenesis was provided by Beere et al. [59] in an elegant experimental study. After ablation of the sinoatrial node in a group of monkeys on atherogenic diet, the heart rate was reduced by about 30%. Monkeys with lowered heart rate were compared with a group whose heart rate was left unchanged. After 6 months of atherogenic diet, the animals were sacrificed, and those in the lower heart rate group had a significantly lower area of coronary atherosclerosis and percentage of stenosis than the group of control. Along the same line of research, Kaplan et al. [60, 61] focused on effect of behavior on coronary atherosclerosis of cynomolgus monkeys and found that aggressive dominant animals developed extensive coronary atherosclerosis. In a second experiment, Kaplan et al. [62] investigated whether treatment with beta-blockers would prevent the increase in coronary lesions in dominant animals. They found that treatment with propranolol actually decreased coronary plaque area only in dominant animals. The pathogenetic role of high heart rate was confirmed by Bassiouny et al. who found a correlation between stress index and the thickness of major atherosclerotic lesions in the infrarenal aorta and iliac arteries in male *Cynomolgus* monkeys [63]. Thus, these animal studies demonstrated that increased heart rate can damage the blood vessels and that heart rate lowering can prevent the atherosclerotic lesions.

More recently, also a study in human beings confirmed those experimental data [64]. In a pooled analysis of four intracoronary ultrasound clinical trials, the volume of coronary atheroma was measured before and after treatment with antihypertensive drugs [64]. In this study, about three quarters of patients were treated with beta-blockers and one quarter with other drugs. Treatment with beta-blockers decreased the volume of coronary atheroma to a larger extent than the other treatments did showing that heart rate reduction can actually reduce coronary atherosclerotic lesions.

Other studies in human beings confirmed the deleterious effects of tachycardia on the coronary arteries. An association between resting heart rate and progression of focal coronary atherosclerosis was described by Huikuri et al. in patients with prior coronary artery bypass surgery [65]. Minimum heart rate measured during 24 h recording was correlated to global severity and rate of progression of coronary atherosclerotic lesions in subjects with myocardial infarction [66].

High heart rate can cause arterial wall lesions and target organ damage also through an increase in arterial stiffness. Heart rate increase with atrial pacing in rats has been shown to produce progressive reduction in carotid distensibility [67]. The same effect was observed in sympathectomized animals suggesting that the increase in heart rate rather than an underlying hyperactivity of the sympathetic nervous system was the responsible factor. The heart rate-arterial stiffness relationship was also shown in human studies which used pulse wave velocity as a marker of stiffness. Albaladejo et al. [68] found a positive correlation between pulse wave velocity and 24 h ambulatory heart rate in subjects with hypertension. In a large multicenter population of normotensive and hypertensive individuals in France, Sa Cunha et al. [69] measured pulse wave velocity and degree of vascular distention at multiple vascular sites. There was a significant correlation of high heart rate with arterial rigidity in the thoracic aorta and lower limbs. The results of studies in which the effect of heart rate manipulation with pacing on pulse wave velocity was evaluated are consistent with the above data. A French [70] and an Australian [71] study showed a progressive increase in carotid-femoral pulse wave velocity with increasing level of heart rate. This effect was independent from the effect of pacing on blood pressure. Also temporal changes in heart rate have been found to be predictive of large artery stiffness [72]. This was shown by Tomiyama et al. in 1795 apparently healthy Japanese subjects (mean age 39 years) in whom heart rate was measured at baseline and also during a 5–6-year follow-up [72]. The authors found that both heart rate at the baseline examination and changes in heart rate during the follow-up period were significantly associated with the corresponding changes in pulse wave velocity even after adjusting for a variety of atherogenic risk factors. These data suggest a synergistic role of high baseline heart rate and of the increase in heart rate during the follow-up in accelerating age-associated increases in arterial stiffness. The stiffening effect of high heart rate on the large arteries is likely to be due to the reduced length of the cardiac cycle associated with tachycardia that does not allow the viscoelastic arterial wall enough time to distend fully [58, 67]. As mentioned above, in addition to low shear stress, each cardiac beat imposes a blood pressure-related tensile stress on the vascular wall. Repeated mechanical load increases the viscosity of the arterial wall which in turn increases the vascular stiffness [67].

There is no doubt that increased vascular stiffness has deleterious effects on the cardiovascular system. This relationship was shown by Laurent et al. [73] in 1980 patients with hypertension followed for an average of 9.3 years. Pulse wave velocity was significantly associated with both all-cause and cardiovascular mortality also in a model adjusted for confounders and risk factors. Similar results were obtained by Willum-Hansen et al. [74] who studied the incidence of fatal and nonfatal cardiovascular endpoints, cardiovascular deaths, and fatal or nonfatal coronary heart disease in a Danish general population followed for 9.4 years. After adjustment for numerous confounders including blood pressure, the pulse wave velocity remained a significant predictor of all endpoints. In a recent meta-analysis [75] of 16 studies involving 17,635 subjects, aortic pulse wave velocity was a highly significant predictor of strokes, coronary artery disease, and all cardiovascular events.

In summary, a body of evidence indicates that increased heart rate exposes the arteries to a larger cumulative stress during the lifetime. The tensile stress induces vascular stiffness, and the low shear stress favors the development of atherosclerotic plaques. As a consequence, people with tachycardia are bound to develop premature and widespread vascular damage.

Not only does elevated heart rate promote development of atherosclerotic plaques and large artery stiffness but it also has a pathogenetic role in precipitating cardiovascular events. This was shown by Heidland and Strauer in a group of patients who underwent two coronary angiograms within 6 months [76]. These authors demonstrated that the hemodynamic stress related to increased heart rate may play a crucial role in coronary plaque disruption [76]. Indeed, after 6 months of follow-up, plaque disruption resulted more common among people with heart rate >80 bpm than in those with lower heart rate. Plaque disruption could be prevented in those subjects who had been administered beta-blockers.

The high sympathetic tone and reduced parasympathetic tone underlying tachycardia can decrease the threshold of ventricular arrhythmias, as demonstrated by Lown and Verrier in dogs with manipulation of autonomic nervous system activity [77]. When sympathetic tone was increased in dogs, the threshold for ventricular fibrillation was reduced, an effect that was abolished by simultaneous vagal stimulation. This mechanism likely accounts for the strong relationship between tachycardia and sudden death found in many epidemiologic studies [78, 79]. An elevated heart rate may facilitate desynchronization of ventricular muscle cells, especially in an ischemic myocardium, increasing oxygen consumption and worsening coronary perfusion [34].

23.6 Should High Heart Rate Be Reduced in Prehypertension?

As mentioned above, elevated heart rate is a common feature in patients with prehypertension and hypertension. Among the young hypertensive subjects participating in the HARVEST study, about one third showed clinical signs of sympathetic predominance at spectral analysis of heart rate variability and increased heart rate [43], a finding consistent with the results obtained in the Tecumseh Study [80]. In the long run, this hemodynamic stress together with the excessive blood pressure load can cause target organ damage. Decreasing blood pressure and heart rate at this point can still reduce the incidence of cardiovascular events, but the underlying atherosclerosis and renal dysfunction will not be reverted. Thus a treatment addressed to prevent target organ damage should be started earlier. As pointed out in a recent document of the European Society of Hypertension, making practical therapeutic suggestions for the hypertensive patients with high heart rate is difficult because of lack of data from clinical trials [81]. In young people with autonomic dysfunction characterized by sympathetic predominance, rather than to merely reduce elevated heart rate and high blood pressure, it would be more rationale to try to restore a normal sympatho-vagal balance. This goal can be achieved by improving subjects' lifestyle.

23.6.1 Lifestyle Measures

Smoking, excessive alcohol consumption, and heavy coffee use increase the sympathetic tone with consequent effects on resting heart rate and blood pressure [34, 82, 83]. Thus improving an unhealthy lifestyle would decrease both these hemodynamic variables. This should be the first goal of a clinician in the management of the hypertensive patient with tachycardia. A dietary intervention addressed to reduce calorie intake in overweight people would improve the tone of the autonomic nervous system and reduce blood pressure and heart rate [84]. Beneficial effects have been shown also by increased consumption of omega-3 fatty acids found in fatty fish and fish oil. Several studies have shown that omega-3 fatty acids may improve parameters of autonomic function including heart rate variability and baroreflex sensitivity [85, 86]. Indeed, omega-3 fatty acids have been reported to cause some beneficial effects on resting heart rate with decreases in the range of 2–4 bpm [85–87].

Besides reducing the consumption of tobacco, alcohol, and caffeinated beverages, a program of regular physical activity should be implemented. Several non-pharmacological interventions have been advocated in people with prehypertension or hypertension such as behavioral therapies (transcendental meditation, other meditation forms, biofeedback, yoga, and other relaxation methods) or non-invasive procedures or devices (acupuncture, device-guided breathing). However, according to a working group of the American Heart Association [88], existing evidence about blood pressure and heart rate lowering exists only for exercise-based regimens. Several studies have shown that dynamic aerobic exercise, dynamic resistance exercise, and even isometric exercise have beneficial effects on blood pressure in hypertension and prehypertension [89, 90]. Regular endurance exercise, in particular, causes a reduction of the sympathetic activity and an increase of vagal tone with a marked reduction in resting heart rate [91–94]. Comparative studies performed with 24 h continuous recording have shown that physically active persons have a ~10 bpm lower heart rate compared to sedentary controls [91]. This effect is comparable to that of beta-blockers. In a study by Meredith et al. [95], hemodynamic changes were associated with a noticeable decrease of sympathetic tone; total norepinephrine spillover to plasma fell by 24%, and the renal norepinephrine spillover decreased by 41%. The antiadrenergic effect of aerobic exercise can explain the effect of regular physical activity on the heart in hypertensive subjects. In a study by Jennings et al., the left ventricular wall thickness decreased by 5.7%, whereas the left ventricle cavity slightly increased [89]. The wall thickness/cavity radius ratio significantly decreased in the exercise group. Several other clinical studies conducted in hypertensive patients have documented a reduction in left ventricular mass and wall thickness after a period of endurance exercise [90]. In the HARVEST study, only 1.7% of the active subjects developed left ventricular hypertrophy during an 8-year follow-up versus 10.3% among the sedentary controls with an adjusted OR of 0.24 (95% CI, 0.07–0.85) [96]. In addition, exercise has a favorable impact on all factors of the insulin resistance syndrome: blood pressure, plasma lipids, serum insulin, and overweight [84, 97]. Regular physical activity has also been found to be associated with a reduction of cardiovascular responsiveness to psychophysiological stressors [98]. In a group of young- to middle-age subjects with stage 1 hypertension, subjects who performed regular physical activity had a smaller blood pressure and heart rate reaction to a psychological stressor and a lower blood pressure increase over time than sedentary subjects [98]. Central autonomic adaptations in response to exercise are likely to be responsible for the reduced hemodynamic responsiveness to psychological stress and might represent a mechanistic pathway for the decreased tendency to develop hypertension in physically active subjects [99]. Thus, adoption of a healthy lifestyle could revert to normal mild elevations of heart rate and blood pressure in young people with hyperkinetic circulation avoiding the use of pharmacological therapy. Exercise thus appears as an important tool for attenuating the negative effect of sympathetic predominance especially in people exposed to high environmental stress. A low-to-moderate exercise intensity program seems to be sufficient for reducing blood pressure in the majority of patients [100]. However, the reduction of heart rate and the favorable metabolic effects of physical training seem to be proportional to the intensity of exercise. For this reason the American

College of Sports Medicine recommends that moderate-to-vigorous activities should be practiced by most healthy individuals [100]. However, low-intensity exercise may be a safer option for many hypertensive patients chiefly for those with a high cardiovascular risk profile.

23.6.2 Pharmacological Treatment

If non-pharmacological measures fail to achieve the desired goal and heart rate remains elevated, a drug treatment addressed to reduce the high heart rate might be considered in hypertensive patients. Unfortunately, the lack of randomized clinical trials on the treatment of high heart rate and the absence of specific recommendations from international guidelines do not allow the clinician to make decisions based on evidence. Another controversial point is the heart rate level that should be used to define tachycardia because the relationship between heart rate and the level of cardiovascular risk in general populations is a continuous one. It follows that the partition level between normal and abnormal values has to be defined according to arbitrary criteria. In most epidemiological studies, a significant increase in risk was found for a heart rate ≥80 bpm [101]. It is therefore obvious that the definition of tachycardia as a heart rate greater than 100 bpm is no longer acceptable for risk stratification. According to some investigators, the upper normal limit for resting heart rate should be the level at which the benefits of treatment outweigh the risks [101]. Unfortunately, no clinical trial has been implemented as yet in hypertension to study the effects of cardiac slowing drugs on morbidity and mortality. Retrospective analyses of patients with myocardial infarction or congestive heart failure have shown that beta-blockers or other bradycardic agents are effective in reducing mortality only in subjects with a high baseline heart rate [102]. Carvedilol has been reported to cause a marked reduction in mortality only in patients with a heart rate >82 bpm [103]. More recent data obtained with the I/f channel antagonist ivabradine indicate that the beneficial effect of this drug can be obtained in patients with heart rate higher than 70 bpm [104, 105]. However, it should be noted that in those studies ivabradine was given on top of beta-blockers, and thus the original heart rate of the patients before treatment was likely to be 10 bpm higher. In summary, the data obtained in epidemiologic studies in general populations and in clinical trials of patients with myocardial infarction or congestive heart failure suggest that the threshold level between normal and high heart rate should be set in the range of 80–85 bpm.

With these caveats in mind, we suggest that cardiac slowing treatment should be considered in hypertensive subjects with high heart rate. As pointed out by a recent document of the European Society of Hypertension, absence of evidence does not mean evidence against the importance of tachycardia as a risk factor for cardiovascular disease [81]. Lifelong exposure to a potentially important risk factor may cause earlier target organ damage and impair the patient's prognosis. Thus, some degree of flexibility with management is expected, and decisions should be made according to the clinical characteristics of the patient and the level of high heart rate.

For these reasons the panel of experts suggested that in some hypertensive patients with tachycardia, especially if they are symptomatic, treatment by available drugs, mostly beta-1 selective beta-blockers, can be considered [81].

References

1. Dyer AR, Persky V, Stamler J, et al. Heart rate as a prognostic factor for coronary heart disease and mortality: findings in three Chicago epidemiological studies. Am J Epidemiol. 1980;112:736–49.
2. Kannel WB, Wilson P, Blair SN. Epidemiological assessment of the role of physical activity and fitness in development of cardiovascular disease. Am Heart J. 1985;109:876–85.
3. Kannel WB, Kannel C, Paffenbarger RS Jr, et al. Heart rate and cardiovascular mortality: the Framingham study. Am Heart J. 1987;113:1489–94.
4. Gillum RF, Makuc DM, Feldman JJ. Pulse rate, coronary heart disease, and death: the NHANES I epidemiological follow-up study. Am Heart J. 1991;121:172–7.
5. Jouven X, Desnos M, Guerot C, et al. Predicting sudden death in the population: the Paris prospective study 1. Circulation. 1999;99:1978–83.
6. Palatini P, Casiglia S, Julius S, et al. Heart rate, a risk factor for cardiovascular mortality in elderly men. Arch Intern Med. 1999;159:585–92.
7. Zhang D, Shen X, Qi X. Resting heart rate and all-cause and cardiovascular mortality in the general population: a meta-analysis. CMAJ. 2016;188:E53–63.
8. Zhang D, Wang W, Li F. Association between resting heart rate and coronary artery disease, stroke, sudden death and noncardiovascular diseases: a meta-analysis. CMAJ. 2016;188:E384–E92.
9. Palatini P, Julius S. Review article: "Heart rate and the cardiovascular risk". J Hypertens. 1997;15:3–17.
10. Ji C, Zheng X, Chen S, et al. Impact of resting heart rate on the progression to hypertension in prehypertension patients. Zhonghua Xin Xue Guan Bing Za Zhi. 2014;42:860–5.
11. Palatini P, Dorigatti F, Zaetta V, et al. Heart rate as a predictor of development of sustained hypertension in subjects screened for stage 1 hypertension: the HARVEST Study. J Hypertens. 2006;24:1873–80.
12. Wang A, Liu X, Guo X, et al. Resting heart rate and risk of hypertension: results of the Kailuan cohort study. J Hypertens. 2014;32:1600–5.
13. Palatini P, Casiglia E, Pauletto P, et al. Relationship of tachycardia with high blood pressure and metabolic abnormalities. A Study with mixture analysis in three populations. Hypertension. 1997;30:1267–73.
14. Farinaro E, Stranges S, Guglielmucci G, et al. Heart rate as a risk factor in hypertensive individuals. The Italian tensiopulse study. Nutr Metab Cardiovasc Dis. 1999;9:196–202.
15. King DE, Everett CJ, Mainous AG, et al. Long-term prognostic value of resting heart rate in subjects with prehypertension. Am J Hypertens. 2006;19:796–800.
16. Ryu M, Bayasgalan G, Kimm H, et al. Association of resting heart rate and hypertension stages on all-cause and cardiovascular mortality among elderly Koreans: the Kangwha cohort study. J Geriatr Cardiol. 2016;13:573–9.
17. Benetos A, Rudnichi A, Thomas F, et al. Influence of heart rate on mortality in a French population. Role of age, gender, and blood pressure. Hypertension. 1999;33:44–52.
18. Gillman MW, Kannel WB, Belanger A, D'Agostino RB. Influence of heart rate on mortality among persons with hypertension: the Framingham study. Am Heart J. 1993;125:1148–54.
19. Saxena A, Minton D, Lee DC, et al. Protective role of resting heart rate on all-cause and cardiovascular disease mortality. Mayo Clin Proc. 2013;88:1420–6.
20. Thomas F, Bean K, Provost JC, et al. Combined effects of pulse pressure and heart rate on cardiovascular mortality. J Hypertens. 2001;19:863–9.

21. Paul L, Hastie CE, Li WS, et al. Resting heart rate pattern during follow-up and mortality in hypertensive patients. Hypertension. 2010;55:567–74.
22. Palatini P, Thijs L, Staessen JA, et al. Predictive value of clinic and ambulatory heart rate for mortality in elderly subjects with systolic hypertension. Arch Intern Med. 2002;162: 2313–21.
23. Okin PM, Kjeldsen SE, Julius S, et al. All-cause and cardiovascular mortality in relation to changing heart rate during treatment of hypertensive patients with electrocardiographic left ventricular hypertrophy. Eur Heart J. 2010;31:2271–9.
24. Kolloch R, Legler UF, Champion A, et al. Impact of resting heart rate on outcomes in hypertensive patients with coronary artery disease: findings from the INternational VErapamil-SR/ trandolapril STudy (INVEST). Eur Heart J. 2008;29:1327–34.
25. Julius S, Palatini P, Kjeldsen S, et al. Usefulness of heart rate to predict cardiac events in treated patients with high-risk systemic hypertension. Am J Cardiol. 2012;109:685–92.
26. Poulter NR, Dobson JE, Sever PS, et al. ASCOT Investigators. Baseline heart rate, antihypertensive treatment, and prevention of cardiovascular outcomes in ASCOT (Anglo-Scandinavian Cardiac Outcomes Trial). J Am Coll Cardiol. 2009;54:1154–61.
27. Böhm M, Schumacher H, Schmieder RE, et al. Resting heart rate is associated with renal disease outcomes in patients with vascular disease: results of the ONTARGET and TRANSCEND studies. J Intern Med. 2015;278:38–49.
28. Salles GF, Cardoso CR, Fonseca LL, et al. Prognostic significance of baseline heart rate and its interaction with beta-blocker use in resistant hypertension: a cohort study. Am J Hypertens. 2013;26:218–26.
29. Palatini P, Reboldi G, Beilin LJ, et al. Predictive value of night-time heart rate for cardiovascular events in hypertension. The ABP-International study. Int J Cardiol. 2013;168:1490–5.
30. Palatini P, Reboldi G, Beilin LJ, et al. Masked tachycardia. A predictor of adverse out come in Hypertension. J Hypertens. 2017;35:487–92.
31. Hozawa A, Inoue R, Ohkubo T, et al. Predictive value of ambulatory heart rate in the Japanese general population: the Ohasama study. J Hypertens. 2008;26:1571–6.
32. Hansen TW, Thijs L, Boggia J, et al. Prognostic value of ambulatory heart rate revisited in 6928 subjects from 6 populations. Hypertension. 2008;52:229–35.
33. Johansen CD, Olsen RH, Pedersen LR, et al. Resting, night-time, and 24 h heart rate as markers of cardiovascular risk in middle-aged and elderly men and women with no apparent heart disease. Eur Heart J. 2013;34:1732–9.
34. Carlson N, Dixen U, Marott JL, et al. Predictive value of casual ECG-based resting heart rate compared with resting heart rate obtained from Holter recording. Scand J Clin Lab Invest. 2014;74:163–9.
35. Palatini P, Julius S. Association of tachycardia with morbidity and mortality: pathophysiological considerations. J Hum Hypertens. 1997;11(S 1):19–27.
36. Menotti A, Mulder I, Nissinen A, et al. Cardiovascular risk factors and 10-year all-cause mortality in elderly European male populations; the FINE study. Finland, Italy, Netherlands, Elderly. Eur Heart J. 2001;22:573–9.
37. Floyd JS, Sitlani CM, Wiggins KL, et al. Variation in resting heart rate over 4 years and the risks of myocardial infarction and death among older adults. Heart. 2015;101:132–8.
38. Cooney MT, Vartiainen E, Laatikainen T, et al. Elevated resting heart rate is an independent risk factor for cardiovascular disease in healthy men and women. Am Heart J. 2010;159:612–9.
39. Jensen MT, Marott JL, Jensen GB. Elevated resting heart rate is associated with greater risk of cardiovascular and all-cause mortality in current and former smokers. Int J Cardiol. 2011;151:148–54.
40. Mancia G, Bousquet P, Elghozi JL, et al. The sympathetic nervous system and the metabolic syndrome. J Hypertens. 2007;25:909–20.
41. Fox K, Borer JS, Camm AJ, et al. Resting heart rate in cardiovascular disease. J Am Coll Cardiol. 2007;50:823–30.
42. Cook S, Togni M, Schaub MC, et al. High heart rate: a cardiovascular risk factor? Eur Heart J. 2006;27:2387–93.

43. Palatini P, Longo D, Zaetta V, et al. Evolution of blood pressure and cholesterol in stage 1 hypertension: role of autonomic nervous system activity. J Hypertens. 2006;24:1375–81.
44. Palatini P, Mos L, Santonastaso M, et al. HARVEST Study Group. Resting heart rate as a predictor of body weight gain in the early stage of hypertension. Obesity (Silver Spring). 2011;19:618–23.
45. Esler M, Straznicky N, Eikelis N, et al. Mechanisms of sympathetic activation in obesity-related hypertension. Hypertension. 2006;48:787–96.
46. Shigetoh Y, Adachi H, Yamagishi S, et al. Higher heart rate may predispose to obesity and diabetes mellitus: 20-year prospective study in a general population. Am J Hypertens. 2009;22:151–5.
47. Licht CM, de Geus EJ, Penninx BW. Dysregulation of the autonomic nervous system predicts the development of the metabolic syndrome. J Clin Endocrinol Metab. 2013;98:2484–93.
48. Carnethon MR, Yan L, Greenland P, et al. Resting heart rate in middle age and diabetes development in older age. Diabetes Care. 2008;31:335–9.
49. Nagaya T, Yoshida H, Takahashi H, et al. Resting heart rate and blood pressure, independent of each other, proportionally raise the risk for type-2 diabetes mellitus. Int J Epidemiol. 2010;39:215–22.
50. Grantham NM, Magliano DJ, Tanamas SK, et al. Higher heart rate increases risk of diabetes among men: the Australian Diabetes Obesity and Lifestyle (AusDiab) Study. Diabet Med. 2013;30:421–7.
51. Bemelmans RH, Wassink AM, van der Graaf Y, et al. SMART Study Group. Risk of elevated resting heart rate on the development of type 2 diabetes in patients with clinically manifest vascular diseases. Eur J Endocrinol. 2012;166:717–25.
52. Jiang X, Liu X, Wu S, et al. Metabolic syndrome is associated with and predicted by resting heart rate: a cross-sectional and longitudinal study. Heart. 2015;101:44–9.
53. Liu X, Luo X, Liu Y, et al. Resting heart rate and risk of metabolic syndrome in adults: a dose-response meta-analysis of observational studies. Acta Diabetol. 2017;54:223–35.
54. Julius S, Pascual AV, London R, et al. Role of parasympathetic inhibition in the hyperkinetic type of borderline hypertension. Circulation. 1971;44:413–8.
55. Julius S, Krause L, Schork NJ, et al. Hyperkinetic borderline hypertension in Tecumseh, Michigan. J Hypertens. 1991;9:77–84.
56. Grassi G, Vailati S, Bertinieri G, et al. Heart rate as marker of sympathetic activity. J Hypertens. 1998;16:1635–9.
57. Bohm R, van Baak M, van Hooff M, et al. Salivary flow in borderline hypertension. Klin Wochenschr. 1985;63(Suppl. 3):154–6.
58. Giannoglou GD, Chatzizisis YS, Zamboulis C, et al. Elevated heart rate and atherosclerosis: an overview of the pathogenetic mechanisms. Int J Cardiol. 2008;126:302–12.
59. Beere PA, Glagov S, Zarins CK. Retarding effect of lowered heart rate on coronary atherosclerosis. Science. 1984;226:180–2.
60. Kaplan JR, Manuck SB, Clarkson TB, et al. Social status, environment, and atherosclerosis in cynomolgus monkeys. Arteriosclerosis. 1982;2:359–68.
61. Kaplan JR, Manuck SB, Clarkson TB, et al. Social stress and atherosclerosis in normocholesterolemic monkeys. Science. 1983;220:733–5.
62. Kaplan JR, Manuck SB, Adams MR, et al. Inhibition of coronary atherosclerosis by propranolol in behaviorally predisposed monkeys fed an atherogenic diet. Circulation. 1987;76:1364–72.
63. Bassiouny HS, Zarins CK, Kadowaki MH, et al. Hemodynamic stress and experimental aortoiliac atherosclerosis. J Vasc Surg. 1994;19:426–34.
64. Sipahi I, Tuzcu EM, Wolski KE, et al. Beta-blockers and progression of coronary atherosclerosis: pooled analysis of 4 intravascular ultrasonography trials. Ann Intern Med. 2007;147:10–8.
65. Huikuri HV, Jokinen V, Syvanne M, et al. Heart rate variability and progression of coronary atherosclerosis. Arterioscler Thromb Vasc Biol. 1999;19:1979–85.
66. Perski A, Olsson G, Laudon C, et al. Minimum heart rate and coronary atherosclerosis: independent relations to global severity and rate of progression of angiographic lesions in men with myocardial infarction at a young age. Am Heart J. 1992;123:609–16.

67. Mangoni AA, Mircoli L, Giannattasio C, et al. Heart rate-dependence of arterial distensibility in vivo. J Hypertens. 1996;14:897–901.
68. Albaladejo P, Asmar R, Safar M, et al. Association between 24 hour ambulatory heart rate and arterial stiffness. J Hum Hypertens. 2000;14:137–41.
69. Sa Cunha R, Pannier B, Benetos A, et al. Association between high heart rate and high arterial rigidity in normotensive and hypertensive subjects. J Hypertens. 1997;15(12 Pt 1):1423–30.
70. Lantelme P, Mestre C, Lievre M, et al. Heart rate: an important confounder of pulse wave velocity assessment. Hypertension. 2002;39:1083–7.
71. Tan I, Spronck B, Kiat H, et al. Heart rate dependency of large artery stiffness. Hypertension. 2016;68:236–42.
72. Tomiyama H, Hashimoto H, Tanaka H, et al. Synergistic relationship between changes in the pulse wave velocity and changes in the heart rate in middle-aged Japanese adults: a prospective study. J Hypertens. 2010;28:687–94.
73. Laurent S, Boutouyrie P, Asmar R, et al. Aortic stiffness is an independent predictor of all-cause and cardiovascular mortality in hypertensive patients. Hypertension. 2001;37:1236–41.
74. Willum-Hansen T, Staessen JA, Torp-Pedersen C, et al. Prognostic value of aortic pulse wave velocity as index of arterial stiffness in the general population. Circulation. 2006;113:664–70.
75. Ben-Shlomo Y, Spears M, Boustred C, et al. Aortic pulse wave velocity improves cardiovascular event prediction: an individual participant meta-analysis of prospective observational data from 17,635 subjects. J Am Coll Cardiol. 2014;63:636–46.
76. Heidland UE, Strauer BE. Left ventricular muscle mass and elevated heart rate are associated with coronary plaque disruption. Circulation. 2001;104:1477–82.
77. Lown B, Verrier RL. Neural activity and ventricular fibrillation. N Engl J Med. 1976;294:1165–7.
78. Schwartz PJ, Priori SG. Sympathetic nervous system and cardiac arrhytmias. In: Zipes DP, Jalife J, editors. Cardiac electrophysiology: from cell to bedside. Philadelphia, PA: WB Saunders Co; 1990. p. 330–43.
79. Hohnloser SH, Klingenheben T, van de Loo A, et al. Reflex versus tonic vagal activity as a prognostic parameter in patients with sustained ventricular tachyardia or ventricular fibrillation. Circulation. 1994;89:1068–73.
80. Julius S, Randall OS, Esler MD, et al. Altered cardiac responsiveness and regulation in the normal cardiac output type of borderline hypertension. Circ Res. 1975;36–37(Suppl. I):I-199–207.
81. Palatini P, Rosei EA, Casiglia E, et al. Management of the hypertensive patient with elevated heart rate: Statement of the Second Consensus Conference endorsed by the European Society of Hypertension. J Hypertens. 2016;34:813–21.
82. Palatini P, Canali C, Graniero GR, et al. Relationship of plasma renin activity with caffeine intake and physical training in mild hypertensive men. HARVEST Study Group. Eur J Epidemiol. 1996;12:485–91.
83. Hering D, Kucharska W, Kara T, et al. Smoking is associated with chronic sympathetic activation in hypertension. Blood Press. 2010;19:152–5.
84. Reid CM, Dart AM, Dewar EM, et al. Interactions between the effects of exercise and weight loss on risk factors, cardiovascular haemodynamics and left ventricular structure in overweight subjects. J Hypertens. 1994;12:291–301.
85. Christensen JH, Korup E, Aarøe J, et al. Fish consumption, n-3 fatty acids in cell membranes, and heart rate variability in survivors of myocardial infarction with left ventricular dysfunction. Am J Cardiol. 1997;79:1670–3.
86. Mozaffarian D, Geelen A, Brouwer IA, et al. Effect of fish oil on heart rate in humans: a meta-analysis of randomized controlled trials. Circulation. 2005;112:1945–52.
87. Dallongeville J, Yarnell J, Ducimetiere P, et al. Fish consumption is associated with lower heart rates. Circulation. 2003;108:820–5.
88. Brook RD, Appel LJ, Rubenfire M, et al. American Heart Association Professional Education Committee of the Council for High Blood Pressure Research, Council on Cardiovascular and Stroke Nursing, Council on Epidemiology and Prevention, and Council on Nutrition, Physical Activity. Beyond medications and diet: alternative approaches to lowering blood pressure: a scientific statement from the American Heart Association. Hypertension. 2013;61:1360–83.

89. Jennings G, Dart A, Meredith I, et al. Effects of exercise and other nonpharmacological measures on blood pressure and cardiac hypertrophy. J Cardiovasc Pharmacol. 1991;17(Suppl 2):S70–4.
90. Palatini P. Cardiovascular effects of exercise in young hypertensives. Int J Sports Med. 2012;33:683–90.
91. Genovesi S, Zaccaria D, Rossi E, et al. Effects of exercise training on heart rate and QT interval in healthy young individuals: are there gender differences? Europace. 2007;9:55–60.
92. Laterza MC, de Matos LD, Trombetta IC, et al. Exercise training restores baroreflex sensitivity in never-treated hypertensive patients. Hypertension. 2007;49:1298–306.
93. Duncan JJ, Farr JE, Upton SJ, et al. The effects of aerobic exercise on plasma catecholamines and blood pressure in patients with mild essential hypertension. JAMA. 1985;254:2609–13.
94. Jennings GL, Chin-Dusting JP, Kingwell BA, et al. Modulation of vascular function by diet and exercise. Clin Exp Hypertens. 1997;19:727–37.
95. Meredith IT, Friberg P, Jennings GL, et al. Exercise training lowers resting renal but not cardiac sympathetic activity in humans. Hypertension. 1991;18:575–82.
96. Palatini P, Visentin P, Dorigatti F, et al. Regular physical activity prevents development of left ventricular hypertrophy in hypertension. Eur Heart J. 2009;30:225–32.
97. Rauramaa R, Halonen P, Vaisanen SB, et al. Effects of aerobic physical exercise on inflammation and atherosclerosis in men: the DNASCO Study: a six-year randomized, controlled trial. Ann Intern Med. 2004;140:1007–14.
98. Palatini P, Bratti P, Palomba D, et al. Regular physical activity attenuates the BP response to public speaking and delays the development of hypertension. J Hypertens. 2010;28:1186–93.
99. O'Sullivan SE, Bell C. The effects of exercise and training on human cardiovascular reflex control. J Auton Nerv Syst. 2000;81:16–24.
100. Garber CE, Blissmer B, Deschenes MR, et al. American College of Sports Medicine. American College of Sports Medicine position stand. Quantity and quality of exercise for developing and maintaining cardiorespiratory, musculoskeletal, and neuromotor fitness in apparently healthy adults: guidance for prescribing exercise. Med Sci Sports Exerc. 2011;43:1334–59.
101. Palatini P. Need for a revision of the normal limits of resting heart rate. Hypertension. 1999;33:622–5.
102. Teo KK, Yusuf S, Furberg CD. Effects of prophylactic antiarrhythmic drug therapy in acute myocardial infarction: an overview of results from randomized controlled trials. JAMA. 1993;270:1589–95.
103. Packer M, Bristow MR, Cohn JN, for the U.S. Carvedilol Heart Failure Study Group. The effect of Carvedilol on morbidity and mortality in patients with chronic heart failure. N Engl J Med. 1996;334:1349–55.
104. Fox K, Ford I, Steg PG, et al. Heart rate as a prognostic risk factor in patients with coronary artery disease and left-ventricular systolic dysfunction (BEAUTIFUL): a subgroup analysis of a randomised controlled trial. Lancet. 2008;372:817–21.
105. Swedberg K, Komajda M, Bohm M, et al. Ivabradine and outcomes in chronic heart failure (SHIFT): a randomised placebo-controlled study. Lancet. 2010;376:875–85.

24 The Role of the Brain in Prehypertension

Stevo Julius

Chronic BP elevation induces changes in the structure and function of cardiovascular organs. Consequently, pathophysiologic studies of advanced hypertension are likely to reveal a mixture of causes and consequences of the high BP. Therefore, we focused on young patients with marginal BP elevation (prehypertension). It was assumed that in these subjects it may be possible to detect mechanisms which precede the evolution of advanced hypertension.

In early studies we used invasive methods for assessment of hemodynamics. A catheter was introduced into the brachial vein and advanced near to or in (80%) the right atrium to inject indocyanine green dye. In parallel a short catheter was placed in the brachial artery to measure the dye dilution curve with a densitometer. The intra-arterial BP was monitored throughout the study.

Using this method, we confirmed previous reports [1–4] that prehypertension is associated with a hyperkinetic state of increased cardiac output and fast heart rates. By year 1976 we accumulated invasive hemodynamic data on 145 participants with prehypertension and 90 healthy normotensive volunteers [5]. About one third of the prehypertensive group had tachycardia (Fig. 24.1). Another graph in the same study showed a similarly skewed distribution of cardiac output in the prehypertension group.

In an early study [6], we compared the hemodynamic characteristics of normotension and borderline hypertension (prehypertension). At rest in a recumbent position, the vascular resistance values of normotension and borderline hypertension groups overlapped. But when the resistance was compared in relation to cardiac output, the borderline hypertensives had higher vascular resistance. In other words, patients with prehypertension were not capable to adequately dilate to accommodate the increased cardiac output. This suggested that the circulation in prehypertension

S. Julius
Michigan Medicine, Frankel Cardiovascular Center, University of Michigan, Ann Arbor, MI, USA
e-mail: sjulius@umich.edu

R. Zimlichman et al. (eds.), *Prehypertension and Cardiometabolic Syndrome*, Updates in Hypertension and Cardiovascular Protection,
https://doi.org/10.1007/978-3-319-75310-2_24

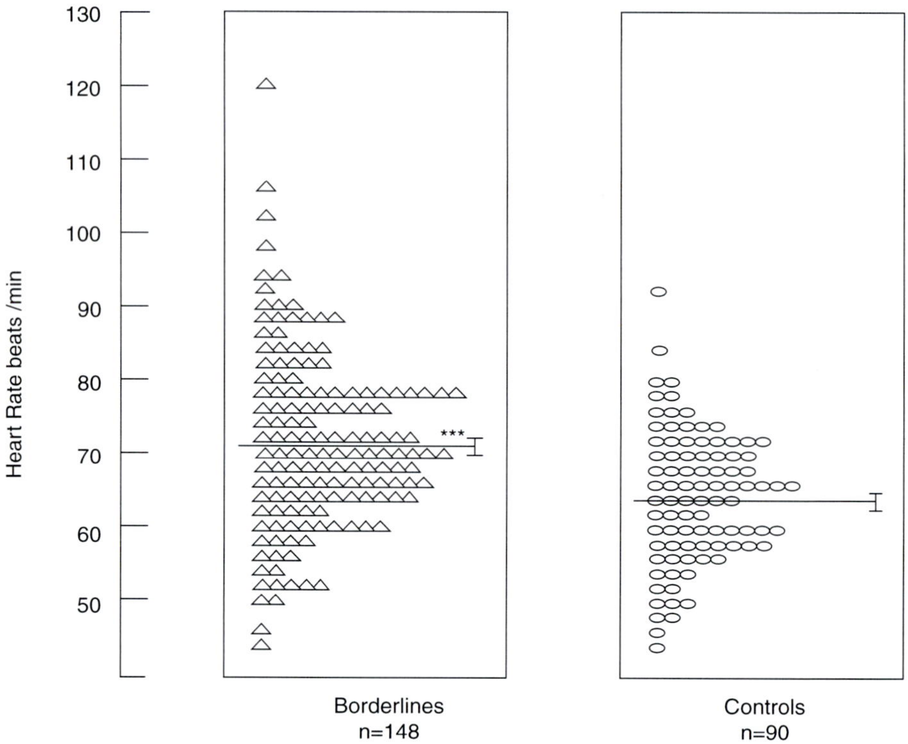

Fig. 24.1 Distribution of the heart rate after 10 min of rest in recumbent position in young men (18–35 years). (Figure reprinted with permission from Julius S, Esler MD, editors. The nervous system in arterial hypertension. Springfield: Charles C Thomas; 1976. Library of Congress Card Number 74-30203, ISBN: 0-398-03377-3)

is not normal and that it resembles the characteristically increased vascular resistance of established hypertension.

In another study [7], we injected intravenously large doses of first propranolol (0.2 mg/kg) and second atropine (0.04 mg/kg) to completely block the autonomic nervous system receptors both in prehypertension and healthy volunteers. Injection of propranolol elicited a larger than normal decrease of heart rate and cardiac output which was indicative of an increased sympathetic tone in prehypertension. After atropine a lesser increase of heart rate and cardiac output was seen in the prehypertension group. Thus the parasympathetic tone in prehypertension was decreased (Fig. 24.2).

The fact that both sympathetic and parasympathetic tones were involved demonstrated that the aberration emanated from the medulla oblongata where the sympathetic and parasympathetic tone are regulated in a reciprocal fashion. Furthermore, the blockade erased the difference in heart rate and cardiac output between the two groups. Thus the hyperkinetic circulation in prehypertension was entirely neurogenic.

However, the blockade did not erase the increase of BP in prehypertension. Prior to injection the BP elevation was associated with a high cardiac output, and after the blockade, it was due to high vascular resistance [8].

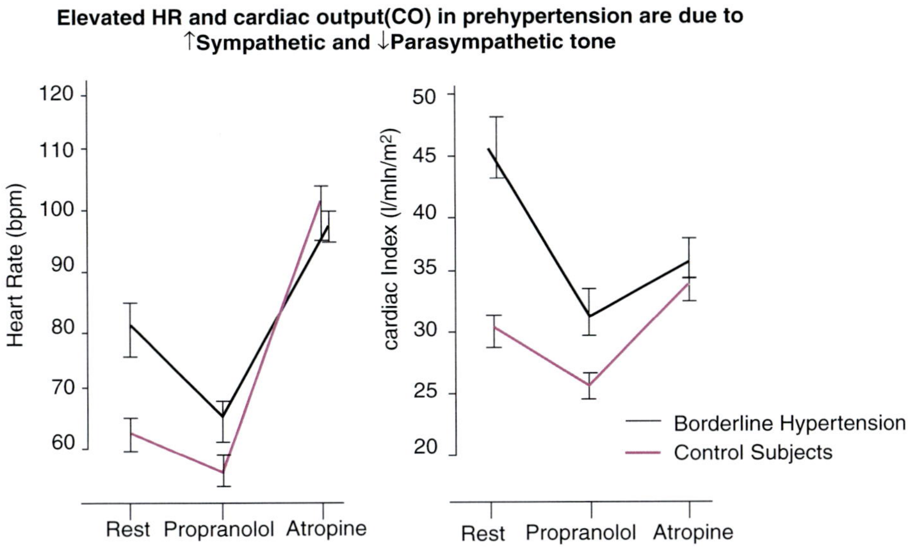

Fig. 24.2 Response to intravenous injection of propranolol (0.2 mg/kg) followed by 0.04 mg/kg of atropine in patients with hyperkinetic borderline hypertension (n = 14, average age 23 years) (n + 88) and in paid volunteers (n = 16, average age 24 years). (Figure reprinted with permission from Julius S, Esler MD, editors. The nervous system in arterial hypertension. Springfield: Charles C Thomas; 1976. Library of Congress Card Number 74-30203, ISBN: 0-398-03377-3)

This hemodynamic plasticity in which the BP level is maintained while the underlying hemodynamic changes is well documented. The comparison of hemodynamic responses to various stressors is shown in Figs. 24.3 and 24.4.

The bold diagonal lines in the graph are iso-resistance lines. The mean BP is represented on the ordinate, and the cardiac output index is shown on the abscissa. Prehypertension is marked by triangle and healthy volunteers are shown by circles. Figure 24.3 shows stressors which increase the cardiac output. The left panel is the response to mild exercise (4 min on a load of 300 kg-m/min), and the right is the effect of expansion of plasma volume by infusion 5% dextran in saline 13 mL/kg over a period of 45 min.

In both instances there was a substantial increase of cardiac index and a decrease of vascular resistance in both groups. The BP in the prehypertension remained elevated, and the response lines of the prehypertension and volunteer groups were perfectly parallel.

Stimuli which increased the vascular resistance are shown in Fig. 24.4. In the left panel, measurements were taken at baseline and 10 min after injection of propranolol. In the right panel, measurements were taken in recumbence and after 4 min of sitting.

Both after propranolol and after sitting, the prehypertension group maintained a higher BP level, and the trends of BP changes in prehypertension and control group were similar. Note the hemodynamic plasticity in the graph. At baseline the higher BP in prehypertension was associated with a high cardiac output. The blockade abolished the difference in cardiac output, and at that point, the higher BP in the prehypertension was linked to an increase of vascular resistance.

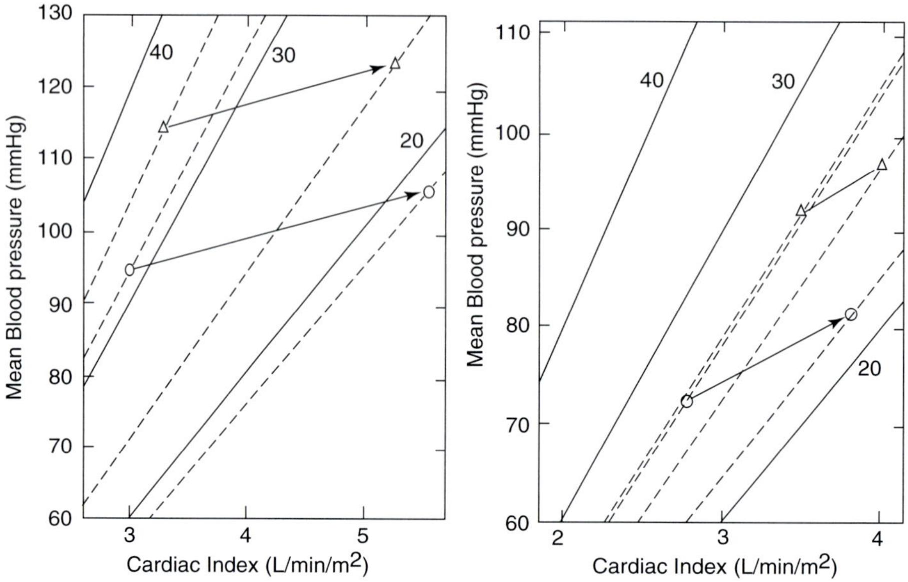

Fig. 24.3 Hemodynamic response to mild exercise and plasma volume expansion in borderline hypertension (n = 77) and in paid volunteers (n = 88). (Figure reprinted with permission from Julius S, Esler MD, editors. The nervous system in arterial hypertension. Springfield: Charles C Thomas; 1976. Library of Congress Card Number 74-30203, ISBN: 0-398-03377-3)

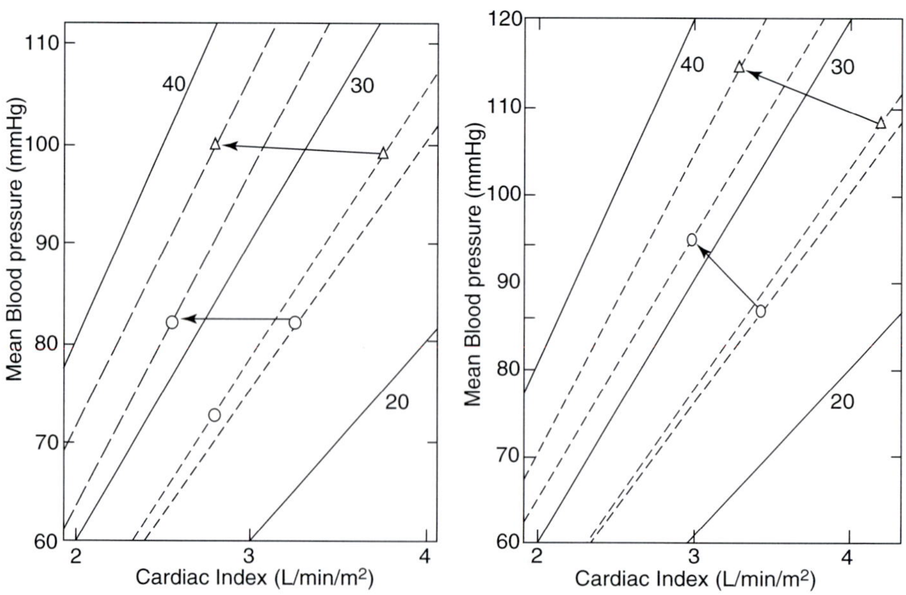

Fig. 24.4 Hemodynamic response to sitting up after recumbent position (right panel) and after injection of propranolol (left panel). (Figure reprinted with permission from Julius S, Esler MD, editors. The nervous system in arterial hypertension. Springfield: Charles C Thomas; 1976. Library of Congress Card Number 74-30203, ISBN: 0-398-03377-3)

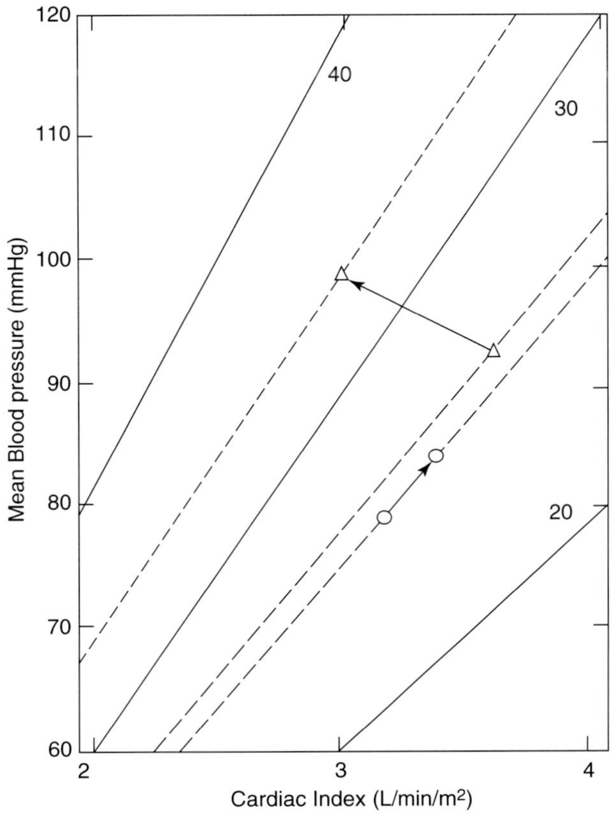

Fig. 24.5 In this experiment subjects remained recumbent and received an injection of propranolol. Circles represent the healthy volunteers (n = 17) and triangles represent the borderline hypertensives (n = 18). Arrows indicate the trends after an injection of atropine was added to propranolol in order to chemically denervate the heart. (Figure reprinted with permission from Julius S, Esler MD, editors. The nervous system in arterial hypertension. Springfield: Charles C Thomas; 1976. Library of Congress Card Number 74-30203, ISBN: 0-398-03377-3)

The effect of total cardiac receptor blockade with propranolol and atropine is shown in Fig. 24.5. There was a remarkable difference in hemodynamic adjustment in the two groups. The prehypertensives maintained the BP elevation by increasing the vascular resistance, whereas the control group responded by a modest increase of cardiac output.

The evidence above proves that the brain seeks a certain preset BP level in the two groups; higher in prehypertension and lower in healthy volunteers. If the BP goal cannot be achieved by changes in cardiac output, it will be attained by a raise of vascular resistance.

This hemodynamic plasticity appears to be the "modus operandi" of the brain under many other circumstances. In a series of experiments, we investigated the BP increase with hindquarter compression in dogs [9]. In these experiments an inflatable suit was placed on the hindquarter of the animals. When inflated, the suit compresses the dog's hind limbs, and this elicited a large increase of mean BP (+30–40 mm Hg). This increase lasted as long as the suit was inflated (up to 3 h), but after deflation the BP instantly returned to normal values. The BP elevation was neurogenic and could be abolished by spinal anesthesia. The BP surge after compression was invariably due to increased vascular resistance. In a group of dogs, we injected the alpha-blocker phenoxybenzamine [10] to prevent

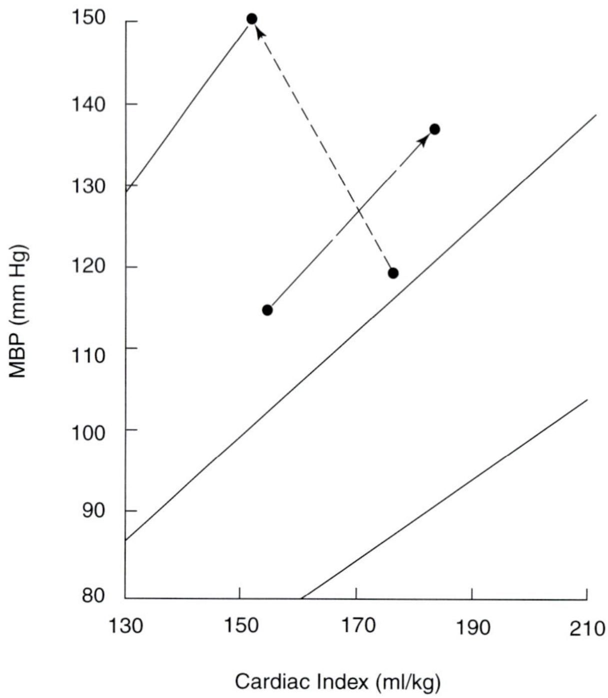

Fig. 24.6 The blood pressure (BP) of eight dogs after hindquarter compression. Compression reproducibly causes huge BP increases (+60 mmHg). The increase is neurogenic since it is abolished with spinal anesthesia. Invariably the compression BP increase is associated with increased vascular resistance (broken line). After vasoconstriction was prevented with alpha adrenergic blockade the BP increase was associated with an increase of cardiac output (solid line). (Figure reprinted with permission from Julius S, Esler MD, editors. The nervous system in arterial hypertension. Springfield: Charles C Thomas; 1976. Library of Congress Card Number 74-30203, ISBN: 0-398-03377-3)

vasoconstriction (Fig. 24.6). The broken line shows that prior to the injection, the increase of BP was associated with an increase of vascular resistance. As the solid line shows, after the alpha-adrenergic, the BP increase blockade did not abolish the BP response, but at that point, the BP surge was linked to an increase of cardiac output.

This hemodynamic plasticity is ubiquitous, and in paper titled "Blood Pressure Seeking Property of the Central Nervous System" [11], we reviewed the ample evidence in the literature that the magnitude of BP increase will be preserved regardless of the underlying hemodynamics.

All evidence about the role of the brain in prehypertension shown so far was obtained by invasive hemodynamic measurement. However, the validity of such findings was challenged already in 1960 by ED Freis [1]. He confirmed that two thirds of patients with hypertension have increased peripheral resistance. He wondered "*whether (in) the remaining one third the elevated cardiac output is the primary hemodynamic fault or whether apprehension associated with the procedure disturbed the basal hemodynamic state*." This notion that the hyperkinetic state is a sign of passing nervousness was embraced by many practicing physicians. Such attitude ignored the contemporary existing solid evidence that transient tachycardia is a predictor of hypertension and of adverse cardiovascular outcomes [12]. Evidence that tachycardia is a strong cardiovascular risk factor continues to accumulate and has been more recently reviewed [13].

The objection that our findings may reflect the stress caused the invasive measurement could not be rejected out of hand. After assessing the validity of various noninvasive methods of measurement of cardiac output [14, 15], we chose the echo-Doppler technique for the Tecumseh field study [16]. The study investigated the evolution of hypertension in a sample of the healthy village population. Of 691 healthy villagers (average age 32.6 years), 99 had a clinic BP reading exceeding 140/90 mm Hg. Thirty-seven percent of these subjects with prehypertension had hyperkinetic circulation.

Besides finding a similar prevalence of hyperkinetic prehypertension with noninvasive as with invasive methods, the field study in Tecumseh provided additional information about the pathophysiology and natural history of the hyperkinetic state. Hyperkinetic prehypertensives had significantly elevated plasma norepinephrine values. Their parents had significantly increased BP levels. We had access to previous BP measurement, and the present hyperkinetic prehypertensives had elevated BP at 5, 8, 21, and 23 years of age. A subgroup with "pure" hyperkinetic state at 32 years of age had tachycardia at 7 and 22 years of age [17]. Thus rather than having a passing BP elevation, individuals with hyperkinetic state had a lifelong increase of BP and heart rate.

In conclusion, one third of young adults have a neurogenic prehypertension characterized by increased BP and tachycardia. In such patients sympathetic stimulation is increased, whereas the parasympathetic inhibition is decreased. This suggests that the aberration emanates from the medulla oblongata where the sympathetic and parasympathetic tones are integrated in a reciprocal fashion. In achieving the higher BP goal, the brain shows a remarkable plasticity; if the stressor is associated with increased cardiac output and that increase is blocked (by beta-blockers), an equal BP increase will be achieved by a higher vascular resistance. Similarly, if the original stressor induced increased vascular resistance and this was blocked (with alpha-blockers), the same degree of BP elevation will be achieved by increased cardiac output.

There is no evidence of increased BP variability in hyperkinetic prehypertension, and such patients are not hyper-responders to various stressors.

Overall these findings prove that the brain plays an important role in the pathophysiology of one third of subjects with prehypertension.

References

1. Freis ED. Hemodynamics of hypertension. Physiol Rev. 1960;40:27–54.
2. Eich RH, Peters RJ, Cuddy RP, et al. The hemodynamics of labile hypertension. Am Heart J. 1962;63:188–95.
3. Widimski J, Fejfarova MH, Fejfar Z. Changes of cardiac output in hypertensive disease. Cardiologia. 1957;31:381–9.
4. Finkielman S, Worcel M, Agrest A. Hemodynamic patterns in essential hypertension. Circulation. 1965;31:356–68.

5. Julius S. Neurogenic component in borderline hypertension. Chapter 14. In: Julius S, Esler MD, editors. The nervous system in arterial hypertension. Springfield: Charles C Thomas Publisher; 1976.
6. Julius S, Conway J. Hemodynamic studies in patients with borderline blood pressure elevation. Circulation. 1968;38:282–8.
7. Julius S, Pascual A, London S. Role of parasympathetic Inhibition in the hyperkinetic type of borderline hypertension. Circulation. 1971;44:413–8.
8. Julius S, Pascual AV, Sannerstedt R, Mitchel C. Relationship between cardiac output and peripheral resistance in borderline hypertension. Circulation. 1971;43:382–90.
9. Osterziel K, Julius S, Brant DO. Blood pressure elevation during hindquarter compression in dogs is neurogenic. J Hypertens. 1984;2:411–7.
10. Julius S, Sanchez R, Brant D. Pressure increase to external hind quarter compression in dogs: a facultative regulatory response. J Hypertens. 1986;4:54–6.
11. Julius S. The blood pressure seeking property of the central nervous system. J Hypertens. 1988;6:177–85. Editorial review.
12. Levy RL, White PD, et al. Transient tachycardia; prognostic significance alone and in association with transient hypertension. Med Press Egypt. 1946;38:207–12.
13. Palatini P, Julius S. Association of tachycardia with morbidity and mortality: pathophysiological considerations. J Hum Hypertens. 1997;11:S19–27.
14. Ferguson RJ, Faulkner JA, Julius S, Conway J. Comparison of cardiac output determined by CO_2 rebreathing and dye dilution methods. J Appl Physiol. 1968;25:450–4.
15. Kiowski W, Randall OS, Steffens TG, Julius S. Reliability of echocardiography in assessing cardiac output. A comparative study with a dye dilution technique. Klin Wochenschr. 1981;59:1115–20.
16. Julius S, Jamerson K, Mejia A, Krause L, Schork N, Jones K. The association of borderline hypertension with target organ changes and higher coronary risk Tecumseh blood pressure study. JAMA. 1990;264:354–8.
17. Julius S, Jamerson K. Sympathetics, insulin resistance and coronary risk in hypertension: the 'chicken-and-egg' question. J Hypertens. 1994;12:495–502. Editorial review.

The Role of the Brain in Neurogenic Prehypertension

25

Gino Seravalle, Dagmara Hering, Guido Grassi, and Krzysztof Narkiewicz

25.1 Introduction

Prehypertension has gained significant recognition over the past decade due to its strong association with an increased risk for CV mortality, mostly from myocardial infarction (MI) and coronary artery disease (CAD). The excess risk for CV events and organ damage has been particularly evident in stage 2 prehypertension (i.e. high-normal BP), the group more likely to develop hypertension when compared to stage 1 prehypertension. The mechanisms underlying the pathophysiology of prehypertension, and the resultant associated risk and poor prognosis remain multifactorial, involving complex interplay between neural mechanisms, haemodynamics, environmental factors and genetics. Evidence indicates that neurogenic component with the activation of the renin-angiotensin system (RAS) and sympathetic nervous system (SNS) lies in the development of prehypertension, its transition to hypertension and adverse CV complications. Patients with prehypertension commonly display the presence of traditional risk factors (i.e. weight gain, hiperinsulinaemia, insulin resistance, dyslipidaemia), circulating markers (i.e. high levels of adipokines, inflammatory cytokines) and underlying metabolic abnormalities which

G. Seravalle
Cardiology Department, Istituto Auxologico Italiano IRCCS Ospedale San Luca, Milano, Italy

D. Hering · K. Narkiewicz (✉)
Department of Hypertension and Diabetology, Medical University of Gdansk, Gdansk, Poland
e-mail: knark@gumed.edu.pl

G. Grassi
Clinica Medica, Department of Medicine and Surgery, University Milano-Bicocca, Milan, Italy

IRCCS Multimedica, Milan, Italy

R. Zimlichman et al. (eds.), *Prehypertension and Cardiometabolic Syndrome*, Updates in Hypertension and Cardiovascular Protection,
https://doi.org/10.1007/978-3-319-75310-2_25

potentiate sympathetic activation, thereby playing a triggering role in BP elevation, subclinical organ damage, progression to hypertension and further disease continuum. In this context, identifying subjects with prehypertension, mainly in the upper end of BP readings and concomitant CV risk, is crucial in prevention of hypertension and CV events.

25.2 Definition

In the past, patients with occasionally elevated BP values were classified as having so-called '*labile* hypertension' and excessive BP variability. Only in the '70, with the absence of clear evidence of a greater BP-related variability, the term 'labile' was replaced with 'borderline hypertension' [1]. The JNC5 (Fifth Joint National Committee on Prevention, Detection, Evaluation, and Treatment of High Blood Pressure) and JNC6 [2] for the first time introduced the term high-normal BP with referring values of 130–139/85–89 mmHg. This term and BP range was also maintained in the European Society of Hypertension (ESH) guidelines [3]. Thus, over the last three decades both definitions with the same BP values have been used.

25.3 Heredity

Starting from the observation that normotensive subjects with a family history of hypertension were characterized by higher BP values and increased adrenergic tone than those observed in subjects without a positive familiar history [4], research was focused on the possible influence of inherited genes.

To this aim, a large cross-sectional study on identical and non-identical twins, their siblings and family members was performed [5]. Prehypertensives had a heritability for systolic BP (44.6%, $p < 0.001$) and demonstrated a significant release in plasma norepinephrine by 65% ($p < 0.001$) and heart rate by 62% ($p < 0.001$). A similar impact was observed for cardiac index and systemic vascular resistance index. As shown in Fig. 25.1 an increase in LV dP/dT max, an index of cardiac contractility is significantly higher in prehypertensive and hypertensive subjects when compared to normotensives suggesting that more than 50% of changes in SBP could be accounted for this haemodynamic parameter. A role of the autonomic nervous system in the pathogenesis of prehypertension and progression to the hypertensive state is well recognized along with genetically determined haemodynamic traits.

Genes are increasingly involved in the pathogenesis of hypertension, however the results are still limited. Although some studies identified numerous causative genes implicated in the progression of the hypertensive state [6–8], there is a need to continue with future human genomic studies

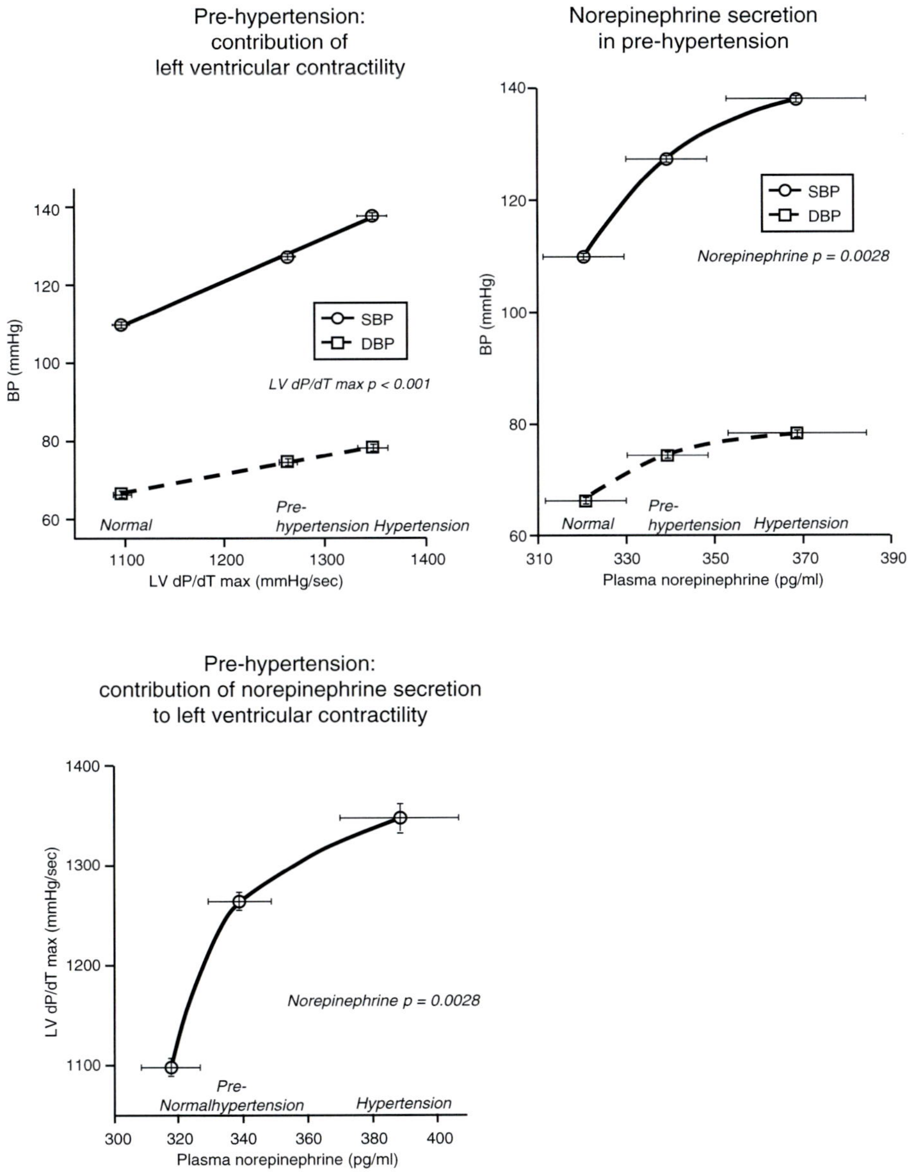

Fig. 25.1 Systolic (S) and diastolic (D) blood pressure (BP) as a function of left ventricular (LV) contractility (max change in pressure divided by change in time) in normotensive, prehypertensive and hypertensive subjects (upper left panel); average plasma norepinephrine levels versus average SBP and DBP in the three groups (upper right panel); average plasma norepinephrine levels versus average LV function (lower panel). Modified from Ref. [5] with the permission

25.4 Prehypertension as a Risk Factor

The relationship between BP and CV risk is well established. Evidence from prospective longitudinal studies documented that the rise in BP from a threshold of 115/75 mmHg increases the risk for premature CV morbidity and mortality, particularly death from cardiac and cerebral events [9]. The Framingham Study has shown that prehypertension is associated with a higher risk of MI and CAD [10]. While the link between prehypertension and atherothrombotic brain infarction (ABI) was not observed in the Framingham Study, in line with previous findings there was a close association between systolic BP and ABI in prehypertensive participants [10].

Further evidence for the relationship between prehypertension and disease progression was examined in the population-based autopsy Hisayama Study [11]. Accordingly, categorized BP levels in the prehypertensive state were significantly associated with the severity of renal arteriosclerosis that was irrespective of the presence or absence of target organ damage, or of the size of intrarenal arteries [11]. These findings suggest that subjects with prehypertension should be considered as high-risk population even in the absence of end-organ damage.

Interestingly, a recent population-based study demonstrated that increased diastolic BP (80–89 mmHg) during late pregnancy (maternal prehypertension at 36 gestational weeks) adversely influences maternal perfusion of the placenta leading to foetal outcomes (i.e. a small-for-gestational-age, stillbirth) when compared to normotensive women (<80 mmHg) [12]. However, the risk of stillbirth was not associated with the rise in diastolic BP from early to late pregnancy.

Given the aforementioned findings it appears that BP levels in the prehypertensive state per se confer an increased prognostic risk with or without the evidence for subclinical organ damage. Subjects with high-normal BP have a greater prevalence of adverse risk factors when compared to normotensives including an increase in body weight or obesity, metabolic syndrome, glycaemic and lipid abnormalities, and are more often smokers [13] which additively and synergistically contribute to established hypertension and CV disease. The presence of organ damage in high-normal BP is not uncommon and includes cardiac (i.e. LVH, diastolic dysfunction, decreased coronary flow reserve), vascular (endothelial dysfunction, arterial stiffness) and renal damage (microalbuminuria, reduced glomerular filtration rate) which are likely to potentiate further risk and disease progression [14]. The Trial of Preventing Hypertension (TROPHY) was first controlled clinical trial that established the safety and efficacy of an angiotensin receptor blocker for reducing BP and preventing or delaying progression to hypertension in subjects with high-normal BP [15]. However, despite available evidence for increased CV risk in stage 2 prehypertension, the initiation of BP lowering therapy in this cohort continues to be under debate.

Although one in three to four adults of the healthy population can be categorized as having high-normal BP, it should be noted that not all individuals with prehypertension are at comparable absolute risk [14]. Further randomized clinical trials are urgently required whether treating high-normal BP may improve CV endpoints in this cohort.

25.5 Tracking Phenomenon

Tracking phenomena is an important longitudinal characteristic of BP changes in response to haemodynamics and metabolic alterations, vascular remodeling and underlying neural mechanisms which play a critical role in BP rise over time; the transition from normal BP values via prehypertensive state to established hypertension. A previous study found that plasma noradrenaline levels predicted subsequent BP elevation and weight gain in lean normotensive men followed annually over 5 years [16] suggesting a cause-and-effect relationship between sympathetic activation and BP. Direct recordings of muscle sympathetic nerve activity (MSNA) measured in subjects with prehypertension have shown that MSNA tracking corresponds with BP changes over time suggesting that tonic activation is likely to influence time-related increase in resting BP and development of sustained hypertension in prehypertension [17]. As illustrated in Fig. 25.2, subjects with prehypertension have increased their systolic BP (Fig. 25.2a) and MSNA (Fig. 25.2b) over an 8-year period and one participant developed hypertension and MI between baseline and follow-up. A separate subject developed hypertension and received antihypertensive treatment over the course of study, and he subsequently had a MI 2 years after study completion (Fig. 25.2a, b). Moreover, in this prehypertensive cohort pulse wave velocity was directly associated with MSNA after 8 years that was independent of BP, body mass index (BMI), heart rate, waist circumference and age suggesting that arterial stiffness and sympathetic activation are possible mechanisms underlying the associated increased risk, likely contributing to poor CV outcomes. This, however, needs to be further explored.

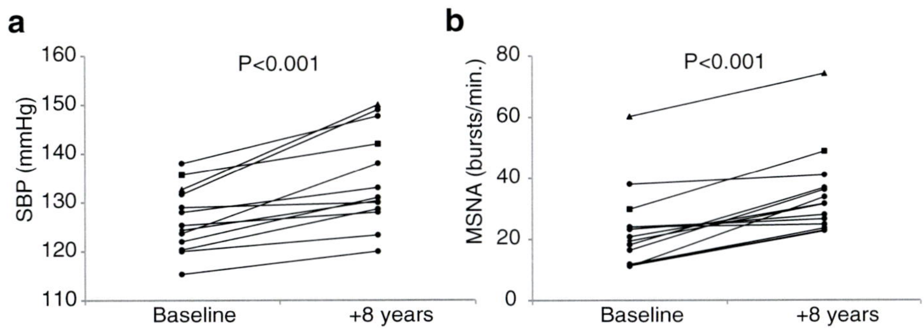

Fig. 25.2 Individual changes in office systolic blood pressure (SBP) at baseline and after 8 years (**a**) and corresponding individual changes in muscle sympathetic nerve activity (MSNA) at baseline and after 8 years in all subjects with prehypertension (**b**). One subject (square) developed hypertension and a MI between baseline and follow-up. A separate subject (triangle) developed hypertension and received antihypertensive treatment (beta-blocker) over the course of the study, and subsequently had a MI 2 years after study completion (at 10 years of follow-up). Modified from Ref. [17] with the permission

25.6 Mechanisms Related to Prehypertension

25.6.1 Autonomic and Reflex Function

The contribution of adrenergic influence to the prehypertensive state has been supported by findings from several studies [5, 18, 19]. While a role of white-coat or masked hypertension has been frequently suggested as a causative factor for the increase in adrenergic tone and BP levels in the prehypertensive state [20–22], other mechanisms including reflex and metabolic appear to be involved with a particular relevance not only in the early stage but also in sustaining its progression to an established condition. As shown in Fig. 25.3 (left panel) prehypertensive state is characterized by BP values greater than those observed in subjects with normal or optimal BP levels and this was associated with a significant increase in sympathetic nerve traffic directly recorded to skeletal muscle (right panel). The dissociation observed between the unchanged heart rate and the peripheral nerve traffic could be related to the fact that the hyperadrenergic tone affects only the peripheral CV system. This hypothesis, however, is not confirmed by the finding that the low-frequency component of the heart rate variability signal is increased in subjects with high-normal BP [23]. It is also possible to speculate that, on the basis of previous studies [24, 25] in hypertension, heart rate may represent an insensitive marker of the overall CV adrenergic activity, due to its predominant parasympathetic control. It is also evident that the baroreflex modulation of the sinus-node activity is already impaired in high-normal BP state suggesting that the baroreflex heart rate control is a very early phenomenon and the effects are already evident with minimal changes in BP values (Fig. 25.4) [18].

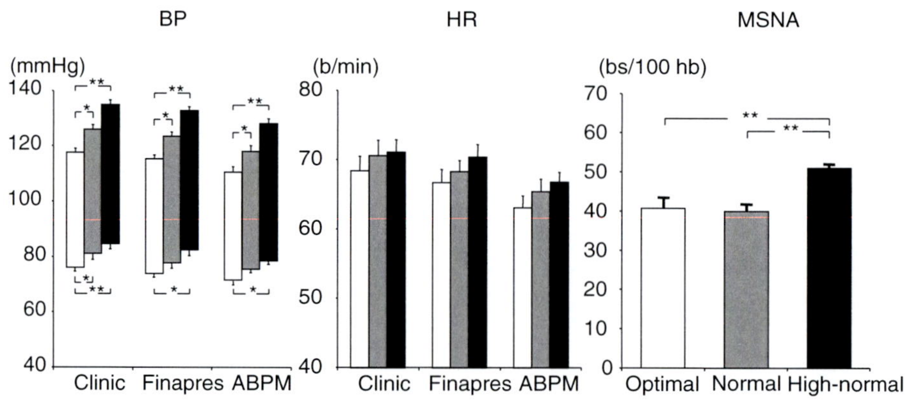

Fig. 25.3 Clinic, beat-to-beat (Finapres) and ambulatory (ABPM) blood pressure (BP) values in optimal (open bars), normal (grey bars) and high-normal (black bars) BP (right panel); Clinic, Finapres and ABPM heart rate in the three groups (middle panel); muscle sympathetic nerve activity corrected for heart rate (MSNAc) in the three groups (left panel). $*p < 0.05$, $**p < 0.01$ refer to the level of statistical significance between groups. Modified from Ref. [9] with the permission

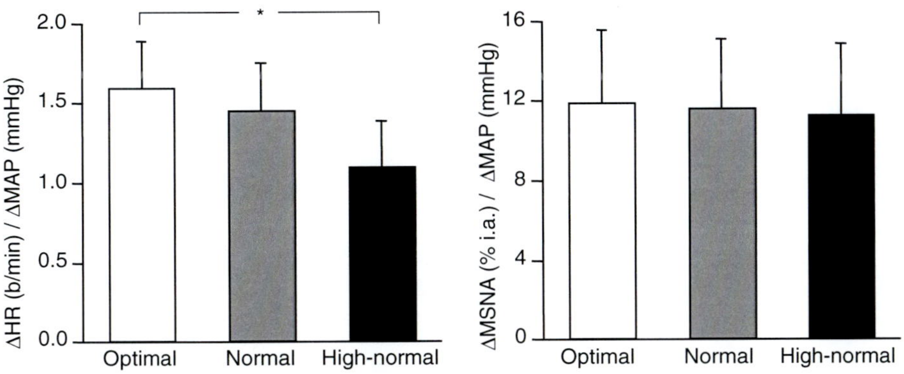

Fig. 25.4 Sensitivities of baroreceptor-heart rate (HR) and baroreceptor-muscle sympathetic nerve activity (MSNA) expressed as average ratios between changes in HR or in MSNA and changes in mean blood pressure (BP) in the three groups of subjects as indicated and explained statistically in Fig. 25.3. Modified from Ref. [9] with the permission

25.6.2 Metabolic Changes

This hyperadrenergic state observed in prehypertensives or high-normal BP subjects is likely to sustain as a result of several confounders including white-coat reaction or masked hypertension, or non-dipping status, or psychological stress [26, 27]. Nevertheless, the factor more involved appears to be a metabolic one indicating that is a greater increase in plasma insulin levels and the relative insulin resistance state (Fig. 25.5) [18]. It has also been observed that among prehypertensives there is a predominance of those with BMI over 25 [28–30], however the potential influence of birth weight and gestational age are still debated [31, 32]. Family history of hypertension and obesity represents a risk of suffering from prehypertension 2.25 times higher compared to the risk in those with a lower BMI. The increase in BMI is associated with hyperinsulinaemia and insulin resistance, and is accompanied by other alterations including hyperleptinaemia, hypercortisolaemia, vascular alterations, activation of the RAS and natriuretic peptide activity [33].

25.6.3 Haemodynamics Characteristics

Old studies have shown that in the earlier stage of the hypertensive state the major haemodynamic determinants were high cardiac output with normal peripheral vascular resistance, often accompanied by an increase in heart rate and inappropriate high oxygen consumption [34–36]. This condition is sustained by the hyperadrenergic tone through stimulation of peripheral metabolic receptors and simultaneous enhancement of α-adrenergic tone. Decreased baroreceptor sensitivity has been hypothesized to be an underlying cause of haemodynamic changes observed in these subjects [4, 18, 37, 38]. Normotensive subjects with persistence of the hyperkinetic state are two or three times more likely to develop hypertension [39]. To explain the

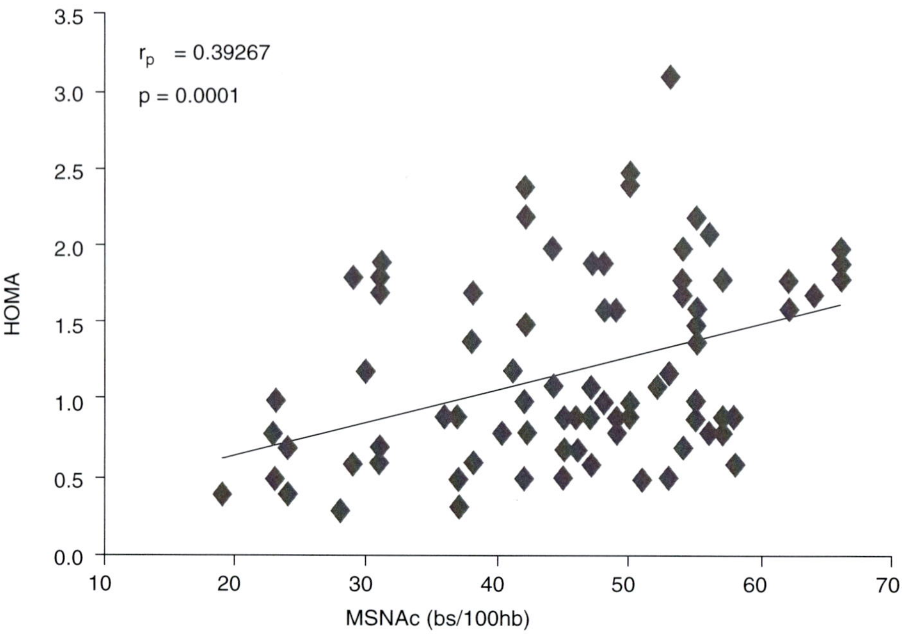

Fig. 25.5 Relationship between muscle sympathetic nerve activity (MSNA) corrected for heart rate and HOMA-IR in the three groups of subjects shown in Fig. 25.3, considered as a whole. Correlation coefficient (*r*) and *P* values are shown. Modified from Ref. [9] with the permission

transition from hyperkinetic state to established hypertension it is necessary to hypothesize a mechanism through which cardiac output decreases and vascular resistance increases with concomitant normalization of markers associated with enhanced adrenergic tone. It is more likely that, starting from hyperkinetic state, the decrease in cardiac output in the course of hypertension depends on both the elevated BP and enhanced sympathetic tone. The enhanced sympathetic tone is also responsible for the down-regulation of cardiac β-adrenergic receptors [40]. The reduction in stroke volume depends on both a decrease in cardiac compliance and an inadequate myocardial relaxation, thereby contributing to a reduction in left ventricular filling [41].

25.6.4 Vascular Changes

Starting from the concept of Folkow [42], it has been show that the development of hypertension is accompanied by a progressive increase in vascular resistance. The vascular hypertrophy is an adaptive phenomenon of the resistance vessels that carry on a progressive thickening of the smooth muscle of the media. This results in an increase in wall/lumen ratio, vascular resistance and hyperresponsiveness to the vasoconstrictive stimuli, thus amplifying the resistance [43–46]. These structural alterations have been shown to be associated with CV functional alterations including an early impairment of the left ventricular diastolic function, a reduced arterial distensibility and an increased vascular inflammation [47]. It has also been shown that high-normal BP state is associated with a cluster of CV and metabolic risk factors including an impaired glucose tolerance and dyslipidemia, conditions that are associated with neurogenic activation [48, 49]. Recent results based on non-invasive evaluation of structural characteristics of retinal microcirculation have shown that in high-normal BP state the alterations of microcirculatory patterns are of early appearance in the clinical course of this condition and systolic BP and pulse pressure appear to be the major determinants of these structural changes. Data obtained from ambulatory BP monitoring have demonstrated the inverse relationship between night-time systolic BP and arteriolar/venular ratio suggesting the relevance of nocturnal BP overload for the microcirculatory vascular alterations [46]. The neurogenic influence to peripheral vessels is well documented in different districts. It consists of vasoconstriction that can selectively or differently increase peripheral vascular resistance maintaining or increasing BP values to allow organs to be adequately perfused in circumstances in which perfusion is required [50, 51]. Removal of sympathetic activity is accompanied by an increase in arterial distensibility indicating that sympathetic activity exerts an influence on the arterial function both in small and large vessels [51].

25.6.5 Brain Mechanisms

There is growing evidence to indicate that the link between hypertension and the brain may be bidirectional [52]. It has been suggested that essential hypertension may influence cerebral functioning early in its course or even that the brain regulatory dysfunction may be a cause of elevated BP [53]. This concept has been supported by magnetic resonance imaging (MRI) studies linking exaggerated BP reactivity to altered brain activation patterns in response to psychological stress in normotensive subjects [54–56]. Very recently, a study which applied fMRI has demonstrated that compensatory functional reorganization (neuroplasticity) in patients with established hypertension may precede structural brain damage [57]. Whether these functional changes are limited to overt clinical hypertension or they can be detected in the group of high-normotensive individuals remain to be elucidated.

Conclusions

Prehypertensive state is characterized by chronic sympathetic activation, likely to contributing to disease progression, adverse CV events in this cohort and preceding the development of established hypertension. Although the transition from prehypertension to hypertension and the strong association with increased CV morbidity and mortality have been well documented, the initiation of BP lowering therapy is not considered in prehypertension, and it is not even recommended in new-onset hypertension with low to moderate CV risk prior to at least 3 months lifestyle modification. Given the alarming increase in the disease burden, randomized clinical trials with prolonged observation are urgently needed to determine the effectiveness of antihypertensive therapy on CV outcomes patients, particularly in subjects with high-normal BP.

Acknowledgments *Conflict of Interest disclosures*: none.

Each author does not have any personal or financial relationships that have any potential to inappropriately influence the manuscript; there are no financial or other potential conflicts of interest including involvement with any organization with a direct financial, intellectual, or other interest in the manuscript. In addition there are no grants and sources of financial support related to the topic of the manuscript.

The authors of this manuscript have certified that they comply with the Principles of Ethical Publishing.

References

1. Julius S, Schork MA. Borderline hypertension—a critical review. J Chronic Dis. 1971;23:723–54.
2. The sixth report of the Joint National Committee on prevention, detection, evaluation, and treatment of high blood pressure. Arch Intern Med. 1997;157:2413–46.
3. Mancia G, De Backer G, Dominiczak A, et al. 2007 Guidelines for the management of arterial hypertension: the task force for the management of arterial hypertension of the European Society of Hypertension (ESH) and the European Society of Cardiology (ESC). J Hypertens. 2007;25:1105–87.
4. Yamada Y, Miyajima E, Tochikubo O, Matsukawa T, Shionoiri H, Ishii M, Kaneko Y. Impaired baroreflex changes in muscle sympathetic nerve activity in adolescents who have a family history of essential hypertension. J Hypertens. 1988;6:S525–8.
5. Davis JT, Rao F, Naqshbandi D, Fung MM, Zhang K, Schork AJ, Nievergelt CM, Ziegler MG, O'Connor DT. Autonomic and hemodynamic origins of prehypertension: central role of heredity. J Am Coll Cardiol. 2012;59:2206–16.
6. Zhang M, Ardile K, Wacholder S, Weich R, Chanock S, O'Brien TR. Genetic variations in CC chemokine receptors and hypertension. Am J Hypertens. 2006;19:67–72.
7. Delles C, McBride MW, Graham D, Padmanabhan S, Dominiczak AF. Genetics of hypertension: from experimental animals to humans. Biochim Biophys Acta. 2010;1802:1299–308.
8. Hottenga JJ, Whitfield JB, de Geus EJ, Booms DI, Martin NG. Heritability and stability of resting blood pressure in Australia twins. Twin Res Hum Genet. 2006;9:205–9.
9. Lewington S, Clarke R, Qizilbash N, Peto R, Collins R, Prospective Studies C. Age-specific relevance of usual blood pressure to vascular mortality: a meta-analysis of individual data for one million adults in 61 prospective studies. Lancet. 2002;360(9349):1903–13.
10. Qureshi AI, Suri MF, Kirmani JF, Divani AA, Mohammad Y. Is prehypertension a risk factor for cardiovascular diseases? Stroke. 2005;36(9):1859–63.
11. Ninomiya T, Kubo M, Doi Y, Yonemoto K, Tanizaki Y, Tsuruya K, et al. Prehypertension increases the risk for renal arteriosclerosis in autopsies: the Hisayama Study. J Am Soc Nephrol. 2007;18(7):2135–42.
12. Wikstrom AK, Gunnarsdottir J, Nelander M, Simic M, Stephansson O, Cnattingius S. Prehypertension in pregnancy and risks of small for gestational age infant and stillbirth. Hypertension. 2016;67(3):640–6.
13. Greenlund KJ, Croft JB, Mensah GA. Prevalence of heart disease and stroke risk factors in persons with prehypertension in the United States, 1999–2000. Arch Intern Med. 2004;164(19):2113–8.
14. Julius S, Nesbitt SD, Egan BM, Weber MA, Michelson EL, Kaciroti N, et al. Feasibility of treating prehypertension with an angiotensin-receptor blocker. N Engl J Med. 2006;354(16):1685–97.
15. Egan BM, Julius S. Prehypertension: risk stratification and management considerations. Curr Hypertens Rep. 2008;10(5):359–66.
16. Masuo K, Kawaguchi H, Mikami H, Ogihara T, Tuck ML. Serum uric acid and plasma norepinephrine concentrations predict subsequent weight gain and blood pressure elevation. Hypertension. 2003;42(4):474–80.

17. Hering D, Kara T, Kucharska W, Somers VK, Narkiewicz K. Longitudinal tracking of muscle sympathetic nerve activity and its relationship with blood pressure in subjects with prehypertension. Blood Press. 2016;25(3):184–92.
18. Seravalle G, Lonati L, Buzzi S, Cairo M, Quarti trevano F, Dell'Oro R, Facchetti R, Mancia G, Grassi G. Sympathetic nerve traffic and baroreflex function in optimal, normal, and high-normal blood pressure states. J Hypertens. 2015;33:1411–7.
19. Julius S, Feldstein CA. Prehypertension: definitions, clinical significance and therapeutic approaches—to treat or not to treat? In: Berbari E, Mancia G, editors. Special issue on hypertension: Springer-Verlag; 2012. p. 3–12.
20. Smith PA, Graham LN, Mackintosh AF, Stoker JB, Mary DA. Sympathetic neural mechanisms in white-coat hypertension. J Am Coll Cardiol. 2002;40:126–33.
21. Grassi G, Seravalle G, Trevano FQ, Dell'Oro R, Bolla GB, Cuspidi C, et al. Neurogenic abnormalities in masked hypertension. Hypertension. 2007;50:537–42.
22. Fagard RH, Stolarz K, Kuznestova T, Seidlerova J, Tikhonoff V, Grodzicki T, et al. Sympathetic activity assessed by power spectral analysis of heart rate variability in white-coat, masked and sustained hypertension versus true normotension. J Hypertens. 2007;25:2280–5.
23. Pal GK, Adithan C, Dutta TK, Amudharaj D, Pravati P, Nandan PG, et al. Assessment of sympathovagal imbalance by spectral analysis of heart rate variability in prehypertensive and hypertensive patients in Indian population. Clin Exp Hypertens. 2011;33:478–83.
24. Grassi G, Esler M. How to assess sympathetic activity in humnans. J Hypertens. 1999;17:719–34.
25. Grassi G, Vailati S, Bertinieri G, Seravalle G, Stella ML, Dell'Oro R, Mancia G. Heart rate as a marker of sympathetic activity. J Hypertens. 1998;16:1635–9.
26. Flaa A, Eide IK, Kjeldsen SE, Rostrup M. Sympathoadrenal stress reactivity is a predictor of future blood pressure: an 18-year follow-up study. Hypertension. 2008;52:336–41.
27. Wilkinson DJ, Thompson JM, Lambert GW, Jennings GL, Schwarz RG, Jefferys D, Turner AG, Esler MD. Sympathetic activity in patients with panic disorder at rest, under laboratory mental stress, and during panic attacks. Arch Gen Psychiatry. 1998;55:511–20.
28. Vasan R, Larson M, Leip E, Kannel W, Levy D. Assessment of frequency of progression to hypertension in non-hypertensive participants in the Framingham Heart Study: a cohort study. Lancet. 2001;358:1682–6.
29. Ishikawa Y, Ishikawa J, Ishikawa S, Kayaba K, Nakamura Y, Shimada K, et al. Prevalence and determinants of prehypertension in a Japanese general population: the Jichi Medical School Cohort Study. Hypertens Res. 2008;31:1323–30.
30. Tirosh A, Afek A, Rudich A, Percik R, Gordon B, Ayalon N, et al. Progression of normotensive adolescents to hypertensive adults. A study of 26980 teenagers. Hypertension. 2010;56:203–9.
31. Barker DJ, Winter PD, Osmond C, Margetts B, Simmonds SJ. Weight in infancy and death from ischemic heart disease. Lancet. 1989;2:577–80.
32. Heijzer-veen MG, Finken MJ, Nauta J, Dekker FW, Hille ET, Frolich M, et al. Is blood pressure increased 19 years after intrauterine growth restriction and preterm birth? A prospective follow-up study in the Netherlands. Pediatrics. 2005;116:725–31.
33. Grassi G, Seravalle G, Cattaneo BM, Bolla GB, Lanfranchi A, Colombo M, Giannattasio C, Brunani A, Cavagnini F, Mancia G. Sympathetic activation in obese normotensive subjects. Hypertension. 1995;25:560–3.
34. Lund-Johansen P. Hemodynamic in early essential hypertension. Acta Med Scand. 1967;482:1–105.
35. Frolich ED, Kozul VJ, Tarazi RC, Dustan HP. Physiological comparison of labile and essential hypertension. Circ Res. 1970;26:55–69.
36. Julius S, Pascual A, Sannerstedt R, Mitchell C. Relationship between cardiac output and peripheral resistance in borderline hypertension. Circulation. 1971;43:382–90.
37. Takeshita A, Tanaka S, Kuroiwa A, Nakamura M. Reduced baroreceptor sensitivity in borderline hepertension. Circulation. 1975;51:738–42.
38. Eckberg DL. Carotid baroreflex function in young men with borderline blood pressure elevation. Circulation. 1979;59:632–6.

39. Levy RL, White PD, Stroud WD, Hillman CC. Transient tachycardia: prognostic significance alone and in association with transient hypertension. JAMA. 1945;129:585–8.
40. Trimarco B, Volpe M, Ricciardelli B, et al. Studies of the mechanisms underlying impairment of beta-adrenoceptor-mediated effects in human hypertension. Hypertension. 1983;5:584–90.
41. Julius S, Randall OS, Esler MD, Kashima T, Ellis CN, Bennett J. Altered cardiac responsiveness and regulation in the normal cardiac output type of borderline hypertension. Circ Res. 1975;36–37(Suppl. I):I-199–207.
42. Folkow B. Physiological aspects of primary hypertension. Physiol Rev. 1982;62:347–503.
43. Mulvany MJ, Hansen PK, Aalkjaer C. Direct evidence that the greater contractility of resistance vessels in spontaneously hypertensive rats is associated with a narrowed lumen, a thickened media, and an increased number of smooth muscle cell layer. Circ Res. 1978;43:854–64.
44. Schiffrin EL. Remodeling of resistance arteries in essential hypertension and effects of antihypertensive treatment. Am J Hypertens. 2004;17:1192–200.
45. Izzard AS, Rizzoni D, Agabiti Rosei E, Heagerty AM. Small artery structure and hypertension: adaptative changes and target organ damage. J Hypertens. 2005;23:247–50.
46. Grassi G, Buzzi S, Dell'Oro R, Mineo C, Dimitriadis K, Seravalle G, Lonati L, Cuspidi C. Structural alterations of the retinal microcirculation in the "prehypertensive" high-normal blood pressure state. Curr Pharmaceutical Des. 2013;19:2375–81.
47. Psaty BM, Arnold AM, Olson J, et al. Association between levels of blood pressure and measures of subclinical disease multiethnic study of atherosclerosis. Am J Hypertens. 2006;19:1110–7.
48. Haffner SM, Miettinen H, Gaskill SP, Stern MP. Metabolic precursors of hypertension. The San Antonio Heart Study. Arch Intern Med. 1996;156:1994–2001.
49. Bo S, Gambino R, Gentile L, et al. High-normal blood pressure is associated with a cluster of cardiovascular and metabolic risk factors: a population-based study. J Hypertens. 2009;27:102–8.
50. Mancia G, Luscher TF, Shepherd JT, Noll G, Grassi G. Cardiovascular regulation: basic considerations. In: Willerson JT, Cohn JN, Wellens HJJ, Holmes Jr DR, editors. Cardiovascular medicine. London: Springer-Verlag; 2007. p. 1525–36.
51. O'Rourke MF. Vascular impedance in studies of arterial and cardiac function. Physiol Rev. 1982;62:570–623.
52. Jennings JR, Zanstra Y. Is the brain the essential in hypertension? Neuroimage. 2009;47(3):914–21.
53. Jennings JR, Heim AF. From brain to behavior: hypertension's modulation of cognition and affect. Int J Hypertens. 2012;2012:701385.
54. Gianaros PJ, Jennings JR, Sheu LK, Derbyshire SW, Matthews KA. Heightened functional neural activation to psychological stress covaries with exaggerated blood pressure reactivity. Hypertension. 2007;49(1):134–40.
55. Gianaros PJ, Sheu LK, Remo AM, Christie IC, Crtichley HD, Wang J. Heightened resting neural activity predicts exaggerated stressor-evoked blood pressure reactivity. Hypertension. 2009;53(5):819–25.
56. Ryan JP, Sheu LK, Gianaros PJ. Resting state functional connectivity within the cingulate cortex jointly predicts agreeableness and stressor-evoked cardiovascular reactivity. Neuroimage. 2011;55(1):363–70.
57. Naumczyk P, Sabisz A, Witkowska M, Graff B, Jodzio K, Gasecki D, et al. Compensatory functional reorganization may precede hypertension-related brain damage and cognitive decline: a functional magnetic resonance imaging study. J Hypertens. 2017;35(6):1252–62.

Part IV

Risk Assessment in Prehypertension

26 Blood Pressure and Atherosclerosis: Subclinical Arteriosclerosis as an Early Sign of Organ Damage

Raimund Erbel, Nils Lehmann, Andreas Stang, Sofia Churzidse, Susanne Moebus, and Karl-Heinz Jöckel

The atherosclerotic continuum, as V Dzau [1, 2] described it, starts with endothelium dysfunction leading to pathological vasomotion followed by early Stary stage I and II lesions, the so-called fatty streaks, followed by intermediate lesions, Stary III [3]. These first stages are regarded as normal aging process variants characterized by the accumulation of lipids in lipid droplets which form more and more a lipid core, creating an atheroma (Stary IV) [4]. With increasing collagen content the atheroma transforms to a fibroatheroma (Stary V).

The coronary artery remodeling process compensates for any luminal narrowing as long as the plaque area does not exceed 40% or 60%, when the vessel circumference is measured according to pathological anatomical studies [5]. According to intravascular ultrasound studies the remodeling threshold for the plaque area can be regarded to be in the range of 45–50% [6–9].

The remodeling phenomenon, today called the Glagov phenomenon, is the main reason why luminograms like coronary angiography are not able to detect early signs of the vessel wall atherosclerosis [5, 6, 10, 11]. Other techniques like scintigraphy, echocardiography, as well as stress electrocardiography remain normal as long as the luminal narrowing is not limiting the coronary flow, meaning the myocardial perfusion [12–16]. When the plaque size exceeds the critical level of 40–50%, coronary angiography can detect some "wall irregularities," often called "minor irregularities" or "nonsignificant" luminal changes. "Significant" coronary stenosis are defined as > 70–75% luminal narrowing in single plane and 90–95% stenosis in biplane quantitative coronary angiography with a minimal luminal

R. Erbel (✉) · N. Lehmann · A. Stang · S. Moebus · K.-H. Jöckel
Institute for Medical Informatics, Biometry and Epidemiology, University Hospital Essen, University Duisburg-Essen, Essen, Germany
e-mail: erbel@uk-essen.de

S. Churzidse
Medizinische Klinik I, Herzzentrum Niederrhein, Helios Hospital Krefeld, Essen, Germany

R. Zimlichman et al. (eds.), *Prehypertension and Cardiometabolic Syndrome*, Updates in Hypertension and Cardiovascular Protection,
https://doi.org/10.1007/978-3-319-75310-2_26

diameter of <1 mm (QCA) [17, 18]. In such lesions the plaque area exceeds 90% related to the vessel area. Even after successful percutaneous coronary interventions (PCI) plaque area remains to be >70% of the vessel size, when balloon angioplasty is used [19, 20].

Acute myocardial infarction, sudden death, and unstable angina are part of the acute coronary syndrome and seem to have an identical pathogenesis. Pathological-anatomical studies have shown that plaque rupture (65%) or erosion (35%) with repetitive micro-emboli and resulting micro-infarcts are leading to the acute events [21, 22]. In few cases calcified noduli are found [23]. Depending on the degree of thrombus formation—mural or occlusive thrombi—non-ST segment or ST segment elevation infarction occurs. If the cardiac biomarkers remain normal, unstable angina is present.

If the lipid core in an eccentric plaque (atheroma or fibroatheroma) reaches >40% in a remodeled segment of an artery, a critical, vulnerable, state is reached, which is usually accompanied by a thinning of the fibrous cap to 60–80 μm or less, reduction of the content of smooth muscle cells but increase of macrophages in the fibrous cap, and neo-revascularization of the adventitia [21–24]. An additional factor has been identified, because plaque hemorrhage of vasa vasorum seems to support plaque progression and instability [25]. Plaque rupture and healing occur repetitively, can be subclinical and explain plaque progression [26]. Multiple signs of rupture and healing are frequently found in sudden death cases [26]. Plaque regression is, however, characterized by a reduction of the lipid content, core and increase of fibrotic tissue, a change of plaque composition [27].

Calcium is found first intracellulary, then extracellulary starting with Stary type III, reaching 10% of the plaque composition. Lipid part present another 10%, fibrotic tissue, however, 70%, and other tissue make up 10% [24]. Calcium in the coronary artery wall can be detected noninvasively, which is known since introduction of chest X-ray and fluoroscopy. Computed tomography (CT) allows not only the detection but also the localization and quantification of coronary artery calcification (CAC) [28]. Thus, CT provides the best available noninvasive technique for detection of signs of subclinical coronary atherosclerosis, even before any symptoms occur due to luminal narrowing.

In the current presentation, the role of subclinical atherosclerosis measured by CT will be analyzed in the context of arterial hypertension based on the results of the Heinz Nixdorf Recall (HNR) study [29–32].

26.1 Coronary Artery Calcification

Previously electronic beam CT was used for CAC imaging worldwide replaced by advanced mechanical CT scanners with up to 624 rows. In the HNR study CAC was assessed from non-contrast enhanced EBCT scans, performed with a C-100 or C-150 scanner (GE Imatron, South San Francisco, USA). Prospective ECG-triggering was done at 80% of the RR-interval [29]. Contiguous 3 mm thick slices from the pulmonary bifurcation to the apex of the heart were obtained in both scans at an image acquisition time of 100 ms. CAC was defined as a focus of at least four contiguous pixels with a CT density ≥130 Hounsfield Units. This density is related to a density factor between 1 and 4 (≥130–199, 200–299, 300–399, ≥400) and multiplied with the area of the plaque. The CAC Agatston score was computed by summing the CAC scores of all foci in the epicardial coronary system. The CT-related X-ray exposure could be measured previously and ranges from 1.0 to 1.3 mSv [33]. Thus, the low X-ray exposure allows the scanning even of healthy individuals, which was necessary in order to obtain data for estimating the natural history and prevalence of CAC.

26.2 Natural History of CAC

The natural history of arteriosclerosis had previously been described in detail [27, 34, 35]. First intracellular then extracellular calcium is a common sign and found not only in advanced atherosclerotic lesions but also in atheroma and fibroatheroma close to the lipid necrotic core, even in young individuals <50 years [34–36]. Typically, the first signs of coronary arteriosclerosis, indicated by plaque formation, are found 2–3 cm from the origin of both the left anterior descending coronary artery [34, 35]. Aging is indicated by the progression of the disease leading to plaque formation also in the distal part of the left anterior descending and circumflex arteries, which was not observed in the same degree in the right coronary artery [35]. Also by coronary angiography including patients with multiple lesions and an average three vessel disease lesions are found in the proximal left artery descending coronary artery followed by the right coronary artery [37, 38]. The natural history of coronary artery sclerosis can be assessed by EBCT in more details, as CAC is part of the vessel wall, whereas angiography is only a luminogram [39–41].

26.3 Prevalence of Coronary Artery Calcification

Already early, it became obvious that coronary artery calcification increases in an exponential curvature related to age in each gender as the population-based cohort of the Heinz Nixdorf Recall Study demonstrated in 4487 participants at the age of 45–75 years [42]. In an Army study, CAC was already found in men at the age of 40–45 years [43]. Very different results were reported, when a cohort of patients with or without symptoms were recruited [42]. The age- and sex-related CAC distribution is very comparable in different cohorts, even in different countries and continents as the multi-ethnic study of atherosclerosis (MESA) demonstrated, which included 6814 participants at the age of 45–80 years [44]. The results are astonishing, as the distribution of risk factors were strikingly different [45]. Meanwhile three observational studies have presented their results: the Heinz Nixdorf Recall study, the MESA, and the Rotterdam study with very similar results in Caucasian participants [44–47]. The percentile distribution of CAC is, however, different in other ethnicities [48, 49], as recently the MESA study confirmed [50].

These percentiles of CAC distribution can be used in order to estimate the individual vascular age, www.recall-Studie.uni-Essen.de, www.mesa-nhlbi.org [41].

Individual CAC values can be compared to this percentile distribution and the difference used to estimate the "vascular age" [41, 44, 45, 51]. In Fig. 26.1

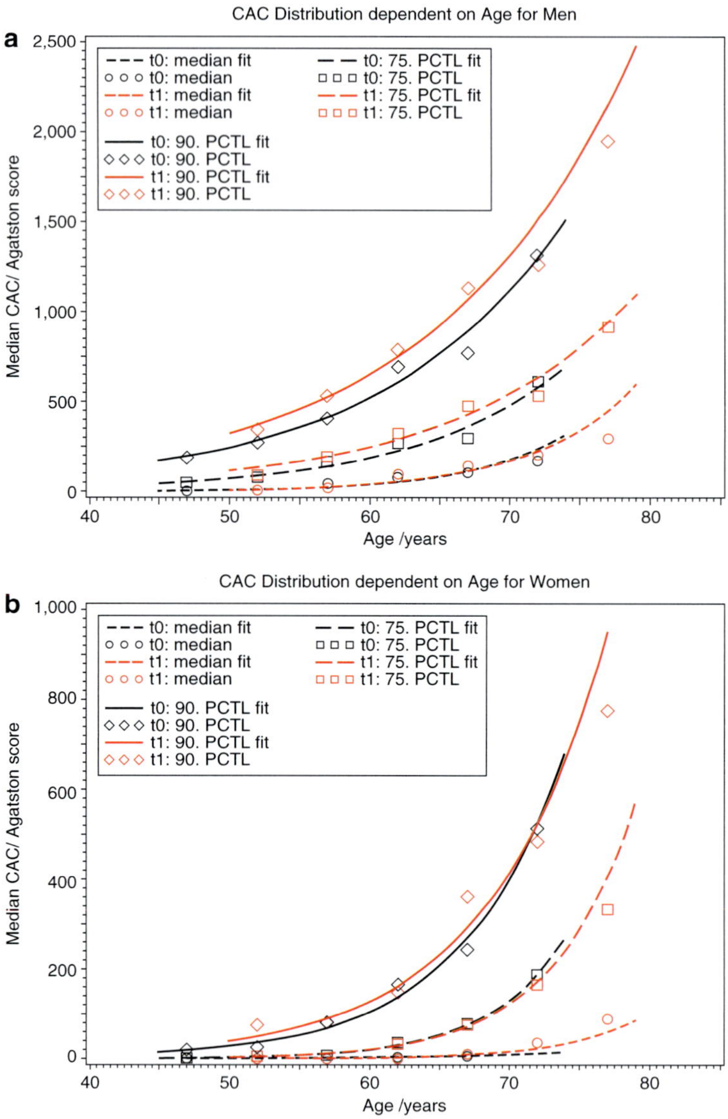

Fig. 26.1 (**a**) Empirical and estimated 50th, 75th, and 90th percentile of the CAC distribution for men by age categories [52]. In black for the baseline values (t0), when the participants (1633 men) were aged between 45 and 74 years, and in red for the 5-year follow-up data (t1), when the cohort was aged 50–79 years. Note the exponential shape of the increase of CAC. Dots represent empirical percentile values for each 5-year age categories, lines show linear quantile regression on a log scale after retransformation. (**b**) Empirical and estimated 50th, 75th, and 90th percentile of the CAC distribution for men by age categories. In black for the baseline values (t0), when the participants (1848 women) were aged between 45 and 74 years, and in red for the 5-year follow-up data (t1), when the cohort was aged 50–79 years. Note the exponential shape of the increase of CAC. Dots represent empirical percentile values for each 5-year age categories, lines show linear quantile regression on a log scale after retransformation. The *y*-axis range in (**a**, **b**) differ by a factor of 2.5 in men compared to women [52]

percentile distribution is shown for men and women, based on the 5 years follow-up data of the HNR study [52]. The follow-up data show in comparison to the baseline data a shift along the given CAC distribution for 5 years without losing the exponential baseline curvature [52]. Based on these analyses a prediction of CAC progression became possible allowing the comparison to the observed change that means a rated CAC progression could differentiate into a progression as predicted, but also into a slow and rapid CAC progression for those showing lower or higher values than predicted [53]. For calculation an App is presented at "CAC Progression."

26.4 Influence of Risk Factors on Coronary Artery Calcification

Traditional and nontraditional cardiovascular risk factors are associated with coronary atherosclerosis. The top four factors are smoking, hypercholesterolemia, diabetes, and hypertension, since the first description by the Framingham study in 1961.

Smoking seems to have a strong influence on CAC and is associated with enhanced CAC yielding a vascular age increase of about 10 years in men and women. For ex-smokers this effect is smaller and reduced to 5 years in men and 2–3 years in women [53, 54]. Passive smoking showed a significant association, too, but this association was is weak [55].

In addition to smoking hyperlipidemia plays a major role and is of great interest, because new medication has been developed to reduce the cholesterol and LDL-cholesterol (LDL-C) level even below 160 and 70 mg/dL, respectively. Elevated levels of total cholesterol and LDL-cholesterol are associated with excessive calcification of coronary arteries. The association between CAC and LDL-C is more pronounced in women than in men [56]. Women with an LDL-cholesterol below 100 mg/dL show nearly no calcification during life, whereas women with an LDL-cholesterol >190 mg/dL demonstrate an excessive calcification process, which starts already very early between 40 and 50 years and yields a vasculature age difference of 17 years [56]. In men the difference is only 4.5 years [56]. However, men with LDL-C have already at the age of 45 years a higher CAC level. The signs of coronary arteriosclerosis give a nice opportunity to analyze whether or not other parameters of the lipoprotein metabolism may improve the association to CAC compared to LDL-C. Apo B shows the highest association to CAC in comparison to all other tested lipoprotein parameters even compared to lipoprotein (a). Neither the ratio LDL-C/HDL-C, nor Apo B/Apo-A1 or non HDL-C yielded stronger associations compared to Apo B or LDL-C. However, the difference to LDL-C is quite small, so that in the clinical field LDL-C remains the most important risk factor for characterizing hyperlipidemia. The association to triglyceride levels was only week and only positive for the highest quartile compared to the lowest in men and women [41, 56].

The age- and sex-dependent distribution of CAC is steeper in those with prediabetes and even more in those with known diabetes mellitus. Again the association for women is more impressive than for men. The vascular age is 13 years higher in those with compared to those without diabetes and 4 years for those with prediabetes. In men the difference is for diabetes 4 years but for prediabetes no difference in relation to the CAC distribution can be detected.

26.5 Influence of Hypertension on Coronary Artery Calcification

Recent years have demonstrated that high blood pressure (BP) is one of the most important risk factors related to cardiovascular mortality including stroke, myocardial infarction, heart failure, aortic diseases, and renal failure [57–59]. The 7th and 8th Joint National Committee on Detection, Evaluation and Treatment of High Blood Pressure have changed the recommendation of treatment and differ in this respect to the European Society of Cardiology (ESC) statements [59, 60]. Parallel to the new 8th JNC recommendation the American Heart Association and American College of Cardiology published the use of a new ASCVD (atherosclerotic cardiovascular disease) score for assessment of CV risk [61]. In addition to the discussion of BP thresholds used for treatment [57, 60, 62], both the ESC and the ACC/AHA recommendation do use the information about organ damage as an important sign of the disease classification already in a subclinical state, but both discuss or nearly neglect the use of CAC in order to detect signs of organ damage at the coronary artery level [63, 64]. However, in the ACC/AHA guideline on the treatment of blood cholesterol to reduce CV risk in adults, a CAC level >300 is recommended to be used for reclassification of individuals with LDL-C between 70 and 189 mg/dL. CAC is recommended in order to improve the clinician–patient discussion, when the ASCVD score is ≥7.5% or 5–7.5%, if a diabetes is present <40 years or LDL <70 mg/dL, or when the patient is $p > 75$ years [63].

As we described earlier [31], epidemiological data show that coronary event rates are highest in those with hypertension, intermediate in those with prehypertension, also called borderline or high normal blood pressure (BP), and lowest in those with normal BP [65–70]. The most common first major events after hypertension onset are hard ischemic heart disease events with acute myocardial infarction and unstable angina in a continuous graded manner with no indication of a critical value [71, 72]. But still a controversy exists whether or not prehypertension can be regarded as a disease entity and should be treated. However, in prehypertension, even an impaired repair capacity of endothelial progenitor cells could be demonstrated [73] as well as retinal vessel narrowing [54] and increased intima-media thickness or even increase of left ventricular mass [75].

In children studied between the age 8 and 18 years and followed until the age of 29–37 years the prevalence of CAC was 30% in men and 10% in women [76]. The risk for CAC was highest for systolic BP in the stepwise multiple logistic regression analysis and higher than for body mass index, HDL-C, and LDL-C. This corresponds to the report of MESA showing that in incidental hypertension CAC can be regarded as a direct sign of target organ damage of the coronary arteries [77].

However, previous studies failed to demonstrate that treatment of prehypertension can be recommended, but demonstrated that it may be more harmful and risky than non-pharmacologic interventions [78–80].

In the HNR study we studied the influence of blood pressure on CAC and tested the association with outcome data of coronary and CV events [31]. We could include 4181 cases between 45 and 75 years between 2000 and 2003, who were followed for 7.18 years (median; Q1–Q3: 6.98–8.24 years). Hard coronary events were defined as fatal and nonfatal myocardial infarction, cardiovascular events as stroke and coronary revascularization. Details on the blood pressure measurements were published previously [81]. Trained technicians took three blood pressure measurements with an automated oscillometric blood pressure device (Omron, HEM-705CP, OMRON Corporation, Hoofdrop, The Netherlands), with appropriate 14 or 16 cm cuff sizes and the participants in the sitting position. The mean of the second and third value of three measurements, recorded with a 3 min interval, was taken in accordance to the Joint National Committee for Prevention Detection and Treatment of High Blood Pressure (JNC 7) guidelines [59]. Participants with systolic/diastolic BP <120/<80 mmHg were categorized as normotensive. Prehypertension was defined as systolic BP 120–139 mmHg or diastolic BP 80–89 mmHg. Hypertension was defined as systolic or diastolic BP ≥140 or ≥90 mmHg, respectively, and subdivided in stage 1 hypertension with either systolic BP 140–159 mmHg or diastolic BP 90–99 mmHg and stage 2 hypertension with either systolic or diastolic BP ≥160 or ≥100 mmHg. Participants were asked to bring their medication in order to verify if antihypertensive medication was used in order to validate some answers in the questionnaire concerning presence of hypertension. Only if antihypertensive medication was verified, we categorized these participants as in hypertension stage 2 [31].

Already prehypertensive participants showed higher prevalence of risk factors. Hypertensive subjects were older, showed higher BMIs and higher cholesterol and triglyceride levels. Prevalence of diabetes increased as well. The Framingham score increased in men from 9.4 ± 5.2 in normotensives to 19.2 ± 5.3% in stage 2 and in women from 3.6 ± 2.0 to 9.7 ± 5.3%. During follow-up of 7.18 years 2.8% ($n = 115$) experienced coronary and 3.6% ($n = 152$) CV events. The time to events decreased in the higher BP categories. This effect was higher for CV than coronary events (Figs. 26.2 and 26.3). In comparison to normotensives, the hazard ratios for the combined endpoint were 1.43 (95%CI 0.82–2.50), $P = 0.21$ for prehypertensives, 1.52 (95%CI 0.85–2.73), $P = 0.16$ for stage 1, and 2.63 (95%CI 1.57–4.43), $P = 0.0003$ for stage 2 hypertensives.

The association between age and CAC scores was strongly dependent on BP categories, but more in women than men (Fig. 26.4). Prehypertensive women had increased CAC score compared to normotensives, which was not obvious in men, but men had roughly a five times higher amount of CAC.

In men, CAC was already found in hypertension stage 2 at the age of 45 years, in women at the age of 50 years, which seems to be related to the lower frequency of hypertension in women compared to men until 45 years of age [82]. Additionally, the prevalence and severity of hypertension increase with age in women, so that

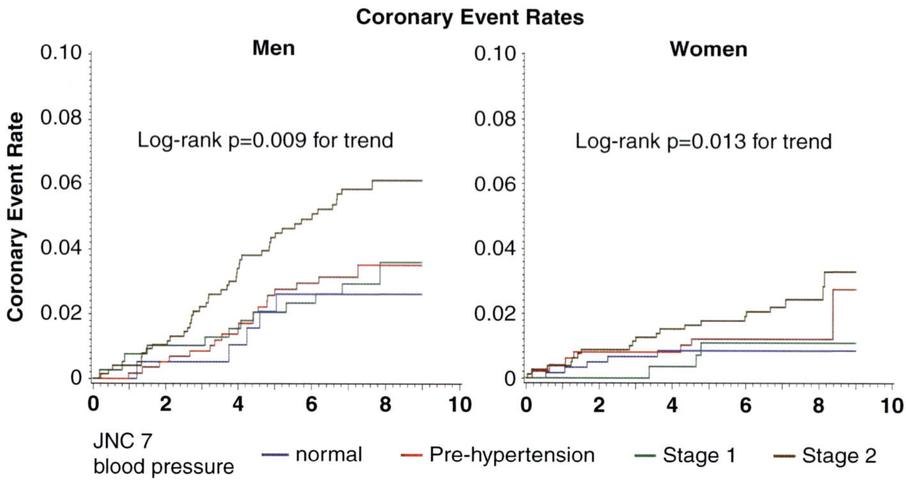

Fig. 26.2 Kaplan-Meier curves of primary coronary events defined as fatal and nonfatal myocardial infarction in JNC 7 blood pressure categories [31]

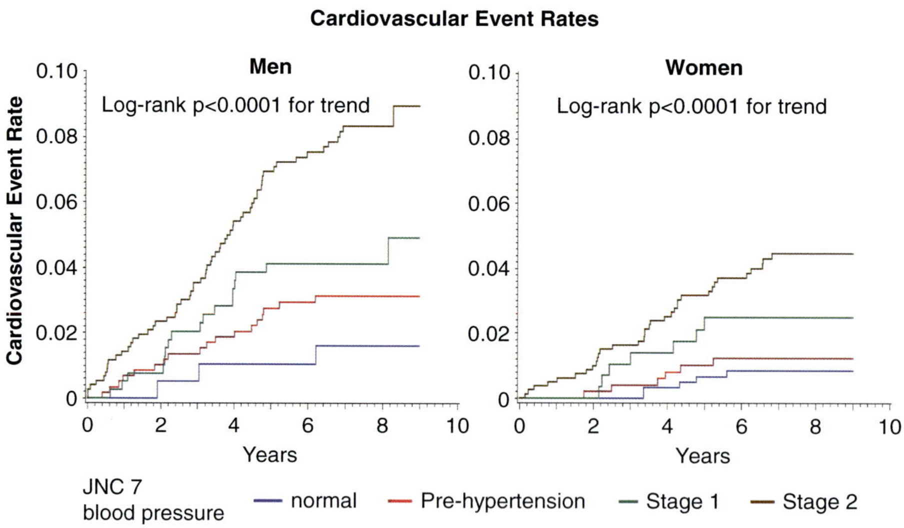

Fig. 26.3 Kaplan-Meier curves of primary cardiovascular events defined as stroke and coronary revascularization in JNC 7 blood pressure categories [31]

beyond 60 years, the majority of women have stage 2 hypertension or receive antihypertensive agents [82, 83]. When CAC is used to estimate "arterial age" [51, 54, 56], it is about 15 years higher in stage 2 hypertensive women than in normotensive women, that is, normotensive women reach any given CAC score many years later than women with stage 2 hypertension. But even for prehypertension and hypertension stage 1, differences of 7–10 years could be demonstrated. In men, however, the

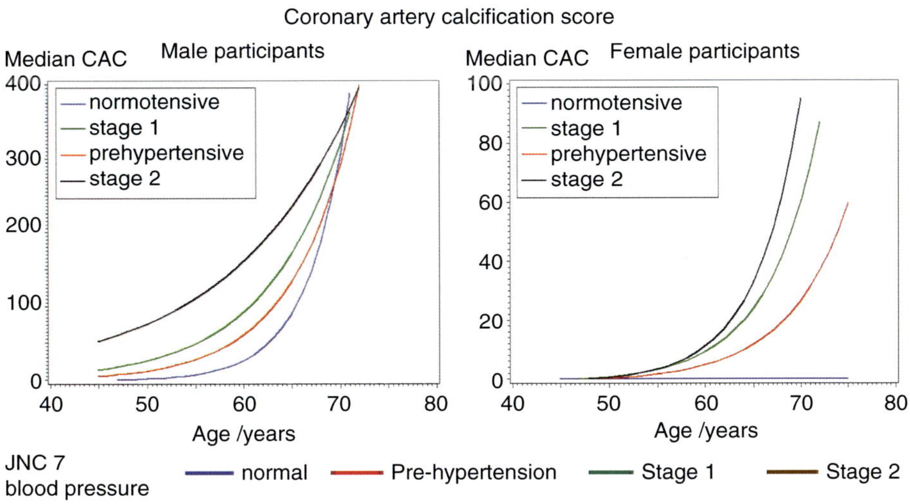

Fig. 26.4 Association of CAC scores with age stratified by JNC 7 blood pressure categories in men and women. Note that the CAC score in normotensive women increases only slightly with age, whereas in prehypertensives and hypertensives a steeper increase with age was observed [31]

differences between the different BP categories were not as striking, but still the estimated vascular age in normotensives was lower than in hypertensives. This may reflect that CAC in men is stronger influenced by other risk factors than BP alone including particularly smoking [84]. Smoking was much more prevalent in men than in women, while in women >60 years smoking also increases systolic BP [85]. CAC percentile distributions in men and women were similar for smokers, former smokers, and never smokers [54]. Yet, men and women with diabetes, prediabetes, and no diabetes showed a similar CAC distribution of percentiles as in this study for BP. This may reflect that CAC in men is stronger influenced by other risk factors than BP alone including particularly smoking [84]. This supports the hypothesis that the higher prevalence of current and former smoking in men compared to women may be the reason for the observed different distribution of CAC percentiles. It presents a typical biological bias [31].

For the total cohort, the factor of increase in (CAC+1) with 10 mmHg systolic BP was very similar in men and women, that is, 1.14 (95%CI: 1.09–1.21), $p < 0.0001$ and 1.13 (95%CI: 1.09–1.18), $p < 0.0001$, respectively, in a full adjusted model [31]. The adjusted HRs (full model using age, sex, diabetes, LDL-C and HDL-C, former and present smoking, lipid-lowering medication, and BMI) for the combined endpoint in comparison to persons without CAC were 1.68 (95%CI 0.90–3.15) for CAC >0–99, 3.09 (95%CI 1.63–5.86) for CAC = 100–399, 7.20 (7.80–13.63) for CAC ≥400, 1.16 (95%CI 1.03–1.29) for 5 years of age, and 1.61 (95%CI 1.08–2.41) for diabetes. In this model presence of lipid-lowering therapy showed no sizeable impact with a HR of 0.93 (95%CI 0.59–1.42), $P = 0.68$. Figure 26.5 presents in a

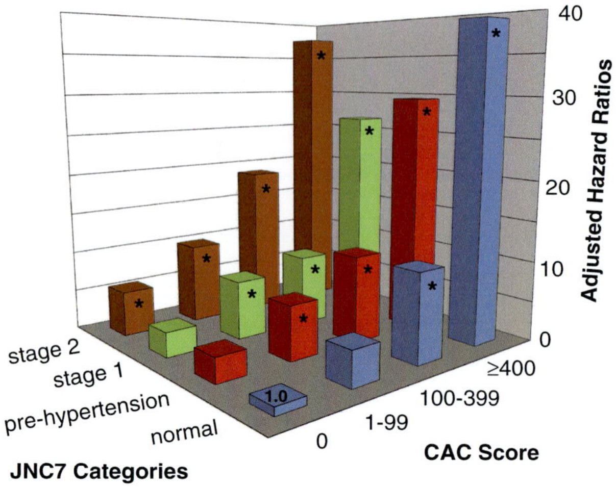

Fig. 26.5 Adjusted hazard ratios of the combined endpoint (fatal and nonfatal myocardial infarction, stroke and coronary revascularization) stratified by CAC score categories and JNC 7 blood pressure categories with normotensives with no CAC as the reference category [59]. *Indicates significant difference from reference

three-dimensional scheme the influence of BP level and CAC score on the event rates. It can be seen that the main influence seems to be the CAC and not the BP level itself.

26.6 CAC Progression and Blood Pressure

Once CAC is found, it will increase over time in an inevitable manner along a given exponential curvature [52]. Related to the baseline measurement the CAC progression can be predicted and compared to the observed increase [53]. In a recent analysis it could be demonstrated that systolic blood pressure in addition to smoking and LDL-C were independent predictors of CAC onset during a follow-up time of 5 years [53]. Currently it is not known if CAC progression adds to our understanding of the influence of risk factors upon outcome.

26.7 Association of Blood Pressure and Outcome Dependent on CAC

The degree of CAC seems to be an excellent prognostic marker for coronary and cardiovascular events [30, 86, 87]. Thresholds of CAC 100 and CAC 400 represent typical levels which correspond to increased and high risk. Interestingly enough, we found a stronger association between BP and secondary than primary endpoints despite strong associations of BP to CAC. This is in line with previous epidemiologic observations showing that hypertension was the most important risk factor in 77% of persons with incidental strokes and in 69% of those with incidental myocardial infarction [88]. The increase in HRs within CAC score categories with

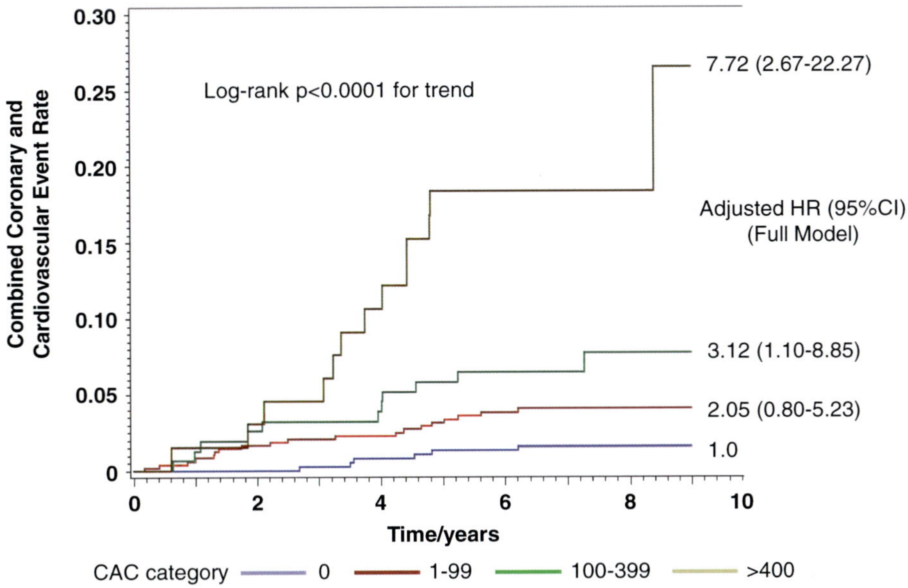

Fig. 26.6 Kaplan-Meier curves of the combined endpoints (fatal and nonfatal myocardial infarction, stroke and revascularization) in prehypertensives only, stratified by CAC score categories [31]

increasing BP is modest, as has been pointed out, except for the increase in risk in cases with stage 2 hypertension (Fig. 26.4). However, within each BP category, the adjusted HRs of the combined coronary and CV endpoints increased by the amount of CAC [31]. The time to events decreased with increasing CAC score categories even among prehypertensives with a gradual and strong relationship of risk with the degree of CAC (Fig. 26.6). In persons with hypertension, that is, stage 1 and stage 2, HRs for the combined endpoint in comparison to persons without CAC were 1.96 (95%CI 1.06–3.63), $P = 0.03$ for CAC 1–99, 3.46 (95%CI 1.84–6.49), $P = 0.0001$ for CAC 100–399, and 7.55 (95%CI 4.03–14.15), $P < 0.0001$ for CAC ≥400 (model 2, full adjustment). Adjusting this relation between CAC and events in hypertensives (stage 1 and 2) further with respect to age, sex, diabetes, LDL-C and HDL-C, former and present smoking, lipid-lowering medication, and BMI confirmed these results. HRs were 1.68 (95%CI 0.90–3.15) for CAC = 0–99, 3.09 (95%CI 1.63–5.86) for CAC = 100–399, 7.20 (7.80–13.63) for CAC ≥400, 1.16 (95%CI 1.03–1.29) for 5 years of age, and 1.61 (95%CI 1.08–2.41) for diabetes.

Conclusion

Our data suggest that coronary atherosclerosis measured by CT as a marker of target organ damage might be considered for further risk stratification. This applies particularly to persons with prehypertension where the clinical significance of antihypertensive medication is controversial. Atherosclerosis imaging may help to guide lifestyle modification and pharmaco-therapeutic therapy to reduce coronary and cardiovascular morbidity and mortality [88]. Interestingly enough, we found a stronger association between BP and secondary than primary endpoints despite strong associations of BP to CAC. This is in line with previous epidemiologic observations showing that hypertension was the most important risk factor in 77% of persons with incidental strokes and in 69% of those with incidental myocardial infarction [89]. The relationship between BP, CAC, and endpoints is supported by previous cross-sectional analyses from MESA and HNR demonstrating that BP was a main determinant of CAC [45]. Similarly, a recent meta-analysis in 73,913 patients demonstrated for intensive blood pressure reduction a positive effect for stroke but not for myocardial infarction in diabetics [90]. Ischemic coronary artery disease based on luminal narrowing can be regarded as a direct consequence of coronary atherosclerosis, and CAC has a high correlation to total plaque burden [91]. Thus, on one hand a strong association with revascularization can be expected, on the other hand a weaker association with coronary events, because the underlying process is not directly related to CAC, but to erosion and plaque rupture of thin cap fibrous atheroma, as visualized at autopsy [25].

CT scans represent the noninvasive method of choice for detection of CAC, which represents a typical sign of subclinical coronary artery disease. For either sex, the amount of CAC increases with an exponential curvature. Risk factor analysis reaches an explained variance of up to 25–30%. That means a great part of the process seems to be genetically determined and heritable, with a strong influence of ethnicity. Systolic blood pressure has been identified as the strongest predictor of CAC in children followed until the young adulthood. The amount of CAC increases depending on the blood pressure level. Between normotensives and hypertension stage 2 a striking difference was found, which was more obvious in women than men. Even in prehypertensives a higher CAC distribution was found in both men and women. In men a biological bias in the elderly was found. The degree of CAC was associated with higher coronary and cardiovascular events in each blood pressure category. Compared to the blood pressure categories the CAC values were much more predictive of events, even in prehypertensives. This coronary sign of subclinical atherosclerosis may be used in the future to preselect those who would benefit from pharmaceutic intervention and avoid treatment in others. Meanwhile, McEvoy JW et al. have proposed CAC as a guide for a personalized risk-based approach to initiation and intensification of antihypertensive therapy [92].

References

1. Dzau VJ, Antman EM, Black HR, Hayes DL, Manson JE, Plutzky J, Popma JJ, Stevenson W. The cardiovascular disease continuum validated: clinical evidence of improved patient outcomes: part I: pathophysiology and clinical trial evidence (risk factors through stable coronary artery disease). Circulation. 2006;114(25):2850–70.
2. Dzau VJ, Antman EM, Black HR, Hayes DL, Manson JE, Plutzky J, Popma JJ, Stevenson W. The cardiovascular disease continuum validated: clinical evidence of improved patient

outcomes: part II: clinical trial evidence (acute coronary syndromes through renal disease) and future directions. Circulation. 2006;114(25):2871–91.

3. Stary HC, Chandler AB, Glagov S, Guyton JR, Insull W Jr, Rosenfeld ME, Schaffer SA, Schwartz CJ, Wagner WD, Wissler RW. A definition of initial, fatty streak, and intermediate lesions of atherosclerosis. A report from the Committee on Vascular Lesions of the Council on Arteriosclerosis, American Heart Association. Circulation. 1994;89(5):2462–78.
4. Stary HC, Chandler AB, Dinsmore RE, Fuster V, Glagov S, Insull W Jr, Rosenfeld ME, Schwartz CJ, Wagner WD, Wissler RW. A definition of advanced types of atherosclerotic lesions and a histological classification of atherosclerosis. A report from the Committee on Vascular Lesions of the Council on Arteriosclerosis, American Heart Association. Circulation. 1995;92(5):1355–74.
5. Glagov S, Weisenberg E, Zarins CK, Stankunavicius R, Kolettis GJ. Compensatory enlargement of human atherosclerotic coronary arteries. N Engl J Med. 1987;316(22):1371–5.
6. Ge J, Erbel R, Zamorano J, Koch L, Kearney P, Görge G, Gerber T, Meyer J. Coronary artery remodeling in atherosclerotic disease: an intravascular ultrasonic study in vivo. Coron Artery Dis. 1993;4:981–6.
7. Gerber TC, Erbel R, Görge G, Ge J, Rupprecht HJ, Meyer J. Extent of atherosclerosis and remodeling of the left main coronary artery determined by intravascular ultrasound. Am J Cardiol. 1994;73:666–71.
8. von Birgelen C, Mintz GS, de Vrey EA, Serruys PW, Kimura T, Nobuyoshi M, Popma JJ, Leon MB, Erbel R, de Feyter PJ. Preintervention lesion remodelling affects operative mechanisms of balloon optimised directional coronary atherectomy procedures: a volumetric study with three dimensional intravascular ultrasound. Heart. 2000;83(2):192–7.
9. Hartmann M, von Birgelen C, Mintz GS, Verhorst PM, Erbel R. Relation between baseline plaque burden and subsequent remodelling of atherosclerotic left main coronary arteries: a serial intravascular ultrasound study with long-term (> or =12 months) follow-up. Eur Heart J. 2006;27(15):1778–84.
10. Isner JM, Kishel J, Kent KM, Ronan JA Jr, Ross AM, Roberts WC. Accuracy of angiographic determination of left main coronary arterial narrowing. Angiographic—histologic correlative analysis in 28 patients. Circulation. 1981;63(5):1056–64.
11. Erbel R, Ge J, Bockisch A, Kearney P, Görge G, Haude M, Schümann D, Zamorano J, Rupprecht HJ, Meyer J. Value of intracoronary ultrasound and Doppler in the differentiation of angiographically normal coronary arteries: a prospective study in patients with angina pectoris. Eur Heart J. 1996;17(6):880–9.
12. Gould KL. Noninvasive assessment of coronary stenoses by myocardial imaging during coronary vasodilation. Part I physiologic principles and experimental validation. Am J Cardiol. 1978;41:267–78.
13. Gould KL, Schelbert HR, Phelps ME, Hoffman EJ. Noninvasive assessment of coronary stenoses with myocardial perfusion imaging during pharmacologic coronary vasodilatation. V. Detection of 47 percent diameter coronary stenosis with intravenous nitrogen-13 ammonia and emission-computed tomography in intact dogs. Am J Cardiol. 1979;43(2):200–8.
14. Gould KL, Schelbert H, Phelps M, Hoffman E. Noninvasive assessment of coronary stenoses by myocardial perfusion imaging during pharmacologic coronary vasodilation. Part V. Detection of 47% diameter coronary stenosis with intravenous 13NH4+ and emission computed tomography in intact dogs. Am J Cardiol. 1979;43:200–8.
15. Gould KL, Kirkeeide RL, Buchi M. Coronary flow reserve as a physiologic measure of stenosis severity. Part I. Relative and absolute coronary flow reserve during changing aortic pressure and cardiac workload and Part II determination from arteriographic stenosis dimensions under standardized conditions. J Am Coll Cardiol. 1990;15:459–74.
16. Gould KL, Johnson NP, Bateman TM, Beanlands RS, Bengel FM, Bober R, Camici PG, Cerqueira MD, Chow BJ, Di Carli MF, Dorbala S, Gewirtz H, Gropler RJ, Kaufmann PA, Knaapen P, Knuuti J, Merhige ME, Rentrop KP, Ruddy TD, Schelbert HR, Schindler TH, Schwaiger M, Sdringola S, Vitarello J, Williams KA Sr, Gordon D, Dilsizian V, Narula J. Anatomic versus physiologic assessment of coronary artery disease. Role of coronary flow

reserve, fractional flow reserve, and positron emission tomography imaging in revascularization decision-making. J Am Coll Cardiol. 2013;62(18):1639–53. https://doi.org/10.1016/j.jacc.2013.07.076.
17. McMahon MM, Brown BG, Cukingnan R, Rolett EL, Bolson E, Frimer M, Dodge HT. Quantitative coronary angiography: measurement of the "critical" stenosis in patients with unstable angina and single-vessel disease without collaterals. Circulation. 1979;60(1):106–13.
18. Wijns W, Serruys PW, Reiber JH, van den Brand M, Simoons ML, Kooijman CJ, Balakumaran K, Hugenholtz PG. Quantitative angiography of the left anterior descending coronary artery: correlations with pressure gradient and results of exercise thallium scintigraphy. Circulation. 1985;71(2):273–9.
19. Gerber TC, Erbel R, Görge G, Ge J, Rupprecht HJ, Meyer J. Classification of morphologic effects of percutaneous transluminal coronary angioplasty assessed by intravascular ultrasound. Am J Cardiol. 1992;70(20):1546–54.
20. Görge G, Haude M, Ge J, Voegele E, Gerber T, Rupprecht HJ, Meyer J, Erbel R. Intravascular ultrasound after low and high inflation pressure coronary artery stent implantation. J Am Coll Cardiol. 1995;26(3):725–30.
21. Falk E, Shah PK, Fuster V. Coronary plaque disruption. Circulation. 1995;92(3):657–71.
22. Davies MJ, Bland JM, Hangartner JR, Angelini A, Thomas AC. Factors influencing the presence or absence of acute coronary artery thrombi in sudden ischaemic death. Eur Heart J. 1989;10(3):203–8.
23. Virmani R, Kolodgie FD, Burke AP, Farb A, Schwartz SM. Lessons from sudden coronary death: a comprehensive morphological classification scheme for atherosclerotic lesions. Arterioscler Thromb Vasc Biol. 2000;20(5):1262–75.
24. Friedewald VE, Ambrose JA, Stone GW, Roberts WC, Willerson JT. The editor's roundtable: the vulnerable plaque. Am J Cardiol. 2008;102(12):1644–53. https://doi.org/10.1016/j.amjcard.2008.09.001.
25. Virmani R, Kolodgie FD, Burke AP, Finn AV, Gold HK, Tulenko TN, Wrenn SP, Narula J. Atherosclerotic plaque progression and vulnerability to rupture: angiogenesis as a source of intraplaque hemorrhage. Arterioscler Thromb Vasc Biol. 2005;25(10):2054–61.
26. Burke AP, Kolodgie FD, Farb A, Weber DK, Malcom GT, Smialek J, Virmani R. Healed plaque ruptures and sudden coronary death: evidence that subclinical rupture has a role in plaque progression. Circulation. 2001;103(7):934–40.
27. Stary HC. The development of calcium deposits in atherosclerotic lesions and their persistence after lipid regression. Am J Cardiol. 2001;88:16E–9E.
28. Agatston AS, Janowitz WR, Hildner FJ, Zusmer NR, Viamonte M Jr, Detrano R. Quantification of coronary artery calcium using ultrafast computed tomography. J Am Coll Cardiol. 1990;15(4):827–32.
29. Schmermund A, Möhlenkamp S, Stang A, Grönemeyer D, Seibel R, Hirche H, Mann K, Siffert W, Lauterbach K, Siegrist J, Jöckel KH, Erbel R. Assessment of clinically silent atherosclerotic disease and established and novel risk factors for predicting myocardial infarction and cardiac death in healthy middle-aged subjects: rationale and design of the Heinz Nixdorf RECALL Study. Risk factors, evaluation of coronary calcium and lifestyle. Am Heart J. 2002;144(2):212–8.
30. Erbel R, Möhlenkamp S, Moebus S, Schmermund A, Lehmann N, Stang A, Dragano N, Grönemeyer D, Seibel R, Kälsch H, Bröcker-Preuss M, Mann K, Siegrist J, Jöckel KH, Heinz Nixdorf Recall Study Investigative Group. Coronary risk stratification, discrimination, and reclassification improvement based on quantification of subclinical coronary atherosclerosis: the Heinz Nixdorf Recall study. J Am Coll Cardiol. 2010;56(17):1397–406. https://doi.org/10.1016/j.jacc.2010.06.030.
31. Erbel R, Lehmann N, Möhlenkamp S, Churzidse S, Bauer M, Kälsch H, Schmermund A, Moebus S, Stang A, Roggenbuck U, Bröcker-Preuss M, Dragano N, Weimar C, Siegrist J, Jöckel KH, Heinz Nixdorf Recall Study Investigators. Subclinical coronary atherosclerosis predicts cardiovascular risk in different stages of hypertension: result of the

Heinz Nixdorf Recall Study. Hypertension. 2012;59(1):44–53. https://doi.org/10.1161/HYPERTENSIONAHA.111.180489.

32. Lehmann N, Erbel R, Mahabadi AA, Kälsch H, Möhlenkamp S, Moebus S, Stang A, Roggenbuck U, Strucksberg KH, Führer-Sakel D, Dragano N, Budde T, Seibel R, Grönemeyer D, Jöckel KH, Investigators HNRS. Accelerated progression of coronary artery calcification in hypertension but also prehypertension. J Hypertens. 2016;34(11):2233–42. https://doi.org/10.1097/HJH.0000000000001080.
33. Hunold P, Vogt FM, Schmermund A, Debatin JF, Kerkhoff G, Budde T, Erbel R, Ewen K, Barkhausen J. Radiation exposure during cardiac CT: effective doses at multi-detector row CT and electron-beam CT. Radiology. 2003;226(1):145–52.
34. Montenegro MR, Eggen DA. Topography of atherosclerosis in the coronary arteries. Lab Invest. 1968;18:586–93.
35. Strong JP. Atherosclerotic lesions. Natural history, risk factors, and topography. Arch Pathol Lab Med. 1992;116:1268–75.
36. Schmermund A, Schwartz RS, Adamzik M, Sangiorgi G, Pfeifer EA, Rumberger JA, Burke AP, Farb A, Virmani R. Coronary atherosclerosis in unheralded sudden coronary death under age 50: histo-pathologic comparison with 'healthy' subjects dying out of hospital. Atherosclerosis. 2001;155(2):499–508.
37. Halon 'DA, Sapoznikov D, Lewis BS, Gotsman MS. Localization of Lesions in the Coronary circulation. Am J Cardiol. 1983;52:921–6.
38. Gotsman M, Rosenheck S, Nassar H, Welber S, Sapoznikov D, Mosseri M, Weiss A, Lotan C, Rozenman Y. Angiographic findings in the coronary arteries after thrombolysis in acute myocardial infarction. Am J Cardiol. 1992;70:715–23.
39. Schmermund A, Möhlenkamp S, Baumgart D, Kriener P, Pump H, Grönemeyer D, Seibel R, Erbel R. Usefulness of topography of coronary calcium by electron-beam computed tomography in predicting the natural history of coronary atherosclerosis. Am J Cardiol. 2000;86:127–32.
40. Schmermund A, Baumgart D, Möhlenkamp S, Kriener P, Pump H, Grönemeyer D, Seibel R, Erbel R. Natural history and topographic pattern of progression of coronary calcification in symptomatic patients: An electron-beam CT study. Arterioscler Thromb Vasc Biol. 2001;21(3):421–6.
41. Erbel R, Mahabadi AA, Kälsch HH. The coronary calcium score for risk prediction. Cardiovasc Med. 2015;18(03):75–82. https://doi.org/10.4414/cvm.2015.00310.
42. Schmermund A, Möhlenkamp S, Berenbein S, Pump H, Moebus S, Roggenbuck U, Stang A, Seibel R, Grönemeyer D, Jöckel KH, Erbel R. Population-based assessment of subclinical coronary atherosclerosis using electron-beam computed tomography. Atherosclerosis. 2006;185(1):177–82.
43. Taylor AJ, Bindeman J, Feuerstein I, Cao F, Brazaitis M, O'Malley PG. Coronary calcium independently predicts incident premature coronary heart disease over measured cardiovascular risk factors: mean three-year outcomes in the Prospective Army Coronary Calcium (PACC) project. J Am Coll Cardiol. 2005;46(5):807–14.
44. McClelland R, Chung H, Detrano R, Post W, Kronmal RA. Distribution of coronary artery calcium by race, gender, and age: results from the Multi-Ethnic Study of Atherosclerosis (MESA). Circulation. 2006;113(1):30–7.
45. Erbel R, Delaney JA, Lehmann N, McClelland RL, Möhlenkamp S, Kronmal RA, Schmermund A, Moebus S, Dragano N, Stang A, Jöckel KH, Budoff MJ, Multi-Ethnic Study of Atherosclerosis, Investigator Group of the Heinz Nixdorf Recall Study. Signs of subclinical coronary atherosclerosis in relation to risk factor distribution in the Multi-Ethnic Study of Atherosclerosis (MESA) and the Heinz Nixdorf Recall Study (HNR). Eur Heart J. 2008;29(22):2782–91. https://doi.org/10.1093/eurheartj/ehn439.
46. Vliegenthart R, Oudkerk M, Hofman A, Oei HH, van Dijck W, van Rooij FJ, Witteman JC. Coronary calcification improves cardiovascular risk prediction in the elderly. Circulation. 2005;112:572–7.

47. Erbel R, Budoff M. Improvement of cardiovascular risk prediction using coronary imaging: subclinical atherosclerosis: the memory of lifetime risk factor exposure. Eur Heart J. 2012;33(10):1201–13. https://doi.org/10.1093/eurheartj/ehs076.
48. Budoff M, Yang TP, Shavelle RM, Lamont DH, Brundage BH. Ethnic differences in coronary atherosclerosis. J Am Coll Cardiol. 2002;39(3):408–12.
49. Lee TC, O'Malley PG, Feuerstein I, Taylor AJ. The prevalence and severity of coronary artery calcification on coronary artery computed tomography in black and white subjects. J Am Coll Cardiol. 2003;41(1):39–44.
50. Bild DE, Detrano R, Peterson D, Guerci A, Liu K, Shahar E, Ouyang P, Jackson S, Saad MF. Ethnic differences in coronary calcification: the Multi-Ethnic Study of Atherosclerosis (MESA). Circulation. 2005;111(10):1313–20.
51. Shaw LJ, Raggi P, Berman DS, Callister TQ. Coronary artery calcium as a measure of biologic age. Atherosclerosis. 2006;188:112–9.
52. Erbel R, Lehmann N, Churzidse S, Rauwolf M, Mahabadi AA, Möhlenkamp S, Moebus S, Bauer M, Kälsch H, Budde T, Montag M, Schmermund A, Stang A, Führer-Sakel D, Weimar C, Roggenbuck U, Dragano N, Jöckel KH, Heinz Nixdorf Recall Study Investigators. Progression of coronary artery calcification seems to be inevitable, but predictable—results of the Heinz Nixdorf Recall (HNR) study. Eur Heart J. 2014;35(42):2960–71. https://doi.org/10.1093/eurheartj/ehu288.
53. Lehmann N, Möhlenkamp S, Mahabadi AA, Schmermund A, Roggenbuck U, Seibel R, Grönemeyer D, Budde T, Dragano N, Stang A, Mann K, Moebus S, Erbel R, Jöckel KH. Effect of smoking and other traditional risk factors on the onset of coronary artery calcification: results of the Heinz Nixdorf recall study. Atherosclerosis. 2014;232(2):339–45. https://doi.org/10.1016/j.atherosclerosis.2013.11.045.
54. Jöckel KH, Lehmann N, Jaeger BR, Moebus S, Möhlenkamp S, Schmermund A, Dragano N, Stang A, Grönemeyer D, Seibel R, Mann K, Volbracht L, Siegrist J, Erbel R. Smoking cessation and subclinical atherosclerosis—results from the Heinz Nixdorf Recall Study. Atherosclerosis. 2009;203:221–7.
55. Peinemann F, Moebus S, Dragano N, Möhlenkamp S, Lehmann N, Zeeb H, Erbel R, Jöckel K-H, Hoffmann B, On Behalf of the Heinz Nixdorf Recall Study Investigative Group. Second-hand smoke exposure and coronary artery calcification among non-smoking participants of a population-based cohort. Environ Health Perspect. 2011;119:1556–61.
56. Erbel R, Lehmann N, Churzidse S, Möhlenkamp S, Moebus S, Mahabadi AA, Schmermund A, Stang A, Dragano N, Grönemeyer D, Seibel R, Kälsch H, Bauer M, Bröcker-Preuss M, Mann K, Jöckel KH, Investigators HNRS. Gender-specific association of coronary artery calcium and lipoprotein parameters: the Heinz Nixdorf Recall Study. Atherosclerosis. 2013;229(2):531–40. https://doi.org/10.1016/j.atherosclerosis.2013.04.015.
57. Mancia G, Fagard R, Narkiewicz K, Redon J, Zanchetti A, Böhm M, Christiaens T, Cifkova R, De Backer G, Dominiczak A, Galderisi M, Grobbee DE, Jaarsma T, Kirchhof P, Kjeldsen SE, Laurent S, Manolis AJ, Nilsson PM, Ruilope LM, Schmieder RE, Sirnes PA, Sleight P, Viigimaa M, Waeber B, Zannad F, Redon J, Dominiczak A, Narkiewicz K, Nilsson PM, Burnier M, Viigimaa M, Ambrosioni E, Caufield M, Coca A, Olsen MH, Schmieder RE, Tsioufis C, van de Borne P, Zamorano JL, Achenbach S, Baumgartner H, Bax JJ, Bueno H, Dean V, Deaton C, Erol C, Fagard R, Ferrari R, Hasdai D, Hoes AW, Kirchhof P, Knuuti J, Kolh P, Lancellotti P, Linhart A, Nihoyannopoulos P, Piepoli MF, Ponikowski P, Sirnes PA, Tamargo JL, Tendera M, Torbicki A, Wijns W, Windecker S, Clement DL, Coca A, Gillebert TC, Tendera M, Rosei EA, Ambrosioni E, Anker SD, Bauersachs J, Hitij JB, Caulfield M, De Buyzere M, De Geest S, Derumeaux GA, Erdine S, Farsang C, Funck-Brentano C, Gerc V, Germano G, Gielen S, Haller H, Hoes AW, Jordan J, Kahan T, Komajda M, Lovic D, Mahrholdt H, Olsen MH, Ostergren J, Parati G, Perk J, Polonia J, Popescu BA, Reiner Z, Rydén L, Sirenko Y, Stanton A, Struijker-Boudier H, Tsioufis C, van de Borne P, Vlachopoulos C, Volpe M, Wood DA. 2013 ESH/ESC guidelines for the management of arterial hypertension: the Task Force for the Management of Arterial Hypertension of the European Society of Hypertension (ESH) and of the European Society of Cardiology (ESC). Eur Heart J. 2013;34(28):2159–219. https://doi.org/10.1093/eurheartj/eht151.

58. Mozaffarian D, Benjamin EJ, Go AS, Arnett DK, Blaha MJ, Cushman M, Das SR, de Ferranti S, Després JP, Fullerton HJ, Howard VJ, Huffman MD, Isasi CR, Jiménez MC, Judd SE, Kissela BM, Lichtman JH, Lisabeth LD, Liu S, Mackey RH, Magid DJ, McGuire DK, Mohler ER 3rd, Moy CS, Muntner P, Mussolino ME, Nasir K, Neumar RW, Nichol G, Palaniappan L, Pandey DK, Reeves MJ, Rodriguez CJ, Rosamond W, Sorlie PD, Stein J, Towfighi A, Turan TN, Virani SS, Woo D, Yeh RW, Turner MB, American Heart Association Statistics Committee, Stroke Statistics Subcommittee. Heart disease and stroke statistics-2016 update: a report from the American Heart Association. Circulation. 2016;133(4):e38–360. https://doi.org/10.1161/CIR.0000000000000350. Erratum in: Circulation. 2016;133(15):e599.
59. Chobanian AV, Bakris GL, Black HR, Cushman WC, Green LA, Izzo JL Jr, Jones DW, Materson BJ, Oparil S, Wright JT Jr, Roccella EJ, Joint National Committee on Prevention, Detection, Evaluation, and Treatment of High Blood Pressure, National Heart, Lung, and Blood Institute, National High Blood Pressure Education Program Coordinating Committee. Seventh report of the Joint National Committee on Prevention, Detection, Evaluation, and Treatment of High Blood Pressure. Hypertension. 2003;42:1206–52.
60. James PA, Oparil S, Carter BL, Cushman WC, Dennison-Himmelfarb C, Handler J, Lackland DT, LeFevre ML, MacKenzie TD, Ogedegbe O, Smith SC Jr, Svetkey LP, Taler SJ, Townsend RR, Wright JT Jr, Narva AS, Ortiz E. 2014 evidence-based guideline for the management of high blood pressure in adults: report from the panel members appointed to the Eighth Joint National Committee (JNC 8). JAMA. 2014;311(5):507–20. https://doi.org/10.1001/jama.2013.284427. Erratum in: JAMA. 2014;311(17):1809.
61. Goff DC Jr, Lloyd-Jones DM, Bennett G, Coady S, D'Agostino RB Sr, Gibbons R, Greenland P, Lackland DT, Levy D, O'Donnell CJ, Robinson JG, Schwartz JS, Shero ST, Smith SC Jr, Sorlie P, Stone NJ, Wilson PW, American College of Cardiology/American Heart Association Task Force on Practice Guidelines. 2013 ACC/AHA guideline on the assessment of cardiovascular risk: a report of the American College of Cardiology/American Heart Association Task Force on Practice Guidelines. J Am Coll Cardiol. 2014;63(25 Pt B):2935–59. https://doi.org/10.1016/j.jacc.2013.11.005. Epub 2013 Nov 12. No abstract available. Erratum in: J Am Coll Cardiol. 2014;63(25 Pt B):3026.
62. Ortiz E, Oparil S, James PA. Guidelines for managing high blood pressure--reply. JAMA. 2014;312(3):295–6. https://doi.org/10.1001/jama.2014.6599.
63. Stone NJ, Robinson JG, Lichtenstein AH, Bairey Merz CN, Blum CB, Eckel RH, Goldberg AC, Gordon D, Levy D, Lloyd-Jones DM, McBride P, Schwartz JS, Shero ST, Smith SC Jr, Watson K, Wilson PW, Eddleman KM, Jarrett NM, LaBresh K, Nevo L, Wnek J, Anderson JL, Halperin JL, Albert NM, Bozkurt B, Brindis RG, Curtis LH, DeMets D, Hochman JS, Kovacs RJ, Ohman EM, Pressler SJ, Sellke FW, Shen WK, Smith SC Jr, Tomaselli GF. American College of Cardiology/American Heart Association Task Force on Practice Guidelines. 2013 ACC/AHA guideline on the treatment of blood cholesterol to reduce atherosclerotic cardiovascular risk in adults: a report of the American College of Cardiology/American Heart Association Task Force on Practice Guidelines. Circulation. 2014;129(25 Suppl 2):S1–45. https://doi.org/10.1161/01.cir.0000437738.63853.7a. Erratum in: Circulation. 2015; 132(25):e396. Circulation. 2014; 129(25 Suppl 2):S46-8.
64. Piepoli MF, Hoes AW, Agewall S, Albus C, Brotons C, Catapano AL, Cooney MT, Corrà U, Cosyns B, Deaton C, Graham I, Hall MS, Hobbs FD, Løchen ML, Löllgen H, Marques-Vidal P, Perk J, Prescott E, Redon J, Richter DJ, Sattar N, Smulders Y, Tiberi M, van der Worp HB, van Dis I, Verschuren WM, Authors/Task Force Members. 2016 European Guidelines on cardiovascular disease prevention in clinical practice: The Sixth Joint Task Force of the European Society of Cardiology and Other Societies on Cardiovascular Disease Prevention in Clinical Practice (constituted by representatives of 10 societies and by invited experts). Developed with the special contribution of the European Association for Cardiovascular Prevention & Rehabilitation (EACPR). Eur Heart J. 2016;37(29):2315–81. https://doi.org/10.1093/eurheartj/ehw106.
65. Julius S, Jamerson K, Mejia A, Krause L, Schork N, Jones K. The association of borderline hypertension with target organ changes and higher coronary risk. Tecumseh blood pressure study. JAMA. 1990;264:354–8.

66. Lloyd-Jones DM, Evans JC, Levy D. Hypertension in adults across the age spectrum: current outcomes and control in the community. JAMA. 2005;294:466–72.
67. Miura K, Daviglus ML, Dyer AR, Liu K, Garside DB, Stamler J, Greenland P. Relationship of blood pressure to 25-year mortality due to coronary heart disease, cardiovascular diseases, and all causes in young adult men: the Chicago Heart Association Detection Project in Industry. Arch Intern Med. 2001;161:1501–8.
68. Vasan RS, Larson MG, Leip EP, Evans JC, O'Donnell CJ, Kannel WB, Levy D. Impact of high-normal blood pressure on the risk of cardiovascular disease. N Engl J Med. 2001;345:1291–7.
69. Russell LB, Valiyeva E, Carson JL. Effects of prehypertension on admissions and deaths: a simulation. Arch Intern Med. 2004;164(19):2119–24. Erratum in: Arch Intern Med. 2005;165:1720.
70. Grotto I, Grossman E, Huerta M, Sharabi Y. Prevalence of prehypertension and associated cardiovascular risk profiles a young Israeli adults. Hypertension. 2006;48:254–9.
71. Lloyd-Jones DM. Ischemic heart disease risk. Chapter B77. In: Izzo JL, Sicca DA, Black HR, editors. Hypertension primer. 4th ed. Philadelphia, PA: Lippincott Williams & Wilkins; 2008. p. 349–53.
72. Kannel WB, PWF W. Cardiovascular risk factors and hypertension. In: Izzo JL, Sicca DA, Black HR, editors. Hypertension Primer. 4th ed. Philadelphia, PA: Lippincott Williams & Wilkins; 2008. p. 244–9.
73. Giannotti G, Doerries C, Mocharla PS, Mueller MF, Bahlmann FH, Horvàth T, Jiang H, Sorrentino SA, Steenken N, Manes C, Marzilli M, Rudolph KL, Lüscher TF, Drexler H, Landmesser U. Impaired endothelial repair capacity of early endothelial progenitor cells in prehypertension: relation to endothelial dysfunction. Hypertension. 2010;55:1389–97.
74. Ikram MK, Witteman JC, Vingerling JR, Breteler MM, Hofman A, de Jong PT. Retinal vessel diameters and risk of hypertension: the Rotterdam Study. Hypertension. 2006;47:189–94.
75. Manios E, Tsivgoulis G, Koroboki E, Stamatelopoulos K, Papamichael C, Toumanidis S, Stamboulis E, Vemmos K, Zakopoulos N. Impact of prehypertension on common carotid artery intima-media thickness and left ventricular mass. Stroke. 2009;40:1515–8.
76. Mahoney LT, Burns TL, Stanford W, Thompson BH, Witt JD, Rost CA, Lauer RM. Coronary risk factors measured in childhood and young adult life are associated with coronary artery calcification in young adults: the Muscatine Study. J Am Coll Cardiol. 1996;27(2):277–84.
77. Peralta CA, Adeney KL, Shlipak MG, Jacobs D Jr, Duprez D, Bluemke D, Polak J, Psaty B, Kestenbaum BR. Structural and functional vascular alterations and incident hypertension in normotensive adults: the Multi-Ethnic Study of Atherosclerosis. Am J Epidemiol. 2010;171:63–71.
78. Julius S, Nesbitt SD, Egan BM, Weber MA, Michelson EL, Kaciroti N, Black HR, Grimm RH Jr, Messerli FH, Oparil S, Schork MA, Trial of Preventing Hypertension (TROPHY) Study Investigators. Feasibility of treating prehypertension with an angiotensin-receptor blocker. N Engl J Med. 2006;354:1685–897.
79. Lüders S, Schrader J, Berger J, Unger T, Zidek W, Böhm M, Middeke M, Motz W, Lübcke C, Gansz A, Brokamp L, Schmieder RE, Trenkwalder P, Haller H, Dominiak P, PHARAO Study Group. The PHARAO study: prevention of hypertension with the angiotensin-converting enzyme inhibitor ramipril in patients with high-normal blood pressure: a prospective, randomized, controlled prevention trial of the German Hypertension League. J Hypertens. 2008;26:1487–96.
80. NAVIGATOR Study Group, McMurray JJ, Holman RR, Haffner SM, Bethel MA, Holzhauer B, Hua TA, Belenkov Y, Boolell M, Buse JB, Buckley BM, Chacra AR, Chiang FT, Charbonnel B, Chow CC, Davies MJ, Deedwania P, Diem P, Einhorn D, Fonseca V, Fulcher GR, Gaciong Z, Gaztambide S, Giles T, Horton E, Ilkova H, Jenssen T, Kahn SE, Krum H, Laakso M, Leiter LA, Levitt NS, Mareev V, Martinez F, Masson C, Mazzone T, Meaney E, Nesto R, Pan C, Prager R, Raptis SA, Rutten GE, Sandstroem H, Schaper F, Scheen A, Schmitz O, Sinay I, Soska V, Stender S, Tamás G, Tognoni G, Tuomilehto J, Villamil AS, Vozár J, Califf RM. Effect of valsartan on the incidence of diabetes and cardiovascular events. N Engl J Med. 2010;362:1477–90.

81. Stang A, Moebus S, Möhlenkamp S, Dragano N, Schmermund A, Beck M, Siegrist J, Erbel R, Jöckel KH, Heinz Nixdorf Recall Study Investigative Group. Algorithms for converting random-zero to automated oscillometric blood pressure values, and vice versa. Am J Epidemiol. 2006;164:85–94.
82. National Center for Health Statistics. Health, United States. With chartbook on trends in the health of Americans. Hyattsville, MD: National Center for Health Statistics; 2007.
83. Westheim A, Klemetsrud T, Tretli S, Stokke HP, Olsen H. Blood pressure levels in treated hypertensive patients in general practice in Norway. Blood Press. 2001;10:37–42.
84. Ong KL, Tso AW, Lam KS, Cheung BM. Gender difference in blood pressure control and cardiovascular risk factors in Americans with diagnosed hypertension. Hypertension. 2008;51:1142–8.
85. Halimi JM, Giraudeau B, Vol S, Cacès E, Nivet H, Tichet J. The risk of hypertension in men: direct and indirect effects of chronic smoking. J Hypertens. 2002;20:187–93.
86. Detrano R, Guerci AD, Carr JJ, Bild DE, Burke G, Folsom AR, Liu K, Shea S, Szklo M, Bluemke DA, O'Leary DH, Tracy R, Watson K, Wong ND, Kronmal RA. Coronary calcium as a predictor of coronary events in four racial or ethnic groups. N Engl J Med. 2008;358:1336–45.
87. Elias-Smale SE, Proença RV, Koller MT, Kavousi M, van Rooij FJ, Hunink MG, Steyerberg EW, Hofman A, Oudkerk M, Witteman JC. Coronary calcium score improves classification of coronary heart disease risk in the elderly: the Rotterdam study. J Am Coll Cardiol. 2010;56:1407–14.
88. Lloyd-Jones D, Adams R, Carnethon M, De Simone G, Ferguson TB, Flegal K, Ford E, Furie K, Go A, Greenlund K, Haase N, Hailpern S, Ho M, Howard V, Kissela B, Kittner S, Lackland D, Lisabeth L, Marelli A, McDermott M, Meigs J, Mozaffarian D, Nichol G, O'Donnell C, Roger V, Rosamond W, Sacco R, Sorlie P, Stafford R, Steinberger J, Thom T, Wasserthiel-Smoller S, Wong N, Wylie-Rosett J, Hong Y, American Heart Association Statistics Committee and Stroke Statistics Subcommittee. Heart disease and stroke statistics—2009 update: a report from the American Heart Association Statistics Committee and Stroke Statistics Subcommittee. Circulation. 2009;119:e21–181.
89. Aronow WS, Fleg JL, Pepine CJ, Artinian NT, Bakris G, Brown AS, Ferdinand KC, Forciea MA, Frishman WH, Jaigobin C, Kostis JB, Mancia G, Oparil S, Ortiz E, Reisin E, Rich MW, Schocken DD, Weber MA, Wesley DJ. ACCF/AHA 2011 Expert Consensus Document on Hypertension in the Elderly: a report of the American College of Cardiology Foundation Task Force on Clinical Expert Consensus Documents. Circulation. 2011;123:2434–506.
90. Reboldi G, Gentile G, Angeli F, Ambrosio G, Mancia G, Verdecchia P. Effects of intensive blood pressure reduction on myocardial infarction and stroke in diabetes: a meta-analysis in 73,913 patients. J Hypertens. 2011;29:1253–69.
91. Rumberger JA, Simons DB, Fitzpatrick LA, Sheedy PF, Schwartz RS. Coronary artery calcium area by electron-beam computed tomography and coronary atherosclerotic plaque area. A histopathologic correlative study. Circulation. 1995;92:2157–62.
92. McEvoy JW, Martin SS, Dardari ZA, Miedema MD, Sandfort V, Yeboah J, Budoff MJ, Goff DC Jr, Psaty BM, Post WS, Nasir K, Blumenthal RS, Blaha MJ. Coronary artery calcium to guide a personalized risk-based approach to initiation and intensification of antihypertensive therapy. Circulation. 2017;135(2):153–65. https://doi.org/10.1161/CIRCULATIONAHA.116.025471.

27 Blood Pressure Measurement, White-Coat and Masked Hypertension

G. Seravalle, G. Grassi, and Giuseppe Mancia

27.1 Introduction

High blood pressure is the most common diagnosis in adult primary care practice and the most important cardiovascular risk factor [1].

While it is quite easy to obtain a blood pressure (BP) measurement, it appears difficult to estimate the correct BP level in a given circumstance [2] and this should be regarded as a surrogate measure for the true BP [3]. Additional modalities capable to overcome the limitations of the clinic BP measurement, the so-called office BP, are now available to physicians wishing to obtain the best BP profile of the patients: automated office BP measurement, home BP monitoring, and ambulatory BP monitoring (ABPM). These new modalities have also allowed to identify two specific phenomena linked to hypertension: the white-coat and masked hypertension. These modalities also allow to evaluate with more accuracy the efficacy of the antihypertensive treatment and are able to correlate with cardiovascular prognosis. These aspects will be considered in this chapter.

G. Seravalle
Cardiology Department, Istituto Auxologico Italiano, IRCCS S. Luca Hospital, Milano, Italy

G. Grassi
Medical Clinic, S. Gerardo Hospital, University Milano-Bicocca, Monza-Milano, Italy

IRCCS Multimedica, Milano, Italy

G. Mancia (✉)
Emeritus Professor of Medicine, University of Milano-Bicocca, Milan, Italy
e-mail: giuseppe.mancia@unimib.it

R. Zimlichman et al. (eds.), *Prehypertension and Cardiometabolic Syndrome*, Updates in Hypertension and Cardiovascular Protection,
https://doi.org/10.1007/978-3-319-75310-2_27

27.2 Automated Measurement: Advantages in Office and Self-Measurement

The automated BP measurement modality allows multiple BP readings being taken with a fully automated device while the patient rests quietly and alone in a room. This could be particularly useful during office detection. An improved accuracy, a reduced digit preference, an absence of observer bias, and a strong relationship with target organ damage are advantage of this modality of BP measurement [4, 5]. It has been shown a high correlation between automated office BP measurements and mean awake ambulatory blood pressure monitoring (ABPM) and target organ damage. This suggests that a replacement of traditional office BP assessment should be advocated. Their use should also be suggested and improved for self-measurement at home.

Home BP monitoring per se shows several advantages: (a) predicts subclinical target organ damage and cardiovascular events similar to ABPM and better than office BP; (b) shows considerable agreement with ABPM in detecting white-coat and masked hypertension; and (c) improves long-term adherence to antihypertensive drug treatment and hypertension control rates in treated hypertensive patients [6]. Thus home BP could have a primary role in the diagnosis and in long-term follow-up [7].

27.3 Ambulatory BP Monitoring

The analysis of 24 h ambulatory BP recordings can yield a rich body of information on different aspects that characterize subjects' BP daily life. This includes quantification of 24 h, daytime and nighttime average BP values, the BP fluctuations between day and night, the difference between clinic and 24 h or daytime average BP and the different components of overall 24 h BP variability. Several studies have shown that these parameters may allow more precise diagnostic and prognostic evaluations of the hypertensive state of our patients [8–10]. Several are the methodological advantages of this measurement: (a) 24 h average BP values are more reproducible than isolated office readings [10]; (b) noninvasive automatic ambulatory BP monitoring, although requiring repeated cuff inflations throughout the day and night and thus unavoidably worsening sleep quality, does not usually prevent the occurrence of a physiological nocturnal BP reduction [11]; (c) automatic and semiautomatic cuff inflations do not trigger any alerting reaction and pressure rise in the patients [12]; and (d) it is largely unaffected by any placebo effect. ABPM enables white-coat hypertension to be ruled out while it facilitates the assessment of BP during sleep-time allowing to find a nondipping pattern and nocturnal hypertension that are strongly associated with increased cardiovascular morbidity and mortality [10].

Some disadvantages should be taken into account. First, the discontinuation nature of the BP readings does not prevent the reliable calculation of the 24 h average BP values and relative BP variability. Second, the accuracy of measurements in ambulant subjects may not be guaranteed even with validated devices. This emphasizes the need for adequate signal editing to remove artifacts before proceeding to data analysis.

27.4 Clinical Value of ABPM

The large diffusion of this technique in a clinical setting has allowed to collect data with an important clinical value. Several studies have shown that the organ damage associated with hypertension is more closely related to 24 h mean [13] and 24 h systolic or diastolic BP has a steeper relationship with cardiovascular morbid or fatal events than the corresponding office BP values (Fig. 27.1) [9, 14–17]. This is particularly true for left ventricular hypertrophy, alterations in left ventricular function, increased number of lacunae at the brain level, renal dysfunction, and alterations in small and large arteries [9, 13, 18]. Data coming from controlled studies have clearly shown that regression of left ventricular hypertrophy was more closely predicted by treatment-induced changes in 24 h average than in clinic BP supporting the prognostic superiority of the former approach [19].

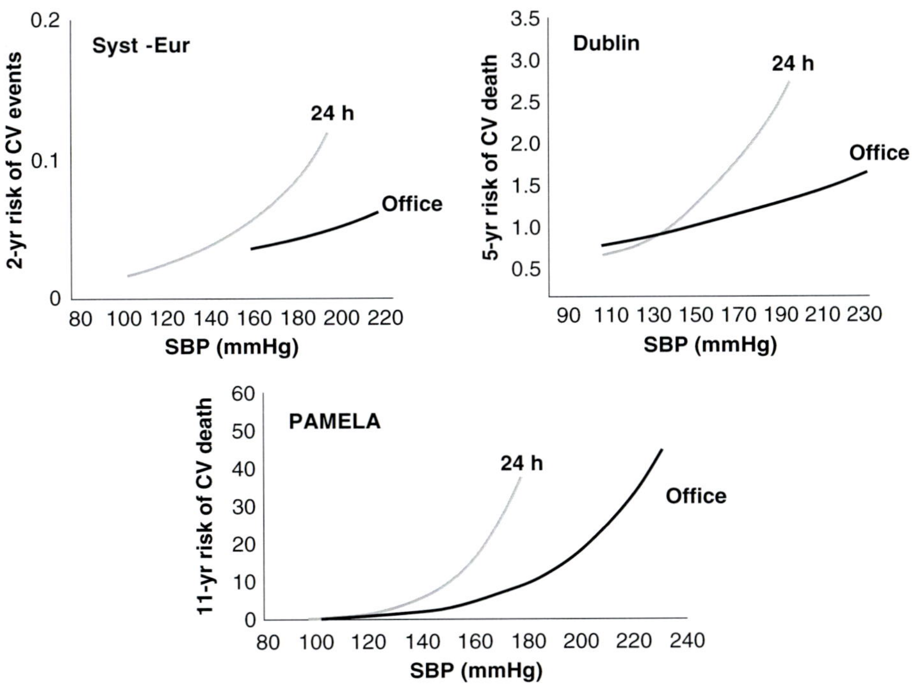

Fig. 27.1 Relationship between office blood pressure (BP) or 24 h average systolic blood pressure (SBP) with cardiovascular (CV) events or mortality in the SYST-EUR study, in the Dublin study, and in the PAMELA study. Figure created with data derived from Refs. [15, 16, and 9], respectively

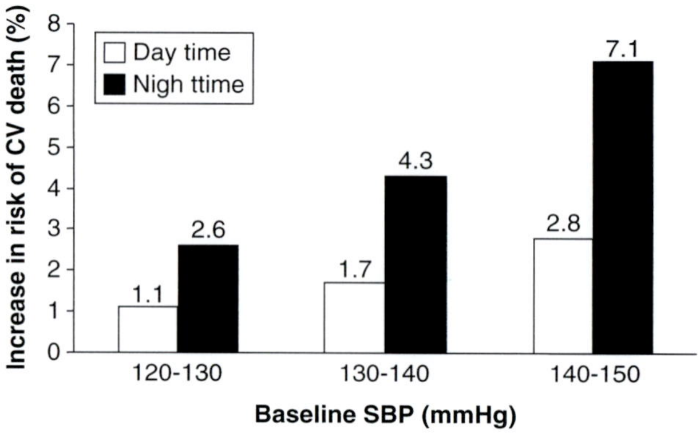

Fig. 27.2 Increase in the risk of cardiovascular (CV) death for a 10 mmHg increase in systolic blood pressure (SBP) at different initial SBP values. Data from the 148-month follow-up in the PAMELA study. Figure created with data derived from Ref. [9]

Additional support to the prognostic importance of the day-night BP cycle comes from the evidence that absolute nighttime BP values are prognostically superior to the daytime ones. In the PAMELA study [9] a 10 mmHg increase of nighttime systolic BP was accompanied by a much greater increase of cardiovascular mortality (Fig. 27.2). This was also evident in the 8.4 years follow-up in the Dublin outcome study [16] showing a 21% increase in cardiovascular mortality for the increase in night systolic BP. The superior prognostic value of nighttime BP has been found to predict also the development of nephropathy [20].

The prognostic importance of the day-night BP reduction has also been documented in population-based longitudinal studies, confirming data obtained in hypertensive population [15, 21]. In the Ohasama study [22] nondipping was associated with a 2.5 increase in cardiovascular mortality than in dippers. This was also evident in the 12 years follow-up of the PAMELA study [23].

In addition to day-night BP changes, 24 h BP monitoring allows to evaluate short-term variations that are particularly marked and frequent during the day and occur in a lesser degree also during the nighttime [24]. These variations largely depend on behavioral activities but other factors may favor or oppose BP changes through the mediation of the autonomic nervous system and vasoactive substances [25]. It has been established that BP variability increases with age and with the progression of the hypertensive state [24, 25]. The limitation due to the intermittent BP readings is improved with the development of devices that are able to measure beat-to-beat ambulatory BP noninvasively, thus allowing a precise quantification of the overall magnitude of the BP variations and an analysis of its patterns.

27.5 White-Coat and Masked Hypertension

The use of ABPM and home BP measurements has allowed to disclose two conditions unknown during office evaluation: white-coat (WC) and masked hypertension [10, 26]. In WCH, out-of-office BP is normal, and BP values in the doctor's office are persistently elevated, whereas in masked is the opposite, that is, out-of-office BP is high, where as office BP is normal (Fig. 27.3). The original definition of WCH is

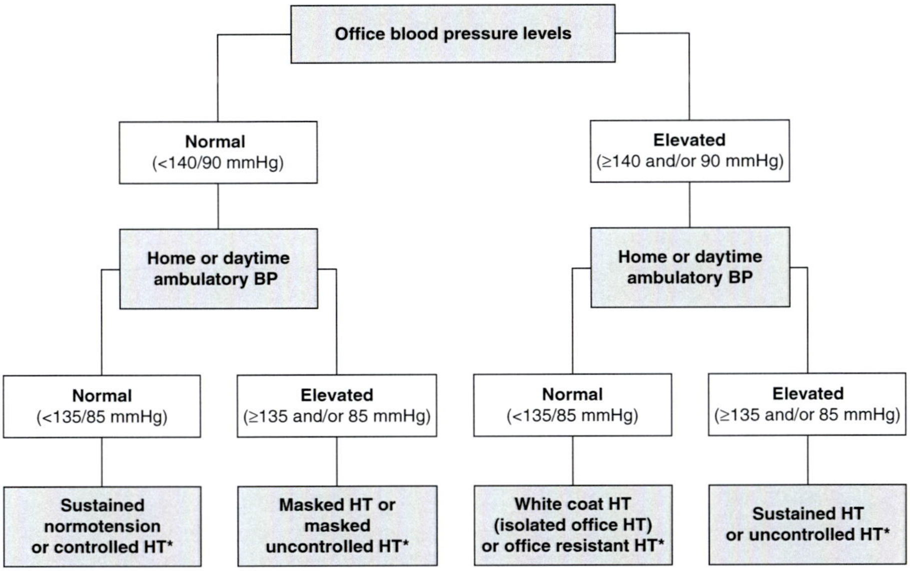

Fig. 27.3 Schematic relationship between office and home or daytime ambulatory blood pressure in treated hypertensive subjects (asterisk). *BP* Blood pressure, *HT* Hypertension

based on the belief that this condition is caused by the alerting reaction and transient BP rise that accompany the doctor's visit but because other factors are involved in frequently the term isolated office hypertension is used [27, 28]. These definitions refer to untreated subjects because in treated patients the BP discrepancy may be caused by specific characteristics of the drugs and patients may have had originally a sustained BP elevation.

27.5.1 White-Coat Hypertension

Although WCH is a consequence of the white-coat effect (WCE), the presence of a significant WCE in a given subject may not necessarily be accompanied by WCH, unless the rise in BP levels during the medical visit is high enough to reach the hypertensive range. In the PIUMA (Progetto Ipertensione Umbria Monitoraggio Ambulatoriale) study [21], conducted in more the 1300 hypertensive subjects, it has been shown that the severity of hypertension was inversely correlated with the prevalence of WCH but directly correlated with the magnitude of WCE. A critical condition for the diagnosis of WCH or isolated office hypertension is the occurrence of a persistent BP elevation at the time of consultation and of normal out-of-office BP levels over time. Thus isolated elevations in office BP values recorded at the beginning of the first visits and that later disappear should be regarded as a temporary BP increase and should not lead to the diagnosis of WCH. In some subjects these transient and non-sustained increases in BP levels may be the result of an increased BP variability.

Also the criteria considered for defining normalcy of BP levels during daytime may lead to over- or underestimation of the frequency of WCH. After the evidence provided by the PAMELA study [29] and other population studies [30, 31] and meta-analyses [32] supporting a threshold value of <130–135/85 mmHg as the upper limit of daytime ambulatory BP normality, the frequency of this phenomenon was reported to range from 9% to 16% in the general population and from 25% to 46% among hypertensive subjects [16, 33, 34]. While the conventional cutoff value for hypertension is an office values of ≥140/90 mmHg, most studies in WCH have used a cutoff value of ≥135/85 mm Hg for out-of-office daytime or home BP and ≥130/80 mmHg for 24 h BP. Due to the importance of nighttime BP levels in predicting cardiovascular outcome and the presence of high BP levels during the night in some subjects with WCH, the new guidelines [10, 26] have expanded the definition of WCH requiring normality not only in awake BP values but also in 24 h (<130/80 mmHg) and sleep (<120/70 mmHg) BP levels.

Several studies have investigated the clinical importance of WCH. These evidences have shown that WCH is frequently associated with cardiac hypertrophy, increased in intima-media thickness or renal damage [35–37]. This was not the case in other studies in which end-organ damage was reported to be similar in WCH and in normotensive subjects [38]. Also longitudinal studies and a recent meta-analysis have reported similar incidence of cardiac and cerebrovascular risk [34, 39, 40]. The observation that the incidence of cerebrovascular events in these patients may begin to rise with a delay greater than 6–8 years indicates however that WCH is not clinically benign. The ten-year follow-up in the Danish study has shown a significant ($p < 0.02$) increase of cardiovascular risk (+25%) [41].

A greater prevalence of metabolic risk factors has been shown in WCH in longer follow-up observation period and this could be associated with the 1.5–2-fold higher risk of developing new-onset diabetes or sustained hypertension [16, 42]. A higher 24 h blood pressure variability with independent and adverse prognostic effects has been observed in WCH than in normotensives and this may contribute to the increased cardiovascular risk of these patients [23].

27.5.2 Masked Hypertension

The prevalence of masked hypertension (normal office BP and elevated ambulatory or home BP values) is thought to be 10–15% of the general population [26]. These subjects should have undergone further examinations because data have clearly suggested that in this condition (a) there is a greater prevalence and severity of metabolic risk factors; (b) common is the relief of subclinical cardiac, vascular, or renal damage; (c) the long-term risk of developing sustained hypertension, diabetes, or left ventricular hypertrophy is 2–3 times greater than that of individuals with normal in- and out-of-office BP; and (d) there is a greater incidence of cardiovascular morbid and fatal events with an overall risk quite closer to established hypertensive subjects [26, 42–46].

27.6 Pathogenetic Mechanisms

As regard the mechanisms, evidences have shown [47–49] that white-coat hypertension is characterized by a marked adrenergic overdrive that appears to be widespread to the whole circulation. It has been shown that muscle sympathetic nerve traffic is about 30% greater in white-coat as compared to age-matched normotensives and that the magnitude of the adrenergic overdrive is almost superimposable to the one characterizing essential hypertension. Direct recordings of sympathetic nerve traffic have shown that the pronounced activation of skin nerves and the concomitant sympathetic inhibition of muscle sympathetic nerve traffic may be similar to a "defense reaction" that has been described in animals. This reaction depends on the activation of superior areas integrating emotional factors [50]. It has been shown that patients with WCH display a higher state of anxiety. Application of laboratory stressors has allowed to show that patients with WCH are not necessarily hyperreactive to all types of emotional stimuli [29]. Microneurographic studies by our group have shown that this adrenergic overactivity observed in essential hypertension and WCH is also associated with an impairment in the baroreflex control of heart rate, but not of sympathetic neural drive [48, 49]. Patients with WCH also display higher circulating levels of asymmetric dimethylarginine, thus suggesting a possible presence of endothelial dysfunction, although not specific for this hypertensive state [51, 52].

Similarly to WCH, masked hypertension is characterized by a hyperadrenergic tone, similar to that observed in WCH and essential hypertension, and by an impairment of baroreflex-mediated cardiovascular control [48]. Some pathophysiological factors have been hypothesized for development of this condition, i.e., increased reactivity to stressor stimuli, smoking, excessive alcohol intake, and endothelial dysfunction; nevertheless the mechanisms responsible for the increase in BP load during ambulatory blood pressure monitoring or at home while office BP remains normal are still unknown [53, 54].

27.7 Prognostic Evidences

The different results of studies on the prognostic value of WCH justify the hypothesis that this condition may have a high prognostic heterogeneity due to its coexistence with metabolic risk factors, subclinical organ damage, and other factors involved in cardiovascular risk. Thus the relationship with an increased incidence of morbid and fatal cerebrovascular and cardiac events may be similar both to normotension and hypertension. Analysis of the PAMELA data has detected two possibilities to differentiate the cardiovascular risk level within the WCH category. One, because in all individuals of this study measurements included both ambulatory and home blood pressure, WC hypertensives were subdivided into those in whom both out-of-office BP values were normal and those in whom one BP was normal while the other was elevated [55]. As shown in Fig. 27.4 the incidence of cardiovascular events was markedly greater in the latter group. The information obtained is

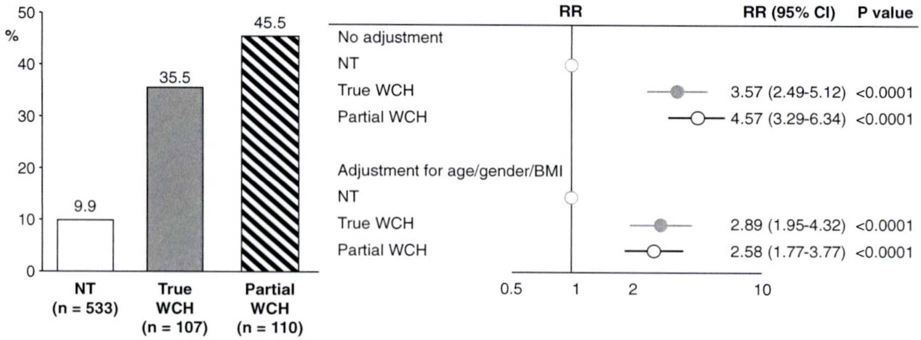

Fig. 27.4 (**a**) Cumulative incidence and (**b**) hazard ratio (HR) for cardiovascular (CV) and all-cause mortality in normotensives (NT), white-coat hypertensives (WCH), and true hypertensives (HT) of PAMELA study over a long follow-up. NT and true HT were defined by office, home, and ambulatory blood pressure normality and elevation, respectively. WCH was defined as true or partial according to whether respectively (1) both ambulatory and home blood pressure were normal and (2) or only one of these pressures was normal. Data were adjusted for age, sex, smoking, blood glucose, serum total cholesterol, body mass index, antihypertensive treatment, and history of cardiovascular events. From Ref. [55], with permission

therefore redundant. The combined use of these two approaches may serve to identify WC hypertensives in whom a substantial increase of cardiovascular risk may justify not only a close follow-up but perhaps also the initiation of antihypertensive treatment. The second possibility is related to the repetition of office blood pressure measurements. WC hypertensive subjects were subdivided into four groups according to whether this condition was found twice or only in one of the office visits. Subjects with stable WCH had an incidence of cardiovascular morbidity and mortality that was greater than that of individuals in whom the office BP elevation was seen one time only.

27.8 Management

Subjects with diagnosis of WCH and masked hypertension need a diagnostic and therapeutic workup to investigate the existence of metabolic risk factors and the presence of target organ damage. They also need frequent follow-up visits and periodical reassessment of risk factors.

While change in lifestyle should be recommended to reduce metabolic abnormalities and the risk of developing diabetes and hypertension, debated is the need of antihypertensive treatment. This issue has never been addressed in specifically designed trials, and large-scale trials on the protective effects of antihypertensive drug treatment have never made use of ambulatory or home-blood pressure measurements except in small subgroups of patients [56]. Because an incorrect diagnosis and treatment of masked hypertension may lead to a worse cardiovascular prognosis, it is fundamental to identify those subjects at higher risk in order to make ambulatory blood pressure monitoring only for those with particular evolution toward diabetes and hypertension or with BP alterations during bedtime due to the fact that even small reductions in out-of-office blood pressure might induce cardiovascular protection.

Conclusions

An improvement on the methods for measuring BP in the doctor's office is needed and should be accompanied with a maintenance of standardized rules. A proper diagnostic approach to the subject who presents with elevated BP levels in the medical office should include implementation of out-of-office BP monitoring for defining whether elevation in BP levels is true or just the result of the white-coat effect. Although ambulatory blood pressure monitoring is considered the reference standard to characterize different subtypes of hypertension, home BP measurements have proved to be similarly effective to discriminate true to false hypertensive or normotensive. The diagnostic approach should be accompanied by the evaluation of metabolic alterations and presence of target organ damage and other factors capable to influence the short- and long-term variability of BP values. While confirmation of WCH would avoid starting antihypertensive treatment in subjects who have otherwise normal out-of-office BP levels, identifying persistent WCH in treated subjects may prevent performing unnecessary and costly additional diagnostic tests, also preventing increasing doses or number of medications. Because of the higher cardiovascular risk of WC and masked hypertensive patients, these deserve a more thorough evaluation and follow-up than normotensive ones.

References

1. Lim SS, Vos T, Flaxman AD, et al. A comparative risk assessment of burden of disease and injury attributable to 67 risk factors and risk factor clusters in 21 regions, 1990–2010: a systematic analysis for the Global Burden of Disease Study 2010. Lancet. 2013;380:2224–60.
2. Turner JR, Viera AJ, Shimbo D. Ambulatory blood pressure monitoring in clinical practice: a review. Am J Med. 2015;128:14–20.
3. Pickering T, Shimbo D, Haas D. Ambulatory blood-pressure monitoring. N Engl J Med. 2006;354:2368–74.
4. Myers MG. Replacing manual sphygmomanometers with automated blood pressure measurement in routine clinical practice. Clin Exp Pharmacol Physiol. 2014;41:46–53.
5. Andreadis EA, Angelopoulos ET, Agaliotis GD, et al. Why use automated office blood pressure measurements in clinical practice? High Blood Press Cardiovasc Prev. 2011;18:89–91.
6. Imai Y. Clinical significance of home blood pressure and its possible practical application. Clin Exp Nephrol. 2014;18:24–40.
7. Stergiou GS, Kollias A, Zeniodi M, et al. Home blood pressure monitoring: primary role in hypertension management. Curr Hypertens Rep. 2014;16:462.
8. Parati G, Mutti E, Ravogli A, et al. Advantages and disadvantages of non-invasive ambulatory blood pressure monitoring. J Hypertens. 1990;8(suppl 6):S33–8.
9. Sega R, Facchetti R, Bombelli M, et al. Prognostic value of ambulatory and home blood pressures compared with office blood pressure in the general population: follow-up results from the Pressioni Arteriose Monitorate e Loro Associazioni (PAMELA) study. Circulation. 2005;111:1777–83.

10. O'Brien E, Parati G, Stergiou G, et al. European Society of Hypertension position paper on ambulatory blood pressure monitoring. J Hypertens. 2013;31:1731–68.
11. Villani A, Parati G, Groppelli A, et al. Noninvasive automatic blood pressure monitoring does not attenuate night-time hypotension. Am J Hypertens. 1992;5:744–7.
12. Parati G, Pomidossi G, Casadei R, Mancia G. Lack of alerting reactions to intermittent cuff inflations during non-invasive blood pressure monitoring. Hypertension. 1985;7:597–601.
13. Mancia G, Parati G. Ambulatory blood pressure monitoring and organ damage. Hypertension. 2000;36:894–900.
14. Redon J, Campos C, Narciso ML, Rodicio JL, Pascual JM, Ruilope LM. Prognostic value of ambulatory blood pressure monitoring in refractory hypertension: a prospective study. Hypertension. 1998;31:712–8.
15. Staessen JA, Thijs L, Fagard R, O'Brien ET, Tuomilehto J, Webster J. Predicting cardiovascular risk using conventional vs ambulatory blood pressure in older patients with systolic hypertension. Systolic Hypertension in Europe Trial Investigators. JAMA. 1999;282:539–46.
16. Dolan E, Stanton A, Thijs L, et al. Superiority of ambulatory over clinic blood pressure measurement in predicting mortality: the Dublin outcome study. Hypertension. 2005;46:156–61.
17. Kikuya M, Hansen TW, Thijs L, et al. International Database on ambulatory blood pressure monitoring in relation to Cardiovascular Outcomes Investigators. Diagnostic thresholds for ambulatory blood pressure monitoring based on 10 year cardiovascular risk. Circulation. 2007;115:2145–52.
18. Zanchetti A, Bond MG, Heening M, et al. On behalf of the ELSA Study group. Risk factors associated with alterations in carotid intima-media thickness in hypertension: baseline data from the European Lacidipine Study on Atherosclerosis. J Hypertens. 1998;16:949–61.
19. Mancia G, Zanchetti A, Agabiti-Rosei et al. for the SAMPLE study group. Ambulatory blood pressure is superiori to clinic blood pressure in predicting treatment-induced regression of left ventricular hypertrophy. Circulation. 1997;95:1464–70.
20. Lurbe E, Redon J, Kesani A, et al. Increase in nocturnal blood pressure and progression to microalbuminuria in type 1 diabetes. N Engl J Med. 2002;347:797–805.
21. Verdecchia P, Porcellati C, Schillaci G, et al. Ambulatory blood pressure. An independent predictor of prognosis in essential hypertension. Hypertension. 1994;24:793–801.
22. Ohkubo T, Imai Y, Tsuji I, et al. Relation between nocturnal decline in blood pressure and mortality. The Ohasama Study. Am J Hypertens. 1997;10:1201–7.
23. Mancia G, Bombelli M, Facchetti R, et al. Long-term prognostic value of blood pressure variability in the general population: results of the Pressioni Arteriose Monitorate e Loro Associazioni Study. Hypertension. 2007;49:1265–70.
24. Mancia G, Parati G, Di Rienzo M, Zanchetti A. Blood pressure variability. In: Zanchetti A, Mancia G, editors. Handbook of hypertension, vol 17: pathophysiology of hypertension. Elsevier, Amsterdam: The Netherlands; 1997. p. 117–69.
25. Mancia G. Short- and long-term blood pressure variability: present and future. Hypertension. 2012;60:512–7.
26. Mancia G, Fagard R, Narkiewicz K, et al. Task Force Members. 2013 ESH/ESC Guidelines for the management of arterial hypertension: the task force for the management of arterial hypertension of the European Society of Hypertension (ESH) and of the European Society of Cardiology (ESC). J Hypertens. 2013;31:1281–357.
27. Mancia G, Bertinieri G, Grassi G, et al. Effects of blood pressure measurement by the doctor on patient's blood pressure and heart rate. Lancet. 1983;2:695–8.
28. Parati G, Bilo G, Mancia G. White coat effect and white coat hypertension: what do they mean? Cardiovasc Rev Rep. 2003;24:477–84.
29. Mancia G, Sega R, Bravi C, et al. Ambulatory blood pressure normality: results from the PAMELA study. J Hypertens. 1995;13:1377–90.
30. Staessen JA, Bieniaszewski L, O'Brien ET, Imai Y, Fagard R. An epidemiological approach to ambulatory blood pressure monitoring: the Belgian Population Study. Blood Press Monit. 1996;1:13–26.

31. Imai Y, Nagai K, Sakuma H, et al. Ambulatory blood pressure of adults in Ohasama. Jpn Hyperten. 1993;22:900–12.
32. Staessen JA, Fagard RH, Lijnen PJ, Thijs L, Van Hoof R, Amery AK. Mean and range of the ambulatory pressure in normotensive subjects from a meta-analysis of 23 studies. Am J Cardiol. 1991;67:723–7.
33. Pickering TG, Hall JE, Appel LJ, et al. Recommendations for blood pressure measurement in humans and experimental animals. Part 1: blood pressure measurement in humans: a statement for professionals from the subcommittee of professionall and public education of the American Heart Association Council on High Blood Pressure Research. Hypertension. 2005;45:142–61.
34. Fagard RH, Cornelissen VA. Incidence of cardiovascular events in white-coat, masked and sustained hypertension versus true normotension: a meta-analysis. J Hypertens. 2007;25:2193–8.
35. Pall D, Juhasz M, Lengyel S, et al. Assessment of target-organ damage in adolescent white-coat and sustained hypertensives. J Hypertens. 2010;28:2139–44.
36. Palatini P, Mormino P, Santonastaso M, et al. Target organ damage in stage I hypertensive subjects with white coat and sustained hypertension. Results from the HARVEST study. Hypertension. 1998;32:377–8.
37. Nakashima T, Yamano S, Sasaki R, et al. White-coat hypertension contributes to the presence of carotid atherosclerosis. Hypertens Res. 2004;27:739–45.
38. Kostis V, Stabouli S. Toumanidis, et al Target organ damage in white-coat and masked hypertension. Am J Hypertens. 2008;21:393–9.
39. Verdecchia P, Reboldi GP, Angeli F, et al. Short- and long-term incidence of stroke in white-coat hypertension. Hypertension. 2005;45:203–8.
40. Kario K, Shimada K, Schwartz JE, et al. Silent and clinically overt stroke in older Japanese subjects with white-coat and sustained hypertension. J Am Coll Cardiol. 2001;38:238–45.
41. Gustavsen PH, Hoegholm A, Bang LE, Kristensen KS. White coat hypertension is a cardiovascular risk factor: a 10 year follow-up study. J Hum Hypertens. 2003;17:811–7.
42. Mancia G, Bombelli M, Facchetti R, et al. Long-term risk of sustained hypertension in white coat or masked hypertension. Hypertension. 2009;54:226–32.
43. Bobrie G, Chatellier G, Genes N, et al. Cardiovascular prognosis of masked hypertension detected by blood pressure self-measurement in elderly treated hypertensive patients. JAMA. 2004;291:1342–9.
44. Angeli F, Reboldi G, Verdecchia P. Masked hypertension: evaluation, prognosis, and treatment. Am J Hypertens. 2010;23:941–8.
45. Pierdomenico SD, Cuccurullo F. Prognostic values of white coat and masked hypertension diagnosed by ambulatory monitoring in initially untreated subjects: an updated meta-analysis. Am J Hypertens. 2011;24:52–8.
46. Ohkubo T, Kikuya M, Metoki H, et al. Prognosis of masked hypertension and white coat hypertension detected by 24-h ambulatory blood pressure monitoring 10 year follow-up from the Ohasama study. J Am Coll Cardiol. 2005;46:508–15.
47. Smith PA, Graham LN, Mackintosh AF, et al. Sympathetic neural mechanisms in white coat hypertension. J Am Coll Cardiol. 2002;40:126–32.
48. Grassi G, Seravalle G, Quarti Trevano F, et al. Neurogenic abnormalities in masked hypertension. Hypertension. 2007;50:537–42.
49. Grassi G, Seravalle G, Buzzi S, et al. Muscle and skin sympathetic nerve traffic during physician and nurse blood pressure measurement. J Hypertens. 2013;31:1131–5.
50. Ogedegbe G, Pickering TG, Clemow L, et al. The misdiagnosis of hypertension: the role of patient anxiety. Arch Intern Med. 2008;168:2459–65.
51. Curgunlu A, Uzun H, Bavunoglu I, et al. Increased circulating concentrations of asymmetric dimethylarginine (ADMA) in white coat hypertension. J Hum Hypertens. 2005;19:629–33.
52. Grassi G. Assessment of sympathetic cardiovascular drive in human hypertension: achievements and perspectives. Hypertension. 2009;54:690–7.
53. Schnall PI, Schwartz JE, Landsbergis PA, Warren K, Pickering TG. Relation between job strain, alcohol, and ambulatory blood pressure. Hypertension. 1992;19:488–94.

54. Mann SJ, James GD, Wang RS, Pickering TG. Elevation of ambulatory systolic blood pressure in hypertesnive smokers. A case-control study. JAMA. 1991;265:2226–8.
55. Mancia G, Bombelli M, Brambilla G, et al. Long-term prognostic value of white coat hypertension: an insight from diagnostic use of both ambulatory and home blood pressure measurements. Hypertension. 2013;62:168–74.
56. Law MR, Morris JK, Wald NJ. Use of blood pressure lowering drugs in the prevention of cardiovascular disease: meta-analysis of 147 randomised trials in the context of expectations from prospective epidemiological studies. BMJ. 2009;338:b1665.

Blood Pressure Variability 28

Gianfranco Parati and Juan Eugenio Ochoa

28.1 Introduction

Blood pressure (BP) values change significantly over time in response to environmental, behavioral, and emotional stimuli. These variations represent a complex phenomenon, and their assessment is possible by means of different BP measurement methodologies over different time windows: from beat to beat [**very short-term** BP variability (BPV)], within 24 h (from minute to minute, hour to hour and from day to night; **short-term** BPV), over different days (**midterm** day-by-day BPV), or between clinic visits performed over weeks, months, seasons, and years (**long-term** BPV) [1]. While in physiological conditions these variations represent an adaptive response to environmental stimulations from daily life, they may also reflect, however, alterations in cardiovascular regulatory mechanisms or underlying pathological conditions. The clinical significance of BPV has been supported by a large body of evidence showing that the BP-related cardiovascular risk may depend not only on average BP levels but also on the degree of BPV. Either in the short-term (24 h), in the midterm (day-by-day), or in the long term (visit-to-visit), increasing values of BPV have been shown to be associated with development, progression, and severity of cardiac, vascular, and renal organ damage and with an increased risk of cardiovascular events and cardiovascular and all-cause mortality (Fig. 28.1). The evidence is limited, however, regarding the question on whether an enhanced BP

G. Parati (✉)
Istituto Auxologico Italiano, IRCCS, Department of Cardiovascular, Neural and Metabolic Sciences, San Luca Hospital, Milan, Italy

Department of Medicine and Surgery, University of Milano-Bicocca, Milan, Italy
e-mail: gianfranco.parati@unimib.it

J. E. Ochoa
Istituto Auxologico Italiano, IRCCS, Department of Cardiovascular, Neural and Metabolic Sciences, San Luca Hospital, Milan, Italy

R. Zimlichman et al. (eds.), *Prehypertension and Cardiometabolic Syndrome*, Updates in Hypertension and Cardiovascular Protection,
https://doi.org/10.1007/978-3-319-75310-2_28

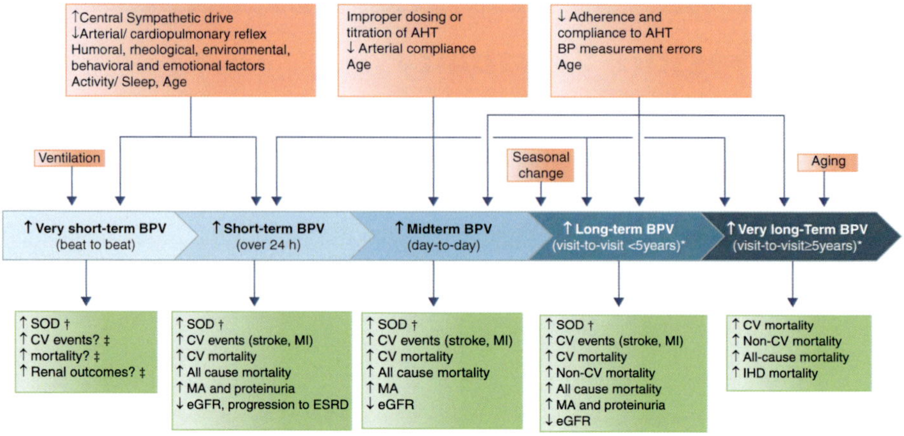

Fig. 28.1 Different types of blood pressure (BP) variability (BPV), their determinants, and prognostic relevance. Taken from [1] by permission. †Cardiac, vascular, and renal SOD; ‡BPV on a beat-by-beat basis has not been routinely measured in population studies. Modified from Parati et al. with permission. *AHT* Antihypertensive treatment, *CV* Cardiovascular, *eGFR* Estimated glomerular filtration rate, *ESRD* End-stage renal disease, *IHD* Ischemic heart disease, *MA* Microalbuminuria, *MI* Myocardial infarction, and *SOD* Subclinical organ damage

variability (considered as an early marker of autonomic dysregulation) may represent also a marker of future hypertension during the prehypertensive (or high normal BP) state. Aim of this chapter is to review the current evidence in the field of BPV regarding its mechanisms, the methodological aspects that should be considered for its assessment, its relevance and significance for cardiovascular prognosis as well as its potential for application in clinical practice. In its last part a brief mention is made on the possible role of BPV as a predictor of future hypertension, as well as on the possibility that the assessment of BPV might contribute to improve the management of subjects with high normal office BP elevation, also defined as prehypertension.

28.2 Very Short-Term and Short-Term BPV

28.2.1 Mechanisms

In physiological conditions, BP fluctuations occurring beat-by-beat and within the 24 h may represent an adaptive response of neural [2–4], humoral, vascular [5–8], and rheological mechanisms to environmental, behavioral, and emotional stimuli of daily life. However, when increases in short-term BPV are sustained, they may also reflect alterations in regulatory mechanisms (i.e., enhanced sympathetic drive and impaired baroreflex function) in the context of pathological conditions or neurological disorders associated with autonomic dysfunction. Among short-term BP variations, alterations in slower changes occurring from day to night (i.e., non-dipping or rising pattern

Table 28.1 Intrinsic cardiovascular mechanisms and extrinsic factors responsible for BP fluctuations occurring in the very short term and in the short term

Intrinsic cardiovascular regulatory mechanisms
• **Neural:** Central sympathetic drive; Arterial and cardiopulmonary reflexes
• **Rheological:** Blood viscosity
• **Humoral:** Catecholamines; Insulin; insulin resistance; angiotensin II; Bradykinin; Endothelin-1; Nitric oxide; endothelial dysfunction
• **Vascular:** viscoelastic properties of large arteries
• **Renal:** salt sensitivity and sodium excretion
• **Genetic susceptibility:** peripheral vasomotor modulation
Extrinsic factors
• **Emotional:** psychosocial stressors
• **Environmental:** seasonal and altitude-related changes
• **Behavioral:** job strain, levels of physical activity, sleep/wakefulness cycles, quality and duration of sleep, postural changes, patterns of sodium intake
Pathological conditions
• Sleep-related breathing disorders (i.e., OSAS)
• Carotid artery disease
• Arterial hypertension
• Chronic kidney disease
• Heart failure
• Diabetes mellitus
• Postural orthostatic tachycardia syndrome
• Parkinson's disease

of BP at night) have shown to be importantly influenced by subject's behavioral factors such as daytime levels of activity, changes in the sleep/wakefulness cycle, alterations in autonomic cardiovascular modulation, increased sympathetic activity during nighttime [4, 9], increased salt sensitivity and reduced sodium excretion [10, 11], sleep-related breathing disorders, obesity, insulin resistance [12], endothelial dysfunction [13], or specific drugs intake [14, 15]. A list of intrinsic cardiovascular mechanisms and extrinsic factors responsible for BP fluctuations occurring in the very short term and in the short term are summarized in Table 28.1.

28.2.2 Methods for Assessment of Different Types of Blood Pressure Variability

An accurate assessment of fast BP fluctuations occurring in the very short term requires implementation of continuous beat-to-beat BP recordings over variable recording periods (i.e., 1 min to 24 h). These recordings not only allow estimation of the standard deviation (SD) of average BP levels (a traditional index of BPV), but also of very low-, low-, and high-frequency components of BP spectra contributing to overall BPV, thus allowing an indirect evaluation of autonomic cardiovascular modulation [16]. However, the difficulties in implementing continuous invasive recordings outside the laboratory setting in a daily life situation on one side and the instability of measurements, the cost, and technical difficulties in performing noninvasive beat-by-beat recordings on the other side have prevented the assessment of beat-by-beat BPV from being widely used in clinical practice. Although continuous beat-to-beat BP recordings would represent the optimal solution also for assessment of short-term BPV, its assessment is also possible through noninvasive, intermittent 24 h ABPM, at intervals between measurements from 15 to 30 min [17, 18]. This allows the straightforward estimation of short-term BPV for the whole 24 h period and separately for the daytime and nighttime subperiods. Table 28.2 summarizes some important aspects regarding the assessment of very short-term and short-term BPV.

Table 28.2 Different components of BPV and methods for their measurement

Characteristic	Very short-term BPV (beat-by-beat)	Short-term BPV (within 24 h)	Midterm BPV (day-by-day)	Long-term BPV (visit-to-visit)
Method for BP measurement	Continuous BP recordings in a laboratory setting or under ambulatory conditions	ABPM	HBPM ABPM over ≥48 h	OBP HBPM ABPM
Measurement intervals	Beat-to-beat	15–20 min intervals for day and night, respectively. A 15-min interval for the whole 24 h time desirable but not always feasible	Day-by-day	Spaced by visits over weeks, months, and years. For treatment changes, allow a 3-month window before estimating BPV
Number of measurements	Variable depending on patients' heart rate and recording duration	Ideally 87–96, at least 72 valid measurements when focusing on BPV	Duplicate BP measurements in the morning and in the evening (1 min apart) for each day over 7 days	At least 2–3 BP measurements during a visit (1 min apart) when using OBP Duplicate BP measurements in the morning and in the evening (1 min apart) for each day over 7 days before each clinic visit when using HBPM. At least 48 valid measurements for ABPM
Time of measurement in treated patients	NA	NA	Morning BP measurements before drug intake	Before drug intake (or maybe drug intake within 24 h before office visit?)

Table 28.2 (continued)

Characteristic	Very short-term BPV (beat-by-beat)	Short-term BPV (within 24 h)	Midterm BPV (day-by-day)	Long-term BPV (visit-to-visit)
Duration of the recording period	Variable recording periods (1 min to 24 h)	24–48 h	Several days, preferably 7 (at least 3 days), over weeks or months	Months to years
Time of measurement	Variable	24 h/daytime/nighttime	Morning and evening	Time of visit when using OBP to be standardized within a study Morning and evening when using HBPM
Main Indices of BPV	SD, CV, AVR Indices of BPV in the frequency domain can be estimated also through spectral analysis (that is, very low-, low-, and high-frequency components). Indices of nonlinear BP changes	SD, CV, ARV, VIM of 24 h, daytime and nighttime BP; time rate of BP changes; 24 h weighted SD Indices of slower BP fluctuations (nighttime BP dipping, morning surge); Slower BP fluctuations and residual components through spectral analysis	SD, CV, ARV, VIM, morning–evening changes, maximum values	SD, CV, ARV, VIM
Stable treatment	NA	Yes	Yes	Not always
Advantages	Beat-to-beat recordings allow assessment of indices of autonomic cardiovascular modulation.	Extensive information on 24 h BP profile (nighttime BP dipping, morning surge). Assessment of efficacy of antihypertensive drug treatment over 24 h.	Appropriate for both midterm and long-term monitoring devoid of the white-coat effect.	Assessment of consistency of BP control by treatment over time. Detection of seasonal BP changes.

(continued)

Table 28.2 (continued)

Characteristic	Very short-term BPV (beat-by-beat)	Short-term BPV (within 24 h)	Midterm BPV (day-by-day)	Long-term BPV (visit-to-visit)
Disadvantages	Stability of measurements might not be guaranteed outside the laboratory setting. Possibility of measurement artifacts.	ABPM: Cannot be repeated frequently. Not well tolerated. Not widely available Difficult to standardize subjects' behavior over 24 h.	Patients' training required for HBPM. 48 h ABPM not well tolerated.	OBP and HBPM provide limited information on diurnal BP profiles. Based on retrospective analysis of available data.

Taken from Parati et al. [1] modified by permission. *BP* Blood pressure, *BPV* Blood pressure variations, *ABPM* Ambulatory blood pressure monitoring, *HBPM* Home blood pressure monitoring, *OBP* Office blood pressure, *SD* Standard deviation, *CV* Coefficient of variation, *ARV* Average real variability, *VIM* Variability independent of the mean

28.2.3 Indices for Estimation of Very Short-Term BPV and Short-Term BPV

In general, indices for assessment of BPV over 24 h can be classified into two main groups: (a) **indices of overall variability**, focusing on faster BP variations occurring reading-to-reading over the 24 h period which assess either the frequency components of BP spectra in the frequency domain, or, in the time domain, the degree of dispersion, the sequence, or the instability of BP values over a certain period of time; and (b) **indices for estimation of specific BPV patterns**, focusing on slower BP variations within 24 h associated with circadian BP changes (i.e., day/night BP profiles) or with other behavioral factors (i.e., "siesta," awakening in the morning) (see Table 28.3).

Assessment of very short-term BPV is only possible from continuous beat-to-beat BP recordings [16]. In addition to calculation of Standard Deviation (SD) and other traditional indices of BPV, continuous BP recordings allow estimation of indices of autonomic cardiovascular modulation by applying power spectral analysis. It decomposes the overall BP Variance or Power into its different components oscillating at different frequencies. The corresponding spectral indices are usually obtained by integrating the BP power spectrum over different frequency bands by focusing on those reported to have a pathophysiological or clinical relevance. This is usually done by computing BP spectral powers over a high-frequency band (HF power, between 0.15 and 0.50 Hz), a low-frequency band (LF power, between 0.15 and 0.07 Hz, centered around 0.1 Hz), and a very low-frequency band (VLF power, <0.07 Hz). These indices yield information on the autonomic control of circulation, on the baroreflex function, and the influence exerted by respiratory activity.

Short-term BPV may be estimated from noninvasive, intermittent 24 h ABP recordings with measurements taken at intervals from 15 to 30 min [17, 18], by

Table 28.3 Indices for estimation of different types of BPV

Overall BPV	
Type of index	Type of BPV assessed
Frequency: – Spectral Indices (HF, LF, VLF) – Residual variability	Short-term BPV Very short-term BPV (spectral analysis)
Dispersion: – Standard Deviation (SD) – Coefficient of variation (CV) – Variability Independent of the Mean (VIM) – Weighted 24 h SD (wSD)[a]	Short-term BPV Midterm BPV Long-term BPV
sequential changes: – Average Real Variability (ARV) – Interval Weighted SD (wSD) – Time rate of BP fluctuations[b]	Short-term BPV Midterm BPV Long-term BPV
Instability: – Range (Maximum-minimum BP) – Peak size (Maximum BP) – Trough size (Mean-minimum BP)	Short-term BPV Midterm BPV
Specific patterns of BPV	
Nocturnal BP fall **Night/day ratio** **Morning Blood Pressure Surge (MBPS)** **Afternoon siesta dipping** **Postprandial Blood Pressure Fall**	Short-term BPV

[a]Assessment of Short-term BPV only
[b]Not for assessment of Short-term BPV

calculating 24 h SD, and also the respective SD for the day- and nighttime subperiods [17, 19]. SD represents the most commonly used index for assessment of short-term BPV and provides a measure of values dispersion over selected time windows (24 h, day and night). SD is affected by trends in BP (e.g., day-night change) and increases with increasing average BP values. In order to account for such a dependence of SD and other absolute measures of BPV on mean BP levels, the coefficient of variation (CV, SD* 100/BP mean) may be computed [19]. **Weighted 24 h SD (wSD)** selectively removes the contribution provided by nighttime BP fall to 24 h SD, by weighting daytime and nighttime BP SD for the duration of the day- and nighttime periods, respectively, and by averaging the SD of these two time subperiods [20]. The corresponding weighted CV may be calculated as well. **Average Real Variability (ARV)** is an index of overall variability based on readings sequence. It is computed as the average of the absolute differences between consecutive BP measurements over 24 h. It focuses on the sequence of BP readings, thus reflecting short-term, reading-to-reading, within-subject variability in BP values [21]. ARV has been shown to be a more specific estimate of 24 h BP variability and a more effective predictor of outcome than SD. Indeed, subjects with different 24 h ABP profiles may have similar SD but different ARV [21–23]. ARV effectively removes the contribution of trends in mean BP to overall BPV and is correlated with mean BP levels. Other indices of overall variability based on reading sequence include **time rate of BP fluctuations** (similar to ARV but quantified as a function of time to provide information also on speed of BP changes) and **interval weighted SD** (similar to SD), both of which take into account the interval between measurements giving larger weight to more distant pairs of readings. **Variability Independent of the Mean (VIM)** excludes the effect of mean BP on BPV by applying nonlinear regression analysis (i.e., plotting SD against mean) [24]. For its estimation, it requires calculation of a factor x from overall population data. Short-term BP variability may also be assessed by estimation of Instability indices that take into account extreme readings of the distribution of BP values within a given time window such as **Range (Maximum-Minimum BP); Peak and Trough values, Peak size (Maximum-Mean BP), and Trough size (Mean-Minimum BP).** Although some studies have demonstrated their clinical value, a major limitation of these indices is that extreme readings have limited reliability within a given distribution of values, including ABPM data, especially when focusing on individual subjects, being unstable and prone to show measurement artifacts more than actual BP values.

It is also possible, from 24 h ambulatory BP recordings, to evaluate **Specific Patterns of BPV** associated with the day/night cycle (representing slower fluctuations within a 24 h time period) or with other behavioral factors (i.e., "siesta"). One of the most common among these indices of BPV estimated from 24 h ABPM is the **nocturnal BP fall**. The reduction in BP during the night can be expressed as percentage of daytime BP [Nocturnal BP fall = (Daytime BP − Nighttime BP)*100/ Daytime BP)] which is mathematically equivalent to the night/day ratio. When considering the degree of nocturnal BP fall (dipping) subjects may be classified into four different categories: (i) normal dipping (fall in nighttime systolic and diastolic BP between 10% and 20%); (ii) non-dipping (or more precisely reduced dipping, with a fall in nighttime systolic and diastolic BP <10%); (iii) rising or "inverted dipping" (increase in nighttime BP compared to daytime values); and (iv) extreme dipping (BP fall during night >20%) [25].

Another index of short-term BPV that can be estimated from 24 h ABPM and which has been suggested to carry a prognostic value is the **morning BP surge (MBPS)**. It is computed in different ways, as a function of the different time points set by the researcher to define wake and sleep time periods. The most commonly employed method is the calculation of the difference between the lowest BP value at night and the highest BP value recorded shortly after awakening. However, when computed in this way, its correlation with nocturnal BP fall may represent a challenge in the interpretation of its impact on outcome data. Other patterns of BP variations that can be evaluated from 24 h ABPM are the **Siesta dipping** (i.e., the BP fall observed in populations where having an afternoon nap (siesta) is a common habit) and the **Postprandial BP fall** which, when excessive, may indicate altered autonomic function. However, up to date, no standards have been provided regarding the calculation of these indices.

28.2.4 Clinical Significance

Several studies have provided evidence supporting the predictive value of short-term BPV either for target organ damage or for cardiovascular events. Most evidence supporting the association of very short- and short-term BPV with target organ damage is derived either from cross-sectional studies reporting on such relationship, or from prospective studies on the predictive value of BPV regarding the development and progression of target organ damage [1]. Early studies implementing intra-arterial beat-to-beat BP recordings in hypertensive subjects showed that at nearly any level of 24 h mean BP, the prevalence and severity of target organ damage was higher in subjects with higher 24 h BPV [26], and that BPV at baseline was a significant predictor of target organ damage, in particular of left ventricular hypertrophy, at the end of follow-up [27]. Regarding the value of short-term BPV as assessed from intermittent ABPM recordings, a recent meta-analysis has shown a significant, although moderate, association between left ventricular mass index and SD of 24 h systolic BP, SD of daytime systolic BP, wSD of 24 h systolic BP, and ARV of 24 h systolic BP [28]. Other studies have shown an independent, although moderate, relationship between short-term BPV and carotid atherosclerosis [29], arterial stiffness, and renal function [7, 30–32]. However, not all studies have reported significant associations [33, 34]. Regarding CV outcomes, several studies and analyses of ABPM registries have confirmed the prognostic role of short-term BPV. An analysis of the International Database on Ambulatory blood pressure in relation to Cardiovascular Outcomes (IDACO) showed a significant predictive value for short-term BPV for most outcomes, ARV of 24 h systolic/diastolic ambulatory BP being a better predictor than SD although the independent additional contribution of BPV to cardiovascular risk was rated as being of minor importance [22]. The analysis of the ABP-International database showed SD of nighttime systolic ambulatory BP to be an independent predictor of cardiovascular events, cardiovascular death, and all-cause mortality in contrast to daytime values [35]. In the Pressioni Arteriose Monitorate e Loro Associazioni (PAMELA) study, there was an independent relationship between the risk of death and SD of 24 h, daytime, and nighttime BP [36]. Moreover, the adjusted risk of cardiovascular death was inversely related to day-night diastolic BP difference and showed a significant positive relationship with residual diastolic BPV, as computed by spectral powers of 24 h ABP recordings, after removing the contribution of day-night BP changes [36]. Accumulating evidence suggests that specific patterns of the diurnal BP variation may indeed have an important prognostic role. Nighttime ambulatory BP carries superior prognostic value as compared to other components of 24 h ABPM [37–39]. In this context, several studies have investigated whether BP fluctuations occurring from day to night or vice versa may have additional prognostic value. More specifically, a non-dipping or even a rising pattern at night have been shown to be associated with increased cardiovascular risk, although recent evidence suggests that it is the nighttime average BP level that mainly matters [38]. Likewise, an increased morning BP surge is associated with a high incidence of cardiovascular events and mortality, but this should be interpreted in the context of the significant relationship between the degree of morning BP surge (carrying high risk) and the degree of nighttime BP fall (carrying low risk), which may affect calculation of the extent of BP rise in the early morning and the interpretation of its prognostic value [40, 41].

Evidence on whether short-term BPV might improve cardiovascular risk stratification over and above average BP levels has been provided by some studies. While in the ABP-International study, the relative integrated discrimination improvement for an increased value of the SD of nighttime systolic BP ranged from 8.5% to 14.5% for cardiovascular and mortality outcomes [35], in the IDACO analysis, ARV added only 0.1% to prediction of the risk of a composite cardiovascular event [22]. This might have depended, however, on the inclusion of data obtained in different populations with different methodology for ambulatory BP monitoring.

Regarding possible threshold values for short-term BPV, evidence has been provided by some outcome studies. An analysis of the ABP-International database showed that a SD of nighttime systolic ambulatory BP ≥12.2 mmHg (compared with SD <12.2 mmHg) was associated with greater risk of cardiovascular events (41%), cardiovascular death (55%), and all-cause mortality (59%) [35]. The corresponding risk estimates for a SD of diastolic BP ≥7.9 mmHg were 48%, 132%, and 77% [35]. The IDACO analysis also presented the risk of total and cardiovascular mortality by fifths of distribution of ARV showing progressively increased risk among quintiles, with higher event rate at systolic/diastolic ARV values of 16.2/12.4 mmHg, respectively [22].

Studies have also been conducted addressing whether short-term BPV may be reduced by specific classes of antihypertensive drugs. In the Natrilix SR Versus Candesartan and Amlodipine in the Reduction of Systolic Blood Pressure in Hypertensive Patients (X-CELLENT) Study, the effect of different antihypertensive agents (candesartan, indapamide sustained release, and amlodipine) as compared to placebo on short-term BPV was examined. Amlodipine and indapamide were the only agents associated with a significantly decreased short-term BPV after a 3-month treatment [42]. Another report in hypertensive subjects showed that subjects treated with Calcium Chanel Blockers (CCBs) or diuretics alone, or in addition to other drugs, had significantly lower SD of 24 h systolic BP compared with those not treated with these drug classes [43].

Since the vast majority of drugs do not have an effect lasting long enough to smootly cover the 24 hours, as shown by their trough-to-peak ratio being significantly lower than 100%, it is expected that their anti-hypertensive action is diminished during nighttime and the early morning hours of next day, when a drug is taken in the morning. This phenomenon may have important implications for subjects with nighttime hypertension, non-dipping profile, and/or pronounced morning surge. However, the concept of restoring a disturbed nighttime BP profile with so-called "chronotherapy," i.e., with administration of antihypertensive drugs in the evening rather than in the morning, needs to be better supported by evidence.

28.3 Midterm BPV

28.3.1 Mechanisms

Behavioral factors such as job strain, levels of physical activity, sleep/wakefulness cycles, quality and duration of sleep, postural changes, patterns of sodium intake are likely to play an important role in determining day-by-day BP fluctuations (see Fig. 28.1). This has been clearly exemplified by some studies in which significant changes in BP levels between working days and the weekend have been reported [44]. Data from several population studies have found a number of factors, such as advanced age, female gender, increased arterial stiffness, elevated mean BP values, reduced body mass index, low heart rate, high heart rate variability, excessive alcohol intake, cigarette smoking, history of peripheral artery disease, cardiovascular disease, diabetes mellitus, diabetic nephropathy, and sedentary lifestyle, to be associated with increased values of day-by-day BPV derived from self-BP measurements performed at subjects' home [8, 45–49]. Studies focusing on treated hypertensive patients have found a higher day-by-day BPV among these individuals compared to untreated subjects [46, 48], also reporting higher values of home BPV in case of treatment with b-blockers [8], short duration of treatment [50], and increasing number of antihypertensive drugs [49]. In such a context a limited adherence of patients to prescribed anti-hypertensive regimen is aslo likely to play a role.

28.3.2 Methods for Assessment

A thorough assessment of midterm BPV can be obtained by performing ABPM over 48 h or repeatedly during a week or a month. However, this approach is limited by the fact that ABPM is neither available in all clinical settings, nor is always well accepted by patients at such a repetition rate. Although HBPM cannot provide extensive information on nighttime BP and 24 h BP profile as ABPM does, it provides enough BP measures for estimation of day-by-day BPV, devoid of the white-coat effect. Besides, HBPM is widely available and well accepted by patients, being thus a feasible alternative for the evaluation of day-by-day BPV, in particular if BP measurements at home are performed according to current guidelines. Overall, HBPM schedule should consist of duplicate morning and evening BP measurements with validated devices for a 7-day period (at least 3 days required) [51]. Because of the large heterogeneity among studies in terms of measurement schedules (number of readings, number of days, morning and/or evening), BP measurement devices and indices of BPV assessed, it has not yet been possible to standardize an evidence-based approach for assessment of home BPV in clinical practice. Table 28.2 resumes some important aspects regarding the assessment of midterm BPV in clinical practice.

28.3.3 Indices for Estimation of Midterm BPV

BP variations in the midterm may be quantified by estimating some of the same indices employed for assessment of short-term BP variability such as SD, CV, VIM, and ARV described in Table 28.3. Also indices of Instability such as Range (Maximum-minimum BP); Peak size (Maximum BP); and Trough size (Mean-minimum BP) can be estimated in order to assess midterm BPV. These indices appear to have different strengths and limitations, and evidence regarding the best index for estimation of BPV in the midterm is still needed.

28.3.4 Clinical Significance

Although evidence has supported the association between midterm BPV and different types of subclinical organ damage, there has not been a single index of BPV nor a marker of target organ damage presenting consistent and independent relationships [33, 34, 52–58] (Fig. 28.1). Regarding CV events, the most solid evidence supporting the prognostic value of midterm BPV comes from the IDHOCO study [59]. An analysis of this database based on day-by-day morning home BP measurements showed all indices of systolic/diastolic BPV (SD, CV, ARV, VIM) to be independently associated with all-cause and cardiovascular mortality [59]. A meta-analysis by Stevens et al. showed similar hazard ratios for all-cause mortality for home day-by-day and for 24 h systolic BPV [HR: 1.12 (95% confidence intervals: 1.05, 1.20); home: 1.15 (1.06, 1.26); 24 h ambulatory: 1.11 (1.04. 1.18)] [60] (see Fig. 28.2).

In addition, it appears that morning day-by-day home BPV has the strongest prognostic value as compared to morning–evening or evening home BPV [61, 62]. Regarding the question on whether midterm BPV may independently add to cardiovascular risk stratification, the IDHOCO analysis revealed only a minor-nonsignificant incremental improvement for home BPV in terms of net reclassification and integrated discrimination improvements [59]. The IDHOCO study also provided some evidence indicating that the risk of cardiovascular morbidity and mortality was steeply increased in the highest decile of systolic/diastolic home BPV (CV ≥11/12.8%, respectively) [59]. Regarding the response of midterm BPV to antihypertensive treatment, a study by Matsui et al. showed that the olmesartan/azelnidipine compared to olmesartan/hydrochlorothiazide combination improved home BPV in addition to home BP reduction, and that the reduction in home BPV was associated with the reduction in the arterial stiffness in the group randomized to azelnidipine [56]. In a study by Hoshide et al. the treatment-induced reduction in urine albumin excretion after a 6-month period of antihypertensive treatment with candesartan (+diuretics) was significantly associated with the reduction of average home BP but was not associated with the reduction in the SD of home systolic BP nor with the reduction in the value of maximum home systolic BP [63].

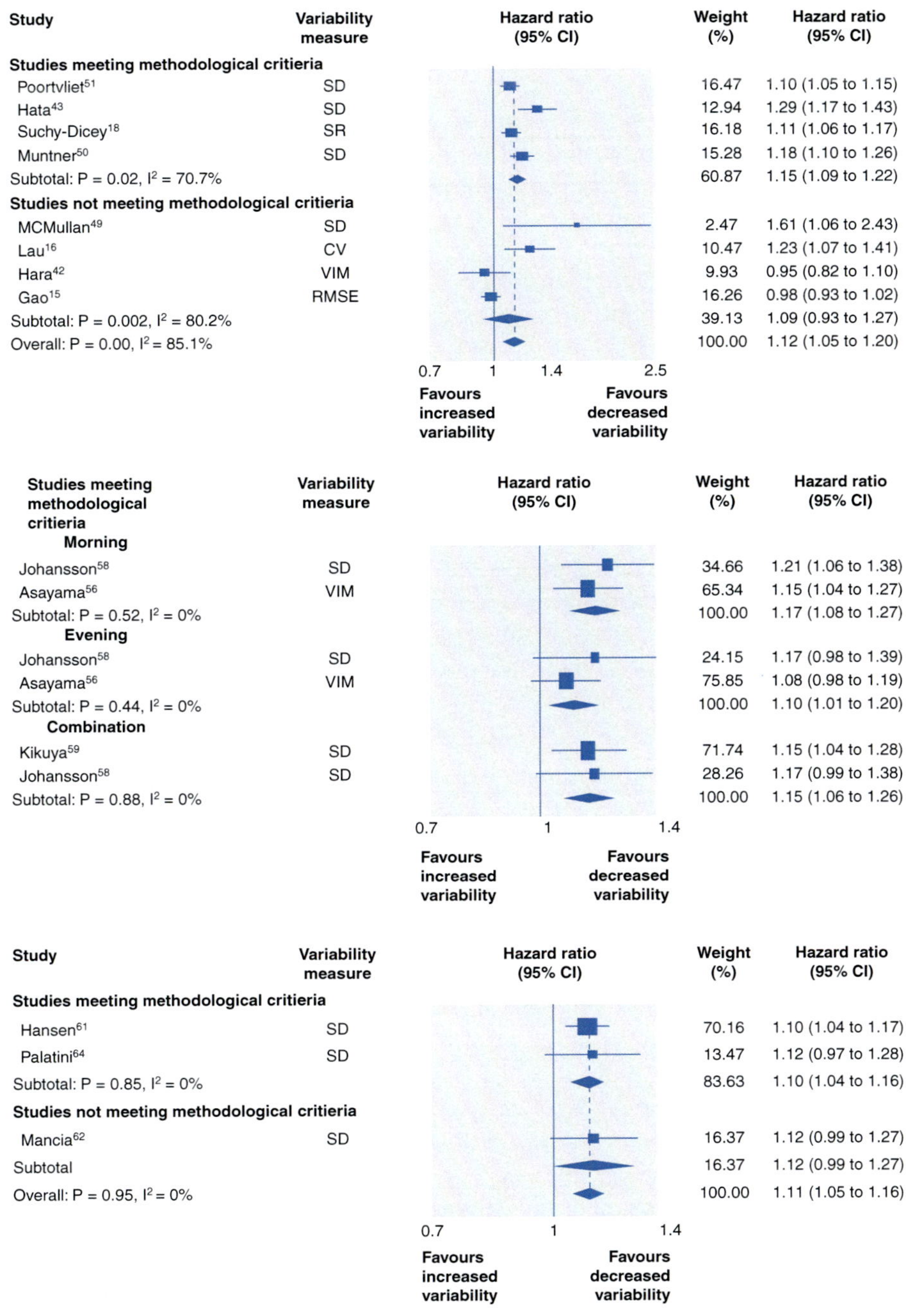

Fig. 28.2 Hazard ratios for all-cause mortality for increases in clinic systolic blood pressure variability (upper panel); in home systolic blood pressure variability (middle panel) or in variability of ambulatory systolic blood pressure (lower panel). Modified from Stevens et al. [60] by permission

28.4 Long-Term BPV

28.4.1 Mechanisms

Although biological and behavioral factors may contribute to visit-to-visit BPV, it may be also importantly affected by treatment-related factors such as inconsistent BP control in subjects receiving treatment for arterial hypertension (Fig. 28.1). In particular, poor patient's adherence to prescribed treatment, improper dosing/titration of antihypertensive drugs, dose omission, or delay in drug intake during the follow-up period, as well as improper BP measurement during assessment of BP control, may all induce important increases in BPV from visit to visit [64]. In the frame of large population studies, long-term BPV has been found to be associated with advanced age, female gender, insomnia and long sleep duration, history of myocardial infarction or stroke, higher mean systolic BP and pulse pressure [24, 65]. Besides, observational studies have shown long-term BPV to be importantly influenced by season-related climatic changes [66, 67], and in particular by changes in outdoor temperature [67, 68]. This has been supported by the finding that BP levels (either office, ambulatory, or home BP) are consistently lower during the summer and higher during the winter [69]. However, not only the changes in outdoor temperature but also an improper downward titration of antihypertensive drugs on the basis of office BP reductions during the summer (with the consequent reduction of the extension of 24 h BP coverage) [68] may lead to a paradoxical increase in nighttime BP levels in the warmer season.

28.4.2 Methods for Assessment

A series of studies in the past decade have indicated that visit-to-visit BPV is a highly reproducible phenomenon with demonstrated predictive value for cardiovascular prognosis [24, 65]. Long-term BPV is most commonly assessed from visit-to-visit by conventional BP measurements obtained in the medical office, which are characterized, however, by several intrinsic limitations such as the "white-coat effect" and may thus not accurately reflect patients' actual BP profile and BPV. Although ABPM performed on repeated visits might represent an ideal approach for the accurate assessment of visit-to-visit BPV in the long-term, this technique is not always available and patients may not easily accept its frequent use on a regular basis. An optimal, alternative approach to overcome the limitations of OBP and ABPM for assessment of long-term BPV might be implementation of HBPM over the days preceding each office visit. Although HBPM cannot provide the extensive information on BP levels over 24 h as ABPM does, it can provide information on BP levels in daily life conditions devoid of the subject's alarm reaction during the medical visit. In recognition of its advantages and prognostic superiority over OBP, the use of HBPM has been recommended for the long-term follow-up of treated hypertensive patients, and might thus be also employed for assessment of long-term BPV [18, 25, 65, 70–72]. Identifying a standard method to obtain reproducible and valid estimates of visit-to-visit BP variability, using either OBP or HBPM, has been difficult due to the inconsistency of the available evidence. However, a higher number of visits considered for the assessment of visit-to-visit BPV has been associated with a greater reproducibility [73] and a stronger prognostic value [24]. Key aspects related to assessment of long-term BPV are presented in Table 28.2.

28.4.3 Indices for Estimation of Long-Term BPV

Several of the indices employed for estimation of short-term BPV may be employed for assessment of long-term BPV (i.e., SD, CV, ARV, VIM) (Table 28.3). Although metrics of long-term BPV are highly correlated to each other, it is not clear which metrics are better representative of true long-term BPV [74, 75]. Most studies have evaluated classical (i.e., SD and CV) but not novel indices of BPV such as ARV or VIM [76]. It is likely that ARV, CV, and SD may reflect different primary determinants of BPV as they are only partly correlated [24]. In the future, clinical trials aimed at establishing the relationship of BPV with cardiovascular outcomes, should ideally evaluate all metrics of overall, ordered and extreme long-term BPV.

28.4.4 Clinical Significance

The prognostic relevance of visit-to-visit BPV was first emphasized by Rothwell et al. [24, 76]. Thereafter, several studies have been conducted supporting the association between long-term BPV with either subclinical organ damage or cardiovascular events. The largest amount of evidence addressing the predictive value of long-term BPV for organ damage comes mainly from studies in diabetic patients in whom the incidence or the progression of renal dysfunction in relation to long-term BPV has been documented [47, 77–81]. In one of these studies, visit-to-visit BPV, assessed by CV of systolic BP, was associated with a significantly increased hazard of developing albuminuria in patients with type 2 diabetes [77]. Visit-to-visit BPV has also been associated with other indices of subclinical organ damage such as left ventricular dysfunction [79, 80], carotid atherosclerosis, and arterial stiffness [47, 80, 81]. Regarding the prognostic value of long-term BPV for cardiovascular events, the evidence is mainly derived from *post hoc* analyses of large randomized trials and meta-analyses [60, 82, 83]. In one of these reports, visit-to-visit BPV independently predicted all-cause mortality (HR 1.12, 95%CI 1.05, 1.20); cardiovascular mortality (HR 1.15, 95%CI 1.03, 1.30); cardiovascular events (HR 1.13, 95%CI 1.04, 1.23); coronary heart disease (HR 1.07, 95%CI 1.00, 1.14); and stroke (HR 1.19, 95%CI 1.11, 1.27) [60] (see Fig. 28.2). These significant associations have led to the question on whether long-term BPV might add to risk stratification over and above average BP levels and baseline cardiovascular risk. In a recent report of the ADVANCE-ON study in patients with type 2 diabetes, addition of SD of systolic clinic BP to the prediction model significantly added to the 8-year risk prediction beyond the contribution of average systolic BP and other traditional risk factors [84]. In another study in patients with cardiovascular disease, addition of CV of systolic BP resulted in a modest but significant improvement in the prediction model [85]. On the contrary, visit-to-visit BPV did not contribute to cardiovascular risk prediction in the ELSA study [86] which however included middle-aged patients with treated, mild to moderate, systolic-diastolic hypertension at relatively low cardiovascular risk [86]. Very recently an analysis of the VALUE (Valsartan Antihypertensive Long-term Use Evaluation) study reported an increased risk of cardiovascular events [HR: 2.1, 95% CI 1.7–2.4; $P < 0.0001$] for patients in the highest quintile of visit-to-visit BPV and a 10% increase in the risk of death (HR 1.10, 95% CI 1.04–1.17; $P = 0.002$) for a 5 mmHg increase in SD of systolic BP [87].

Despite the large amount of evidence on the prognostic value of long-term BPV, there is no specific suggestion of thresholds for its clinical application, at present. The largest study addressing the clinical value of long-term BPV reported the risk of cardiovascular events among quartiles of SD of SBP with an incremental risk for SD quartiles 2 through 4 for all-cause mortality, coronary heart disease, stroke, and end-stage renal disease [88]. The SD of systolic BP which corresponded to the highest quartile was 15.6 mmHg [88].

The question on whether long-term BPV might be modulated by antihypertensive treatment and whether this might be translated into improved CV prognosis has been addressed by *post hoc* analyses of randomized clinical trials. Overall, these reports have indicated a favorable effect of CCBs versus other drugs, especially beta-blockers, in reducing visit-to-visit BPV and the risk of stroke. In particular, the *post hoc* analysis of the Anglo-Scandinavian Cardiac Outcomes Trial Blood Pressure Lowering Arm (ASCOT-BPLA) showed that amlodipine-based compared to atenolol-based regimen was associated with a greater reduction in outcome, with a greater effect of CCBs versus other drugs, especially beta-blockers, in reducing visit-to-visit BPV [76]. In addition, a meta-analysis by Webb et al. [89] showed that compared to other drugs, interindividual variability in systolic BP was reduced by CCBs and by non-loop diuretic drugs, and increased by renin-angiotensin system blockers and beta-blockers [89]. This finding is of interest, although reduction in interindividual BPV cannot be considered as an acceptable surrogate for a reduction in within-individual BPV. Compared to placebo, CCBs were the most effective drug class to reduce interindividual variability in systolic BP [89]. In another recent meta-analysis of five studies, amlodipine was found to be more effective than other active comparators in reducing intra-individual visit-to-visit BPV [90]. The benefits of treatment-induced changes in BPV were reported in the ASCOT-BLA study, in which the reduction in the risk of stroke was partly attributed to the reduction of BPV [76]. In the same line, in the meta-analysis by Webb et al. the reduction in the risk of stroke was attributed not only to the reduction of average systolic BP, but also to the reduction of inter-individual systolic BPV [89].

28.5 Blood Pressure Variability and Prehypertension

Many of the mechanisms associated with an increased BPV (i.e., Autonomic dysfunction, RAAS system dysregulation) have also been reported to be present with a higher frequency in subjects with prehypertension (high normal BP) than in subjects with normotension. Compared to normotensives, subjects with prehypertension or high normal office BP are characterized by a higher number of abnormally elevated BP readings (i.e., a higher BP load) in ambulatory conditions, in spite of the finding of office BP values still within normal ranges. Besides, patients with a higher degree of BP elevation in response to the alarm reaction elicited by the medical visit (i.e., white-coat effect) and those with white-coat hypertension (high office BP levels, but normal out of office BP levels) have been shown to be at a higher risk of developing sustained hypertension as indicated by several population studies [91, 92] leading to consider this condition as a prehypertensive state [93]. Clinical and experimental studies have also indicated that the magnitude of the BP response to static muscle contraction in prehypertensive subjects is exaggerated compared to normotensive subjects [94] and most (but not all) studies have shown an excessive BP rise during exercise to be predictive of development of hypertension independently of BP at rest [95, 96]. Along this line of thinking, it is likely that increases in BP variability and the associated alterations in BP regulation might predict development of future hypertension, in particular in prehypertensive subjects. Identification of subjects with normal office and/or average ABP values but with increased BPV, who could theoretically be at a higher risk of future sustained hypertension as compared to subjects with sustained normotension, might allow implementation of early interventions aimed at improving subjects' lifestyle and at detecting/preventing subclinical organ damage at an early stage [97, 98]. However, the evidence from studies directly aimed at evaluating the predictive value of an increased BPV for development of hypertension is limited if not absent. Besides, if considered that average BP levels and BPV are affected by significant collinearity (i.e., increasing average BP levels are associated with increasing BPV), determining whether an increased BPV precedes BP elevation or vice versa becomes a challenge based on the available studies. Finally, it has to be considered that in the recent 2017 American Heart Association/American College of Cardiology guidelines for hypertension management, the condition formerly defined as "prehypertension" is now defined as "stage 1 hypertension," because of the evidence of an increased risk of events in such a BP range [99], which may imply the need for a re-assessment also of the possible role of BPV in this context.

Conclusions

Accumulating evidence supports the concept that an increased BPV may contribute to cardiovascular risk prediction over and above the impact of average BP levels. These findings suggest the possible usefulness of assessing BPV in clinical practice and of considering an elevated BPV as a possible target for treatment to further improve prognosis. However, although several indices of BPV have been shown to be of prognostic value, no interventional longitudinal outcome study has yet been conducted specifically addressing a number of important issues in this field, namely which the best BPV index to be considered in clinical practice could be, what BPV levels should be regarded as normal, or which BPV level should be achieved by antihypertensive treatment. Similarly, no intervention study has yet explored the key question of whether a reduction in BPV by treatment translates into a better outcome. Regarding the type of BPV that should be considered in clinical practice (short term, midterm, or long term), the poor correlation and agreement between indices of short-term (24 h) and long-term variability indicate that they may reflect different pathophysiological and clinical phenomena and may thus not be interchangeable, but rather represent complementary variables to be separately quantified. Whether assessing BPV could improve the prediction of future hypertension, thus improving the management of subjects with high normal office BP elevation/prehypertension is still a question to be properly evaluated in future studies, too.

In conclusion, although an increased BPV, in the different time windows considered in this paper, represents a phenomenon characterizing daily clinical practice which should not be disregarded, it is not yet possible to provide clear recommendations regarding its interpretation either as an additional independent risk predictor nor as a possible new target for treatment. More research is therefore still needed in this field, and the importance to further explore these issues is clearly emphasized by the huge amount of data on the association between increase in size of different BPV indices and adverse outcome provided by available experimetnal studies in animals, observational studies in humans and meta-analyses of randomized clinical trials.

References

1. Parati G, Ochoa JE, Lombardi C, Bilo G. Assessment and management of blood-pressure variability. Nat Rev Cardiol. 2013;10(3):143–55.
2. Mancia G, Parati G, Pomidossi G, Casadei R, Di Rienzo M, Zanchetti A. Arterial baroreflexes and blood pressure and heart rate variabilities in humans. Hypertension. 1986;8(2):147–53.
3. Parati G, Saul JP, Di Rienzo M, Mancia G. Spectral analysis of blood pressure and heart rate variability in evaluating cardiovascular regulation. A critical appraisal. Hypertension. 1995;25(6):1276–86.
4. Narkiewicz K, Winnicki M, Schroeder K, Phillips BG, Kato M, Cwalina E, et al. Relationship between muscle sympathetic nerve activity and diurnal blood pressure profile. Hypertension. 2002;39(1):168–72.
5. Parati G, Faini A, Valentini M. Blood pressure variability: its measurement and significance in hypertension. Curr Hypertens Rep. 2006;8(3):199–204.
6. Kotsis V, Stabouli S, Karafillis I, Papakatsika S, Rizos Z, Miyakis S, et al. Arterial stiffness and 24 h ambulatory blood pressure monitoring in young healthy volunteers: the early vascular ageing Aristotle University Thessaloniki Study (EVA-ARIS Study). Atherosclerosis. 2011;219(1):194–9.
7. Schillaci G, Bilo G, Pucci G, Laurent S, Macquin-Mavier I, Boutouyrie P, et al. Relationship between short-term blood pressure variability and large-artery stiffness in human hypertension: findings from 2 large databases. Hypertension. 2012;60(2):369–77.

8. Okada H, Fukui M, Tanaka M, Inada S, Mineoka Y, Nakanishi N, et al. Visit-to-visit variability in systolic blood pressure is correlated with diabetic nephropathy and atherosclerosis in patients with type 2 diabetes. Atherosclerosis. 2012;220(1):155–9.
9. Grassi G, Seravalle G, Quarti-Trevano F, Dell'Oro R, Bombelli M, Cuspidi C, et al. Adrenergic, metabolic, and reflex abnormalities in reverse and extreme dipper hypertensives. Hypertension. 2008;52(5):925–31.
10. Fujii T, Uzu T, Nishimura M, Takeji M, Kuroda S, Nakamura S, et al. Circadian rhythm of natriuresis is disturbed in nondipper type of essential hypertension. Am J Kidney Dis. 1999;33(1):29–35.
11. Verdecchia P, Schillaci G, Gatteschi C, Zampi I, Battistelli M, Bartoccini C, et al. Blunted nocturnal fall in blood pressure in hypertensive women with future cardiovascular morbid events. Circulation. 1993;88(3):986–92.
12. Haynes WG. Role of leptin in obesity-related hypertension. Exp Physiol. 2005;90(5):683–8.
13. Quinaglia T, Martins LC, Figueiredo VN, Santos RC, Yugar-Toledo JC, Martin JF, et al. Non-dipping pattern relates to endothelial dysfunction in patients with uncontrolled resistant hypertension. J Hum Hypertens. 2011;25(11):656–64.
14. Holt-Lunstad J, Steffen PR. Diurnal cortisol variation is associated with nocturnal blood pressure dipping. Psychosom Med. 2007;69(4):339–43.
15. Panarelli M, Terzolo M, Piovesan A, Osella G, Paccotti P, Pinna G, et al. 24-hour profiles of blood pressure and heart rate in Cushing's syndrome. Evidence for differential control of cardiovascular variables by glucocorticoids. Ann Ital Med Int. 1990;5(1):18–25.
16. Mancia G, Parati G, di Rienzo M, Zanchetti A. Blood pressure variability. In: Mancia G, Zanchetti A, editors. Handbook of hypertension: pathophysiology of hypertension. Amsterdam: Elsevier Science; 1997. p. 117–69.
17. Mancia G, Di Rienzo M, Parati G. Ambulatory blood pressure monitoring use in hypertension research and clinical practice. Hypertension. 1993;21(4):510–24.
18. Parati G, Ochoa JE, Bilo G. Blood pressure variability, cardiovascular risk, and risk for renal disease progression. Curr Hypertens Rep. 2012;14(5):421–31.
19. di Rienzo M, Grassi G, Pedotti A, Mancia G. Continuous vs intermittent blood pressure measurements in estimating 24-hour average blood pressure. Hypertension. 1983;5(2):264–9.
20. Bilo G, Giglio A, Styczkiewicz K, Caldara G, Maronati A, Kawecka-Jaszcz K, et al. A new method for assessing 24-h blood pressure variability after excluding the contribution of nocturnal blood pressure fall. J Hypertens. 2007;25(10):2058–66.
21. Mena L, Pintos S, Queipo NV, Aizpurua JA, Maestre G, Sulbaran T. A reliable index for the prognostic significance of blood pressure variability. J Hypertens. 2005;23(3):505–11.
22. Hansen TW, Thijs L, Li Y, Boggia J, Kikuya M, Bjorklund-Bodegard K, et al. Prognostic value of reading-to-reading blood pressure variability over 24 hours in 8938 subjects from 11 populations. Hypertension. 2010;55(4):1049–57.
23. O'Brien E, Parati G, Stergiou G, Asmar R, Beilin L, Bilo G, et al. European Society of Hypertension position paper on ambulatory blood pressure monitoring. J Hypertens. 2013;31(9):1731–68.
24. Rothwell PM, Howard SC, Dolan E, O'Brien E, Dobson JE, Dahlof B, et al. Prognostic significance of visit-to-visit variability, maximum systolic blood pressure, and episodic hypertension. Lancet. 2010;375(9718):895–905.
25. Pickering TG, Hall JE, Appel LJ, Falkner BE, Graves J, Hill MN, et al. Recommendations for blood pressure measurement in humans and experimental animals: Part 1: blood pressure measurement in humans: a statement for professionals from the Subcommittee of Professional and Public Education of the American Heart Association Council on High Blood Pressure Research. Hypertension. 2005;45(1):142–61.
26. Parati G, Pomidossi G, Albini F, Malaspina D, Mancia G. Relationship of 24-hour blood pressure mean and variability to severity of target-organ damage in hypertension. J Hypertens. 1987;5(1):93–8.
27. Frattola A, Parati G, Cuspidi C, Albini F, Mancia G. Prognostic value of 24-hour blood pressure variability. J Hypertens. 1993;11(10):1133–7.

28. Madden JM, O'Flynn AM, Fitzgerald AP, Kearney PM. Correlation between short-term blood pressure variability and left-ventricular mass index: a meta-analysis. Hypertens Res. 2016;39(3):171–7.
29. Mancia G, Parati G, Hennig M, Flatau B, Omboni S, Glavina F, et al. Relation between blood pressure variability and carotid artery damage in hypertension: baseline data from the European Lacidipine Study on Atherosclerosis (ELSA). J Hypertens. 2001;19(11):1981–9.
30. Shintani Y, Kikuya M, Hara A, Ohkubo T, Metoki H, Asayama K, et al. Ambulatory blood pressure, blood pressure variability and the prevalence of carotid artery alteration: the Ohasama study. J Hypertens. 2007;25(8):1704–10.
31. Tatasciore A, Renda G, Zimarino M, Soccio M, Bilo G, Parati G, et al. Awake systolic blood pressure variability correlates with target-organ damage in hypertensive subjects. Hypertension. 2007;50(2):325–32.
32. Manios E, Tsagalis G, Tsivgoulis G, Barlas G, Koroboki E, Michas F, et al. Time rate of blood pressure variation is associated with impaired renal function in hypertensive patients. J Hypertens. 2009;27(11):2244–8.
33. Veloudi P, Blizzard CL, Head GA, Abhayaratna WP, Stowasser M, Sharman JE. Blood pressure variability and prediction of target organ damage in patients with uncomplicated hypertension. Am J Hypertens. 2016;29(9):1046–54.
34. Wei FF, Li Y, Zhang L, Xu TY, Ding FH, Wang JG, et al. Beat-to-beat, reading-to-reading, and day-to-day blood pressure variability in relation to organ damage in untreated Chinese. Hypertension. 2014;63(4):790–6.
35. Palatini P, Reboldi G, Beilin LJ, Casiglia E, Eguchi K, Imai Y, et al. Added predictive value of night-time blood pressure variability for cardiovascular events and mortality: the Ambulatory Blood Pressure-International Study. Hypertension. 2014;64(3):487–93.
36. Mancia G, Bombelli M, Facchetti R, Madotto F, Corrao G, Trevano FQ, et al. Long-term prognostic value of blood pressure variability in the general population: results of the Pressioni Arteriose Monitorate e Loro Associazioni Study. Hypertension. 2007;49(6):1265–70.
37. Niiranen TJ, Maki J, Puukka P, Karanko H, Jula AM. Office, home, and ambulatory blood pressures as predictors of cardiovascular risk. Hypertension. 2014;64(2):281–6.
38. Hansen TW, Li Y, Boggia J, Thijs L, Richart T, Staessen JA. Predictive role of the nighttime blood pressure. Hypertension. 2011;57(1):3–10.
39. Fagard RH, Celis H, Thijs L, Staessen JA, Clement DL, De Buyzere ML, et al. Daytime and nighttime blood pressure as predictors of death and cause-specific cardiovascular events in hypertension. Hypertension. 2008;51(1):55–61.
40. Metoki H, Ohkubo T, Kikuya M, Asayama K, Obara T, Hashimoto J, et al. Prognostic significance for stroke of a morning pressor surge and a nocturnal blood pressure decline: the Ohasama study. Hypertension. 2006;47(2):149–54.
41. Kario K, Pickering TG, Umeda Y, Hoshide S, Hoshide Y, Morinari M, et al. Morning surge in blood pressure as a predictor of silent and clinical cerebrovascular disease in elderly hypertensives: a prospective study. Circulation. 2003;107(10):1401–6.
42. Zhang Y, Agnoletti D, Safar ME, Blacher J. Effect of antihypertensive agents on blood pressure variability: the Natrilix SR versus candesartan and amlodipine in the reduction of systolic blood pressure in hypertensive patients (X-CELLENT) study. Hypertension. 2011;58(2):155–60.
43. Levi-Marpillat N, Macquin-Mavier I, Tropeano AI, Parati G, Maison P. Antihypertensive drug classes have different effects on short-term blood pressure variability in essential hypertension. Hypertens Res. 2014;37(6):585–90.
44. Murakami S, Otsuka K, Kubo Y, Shinagawa M, Matsuoka O, Yamanaka T, et al. Weekly variation of home and ambulatory blood pressure and relation between arterial stiffness and blood pressure measurements in community-dwelling hypertensives. Clin Exp Hypertens. 2005;27:231–9.
45. Niiranen TJ, Hanninen MR, Johansson J, Reunanen A, Jula AM. Home-measured blood pressure is a stronger predictor of cardiovascular risk than office blood pressure: the Finn-Home study. Hypertension. 2010;55(6):1346–51.

46. Thijs L, Staessen JA, Celis H, Fagard R, De Cort P, de Gaudemaris R, et al. The international database of self-recorded blood pressures in normotensive and untreated hypertensive subjects. Blood Press Monit. 1999;4(2):77–86.
47. Nagai M, Hoshide S, Ishikawa J, Shimada K, Kario K. Visit-to-visit blood pressure variations: new independent determinants for carotid artery measures in the elderly at high risk of cardiovascular disease. J Am Soc Hypertens. 2011;5(3):184–92.
48. Niiranen TJ, Asayama K, Thijs L, Johansson JK, Ohkubo T, Kikuya M, et al. Outcome-driven thresholds for home blood pressure measurement: international database of home blood pressure in relation to cardiovascular outcome. Hypertension. 2013;61(1):27–34.
49. Okada T, Nakao T, Matsumoto H, Nagaoka Y, Tomaru R, Iwasawa H, et al. [Day-by-day variability of home blood pressure in patients with chronic kidney disease]. Nihon Jinzo Gakkai Shi 2008;50(5):588–596.
50. Ishikura K, Obara T, Kato T, Kikuya M, Shibamiya T, Shinki T, et al. Associations between day-by-day variability in blood pressure measured at home and antihypertensive drugs: the J-HOME-Morning study. Clin Exp Hypertens. 2012;34(4):297–304.
51. Parati G, Stergiou GS, Asmar R, Bilo G, de Leeuw P, Imai Y, et al. European Society of Hypertension guidelines for blood pressure monitoring at home: a summary report of the Second International Consensus Conference on Home Blood Pressure Monitoring. J Hypertens. 2008;26(8):1505–26.
52. Stergiou GS, Ntineri A, Kollias A, Ohkubo T, Imai Y, Parati G. Blood pressure variability assessed by home measurements: a systematic review. Hypertens Res. 2014;37(6):565–72.
53. Shibasaki S, Hoshide S, Eguchi K, Ishikawa J, Kario K, Japan Morning Surge-Home Blood Pressure Study Group. Increase trend in home blood pressure on a single occasion is associated with B-type natriuretic peptide and the estimated glomerular filtration rate. Am J Hypertens. 2015;28(9):1098–105.
54. Ushigome E, Fukui M, Hamaguchi M, Tanaka T, Atsuta H, Mogami S, et al. Maximum home systolic blood pressure is a useful indicator of arterial stiffness in patients with type 2 diabetes mellitus: post hoc analysis of a cross-sectional multicenter study. Diabetes Res Clin Pract. 2014;105(3):344–51.
55. Liu Z, Zhao Y, Lu F, Zhang H, Diao Y. Day-by-day variability in self-measured blood pressure at home: effects on carotid artery atherosclerosis, brachial flow-mediated dilation, and endothelin-1 in normotensive and mild-moderate hypertensive individuals. Blood Press Monit. 2013;18(6):316–25.
56. Matsui Y, O'Rourke MF, Hoshide S, Ishikawa J, Shimada K, Kario K. Combined effect of angiotensin II receptor blocker and either a calcium channel blocker or diuretic on day-by-day variability of home blood pressure: the Japan Combined Treatment With Olmesartan and a Calcium-Channel Blocker Versus Olmesartan and Diuretics Randomized Efficacy Study. Hypertension. 2012;59(6):1132–8.
57. Ushigome E, Fukui M, Hamaguchi M, Senmaru T, Sakabe K, Tanaka M, et al. The coefficient variation of home blood pressure is a novel factor associated with macroalbuminuria in type 2 diabetes mellitus. Hypertens Res. 2011;34(12):1271–5.
58. Matsui Y, Ishikawa J, Eguchi K, Shibasaki S, Shimada K, Kario K. Maximum value of home blood pressure: a novel indicator of target organ damage in hypertension. Hypertension. 2011;57(6):1087–93.
59. Juhanoja EP, Niiranen TJ, Johansson JK, Puukka PJ, Thijs L, Asayama K, et al. Outcome-driven thresholds for increased home blood pressure variability. Hypertension. 2017;69(4):599–607.
60. Stevens SL, Wood S, Koshiaris C, Law K, Glasziou P, Stevens RJ, et al. Blood pressure variability and cardiovascular disease: systematic review and meta-analysis. BMJ. 2016;354:i4098.
61. Johansson JK, Niiranen TJ, Puukka PJ, Jula AM. Prognostic value of the variability in home-measured blood pressure and heart rate: the Finn-Home Study. Hypertension. 2012;59(2):212–8.
62. Ohkubo T, Asayama K, Kikuya M, Metoki H, Hoshi H, Hashimoto J, et al. How many times should blood pressure be measured at home for better prediction of stroke risk? Ten-year follow-up results from the Ohasama study. J Hypertens. 2004;22(6):1099–104.

63. Hoshide S, Yano Y, Shimizu M, Eguchi K, Ishikawa J, Kario K. Is home blood pressure variability itself an interventional target beyond lowering mean home blood pressure during antihypertensive treatment? Hypertens Res. 2012;35(8):862–6.
64. Mancia G, Facchetti R, Parati G, Zanchetti A. Visit-to-visit blood pressure variability in the European Lacidipine Study on Atherosclerosis: methodological aspects and effects of antihypertensive treatment. J Hypertens. 2012;30(6):1241–51.
65. Muntner P, Shimbo D, Tonelli M, Reynolds K, Arnett DK, Oparil S. The relationship between visit-to-visit variability in systolic blood pressure and all-cause mortality in the general population: findings from NHANES III, 1988 to 1994. Hypertension. 2011;57(2):160–6.
66. Myers MG, Godwin M, Dawes M, Kiss A, Tobe SW, Grant FC, et al. Conventional versus automated measurement of blood pressure in primary care patients with systolic hypertension: randomised parallel design controlled trial. BMJ. 2011;342:d286.
67. Stergiou GS, Myrsilidi A, Kollias A, Destounis A, Roussias L, Kalogeropoulos P. Seasonal variation in meteorological parameters and office, ambulatory and home blood pressure: predicting factors and clinical implications. Hypertens Res. 2015;38(12):869–75.
68. Modesti PA, Morabito M, Bertolozzi I, Massetti L, Panci G, Lumachi C, et al. Weather-related changes in 24-hour blood pressure profile: effects of age and implications for hypertension management. Hypertension. 2006;47(2):155–61.
69. Sega R, Cesana G, Bombelli M, Grassi G, Stella ML, Zanchetti A, et al. Seasonal variations in home and ambulatory blood pressure in the PAMELA population. Pressione Arteriose Monitorate E Loro Associazioni. J Hypertens. 1998;16(11):1585–92.
70. Mancia G, De Backer G, Dominiczak A, Cifkova R, Fagard R, Germano G, et al. Guidelines for the Management of Arterial Hypertension: The Task Force for the Management of Arterial Hypertension of the European Society of Hypertension (ESH) and of the European Society of Cardiology (ESC). J Hypertens. 2007;25(6):1105–87.
71. Chobanian AV, Bakris GL, Black HR, Cushman WC, Green LA, Izzo JL Jr, et al. Seventh report of the Joint National Committee on Prevention, Detection, Evaluation, and Treatment of High Blood Pressure. Hypertension. 2003;42(6):1206–52.
72. O'Brien E, Asmar R, Beilin L, Imai Y, Mallion JM, Mancia G, et al. European Society of Hypertension recommendations for conventional, ambulatory and home blood pressure measurement. J Hypertens. 2003;21(5):821–48.
73. Muntner P, Joyce C, Levitan EB, Holt E, Shimbo D, Webber LS, et al. Reproducibility of visit-to-visit variability of blood pressure measured as part of routine clinical care. J Hypertens. 2011;29(12):2332–8.
74. Levitan EB, Kaciroti N, Oparil S, Julius S, Muntner P. Relationships between metrics of visit-to-visit variability of blood pressure. J Hum Hypertens. 2013;27(10):589–93.
75. Levitan EB, Kaciroti N, Oparil S, Julius S, Muntner P. Blood pressure measurement device, number and timing of visits, and intra-individual visit-to-visit variability of blood pressure. J Clin Hypertens (Greenwich). 2012;14(11):744–50.
76. Rothwell PM, Howard SC, Dolan E, O'Brien E, Dobson JE, Dahlof B, et al. Effects of beta blockers and calcium-channel blockers on within-individual variability in blood pressure and risk of stroke. Lancet Neurol. 2010;9(5):469–80.
77. Okada H, Fukui M, Tanaka M, Matsumoto S, Mineoka Y, Nakanishi N, et al. Visit-to-visit blood pressure variability is a novel risk factor for the development and progression of diabetic nephropathy in patients with type 2 diabetes. Diabetes Care. 2013;36(7):1908–12.
78. Parati G, Liu X, Ochoa JE. Clinical relevance of visit-to-visit blood pressure variability: impact on renal outcomes. J Hum Hypertens. 2014;28(7):403–9.
79. Masugata H, Senda S, Murao K, Inukai M, Hosomi N, Iwado Y, et al. Visit-to-visit variability in blood pressure over a 1-year period is a marker of left ventricular diastolic dysfunction in treated hypertensive patients. Hypertens Res. 2011;34(7):846–50.
80. Okada R, Okada A, Okada T, Nanasato M, Wakai K. Visit-to-visit blood pressure variability is a marker of cardiac diastolic function and carotid atherosclerosis. BMC Cardiovasc Disord. 2014;14:188.

81. Tedla YG, Yano Y, Carnethon M, Greenland P. Association between long-term blood pressure variability and 10-year progression in arterial stiffness: the multiethnic study of atherosclerosis. Hypertension. 2017;69(1):118–27.
82. Wang J, Shi X, Ma C, Zheng H, Xiao J, Bian H, et al. Visit-to-visit blood pressure variability is a risk factor for all-cause mortality and cardiovascular disease: a systematic review and meta-analysis. J Hypertens. 2017;35(1):10–7.
83. Diaz KM, Tanner RM, Falzon L, Levitan EB, Reynolds K, Shimbo D, et al. Visit-to-visit variability of blood pressure and cardiovascular disease and all-cause mortality: a systematic review and meta-analysis. Hypertension. 2014;64(5):965–82.
84. Ohkuma T, Woodward M, Jun M, Muntner P, Hata J, Colagiuri S, et al. Prognostic value of variability in systolic blood pressure related to vascular events and premature death in type 2 diabetes mellitus: the ADVANCE-ON study. Hypertension. 2017;70(2):461–8.
85. Blacher J, Safar ME, Ly C, Szabo de Edelenyi F, Hercberg S, Galan P. Blood pressure variability: cardiovascular risk integrator or independent risk factor? J Hum Hypertens. 2015;29(2):122–6.
86. Mancia G, Facchetti R, Parati G, Zanchetti A. Visit-to-visit blood pressure variability, carotid atherosclerosis, and cardiovascular events in the European Lacidipine Study on Atherosclerosis. Circulation. 2012;126(5):569–78.
87. Mehlum MH, Liestol K, Kjeldsen SE, Julius S, Hua TA, Rothwell PM, et al. Blood pressure variability and risk of cardiovascular events and death in patients with hypertension and different baseline risks. Eur Heart J. 2018. https://doi.org/10.1093/eurheartj/ehx760.
88. Gosmanova EO, Mikkelsen MK, Molnar MZ, Lu JL, Yessayan LT, Kalantar-Zadeh K, et al. Association of systolic blood pressure variability with mortality, coronary heart disease, stroke, and renal disease. J Am Coll Cardiol. 2016;68(13):1375–86.
89. Webb AJ, Fischer U, Mehta Z, Rothwell PM. Effects of antihypertensive-drug class on interindividual variation in blood pressure and risk of stroke: a systematic review and meta-analysis. Lancet. 2010;375(9718):906–15.
90. Wang JG, Yan P, Jeffers BW. Effects of amlodipine and other classes of antihypertensive drugs on long-term blood pressure variability: evidence from randomized controlled trials. J Am Soc Hypertens. 2014;8(5):340–9.
91. Mancia G, Bombelli M, Facchetti R, Madotto F, Quarti-Trevano F, Polo Friz H, et al. Long-term risk of sustained hypertension in white-coat or masked hypertension. Hypertension. 2009;54(2):226–32.
92. Siven SS, Niiranen TJ, Kantola IM, Jula AM. White-coat and masked hypertension as risk factors for progression to sustained hypertension: the Finn-Home study. J Hypertens. 2016;34(1):54–60.
93. Bidlingmeyer I, Burnier M, Bidlingmeyer M, Waeber B, Brunner HR. Isolated office hypertension: a prehypertensive state? J Hypertens. 1996;14(3):327–32.
94. Kim KA, Stebbins CL, Choi HM, Nho H, Kim JK. Mechanisms Underlying Exaggerated Metaboreflex Activation in Prehypertensive Men. Med Sci Sports Exerc. 2015;47(8):1605–12.
95. Le VV, Mitiku T, Sungar G, Myers J, Froelicher V. The blood pressure response to dynamic exercise testing: a systematic review. Prog Cardiovasc Dis. 2008;51(2):135–60.
96. Holmqvist L, Mortensen L, Kanckos C, Ljungman C, Mehlig K, Manhem K. Exercise blood pressure and the risk of future hypertension. J Hum Hypertens. 2012;26(12):691–5.
97. Zachariah PK, Sheps SG, Bailey KR, Wiltgen CM, Moore AG. Age-related characteristics of ambulatory blood pressure load and mean blood pressure in normotensive subjects. JAMA. 1991;265(11):1414–7.
98. White WB. Blood pressure load and target organ effects in patients with essential hypertension. J Hypertens Suppl. 1991;9(8):S39–41.
99. Whelton PK, Carey RM, Aronow WS, Casey DE Jr, Collins KJ, Dennison Himmelfarb C, et al. 2017 ACC/AHA/AAPA/ABC/ACPM/AGS/APhA/ASH/ASPC/NMA/PCNA Guideline for the Prevention, Detection, Evaluation, and Management of High Blood Pressure in Adults: a report of the American College of Cardiology/American Heart Association Task Force on Clinical Practice Guidelines. Hypertension. 2017. https://doi.org/10.1161/HYP.0000000000000065.

Home Blood Pressure Monitoring in Prehypertension and Hypertension

29

Angeliki Ntineri, Anastasios Kollias, and George S. Stergiou

29.1 Introduction

In the last two decades, considerable evidence on home blood pressure (BP) monitoring has accumulated, and current guidelines recommend its wide application in clinical practice. Although conventional BP measurement in the office remains the basis for hypertension diagnosis and management, it is recognized that this method might often be misleading in both untreated and treated subjects, mainly due to the white-coat and masked hypertension phenomena [1–5]. Thus, for a reliable assessment of BP status, the evaluation of out-of-office BP is necessary. These methods are ambulatory and home BP monitoring, which both provide multiple measurements taken in the individual's usual environment. However, they have also important differences in their role in the clinical management of hypertension and are therefore regarded as complementary rather than interchangeable methods.

This chapter presents the considerable potential of home BP monitoring as a tool for the initial evaluation of BP levels, for treatment initiation and adjustment, as well as for long-term follow-up of treated individuals [1–5].

29.2 Advantages and Disadvantages

29.2.1 Advantages

There are important advantages of home BP monitoring compared to the conventional office measurements and in some aspects also to ambulatory monitoring

A. Ntineri · A. Kollias · G. S. Stergiou (✉)
Hypertension Center STRIDE-7, National and Kapodistrian University of Athens, School of Medicine, Third Department of Medicine, Sotiria Hospital, Athens, Greece
e-mail: gstergi@med.uoa.gr

R. Zimlichman et al. (eds.), *Prehypertension and Cardiometabolic Syndrome*, Updates in Hypertension and Cardiovascular Protection,
https://doi.org/10.1007/978-3-319-75310-2_29

Table 29.1 Advantages of home blood pressure

Advantages of home compared to office blood pressure
• Multiple measurements in several days, weeks, or months and in usual environment
• Detection of white-coat and masked hypertension phenomena
• Superior reproducibility—improves power of clinical trials
• Devoid of observer error and bias (automated devices with memory or PC link capacity or home blood pressure tele-monitoring)
• Devoid of placebo effect
• Superior prognostic value for preclinical organ damage and cardiovascular disease
• More widely available
• Improve patients' compliance with antihypertensive drug therapy
• Improve hypertension control rates
• Potential for automated home blood pressure monitoring during nighttime sleep
• Cost-effectiveness
Advantages of home compared to ambulatory blood pressure
• More widely available
• Good acceptance and preferred by users
• Less discomfort and minimal restriction of daily activities and sleep
• Less costly

(Table 29.1). As is the case with ambulatory BP monitoring, home monitoring provides more detailed information on BP behavior by obtaining multiple readings taken in the usual environment of each individual, away from the stressful office setting. Thus, home BP can detect the white-coat and masked hypertension phenomena, which are major limitations of the conventional office BP [1, 3, 6]. Home and ambulatory BP monitoring are devoid of the placebo effect, which limits the reliability of office BP measurements to accurately quantify treatment-induced BP changes in clinical research and in practice [7]. Furthermore, using automated electronic BP devices and the oscillometric technique, the intra- and interobserver error (including the terminal digit preference, usually 5 or 0) and the observer prejudice and bias (the observer adjusts the recorded BP according to his/her expectations), which are known drawbacks of auscultatory office BP measurements, are all avoided [8]. In addition, home BP readings can be obtained over a period of several days, weeks, or even months in the long-term follow-up of treated hypertensives, whereas ambulatory BP monitoring is crowded into 24 h and is rather difficult to perform in repeated sessions.

Studies have shown that home BP have similar reproducibility to ambulatory BP and superior to that of office BP, a characteristic that increases the statistical power of clinical trials allowing the inclusion of a smaller sample size than when using office BP measurements [9]. Home BP appears to have similar diagnostic ability as ambulatory BP, with the observed diagnostic disagreement between the two methods mainly due to the imperfect reproducibility of the two methods [10].

Home BP monitoring is well accepted by most patients and preferred to ambulatory monitoring, as it entails less discomfort and minimal restrictions on daily activities and particularly during sleep [11, 12]. Studies have shown that home BP monitoring can improve hypertension control rates by improving patients' long-term compliance with antihypertensive drug treatment [13, 14]. These features, together with the wider availability and the lower cost of the method compared to office and ambulatory BP monitoring, render it the most cost-effective method for long-term BP monitoring [15, 16].

29.2.2 Disadvantages

An important limitation of home BP monitoring is the potential for reporting bias with over- or underreporting of home BP readings which is the "Achilles' heel" of the method and might lead in over- or undertreatment, especially in high-risk hypertensives or those with high BP variability (Table 29.2) [17]. This can be prevented by using devices with automated memory or PC link capacity or with home BP telemonitoring [17]. Another important concern is that home BP monitoring might induce anxiety and obsessive behavior in some patients. Careful training and medical supervision are required in order to obtain reliable BP measurements and feel comfortable with the process of home monitoring and make sensible use of it. It should be mentioned that even if home BP monitoring is carefully performed according to the current recommendations, it only provides seated BP readings only at home, not at work or during other usual activities, under standardized conditions and thus not representing the dynamic behavior of BP during usual daily challenges [1–5]. Ambulatory BP monitoring is regarded as advantageous compared to home BP monitoring because it allows the evaluation of BP during nighttime sleep, which is important particularly in patients with diabetes, kidney disease, or sleep apnea. However, some novel low-cost home BP monitors allow reliable nocturnal BP evaluation and the detection of non-dippers, which is comparable to ambulatory BP monitoring [18, 19].

Table 29.2 Disadvantages of home blood pressure compared to office measurements and ambulatory monitoring

- Reporting bias of home measurements (avoidable with automated devices having memory or PC link capacity or home blood pressure tele-monitoring)
- Inability to monitor asleep blood pressure (possible with some novel home monitors)
- Measurements do not reflect usual daily activities
- Questionable accuracy of oscillometric devices in the presence of arrhythmias
- Devices often not properly validated for blood pressure measurement accuracy
- Potential to induce anxiety and excessive blood pressure monitoring
- Some patients may self-modify their drug treatment on the basis of casual blood pressure readings
- Need for training (minimal with automated devices) and medical supervision

29.3 Clinical Indications

Ambulatory and home BP monitoring are regarded as indispensable tools adjunct to the classic office BP measurements for screening, diagnosis, and management of hypertension. Although ambulatory BP monitoring remains the reference out-of-office BP monitoring method, in most cases the two methods might be considered interchangeable. Indeed, these methods should be regarded as complementary rather than competitive tools in the assessment of hypertensive patients. When deciding which method to use, equipment availability and patients' characteristics and preference should be taken into account. Home BP monitoring may be more suitable in the initial assessment of subjects with suspected hypertension whereas home BP monitoring for the long-term follow-up of treated hypertensives.

The main clinical indications for home BP monitoring include (1) the suspicion of white-coat and (2) masked hypertension; (3) identification of white-coat reaction and masked hypertension effect in treated hypertensives; (4) considerable variability of office BP over the same or different visits; (5) identification of true and false resistant hypertension; (6) autonomic, postural, postprandial, siesta- and drug-induced hypotension; and (7) elevated office BP or suspected preeclampsia in pregnant women [2, 3]. Thus, the major value of home BP monitoring is its usefulness in detecting the white-coat and masked hypertension phenomena, which remain undiagnosed and inadequately treated when considering using exclusively office BP measurements [2, 3]. White-coat hypertension is defined by normal home BP monitoring (<135/85 mmHg, systolic/diastolic) and elevated office BP values (≥140/90 mmHg), thus not truly reflecting the "true" BP of an individual. These subjects should not be considered as normotensives, as they present higher out-of-office BP than truly normotensives, frequently have dysmetabolic risk factors or asymptomatic organ damage, are more likely to develop progress to sustained hypertension within the next years, and, thus, carry intermediate cardiovascular risk between normotensives and hypertensives [20–22]. Factors that raise the possibility of white-coat hypertension are mildly elevated office BP, older age, female gender, and non-smoking habit [23]. In addition, high-normal office BP in low cardiovascular risk individuals without asymptomatic organ damage is a condition that white-coat hypertension is most likely and should be ruled out. On the other hand, masked hypertensives have elevated home BP (≥135/85 mmHg) but normal office BP (<140/90 mmHg) and present higher prevalence of preclinical target organ damage and increased cardiovascular risk, which is close to that of the sustained hypertensives [22, 24, 25]. High-normal office BP and normal office BP in individuals with high cardiovascular risk or asymptomatic organ damage are considered as conditions that might be associated with the presence of masked hypertension. Other predictors of the phenomenon are the male gender, younger (and older) age, smoking habit, increased body mass index, occasional elevation of office BP, or the presence of concomitant disease (diabetes mellitus type 2, end-stage renal disease, cardiac hypertrophy, peripheral arterial disease, obstructive sleep apnea) [26–28]. The masked hypertension phenomenon is also frequent in treated hypertensives (masked uncontrolled hypertension). When the diagnosis of these phenomena is confirmed, treatment adjustment should be considered, particularly in subjects with high cardiovascular risk [2].

29.3.1 Home Blood Pressure Monitoring in Prehypertension

A considerable proportion of subjects in the general population assessed with different BP measurement methods (office, home, or ambulatory BP measurements) cluster close to the diagnostic BP thresholds of hypertension (differ less than 5 mmHg) entailing diagnostic uncertainty and confusion. A study that investigated the level of agreement between ambulatory and home BP in the diagnosis of masked hypertension (Fig. 29.1) showed that, in subjects attending a hypertension clinic, when assessing participants with office BP measurements, there is a high proportion with high-normal office BP (possible masked hypertension) or stage 1 office hypertension (possible white-coat hypertension) among both untreated and treated subjects. All of them should undergo out-of-office BP evaluation in order to reveal the true BP phenotype. By combining office and out-of-office BP measurements, about 2/3 of subjects with high-normal office BP will exhibit high-normal BP also in the home BP monitoring and confirm the diagnosis of prehypertension, yet the rest 1/3 of them will be diagnosed with masked hypertension [29]. Similarly, all individuals with stage 1 office hypertension should be offered out-of-office BP monitoring in order to exclude the diagnosis of white-coat hypertension and avoid unnecessary treatment initiation or titration. It is important to note that even in these tricky cases

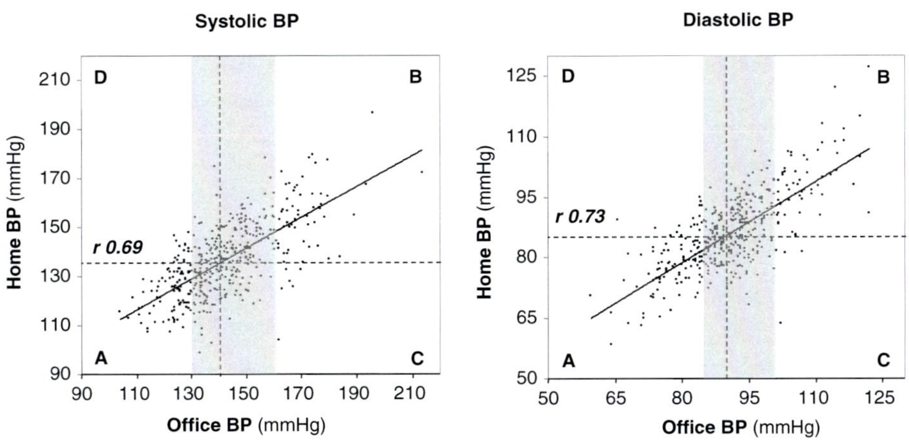

Fig. 29.1 Relationship of office with home blood pressure measurements and hypertension phenotypes (Group *A*, normotensives; *B*, hypertensives; *C*, subjects with white-coat phenomenon; *D*, subjects with masked hypertension phenomenon). Gray zone indicates high-normal office blood pressure and office hypertension stage 1 range, where masked and white-coat hypertension, respectively, are particularly common and out-of-office blood pressure monitoring is mandatory (Modified from [29]). *BP* blood pressure, *r* correlation coefficient

within the gray zones of uncertainty (BP close to the diagnostic threshold), home BP monitoring is regarded as having similar diagnostic value with ambulatory BP monitoring with the disagreement between them being rather uncommon and in most cases clinically irrelevant [29].

29.4 Clinical Value

29.4.1 Diagnostic Value

Several studies during the last decade have demonstrated the efficiency of home BP monitoring in the accurate diagnosis of hypertension. These studies investigated the diagnostic performance of home BP monitoring by determining the sensitivity, specificity, positive and negative diagnostic values, and diagnostic agreement by considering ambulatory BP monitoring as reference method [1]. Most of these studies have examined particular diagnostic phenotypes of hypertension (sustained, white-coat, masked, or resistant) and included populations with different characteristics (untreated subjects, treated hypertensives, patients with type 2 diabetes, chronic kidney disease, children). The available data suggest considerable diagnostic agreement between the two methods ranging from about 70 to 90%, with home BP monitoring being more efficient in identifying normotensive individuals, yet less accurate in detecting truly hypertensives, as it was associated with high specificity and negative predictive value (>80%) but relatively lower sensitivity and positive predictive value (60–70%) [30]. One of these studies examined the diagnostic accuracy of home BP monitoring separately in 613 untreated and treated subjects and reported that the sensitivity for hypertension diagnosis varied between 48–100% in untreated subjects and 52–97% in treated subjects and specificity between 44–93% and 63–84%, respectively [31]. Another study in resistant hypertension also showed that home BP monitoring was a reliable alternative diagnostic method to ambulatory BP monitoring [32]. These conclusions are based on the assumption that ambulatory BP monitoring is perfectly reproducible and reliable, which certainly is not the case. Moreover, the diagnostic disagreement between the two methods in several cases was "arithmetical" and clinically irrelevant (within 5 mmHg) and mostly present in subjects whose BP levels were close to the diagnostic thresholds and, therefore, is probably attributed, to a great extent, to the imperfect reproducibility of all BP measurement methods [1, 29].

29.4.2 Prognostic Value

29.4.2.1 Association with Preclinical Target Organ Damage

Preclinical target organ damage is recognized as an intermediate stage in the sequence of cardiovascular disease development, and its presence in asymptomatic hypertensive subjects indicates increased risk of future cardiovascular events [2].

Several cross-sectional studies have investigated the association of home BP monitoring with indices of preclinical target organ damage at the level of the heart, the large arteries, and the kidneys and showed superiority compared to the conventional office measurements and similar correlations as with ambulatory BP measurements. A meta-analysis compared the association of home vs. office and ambulatory BP monitoring with indices of organ damage, and the most extensively studied marker was echocardiographic left ventricular mass index [33]. Analysis of ten studies revealed stronger correlation coefficients for home vs. office BP (systolic/diastolic, pooled $r = 0.46/0.28$ vs. 0.23/0.19, respectively), whereas data from nine studies indicated similar coefficients for home and ambulatory BP monitoring [33]. There is weaker evidence for carotid intima-media thickness, pulse wave velocity, and urine protein excretion, with a consistent trend toward stronger coefficients for home than office BP, with the latter not reaching statistical significance [33]. Another meta-analysis showed that home BP is superior to office BP in determining proteinuria [34].

29.4.2.2 Prediction of Cardiovascular Outcome

Further to the abovementioned studies assessing surrogate endpoints, current guidelines for hypertension in adults are mainly based on large, long-term observational and interventional outcome studies with hard endpoints of cardiovascular morbidity and mortality [2, 35].

Two meta-analyses (Table 29.3) have investigated the evidence sourced from outcome trials in the general population, in primary care, and in hypertensive patients and assessed the prognostic ability of home compared to office BP measurements [36, 37]. Both were based on data from 8 prospective studies and 17,688 patients followed for 3.2–10.9 years, which resulted in the availability of information based on almost 100,000 person/years of follow-up, and showed home to be superior to office BP measurements, with this difference being beyond chance for systolic BP [36, 37]. Moreover, in the meta-analysis by Ward et al., home BP remained a significant predictor of cardiovascular mortality and cardiovascular events even after adjustment for office BP, suggesting its independent prognostic value over and beyond that of office BP [37]. However, one major limitation of the abovementioned meta-analyses was that these were based on aggregate data.

In 2014 the International Database of HOme BP in relation to Cardiovascular Outcome (IDHOCO) including individual participants' data of five population

Table 29.3 Meta-analyses of studies on prognostic value of home versus office blood pressure (random-effects estimates)

	Systolic blood pressure		Diastolic blood pressure	
	Home	Office	Home	Office
Stergiou et al. [36]	1.15 (1.10–1.20)	1.07 (1.04–1.11)	1.12 (1.09–1.16)	1.08 (1.02–1.14)
Ward et al. [37]	1.14 (1.09–1.20)	1.10 (1.06–1.15)	1.13 (1.08–1.18)	1.07 (0.99–1.16)

Hazard ratios for cardiovascular events per 10 mmHg increase in systolic or 5 mmHg diastolic office and home blood pressure (adjusted hazard ratios with 95% confidence intervals in parentheses)

studies (n = 5008, mean follow-up 8.3 years, 46,593 person-years) showed that home BP substantially refined risk stratification at office BP levels assumed to carry no or only mildly increased risk, in particular in the presence of masked hypertension [38]. More specifically, in participants with optimal or normal office BP, hazard ratios for a composite cardiovascular endpoint associated with a 10 mmHg higher systolic home BP were 1.28 and 1.22, respectively [38]. At high-normal office BP and in mild hypertension, the hazard ratios were at about 1.20 for all cardiovascular events and 1.30 for stroke [38]. In contrast, in severe hypertension, self-measured home BP did not improve the prediction of death or cardiovascular complications. A further analysis of the same dataset was performed separately in untreated and treated subjects [22]. Among untreated subjects, cardiovascular risk was higher in those with white-coat hypertension (adjusted hazard ratio 1.42), masked hypertension (1.55), and sustained hypertension (2.13) compared with normotensive subjects [22]. Among treated patients, only masked uncontrolled hypertension but not white-coat hypertension assessed by home measurements was demonstrated as a cardiovascular risk factor, probably because the latter receives effective treatment on the basis of elevated office BP, whereas the former probably remains undertreated because of low office BP.

Another important point is the prognostic information that is provided by home BP monitoring independently of that obtained from ambulatory BP monitoring. This was clearly demonstrated in two population outcome studies (PAMELA, Ohasama) where subjects with elevated ambulatory but low home BP or the reverse were at increased cardiovascular risk compared to normotensives (low home and ambulatory BP), rendering the two methods not fully interchangeable [39, 40].

29.4.3 Role in Treatment Adjustment

Home BP monitoring is very often used in clinical practice in decision-making for antihypertensive drug treatment initiation and titration. Because of its superior reproducibility, home BP can evaluate accurately the magnitude of the antihypertensive drug action and can thereby identify treatment-induced changes in BP more reliably than the office measurements [9]. Moreover, morning home BP measured before drug intake reflects the trough BP lowering effect of antihypertensive drugs and evening home BP the plateau effect. Thus, the use of the morning/evening home BP ration provides similar information on the duration of antihypertensive drug effect though the 24 h period as the trough: peak ratio assessed by 24 h ambulatory BP monitoring [41].

Two studies investigated the association between treatment-induced changes in home, ambulatory, and office BP and treatment-induced changes in indices of preclinical organ damage. In the Study on Ambulatory Monitoring of Blood Pressure and Lisinopril Evaluation (SAMPLE) in 206 hypertensives followed for 12 months, the treatment-induced regression in left ventricular hypertrophy was more closely associated with treatment-induced changes in ambulatory than in office or home BP [42]. However, only two home readings were obtained in this study, and, therefore, in that study the potential of home BP monitoring has not been exhausted. Another study in 116 hypertensives, with 13.4-month follow-up, showed that treatment-induced changes in both 24 h ambulatory and 7-day home BP monitoring were more closely related than office BP measurements with treatment-induced changes in organ damage (left ventricular mass index, pulse wave velocity, albuminuria) [43]. Interestingly, there were differences between home and ambulatory BP monitoring in their associations with the changes in different indices of organ damage, which implies that these methods are complementary rather than interchangeable in monitoring the effects of antihypertensive treatment on target organ damage [43].

Nine randomized studies assessed treatment adjustment based on home compared to office BP (seven studies) [44–50] or ambulatory BP monitoring (two studies) [51, 52]. These studies differed in their inclusion criteria, population characteristics, BP measurement methodology, BP goals, and duration of follow-up. Three of the studies used the same threshold for office and home BP, which is not in line with current guidelines and led to inferior BP control with home BP monitoring [45, 46, 48]. Four other studies showed larger BP decline with treatment adjustment based on home rather than office BP measurements [44, 47, 49, 50]. Two studies compared home vs. ambulatory BP for treatment adjustment. The first in 98 subjects followed for 6 months found no difference in BP control when using home or ambulatory BP monitoring [51]. The second one randomized 116 subjects to treatment initiation based either on home BP alone or on combined use of office BP and ambulatory BP monitoring [52]. After an average follow-up of 13.4 months, there was no difference between the two arms in BP decline and hypertension control assessed by home or ambulatory BP monitoring, and, more importantly, there was no difference in treatment-induced changes in several indices of preclinical target organ damage [52].

29.4.4 Role in Long-Term Follow-Up and Benefits

The long-term use of home BP monitoring by patients treated for hypertension is recommended by current guidelines. Home BP measurements have the unique advantage compared to office and ambulatory BP monitoring to enable hypertensive individuals to check their BP levels not only through a period of days but during weeks, months, and even years and at minimal cost. Thus, this method increases their awareness motivating for active participation in their follow-up in cooperation with the health-care provider.

Several randomized controlled trials have shown that treated hypertensives who perform home BP measurements have improved long-term adherence to drug therapy and thereby higher hypertension control rates [14, 53]. In addition, home BP monitoring prevents them from adhering to therapy only before an office visit, a phenomenon known as "white-coat adherence," which is associated with increased cardiovascular risk [2, 3]. A systematic review of 72 randomized controlled trials that evaluated the effectiveness of several interventions aiming to improve BP control (home BP monitoring, educational interventions, pharmacist- or nurse-led care, organizational interventions, appointment reminder systems) showed home BP monitoring to be the most efficient method [54]. The MONITOR study in treated uncontrolled hypertensives showed that a 2-month home BP monitoring protocol without medication titration led to superior ambulatory BP monitoring control than the usual care control group [55]. Another study in 1350 hypertensive patients attending a BP clinic showed that those using home BP measurements had higher BP control rates [56].

29.5 Nocturnal Home Blood Pressure

Nighttime ambulatory BP carries superior prognostic value in terms of cardiovascular risk compared to daytime ambulatory, home, or office BP [57, 58]. Novel time-equipped home BP monitors allow automated BP monitoring during nighttime sleep and rendered nocturnal home BP monitoring a feasible method, alternative to ambulatory BP monitoring for the evaluation of nighttime BP and detection.

A recently published systematic review and meta-analysis identified a few studies providing comparative data between nighttime home and ambulatory BP monitoring regarding their differences as well as their association with indices of preclinical target organ damage [59]. Six studies, mainly including hypertensives, reported similar and strongly correlated values for nighttime home and ambulatory BP [19, 60–64]. As shown in two studies, the two methods have close agreement (77.3%) in detecting non-dippers [19, 60]. Three studies reported data on the association of systolic nighttime home and ambulatory BP with left ventricular mass index and two studies on their association with common carotid intima-media thickness with the pooled correlation coefficients being comparable [59, 60, 63]. Two studies reported on the association of urinary albumin excretion with systolic nighttime home and nighttime ambulatory BP suggesting stronger relationship with the former [59, 60, 62]. In conclusion, preliminary data suggest that nighttime home BP seems to be at least as reliable as nighttime ambulatory BP monitoring in determining preclinical target organ damage. However, these data are cross-sectional, and outcome studies are needed to confirm the value of nighttime home BP in predicting cardiovascular morbidity and mortality.

29.6 Cost-Effectiveness

Home BP monitoring has the potential for significant cost savings through the prevention of unnecessary treatment in subjects with white-coat phenomenon, the lesser need for office visits, and the optimal treatment of masked hypertensives that is expected to reduce the incidence of cardiovascular complications [4, 30]. On the other hand, there are several costs, such as that for purchasing home BP devices which is usually covered by the patients themselves; the cost for the time required for patients' training by the physicians or medical staff on the appropriate use of the method, which required for the necessary validation of devices; and also costs for the physician time for data interpretation and consultation to patients regarding changes in treatment [4, 30].

An old review showed that the estimated annualized resource cost of home BP monitoring was less than half of that of ambulatory BP monitoring [65]. A decision tree model based on data from the Ohasama home BP outcome study applied on a Japanese national database concluded that the introduction of home BP monitoring for the diagnosis and treatment of hypertension would be very effective to save costs [66, 67]. This was mainly attributed to avoidance of treatment of white-coat hypertensives and improvement of prognosis due to better control of hypertension [66, 67]. A recent study in 116 untreated hypertensive subjects who were randomized to use home or office/ambulatory BP monitoring for antihypertensive treatment initiation and titration showed that the cost related to health resources utilized within 12-month follow-up was lower in the home BP monitoring arm [16]. Interestingly, this difference in favor of home BP monitoring became more evident in a 5-year projection [16]. Another study performed a cost-benefit analysis from the perspective of the insurer by using a decision-analytic model that simulated the transitions among health states from initial physician visit to hypertension diagnosis, to treatment, to hypertension-related cardiovascular diseases, and to patient death or resignation from the plan [15]. This study concluded that reimbursement of home BP monitoring is cost beneficial from an insurer's perspective for diagnosing and treating hypertension [15].

29.7 Clinical Application

29.7.1 Devices and Cuffs

Validated automated electronic upper-arm-cuff devices, especially those using an oscillometric algorithm, are currently recommended for home BP monitoring, as they are easy to use, relatively accurate, and devoid of the observer bias [3]. Aneroid or hybrid auscultatory devices might also be used but require skills, training, and more regular calibration, which often are not feasible in general practice. Wrist devices are regarded as less accurate than upper-arm devices, mainly because of anatomical differentiations of the wrist and of difficulty in following the correct wrist position (at heart level and relaxed) [3]. The accuracy of electronic BP monitors should have been tested against conventional mercury sphygmomanometry according to established validation protocols [68–71]. The use of cuffs of appropriate inflatable bladder size (length should cover 80–100% of the arm circumference, and the width should be about half of the length) is of major importance in order to avoid over- or underestimation of BP. The use of monitors with automated memory or PC link capacity is also recommended to prevent misreporting of self-BP readings by patients (Table 29.4).

Table 29.4 Recommendations for optimal application of home blood pressure monitoring

Devices and cuffs	Automated electronic (oscillometric) upper-arm devices validated according to an established protocol and equipped with automated memory (or PC link capacity) Cuff (bladder) size according to individual arm circumference
Conditions	Measurements in a quiet room after 5 min sitting rest with back supported and arm resting at heart level
Monitoring schedule	Monitoring for 7 days before each office visit with duplicate (1 min intervals) morning (before drug intake) and evening measurements. Not fewer than 3 days (12 readings)
Evaluation	Calculation of average blood pressure of all readings after discarding the first day
Diagnostic thresholds	Normal home blood pressure, <130/80 mmHg; hypertension, ≥135/85 mmHg, intermediate levels are considered borderline
Long-term follow-up	1–2 duplicate measurements per week

29.7.2 Conditions and Procedure

The patient should be seated, with the back supported, without crossing legs, in a quiet room at a comfortable temperature, and at least 5 min of rest should precede the measurement [3]. Talking during the measurement and coffee or smoking for at least 30 min before the measurement should be discouraged [3]. The cuff should be placed at heart level with the center of the bladder over the brachial artery [3]. In individuals without a consistent between-arm difference as checked in the office on repeated measurements, home BP measurements should be performed sequentially on the same, usually the non-dominant, arm [3].

29.7.3 Monitoring Schedule

For the initial evaluation of BP levels (untreated subjects) and before each visit to the physician (for treated hypertensives), a standard monitoring schedule which includes duplicate measurements (with 1 min interval) in the morning (before drug intake if treated), and the evening, for 7 routine work days (not less than 3 days) is recommended [3]. In any case, 12 home BP readings obtained as described above seem to be the minimum acceptable sample [3]. For the long-term follow-up of treated hypertensives, home BP measurements once or twice per week might seem to be appropriate to ensure maintenance of adequate BP control.

29.7.4 Diagnostic Threshold and Interpretation

Home BP readings of the first monitoring day should be better discarded, as they are typically higher and more variable than of the next days [3]. Based on evidence derived from meta-analyses, cross-sectional, and also long-term observational studies, the current guidelines recommend a hypertension threshold for average home

BP at 135/85 mmHg (the same as for awake ambulatory BP) [3, 4]. Levels exceeding this threshold are considered elevated. Home BP levels ranging between 130–135 mmHg for systolic and 80–85 mmHg for diastolic BP are regarded as borderline (prehypertension range) and those <130/80 mmHg as normal [3].

29.8 Summary

Increasing evidence suggests that self-home BP monitoring has primary role for most patients with hypertension in both the diagnosis and the long-term management. Recent European guidelines recommend home BP monitoring for out-of-office BP evaluation in clinical practice to have similar clinical indications as ambulatory BP monitoring and the choice between them in each case to be depended on their availability and on patients' special characteristics and preference. Particularly in untreated or treated individuals with office BP levels close to the diagnostic thresholds (prehypertension, office hypertension stage 1), home BP monitoring is mandatory for the optimal decision-making, as it allows the identification of intermediate phenotypes of hypertension (white-coat and masked hypertension).

References

1. Stergiou GS, Kollias A, Zeniodi M, Karpettas N, Ntineri A. Home blood pressure monitoring: primary role in hypertension management. Curr Hypertens Rep. 2014;16:462.
2. Mancia G, Fagard R, Narkiewicz K, Redon J, Zanchetti A, Bohm M, Christiaens T, Cifkova R, De Backer G, Dominiczak A, Galderisi M, Grobbee DE, Jaarsma T, Kirchhof P, Kjeldsen SE, Laurent S, Manolis AJ, Nilsson PM, Ruilope LM, Schmieder RE, Sirnes PA, Sleight P, Viigimaa M, Waeber B, Zannad F. 2013 ESH/ESC Guidelines for the management of arterial Hypertension: the Task Force for the Management of Arterial Hypertension of the European Society of Hypertension (ESH) and of the European Society of Cardiology (ESC). J Hypertens. 2013;31:1281–357.
3. Parati G, Stergiou GS, Asmar R, Bilo G, de Leeuw P, Imai Y, Kario K, Lurbe E, Manolis A, Mengden T, O'Brien E, Ohkubo T, Padfield P, Palatini P, Pickering T, Redon J, Revera M, Ruilope LM, Shennan A, Staessen JA, Tisler A, Waeber B, Zanchetti A, Mancia G. European Society of Hypertension guidelines for blood pressure monitoring at home: a summary report of the second international consensus conference on home blood pressure monitoring. J Hypertens. 2008;26:1505–26.
4. Pickering TG, Miller NH, Ogedegbe G, Krakoff LR, Artinian NT, Goff D. Call to action on use and reimbursement for home blood pressure monitoring: a joint scientific statement from the American Heart Association, American Society Of Hypertension, and Preventive Cardiovascular Nurses Association. Hypertension. 2008;52:10–29.
5. Stergiou GS, Kollias A. Home monitoring of blood Pressure. In: Bakris LG, Sorrentino MJ, editors. Hypertension: a companion to Braunwald's heart disease. 3rd ed. Philadelphia, PA: Elsevier; 2018. p. 89–95.
6. Parati G, Stergiou GS. Self measured and ambulatory blood pressure in assessing the 'white-coat' phenomenon. J Hypertens. 2003;21:677–82.
7. Vaur L, Dubroca II, Dutrey-Dupagne C, Genes N, Chatellier G, Bouvier-d'Yvoire M, Elkik F, Menard J. Superiority of home blood pressure measurements over office measurements for testing antihypertensive drugs. Blood Press Monit. 1998;3:107–14.

8. Rose G. Standardisation of observers in blood-pressure measurement. Lancet. 1965;1:673–4.
9. Stergiou GS, Baibas NM, Gantzarou AP, Skeva II, Kalkana CB, Roussias LG, Mountokalakis TD. Reproducibility of home, ambulatory, and clinic blood pressure: implications for the design of trials for the assessment of antihypertensive drug efficacy. Am J Hypertens. 2002;15:101–4.
10. Stergiou GS, Ntineri A. The optimal schedule for self-home blood pressure monitoring. J Hypertens. 2015;33:693–7.
11. Little P, Barnett J, Barnsley L, Marjoram J, Fitzgerald-Barron A, Mant D. Comparison of acceptability of and preferences for different methods of measuring blood pressure in primary care. BMJ. 2002;325:258–9.
12. Nasothimiou EG, Karpettas N, Dafni MG, Stergiou GS. Patients' preference for ambulatory versus home blood pressure monitoring. J Hum Hypertens. 2014;28:224–9.
13. Cappuccio FP, Kerry SM, Forbes L, Donald A. Blood pressure control by home monitoring: meta-analysis of randomised trials. BMJ. 2004;329:145.
14. Ogedegbe G, Schoenthaler A. A systematic review of the effects of home blood pressure monitoring on medication adherence. J Clin Hypertens (Greenwich). 2006;8:174–80.
15. Arrieta A, Woods JR, Qiao N, Jay SJ. Cost-benefit analysis of home blood pressure monitoring in hypertension diagnosis and treatment: an insurer perspective. Hypertension. 2014;64:891–6.
16. Boubouchairopoulou N, Karpettas N, Athanasakis K, Kollias A, Protogerou AD, Achimastos A, Stergiou GS. Cost estimation of hypertension management based on home blood pressure monitoring alone or combined office and ambulatory blood pressure measurements. J Am Soc Hypertens. 2014;8:732–8.
17. Myers MG, Stergiou GS. Reporting bias: Achilles' heel of home blood pressure monitoring. J Am Soc Hypertens. 2014;8:350–7.
18. Hosohata K, Kikuya M, Ohkubo T, Metoki H, Asayama K, Inoue R, Obara T, Hashimoto J, Totsune K, Hoshi H, Satoh H, Imai Y. Reproducibility of nocturnal blood pressure assessed by self-measurement of blood pressure at home. Hypertens Res. 2007;30:707–12.
19. Stergiou GS, Nasothimiou EG, Destounis A, Poulidakis E, Evagelou I, Tzamouranis D. Assessment of the diurnal blood pressure profile and detection of non-dippers based on home or ambulatory monitoring. Am J Hypertens. 2012;25:974–8.
20. Kollias A, Ntineri A, Stergiou GS. Is white-coat hypertension a harbinger of increased risk? Hypertens Res. 2014;37:791–5.
21. Briasoulis A, Androulakis E, Palla M, Papageorgiou N, Tousoulis D. White-coat hypertension and cardiovascular events: a meta-analysis. J Hypertens. 2016;34:593–9.
22. Stergiou GS, Asayama K, Thijs L, Kollias A, Niiranen TJ, Hozawa A, Boggia J, Johansson JK, Ohkubo T, Tsuji I, Jula AM, Imai Y, Staessen JA, International Database on HOme blood pressure in relation to Cardiovascular Outcome (IDHOCO) Investigators. Prognosis of white-coat and masked hypertension: International Database of HOme blood pressure in relation to Cardiovascular Outcome. Hypertension. 2014;63:675–82.
23. Dolan E, Stanton A, Atkins N, Den Hond E, Thijs L, McCormack P, Staessen J, O'Brien E. Determinants of white-coat hypertension. Blood Press Monit. 2004;9:307–9.
24. Cuspidi C, Sala C, Tadic M, Rescaldani M, Grassi G, Mancia G. Untreated masked hypertension and subclinical cardiac damage: a systematic review and meta-analysis. Am J Hypertens. 2015;28:806–13.
25. Bobrie G, Chatellier G, Genes N, Clerson P, Vaur L, Vaisse B, Menard J, Mallion JM. Cardiovascular prognosis of "masked hypertension" detected by blood pressure self-measurement in elderly treated hypertensive patients. JAMA. 2004;291:1342–9.
26. Barochiner J, Cuffaro PE, Aparicio LS, Alfie J, Rada MA, Morales MS, Galarza CR, Waisman GD. Predictors of masked hypertension among treated hypertensive patients: an interesting association with orthostatic hypertension. Am J Hypertens. 2013;26:872–8.
27. Hänninen MR, Niiranen TJ, Puukka PJ, Mattila AK, Jula AM. Determinants of masked hypertension in the general population: the Finn-Home study. J Hypertens. 2011;29:1880–8.
28. Sheppard JP, Fletcher B, Gill P, Martin U, Roberts N, McManus RJ. Predictors of the home-clinic blood pressure difference: a systematic review and meta-analysis. Am J Hypertens. 2016;29:614–25.

29. Stergiou GS, Salgami EV, Tzamouranis DG, Roussias LG. Masked hypertension assessed by ambulatory blood pressure versus home blood pressure monitoring: is it the same phenomenon? Am J Hypertens. 2005;18:772–8.
30. Stergiou GS, Bliziotis IA. Home blood pressure monitoring in the diagnosis and treatment of hypertension: a systematic review. Am J Hypertens. 2011;24:123–34.
31. Nasothimiou EG, Tzamouranis D, Rarra V, Roussias LG, Stergiou GS. Diagnostic accuracy of home vs. ambulatory blood pressure monitoring in untreated and treated hypertension. Hypertens Res. 2012;35:750–5.
32. Nasothimiou EG, Tzamouranis D, Roussias LG, Stergiou GS. Home versus ambulatory blood pressure monitoring in the diagnosis of clinic resistant and true resistant hypertension. J Hum Hypertens. 2012;26:696–700.
33. Bliziotis IA, Destounis A, Stergiou GS. Home versus ambulatory and office blood pressure in predicting target organ damage in hypertension: a systematic review and meta-analysis. J Hypertens. 2012;30:1289–99.
34. Fuchs SC, Mello RG, Fuchs FC. Home blood pressure monitoring is better predictor of cardiovascular disease and target organ damage than office blood pressure: a systematic review and meta-analysis. Curr Cardiol Rep. 2013;15:413.
35. Lewington S, Clarke R, Qizilbash N, Peto R, Collins R. Age-specific relevance of usual blood pressure to vascular mortality: a meta-analysis of individual data for one million adults in 61 prospective studies. Lancet. 2002;360:1903–13.
36. Stergiou GS, Siontis KC, Ioannidis JP. Home blood pressure as a cardiovascular outcome predictor: it's time to take this method seriously. Hypertension. 2010;55:1301–3.
37. Ward AM, Takahashi O, Stevens R, Heneghan C. Home measurement of blood pressure and cardiovascular disease: systematic review and meta-analysis of prospective studies. J Hypertens. 2012;30:449–56.
38. Asayama K, Thijs L, Brguljan-Hitij J, Niiranen TJ, Hozawa A, Boggia J, Aparicio LS, Hara A, Johansson JK, Ohkubo T, Tzourio C, Stergiou GS, Sandoya E, Tsuji I, Jula AM, Imai Y, Staessen JA, International Database of Home Blood Pressure in Relation to Cardiovascular Outcome (IDHOCO) investigators. Risk stratification by self-measured home blood pressure across categories of conventional blood pressure: a participant-level meta-analysis. PLoS Med. 2014;e1001591:11.
39. Mancia G, Facchetti R, Bombelli M, Grassi G, Sega R. Long-term risk of mortality associated with selective and combined elevation in office, home, and ambulatory blood pressure. Hypertension. 2006;47:846–53.
40. Satoh M, Asayama K, Kikuya M, Inoue R, Metoki H, Hosaka M, Tsubota-Utsugi M, Obara T, Ishiguro A, Murakami K, Matsuda A, Yasui D, Murakami T, Mano N, Imai Y, Ohkubo T. Long-term stroke risk due to partial white-coat or masked hypertension based on home and ambulatory blood pressure measurements: The Ohasama Study. Hypertension. 2016;67:48–55.
41. Stergiou GS, Efstathiou SP, Skeva II, Baibas NM, Roussias LG, Mountokalakis TD. Comparison of the smoothness index, the trough: peak ratio and the morning: evening ratio in assessing the features of the antihypertensive drug effect. J Hypertens. 2003;21:913–20.
42. Mancia G, Zanchetti A, Agabiti-Rosei E, Benemio G, De Cesaris R, Fogari R, Pessina A, Porcellati C, Rappelli A, Salvetti A, Trimarco B. Ambulatory blood pressure is superior to clinic blood pressure in predicting treatment-induced regression of left ventricular hypertrophy. SAMPLE Study Group. Study on Ambulatory Monitoring of Blood Pressure and Lisinopril Evaluation. Circulation. 1997;95:1464–70.
43. Karpettas N, Destounis A, Kollias A, Nasothimiou E, Moyssakis I, Stergiou GS. Prediction of treatment-induced changes in target-organ damage using changes in clinic, home and ambulatory blood pressure. Hypertens Res. 2014;37:543–7.
44. Zarnke KB, Feagan BG, Mahon JL, Feldman RD. A randomized study comparing a patient-directed hypertension management strategy with usual office-based care. Am J Hypertens. 1997;10:58–67.
45. Broege PA, James GD, Pickering TG. Management of hypertension in the elderly using home blood pressures. Blood Press Monit. 2001;6:139–44.

46. Staessen JA, Den Hond E, Celis H, Fagard R, Keary L, Vandenhoven G, O'Brien ET, Treatment of Hypertension Based on Home or Office Blood Pressure (THOP) Trial Investigators. Treatment of Hypertension Based on Home or Office Blood Pressure (THOP) Trial Investigators. Antihypertensive treatment based on blood pressure measurement at home or in the physician's office: a randomized controlled trial. JAMA. 2004;291:955–64.
47. Halme L, Vesalainen R, Kaaja M, Kantola I, HOme MEasuRement of blood pressure study group. Self-monitoring of blood pressure promotes achievement of blood pressure target in primary health care. Am J Hypertens. 2005;18:1415–20.
48. Verberk WJ, Kroon AA, Lenders JW, Kessels AG, van Montfrans GA, Smit AJ, van der Kuy PH, Nelemans PJ, Rennenberg RJ, Grobbee DE, Beltman FW, Joore MA, Brunenberg DE, Dirksen C, Thien T, de Leeuw PW, Home Versus Office Measurement, Reduction of Unnecessary Treatment Study Investigators. Home versus office measurement, reduction of unnecessary treatment study investigators. Self-measurement of blood pressure at home reduces the need for antihypertensive drugs: a randomized, controlled trial. Hypertension. 2007;50:1019–25.
49. Tobe SW, Hunter K, Geerts R, Raymond N, Pylypchuk G, Canadian Hypertension Society. IMPPACT: Investigation of Medical Professionals and Patients Achieving Control Together. Can J Cardiol. 2008;24:205–8.
50. McManus RJ, Mant J, Bray EP, Holder R, Jones MI, Greenfield S, Kaambwa B, Banting M, Bryan S, Little P, Williams B, Hobbs FD. Telemonitoring and self-management in the control of hypertension (TASMINH2): a randomized controlled trial. Lancet. 2010;376:163–72.
51. Niiranen TJ, Kantola IM, Vesalainen R, Johansson J, Ruuska MJ. A comparison of home measurement and ambulatory monitoring of blood pressure in the adjustment of antihypertensive treatment. Am J Hypertens. 2006;19:468–74.
52. Stergiou GS, Karpettas N, Destounis A, Tzamouranis D, Nasothimiou E, Kollias A, Roussias L, Moyssakis I. Home blood pressure monitoring alone vs. combined clinic and ambulatory measurements in following treatment-induced changes in blood pressure and organ damage. Am J Hypertens. 2014;27:184–92.
53. Agarwal R, Bills JE, Hecht TJ, Light RP. Role of home blood pressure monitoring in overcoming therapeutic inertia and improving hypertension control: a systematic review and meta-analysis. Hypertension. 2011;57:29–38.
54. Glynn LG, Murphy AW, Smith SM, Schroeder K, Fahey T. Self-monitoring and other non-pharmacological interventions to improve the management of hypertension in primary care: a systematic review. Br J Gen Pract. 2010;60:e476–88.
55. Fuchs SC, Ferreira-da-Silva AL, Moreira LB, Neyeloff JL, Fuchs FC, Gus M, Wiehe M, Fuchs FD. Efficacy of isolated home blood pressure monitoring for blood pressure control: randomized controlled trial with ambulatory blood pressure monitoring – MONITOR study. J Hypertens. 2012;30:75–80.
56. Cuspidi C, Meani S, Fusi V, Salerno M, Valerio C, Severgnini B, Catini E, Leonetti G, Magrini F, Zanchetti A. Home blood pressure measurement and its relationship with blood pressure control in a large selected hypertensive population. J Hum Hypertens. 2004;18:725–31.
57. O'Brien E, Parati G, Stergiou G, Asmar R, Beilin L, Bilo G, Clement D, de la Sierra A, de Leeuw P, Dolan E, Fagard R, Graves J, Head GA, Imai Y, Kario K, Lurbe E, Mallion JM, Mancia G, Mengden T, Myers M, Ogedegbe G, Ohkubo T, Omboni S, Palatini P, Redon J, Ruilope LM, Shennan A, Staessen JA, vanMontfrans G, Verdecchia P, Waeber B, Wang J, Zanchetti A, Zhang Y. European Society of Hypertension position paper on ambulatory blood pressure monitoring. J Hypertens. 2013;31:1731–68.
58. Hansen TW, Li Y, Boggia J, Thijs L, Richart T, Staessen JA. Predictive role of the nighttime blood pressure. Hypertension. 2011;57:3–10.
59. Kollias A, Ntineri A, Stergiou GS. Association of night-time home blood pressure with night-time ambulatory blood pressure and target-organ damage: a systematic review and meta-analysis. J Hypertens. 2017;35:442–52.
60. Andreadis EA, Agaliotis G, Kollias A, Kolyvas G, Achimastos A, Stergiou GS. Night-time home versus ambulatory blood pressure in determining target organ damage. J Hypertens. 2016;34:438–44; discussion 444.

61. Ushio H, Ishigami T, Araki N, Minegishi S, Tamura K, Okano Y, Uchino K, Tochikubo O, Umemura S. Utility and feasibility of a new programmable home blood pressure monitoring device for the assessment of nighttime blood pressure. Clin Exp Nephrol. 2009;13(5):480.
62. Ishikawa J, Hoshide S, Eguchi K, Ishikawa S, Shimada K, Kario K, Japan Morning Surge-Home Blood Pressure Study Investigators Group. Nighttime home blood pressure and the risk of hypertensive target organ damage. Hypertension. 2012;60:921–8.
63. Lindroos AS, Johansson JK, Puukka PJ, Kantola I, Salomaa V, Juhanoja EP, Sivén SS, Jousilahti P, Jula AM, Niiranen TJ. The association between home versus ambulatory night-time blood pressure and end-organ damage in the general population. J Hypertens. 2016;34:1730–7.
64. Ishikawa J, Shimizu M, Sugiyama Edison E, Yano Y, Hoshide S, Eguchi K, Kario K, J-TOP (Japan Morning Surge-Target Organ Protection) Study Investigators Group. Assessment of the reductions in night-time blood pressure and dipping induced by antihypertensive medication using a home blood pressure monitor. J Hypertens. 2014;32:82–9.
65. Appel LJ, Stason WB. Ambulatory blood pressure monitoring and blood pressure self-measurement in the diagnosis and management of hypertension. Ann Intern Med. 1993;118:867–82.
66. Funahashi J, Ohkubo T, Fukunaga H, Kikuya M, Takada N, Asayama K, Metoki H, Obara T, Inoue R, Hashimoto J, Totsune K, Kobayashi M, Imai Y. The economic impact of the introduction of home blood pressure measurement for the diagnosis and treatment of hypertension. Blood Press Monit. 2006;11:257–67.
67. Fukunaga H, Ohkubo T, Kobayashi M, Tamaki Y, Kikuya M, Obara T, Nakagawa M, Hara A, Asayama K, Metoki H, Inoue R, Hashimoto J, Totsune K, Imai Y. Cost-effectiveness of the introduction of home blood pressure measurement in patients with office hypertension. J Hypertens. 2008;26:685–90.
68. Association for the Advancement of Medical Instrumentation. American National Standard. Electronic or automated sphygmomanometers ANSI/AAMI SP10-1987. 3330 Washington Boulevard, Suite 400, Arlington, VA 22201-4598. USA: AAMI; 1987.
69. O'Brien E, Petrie J, Littler W, de Swiet M, Padfield PL, O'Malley K, Jamieson M, Altman D, Bland M, Atkins N. The British Hypertension Society Protocol for the evaluation of automated and semi-automated blood pressure measuring devices with special reference to ambulatory systems. J Hypertens. 1990;8:607–19.
70. O'Brien E, Pickering T, Asmar R, Myers M, Parati G, Staessen J, Mengden T, Imai Y, Waeber B, Palatini P, Gerin W, Working Group on Blood Pressure Monitoring of the European Society of Hypertension. Working Group on Blood Pressure Monitoring of the European Society of Hypertension International Protocol for validation of blood pressure measuring devices in adults. Blood Press Monit. 2002;7:3–17.
71. O'Brien E, Atkins N, Stergiou G, Karpettas N, Parati G, Asmar R, Imai Y, Wang J, Mengden T, Shennan A. European Society of Hypertension International Protocol revision 2010 for the validation of blood pressure measuring devices in adults. Blood Press Monit. 2010;15:23–38.

Morning Surge of Blood Pressure in Prehypertension and Hypertension

30

Uday M. Jadhav and Onkar C. Swami

30.1 Introduction

Cardiovascular (CV) disease is an important cause of morbidity and mortality worldwide. It has been long accepted that hypertension is a key risk factor for CV disease [1]. The management of hypertension and associated adverse CV outcomes has always been at the forefront of prevention-based strategy [2]. Absolute blood pressure (BP) values are considered as an important determinant of adverse CV outcomes; however, these outcomes may depend on increased BP variability [3].

Morning blood pressure surge (MBPS) is a part of diurnal BP variability [4]. Recent studies have reported that an exaggerated MBPS is a CV risk in both the normotensive and hypertensive subjects. MBPS is linked with target organ damage and subsequently increased CV risk in patients with hypertension [5–7]. With every 10 mm Hg increase in the early-morning systolic BP surge, the risk of stroke increases by 22% [8]. Incidence of ischemic stroke is four times higher in the morning period. Similarly, the risk of sudden cardiac death is 70% higher between 7 and 9 AM compared to other times of the day. There is 2.5-fold greater risk of sudden cardiac death at 11 AM in an hour-by-hour analysis [9].

The clinical relevance and prognostic implications of MBPS can vary substantially based on the method and time interval of assessment. There are many definitions and different pathophysiological mechanisms proposed for MBPS [3]. An improved understanding of this phenomenon is required. In this chapter, we assessed the recently available data on MBPS with special emphasis on its definition, etiology, clinical outcomes, diagnostic evaluation, and treatment strategy.

U. M. Jadhav (✉)
Cardiology Department, MGM New Bombay Hospital, New Mumbai, India

O. C. Swami
Pune, India

R. Zimlichman et al. (eds.), *Prehypertension and Cardiometabolic Syndrome*, Updates in Hypertension and Cardiovascular Protection,
https://doi.org/10.1007/978-3-319-75310-2_30

Table 30.1 MBPS definitions

Morning BP surge description	Definition
Sleep-through surge	Difference between morning BP (average of 2 h of readings after wake-up) and the lowest night-time reading (average of the lowest night-time reading and the two adjacent readings before and after)
Pre-waking surge	Difference between morning BP (average of 2 h of readings after wake-up) and the pre-awake BP (average of 2 h of readings before wake-up)
Rising surge	Difference between BP on rising (single reading after wake-up) and BP before wake-up (single reading before wake-up)
Morning night-time difference	Difference between two morning BP readings (after 7 am) and the average night-time BP
Morning BP	Average morning BP for 2 h after wake-up
Morning-evening difference	Difference between morning BP (average of self-monitored BP readings taken in the morning) and evening BP (average of self-monitored BP readings taken in the evening)

Note: Data adapted from a previous study [11]. *MBPS* morning blood pressure surge, *BP* blood pressure

30.2 Definition of Morning BP Surge

Presently there is a discrepancy on the definition of MBPS [10]. There are several definitions of MBPS (Table 30.1) [8, 11]. Two main definitions of the morning surge in BP are illustrated in the literature. One is "sleep-through morning surge," and the second is "pre-waking morning surge" [4, 12]. Kario K et al. first defined sleep-through and pre-waking morning surge and evaluated the association between excess MBPS and the risk of cerebrovascular diseases [13]. Stergiou GS et al. assessed the reliability of different definitions of MBPS; they anticipated the difference between BP readings 2 h after rising and the average of all readings during sleep as the most reliable approach for assessing the MBPS [14].

30.3 Mechanisms of Morning BP Surge

An increase in BP after waking is a physiological phenomenon; however, a marked and rapid MBPS is associated with increased CV risk [12]. The pathophysiology of the morning surge in BP is unspecified. Insight in underlying mechanisms of morning surge, particularly in patients with hypertension, will be helpful in detecting new therapeutic strategies [10].

Elevated MBPS is believed to be associated with small and large arterial diseases [15]. There is a curvilinear association between contraction of the resistance arteries and vascular resistance, which explicates the acceleration of hypertension (Fig. 30.1) [16, 17]. The difference in vascular resistance between small arteries with and without remodeling is augmented in the morning when the vascular tone is increased as compared to sleep [18].

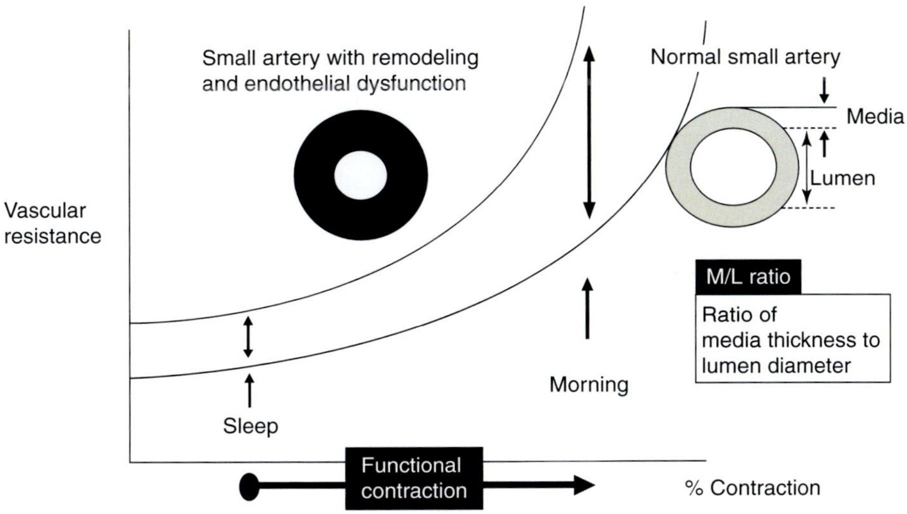

Fig. 30.1 Mechanism of elevated morning blood pressure surge in patients with small artery disease. Note: Data reproduced from a previous study [16]

Table 30.2 Factors influencing the morning surge in BP

Increase in sympathetic activity	Increase in aortic stiffness
Increase in renin-angiotensin system activity	Microvascular dysfunction
Decrease in baroreflex sensitivity	Heavy drinking
Endothelial dysfunction	Smoking
Circadian rhythm	Sleep apnea
Increase in platelet aggregation	Insufficient efficacy of antihypertensive drugs
Oxidative stress	Sodium/caffeine ingestion
Plasma cortisol	Age (>70 years), Monday/winter

Note: Data adapted from previous study [20, 21]. *BP* blood pressure

There is activation of the sympathetic nervous system and the renin-angiotensin system early in the morning [4]. The augmented activity of sympathetic nervous system and the renin-angiotensin system (RAS) may be possible mechanisms to increase in vascular resistance and the morning BP surge [12]. Predominantly, an activity of α-adrenergic component is increased [17], which increases the vascular tone of the small resistance arteries and may contribute to MBPS. Additionally, plasma renin activity, angiotensin II, and aldosterone levels are increased before awakening [19]. There are several factors which possibly influences the morning surge in BP (Table 30.2) [20, 21].

Alpha-adrenergic vasoconstrictor response of small resistance vessels and progressive remodeling of the small vessels are predominant determinants of the rise in BP on awakening. Various risk factors for morning hypertension consist of older age, excessive alcohol intake, tobacco consumption, longer sleep, and later awakening times. Amplified arousal response of BP is the possible reason for the rise in BP immediately after wake up and is commonly noted in elderly with hypertension, whereas the morning surge beginning gradually during sleep is more common in younger individuals with hypertension [10].

The link between MBPS, short-term BP variability, and arterial stiffness in untreated patients with hypertension has been evaluated by Pucci G et al. Sleep-through MBPS was found to be directly related to aortic stiffness, mediated by an increased average real variability of 24 h SBP. Adverse effects of MBPS may be partly explained by its association with arterial stiffness, mediated by short-term SBP variability [22].

Patients with hypertension are more prone for morning surge in BP as compared to normotensives. Head GA et al. investigated 24 h recordings by a new logistic curve method, which exposed distinct asymmetric circadian patterns of cardiovascular changes in normotensive and hypertensive subjects. The method detected a 30–40% greater rate of increase in BP in the hypertensive subjects [23].

30.4 Morning BP Surge and CV Outcomes

Morning is considered as the peak time for a range of adverse CV events. There is mounting evidence suggesting significant associations between MBPS and cardiac, cerebral, renal, and vascular damage (Fig. 30.2) [18]. Jaewon Oh et al. recently evaluated an association of morning hypertension subtype (with nocturnal hypertension) by means of vascular target organ damage and central hemodynamics in patients with high CV risk. Increased arterial stiffness and high central BP were prominently detected [5]. Association of MBPS with adverse CV outcomes may be due to the hemodynamic effects of the high BP on the arterial wall and the associated neurohumoral activation [10]. MBPS is associated with left ventricular

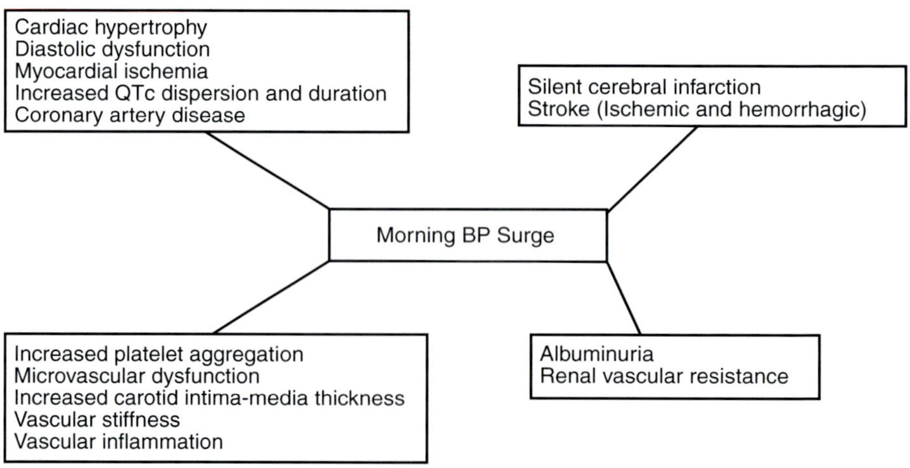

Fig. 30.2 Associations between morning blood pressure surge and cardiovascular diseases. Note: Data adapted from a previous study [18]. *BP* blood pressure

hypertrophy, carotid atherosclerosis, arterial stiffness, albuminuria, and silent cerebrovascular disease [17].

The clinical implication of MBPS as a risk for triggering CV events is increased in patients with the advanced vascular disease. Kario K et al. recently proposed the concept of a vicious cycle between hemodynamic stress and vascular disease that damages organs and plays a role in CV events such as systemic hemodynamic atherothrombotic syndrome (SHATS) [24]. In the following section, some of the CV outcomes of exaggerated MBPS in hypertension and prehypertension are elucidated.

Vascular disease and inflammation: MBPS is linked with carotid atherosclerosis in untreated patients with hypertension [25–27]. Plaque instability can be induced due to its association with increased vascular inflammation. Newly diagnosed and never-treated patients with higher sleep-through MBPS have higher carotid intima-media thickness as reported in a study involving compromising untreated middle-aged 241 patients with hypertension [28]. Alpaydin S et al. evaluated the association between the rate of BP variation and carotid intima-media thickness in patients with prehypertension and demonstrated an independent association of elevated MBPS with carotid intima-media thickness in such patients [29].

Hypertensive heart disease: Published evidence reported that an elevated MBPS is associated with hypertensive heart disease. MBPS augments cardiac afterload and arterial stiffness, contributing to left ventricular hypertrophy [18].

Stroke: Kario K et al. first reported that patients in the high sleep-through morning surge group have a high stroke incidence [8]. Silent cerebral infarction (SCI) is the strongest surrogate marker of clinical stroke, particularly in those with increased C-reactive protein levels [30]. Increased risk of SCI was observed in the morning surge group in elderly hypertensives [8]. The association between elevated MBPS and SCI is slightly influenced by low-grade inflammation [31]. Morning hypertension is an important risk for stroke in the Asian population [32].

Chronic kidney disease: Positive association between MBPS and renal disease has been reported [33, 34]. Elevated MBPS is associated with deterioration of kidney function and development of chronic kidney disease (CKD). Turak O et al. investigated the association between elevated MBPS and the development of incident CKD in 622 patients with essential hypertension. Patients underwent ambulatory BP measurements and were followed for a median of 3.33 years. During follow-up, 32 patients developed CKD. Higher MBPS was associated with incident CKD in all models [35].

CV mortality: Morning BP surge was associated with mortality in a study of 632 hypertensive patients by Amodeo C et al. Patients with MBPS of 41 mm Hg were associated with a higher risk for mortality [36].

All-cause mortality: Xie JC et al. evaluated the predictive value of MBPS for future CV events, stroke, and all-cause mortality. Excess sleep-through surge found to be a strong predictor of mortality. Individuals for future all-cause with higher pre-waking surge showed a tendency for increased risk of CV outcomes, but the differences were insignificant [13].

Morning BP surge, an indicator of prehypertension: An exaggerated morning rise in BP may be one of the indicators of a prehypertensive status with advanced small artery remodeling. Various pathophysiological factors affect arterial wall structure and endothelial function which may lead to prehypertension followed by hypertension and cardiovascular disease. Reported evidence suggests the significant association between a morning BP surge and small artery remodeling which would begin even in case of normotension [37].

Stress hypertension, orthostatic hypertension, ambulatory BP surge, sleep apnea-related midnight surge, etc. are few of the surges other than morning BP surge reported to be a risk for developing cardiovascular disease. These BP surges may partly be related to each other on the basis of sympathetic hyperactivity and can be considered as indicative of a prehypertensive status [37].

30.5 Diagnostic Evaluation of MBPS

Evidence from ambulatory BP monitoring (ABPM) or home BP monitoring (HBPM) studies has pointed out that MBPS is more closely associated with the CV risk [38].

Home BP monitoring was the best predictor of stroke event in a nationwide Japan Morning Surge-Home BP (JHOP) Study [39]. The Ohasama Study and FinHome Study in Finland reported that day-by-day variability of blood pressures based on home blood pressure has a prognostic significance for CVD [40]. Intermittent BP measurement at fixed intervals would undervalue the CV risk of MBPS. Ideally, beat-by-beat continuous BP monitoring is the best means of assessing BP variability. Kario K developed a new hypoxia-triggered home nocturnal BP monitoring system, in which severe desaturation continuously monitored by pulse oximetry sends the signal of BP measurement to the device [41].

Common approach to evaluate the morning increase in blood pressure has been to synchronize records relative to the time of waking [42]. The morning BP-guided approach using HBPM is the first step toward perfect 24 h BP control [12]. Head GA and Lukoshkova EV described a novel method for determining the individual changes using a double logistic equation fitted to the individual pattern of blood pressure change [9].

30.6 Antihypertensive Strategy Targeting MBPS

Morning BP could be an important target of antihypertensive treatment [43]. Control of morning hypertension can be regarded as the first step to strict 24 h BP control [44]. Suppression of elevated MBPS, strict BP control of <130/80 mm Hg for 24 h, and adequate circadian rhythm (dipper type; 10–20% of nocturnal BP fall) are key components of perfect 24 h BP control [45]. Asians show greater MBPS [39]; it is particularly important to control morning BP as the first step toward achieving perfect 24 h BP control [38].

Till recently, there has been a difference of opinion on specific treatments for early-morning hypertension [46]. More definite treatment for MBPS may be achieved using antihypertensive drugs that reduce the pressor effect of the neurohumoral factors, which is potentiated in the morning, such as inhibitors of sympathetic activity [47]. Conceptually, specific treatments could include inhibition of the sympathetic nervous system and the RAS [46]. A chronotherapeutic approach, such as bedtime dosing and a drug delivery system that incorporates extended-release or delayed-onset antihypertensive agents, is useful for reducing MBPS [20, 46].

Selection of antihypertensive drugs including a specific class (e.g., sympatholytics or RAS inhibitors) and timing of doses are important factors. Bedtime dosing of the antihypertensive drug, especially calcium channel blocker, alpha blocker, and RAS inhibitors, may suppress exaggerated MBPS without excessive nocturnal hypotension during sleep. Persistent reduction in sleep BP results in the reduction in nocturnal hypertension type of MBPS [47].

The MAPEC (Ambulatory BP Monitoring for Prediction of Cardiovascular Events) study showed that bedtime chronotherapy with ≥1 antihypertensives exerted better BP control and CVD risk reduction than conventional therapy. In this study, participants taking bedtime administration of at least one medication had significantly lower incidence of CV events (Fig. 30.3) [48]. Participating physicians were given the choice of prescribing, at least one medication of the recommended therapeutic classes, (angiotensin receptor blockers, angiotensin-converting enzyme inhibitors, calcium channel blockers, β-blockers) during the study [48].

Alpha-adrenergic blockade at bedtime may be an effective means to reduce the morning BP rise in patients with uncontrolled morning hypertension [49]. RAS-blocking agents that maintain pharmacodynamic effects into the early-morning period may be of help in individuals with the exaggerated rise in morning BP [50].

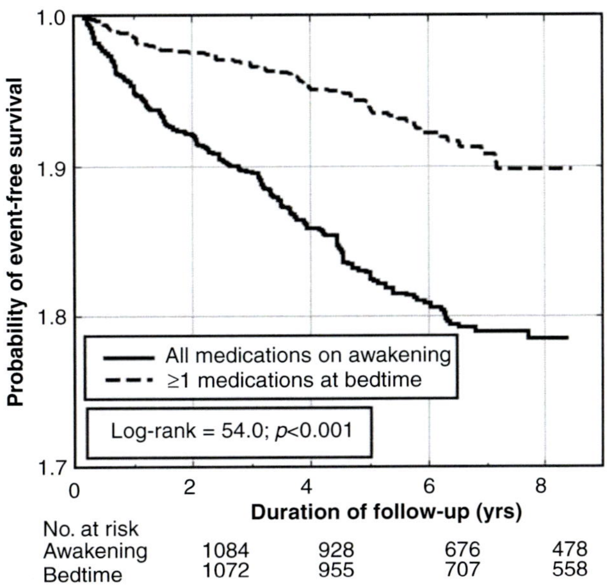

Fig. 30.3 Kaplan-Meier survival curves for subjects ingesting either all their medications upon awakening or ≥1 medications at bedtime. Note: Data reproduced from a previous study [48]

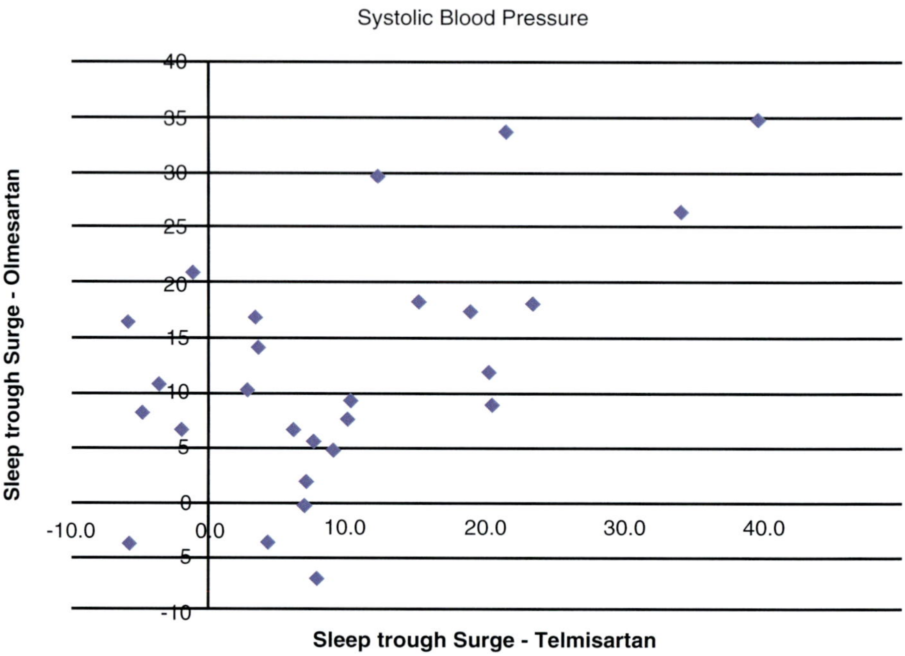

Fig. 30.4 Sleep-through surge with olmesartan and telmisartan. Note: Data reproduced from a previous study [51]

Jadhav UM et al. evaluated the comparative efficacy of angiotensin receptor blockers on MBPS in hypertension. Olmesartan and telmisartan showed the beneficial and similar effect on the MBPS measured by different parameters on the 24 h ABPM (Fig. 30.4) [51].

Lifestyle modifications, such as better night-time sleep and moderation in alcohol intake, are the important part of the essential approach to suppress MBPS along with long-acting antihypertensive drugs, such as long-acting calcium channel blockers or inhibitors of the RAS [20]. Renal denervation is also an effective therapy for reducing morning surge of BP [47].

Morning BP guided approach by using home BP monitoring is the most promising step for effective antihypertensive treatment [12]. Kario K has suggested a strategy for the morning BP guided management of hypertension using home BP monitoring with three steps; first achieve the level of morning systolic BP as <145 mm Hg, then the morning systolic BP level of 135 mm Hg should be attained, and finally about 125 mm Hg or less should be achieved and maintained [45].

Therapeutic approaches to be considered: Reported evidence shown that long-acting antihypertensive medications have advantages in controlling BP over 24 h in contrast to short-acting or intermediate-acting drugs. Hypertension guidelines have suggested the use of full dose or maximum dose of antihypertensive drugs, regardless of combination or monotherapy. Combination therapy of an angiotensin receptor blocker or angiotensin-converting enzyme inhibitor and a calcium channel

Table 30.3 Summary of some important studies on therapeutic approaches for the treatment of elevated MBPS in hypertension

Study, design, sample size	Study medication (mg/day)	Study conclusion
Long-acting vs. short-acting antihypertensives		
Ferrucci et al. [52], crossover, 40	Amlodipine vs. nifedipine	Amlodipine had greater antihypertensive efficacy vs. nifedipine
White et al. [53], parallel group, 490	Telmisartan vs. valsartan	Telmisartan achieved greater antihypertensive effect vs. valsartan during the early-morning period
Full dose vs. low dose of antihypertensive drugs		
Bilo et al. [54], parallel group, 626	Amlodipine 5 vs. olmesartan/amlodipine 10/5 vs. 20/5 vs. 40/5	Olmesartan/amlodipine combination has better 24 h dose-related improvement in BP lowering vs. amlodipine alone
Kai et al. [55], parallel group, 110	Losartan 50/HCTZ 12.5 vs. losartan 50. Control rate of both morning and evening hypertension (<135/85 mm Hg): 54.5 vs. 29.1%	Losartan/HCTZ combination was superior to high-dose losartan in treating both types of morning hypertension
Combination vs. monotherapy of antihypertensive drugs		
Shimada et al. [56], parallel group, 862	Olmesartan/azelnidipine vs. olmesartan vs. azelnidipine	Combination therapy was associated with significant reduction in MBPS vs. monotherapy of either agents
Miyauchi et al. [57], parallel group, 263	Amlodipine/ARB vs. high-dose ARB	Amlodipine combination regimen provides better antihypertensive effect vs. ARB alone.
Bilo et al. [54], parallel group, 626	Olmesartan/amlodipine vs. amlodipine	Combination therapy was effective in lowering 24 h BP vs. amlodipine monotherapy.
Timed dosing of long-acting antihypertensive drugs		
Qiu et al. [58], crossover, 62	Morning vs. evening dosing of amlodipine 5 and 10 mg	Morning administered amlodipine had a better effect on the circadian BP compared with evening administered amlodipine in mild-to-moderate essential hypertension
Drugs of specific mechanisms		
Kario K et al. [59], parallel group, 611	Doxazosin	Adding a bedtime dose of an alpha-adrenergic blocker in patients with uncontrolled morning hypertension significantly reduced BP and urinary albumin excretion rate

Data adapted from a previous study [60]. *MBPS* morning blood pressure surge, *BP* blood pressure, *vs.* versus, *ARB* angiotensin receptor blocker

blocker or diuretic may improve 24 h BP control, especially during the trough effect morning hours. Therapeutic use of antihypertensive drugs of specific mechanisms can be one of the preferable targeted approaches (Table 30.3) [60].

CV benefits from the suppression of an exaggerated MBPS are still to be well established. Interventional studies to examine whether or not a reduction in MBPS, with pharmacologic or nonpharmacologic therapy, can lead to an improvement of

Table 30.4 What is known and new about MBPS

What is already known about MBPS
• MBPS is a part of diurnal BP variability [4] • Excessive MPBS is a predictor of subsequent stroke events in elderly hypertensive patients [45] • utomatic measurements of BP by ambulatory monitoring are required to closely examine the sleep/awake differences [61] • Long-acting drugs are part of the non-specific therapy for controlling morning hypertension [45]
What is new about MBPS
• Morning BP may be an independent predictor of CV events [60] • Importance of HBPM for the cardiovascular prognosis of hypertensive individuals is recently revealed [61] • Morning HBPM can be the best predictor of stroke event [39] • Asians shows greater MBPS [39] • Evidence proposed three-step strategy for the morning BP-guided management of hypertension using HBPM [7] • Once-daily dosing antihypertensive agents are now widely used as conventional antihypertensive medication [62] • Renal denervation is effective for reducing morning BP [50] • Specific treatment includes the time of dosing of antihypertensive drugs and selecting the specific class of antihypertensive drugs, such as inhibitors of sympathetic activity or renin-angiotensin system [46] • Current hypertension guidelines had some forms of recommendations on the measurement of morning BP [63] • Masked morning hypertension, as the other forms of masked hypertension, is the emerging concept as the Japanese guidelines defined it [64] • To improve the management of hypertension in general, and morning hypertension in particular, long-acting antihypertensive drugs should be used in appropriate often full dosages and in proper combinations [60]

MBPS morning blood pressure surge, *BP* blood pressure, *CV* cardiovascular, *HBPM* home blood pressure monitoring

CV morbidity and mortality in hypertensive patients independently of 24 h BP reduction are required. In addition, whether titrating of the home BP level in the morning as a means of preventing CV events is superior versus clinic BP has not been established. Some of the key known and new aspects regarding MBPS are represented in following table (Table 30.4).

Conclusions

BP variability in the form of MBPS is an independent risk factor for CV events. There are various pathophysiological mechanisms suggested for MBPS including vascular damage of small and large arteries. Home BP monitoring can be a useful tool for assessment of MBPS. MBPS needs to be controlled for preventing CV events. Long-acting antihypertensives, inhibitors of sympathetic activity, or the RAS system administered at bedtime will be a useful strategy in control of elevated MBPS and more effective prevention of CV events.

References

1. Bromfield S, Muntner P. High blood pressure: the leading global burden of disease risk factor and the need for worldwide prevention programs. Curr Hypertens Rep. 2013;15(3):134–6.
2. Patel PV, Wong JL, Arora R. The morning blood pressure surge: therapeutic implications. J Clin Hypertens (Greenwich). 2008;10(2):140–5.
3. Parati G, Ochoa JE, Lombardi C, Bilo G. Assessment and management of blood-pressure variability. Nat Rev Cardiol. 2013;10(3):143–55.
4. Kario K, Shimada K, Pickering TG. Clinical implication of morning blood pressure surge in hypertension. J Cardiovasc Pharmacol. 2003;42(Suppl 1):S87–91.
5. Jaewon O, Lee CJ, Kim I-C, Lee S-H, Kang S-M, Choi D, et al. Association of morning hypertension subtype with vascular target organ damage and central hemodynamics. J Am Heart Assoc. 2017;6:e005424.
6. Hoshide S, Kario K, Yano Y, Haimoto H, Yamagiwa K, Uchiba K, et al. Association of morning and evening blood pressure at home with asymptomatic organ damage in the J-HOP Study. Am J Hypertens. 2014;27:939–47.
7. Kario K, Saito I, Kushiro T, Teramukai S, Tomono Y, Okuda Y, Shimada K. Morning home blood pressure is a strong predictor of coronary artery disease: the HONEST Study. J Am Coll Cardiol. 2016;67:1519–27.
8. Kario K, Pickering TG, Umeda Y, Hoshide S, Hoshide Y, Morinari M, et al. Morning surge in blood pressure as a predictor of silent and clinical cerebrovascular diseases in elderly hypertensives: a prospective study. Circulation. 2003;107:1401–6.
9. Head GA, Lukoshkova EV. Understanding the morning rise in blood pressure. Clin Exp Pharmacol Physiol. 2008;35(4):516–21.
10. Palatini P, Grassi G. The morning blood pressure surge: a dynamic and challenging concept. J Hypertens. 2011;29(12):2316–9.
11. Sheppard JP, Hodgkinson J, Riley R, Martin U, Bayliss S, McManus RJ. Prognostic significance of the morning blood pressure surge in clinical practice: a systematic review. Am J Hypertens. 2015;28(1):30–41.
12. Kario K. Evidence and perspectives on the 24-hour management of hypertension: hemodynamic biomarker-initiated 'anticipation medicine' for zero CV event. Prog Cardiovasc Dis. 2016;59(3):262–81.
13. Xie JC, Yan H, Zhao YX, Liu XY. Prognostic value of morning blood pressure surge in clinical events: a meta-analysis of longitudinal studies. J Stroke Cerebrovasc Dis. 2015;24(2):362–9.
14. Stergiou GS, Mastorantonakis SE, Roussias LG. Morning blood pressure surge: the reliability of different definitions. Hypertens Res. 2008;31(8):1589–94.
15. Kario K. Vascular damage in exaggerated morning surge in blood pressure. Hypertension. 2007;49:771–2.
16. Folkow B. Physiological aspects of primary hypertension. Physiol Rev. 1982;62:347–504.
17. Kario K. Morning surge in blood pressure in hypertension: clinical relevance, prognostic significance, and therapeutic approach. In: Berbari AE, Mancia G, editors. Special issues in hypertension. Milano: Springer Milan; 2012. p. 71–89.
18. Yano Y, Kario K. Nocturnal BP, morning BP surge, and cerebrovascular events. Curr Hypertens Rep. 2012;14(3):219–27.
19. Panza JA, Epstein SE, Quyyumi AA. Circadian variation in vascular tone and its relation to alpha-sympathetic vasoconstrictor activity. N Engl J Med. 1991;325:986–90.
20. Brandenberger G, Follenius M, Goichot B, et al. Twenty-four-hour profiles of plasma renin activity in relation to the sleep-wake cycle. J Hypertens. 1994;12:277–83.
21. Patel PV, Wong JL, Arora R. The morning BP surge: therapeutic implications. J Clin Hypertens (Greenwich). 2008;10(2):140–5.
22. Pucci G, Battista F, Anastasio F, Schillaci G. Morning pressor surge, BP variability, and arterial stiffness in essential hypertension. J Hypertens. 2017;35(2):272–8.

23. Head GA, Reid CM, Shiel LM, Jennings GL, Lukoshkova EV. Rate of morning increase in BP is elevated in hypertensives. Am J Hypertens. 2006;19(10):1010–7.
24. Kario K. New insight of morning BP surge into the triggers of cardiovascular disease-synergistic resonance of BP variability. Am J Hypertens. 2016;29(1):14–6.
25. Zakopoulos NA, Tsivgoulis G, Barlas G, et al. Time rate of BP variation is associated with increased common carotid artery intima-media thickness. Hypertension. 2005;45:505–12.
26. Marfella R, Siniscalchi M, Nappo F, et al. Regression of carotid atherosclerosis by control of morning BP peak in newly diagnosed hypertensive patients. Am J Hypertens. 2005;18:308–18.
27. Marfella R, Siniscalchi M, Portoghese M, et al. MBPS as a destabilizing factor of atherosclerotic plaque: role of ubiquitin-proteasome activity. Hypertension. 2007;49:784–91.
28. Pręgowska-Chwała B, Prejbisz A, Kabat M, Puciłowska B, Paschalis-Purtak K, Florczak E, et al. Morning blood pressure surge and markers of cardiovascular alterations in untreated middle-aged hypertensive subjects. J Am Soc Hypertens. 2016;10(10):790–798.e2.
29. Alpaydin S, Turan Y, Caliskan M, Caliskan Z, Aksu F, Ozyildirim S, et al. Morning blood pressure surge is associated with carotid intima-media thickness in prehypertensive patients. Blood Press Monit. 2017;22(3):131–6.
30. Kario K, Shimada K, Matsuo T, et al. Silent and clinically overt stroke in older Japanese subjects with white-coat and sustained hypertension. J Am Coll Cardiol. 2001;38:238–45.
31. Ishikawa J, Tamura Y, Hoshide S, Eguchi K, et al. Low-grade inflammation is a risk factor for clinical stroke events in addition to silent cerebral infarcts in Japanese older hypertensives. The Jichi medical school ABPM study, wave 1. Stroke. 2007;38:911–7.
32. Shimizu M, Ishikawa J, Yano Y, et al. The relationship between the morning bloodpressure surge and low-grade inflammation on silent cerebral infarct and clinical stroke events. Atherosclerosis. 2011;219:316–21.
33. Hoshide S, Kario K, Yano Y, Haimoto H, Yamagiwa K, Uchiba K, et al. Morning hypertension is an important risk for stroke in Asian population. From J-HOP study. J Hypertens. 2015;33(Suppl 1):e126.
34. Kimura G. Kidney and circadian BP rhythm. Hypertension. 2008;51:827–828 34.
35. Turak O, Afsar B, Siriopol D, Ozcan F, Cagli K, Yayla C, et al. Morning BP surge as a predictor of development of chronic kidney disease. J Clin Hypertens (Greenwich). 2016;18(5):444–8.
36. Amodeo C, Guimarães GG, Picotti JC, dos Santos CC, Bezzerra Fonseca KD, Matins RF, et al. Morning blood pressure surge is associated with death in hypertensive patients. Blood Press Monit. 2014;19(4):199–202.
37. Kario K. Preceding linkage between a morning surge in BP and small artery remodeling: an indicator of prehypertension? J Hypertens. 2007;25(8):1573–5.
38. Redon J, Bertolin V, Giner V, Lurbe E. Assessment of blood pressure early morning rise. Blood Press Monit. 2001;6:207–10.
39. Hoshide S, Yano Y, Haimoto H, Yamagiwa K, Uchiba K, Nagasaka S, et al. Morning and evening home blood pressure and risks of incident stroke and coronary artery disease in the Japanese general practice population the Japan morning surge-home blood pressure study. Hypertension. 2016;68:54–61.
40. Fukuda M, Mizuno M, Yamanaka T, et al. Patients with renal dysfunction require a longer duration until BP dips during the night. Hypertension. 2008;52:1155–60.
41. Kario K. Essential manual of 24-hour blood pressure management from morning to nocturnal hypertension. London: Wiley-Blackwell; 2015. p. 1–138.
42. Kario K. Morning hypertension: a pitfall of current hypertensive management. JMAJ. 2005;48(5):234–40.
43. The Japanese Society of Hypertension Guidelines for the Management of Hypertension (JSH 2009). Chapter 2. Measurement and clinical evaluation of blood pressure. Hypertens Res. 2014;37:266–78.
44. Matsui Y, Eguchi K, Shibasaki S, Ishikawa J, Hoshide S, Pickering TG, et al. Effect of doxazosin on the left ventricular structure and function in morning hypertensive patients: the Japan morning surge 1 study. J Hypertens. 2008;26:1463–71.

45. Kario K. Assessment and treatment of morning hypertension: update. J Hypertens. 2016;34(Suppl 1):ISH 2016 Abstract Book:e29.
46. White WB, Weber MA, Davidai G, Neutel JM, Bakris GL, Giles T. Ambulatory blood pressure monitoring in the primary care setting: assessment of therapy on the circadian variation of blood pressure from the MICCAT-2 trial. Blood Press Monit. 2005;10:157–63.
47. Hoshide S, Kario K. Early morning hypertension: a narrative review. Blood Press Monit. 2013;18(6):291–6.
48. Hermida RC, Ayala DE, Mojón A, Fernández JR. Influence of circadian time of hypertension treatment on cardiovascular risk: results of the MAPEC study. Chronobiol Int. 2010;27(8):1629–51.
49. Kario K, Pickering TG, Hoshide S, et al. MBPS and hypertensive cerebrovascular disease: role of the alpha-adrenergic sympathetic nervous system. Am J Hypertens. 2004;17:668–75.
50. Kario K, Bhatt DL, Brar S, Cohen SA, Fahy M, Bakris GL. Effect of catheter-based renal denervation on morning and nocturnal blood pressure: insights from SYMPLICITY HTN-3 and SYMPLICITY HTN-Japan. Hypertension. 2015;66(6):1130–7.
51. Jadhav UM, Kulkarni A. Comparative efficacy of angiotensin receptor antagonist olmesartan and telmisartan on morning blood pressure surge in hypertension. J Am Soc Hypertens. 2016;10(4S):e19–38.
52. Ferrucci A, Marcheselli A, Strano S, Ciavarella GM, Messa F, Calcagnini G. 24-h blood pressure profiles in patients with hypertension treated with amlodipine or nifedipine GITS. Clin Drug Invest. 1997;13(Suppl 1):67–72.
53. White WB, Lacourciere Y, Davidai G. Effects of the angiotensin II receptor blockers telmisartan versus valsartan on the circadian variation of blood pressure: impact on the early morning period. Am J Hypertens. 2004;17:347–53.
54. Bilo G, Koch W, Hoshide S, Parati G. Efficacy of olmesartan/amlodipine combination therapy in reducing ambulatory blood pressure in moderate-to-severe hypertensive patients not controlled by amlodipine alone. Hypertens Res. 2014;37:836–44.
55. Kai H, Ueda T, Uchiwa H, Iwamoto Y, Aoki Y, Anegawa T, et al., MAPPY Study Investigators. Benefit of losartan/hydrochlorothiazide fixed dose combination treatment for isolated morning hypertension: the MAPPY study. Clin Exp Hypertens. 2015;37:473–81.
56. Shimada K, Ogihara T, Saruta T, Kuramoto K. Effects of combination olmesartan medoxomil plus azelnidipine versus monotherapy with either agent on 24-h ambulatory blood pressure and pulse rate in Japanese patients with essential hypertension: additional results from the REZALT study. Clin Ther. 2010;32:861–81.
57. Miyauchi K, Yamazaki T, Watada H, Tanaka Y, Kawamori R, Imai Y, et al. Management of home blood pressure by amlodipine combined with angiotensin II receptor blocker in type 2 diabetes. Circ J. 2012;76:2159–66.
58. Qiu YG, Chen JZ, Zhu JH, Yao XY. Differential effects of morning or evening dosing of amlodipine on circadian blood pressure and heart rate. Cardiovasc Drugs Ther. 2003;17:335–41.
59. Kario K, Matsui Y, Shibasaki S, Eguchi K, Ishikawa J, Hoshide S, et al. An alpha-adrenergic blocker titrated by self-measured blood pressure recordings lowered blood pressure and microalbuminuria in patients with morning hypertension: the Japan Morning Surge-1 Study. J Hypertens. 2008;26:1257–65.
60. Wang JG, Kario K, Park JB, Chen CH. Morning blood pressure monitoring in the management of hypertension. J Hypertens. 2017;35(8):1554–63.
61. Kaplan NM. Morning surge in blood pressure. Circulation. 2003;107(10):1347.
62. Kario K. Prognosis in relation to blood pressure variability: pro side of the argument. Hypertension. 2015;65(6):1163–9.
63. Chiang CE, Wang TD, Ueng KC, Lin TH, Yeh HI, Chen CY, et al. Guidelines of the Taiwan Society of Cardiology and the Taiwan Hypertension Society for the management of hypertension. J Chin Med Assoc. 2015;78:1–47.
64. Shimamoto K, Ando K, Fujita T, Hasebe N, Higaki J, Horiuchi M, et al. The Japanese Society of Hypertension guidelines for the management of hypertension (JSH 2014). Hypertens Res. 2014;37:253–387.

Physical Activity and Exercise Training as Important Modifiers of Vascular Health

31

Arno Schmidt-Trucksäss

The world is in a permanent process of increasing automation and reduction of physical activity during daily work. Machines and robots take over man's work and thereby reduce daily energy expenditure and increase sitting time. Prolonged sitting without interruption, predominantly in front of a PC screen, is an independent risk factor for cardiovascular events, increasing prevalence of chronic diseases and all-cause mortality [1]. Nowadays, sitting time by far exceeds time spent with physical activity in the western countries [2]. Compensation of the reduced work-associated physical activity through an increase in leisure-time physical activity and exercise training provides various health benefits and is recommended for industrialized societies. This was inconceivable almost 100 years ago when it was still a privilege not having to be involved in strenuous physical work.

The prevalence of physical inactivity has reached almost one-third in the westernized countries and life expectancy of the world's population would increase by 0.68 years if physical inactivity were eliminated [3]. It is now among the top ten risk factors causing disability-adjusted life years as the sum of life years lost plus years suffering from disability [4]. Although the relative risk attributable to physical inactivity is lower than that for smoking, the higher prevalence of physical inactivity in the population results in similar population-attributable fractions of both risk factors creating the slogan: physical inactivity is the new smoking [3].

A. Schmidt-Trucksäss
Division of Sports and Exercise Medicine, Department of Sport, Exercise and Health, University of Basel, Basel, Switzerland
e-mail: arno.schmidt-trucksaess@unibas.ch

R. Zimlichman et al. (eds.), *Prehypertension and Cardiometabolic Syndrome*, Updates in Hypertension and Cardiovascular Protection,
https://doi.org/10.1007/978-3-319-75310-2_31

31.1 Diversity of Physical Activity and Exercise

To understand the effect of physical activity and exercise on vascular health it is necessary to, first of all, give a definition. According to Caspersen et al., physical activity is defined as "any bodily movement produced by skeletal muscles which results in energy expenditure" [5]. Types of physical activity can be occupational, sports, conditioning, household, or other activities. Physical activity with the exception of exercise grossly classifies a behavior [5]. It is preferably implemented into daily life. A potentially significant component of weekly physical activity could be the active commute to work by foot or by bicycle [6–8]. At the work place, even small interruptions of permanent sitting and standing have shown to be beneficial for the glucose metabolism [9]. The recommended amount of physical activity per week is ≥150 min of moderate physical activity or 75 min of vigorous physical activity or any combination of the two with at least 10 min of uninterrupted activity per activity bout [10–12].

"Exercise is a subset of physical activity that is planned, structured, and repetitive and has as a final or an intermediate objective the improvement or maintenance of physical fitness" [5]. The types of exercise are mainly divided into endurance and strength exercises. Typical endurance exercises for health are running, walking, bicycling, or swimming. Strength exercises to preserve or increase skeletal musculature are done with the own body weight or with additional loads exerted by free weights or in a weight circuit. Several exercise disciplines are a mixture of both components. Popular lifelong activities/sports for health prevention are tennis, golf, football, or basketball [10]. Exercise training yields benefits for cardiovascular health that are additional to those of habitual physical activity. Leisure-time physical activity—and not occupational activity—contributes mainly to the conditioning of the cardiocirculatory system [13].

Physical fitness is associated with physical activity. It is defined as "a set of attributes that people have or achieve that relates to the ability to perform physical activity" [5]. Vigorous physical activity contributes to an increase in physical fitness of 4–5 mL/kg/min in maximal oxygen uptake in previously inactive individuals [14]. This confers to an enormous mortality risk reduction of 25–30% [15].

31.2 Effect of Physical Activity on the Population Level

Increasing physical activity and exercise is thus a most important aim of public health initiatives to win the fight against the chronic disease epidemic [3], which is especially true for cardiometabolic diseases [16, 17]. Both prospective and retrospective, large cohort studies have frequently shown a reduction of cardiovascular events and mortality in more active people [18]. A dose-dependent effect, increasing with higher volume and higher intensity of physical activity and exercise, has shown a reduction of cardiovascular and all-cause mortality of up to 45% compared to physical inactivity [3, 19]. In this context, only one-fourth of the time is required when exercising with vigorous intensity (jogging) compared to moderate intensity (walking) to gain a similar effect in cardiovascular event reduction [20]. Running for 20–40 min only one to two times per week was associated with an approximately 40–50% risk reduction for future cardiovascular events and all-cause mortality [21]. Even weekend warriors, accumulating all exercise at the weekend or by a leisure-time physical activity pattern characterized by one or two sessions per week may reduce all-cause and cardiovascular mortality by almost 40% [22]. Thus, interruption of exercise for more than 3 days still provides a health benefit which has not been sufficiently acknowledged in current exercise prescriptions for health. Although studies comparing the effect of exercise training and drug treatment on cardiovascular and all-cause mortality as endpoints are rare, physical activity has been shown to be superior or at least equal to a treatment with antihypertensive or lipid-lowering drugs in a meta-analytic approach (339,274 subjects in 305 randomized controlled trials (RCT)). This meta-analysis showed an odds ratio for drugs versus exercise of 1.34 and 8.66 in favor of exercise for prediabetes and stroke mortality, respectively, and an almost equal odds ratio for coronary heart disease (0.94) and heart failure (0.99) [23].

31.3 Physical Activity and Exercise—Indirect Pathways to Vascular Health

Traditional risk factors for atherosclerosis are known to be positively affected by an increase in physical activity and exercise, which is thought to be the dominant way to achieve benefits in vascular health. Single effects on risk factors are rather small. Blood pressure reduction following endurance [24] or resistance [25] exercise were −3.0/−2.4 mmHg (systolic) and −3.9/−3.9 mmHg (diastolic) in normotensive and −6.9/−4.9 (systolic) and −4.1/−1.5 mmHg (diastolic; not significant) in hypertensive individuals, respectively. No effects on LDL-, HDL-cholesterol and only small effects on triglycerides (−6 mg/dL) have been shown [26]. In summation, the "polypill" physical activity may have a bigger anti-arteriosclerotic effect. Going beyond classical risk factors, additional benefits arise from anti-inflammatory mechanisms, increased insulin sensitivity, improved hemostasis, reduction of the sympathetic drive, and antidepressive or other psychic effects. Taking together these multiple ways of action, approximately one-third of risk reduction is not explained by the indirect effects of physical activity and exercise which has been largely overlooked in the past [27]. Thus, direct effects of exercise are most likely to at least partially close the gap [28]. Among them, the increases in blood flow and to a smaller extent the exercise-associated increase in blood pressure are thought to be beneficial for the vascular wall (Fig. 31.1).

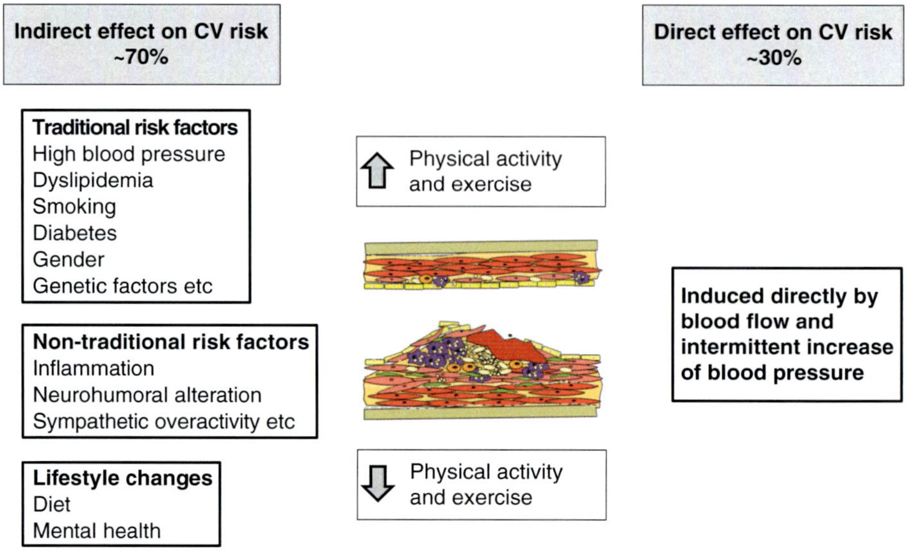

Fig. 31.1 The indirect effects of physical activity or inactivity via traditional, nontraditional risk factors and lifestyle changes, respectively, explain approximately 70% of the vascular health. Around 30% of the "polypill" physical activity and exercise seems to be the direct effect of exercise-increased blood flow and intermittent increase in blood pressure. The upward pointing arrow indicates an increase in physical activity and exercise and vice versa

31.4 Blood Flow and Vascular Properties

Blood flow increases occur mainly in endurance-type exercises. During maximal endurance exercise, cardiac output increases 4- to 5-fold in untrained individuals and 7- to 8-fold in elite endurance athletes [29]. At the same time, blood flow in conducting arteries that lead to the working musculature increases 10- to 15-fold [30, 31] while arteries leading to the brain show only a mild increase of up to 1.3-fold [32, 33]. In contrast, the blood flow increase during maximal strength exercise is nearly completely restricted above an intensity of 30% of the one repetition maximum (1RM). This is why especially endurance exercise is associated with an increase in arterial shear stress and thus with the release of nitric oxide (NO) by endothelial cells in a dose-dependent manner. In general terms, the higher the blood flow, the higher the shear stress, the higher the endothelial NO release. NO is the most important mediator of a normal endothelial function [34]. NO acts as a strong vasodilator by itself and induces a strong anti-atherosclerotic effect in the arteries [35]. However, only an intact endothelium is able to produce NO, which is synthesized by the endothelial NO synthase (eNOS or NOS III) via the interaction of different neurohumoral mediators such as acetylcholine [36, 37].

Chronically increased blood flow to the working musculature as typically seen in endurance athletes is initially associated with an increased arterial shear stress triggering an adaptive growth of vascular wall cells that normalize the shear stress to a pretraining level [38, 39]. The diameter of conducting arteries leading to the working musculature is typically higher in endurance athletes compared to their sedentary peers [38, 40, 41]. The adaptive vascular responses are depicted in Fig. 31.2.

This adaptation is not visible in arteries without a significant exercise-induced increase in blood flow and shear stress [42]. The ideal human model for this phenomenon is tennis players with an increased diameter only of the brachial artery of the playing arm [40]. Immobilization, on the opposite, is associated with missing intermittent increase of blood flow and adequate stimulus of wall property preservation. This is also associated with impaired endothelial function, visible in arteries of immobilized extremities as a consequence of traumatic injury, paraplegia, or bed rest [38, 43, 44].

Areas of the arterial tree with reduced shear stress are the arterial branches which as a consequence are prone to develop arterial plaques [45]. Typical sites are the carotid bifurcation or the rectangular branches of the medial cerebral artery where flow obstructions occur frequently [46].

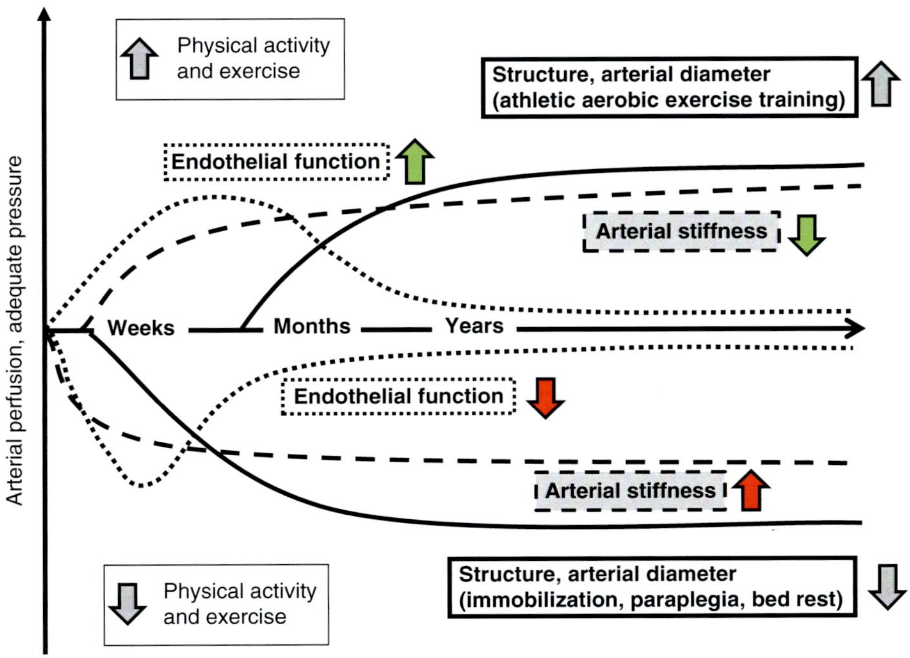

Fig. 31.2 Shows the functional and structural adaptations to increased or reduced blood flow and blood pressure induced by increased physical activity or exercise training versus physical inactivity. Endothelial function nearly normalizes to pretraining or de-training level while arterial stiffness and the change of arterial diameter seems to be permanent changes. Note the different time courses of functional and structural vascular adaptations. The arrows indicate the direction of change. The green color stands for the improve and red color for the deterioration of the function

31.5 Blood Pressure and Vascular Properties

During endurance exercise, invasively measured systolic blood pressure increases by 50–60% and diastolic blood pressure by 10–20% [47]. Subsequently, the arterial diameter increases during the systole and decreases during the diastole. If transmural pressure and thus circumferential stress (calculated as blood pressure × arterial diameter/wall thickness) is chronically increased, i.e., in hypertension or during high load exercise training, the arterial wall compensates through hypertrophy of vascular smooth muscle cells and proliferation of the endothelium [48, 49]. The mechanical stimuli for the endothelium are converted into chemical signals that trigger cell adaptation [50, 51]. The consequence is either a physiologic adaptation or an adverse change of the arterial wall. The latter is characterized by hypertrophy of vascular smooth muscle cells, disruption of elastin lamellae, increased storage of collagen, and stiffening of the arterial wall (arteriosclerosis) and/or plaque formation (atherosclerosis) [52, 53]. This is strongly driven by increased production of reactive oxygen species (ROS) [54]. Since exercise sessions usually have durations of less than 2 h, this temporary increase in circumferential stress and thus increased production of ROS by the endothelium does not seem to harm the arterial wall [55]. Adverse effects on the arterial wall are to be expected, however, if the pressure is chronically increased due to an unfavorable risk factor profile.

Comparing the effects of endurance- and resistance-type exercise, endurance exercise with laminar flow conditions and steady increase of shear stress is able to reduce the concentration of ROS and preserve and enhance endothelial function. Strength exercise with low or no increase of blood flow does not exert a significant NO-stimulating effect on the endothelial cell. The temporary increase in blood pressure and thus circumferential stress associated with either endurance or strength exercise training does not seem to have lasting negative effects on arterial wall properties and thus for vascular health.

31.6 Impact of Physical Activity on the Arterial Structure

Arteriosclerosis is a process beginning at its earliest stage with endothelial dysfunction and ending with an atherosclerotic plaque with or without obstruction of the blood flow [56, 57]. Halfway between mild to severe stages of arteriosclerosis are the changes of the vascular wall without plaque formation but with thickening of the wall. The attraction to assess vascular wall thickening and plaque as biomarkers or indicators of vascular health lies in the possibility to visualize these changes noninvasively by high-resolution ultrasound [58, 59]. Although wall thickening is sometimes thought to be a precursor of plaque formation, both carotid intima-media thickness (IMT) and plaque presence provide complementary prognostic information [60]. The carotid artery is the site where both features of the atherosclerotic process are most commonly and easily accessed.

31.7 Clinical Relevance of Carotid Artery Wall Thickness

The carotid IMT is a well-established predictor of cardiovascular events such as myocardial infarction and/or stroke. An increase of 0.1 mm from baseline IMT was associated with an increase of age and sex-adjusted relative risk of 16% for cardiovascular events in a meta-analysis that included 16 studies with 36,984 participants [61]. The risk prediction based on carotid IMT has been shown to be equivalent to the Framingham risk score. However, the net reclassification index (NRI) to allocate the risk to a higher or lower risk group based on the measurement of the carotid IMT is rather small with around 3–4% [62]. In contrast to carotid IMT, carotid plaque is better-suited for risk assessment with a NRI of 8.1% for individuals without CV disease at baseline. The combination of both achieves a clinical NRI of 21.7% in individuals with intermediate risk [63]. Increasing wall thickness of peripheral arteries principally has a similar association with cardiovascular risk, but in clinical practice the assessment has not yet asserted itself.

31.8 Physical Activity and Carotid IMT

Carotid IMT is not uniformly associated with the level of physical activity. In men and women at the age of 44 ± 8 years ($N = 614$), without carotid arteriosclerosis and without increased coronary heart disease risk, an inverse association of time spent in sedentary activity and carotid IMT was shown after adjustment for age and the established risk factors [64]. At the 3-year follow-up ($N = 495$), the increase in carotid IMT was not stopped, but carotid IMT showed a significantly lower progression in individuals engaged in vigorous physical activity compared to those engaged in light or moderate physical activity [64].

A similar finding was shown in the Los Angeles Atherosclerosis Study (age 50 ± 5 years) in which only vigorous aerobic physical activity ≥3.5 times per week slowed carotid IMT progression [65]. The sedentary group showed a threefold higher progression rate than the regularly active group which persisted after adjustment for several classical and lifestyle-dependent risk factors. This suggests an anti-atherosclerotic effect of vigorous activity independent of traditional risk factors. It is noteworthy that the rate of progression of IMT was not associated with workplace activity implying no benefit for vascular health. The finding is in line with a recent study investigating the effect of occupational versus leisure-time physical activity on maximal oxygen uptake in which only conditioning leisure-time physical activity, but not occupational physical activity was associated with an increased maximal aerobic capacity [13].

Based on the observed progression rate in healthy individuals, structural changes of the carotid IMT take at least 1 year [66–68]. The only RCT that was exclusively based on exercise training and took this into consideration was conducted in middle-aged Finnish men (57.2, age range 56.6–57.9 years) with an intervention phase of 6 years [69]. The intervention group expended an additional 1515 kcal per week through light to moderate-intensity walking that corresponded to 40–60% of maximal oxygen uptake leading to a 16% increase of the ventilatory aerobic threshold compared to a 3.5% decrease in the control group. Despite this remarkable increase in aerobic capacity, the progression of carotid IMT slowed only in the subgroup of men not taking statins. This "insufficient effect" of moderate physical activity on vascular structure gives support to thve use of vigorous-intensity physical activity in health prevention.

Another long-term intervention of 4 years duration in premenopausal women (353 women, age 44–50 years) aimed at slowing the known accelerated progression of atherosclerosis in the transition from premenopause to postmenopause [70]. This intervention based on lifestyle changes including dietary advice and increase in leisure-time physical activity, equivalent to an energy expenditure of 1000–1500 kcal/week, was able to significantly slow the progression of carotid IMT. Although the additional energy expenditure was even less than in the Finnish intervention trial, one may hypothesize that multidimensional interventions may amplify the effects of the single components.

These results are in line with a lifestyle intervention study in Germany in 618 middle-aged individuals (47.0 years at average) free of clinical cardiovascular disease [71]. The intervention with a mean follow-up of 2.4 years was comprised of weekly sessions of structured exercise, dietary education, and mental stress reduction. Of the 618 participants, 196 participated in the structured program for the first 6 months, 175 participated for the entire study duration, and 239 participated in no structured intervention. The progression of the carotid IMT was significant in participants participating in the 6-month intervention (+0.0159 mm, CI +0.0064 to +0.0253) and in those participating in no intervention (+0.0127 mm, CI +0.0046 to +0.0208), but stopped in participants who participated for the entire duration of the study (+0.0060 mm, −0.0036 to +0.0156) [71]. The results indicate the need for a continuously running intervention in the primary prevention of vascular disease.

A recent exercise intervention study over 12 months in patients (N = 123) with coronary artery disease and diabetes (63.1 ± 7.9 years) showed no effect of combined endurance ($\frac{2}{3}$ of sessions) and resistance training ($\frac{1}{3}$ of sessions) on carotid IMT [72] although the total exercise volume prescribed was 150 min/week including parts of high-intensity interval training (RPE ≥ 15). However, the patients with no atherosclerotic plaque (N = 65) showed a reduction of carotid IMT compared to control (−0.034 mm, CI −0.060 to −0.008 vs. 0.013 mm, −0.011 to 0.038). The authors interpret these findings as a potentially weaker NO-mediated effect of exercise in areas with plaques, and thus exercise may have only an effect in patients with less severe atherosclerotic diseases. All successful interventions attenuating the progression of carotid IMT were based dominantly on endurance-type exercise. Resistance-type exercise showed no effect in healthy volunteers [73].

In children and adolescents the carotid IMT is the only structural vascular biomarker to visualize the effect of an increased risk factor burden because more advanced stages of atherosclerosis in shape of plaques are not yet present. Further, the carotid IMT seems to be more sensitive to changes in the arterial milieu. This has been shown in children with an acute infectious disease where a normalization of the "swollen" carotid IMT was visible within 3 months after the infection [74]. Therefore, it is no surprise that a recent meta-analysis of 6 RCTs in an obese pediatric population (6–18 years, $N = 303$) showed a small-to-moderate reduction of carotid IMT following exercise training with a duration of 12–24 weeks [75]. All interventions were of endurance type, half of them with additional resistant-type exercise. The duration of the intervention in weeks or the minutes of exercise per week seemed to be the general conditions of success, meaning that longer duration of the intervention and higher volume of exercise increases the effect on carotid IMT.

A promising parameter of carotid structure assessed with noninvasive ultrasound seems to be the irregularity of the IMT, the IM-roughness, representing an early sign of atherosclerotic carotid wall changes [76]. IM-roughness can be automatically quantified and discriminates better between clinically healthy elderly individuals and patients with coronary artery disease [77]. The IM-roughness has been shown to be inversely associated with maximal oxygen uptake in healthy lifelong physically active men (64.48 ± 3.45 years; $N = 51$), meaning that fitter men have a smoother arterial wall [78]. A recent study in 602 healthy German school children (aged 8–18 years) showed that carotid IM-roughness was significantly and negatively correlated with physical fitness ($r = -0.212, p < 0.0001$). Low physical fitness seems to be a strong predictor for the carotid IM-roughness increase [79].

To summarize, endurance-based exercise interventions seem to mitigate the progression of carotid IMT in a middle-aged to elderly population. The few trials and prospective cohort studies with sufficient duration of at least 12 months indicate that vigorous intensity seems to be more effective than lower intensity, especially in individuals with a lower atherosclerotic disease burden (Fig. 31.3). In children and adolescents, carotid IMT might be sensitive to the effects of physical activity and change of fitness. Carotid IM-roughness is associated with higher cardiorespiratory fitness across the age-span.

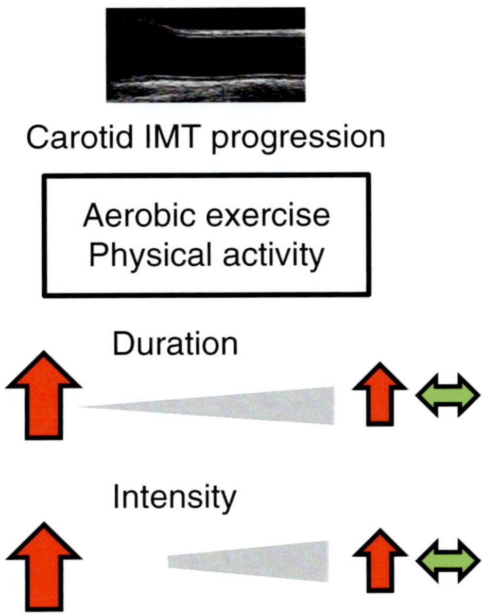

Fig. 31.3 Shows the effect of aerobic exercise/physical activity on the progression of the carotid intima-media thickness (IMT). Longer duration and higher intensity seems to reduce or even stop the increase of carotid IMT. Higher intensity exercise seems to be superior to low and moderate intensity exercise. The upward pointing arrow indicates an increase in IMT, the horizontal arrow indicates stagnation of progression

31.9 Impact of Physical Activity on the Arterial Function

The arterial function is dependent on the regulatory capacity of the endothelium to release endocrine hormones (among which NO is one of the most potent one [80]), the tonicity of the smooth muscle cells, and the passive properties of elastic fibers and connective tissue. All these components contribute to arterial stiffness. Arterial stiffness is influenced by ventricular stroke volume, the buffering capacity of the arterial tree (Windkessel), and the peripheral wave reflection [81]. Arterial wall stiffness increases from the aorta to large elastic arteries and to the peripheral muscular conduit arteries. Lumen narrowing of the aorta and the peripheral arteries and local arterial branching create an impedance mismatch causing wave reflections traveling back to the central aorta and superimpose with central blood pressure [81, 82]. The higher the arterial stiffness of central conduit arteries, the faster is the propagating and reflecting wave. In an elastic aorta, the reflecting pressure wave arrives during diastole augmenting the coronary artery blood flow mainly during diastole [83]. In a stiffer aorta, the reflecting pressure wave superimposes with the central pressure already during systole causing an increased cardiac afterload with subsequent increased cardiac muscle oxygen consumption [84]. In the mid to long-term, the consequence is left ventricular hypertrophy as an established risk factor for future cardiovascular events and heart failure. Endothelial dysfunction contributes partially to an increase in arterial stiffness, which has been shown by in vivo blockade of NO in the iliac artery [85]. From the clinical point of view, it is important to prevent the arterial tree from early arterial stiffening in order to preserve cardiac function.

31.10 Pulse Wave Velocity

Pulse wave velocity (PWV) is defined as the velocity of the pulse as it travels from the heart to the carotid, the femoral artery or the arteries of the lower leg. An increase of the PWV is the result primarily from stiffening of the arterial wall with a loss of elastic properties by various processes such as calcification of the media and internal elastic lamina [86]. The carotid-femoral PWV is usually considered the "gold standard" measuring PWV tonometrically as the distance from the measuring site over the time delay of the two waveforms (see Fig. 31.4). The beginning of the waveforms is termed the foot and the velocity the "foot-to-foot" velocity [87]. The brachial-ankle PWV is measured with cuffs wrapped around both upper arms and ankles of the subjects lying in a supine position. The cuffs are connected to plethysmographic and oscillometric sensors. The brachial-ankle PWV is measured as the path lengths from the suprasternal notch to the brachial cuff and from the suprasternal notch to the ankle cuff corrected for the height of the individual [88].

The PWV has an independent predictive value for cardiovascular events and all-cause as well as CV mortality. One standard deviation increase in carotid-femoral PWV was associated with a 30% increase in cardiovascular disease events after

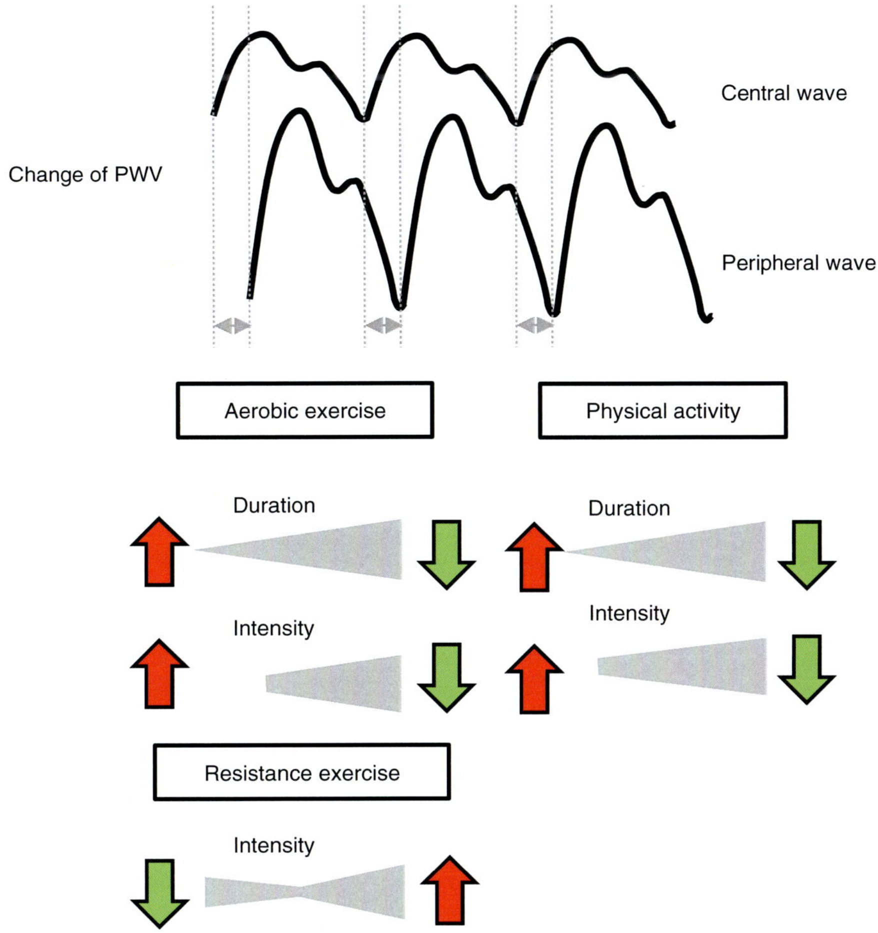

Fig. 31.4 Shows the effect of aerobic and resistance exercise and physical activity on pulse wave velocity (PWV). The positive effect of aerobic exercise on PWV increases with increasing duration and intensity. Resistance exercise has a small reducing effect at low to moderate intensity but increases PWV unfavorably at higher loads of >80% of the one repetition maximum. Physical activity decreases PWV stronger with longer duration and intensity. Even low intensities seem to have a beneficial effect in elderly people. Sedentarism regarding aerobic exercise or physical activity increases PWV. The downward pointing arrow indicates a decrease in PWV and vice versa. The green color stands for the improve and red color for the deterioration of the function

adjustment for traditional risk factors [89]. The 5-year overall NRI for coronary heart disease and stroke in intermediate risk individuals was 14.8% and 19.2%, respectively, and thus better than for carotid IMT and carotid plaque [89]. An increase in brachial-ankle PWV by 1 m/s was associated with an increase by 12% in cardiovascular events and 13% in cardiovascular mortality adjusted for traditional risk factors [90]. The ease of use and the independent predictive value are arguments among others for the broader usage of PWV in research and clinical practice. For both methods, it still has to be proven that their use improves clinical outcomes in addition to and beyond established treatment strategies [60].

31.11 Physical Activity and Arterial Stiffness

Arterial stiffness is determined by functional components promising a faster adaptation to exercise training or to change of physical activity. In contrast to endothelial function [28] there are no indications that arterial stiffness will normalize (reverse) after structural adaptation has occurred.

Only few population-based studies investigating the association of physical activity and arterial stiffness exist. In 198 men and women higher habitual physical activity (>6600 steps/day and/or exercised for more than 16 min/day at an intensity >3 METs) was associated with lesser stiffening of central arteries [91]. In 538 healthy Japanese men and women carotid-femoral PWV was lower (better) (9.45 ± 19 m/s vs. 8.82 ± 0.16 m/s; $P < 0.01$) in elderly individuals (63 ± 0.3 years) with a higher amount of light physical activity (~700 min/day vs. ~500 min/day at an intensity <38% VO_{2max}). Since it may be easier to promote the replacement of inactivity by light physical activity, such as household tasks and other unstructured activities especially in inactive individuals due to a lower threshold, this study is of high importance for public health by preventing age-related arterial stiffening [92]. In the Swiss Cohort Study on Air Pollution and Lung and Heart Diseases in Adults (SAPALDIA) high versus no vigorous physical activity (2880 MET min/week vs. 0 MET min/week) was associated with lower brachial-ankle PWV in elderly individuals (63.3 years on average) [93]. Moderate and low-intensity physical activity was not associated with different PWV. This finding is in contrast to the Japanese study [92]. However, ethnic differences might account for that. Another study in the SAPALDIA cohort was conducted to analyze potential changes in physical activity and their effect on PWV [94]. Men increasing the amount of moderate-to-vigorous physical activity to a sufficient level (>150 min/week) from SAPALDIA 2 to SAPALDIA 3 (time interval 8.3 years) had a significantly lower PWV than those with no change. However, men and women who were permanently sufficiently active presented the best arterial stiffness values [94]. In summary, staying active or increasing physical activity to a sufficient level at an advanced adult age is good for vascular health measured as arterial stiffness. The recommended intensity of physical activity is not completely clear but any activity seems to be better than complete physical inactivity.

Aerobic endurance exercise training has a significant reducing effect on central and peripheral PWV. This effect is visible in healthy individuals and in patients with chronic diseases such as hypertension or type 2 diabetes. A tendency to a lesser or no change is visible in diseases with a more pronounced atherosclerotic progression such as chronic kidney disease [95, 96].

Already 4–8 weeks of endurance training were associated with a small reduction of PWV (−0.35, CI −0.68 to −0.02) and the effect nearly doubled with a twice as long intervention duration of 9–16 weeks (−0.69, CI −1.13 to −0.25) and even further increased with an even longer intervention time (>16 weeks, −1.19, CI −1.92 to −0.47). A second influencing factor on PWV was a relative improvement in aerobic capacity measured as VO_{2max}. Even low improvements (<10%) were associated with significant decreases in PWV (−0.40, CI −0.52 to −0.28), while every additional 5% improvement in VO_{2max} led to further 0.4 to 0.5 decreases in PWV [95] (Fig. 31.4).

In contrast to aerobic exercise, resistance exercise does not exhibit such uniform effects on PWV (Fig. 31.4). The ideal resistance training should provide strengthening of the musculature without health hazards to the vasculature. However, this does not seem to be true for all types of resistance training. The existing RCTs varied in training frequency (in average 2–3 weekly sessions) and intensity ranging from 20% to 100% of the 1RM [96]. Most programs consisted of concentric-type exercises for several large muscle groups of the whole body. Light (≤50% 1RM) to moderate intensity (>50–70% of 1RM) showed a reduction of PWV of around 5% [96] while high-intensity (≥80% 1RM) resistance exercise was associated with a noticeable stiffening of up to 30% [97]. One RCT compared lower limb with upper limb resistance training, with an increase in PWV of 12.2% (CI 5.6% to 18.8%) for upper limb exercise and no effect for lower limb resistance training with an intensity of 80% of 1RM in young healthy individuals [98]. Further, eccentric-type resistance training at 100% of 1RM resulted in a slight decrease of PWV (−3.9%, CI, −6.6% to −1.2%) while concentric-type resistance training led to increase in PWV (9.9%, CI 7.2% to 12.6%) [99].

Several training programs combine aerobic endurance exercise with resistance exercise. In those studies, the training frequency amounted to 3 weekly sessions with an intensity range of 50–80% of 1RM and 60–90% of maximal heart rate (moderate to high-intensity aerobic exercise) [96]. If endurance training directly follows resistance training, no change in PWV will occur, suggesting that combined exercise may be of particular relevance for the prevention of sarcopenia in elderly individuals with a prevalence of hypertension of almost 70–80% beyond the age of 70 years [100]. However, single studies suggest that the resistance training-induced protein complex (mTORC1) which controls protein synthesis and regulates muscle mass may be downregulated by aerobic training thus impairing the effect of resistance training on muscle hypertrophy [101]. Therefore, the ultimate aim should be to find a favorable type of strength training that sufficiently increases muscular strength but does not cause any increases in PWV and thus an increased cardiac burden.

To summarize, endurance exercise interventions are most likely to reduce arterial stiffness in a healthy population and in patients with several chronic diseases. Because of the "functional" nature of arterial stiffness, the positive effects are visible within a shorter time frame of only a couple of months and increase with duration and intensity of the program. Resistance exercise training has inhomogeneous effects on arterial stiffness with an adverse increase following high-intensity training and upper limb training and small beneficial effects following low-intensity training and lower limb muscle groups.

References

1. Chau JY, Grunseit AC, Chey T, Stamatakis E, Brown WJ, Matthews CE, Bauman AE, van der Ploeg HP. Daily sitting time and all-cause mortality: a meta-analysis. PLoS One. 2013;8:e80000.
2. Biswas A, Oh PI, Faulkner GE, Bajaj RR, Silver MA, Mitchell MS, Alter DA. Sedentary time and its association with risk for disease incidence, mortality, and hospitalization in adults: a systematic review and meta-analysis. Ann Intern Med. 2015;162:123–32.
3. Lee IM, Shiroma EJ, Lobelo F, Puska P, Blair SN, Katzmarzyk PT, Lancet Physical Activity Series Working, G. Effect of physical inactivity on major non-communicable diseases worldwide: an analysis of burden of disease and life expectancy. Lancet. 2012;380:219–29.
4. Lim SS, Vos T, Flaxman AD, Danaei G, Shibuya K, Adair-Rohani H, Amann M, Anderson HR, Andrews KG, Aryee M, Atkinson C, Bacchus LJ, Bahalim AN, Balakrishnan K, Balmes J, Barker-Collo S, Baxter A, Bell ML, Blore JD, Blyth F, Bonner C, Borges G, Bourne R, Boussinesq M, Brauer M, Brooks P, Bruce NG, Brunekreef B, Bryan-Hancock C, Bucello C, Buchbinder R, Bull F, Burnett RT, Byers TE, Calabria B, Carapetis J, Carnahan E, Chafe Z, Charlson F, Chen H, Chen JS, Cheng AT, Child JC, Cohen A, Colson KE, Cowie BC, Darby S, Darling S, Davis A, Degenhardt L, Dentener F, des Jarlais DC, Devries K, Dherani M, Ding EL, Dorsey ER, Driscoll T, Edmond K, Ali SE, Engell RE, Erwin PJ, Fahimi S, Falder G, Farzadfar F, Ferrari A, Finucane MM, Flaxman S, Fowkes FG, Freedman G, Freeman MK, Gakidou E, Ghosh S, Giovannucci E, Gmel G, Graham K, Grainger R, Grant B, Gunnell D, Gutierrez HR, Hall W, Hoek HW, Hogan A, Hosgood HD 3rd, Hoy D, Hu H, Hubbell BJ, Hutchings SJ, Ibeanusi SE, Jacklyn GL, Jasrasaria R, Jonas JB, Kan H, Kanis JA, Kassebaum N, Kawakami N, Khang YH, Khatibzadeh S, Khoo JP, Kok C, Laden F, et al. A comparative risk assessment of burden of disease and injury attributable to 67 risk factors and risk factor clusters in 21 regions, 1990–2010: a systematic analysis for the Global Burden of Disease Study 2010. Lancet. 2012;380:2224–60.
5. Caspersen CJ, Powell KE, Christenson GM. Physical activity, exercise, and physical fitness: definitions and distinctions for health-related research. Public Health Rep. 1985;100:126–31.
6. Grontved A, Koivula RW, Johansson I, Wennberg P, Ostergaard L, Hallmans G, Renstrom F, Franks PW. Bicycling to work and primordial prevention of cardiovascular risk: a cohort study among Swedish men and women. J Am Heart Assoc. 2016;5:e004413.
7. Hoechsmann, C., Meister, S., Gehrig, D., Gordon, E., Li, Y., Nussbaumer, M., Rossmeissl, A., Hanssen, H., Schmidt-Trucksäss, A. Effect of e-bike versus bike commuting on cardiorespiratory fitness in overweight adults: a 4-week randomized pilot study. Clin J Sport Med. 2017. https://doi.org/10.1097/JSM.0000000000000438
8. Lusk AC, Mekary RA, Feskanich D, Willett WC. Bicycle riding, walking, and weight gain in premenopausal women. Arch Intern Med. 2010;170:1050–6.
9. Dunstan DW, Kingwell BA, Larsen R, Healy GN, Cerin E, Hamilton MT, Shaw JE, Bertovic DA, Zimmet PZ, Salmon J, Owen N. Breaking up prolonged sitting reduces postprandial glucose and insulin responses. Diabetes Care. 2012;35:976–83.
10. Garber CE, Blissmer B, Deschenes MR, Franklin BA, Lamonte MJ, Lee IM, Nieman DC, Swain DP, American College of Sports, M. American College of Sports Medicine position stand. Quantity and quality of exercise for developing and maintaining cardiorespiratory, musculoskeletal, and neuromotor fitness in apparently healthy adults: guidance for prescribing exercise. Med Sci Sports Exerc. 2011;43:1334–59.
11. Vanhees L, de Sutter J, Gelada SN, Doyle F, Prescott E, Cornelissen V, Kouidi E, Dugmore D, Vanuzzo D, Borjesson M, Doherty P, EACPR. Importance of characteristics and modalities of physical activity and exercise in defining the benefits to cardiovascular health within the general population: recommendations from the EACPR (Part I). Eur J Prev Cardiol. 2012;19:670–86.
12. Vanhees L, Geladas N, Hansen D, Kouidi E, Niebauer J, Reiner Z, Cornelissen V, Adamopoulos S, Prescott E, Borjesson M, Bjarnason-Wehrens B, Bjornstad HH, Cohen-Solal A, Conraads

V, Corrado D, de Sutter J, Doherty P, Doyle F, Dugmore D, Ellingsen O, Fagard R, Giada F, Gielen S, Hager A, Halle M, Heidbuchel H, Jegier A, Mazic S, Mcgee H, Mellwig KP, Mendes M, Mezzani A, Pattyn N, Pelliccia A, Piepoli M, Rauch B, Schmidt-Trucksäss A, Takken T, Van Buuren F, Vanuzzo D. Importance of characteristics and modalities of physical activity and exercise in the management of cardiovascular health in individuals with cardiovascular risk factors: recommendations from the EACPR. Part II. Eur J Prev Cardiol. 2012;19:1005–33.

13. Mundwiler J, Schupbach U, Dieterle T, Leuppi JD, Schmidt-Trucksäss A, Wolfer DP, Miedinger D, Brighenti-Zogg S. Association of occupational and leisure-time physical activity with aerobic capacity in a working population. PLoS One. 2017;12:e0168683.
14. Aspenes ST, Nauman J, Nilsen TI, Vatten LJ, Wisloff U. Physical activity as a long-term predictor of peak oxygen uptake: the HUNT Study. Med Sci Sports Exerc. 2011;43:1675–9.
15. Myers J, Kaykha A, George S, Abella J, Zaheer N, Lear S, Yamazaki T, Froelicher V. Fitness versus physical activity patterns in predicting mortality in men. Am J Med. 2004;117:912–8.
16. Hahn V, Halle M, Schmidt-Trucksäss A, Rathmann W, Meisinger C, Mielck A. Physical activity and the metabolic syndrome in elderly German men and women: results from the population-based KORA survey. Diabetes Care. 2009;32:511–3.
17. Jeon CY, Lokken RP, Hu FB, Van Dam RM. Physical activity of moderate intensity and risk of type 2 diabetes: a systematic review. Diabetes Care. 2007;30:744–52.
18. Manson JE, Greenland P, Lacroix AZ, Stefanick ML, Mouton CP, Oberman A, Perri MG, Sheps DS, Pettinger MB, Siscovick DS. Walking compared with vigorous exercise for the prevention of cardiovascular events in women. N Engl J Med. 2002;347:716–25.
19. Powell KE, Paluch AE, Blair SN. Physical activity for health: what kind? How much? How intense? On top of what? Annu Rev Public Health. 2011;32:349–65.
20. Wen CP, Wai JP, Tsai MK, Yang YC, Cheng TY, Lee MC, Chan HT, Tsao CK, Tsai SP, Wu X. Minimum amount of physical activity for reduced mortality and extended life expectancy: a prospective cohort study. Lancet. 2011;378:1244–53.
21. Lee DC, Pate RR, Lavie CJ, Sui X, Church TS, Blair SN. Leisure-time running reduces all-cause and cardiovascular mortality risk. J Am Coll Cardiol. 2014;64:472–81.
22. O'donovan G, Lee IM, Hamer M, Stamatakis E. Association of "weekend warrior" and other leisure time physical activity patterns with risks for all-cause, cardiovascular disease, and cancer mortality. JAMA Intern Med. 2017;177:335–42.
23. Naci H, Ioannidis JP. Comparative effectiveness of exercise and drug interventions on mortality outcomes: metaepidemiological study. BMJ. 2013;347:f5577.
24. Cornelissen VA, Fagard RH. Effects of endurance training on blood pressure, blood pressure-regulating mechanisms, and cardiovascular risk factors. Hypertension. 2005;46:667–75.
25. Cornelissen VA, Fagard RH, Coeckelberghs E, Vanhees L. Impact of resistance training on blood pressure and other cardiovascular risk factors: a meta-analysis of randomized, controlled trials. Hypertension. 2011;58:950–8.
26. Kelley GA, Kelley KS, Roberts S, Haskell W. Comparison of aerobic exercise, diet or both on lipids and lipoproteins in adults: a meta-analysis of randomized controlled trials. Clin Nutr. 2012;31:156–67.
27. Mora S, Cook N, Buring JE, Ridker PM, Lee IM. Physical activity and reduced risk of cardiovascular events: potential mediating mechanisms. Circulation. 2007;116:2110–8.
28. Green DJ, Hopman MT, Padilla J, Laughlin MH, Thijssen DH. Vascular adaptation to exercise in humans: role of hemodynamic stimuli. Physiol Rev. 2017;97:495–528.
29. Joyner MJ, Casey DP. Regulation of increased blood flow (hyperemia) to muscles during exercise: a hierarchy of competing physiological needs. Physiol Rev. 2015;95:549–601.
30. Calbet JA, Gonzalez-Alonso J, Helge JW, Sondergaard H, Munch-Andersen T, Boushel R, Saltin B. Cardiac output and leg and arm blood flow during incremental exercise to exhaustion on the cycle ergometer. J Appl Physiol (1985). 2007;103:969–78.
31. Harrison PR, Affara N, Mcnab A, Paul J. Erythroid differentiation in a friend erythroleukemic cell X lymphoma hybrid cell line is limited, possibly due to reduced hem levels. Exp Cell Res. 1977;109:237–46.

32. Hellstrom G, Fischer-Colbrie W, Wahlgren NG, Jogestrand T. Carotid artery blood flow and middle cerebral artery blood flow velocity during physical exercise. J Appl Physiol (1985). 1996;81:413–8.
33. Sato K, Ogoh S, Hirasawa A, Oue A, Sadamoto T. The distribution of blood flow in the carotid and vertebral arteries during dynamic exercise in humans. J Physiol. 2011;589:2847–56.
34. Furchgott RF. The 1996 Albert Lasker medical research awards. The discovery of endothelium-derived relaxing factor and its importance in the identification of nitric oxide. JAMA. 1996;276:1186–8.
35. Napoli C, Ignarro LJ. Nitric oxide and atherosclerosis. Nitric Oxide. 2001;5:88–97.
36. Davies PF. Flow-mediated endothelial mechanotransduction. Physiol Rev. 1995;75:519–60.
37. Moncada S, Higgs A. The L-arginine-nitric oxide pathway. N Engl J Med. 1993;329:2002–12.
38. Schmidt-Trucksäss A, Schmid A, Brunner C, Scherer N, Zach G, Keul J, Huonker M. Arterial properties of the carotid and femoral artery in endurance-trained and paraplegic subjects. J Appl Physiol (1985). 2000;89:1956–63.
39. Tinken TM, Thijssen DH, Hopkins N, Dawson EA, Cable NT, Green DJ. Shear stress mediates endothelial adaptations to exercise training in humans. Hypertension. 2010;55:312–8.
40. Huonker M, Schmid A, Schmidt-Trucksäss A, Grathwohl D, Keul J. Size and blood flow of central and peripheral arteries in highly trained able-bodied and disabled athletes. J Appl Physiol (1985). 2003;95:685–91.
41. Rowley NJ, Dawson EA, Hopman MT, George KP, Whyte GP, Thijssen DH, Green DJ. Conduit diameter and wall remodeling in elite athletes and spinal cord injury. Med Sci Sports Exerc. 2012;44:844–9.
42. Huonker M, Schmid A, Sorichter S, Schmidt-Trucksab A, Mrosek P, Keul J. Cardiovascular differences between sedentary and wheelchair-trained subjects with paraplegia. Med Sci Sports Exerc. 1998;30:609–13.
43. Giannattasio C, Failla M, Grappiolo A, Bigoni M, Carugo S, Denti M, Mancia G. Effects of prolonged immobilization of the limb on radial artery mechanical properties. Hypertension. 1998;32:584–7.
44. van Duijnhoven NT, Green DJ, Felsenberg D, Belavy DL, Hopman MT, Thijssen DH. Impact of bed rest on conduit artery remodeling: effect of exercise countermeasures. Hypertension. 2010;56:240–6.
45. Cunningham KS, Gotlieb AI. The role of shear stress in the pathogenesis of atherosclerosis. Lab Investig. 2005;85:9–23.
46. Glagov S, Zarins C, Giddens DP, Ku DN. Hemodynamics and atherosclerosis. Insights and perspectives gained from studies of human arteries. Arch Pathol Lab Med. 1988;112:1018–31.
47. Robinson TE, Sue DY, Huszczuk A, Weiler-Ravell D, Hansen JE. Intra-arterial and cuff blood pressure responses during incremental cycle ergometry. Med Sci Sports Exerc. 1988;20:142–9.
48. Boutouyrie P, Bussy C, Lacolley P, Girerd X, Laloux B, Laurent S. Association between local pulse pressure, mean blood pressure, and large-artery remodeling. Circulation. 1999;100:1387–93.
49. Roman MJ, Pickering TG, Schwartz JE, Pini R, Devereux RB. Relation of arterial structure and function to left ventricular geometric patterns in hypertensive adults. J Am Coll Cardiol. 1996;28:751–6.
50. Davies PF. Hemodynamic shear stress and the endothelium in cardiovascular pathophysiology. Nat Clin Pract Cardiovasc Med. 2009;6:16–26.
51. Johnson BD, Mather KJ, Wallace JP. Mechanotransduction of shear in the endothelium: basic studies and clinical implications. Vasc Med. 2011;16:365–77.
52. Cai H, Harrison DG. Endothelial dysfunction in cardiovascular diseases: the role of oxidant stress. Circ Res. 2000;87:840–4.
53. Malek AM, Alper SL, Izumo S. Hemodynamic shear stress and its role in atherosclerosis. JAMA. 1999;282:2035–42.
54. Munzel T, Camici GG, Maack C, Bonetti NR, Fuster V, Kovacic JC. Impact of oxidative stress on the heart and vasculature: part 2 of a 3-part series. J Am Coll Cardiol. 2017;70:212–29.

55. Spescha RD, Glanzmann M, Simic B, Witassek F, Keller S, Akhmedov A, Tanner FC, Luscher TF, Camici GG. Adaptor protein p66(Shc) mediates hypertension-associated, cyclic stretch-dependent, endothelial damage. Hypertension. 2014;64:347–53.
56. Stary HC, Chandler AB, Dinsmore RE, Fuster V, Glagov S, Insull W Jr, Rosenfeld ME, Schwartz CJ, Wagner WD, Wissler RW. A definition of advanced types of atherosclerotic lesions and a histological classification of atherosclerosis. A report from the Committee on Vascular Lesions of the Council on Arteriosclerosis, American Heart Association. Circulation. 1995;92:1355–74.
57. Stary HC, Chandler AB, Glagov S, Guyton JR, Insull W Jr, Rosenfeld ME, Schaffer SA, Schwartz CJ, Wagner WD, Wissler RW. A definition of initial, fatty streak, and intermediate lesions of atherosclerosis. A report from the Committee on Vascular Lesions of the Council on Arteriosclerosis, American Heart Association. Circulation. 1994;89:2462–78.
58. Bauer M, Caviezel S, Teynor A, Erbel R, Mahabadi AA, Schmidt-Trucksäss A. Carotid intima-media thickness as a biomarker of subclinical atherosclerosis. Swiss Med Wkly. 2012;142:w13705.
59. Touboul PJ, Hennerici MG, Meairs S, Adams H, Amarenco P, Bornstein N, Csiba L, Desvarieux M, Ebrahim S, Hernandez Hernandez R, Jaff M, Kownator S, Naqvi T, Prati P, Rundek T, Sitzer M, Schminke U, Tardif JC, Taylor A, Vicaut E, Woo KS. Mannheim carotid intima-media thickness and plaque consensus (2004–2006–2011). An update on behalf of the advisory board of the 3rd, 4th and 5th watching the risk symposia, at the 13th, 15th and 20th European Stroke Conferences, Mannheim, Germany, 2004, Brussels, Belgium, 2006, and Hamburg, Germany, 2011. Cerebrovasc Dis. 2012;34:290–6.
60. Vlachopoulos C, Xaplanteris P, Aboyans V, Brodmann M, Cifkova R, Cosentino F, de Carlo M, Gallino A, Landmesser U, Laurent S, Lekakis J, Mikhailidis DP, Naka KK, Protogerou AD, Rizzoni D, Schmidt-Trucksäss A, Van Bortel L, Weber T, Yamashina A, Zimlichman R, Boutouyrie P, Cockcroft J, O'Rourke M, Park JB, Schillaci G, Sillesen H, Townsend RR. The role of vascular biomarkers for primary and secondary prevention. A position paper from the European Society of Cardiology Working Group on peripheral circulation: Endorsed by the Association for Research into Arterial Structure and Physiology (ARTERY) Society. Atherosclerosis. 2015;241:507–32.
61. Lorenz MW, Polak JF, Kavousi M, Mathiesen EB, Volzke H, Tuomainen TP, Sander D, Plichart M, Catapano AL, Robertson CM, Kiechl S, Rundek T, Desvarieux M, Lind L, Schmid C, Dasmahapatra P, Gao L, Ziegelbauer K, Bots ML, Thompson SG, Group P-IS. Carotid intima-media thickness progression to predict cardiovascular events in the general population (the PROG-IMT collaborative project): a meta-analysis of individual participant data. Lancet. 2012;379:2053–62.
62. den Ruijter HM, Peters SA, Anderson TJ, Britton AR, Dekker JM, Eijkemans MJ, Engstrom G, Evans GW, de Graaf J, Grobbee DE, Hedblad B, Hofman A, Holewijn S, Ikeda A, Kavousi M, Kitagawa K, Kitamura A, Koffijberg H, Lonn EM, Lorenz MW, Mathiesen EB, Nijpels G, Okazaki S, O'leary DH, Polak JF, Price JF, Robertson C, Rembold CM, Rosvall M, Rundek T, Salonen JT, Sitzer M, Stehouwer CD, Witteman JC, Moons KG, Bots ML. Common carotid intima-media thickness measurements in cardiovascular risk prediction: a meta-analysis. JAMA. 2012;308:796–803.
63. Polak JF, Szklo M, Kronmal RA, Burke GL, Shea S, Zavodni AE, O'leary DH. The value of carotid artery plaque and intima-media thickness for incident cardiovascular disease: the multi-ethnic study of atherosclerosis. J Am Heart Assoc. 2013;2:e000087.
64. Kozakova M, Palombo C, Morizzo C, Nolan JJ, Konrad T, Balkau B, Investigators, R. Effect of sedentary behaviour and vigorous physical activity on segment-specific carotid wall thickness and its progression in a healthy population. Eur Heart J. 2010;31:1511–9.
65. Nordstrom CK, Dwyer KM, Merz CN, Shircore A, Dwyer JH. Leisure time physical activity and early atherosclerosis: the Los Angeles Atherosclerosis Study. Am J Med. 2003;115:19–25.
66. Homma S, Hirose N, Ishida H, Ishii T, Araki G. Carotid plaque and intima-media thickness assessed by b-mode ultrasonography in subjects ranging from young adults to centenarians. Stroke. 2001;32:830–5.

67. Rosvall M, Persson M, Ostling G, Nilsson PM, Melander O, Hedblad B, Engstrom G. Risk factors for the progression of carotid intima-media thickness over a 16-year follow-up period: the Malmo Diet and Cancer Study. Atherosclerosis. 2015;239:615–21.
68. Schmidt-Trucksäss A, Grathwohl D, Schmid A, Boragk R, Upmeier C, Keul J, Huonker M. Structural, functional, and hemodynamic changes of the common carotid artery with age in male subjects. Arterioscler Thromb Vasc Biol. 1999;19:1091–7.
69. Rauramaa R, Halonen P, Vaisanen SB, Lakka TA, Schmidt-Trucksäss A, Berg A, Penttila IM, Rankinen T, Bouchard C. Effects of aerobic physical exercise on inflammation and atherosclerosis in men: the DNASCO Study: a six-year randomized, controlled trial. Ann Intern Med. 2004;140:1007–14.
70. Wildman RP, Schott LL, Brockwell S, Kuller LH, Sutton-Tyrrell K. A dietary and exercise intervention slows menopause-associated progression of subclinical atherosclerosis as measured by intima-media thickness of the carotid arteries. J Am Coll Cardiol. 2004;44:579–85.
71. Mang C. Effect of complex lifestyle intervention on common carotid intima-media thickness. Doctoral thesis, University of Freiburg; 2013.
72. Byrkjeland R, Stensaeth KH, Anderssen S, Njerve IU, Arnesen H, Seljeflot I, Solheim S. Effects of exercise training on carotid intima-media thickness in patients with type 2 diabetes and coronary artery disease. Influence of carotid plaques. Cardiovasc Diabetol. 2016;15:13.
73. Olson TP, Dengel DR, Leon AS, Schmitz KH. Moderate resistance training and vascular health in overweight women. Med Sci Sports Exerc. 2006;38:1558–64.
74. Liuba P, Persson J, Luoma J, Yla-Herttuala S, Pesonen E. Acute infections in children are accompanied by oxidative modification of LDL and decrease of HDL cholesterol, and are followed by thickening of carotid intima-media. Eur Heart J. 2003;24:515–21.
75. Garcia-Hermoso A, Gonzalez-Ruiz K, Triana-Reina HR, Olloquequi J, Ramirez-Velez R. Effects of exercise on carotid Arterial Wall thickness in obese pediatric populations: a meta-analysis of randomized controlled trials. Child Obes. 2017;13:138–45.
76. Belcaro G, Nicolaides AN, Laurora G, Cesarone MR, de Sanctis M, Incandela L, Barsotti A. Ultrasound morphology classification of the arterial wall and cardiovascular events in a 6-year follow-up study. Arterioscler Thromb Vasc Biol. 1996;16:851–6.
77. Schmidt-Trucksäss A, Sandrock M, Cheng DC, Muller HM, Baumstark MW, Rauramaa R, Berg A, Huonker M. Quantitative measurement of carotid intima-media roughness--effect of age and manifest coronary artery disease. Atherosclerosis. 2003;166:57–65.
78. Sandrock M, Schulze C, Schmitz D, Dickhuth HH, Schmidt-Trucksaess A. Physical activity throughout life reduces the atherosclerotic wall process in the carotid artery. Br J Sports Med. 2008;42:839–44.
79. Dalla Pozza R, Pirzer R, Beyerlein A, Weberruss H, Oberhoffer R, Schmidt-Trucksäss A, Netz H, Haas N. Beyond intima-media-thickness: analysis of the carotid intima-media-roughness in a paediatric population. Atherosclerosis. 2016;251:164–9.
80. Ghasemi A, Zahediasl S. Is nitric oxide a hormone? Iran Biomed J. 2011;15:59–65.
81. Avolio A. Arterial stiffness. Pulse (Basel). 2013;1:14–28.
82. London GM, Pannier B. Arterial functions: how to interpret the complex physiology. Nephrol Dial Transplant. 2010;25:3815–23.
83. Weber T, Auer J, O'rourke MF, Kvas E, Lassnig E, Berent R, Eber B. Arterial stiffness, wave reflections, and the risk of coronary artery disease. Circulation. 2004;109:184–9.
84. O'rourke MF, Staessen JA, Vlachopoulos C, Duprez D, Plante GE. Clinical applications of arterial stiffness; definitions and reference values. Am J Hypertens. 2002;15:426–44.
85. Schmitt M, Avolio A, Qasem A, Mceniery CM, Butlin M, Wilkinson IB, Cockcroft JR. Basal NO locally modulates human iliac artery function in vivo. Hypertension. 2005;46:227–31.
86. Fishbein MC, Fishbein GA. Arteriosclerosis: facts and fancy. Cardiovasc Pathol. 2015;24:335–42.
87. Cavalcante JL, Lima JA, Redheuil A, Al-Mallah MH. Aortic stiffness: current understanding and future directions. J Am Coll Cardiol. 2011;57:1511–22.

88. Munakata M. Brachial-ankle pulse wave velocity: background, method, and clinical evidence. Pulse (Basel). 2016;3:195–204.
89. Ben-Shlomo Y, Spears M, Boustred C, May M, Anderson SG, Benjamin EJ, Boutouyrie P, Cameron J, Chen CH, Cruickshank JK, Hwang SJ, Lakatta EG, Laurent S, Maldonado J, Mitchell GF, Najjar SS, Newman AB, Ohishi M, Pannier B, Pereira T, Vasan RS, Shokawa T, Sutton-Tyrell K, Verbeke F, Wang KL, Webb DJ, Willum Hansen T, Zoungas S, Mceniery CM, Cockcroft JR, Wilkinson IB. Aortic pulse wave velocity improves cardiovascular event prediction: an individual participant meta-analysis of prospective observational data from 17,635 subjects. J Am Coll Cardiol. 2014;63:636–46.
90. Vlachopoulos C, Aznaouridis K, Stefanadis C. Prediction of cardiovascular events and all-cause mortality with arterial stiffness: a systematic review and meta-analysis. J Am Coll Cardiol. 2010;55:1318–27.
91. Aoyagi Y, Park H, Kakiyama T, Park S, Yoshiuchi K, Shephard RJ. Yearlong physical activity and regional stiffness of arteries in older adults: the Nakanojo Study. Eur J Appl Physiol. 2010;109:455–64.
92. Gando Y, Yamamoto K, Murakami H, Ohmori Y, Kawakami R, Sanada K, Higuchi M, Tabata I, Miyachi M. Longer time spent in light physical activity is associated with reduced arterial stiffness in older adults. Hypertension. 2010;56:540–6.
93. Endes S, Schaffner E, Caviezel S, Dratva J, Autenrieth CS, Wanner M, Martin B, Stolz D, Pons M, Turk A, Bettschart R, Schindler C, Kunzli N, Probst-Hensch N, Schmidt-Trucksäss A. Physical activity is associated with lower arterial stiffness in older adults: results of the SAPALDIA 3 Cohort Study. Eur J Epidemiol. 2016;31:275–85.
94. Endes S, Schaffner E, Caviezel S, Dratva J, Autenrieth CS, Wanner M, Martin B, Stolz D, Pons M, Turk A, Bettschart R, Schindler C, Kunzli N, Probst-Hensch N, Schmidt-Trucksäss A. Long-term physical activity is associated with reduced arterial stiffness in older adults: longitudinal results of the SAPALDIA cohort study. Age Ageing. 2016;45:110–5.
95. Huang C, Wang J, Deng S, She Q, Wu L. The effects of aerobic endurance exercise on pulse wave velocity and intima media thickness in adults: a systematic review and meta-analysis. Scand J Med Sci Sports. 2016;26:478–87.
96. Li Y, Hanssen H, Cordes M, Rossmeissl A, Endes S, Schmidt-Trucksäss A. Aerobic, resistance and combined exercise training on arterial stiffness in normotensive and hypertensive adults: a review. Eur J Sport Sci. 2015;15:443–57.
97. Miyachi M, Kawano H, Sugawara J, Takahashi K, Hayashi K, Yamazaki K, Tabata I, Tanaka H. Unfavorable effects of resistance training on central arterial compliance: a randomized intervention study. Circulation. 2004;110:2858–63.
98. Okamoto T, Masuhara M, Ikuta K. Upper but not lower limb resistance training increases arterial stiffness in humans. Eur J Appl Physiol. 2009;107:127–34.
99. Okamoto T, Masuhara M, Ikuta K. Effects of eccentric and concentric resistance training on arterial stiffness. J Hum Hypertens. 2006;20:348–54.
100. Kearney PM, Whelton M, Reynolds K, Muntner P, Whelton PK, He J. Global burden of hypertension: analysis of worldwide data. Lancet. 2005;365:217–23.
101. Ogasawara R, Sato K, Matsutani K, Nakazato K, Fujita S. The order of concurrent endurance and resistance exercise modifies mTOR signaling and protein synthesis in rat skeletal muscle. Am J Physiol Endocrinol Metab. 2014;306:E1155–62.

Role of Ambulatory Blood Pressure Monitoring in Prehypertension

32

Giacomo Pucci, Gianpaolo Reboldi, Fabio Angeli, Dario Turturiello, and Paolo Verdecchia

32.1 Introduction

The term prehypertension appeared for the first time in the Seventh Report of the Joint National Committee (JNC-VII) on Prevention, Detection, Evaluation and Treatment of High Blood Pressure in 2003 [1]. This category included subjects with office systolic BP (SBP) between 120 and 139 mmHg or diastolic BP (DBP) between 80 and 90 mmHg. The choice to reclassify what was previously conceived just as normal or borderline BP found its rationale on two levels of evidence: first, subjects included in this BP category, as compared with subjects with normal or optimal BP (BP < 120/80 mmHg), were shown to be at increased risk to became truly hypertensives [2]. Second, the CV risk associated with BP values begins to increase after 115/75 mmHg, as shown by a large-scale meta-analysis published in 2001 [3]. The Committee thus recommended close follow-up and possible

G. Pucci (✉)
Department of Medicine, University of Perugia, Perugia, Italy

Unit of Internal Medicine, Terni University Hospital, Terni, Italy
e-mail: giacomo.pucci@unipg.it

G. Reboldi
Department of Medicine, University of Perugia, Perugia, Italy

F. Angeli
Department of Cardiology and Cardiovascular Pathophysiology, Hospital and University of Perugia, Perugia, Italy

D. Turturiello
Department of Medicine, Hospital of Assisi, Perugia, Italy

P. Verdecchia
Department of Medicine, Hospital of Assisi, Assisi, Italy

Fondazione Umbra Cuore ed Ipertensione - AUCI ONLUS, Perugia, Italy

R. Zimlichman et al. (eds.), *Prehypertension and Cardiometabolic Syndrome*, Updates in Hypertension and Cardiovascular Protection,
https://doi.org/10.1007/978-3-319-75310-2_32

non-pharmacologic intervention for individuals in this category to reduce the progression toward sustained hypertension.

Among the large efforts made to describe the main characteristics of subjects with prehypertension, and the causes of the associated increased CV risk, ambulatory blood pressure monitoring (ABPM) played a decisive role. ABPM, in the setting of hypertension and other clinical contexts, was a paradigm shift in the diagnosis and management of individuals with elevated BP values. 24 h average BP, or other out-of-office BP measurements obtained by multiple readings and including a dynamic behaviour, are well acknowledged as the most accurate and representative measures of individual's usual BP. ABPM-derived BP values are more reproducible than casual BP [4], less prone to observer bias, more strongly related to target organ damage [5], and its prognostic value is clearly superior to that of office BP [6–8].

A number of studies demonstrated that subjects with prehypertension are likely to exhibit 24 h BP values that often fall in the range of true hypertension. This phenomenon has been named "masked hypertension". The prevalence of masked hypertension is definitely higher in subjects with prehypertension than in normotensive subjects, and this could in part explain the increased CV risk observed in this particular patient category.

Usually, drug treatment in prehypertension is not recommended; however, patients with prehypertension and associated masked hypertension more frequently develop target organ damage and cardiovascular (CV) events. Therefore, subjects with prehypertension and masked hypertension should be well characterized and, once the diagnosis is confirmed, they could benefit from drug treatment to reduce their overall CV risk. The next section will narratively review the existing evidence supporting an increased CV risk in subjects with prehypertension and masked hypertension.

32.2 Relationship Between Office and Out-of-Office BP Values

In each subject, office BP and corresponding out-of-office BP values are closely associated. At the population level, when values of office BP are plotted against ABPM-derived 24 h BP, it could easily be observed that values are almost completely displayed around a straight regression line (Fig. 32.1) [9].

The degree of correlation between these two measures, calculated as Pearson's correlation coefficient, is about 0.6. Similar results were found also with home BP monitoring (HBPM) [10]. In statistical terms, that means that less than half of the total variance (R-squared) of office BP is explained by out-of-office BP, and the remaining variance is equally scattered around the line of predicted BP values: half of subjects are therefore characterized to have out-of-office BP higher than values predicted from office BP, and half of subjects have out-of-office BP lower than office BP-predicted values.

As widely acknowledged, BP measurement is subjected to random error, and repeated BP measurement performed on the same subject show the phenomenon of

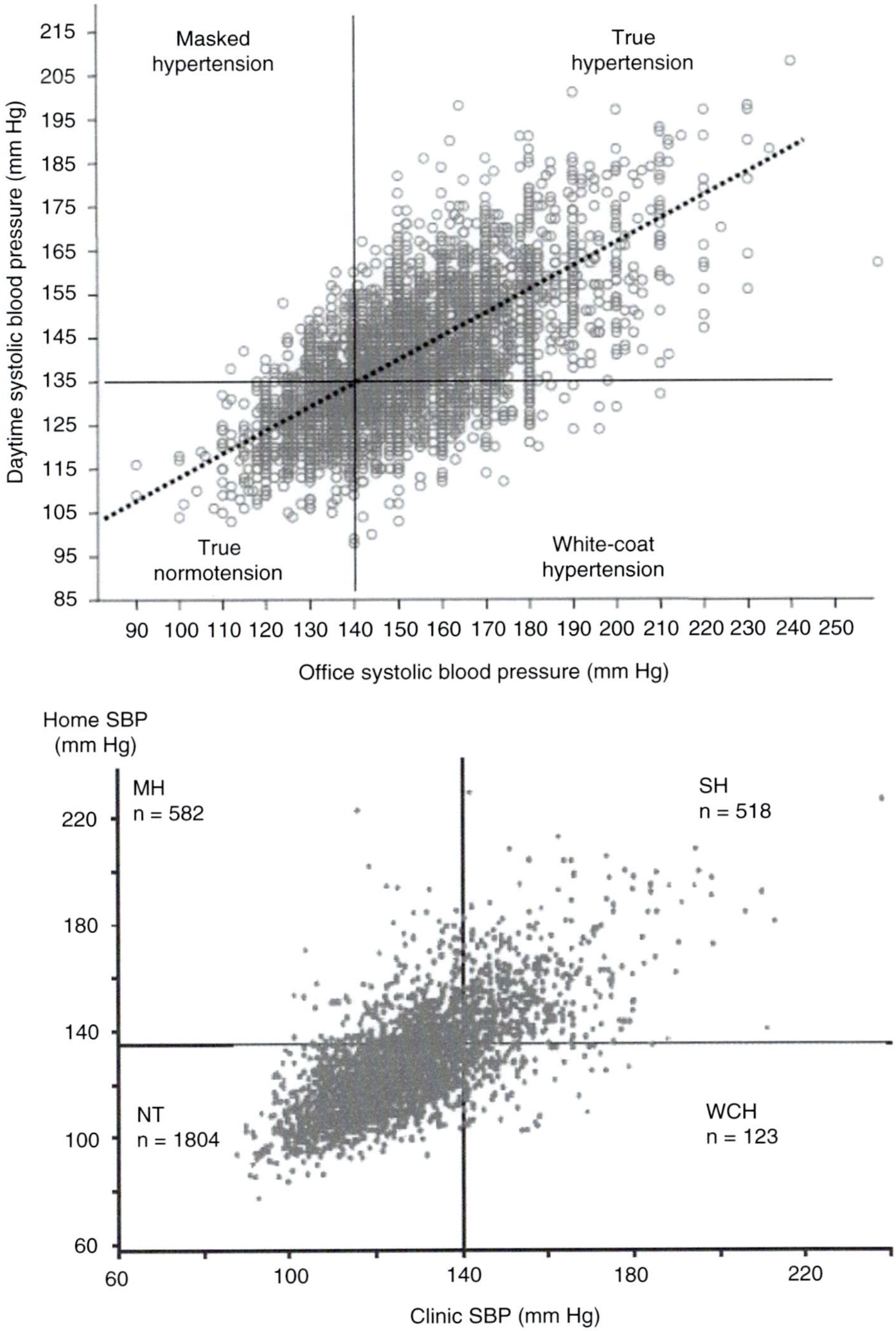

Fig. 32.1 Scatterplots of office systolic blood pressure vs daytime systolic blood pressure (evaluated from 24 h ambulatory blood pressure monitoring (*upper side*), and home SBP (*lower side*). From Angeli F et al. [9] (*upper side*) and Tientcheu D et al. [10] (*lower side*)

the regression to the mean [11]. Since the number of out-of-office BP measures is by definition higher than casual BP readings obtained in the office setting, the relative weight of the regression to the mean effect on average BP obtained from out-of-office measurement becomes more noticeable than on casual BP readings. As a consequence, the slope of the regression line between office BP (X-axis) and 24 h BP (Y-axis) tends to be lower than the unit order, and the intercept line usually crosses the ordinate at values higher than zero. This means that at increasing office BP values, the absolute difference between office BP and out-of-office BP statistically tend to increase. Similarly, at decreasing office BP values, the difference between office and out-of-office BP tend to lower. As a matter of fact, 24 h BP values in the range of normotension have been shown to be higher than office BP [12].

Nevertheless, there is a wide-held belief that, in absolute terms, ABPM values are constantly lower than office BP. Prospective data from the International Database on Ambulatory Blood Pressure Monitoring in Relation to Cardiovascular Outcomes (IDACO) study suggested that outcome-driven thresholds of ABPM yielding the same 10-year cardiovascular risk of office BP corresponding to 140/90 are about 10 mmHg lower (131/79 mmHg) [13]. This was acknowledged in the recent international guidelines [14–16], leading to the consensus values for the diagnosis of hypertension based on 24 h BP fixed values (Table 32.1), as 24 h SBP/DBP > 130/80 mmHg, daytime SBP/DBP > 135/85 mmHg, or night-time SBP/DBP >120/70 mmHg.

As the direct consequence of fixed BP thresholds for the diagnosis of hypertension based on 24 h BP values, the proportion of subjects that, in the range of prehypertension, display 24 h BP values higher than normal (>130/80 mmHg) is directly related to office-BP cutpoint: the higher will be office BP, the higher the prevalence of masked hypertension. A number of studies showed that the prevalence of masked hypertension is directly related to office BP values. In the IDACO study, a population-based study including 11 randomly recruited population cohorts for a total of 12.148 participants, the prevalence of masked hypertension was 7.5% among normotensives, and 29.3% among prehypertensives [13]. In the Jackson Heart Study, a population-based survey exploring the prevalence of masked hypertension among 942 African American patients with normal or high-normal BP undergoing ABPM, the overall proportion of masked hypertension was 25.9%. Interestingly, the prevalence of masked hypertension had an exponential rather than linear increase at increasing categories of office BP, being 15.4% among subjects with office BP <100/70 mmHg, 18.1% among subjects with 100–109/70–74 mmHg, 20.5% among subjects with 110–119/75–79 mmHg, 36.8% among subjects with

Table 32.1 Consensus definition of masked hypertension

Office BP < 140/90 mmHg AND
Daytime BP > 135/85 mmHg
Night-time BP >120/70 mmHg
24 h BP > 130/80 mmHg
Home BP > 135/85 mmHg

This definition is related only to untreated patients. If the same condition is found among treated patients, the adopted definition is masked uncontrolled hypertension

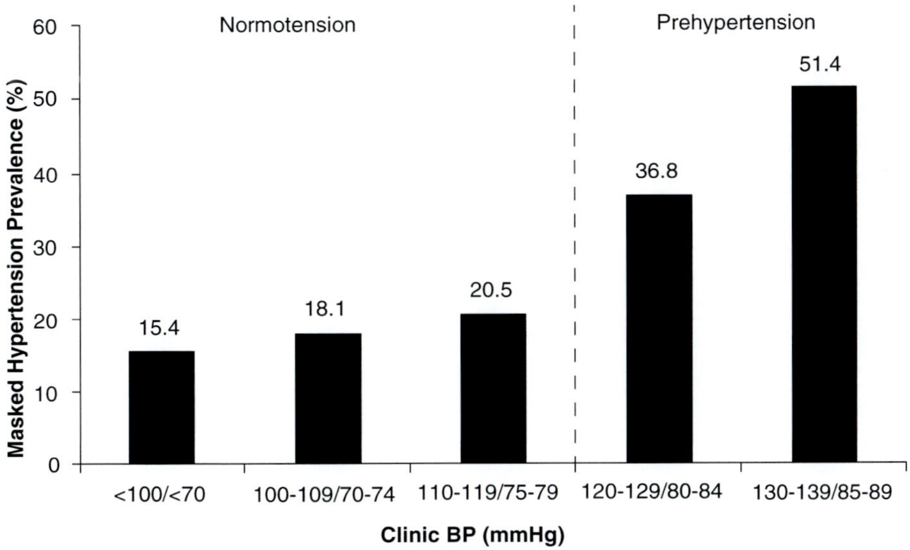

Fig. 32.2 Results from the Jackson Heart Study [17] show how the prevalence of masked hypertension among office BP categories follows an exponential distribution

120–130/80–84 mmHg, and 51.4% among subjects with 130–139/85–89 mmHg (Fig. 32.2) [17].

Similarly, in the Masked Hypertension Study, among normotensives or untreated hypertensive subjects whose mean office BP was 116/75 mmHg, the prevalence of masked hypertension was 14.9%. In the entire cohort, the average 24 h BP was significantly higher than office BP, and 24 h BP values exceeded office BP more frequently than office BP exceeded 24 h BP. As a confirmatory finding, even in this study, the probability of having masked hypertension increased at increasing office BP values, being 10% in subjects with office SBP between 120 and 130 mmHg, 34% in those with office SBP between 130 and 135 mmHg, and 50% between 135 and 140 mmHg. Similar trends were observed also for DBP [12]. On a different level, among subjects with masked hypertension, prehypertension was found in the 84% of the entire cohort [18]. Recently, pooled data from the Masked Hypertension Study and the National Health and Nutrition Examination Survey (NHANES; 2005–2010) were used to impute the ABPM-derived hypertension status for NHANES participants and estimate prevalence of masked hypertension among US adults with non-elevated clinic BP, no history of overt cardiovascular disease, and no use of antihypertensive medication. The prevalence of masked hypertension among 139 million US adults with office-BP lower than 140/90 mmHg was 12.3%, corresponding to 17.1 million adults misclassified as not having hypertension [19].

When home BP replaced ABPM for the evaluation of out-of-office hypertension, the proportion of subjects with masked hypertension, defined as those with average HBPM>135/85 mmHg and office BP < 140/90 mmHg, still varied as a function of office BP levels. In the International Database of Home Blood Pressure in Relation to Cardiovascular Outcome (IDHOCO) study, an individual-participant meta-analysis of more than 5000 participants recruited from six populations, the prevalence of masked hypertension was 5% among participants with optimal office BP (<120/80 mmHg), 18.4% among subjects with office BP between 120/80 and 129/84 mmHg, and 30.4% among subjects with office BP between 130/85 and 140/90 mmHg [20].

The diagnosis of masked hypertension is not only referred to 24 h or home average BP values, but also include patients with elevated BP only in the awake or asleep period, defined as daytime BP > 135/85 or night-time BP > 120/70 mmHg, respectively.

Although the term "masked hypertension" is generally referred only to treatment-naïve patients, when elevated 24 h BP among treated hypertensives is found at face of controlled office BP (<140/90 mmHg), they are classified as having "masked uncontrolled hypertension". Interestingly, the prevalence of masked uncontrolled hypertension is higher than masked hypertension. Part of this finding is explained by a higher treatment-induced BP reduction on office BP than on 24 h BP, as it was demonstrated in a meta-analysis including 44 studies [21].

In the large dataset of the Spanish Society of Hypertension Ambulatory Blood Pressure Monitoring, including more than 62,700 patients, the prevalence of masked uncontrolled hypertension was 31.1%. Among subjects with masked uncontrolled hypertension, the proportion of nocturnal masked hypertension (normal 24 h daytime BP values and elevated 24 h nocturnal BP values) was 28% and almost doubled the proportion of subjects with masked daytime hypertension (elevated 24 h daytime BP values and normal 24 h nocturnal BP values) [22]. This suggest that the diagnosis of masked hypertension (or masked uncontrolled hypertension) is sensitive to BP thresholds adopted, and also that ABPM, as compared to other methods for the evaluation of out-of-office BP not properly suited for nocturnal BP measurement, may be more sensitive in capturing a relatively higher proportion of subjects with masked hypertension due to increased BP levels only in the nocturnal interval.

32.3 Reproducibility of the Diagnosis of Masked Hypertension

The diagnosis of masked hypertension is based on two BP measures: the office and the out-of-office (ABPM or HBPM) BP. Therefore, the reproducibility of the diagnosis is inherently dependent upon the reproducibility of each assessment. Some studies addressed this issue on patients undergoing repeated measures of office BP and ABPM. In a small study, the reproducibility of masked hypertension was tested in 82 subjects undergoing repeated ABPM assessment for standard clinical indications. Masked hypertension was diagnosed by means of awake BP (>135/85 mmHg). Office DBP significantly changed between the first and the second assessment (153/85 vs. 149/82 mmHg, p for DBP change <0.05), while awake BP demonstrated a more stable behaviour (141/82 vs. 139/81, p for SBP/DBP changes = n.s.). The test-retest correlation coefficients confirmed that office SBP correlation was significantly inferior to awake SBP. Masked hypertension was diagnosed in seven patients at first visit; of those, only four confirmed this status at the second visit. The number of subjects with masked hypertension at visit 2 was 15, and most of these patients had initially sustained hypertension [23].

Another study tested the short-term reproducibility of the diagnosis of masked hypertension using office and home BP readings performed about 2 weeks apart in a cohort of hypertensive patients under-treated with an angiotensin II receptor blocker. The prevalence of masked (uncontrolled?) hypertension increased from 8% at the first visit to 18% at the second visit. The main determinant of such findings was a significant change in office BP between the two visits, whereas HBPM values did not significantly change [24]. The long-term reproducibility of masked hypertension was recently assessed in a cohort of 839 untreated patients undergoing repeated office BP and ABPM during a period of 3 months. As compared to normotension, white-coat hypertension and sustained hypertension, masked hypertension showed the least proportion of reproducibility, being confirmed in only 47% of subjects. Interestingly 33% of masked developed sustained hypertension, and a higher office DBP at first evaluation was the unique determinant of this progression [25].

Taken together, these results show that masked hypertension is a poorly reproducible condition both in the short-term and long-term. This is in large part due to the short-term and long-term variability of office-BP. This finding is opened to a number of interpretation; nevertheless, it seems to add a point in favour of those supporting an ABPM-based approach for hypertension diagnosis and management [26].

32.4 Risk Factors for Masked Hypertension

The factors associated with the occurrence of masked hypertension among normotensives and prehypertensives are still the focus of active research. The importance of correctly stratifying the risk of masked hypertension could have important clinical and practical implications, including a compelling indication for ABPM or HBPM screening despite normal office BP levels.

Several studies suggest that the risk of masked hypertension is higher in young subjects and progressively decreases with ageing, as the result of a steeper trajectory of office BP with ageing as compared with ABPM. A potential confounding factor, in part related to this finding, is that young subjects are more physically active than older counterparts, and therefore more exposed to exercise-induced BP fluctuations [27]. However, to the best of our knowledge, no studies compared the prevalence of masked hypertension among different age categories with similar values of office BP.

An interesting study showed that, during a brief low-level cycling exercise (60–70% of age-predicted maximal heart rate), subjects with masked hypertension reach significantly higher SBP values than normotensive subjects. An exercise SBP higher than 175 mmHg during low-level physical activity was able to identify subjects with masked hypertension with 74% sensitivity and 67% specificity. Therefore, subjects with masked hypertension are characterized by an increased pressor response to low-level exercise [28]. However, it should be pointed out that the group of subjects with masked hypertension had significantly higher office BP levels as compared with normotensive group.

Masked hypertension was also associated with job strain in "white-collar" men. The risk of masked hypertension was doubled (adjusted odds ratio, 2.07; 95% confidence interval, 1.30–3.31) for men in the active group characterized by high psychological demands and high decision latitude [29]. Taken together, these findings suggest that masked hypertension could be the result of more pronounced and repeated BP responses to physical and mental stressors.

Smoking status and alcohol consumption were also associated with an increased risk of masked hypertension. In fact, both smoking exposure and alcohol consumption elicit acute pressor effects that could last for many hours after the exposure, and are therefore more easily captured by out-of-office BP measurement [17, 30, 31].

Obesity and associated metabolic disorders are frequently found among subjects with masked hypertension. The prevalence of masked hypertension among subjects with the metabolic syndrome was evaluated in the Finn-Home study, a population-based nationwide registry enrolling 1582 subjects undergoing office and out-of-office BP evaluation. As compared to normotensives and white-coat hypertensives, subjects with masked hypertension had nearly doubled odds for the metabolic syndrome and insulin resistance. Consistent results were found when home BP replaced average 24 h BP. Among the components of the metabolic syndrome, increased body mass index and waist circumference were the major determinants of masked hypertension [32].

Masked hypertension had often been found in subjects with obstructive sleep apnoea [33, 34], a commonly associated condition in patients with hypertension and obesity. Usually, in these patients, masked hypertension is due to nocturnal BP increases, in turn a consequence of the repeated sympathetic activations induced by apnea-hypopnea episodes [35]. Interestingly, a relationship between masked hypertension and poor sleep quality has been recently reported. The study demonstrated impaired sleep quality, measured by the Pittsburgh Sleep Quality Index, in subjects with masked hypertension, particularly those with a non-dipper pattern [36].

The prevalence of masked hypertension is also increased in patients with diabetes mellitus and chronic kidney disease. Among normotensive subjects enrolled in the IDACO study, the prevalence of masked hypertension was found to be 29.3% in diabetic patients, and 18.8% in non-diabetics. The authors also showed that the CV risk of subjects with diabetes mellitus and masked hypertension was almost comparable to untreated stage I hypertensive subjects. Based on author's perspective, this would require specific attention, because the increased risk of masked hypertension among diabetic individuals could justify the routine assessment of 24 h BP in this high-risk group. However, it should also be noted that the group of untreated diabetic subjects, where the increased prevalence of masked hypertension was found, had higher average office BP values as compared to non-diabetic individuals (129/76 vs. 120/72 mmHg) [37].

In chronic kidney disease (CKD), the prevalence of masked hypertension ranged between 16% and 20% [38, 39]. In a meta-analysis of 54 cross-sectional studies evaluating out-of-office BP in CKD patients through home BP or 24 h BP, the prevalence of masked hypertension among normotensive subjects varied between 4.7 and 31.3% due to different threshold classifications adopted for the diagnosis. When studies were selected based on stricter definitions, the average weighted prevalence of masked hypertension was 19.8% [40]. Another recent meta-analysis, based on 70 studies reporting values of office BP and out-of-office BP for a total of 86,167 subjects included in the final analysis, provided a unique opportunity to describe the risk associated with the main determinants of masked hypertension in a large-scale setting. In keeping with previous evidence, the study showed that masked hypertension, either diagnosed by ABPM or HBPM, was associated with male sex (OR 1.47), body mass index (OR 1.07 per 1 Kg/m^2 increase), smoking status (OR 1.32), and systolic office BP (OR 1.10 per 1 mmHg increase) [41].

The main characteristics associated with an increased risk of having masked hypertension are reported in Table 32.2.

In summary, an increased risk is found in young subjects with prehypertension, smokers or heavy drinkers, obese subjects with metabolic syndrome or overt type II diabetes, sleep apnoea or sleep disturbances, or with chronic kidney disease. A

Table 32.2 Main predictors of masked hypertension. References for each category are reported in the text

Predictors of masked hypertension
Prehypertension
High physical or mental stress at work/home
Smoking, excessive alcohol consumption
Metabolic syndrome
Diabetes
Chronic kidney disease
Obstructive sleep apnea
Poor exercise tolerance

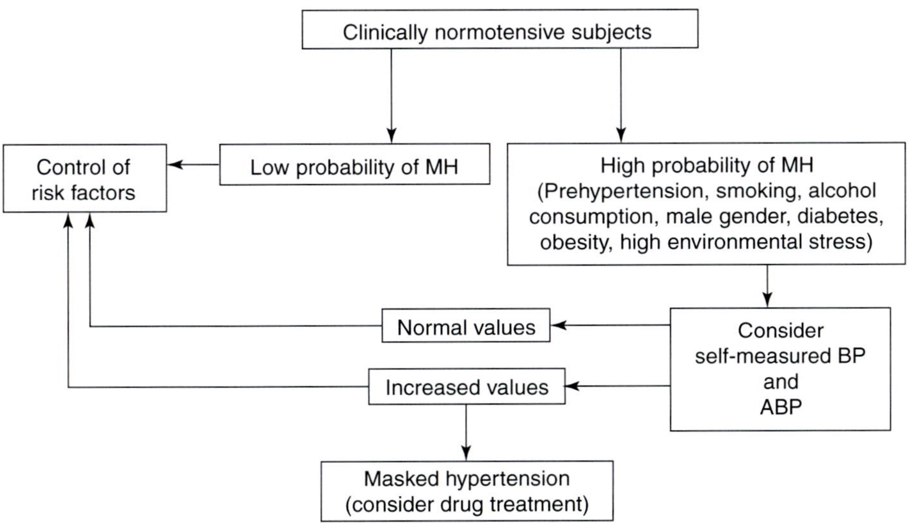

Fig. 32.3 Suggested algorithm for the identification and management of subjects with masked hypertension. *ABP* ambulatory blood pressure, *BP* blood pressure, *MH* masked hypertension. From Angeli F et al. [9]

previously published algorithm [9] for the identification and management of subjects with masked hypertension is reported in Fig. 32.3.

32.5 Masked Hypertension and Target Organ Damage

The association between masked hypertension and markers of hypertension-related target organ damage had been reported in several studies. Most studies showed a stronger association between 24 h BP over office BP with target organ damage, a finding that was consistently reported across different clinical conditions [42]. The presence of target organ damage in masked hypertension may also explain the increased CV risk of this population. The strength of the association and the number and type of organ damage associated with masked hypertension are therefore of high clinical relevance.

In a seminal study by Liu JE et al., echocardiography and arterial ultrasonography were performed in a cohort of 359 subjects, classified as sustained normotensives (office BP < 140/90 and awake BP <134/90, n. 234), sustained hypertensives (office BP > 140/90 and awake BP >134/90, n. 64), and white-coat normotensives (n. 61), a different term defining subjects with normal office BP (<140/90 mmHg) and elevated awake BP (>134/90 mmHg). As compared to sustained normotensives, patients with white-coat normotension (or masked hypertension) showed significantly increased values of left ventricular mass (LVM) and relative wall thickness, while no difference were found in comparison to sustained hypertensives. Similarly, common carotid intima-media thickness (c-IMT) in white-coat normotensives was not different from what was observed among sustained hypertensives [43].

Results from the Jackson Heart Study were confirmatory and strongly supported this view: subjects with masked hypertension had increased left ventricular mass as compared with normotensives, even after adjustment for a number of confounding factors such as age, sex and other cardiovascular risk factors (82 vs. 75 g/m^2, $p < 0.001$). Values found among sustained hypertensives (81 g/m^2) were generally in line with those found among masked hypertensives. Carotid Intima Media Thickness (c-IMT) showed the same behaviour: after adjustment for covariates, c-IMT was found to be significantly higher in subjects with masked hypertension than in normotensives (0.75 vs. 0.72 mm, $p < 0.05$). Among sustained hypertensives, c-IMT was slightly higher than masked hypertension (0.78 mm), although this difference was not formally tested. In the same study, the authors also observed increased values of microalbuminuria in masked hypertensives versus normotensives [17]. In a meta-analysis enrolling 2752 untreated subjects aimed at exploring the relationship between c-IMT and hypertension categories, a progressive increase in c-IMT was shown from normotension (0.68 mm) to masked hypertension (0.76 mm, $p < 0.01$ vs. normotensives) to sustained hypertension (0.79 mm, $p < 0.01$ vs. normotensives). Of note, after adjustment for publication bias the statistical difference between groups was attenuated [44].

The Masked Hypertension Study added novel findings to the relationship between masked hypertension, prehypertension, and cardiac target organ damage.

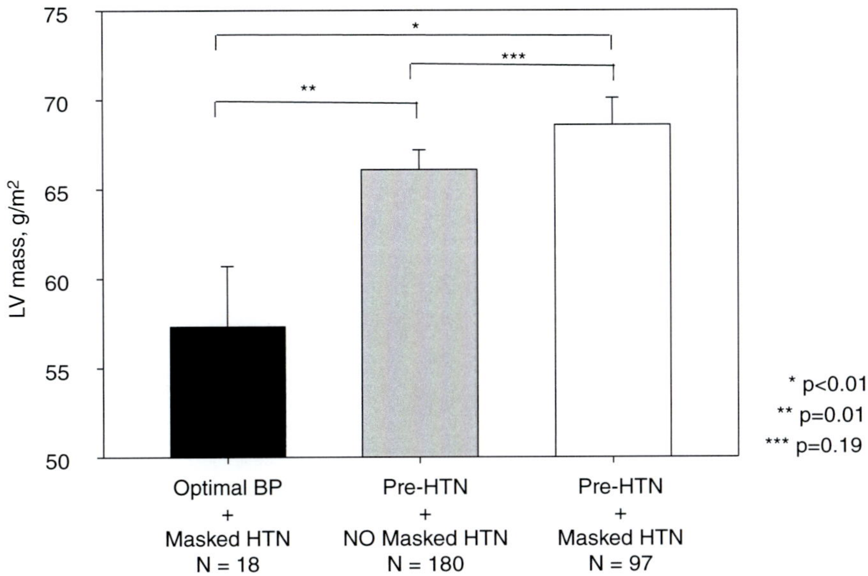

Fig. 32.4 Left ventricular mass levels according to categories of office and 24 h BP. *BP* blood pressure, *LV* left ventricular, *HTN* hypertension. Adapted from Shimbo F et al. [18]

Subjects with office BP <140/90 mmHg were divided into three categories: subjects with optimal BP and masked hypertension, prehypertensives without masked hypertension, and prehypertensives with masked hypertension. The three groups, as expected, showed slight differences in BP and other clinical characteristics. In a multivariable analysis, after adjustment for age, sex, BMI, race, current smoking, hypercholesterolemia, diabetes, family history of hypertension and physical activity, LV mass in patients with optimal BP and masked hypertension (57 g/m^2) was significantly lower than both subjects with prehypertension without masked hypertension (66 g/m^2) and subjects with prehypertension and masked hypertension (69 g/m^2, Fig. 32.4). The difference between prehypertensive subjects with and without masked hypertension was not significant. The authors concluded that subjects with optimal BP, despite masked hypertension, are not prone to develop target organ damage, and a 24 h BP evaluation in these patients might not be warranted. However, it should be noted that the conclusions are weakened by the limited number of patients with optimal BP and masked hypertension ($n = 18$) [18].

Findings from the Masked Hypertension Study also disclosed that subjects with masked hypertension share the same degree of diastolic dysfunction, evaluated through cardiac tissue Doppler, than patients with sustained hypertension. Compared to normotensives, these participants were characterized by a significant increase of E/E' ratio (6.20 for masked hypertension, 6.57 for sustained hypertension, $p = 0.47$, both $p < 0.05$ vs. normotensives) [45]. Interestingly, the same relationship was found in a cohort study of treated hypertensive patients, with at least one CV risk factor, undergoing cardiac Doppler evaluation. Among patients with masked uncontrolled hypertension, the E/E' ratio was significantly higher than in subjects with controlled hypertension (8.3 vs. 7.3, $p = 0.02$), without any statistically significant difference with the group of subjects with uncontrolled hypertension (8.3 vs. 8.3) [46]. Confirmatory results were shown among diabetic subjects [47] and in general population [48].

The strong relationship between masked hypertension and markers of target organ damage was also found when the diagnosis was made according to home BP monitoring. In the Finn-Home study, subjects with masked hypertension, defined as office BP <140/90 mmHg and home BP > 135/85 mmHg, showed increased odds for having left ventricular hypertrophy, evaluated through ECG as the Cornell voltage criteria. After adjustment for sex, age and other covariates, the Cornell voltage in the group of masked hypertensives was similar to sustained hypertensive and significantly higher to both normotensives and white-coat hypertensives [49]. In the Hisayama study, a cross-sectional survey of about 3000 community-dwelling Japanese subjects undergoing office- and home-BP evaluation, c-IMT and the burden of carotid plaques found among masked hypertensives were comparable to those observed in sustained hypertensives, and significantly higher than values observed in the normotensive group [50].

Some interesting observations shed lights on the occurrence of organ damage in prehypertension. In an untreated population of 807 subjects, higher values of c-IMT were found among prehypertensives as compared to normotensives. However, when prehypertensives were split according to the presence of masked hypertension, the group of prehypertensives without masked hypertension showed similar degrees of organ damage as normotensives (0.65 mm in normotensives, 0.65 mm in prehypertensives without masked hypertension); these values were significantly lower than what were found among prehypertensives with masked hypertension (0.71 mm) [51]. Another finding from the Jackson Heart Study came to the same results by analysing values of left ventricular mass in a mixed population of 909 hypertensives. The authors described that masked hypertension carried an increased risk of higher LV mass, even after adjustment for prehypertensive status [52].

Overall, the previous results unremarkably demonstrated the need to perform ABPM or other out-of-office BP assessment among prehypertensives in order to better refine the risk of organ damage.

The association of masked hypertension with arterial stiffness deserves special attention, because, especially when expressed as carotid-to-femoral pulse wave velocity (cf-PWV), arterial stiffness is critically dependent from blood pressure measured at the time of evaluation. Therefore, the evaluation of pulse wave velocity is dependent on instantaneous blood pressure. Based on this evidence, one might expect that subjects with normal or near-normal office BP should have lower cf-PWV values as compared with both sustained and white-coat hypertension. In a population of 539 never-treated Italian hypertensives, Schillaci et al. reported increased values of cf-PWV in subjects with white-coat hypertension as compared to normotensives, after adjustment for age, sex and heart rate (9.3 m/s vs. 8.3 m/s, $p < 0.05$). However, when the entire population was split according to the difference between office and 24 h BP, subjects whose 24 h BP was higher than predicted from office-BP showed increased values of cf-PWV than subjects with 24 h BP lower than predicted (9.9 m/s vs. 9.5 m/s, $p < 0.05$). This resulted despite the two groups shared, by definition, the same office-BP values. These results suggest that chronic hypertension-related structural damage to the arterial wall result in an increased pressure-independent component of arterial stiffness [53]. Therefore, subjects with masked hypertension, as compared to normotensives, could be at risk of having increased pressure-independent arterial stiffness.

Some studies confirmed this hypothesis. Among 414 diabetic patients undergoing clinical evaluation for the diagnosis of masked hypertension, subjects with normal office BP and masked nocturnal hypertension showed increased cf-PWV values than patients with nocturnal normotension (10.2 m/s vs. 9.4 m/s, $p = 0.03$) [54]. In the subgroup of untreated patients from the Dallas Heart Study, a multi-ethnic population cohort, subjects with masked hypertension and with white-coat hypertension were both characterized by increased values of cf-PWV as compared to normotensives (5.53 m/s in white-coat hypertensives, 5.39 m/s in masked hypertensives, 4.56 in normotensives, $p < 0.01$), even after adjustment for confounders [10]. Another study, by confirming the same results, showed a gender-specific association between masked hypertension and target organ damage, being stronger in the female sex than in men [55].

32.6 Prognostic Significance of Masked Hypertension in Prehypertension

The prognostic implications of masked hypertension had been addressed by several prospective studies, most of which did not stratify subjects based on the presence of prehypertension. However, from a broader perspective, the main aim of these studies was to test whether subjects exposed to an increased BP load, irrespective of office BP values, are at increased risk of developing cardiovascular events. In other terms, if it is demonstrated that the relationship between out-of-office BP with cardiovascular morbidity and mortality is stronger than office BP, this indirectly support the usefulness of 24 h pressure load in prehypertension [56].

Bjorklund et al., in 2003, were among the first to demonstrate, in untreated elderly men, that subjects classified as having "isolated ambulatory hypertension" (office BP < 140/90 mmHg and daytime BP >135/85 mmHg, a definition that correspond to masked hypertension) were at increased risk of developing cardiovascular morbidity over a period of 8.4 years. Interestingly, the risk associated with this condition (hazard ratio -HR- 2.77) was of the same magnitude of that associated with sustained hypertension (HR 2.94), even though this was not formally tested. Moreover, when ambulatory daytime SBP was introduced as a continuous variable, the association was independent from office SBP [57]. Confirmatory results were described in the Ohasama study, where 1.332 subjects from general population underwent office and 24 h BP evaluation, and were prospectively followed for 10 years. The adjusted risk for CV events for masked hypertension was 2.13, and it was consistent with the estimate for sustained hypertension (HR 2.26), whereas the risk associated with white-coat hypertension did not differ from normotension [58] (Fig. 32.5).

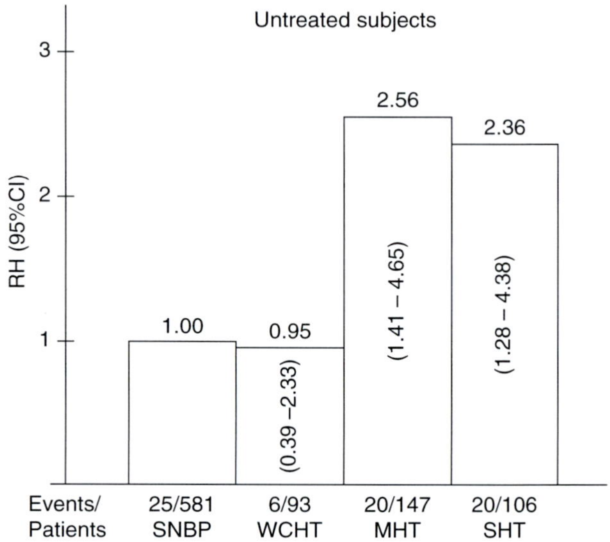

Fig. 32.5 Relative hazards (RH) and 95% confidence intervals (CI) of sustained normal blood pressure (SNBP), white-coat hypertension (WCHT), masked hypertension (MHT), and sustained hypertension (SHT) for risk of the composite of cardiovascular disease (CVD) mortality/stroke morbidity. The SNBP group was treated as the reference category. From Ochubo T et al. [58]

In The IDACO study, an international database made of 7030 individuals from 4 countries, subjects were followed for an average period of 9.5 years. Patients with masked hypertension, irrespective of which daytime BP threshold was adopted for the diagnosis (130/80 or 135/85 mmHg), showed increased odds for cardiovascular and cerebrovascular events, as compared to both normotensives and white-coat hypertensives. The study was the first to demonstrate that the risk for CV events associated with masked hypertension (HR 2.11) and sustained hypertension (HR 2.08) were of the same order of magnitude. Furthermore, when office BP was forced along with 24 h BP and other covariates in a Cox-regression model, both office SBP and DBP lost their predictive value, while 24 h SBP and DBP retained their prognostic significance [7].

Masked uncontrolled hypertension also confers an increased risk of CV events. In a cohort of 742 treated hypertensives, the CV risk associated with masked uncontrolled hypertension (defined as treated office BP < 140/90 mmHg and daytime BP >135/85 mmHg) was significantly higher than controlled hypertension (RR 2.28), while the risk associated with resistant hypertension was of a greater extent (RR 2.94).

A worse prognosis was also found when masked hypertension was diagnosed according to home BP values. In a cohort of 4939 elderly treated hypertensives, as compared to subjects with controlled hypertension, individuals with masked uncontrolled hypertension had a nearly doubled risk of adverse cardiovascular outcome (HR 2.06), after adjustment for confounding factors. The study also confirmed that home BP, but not office BP, was significantly associated with adverse prognosis (RR 1.17 for any increase in 1 SD of SBP, RR = 1.12 for any increase in 1SD of DBP) [59]. A large-scale prospective observational study which enrolled 21.591

hypertensive Japanese patients treated with olmesartan, came to similar conclusions by observing that subjects with elevated morning home SBP (>145 mmHg) and normal office SBP (<130 mmHg) had an increased risk of cardiovascular events as compared to individuals with normal morning home SBP (<125 mmHg) and normal office SBP (<130 mmHg). In this population, the cut-off values for both home and office BP were derived from spline regression analysis as those corresponding to maximum and minimum CV risk [60].

Stergiou et al. investigated the prognostic meaning of masked hypertension evaluated by HBPM in the International Database of HOme blood pressure in relation to Cardiovascular Outcomes (IDHOCO) study, a population-based international database enrolling subjects from five populations. Among untreated subjects (n = 5007), the risk of adverse CV events was found increased in masked hypertensives (adjusted HR 1.57) and in white-coat hypertensives (adjusted HR 1.42); the risk associated with sustained hypertension was significantly higher (adjusted HR 2.13). The two novel findings from this study were that the risk associated with masked hypertension was consistently lower than sustained hypertension, and that white-coat hypertension, diagnosed by HBPM, was associated with an adverse outcome. Given that the threshold levels for both office and home BP were in line with previous report, the authors suggested that part of the risk associated with white-coat hypertension was related to relatively higher levels of home BP (although in the range of normality) in this category as compared to normotensives.

Similar results were found in the Dallas Heart Study: after a median follow-up of 9 years, the risk associated with masked hypertension for developing adverse CV outcomes was significantly higher than normotensive, and also comparable to the risk observed in the population of individuals with white-coat hypertension (HR 2.03 and HR 2.09, respectively) [10].

In a meta-analysis enrolling 13,526 patients from 8 studies, masked hypertension was confirmed to be associated with worse CV prognosis, both if evaluated through ABPM (HR 2.0, 95% C.I. 1.54–2.60) and through HBPM (HR 2.13, 95% C.I. 1.35–3.35, Fig. 32.6) [9]. At present, however, there are no convincing evidences supporting the prognostic superiority of masked hypertension as diagnosed by ambulatory 24 h or home BP.

Masked hypertension was associated with a worse CV outcome even among diabetic subjects and among patients with chronic kidney disease. In a subpopulation of 229 untreated diabetics from the IDACO study, the risk of CV events associated with masked hypertension tended to be higher than the risk associated with normotension (HR 1.96, $p = 0.059$), and was on the same degree of the risk associated with grade-1 hypertensives (HR 1.07, $p = 0.82$) [37]. In a group of 588 patients with non-dialysis chronic kidney disease undergoing office and 24 h BP evaluation, individuals with masked hypertension (20.6% of the entire cohort) showed increased risk of cardiac and cerebrovascular events, total mortality and renal events, although the relative low sample size is a limitation to the generalizability of results [39].

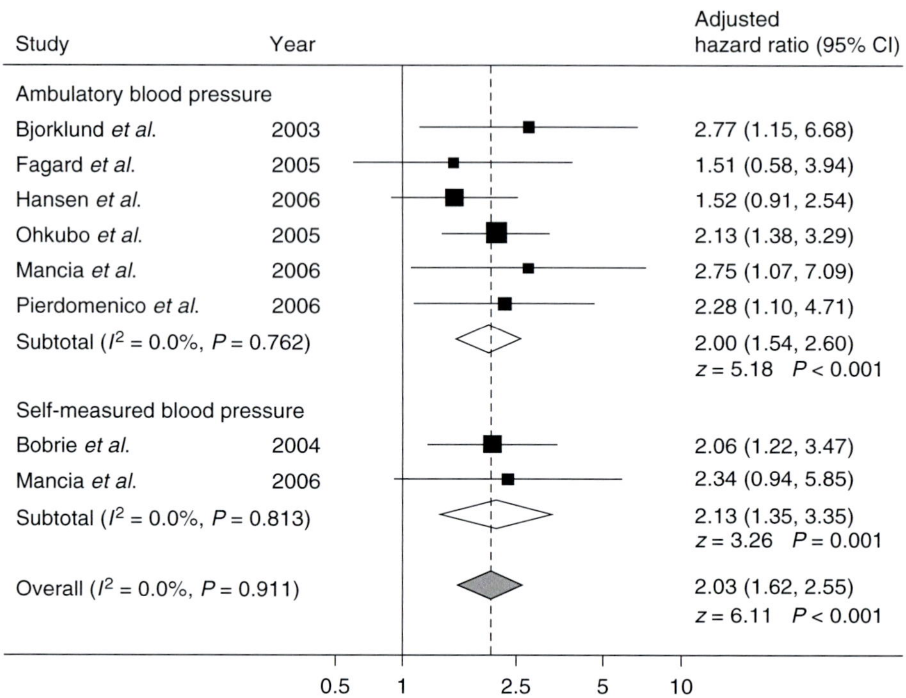

Fig. 32.6 Overview of longitudinal studies addressing the prognostic impact of masked hypertension diagnosed by ABPM and HBPM. See the text for details

32.7 Treatment Strategies in Prehypertension with Masked Hypertension

We previously speculated that subjects with masked hypertension are at increased risk of developing intermediate target organ damage and overt cardiovascular events. From a theoretical standpoint, individuals with masked hypertension might benefit from an effective pharmacologic antihypertensive approach aimed at reducing the increased BP load. Moreover, subjects with masked hypertension are often exposed to additional cardiovascular risk due to the increased prevalence, within their clinical phenotype, of diabetes, chronic kidney disease, and obstructive sleep apnoea. Therefore, the optimal strategy for CV risk reduction should take into account the effective management of concomitant conditions.

Unluckily, to date there is no substantive evidence, either on intermediate outcomes or on hard endpoints, supporting the efficacy of drug treatment for masked hypertension. Moreover, there is no demonstration that drug treatment in patients with masked hypertension will provide a relative risk reduction consistent with that observed in subjects with sustained hypertension. Despite reasons supporting treatment of masked hypertension appear rational, it should be remembered that masked hypertension is a poorly reproducible condition. Therefore the risk of overdiagnosis and overtreatment should be thoroughly considered and monitored. Another issue fuelling the controversy on how this condition should be diagnosed and managed depends on whether the definition should be based on home or 24 h BP, daytime or night-time (or both) BP thresholds. This is another "grey area" in urgent need of sound evidence.

The European Guidelines for the Management of arterial hypertension add more uncertainty to the field, since the recommendation to treat subjects with masked hypertension with both lifestyle measures and antihypertensive drugs has been reported with the class of recommendation IIa (Weight of evidence/opinion in favour of usefulness/efficacy) and the lowest level of evidence (grade C, corresponding to expert opinion and result from small studies or registries) [61].

There are at least two planned prospective studies aiming to provide definitive answers to these questions. The first trial, which is named "MASked and masked-unconTrolled hypERtension managed based on office BP or out-of-office BP measurements" (MASTER) Study, is a prospective, randomized, blinded-end-point (PROBE design) study, which will randomize participants to an office BP-guided treatment or to an ABPM- or Home BP-guided treatment (registered at clinicaltrials.gov as NCT02804074). The study will explore if tailoring of antihypertensive treatment based on office or out-of-office BP will be associated with a different incidence in intermediate outcomes, including cardiovascular and renal endpoints (LV mass and albumin/creatinine ratio) at 1 year, a different occurrence in cardiovascular events during a period of 4 years, and changes in a number of BP-related variables through the study. The planned sample size of study is set at 1240 subjects to be recruited in 30 centres, taking into account a dropout rate of 15%.

A second study with similar aim will assess whether antihypertensive treatment in masked hypertension will be associated with a conversion to the controlled hypertension category. The study also aims to explore the effect of drug treatment of masked hypertension on the occurrence of target organ damage, such as left ventricular hypertrophy and proteinuria (registered at clinicaltrials.gov as NCT02142881). The study is planned to collect data for the primary outcome measure by December 2018.

Conclusions

The need for an out-of-office evaluation in patients with prehypertension is justified by the likelihood to detect masked hypertension, a condition characterized by sustained increased BP load and a higher probability of target organ damage. Masked hypertension is frequent among prehypertensive subjects, and its prevalence increases with office BP. A clinical phenotype characterized by male gender, increased BP response to physical and mental stressors, obesity, diabetes, metabolic syndrome, smoking, and obstructive sleep apnoea is often associated with masked hypertension. In these subjects, an out-of-office BP evaluation can be justified.

The prevalence and reproducibility of masked hypertension is critically dependent from the cut-off BP levels adopted for the diagnosis. At present, there are at least four BP combinations (daytime BP, night-time BP, 24 h BP and home BP) proposed for the diagnosis of masked hypertension. Longitudinal outcome studies are needed to compare of the specific prognostic implications of each of these categories.

There is general consensus that subjects with masked hypertension and patients with sustained hypertension share a similar relative risk of CV events. This holds for Grade I hypertension confirmed at the out-of-office BP evaluation. Studies relying on home-BP measurement for the diagnosis of masked hypertension are consistent. There is urgent need of ad hoc designed prospective studies to ascertain the hypothesized beneficial effects of treating masked hypertension with lifestyle intervention measures and/or antihypertensive medications.

References

1. The Seventh Report of the Joint National Committee on Prevention, Detection, Evaluation, and Treatment of High Blood Pressure. National High Blood Pressure Education Program. Bethesda (MD): National Heart, Lung, and Blood Institute (US); 2004 Aug. Report No.: 04-5230.
2. Vasan RS, Larson MG, Leip EP, Kannel WB, Levy D. Assessment of frequency of progression to hypertension in non-hypertensive participants in the Framingham heart study: a cohort study. Lancet. 2001;358:1682–6.
3. Lewington S, Clarke R, Qizilbash N, Peto R. Collins R; prospective studies collaboration. Age-specific relevance of usual blood pressure to vascular mortality: a meta-analysis of individual data for one million adults in 61 prospective studies. Lancet. 2002;360:1903–13.
4. van der Steen MS, Lenders JW, Graafsma SJ, den Arend J, Thien T. Reproducibility of ambulatory blood pressure monitoring in daily practice. J Hum Hypertens. 1999;13:303–8.
5. Hara A, Tanaka K, Ohkubo T, et al. Ambulatory versus home versus clinic blood pressure: the association with subclinical cerebrovascular diseases: the Ohasama study. Hypertension. 2012;59:22–8.
6. O'Brien E, Atkins N, Stergiou G, Karpettas N, Parati G, Asmar R, et al. European Society of Hypertension Working Group on blood pressure monitoring. Practice guidelines of the European Society of Hypertension for clinic, ambulatory and self blood pressure measurement. J Hypertens. 2005;23:697–701.
7. Hansen TW, Kikuya M, Thijs L, Bjorklund-Bodega K, Kuznetsova T, Ohkubo T, et al. Prognostic superiority of daytime ambulatory over conventional blood pressure in four populations: a meta-analysis of 7,030 individuals. J Hypertens. 2007;25:1554–64.
8. Verdecchia P, Porcellati C, Schillaci G, Borgioni C, Ciucci A, Battistelli M, Guerrieri M, Gatteschi C, Zampi I, Santucci A, Santucci C, Reboldi G. Ambulatory blood pressure. An independent predictor of prognosis in essential hypertension. Hypertension. 1994;24:793–801.
9. Angeli F, Reboldi G, Verdecchia P. Masked hypertension: evaluation, prognosis, and treatment. Am J Hypertens. 2010;23:941–8.
10. Tientcheu D, Ayers C, Das SR, McGuire DK, de Lemos JA, Khera A, Kaplan N, Victor R, Vongpatanasin W. Target organ complications and cardiovascular events associated with masked hypertension and white-coat hypertension: analysis from the Dallas heart study. J Am Coll Cardiol. 2015;66:2159–69.
11. Barnett AG, van der Pols JC, Dobson AJ. Regression to the mean: what it is and how to deal with it. Int J Epidemiol. 2005;34:215–20.

12. Schwartz JE, Burg MM, Shimbo D, Broderick JE, Stone AA, Ishikawa J, Sloan R, Yurgel T, Grossman S, Pickering TG. Clinic blood pressure underestimates ambulatory blood pressure in an untreated employer-based US population: results from the masked hypertension study. Circulation. 2016;134:1794–807.
13. Kikuya M, Hansen TW, Thijs L, Bjorklund-Bodegaard K, Kuznetsova T, Ohkubo T, et al. International database on ambulatory blood pressure monitoring in relation to cardiovascular outcomes investigators. Diagnostic thresholds for ambulatory blood pressure monitoring based on 10-year cardiovascular risk. Circulation. 2007;24:2145–52.
14. National Institute for Health and Clinical Excellence (NICE). Hypertension. The clinical management of primary hypertension in adults. Clinical Guideline. 2011;127. www.nice.org.uk/guidance/CG127.
15. Chobanian AV, Bakris GL, Black HR, Cushman WC, Green LA, Izzo JL Jr, et al., Joint National Committee on Prevention, Detection, Evaluation, and Treatment of High Blood Pressure. National Heart, Lung, and Blood Institute; National High Blood Pressure Education Program Coordinating Committee. Seventh report of the Joint National Committee on prevention, detection, evaluation, and treatment of high blood pressure. Hypertension. 2003;42:1206–52.
16. Mancia G, Fagard R, Narkiewicz K, Redon J, Zanchetti A, Bohm M, et al. The Task Force for the management of arterial hypertension of the European Hypertension Society (ESH) and of the European Society of Cardiology (ESC). 2013 ESH/ESC Guidelines for the management of arterial hypertension. J Hypertens. 2013;22:193–278.
17. Diaz KM, Veerabhadrappa P, Brown MD, Whited MC, Dubbert PM, Hickson DA. Prevalence, determinants, and clinical significance of masked hypertension in a population-based sample of African Americans: The Jackson Heart Study. Am J Hypertens. 2015;28:900–8.
18. Shimbo D, Newman JD, Schwartz JE. Masked hypertension and prehypertension: diagnostic overlap and interrelationships with left ventricular mass: the masked hypertension study. Am J Hypertens. 2012;25:664–71.
19. Wang YC, Shimbo D, Muntner P, Moran AE, Krakoff LR, Schwartz JE. Prevalence of masked hypertension among US adults with nonelevated clinic blood pressure. Am J Epidemiol. 2017;185:194–202.
20. Asayama K, Thijs L, Brguljan-Hitij J, Niiranen TJ, Hozawa A, Boggia J, Aparicio LS, Hara A, Johansson JK, Ohkubo T, Tzourio C, Stergiou GS, Sandoya E, Tsuji I, Jula AM, Imai Y, Staessen JA. Risk stratification by self-measured home blood pressure across categories of conventional blood pressure: a participant-level meta-analysis. PLoS Med. 2014;11:e1001591.
21. Mancia G, Parati G. Office compared with ambulatory blood pressure in assessing response to antihypertensive treatment: a meta-analysis. J Hypertens. 2004;22:435–45.
22. Banegas JR, Ruilope LM, de la Sierra A, de la Cruz JJ, Gorostidi M, Segura J, Martell N, García-Puig J, Deanfield J, Williams B. High prevalence of masked uncontrolled hypertension in people with treated hypertension. Eur Heart J. 2014;35:3304–12.
23. Ben-Dov IZ, Ben-Arie L, Mekler J, Bursztyn M. In clinical practice, masked hypertension is as common as isolated clinic hypertension: predominance of younger men. Am J Hypertens. 2005;18:589–93.
24. Bobrie G, Clerson P, Cuchet A, Mahmoudi A, Postel-Vinay N, Chatellier G. Prevalence and mechanism of masked hypertension: the ol'mesures survey. Arch Mal Coeur Vaiss. 2006;99:760–3.
25. de la Sierra A, Vinyoles E, Banegas JR, Parati G, de la Cruz JJ, Gorostidi M, Segura J, Ruilope LM. Short-term and long-term reproducibility of hypertension phenotypes obtained by office and ambulatory blood pressure measurements. J Clin Hypertens (Greenwich). 2016;18:927–33.
26. Lovibond K, Jowett S, Barton P, Caulfield M, Heneghan C, Hobbs FD, Hodgkinson J, Mant J, Martin U, Williams B, Wonderling D, McManus RJ. Cost-effectiveness of options for the diagnosis of high blood pressure in primary care: a modelling study. Lancet. 2011;378:1219–30.
27. Leary AC, Donnan PT, MacDonald TM, Murphy MB. The influence of physical activity on the variability of ambulatory blood pressure. Am J Hypertens. 2000;13:1067–73.
28. Schultz MG, Hare JL, Marwick TH, Stowasser M, Sharman JE. Masked hypertension is "unmasked" by low-intensity exercise blood pressure. Blood Press. 2011;20:284–9.

29. Trudel X, Brisson C, Milot A. Job strain and masked hypertension. Psychosom Med. 2010;72:786–93.
30. Seki M, Inoue R, Ohkubo T, Kikuya M, Hara A, Metoki H, Hirose T, Tsubota-Utsugi M, Asayama K, Kanno A, Obara T, Hoshi H, Totsune K, Satoh H, Imai Y. Association of environmental tobacco smoke exposure with elevated home blood pressure in Japanese women: the Ohasama study. J Hypertens. 2010;28:1814–20.
31. Ohira T, Tanigawa T, Tabata M, Imano H, Kitamura A, Kiyama M, Sato S, Okamura T, Cui R, Koike KA, Shimamoto T, Iso H. Effects of habitual alcohol intake on ambulatory blood pressure, heart rate, and its variability among Japanese men. Hypertension. 2009;53:13–9.
32. Hänninen MR, Niiranen TJ, Puukka PJ, Jula AM. Metabolic risk factors and masked hypertension in the general population: the Finn-Home study. J Hum Hypertens. 2014;28:421–6.
33. Baguet JP, Lévy P, Barone-Rochette G, Tamisier R, Pierre H, Peeters M, Mallion JM, Pépin JL. Masked hypertension in obstructive sleep apnea syndrome. J Hypertens. 2008;26: 885–92.
34. Drager LF, Diegues-Silva L, Diniz PM, Bortolotto LA, Pedrosa RP, Couto RB, Marcondes B, Giorgi DM, Lorenzi-Filho G, Krieger EM. Obstructive sleep apnea, masked hypertension, and arterial stiffness in men. Am J Hypertens. 2010;23:249–54.
35. Lee S, Thomas RJ, Kim H, Seo HS, Baik I, Yoon DW, Kim SJ, Lee SK, Shin C. Association between high nocturnal blood pressure and white matter change and its interaction by obstructive sleep apnoea among normotensive adults. J Hypertens. 2014;32:2005–12.
36. Erdem F, Cakır U, Yıldırım O, Alcelik A, Donmez I, Tuman TC, Caglar SO, Erdem A, Yazıcı M. A new diagnostic tool for masked hypertension: impaired sleep quality. Arch Med Sci. 2016;12:1207–13.
37. Franklin SS, Thijs L, Li Y, Hansen TW, Boggia J, Liu Y, Asayama K, Björklund-Bodegård K, Ohkubo T, Jeppesen J, Torp-Pedersen C, Dolan E, Kuznetsova T, Stolarz-Skrzypek K, Tikhonoff V, Malyutina S, Casiglia E, Nikitin Y, Lind L, Sandoya E, Kawecka-Jaszcz K, Filipovsky J, Imai Y, Wang J, Ibsen H, O'Brien E, Staessen JA. Masked hypertension in diabetes mellitus: treatment implications for clinical practice. Hypertension. 2013;61:964–71.
38. Tang H, Gong WY, Zhang QZ, Zhang J, Ye ZC, Peng H, Wang C, Lou T. Prevalence, determinants, and clinical significance of masked hypertension and white-coat hypertension in patients with chronic kidney disease. Nephrology (Carlton). 2016;21:841–50.
39. Wang C, Zhang J, Li Y, Ma X, Ye Z, Peng H, Lou T. Masked hypertension, rather than white-coat hypertension, has a prognostic role in patients with non-dialysis chronic kidney disease. Int J Cardiol. 2017;230:33–9.
40. Bangash F, Agarwal R. Masked hypertension and white-coat hypertension in chronic kidney disease: a meta-analysis. Clin J Am Soc Nephrol. 2009;4:656–64.
41. Sheppard JP, Fletcher B, Gill P, Martin U, Roberts N, McManus RJ. Predictors of the home-clinic blood pressure difference: a systematic review and meta-analysis. Am J Hypertens. 2016;29:614–25.
42. Dolan E, Stanton A, Thijs L, Hinedi K, Atkins N, McClory S, Den Hond E, McCormack P, Staessen JA, O'Brien E. Superiority of ambulatory over clinic blood pressure measurement in predicting mortality: the Dublin outcome study. Hypertension. 2005;46:156–61.
43. Liu JE, Roman MJ, Pini R, Schwartz JE, Pickering TG, Devereux RB. Cardiac and arterial target organ damage in adults with elevated ambulatory and normal office blood pressure. Ann Intern Med. 1999;131:564–72.
44. Cuspidi C, Sala C, Tadic M, Rescaldani M, De Giorgi GA, Grassi G, Mancia G. Untreated masked hypertension and carotid atherosclerosis: a meta-analysis. Blood Press. 2015;24: 65–71.
45. Oe Y, Shimbo D, Ishikawa J, Okajima K, Hasegawa T, Diaz KM, Muntner P, Homma S, Schwartz JE. Alterations in diastolic function in masked hypertension: findings from the masked hypertension study. Am J Hypertens. 2013;26:808–15.
46. Komori T, Eguchi K, Kabutoya T, Ishikawa J, Hoshide S, Kario K. Left ventricular diastolic function evaluated by the E/e' ratio is impaired in patients with masked uncontrolled hypertension. Clin Exp Hypertens. 2014;36:538–44.

47. Marchesi C, Maresca AM, Solbiati F, Franzetti I, Laurita E, Nicolini E, Gianni M, Guasti L, Marnini P, Venco A, Grandi AM. Masked hypertension in type 2 diabetes mellitus. Relationship with left-ventricular structure and function. Am J Hypertens. 2007;20:1079–84.
48. Sega R, Trocino G, Lanzarotti A, Carugo S, Cesana G, Schiavina R, Valagussa F, Bombelli M, Giannattasio C, Zanchetti A, Mancia G. Alterations of cardiac structure in patients with isolated office, ambulatory, or home hypertension: data from the general population (Pressione Arteriose Monitorate E Loro Associazioni [PAMELA] Study). Circulation. 2001;104:1385–92.
49. Hänninen MR, Niiranen TJ, Puukka PJ, Kesäniemi YA, Kähönen M, Jula AM. Target organ damage and masked hypertension in the general population: the Finn-Home study. J Hypertens. 2013;31:1136–43.
50. Fukuhara M, Arima H, Ninomiya T, Hata J, Hirakawa Y, Doi Y, Yonemoto K, Mukai N, Nagata M, Ikeda F, Matsumura K, Kitazono T, Kiyohara Y. White-coat and masked hypertension are associated with carotid atherosclerosis in a general population: the Hisayama study. Stroke. 2013;44:1512–7.
51. Manios E, Michas F, Tsivgoulis G, Stamatelopoulos K, Tsagalis G, Koroboki E, Alexaki E, Papamichael C, Vemmos K, Zakopoulos N. Impact of prehypertension on carotid artery intima-media thickening: actual or masked? Atherosclerosis. 2011;214:215–9.
52. Redmond N, Booth JN 3rd, Tanner RM, Diaz KM, Abdalla M, Sims M, Muntner P, Shimbo D. Prevalence of masked hypertension and its association with subclinical cardiovascular disease in African Americans: results from the Jackson Heart Study. J Am Heart Assoc. 2016;5:e002284.
53. Schillaci G, Pucci G, Pirro M, Settimi L, Hijazi R, Franklin SS, Mannarino E. Combined effects of office and 24-h blood pressure on aortic stiffness in human hypertension. J Hypertens. 2011;29:869–75.
54. Wijkman M, Länne T, Engvall J, Lindström T, Ostgren CJ, Nystrom FH. Masked nocturnal hypertension--a novel marker of risk in type 2 diabetes. Diabetologia. 2009;52(7):1258–64. https://doi.org/10.1007/s00125-009-1369-9. Epub 2009 Apr 25
55. Scuteri A, Morrell CH, Orru' M, AlGhatrif M, Saba PS, Terracciano A, Ferreli LA, Loi F, Marongiu M, Pilia MG, Delitala A, Tarasov KV, Schlessinger D, Ganau A, Cucca F, Lakatta EG. Gender specific profiles of white coat and masked hypertension impacts on arterial structure and function in the SardiNIA study. Int J Cardiol. 2016;217:92–8.
56. Verdecchia P, Reboldi G, Porcellati C, Schillaci G, Pede S, Bentivoglio M, Angeli F, Norgiolini S, Ambrosio G. Risk of cardiovascular disease in relation to achieved office and ambulatory blood pressure control in treated hypertensive subjects. J Am Coll Cardiol. 2002;39:878–85.
57. Björklund K, Lind L, Zethelius B, Andrén B, Lithell H. Isolated ambulatory hypertension predicts cardiovascular morbidity in elderly men. Circulation. 2003;107:1297–302.
58. Ohkubo T, Kikuya M, Metoki H, Asayama K, Obara T, Hashimoto J, Totsune K, Hoshi H, Satoh H, Imai Y. Prognosis of "masked" hypertension and "white-coat" hypertension detected by 24-h ambulatory blood pressure monitoring 10-year follow-up from the Ohasama study. J Am Coll Cardiol. 2005;46:508–15.
59. Bobrie G, Chatellier G, Genes N, Clerson P, Vaur L, Vaisse B, Menard J, Mallion JM. Cardiovascular prognosis of "masked hypertension" detected by blood pressure self-measurement in elderly treated hypertensive patients. JAMA. 2004;291:1342–9.
60. Kario K, Saito I, Kushiro T, Teramukai S, Ishikawa Y, Mori Y, Kobayashi F, Shimada K. Home blood pressure and cardiovascular outcomes in patients during antihypertensive therapy: primary results of HONEST, a large-scale prospective, real-world observational study. Hypertension. 2014;64:989–96.
61. Mancia G, Fagard R, Narkiewicz K, Redón J, Zanchetti A, Böhm M, Christiaens T, Cifkova R, De Backer G, Dominiczak A, Galderisi M, Grobbee DE, Jaarsma T, Kirchhof P, Kjeldsen SE, Laurent S, Manolis AJ, Nilsson PM, Ruilope LM, Schmieder RE, Sirnes PA, Sleight P, Viigimaa M, Waeber B, Zannad F. 2013 ESH/ESC Guidelines for the management of arterial hypertension: the task force for the management of arterial hypertension of the European Society of Hypertension (ESH) and of the European Society of Cardiology (ESC). J Hypertens. 2013;31:1281–357.

33 Sympathoadrenal Reactivity to Stress as a Predictor of Cardiovascular Risk Factors

Arnljot Flaa, Morten Rostrup, Sverre E. Kjeldsen, and Ivar Eide

33.1 Introduction

Hypertension is an independent cardiovascular risk factor, but is also strongly associated with other risk factors like obesity, insulin resistance, and dyslipidemia. We have for many years focused on the pathophysiology underlying these conditions in young, healthy subjects with special attention to the sympathoadrenal system.

A. Flaa
Department of Cardiology, Oslo University Hospital, Ullevaal, Oslo, Norway

Section of Cardiovascular and Renal Research, Medical Clinic, Oslo University Hospital, Ullevaal, Oslo, Norway

M. Rostrup
Section of Cardiovascular and Renal Research, Medical Clinic, Oslo University Hospital, Ullevaal, Oslo, Norway

Department of Acute Medicine, Oslo University Hospital, Ullevaal, Oslo, Norway

Faculty of Medicine, Institute for Clinical Medicine, University of Oslo, Oslo, Norway

S. E. Kjeldsen (✉)
Department of Cardiology, Oslo University Hospital, Ullevaal, Oslo, Norway

Section of Cardiovascular and Renal Research, Medical Clinic, Oslo University Hospital, Ullevaal, Oslo, Norway

Faculty of Medicine, Institute for Clinical Medicine, University of Oslo, Oslo, Norway
e-mail: s.e.kjeldsen@medisin.uio.no; sverrkj@online.no

I. Eide
Section of Cardiovascular and Renal Research, Medical Clinic, Oslo University Hospital, Ullevaal, Oslo, Norway

Faculty of Medicine, Institute for Clinical Medicine, University of Oslo, Oslo, Norway

Department of Nephrology, Oslo University Hospital, Ullevaal, Oslo, Norway

R. Zimlichman et al. (eds.), *Prehypertension and Cardiometabolic Syndrome*, Updates in Hypertension and Cardiovascular Protection,
https://doi.org/10.1007/978-3-319-75310-2_33

Since the 1980s we have selected young men according to their blood pressure at the military draft screening for laboratory examinations, and have demonstrated an association between blood pressure and hyperreactivity to mental stress (intense arithmetical calculations) [1]. Moreover, the apparently consistent covariation between sympathoadrenal activity on one side and total cholesterol, high density lipoprotein (HDL), insulin resistance, left ventricle mass, and platelet activation on the other [2, 3] lead to the interest in sympathoadrenal hyperreactivity to mental stress as a possible important predictor of future cardiovascular risk factors.

33.1.1 The Sympathoadrenal System

The autonomic nervous system regulates body functions in general without our consciousness, and its main goal is to maintain homeostasis in the body. It consists of the sympathoadrenal and parasympathetic nervous system. The central regulation of the autonomic nervous system is extremely complex, where the hypothalamus acts as a control center. It receives afferent signals from the body in addition to stimulation from the limbic system and the cortex. The efferent signals are mediated direct and indirect to the preganglionic neurons. These preganglionic axons leave the central nervous system via cranial nerves or ventral roots to synapse in specialized ganglia with the postganglionic nerves that innervate the target organs. Most organs are regulated by both systems, and they are mainly regulated in a reciprocal manner [4].

The peripheral sympathetic nervous system originates in the spinal cord at the level of T1-L2, where the preganglionic neurons are located in the intermediolateral cell column (see Fig. 33.1). These preganglionic nerves travel a short distance and enter the sympathetic ganglia, mainly arranged in two chains located alongside the vertebral bodies. The sympathetic ganglionic chains extend from the cervical to the sacral region, and the short preganglionic nerves enter the chain and make a synapse with the postganglionic nerves, which reach the effector organs. Some preganglionic fibers do not synapse in the sympathetic chains but terminate in separate cervical or abdominal ganglia, and some even synapse directly with chromaffin cells in the adrenal medulla [5].

The sympathetic postganglionic nerves are widely distributed in the blood vessel walls and in most organs, especially the heart, spleen, and salivary glands. Sympathetic activation increases the heart rate, cardiac output, and blood pressure, and redistributes the blood by constricting or dilating arterioles in the skin, splanchnic organs, and skeletal muscle. Moreover, pupils are widened, bronchi are dilated, and sphincters constricted. Metabolic changes include mobilization of fat and glycogen [5]. The effect may be highly differentiated. Preganglionic activation of the adrenal medulla, on the other hand, leads to secretion of adrenaline and noradrenaline into the circulation, thus producing a far-reaching hormonal effect instead of the local effect made by the sympathetic nerves [4].

The catecholamines act predominantly on adrenergic receptors, located in the membrane of the effector cells. The different effects of the various catecholamines on the heart and smooth muscle cells are caused by different types of adrenoceptors,

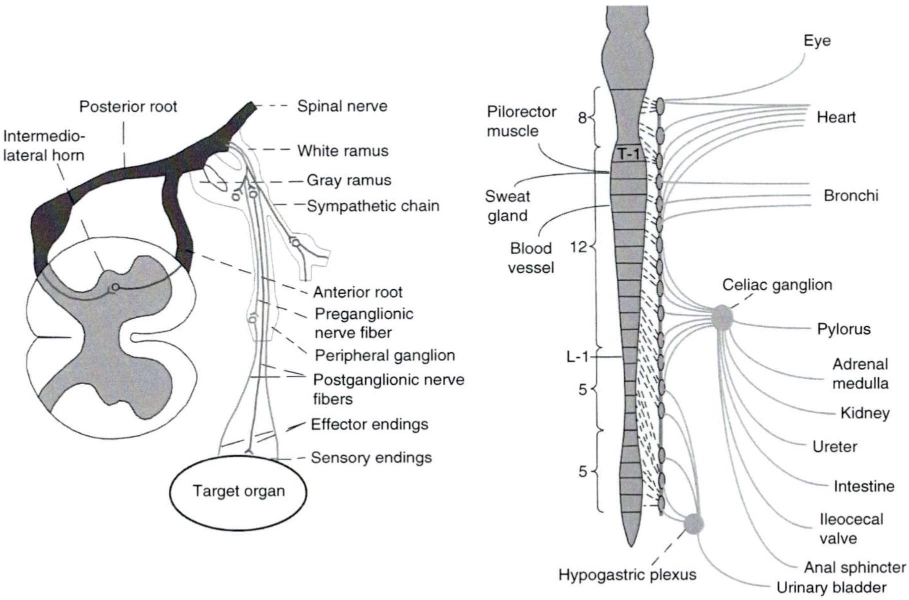

Fig. 33.1 The sympathetic nervous system

of which there are two groups, the α- and the β-receptors, and at least five different subtypes [5]:

- α_1-Adrenoceptor is located in smooth muscle, particularly in blood vessels in the skin and the gastrointestinal system. The principal effect of stimulation of these receptors in blood vessels is vasoconstriction.
- α_2-Adrenoceptor is a pre- and postsynaptic receptor, and mediates synaptic transmission.
- β_1-Adrenoceptor stimulation in the heart increases the contractility and heart rate, while stimulation of these receptors in the juxtaglomerular cells in the kidneys results in renin release, augmenting the conversion of angiotensin II.
- β_2-Adrenoceptors are mainly situated in the vascular and bronchial smooth muscles, where agonists dilate the vessels and bronchi.
- β_3-Adrenoceptors mediate lipolytic and thermic responses in brown and white adipose tissue [6]. In the heart, they are believed to have the opposite effect to the other β-adrenoceptors, and their negative inotropic effects might play a role as a "safety-valve" during intense adrenergic stimulation. In vessels, they mediate vasodilatation [7].

We use the term "sympathoadrenal system" and not "sympathetic system" to emphasize the fact that the sympathoadrenal system consists of two different elements which not necessarily act as a unit [8]. Due to the highly differentiated activity in different parts of the sympathetic system, activity in the adrenal medulla may show reciprocal alterations compared to measurements of overall sympathetic activity, even though medullary activity is stimulated by preganglionic sympathetic nerves. The sympathoadrenal system is probably most known for the ability to prepare the body for fear, flight, and fight situations, but it also participates in several other settings like cold exposure, eating, standing up, sexual activity, and pain. These different settings involve differentiated patterns of sympathoadrenal activity. Still, we use the expression "sympathoadrenal activity" although it is not a strictly defined term.

33.1.2 Sympathoadrenal Activity and Development of Cardiovascular Disease

The first report suggesting an association between transient tachycardia and development of hypertension was published in 1945 [9]. Levy et al. followed 22,741 US army officers from 1 to more than 25 years and found that subjects with a heart rate of 100 beats per minute or above had increased risk of developing sustained hypertension. Likewise, they found that sustained hypertension developed more frequently in those with previous transient hypertension than in those who never showed an elevation of blood pressure [10]. Although heart rate is dependent on both parasympathetic and sympathoadrenal activity, there are close correlations between heart rate and indices of sympathetic activity like electric activity in sympathetic fibers and noradrenaline plasma concentrations [11], and these early reports indicated that increased sympathoadrenal reactivity could be a causal factor in hypertension.

The sympathoadrenal system affects the function of nearly all the internal organs of the body and represents an important tool for the central nervous system to maintain homeostasis during acute and chronic changes in the physiological state [12]. However, chronic inappropriate activations over time are thought to initiate and accelerate cardiovascular disease [13]. The simplified overview in Fig. 33.2 illustrates the complex relations between sympathoadrenal activity and development of cardiovascular disease.

The metabolic syndrome is a clustering of risk factors linked to cardiovascular morbidity and mortality [14], and there is a positive relationship between the cardiovascular risk and the number of components of the metabolic syndrome that is present [15]. There are several definitions of the metabolic syndrome, but the usual risk factors included in the definitions are visceral obesity (increased waist circumference), elevated triglycerides, reduced HDL, insulin resistance, and high blood pressure [16, 17]. One theory is that lipolysis in excessive visceral adipose tissue accompanying obesity is the key feature of the metabolic syndrome. Other possible underlying mechanisms behind the syndrome are insulin resistance, atherogenic dyslipidemia, and chronic low grade inflammation [18–20]. There seems to be, however, consensus that insulin resistance is perhaps the most important pathophysiological feature of the metabolic syndrome, leading to increased secretion of insulin and hyperinsulinemia, which may account for all the changes in the metabolic syndrome

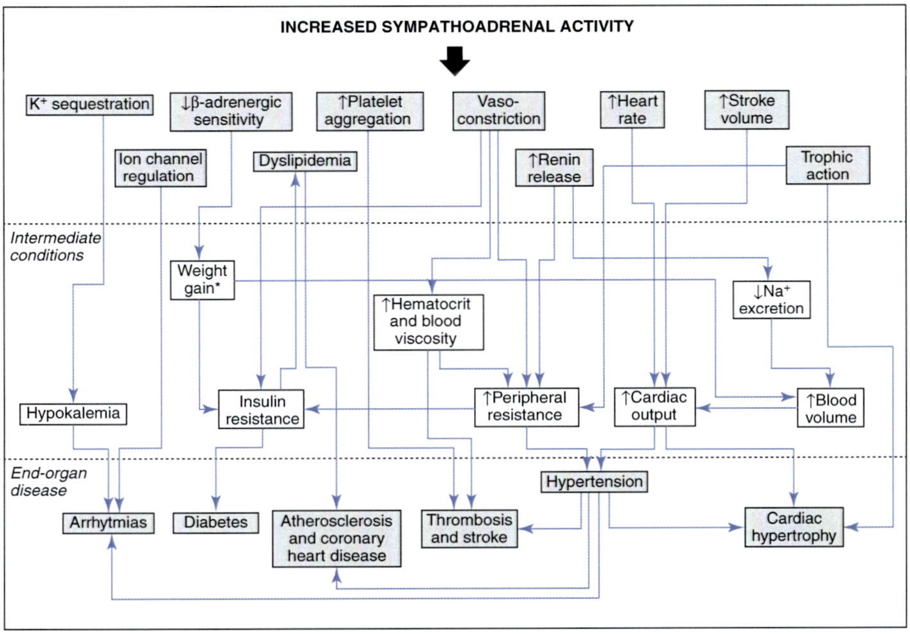

Fig. 33.2 Effects of increased sympathoadrenal activity. * While increased sympathetic activity may reduce adrenergic sensitivity and thereby increase body weight, there are also reports suggesting a negative relationship between sympathoadrenal activity and weight gain in longitudinal studies

[15]. Then the question arises: "What causes insulin resistance?" Data indicate that sympathoadrenal hyperactivity may in fact constitute the "core" of the metabolic syndrome, and the above mechanisms may be explained by a common pathogenic background in the sympathoadrenal system (Fig. 33.3) [21, 22]. This hypothesis is based on three findings [15]:

1. Sympathetic activity reduces insulin sensitivity, probably through hemodynamic and possibly cellular effects.
2. Several components of the metabolic syndrome are accompanied by increased activity in the sympathoadrenal system.
3. Sympathoadrenal activity is able, directly or indirectly, to favor the development and progression of organ damage associated with the metabolic syndrome.

33.1.2.1 Sympathoadrenal Activity and Hypertension

There is much uncertainty about the pathophysiology of essential hypertension, and there are probably a large number of factors contributing to the elevated blood pressure [23]. One possible cause may be alterations in the autonomic nervous system, which plays an important role in the normal physiological regulation of pressure.

Several cross-sectional studies demonstrate increased sympathetic activity among hypertensives compared to normotensives [24–27], and about 30% of young

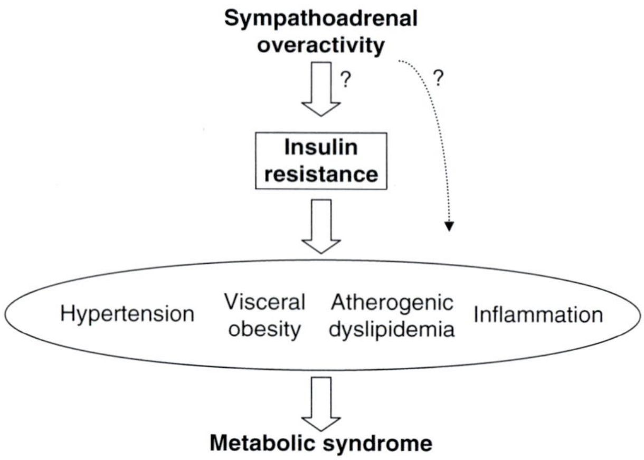

Fig. 33.3 Possible pathogenic mechanisms of the metabolic syndrome

subjects with borderline hypertension have a hyperkinetic circulation with tachycardia, high cardiac output and elevated noradrenaline levels in plasma, while the total peripheral resistance is fairly normal [28, 29]. Data indicate that some of the sympathoadrenal activation in young hypertensives may be due to the awareness of hypertension [30–32]. These subjects differ from older patients with established hypertension, who show a hemodynamic pattern characterized by normalization of the cardiac output and an elevated total peripheral resistance [29]. In other words, there seems to be a hemodynamic transition from a hyperkinetic state to increased total peripheral resistance. There are at least two main hypotheses behind this finding. The theory of autoregulation proposes that increased intravascular volume and increased cardiac output will lead to an over-perfusion, exceeding the metabolic needs of the tissues. To maintain normal perfusion, the total vascular resistance would increase [33]. Julius, however, claims there is no evidence of volume expansion in hyperkinetic hypertension [28]. Furthermore, the cardiac output does probably not exceed the metabolic need. As data indicate that increased sympathetic activity may reduce chronotropic and inotropic β-adrenergic responsiveness, he therefore suggests that the responsiveness in the heart decreases, involving downregulation of β-adrenergic receptors, while in the vascular beds the responsiveness increases during the course of hypertension, due to structural changes in the arteriolar wall described by Folkow [34]. This could lead to the observed normalization of cardiac output accompanied by increase of vascular resistance (Figs. 33.4 and 33.5).

The reason why activity in the sympathetic nervous system eventually decreases with age is not known, but one possible explanation could be that as total peripheral resistance increases due to structural changes, less sympathetic activity is needed to maintain a certain level of blood pressure [35].

As most of the studies on sympathoadrenal activity and hypertension have been cross-sectional, the data do not allow any causal conclusions. There are only a few

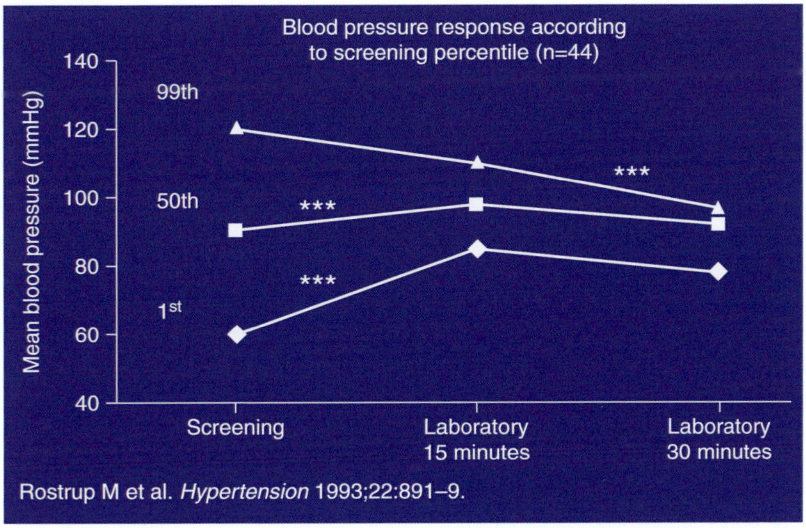

Fig. 33.4 Blood pressures in young men from 1st, 50th, and 99th percentiles at screening, seated in the laboratory for 15 min and resting supine in the laboratory for 30 min prior to stress testing

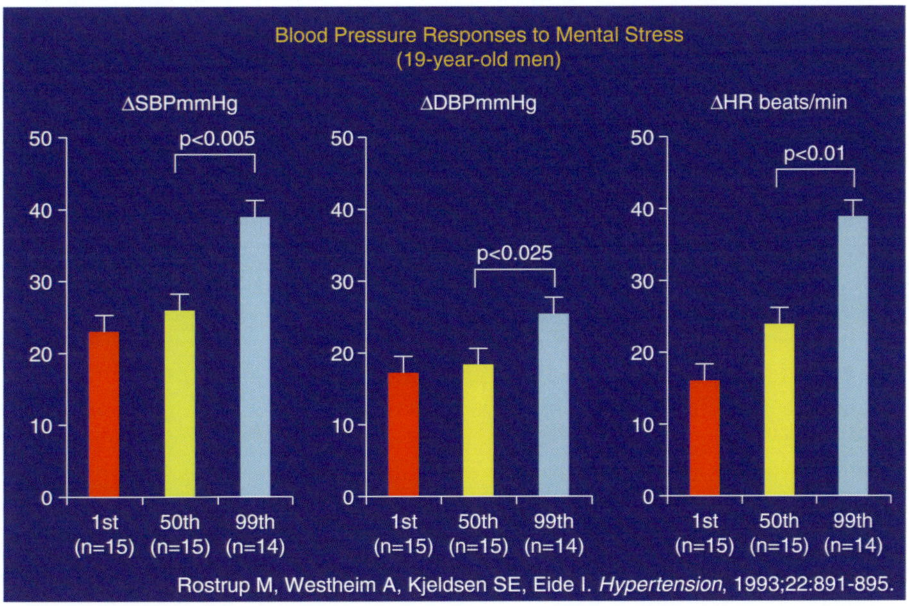

Fig. 33.5 Blood pressure and heart rate responses to mental stress test in young men from 1st, 50th, and 99th percentiles

available prospective longitudinal studies assessing the predictive power. Bohm et al. found higher resting noradrenaline concentration at rest in subjects who developed hypertension, compared to those who remained normotensive or borderline hypertensive [36]. Another study found that mental stress-induced blood pressure responses together with plasma noradrenaline response to bicycle ergometry and psychological factors were relatively weak predictors of future blood pressure classification over 2.5 years [37]. Finally, Masuo et al. demonstrated that resting noradrenaline concentration was a predictor of mean blood pressure increase over 5 years in Japanese subjects [38].

33.1.2.2 Sympathoadrenal Activity and Obesity

Genetic factors may account for 25–40% of the variability in human body weight [39], and the sympathoadrenal system and β-adrenergic receptors are thought to play an important role [40–42]. However, whether alterations in the sympathoadrenal system contribute to obesity or, rather, are consequences of it, is still an unresolved issue [43]. There has been an intense debate on the relationship between obesity and the sympathoadrenergic system. At the beginning of the 90s, based on urine catecholamines in cross-sectional studies, there was a consensus of a reduced activity in the sympathetic nervous and adrenal medullary system in obesity. However, more sophisticated and accurate methods such as sympathetic nerve recording techniques and isotope dilution methodology measuring noradrenaline release from sympathetic nerves, later demonstrated that human obesity was, in fact, accompanied by an activation of the sympathetic nervous system, which was believed to be an adaptation to the increased weight [42].

Few longitudinal studies have addressed this issue. Tataranni et al. studied 44 Pima Indians over a period of 3.3 years and found that urine adrenaline and noradrenaline excretion rates correlated negatively with changes in waist-to-thigh circumference ratio and body weight, respectively [44]. Masuo et al. on the other hand, found resting plasma noradrenaline to be a positive predictor of changes in body mass index (BMI) over a 5-year period in 433 Japanese subjects [38]. Hence, the available data are contradictory, and the follow-up periods are short.

33.1.2.3 Sympathoadrenal Activity and Insulin Resistance

Insulin is a powerful determinant of sympathetic activity. Fasting suppresses [8] and overfeeding stimulates [45] the sympathetic nervous system through insulin-mediated signals, in order to regulate diet-induced thermogenesis [46]. Landsberg hypothesized in 1986 that insulin-stimulated sympathetic activity in obese subjects, which is supposed to increase thermogenesis and thereby energy production and weight reduction, would unintendedly increase blood pressure, explaining the clustering of obesity, insulin resistance, hypertension, and increased sympathetic activity in the metabolic syndrome [47]. Likewise, Reaven et al. asserted that insulin resistance and hyperinsulinemia are the primary events, with subsequent enhancement of the sympathetic activity [48]. Julius, among others, postulated on the other hand that insulin resistance follows changes in muscle blood flow based on a raised activity in the sympathetic nervous system as the primary cause [49]. Sympathetic vasoconstriction may induce insulin resistance by decreasing the number of open capillaries in the skeletal muscles. To compensate for hyperglycemia caused by decreased glucose extraction, the pancreas secretes more insulin.

The fact that insulin resistance and sympathetic activity are related in a positive feedback fashion leading to their reciprocal reinforcement [50] makes it difficult to identify which of the two precedes the other. Although there have been a large number of studies addressing this issue, the cross-sectional design of the studies has made it difficult to solve the "chicken-and-egg" puzzle. Only one longitudinal study has been performed prior to our study, and they demonstrated that the sympathetic activity seemed to precede hyperinsulinemia through a 10-year follow-up in Japanese subjects [51].

33.2 Aims

Based on our previous observations, we hypothesized that resting blood pressure was related to arterial plasma catecholamines, cardiovascular and sympathetic reactivity, and cardiovascular risk factors in a cross-sectional study in young men with low, normal, and high blood pressure who were unaware of their blood pressure status [52]. In a follow-up study over 18 years, we hypothesized that initial sympathoadrenal reactivity to stress at 19 years of age was related to the development of future cardiovascular risk factors such as (a) blood pressure [53], (b) obesity [54], and (c) insulin resistance [55]. Furthermore, we examined whether reactivity to the cold pressor test and the mental stress test differed in predictive power [53–55].

33.3 Subjects and Methods

33.3.1 Subjects

The data for the cross-sectional study [52] was collected in 1986–1989. All subjects were initially selected from the military draft procedures in 1986 and 1987, which is compulsory to all young men in Norway. In 1986 the number of screened subjects was 3861, while 4123 were screened in 1987. Blood pressure measurements on all the subjects attending in Oslo were undertaken once after 5 min of sitting. Mean blood pressure was thereafter calculated as diastolic blood pressure + pulse pressure/3. None of the subjects were informed about the results of the blood pressure recordings at this stage, to avoid effects of hypertension labelling on responses to the forthcoming stress tests [30, 31]. We have previously published a cross-sectional study on subjects with low, normal, and high screening blood pressure and demonstrated a clear tendency of normalization of the blood pressure in the high blood pressure group when reexamined after 30 min of rest in our laboratory [32]. Thus, in order to secure and reassess differences in resting blood pressure [52], the subjects were reexamined in our laboratory on a separate day before final inclusion.

Subjects belonging to the 98th to 99th percentile of the military screening blood pressure distribution were included if the mean blood pressure at reexamination exceeded the population blood pressure + 1 SD. Subjects of the 50th percentile were included if their mean blood pressure was within mean screening blood pressure ± 1 SD. Subjects of the 1st percentile were included if their mean blood pressure was lower than mean screening blood pressure −1 SD. As these data were not published immediately after the examination, we published them at the time of reexamination 18 years later.

In the follow-up study performed in 2005–2006 [53–55] we selected subjects from the 1st percentile, the 50th percentile, and the 95th–99th percentiles of the mean blood pressure distribution of the initial military screening, some of them were also included in the previous analyses [52]. All were previously healthy and of Caucasian origin except one who was half Asian and half Caucasian. 99 of the subjects from entry had satisfactory examinations and were suitable for follow-up. Out of these, 81 (82%) subjects were available for examination at follow-up, and a total of eighteen were not reexamined; one was excluded due to probable i.v. drug addiction, two lived abroad and were not able to attend, four did not answer any letters or calls, and eleven did not want to participate. The subjects that were not eligible for follow-up did not differ from eligible subjects in resting blood pressure, heart rate, BMI, waist circumference, or catecholamine stress responses at entry. One subject who was reexamined had ulcerative colitis and had to be excluded from further analyses due to a previous colectomy and an excessive intake of water and salt. At follow-up, 21 subjects (25.9%) reported having one or more of the following diseases: hypertension (9 subjects), hypercholesterolemia [12], diabetes mellitus [3], and previous myocardial infarction [1]. Eight of these subjects used one or more of the following medications regularly: angiotensin receptor blockers [3], β-blockers [3], ACE inhibitor [1], statins [2], antidiabetics [3], and acetylsalicylic acid [1] (Fig. 33.6).

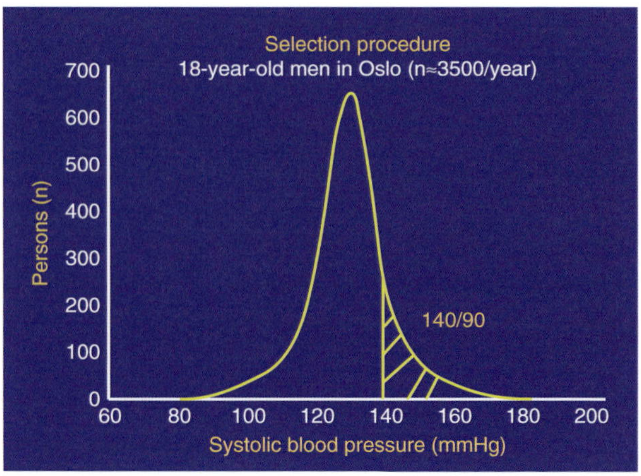

Fig. 33.6 Distribution of blood pressure at screening

33.3.2 Methods

33.3.2.1 Blood Pressure Measurements

Screening measurements at military draft procedures in 1986 and resting measurements in the laboratory were determined by an automatic auscultatory device (Boso-digital II S, Bosh & Sohn GmbH u Co, Jungingen, Germany) validated against a sphygmomanometer, and a hidden printer, to serve as an unbiased measurement. However, the diastolic blood pressure distribution of the 3861 men at screening was skewed to the left, suggesting an underestimating in some subjects. Thus, in 1987 we decided to use a standard sphygmomanometer.

Blood pressures during the stress tests in the laboratory at entry were monitored directly by a canula in the brachial artery of the nondominant arm. All subjects were unaware of their blood pressure status, previously shown to be a confounding factor [1, 30, 31].

At follow-up, resting blood pressure was measured three times with a mercury sphygmomanometer on the left arm after at least 15 min of sitting, and was calculated as mean of the last two measurements.

33.3.2.2 Plasma Catecholamines

Arterial plasma catecholamines were measured by a radioenzymatic technique [56, 57] as previously reported [24, 31]. All the blood samples were analyzed by the same technician at entry and at follow-up. The assay has been used for over 20 years in our laboratory, and is also precise at low plasma concentrations.

33.3.2.3 Insulin Resistance

Insulin resistance at follow-up [55] was quantified using the homeostasis model assessment for insulin resistance (HOMA-IR). HOMA-IR was calculated in fasting conditions as serum glucose (mmol/L) multiplied by serum insulin (pmol/L) and divided with 135, as described by Matthews et al. [58].

33.3.2.4 Stress Tests

Stress tests are designed to examine autonomic responses to different stimuli. We used three stress tests in the present work to activate the sympathoadrenal system. We sampled plasma catecholamines and measured blood pressure and heart rate before, during, and after the stress tests. The response to stress was defined as the mean values during the tests minus the baseline value or the absolute value during the tests [53].

Mental Stress Test

The mental arithmetic stress test has been widely used. In our studies, the subjects were asked to subtract the number "13" repetitively starting from "1079" for 5 min, while a metronome made noise at a frequency of 2 Hz. The subjects had to calculate loudly, and feedback was given at any miscalculation. Mental stress test is known to elicit a fight and flight reaction, and is a classic example of a β-adrenergic response, where the increased blood pressure is mediated primarily via an increase of cardiac output [59, 60]. Total peripheral resistance shows little change during the test (Fig. 33.7).

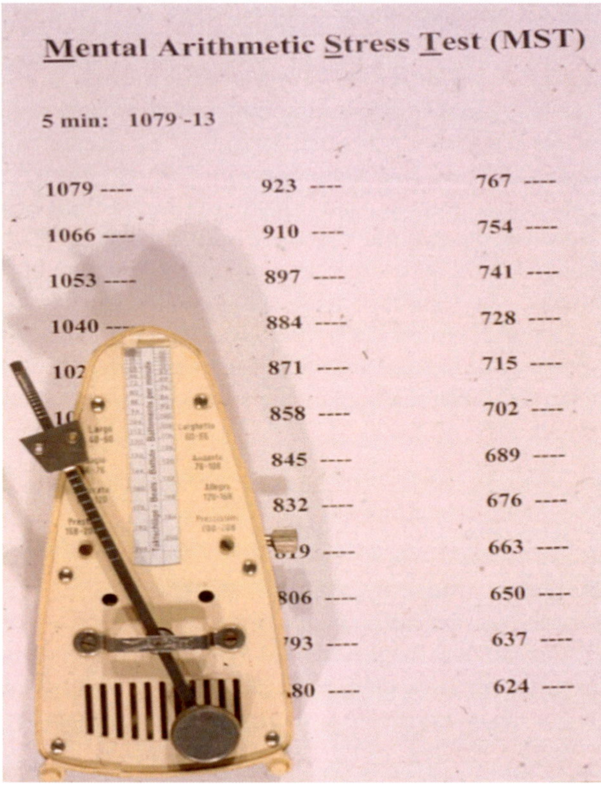

Fig. 33.7 Work sheet and metronome used during mental stress testing of young men

Cold Pressor Test

Hines and Brown introduced this test in 1932 [61], where one hand is completely immersed in ice water (0–2 °C) for 1–6 min. We used 1 min in our studies. In contrast to the mental stress test, the cold pressor test elicits a response that is predominantly mediated by α-adrenergic vasoconstriction [60]. This means that the observed increase in blood pressure mainly is due to an increased total peripheral resistance.

Orthostatic Test

The subjects were asked to stand up for 2 min from the supine position for the orthostatic stress test [52]. After standing up, pooling of the blood takes place in the legs. A transient reduction in cardiac output elicits a reflex increase in sympathetic activity [62].

Statistics

The data were analyzed using the statistical package SPSS version 12.0 [52] and 14.0 [53–55] for Windows (SPSS Inc., Chicago, IL). Parametric tests were used for normally distributed data and nonparametric when normality was not achieved by natural log transformation.

One way analysis of variance (ANOVA) with trend analysis or Kruskal-Wallis test was used to compare differences between the initial screening groups [52]. Subsequent Student's t-tests without adjustments were carried out if there was any significant group interaction. The effect of stress tests on blood pressure and plasma catecholamines was additionally analyzed by repeated-measures ANOVA, and group differences were analyzed by effect*group interaction, with subsequent t-tests [52].

Associations between continuous variables were assessed using Pearson's correlations or Spearman's rank correlation, while Chi-Square testing with linear-by-linear association was used for dichotomous. In order to adjust for possible confounders, linear regression analysis was performed. Due to a large number of univariate correlation analyses [53], the Bonferroni correction was used to reduce the risk of Type 1 errors.

Paired samples T-tests or the Wilcoxon test were used to analyze possible changes in normally distributed continuous variables from entry to follow-up [53–55], while categorical variables were analyzed by sign test.

33.4 Results

33.4.1 Cross-Sectional Associations Between Resting Blood Pressure and Sympathoadrenal Activity and Stress Reactivity

Differences in resting blood pressure among the 19-year-old men were reflected by a similar pattern in both arterial adrenaline and noradrenaline concentration at rest. Mental stress test, cold pressor test, and orthostatic test evoked significant cardiovascular and catecholamine responses in all blood pressure groups [52]. However, mental stress test was the only test that induced differential responses between the three blood pressure groups, where the high blood pressure group showed the most and the low blood pressure group the least pronounced response in blood pressure, heart rate, and plasma catecholamines [52]. The present study also showed that lower blood pressure was associated with a better lipoprotein profile and a lower fructosamine concentration and waist-hip ratio (Fig. 33.8).

33.4.2 Sympathoadrenal Reactivity as a Predictor of Future Blood Pressure

The adrenaline and noradrenaline concentrations during mental stress test were significant predictors of future systolic blood pressure, while the plasma catecholamine levels at rest and during the cold pressor test did not show significant associations with later blood pressure [53]. Together, in the multiple regression model, adrenaline and noradrenaline levels during mental stress explained 12.7% of the variation of future systolic blood pressure [53], after adjusting for resting blood pressure, family history, BMI at entry, and systolic blood pressure during stress (Adj.R^2 for the whole model: 0.65) (Fig. 33.9).

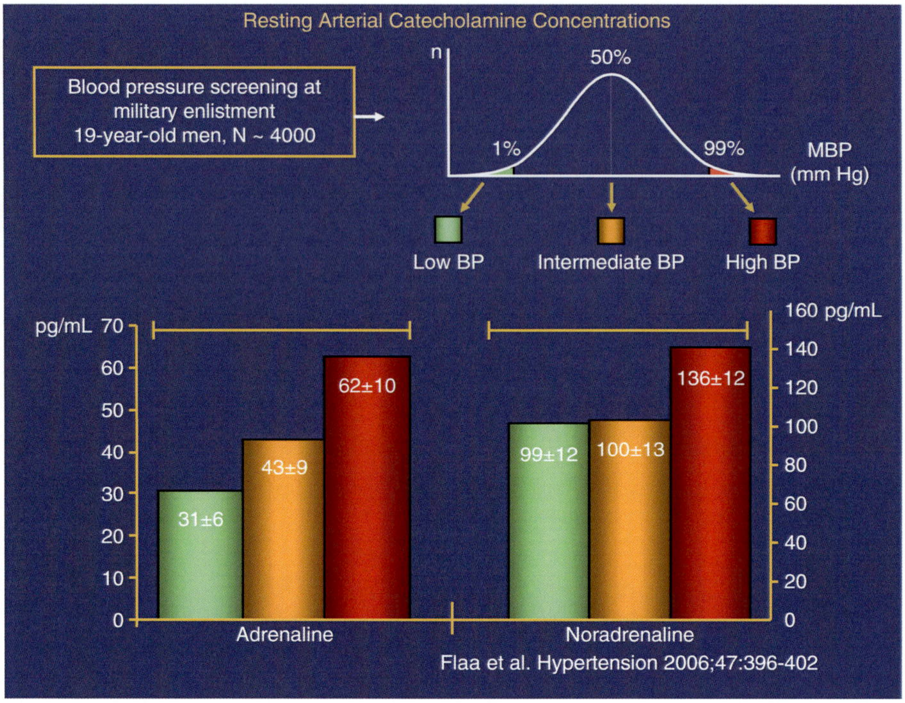

Fig. 33.8 Arterial plasma catecholamines in young men from 1st, 50th, and 99th percentiles of blood pressure at screening

33.4.3 Sympathoadrenal Reactivity as a Predictor of Future Body Fat

The adrenaline response to mental stress was negatively related to changes in BMI and waist circumference during the follow-up in univariate analyses [54]. In supplementary multiple regression analyses, the adrenaline response was a highly consistent negative predictor of future BMI, waist circumference, and triceps skinfold thickness after adjusting for exercise level and initial BMI, waist circumference, or triceps skinfold [54]. The noradrenaline response to mental stress was a weak positive predictor for future waist circumference, and did not significantly predict BMI and triceps skinfold thickness [54]. None of the other adrenaline or noradrenaline parameters during rest or cold pressor test were significantly related to changes in BMI, waist circumference, or triceps skinfold thickness (Fig. 33.10).

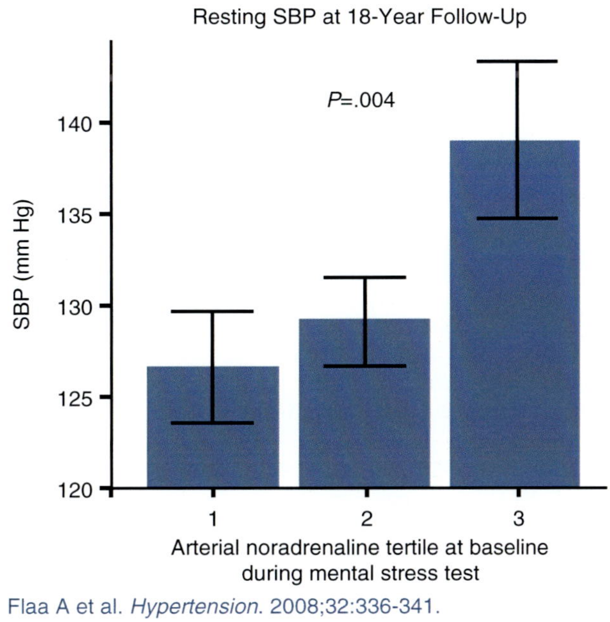

Fig. 33.9 Arterial plasma noradrenaline measured during mental stress test predicts systolic blood pressure at 18-year follow-up

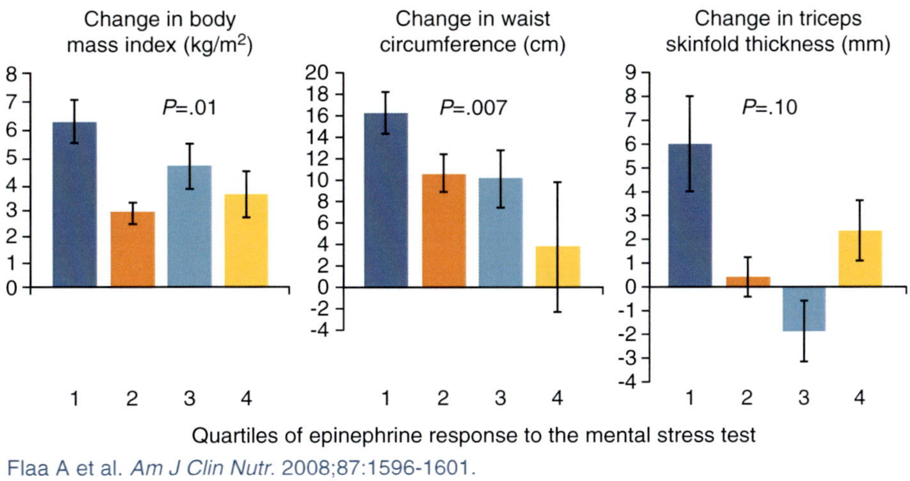

Fig. 33.10 Arterial plasma adrenaline measured during mental stress negatively predicts changes in body built at 18-year follow-up

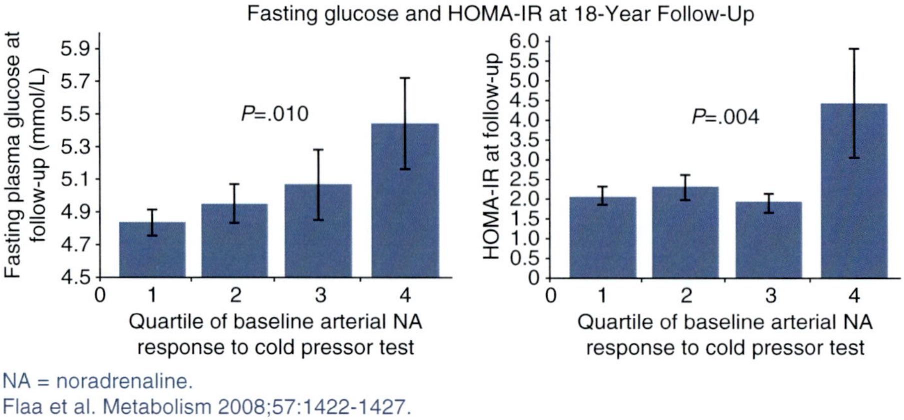

Fig. 33.11 Arterial plasma noradrenaline responses to cold pressor test predict glucose and HOMA-index at 18-year follow-up

33.4.4 Sympathoadrenal Reactivity as a Predictor of Future Insulin Resistance

The noradrenaline response to the cold pressor test was positively related to fasting plasma glucose and HOMA-IR at follow-up in univariate analyses [55]. In the multiple regression analyses, the noradrenaline response was an independent positive predictor of HOMA-IR [55]. There were no significant associations with plasma catecholamines at rest or during mental stress (Fig. 33.11).

33.5 Discussion

33.5.1 Methodological Aspects

33.5.1.1 Subjects

The participants were recruited from the military draft procedures in Oslo, securing a homogenous sample of subjects at the same age, race, and gender, thus reducing the biological and statistical variance. However, this advantage also implies a limited ability to generalize the present results to older subjects, other ethnicities and women.

We did not include a randomized sample from military screening, but rather a stratified selection which leads to an overrepresentation of subjects with extreme low and high blood pressure. However, we had a moderate sample size due to our resource demanding invasive examinations, and the blood pressure criteria ensured a satisfying dispersion of the blood pressure range, which makes it easier to demonstrate relationships.

The military blood pressure screening was based on one blood pressure recording in the sitting position after 5 min of rest. These measurements involve elements of both rest and stress, and are not fulfilling the normal guidelines on blood pressure measurements. It may be questioned whether one screening blood pressure value is representative for the subject's true blood pressure level, as current guidelines recommend several measurements taken over separate occasions over a period of time, due to spontaneous variations both during days and between days [63]. Nevertheless, blood pressure was determined according to the guidelines later in laboratory on the selected individuals, ensuring resting conditions.

We compared the three blood pressure groups on their response to the three different stress tests in a cross-sectional study [52]. The selection procedure (military enlistment) may be regarded as a psychological stress situation, raising the question whether subjects with high blood pressure were partly preselected to respond vigorously to the mental stress test. However, there is evidence that hypertension and high normal blood pressure are associated with increased cardiovascular and sympathoadrenal reactivity to mental stress compared to physical stress, such as orthostatic and cold pressor test [64]. The sample groups were rather small in this study ($n = 15$, 15 and 13 in the low (gr. 1), normal (gr. 2) and high blood pressure group (gr. 3), respectively), and the lack of significant findings during the cold pressor test and orthostatic test could be due to insufficient power. However, the statistical power to detect a similar difference during cold pressor test and orthostatic test as during mental stress test was above 80% for adrenaline, noradrenaline, mean blood pressure and heart rate between gr. 1 and 3, indicating sufficient sample sizes.

At follow-up [53–55], we were able to analyze 80 subjects of the original 99 at entry. This is a remarkably high attendance rate after so many years, and the fact that subjects not eligible for follow-up had similar resting blood pressure, heart rate, BMI, waist circumference, and catecholamine stress responses at entry as the 80 eligible subjects, decreases the risk of sample bias. Due to certain diseases among the subjects at follow-up, analyses and interpretations were performed with precautions. When examining development of blood pressure, we excluded five subjects using blood pressure lowering treatment. β-Blockers may affect body weight, but including this parameter in the analyses of weight development did not alter the results, and we chose to remove the variable from the final analyses as there were only three subjects using them. Regarding development of insulin resistance, some would possibly argue that the three subjects with type 2 diabetes should be excluded from the analyses. However, they represent a true and important part of the blood glucose distribution in the population. Furthermore, they took oral antidiabetics, and as none of them took insulin, HOMA-IR was a suitable measure of insulin resistance in these subjects.

According to the selection procedure at entry, we could have assessed the prevalence of the various risk factors at follow-up in the three original blood pressure groups. Even though there are close cross-sectional relationship between these groups and catecholamine levels as demonstrated [52], we chose to focus our attention on the cardiovascular and catecholamine parameters independently of the initial blood pressure groups, making it possible to study the various components of the sympathoadrenal system during rest and stress tests in more detail. Moreover, even though they originally represented three different groups of blood pressure at screening, their blood pressure showed a normal distribution when reexamined in laboratory due to the regression to the mean.

33.5.1.2 Reproducibility and Generalizability of Stress Tests

There are several methods available to test reactivity to stress, and to better standardize and measure reactivity certain laboratory stress tests have been developed. Test-retest reproducibility varies, but stability has been found to increase when the number of measurements during stress tests increases [65]. Due to continuous intra-arterial blood pressure and heart rate monitoring during the stress tests, we were able to perform more measurements and calculate the mean during each stress test. There are, however, no data available on reproducibility on catecholamine reactivity.

Another aspect is whether these tests performed in an artificial setting elicit responses which are in correspondence with real life stress. If individual differences in stress reactivity do not reflect stress responses outside the laboratory, they become less plausible as a cause of disease, although they may serve as a risk factor [66]. The literature on generalizability is inconsistent. Some have observed significant correlations between blood pressure reactions to mental stress tests and blood pressure variability during waking hours [67] and between systolic blood pressure response to cognitive tasks and waking and sleeping systolic blood pressure levels [68]. Others, on the other hand, have found only moderate relation between systolic and diastolic blood pressure reactions to several stressors and ambulatory systolic blood pressure [69]. One study found that type A and type B subjects differed in their heart rate and blood pressure responses to a cognitive task while there were no differences in the daily life [70]. van Doornen and van Blokland compared responses to two "active coping tasks" and a "passive coping task" (the cold pressor test) with the responses while anticipating a strong and well-defined stressor: the public defense of their PhD thesis [71]. They found that heart rate response to a reaction time task and the cold pressor test added significantly to the prediction of real life blood pressure levels and responses more than the prediction in the basis of pretask baselines. The clear relationship between screening blood pressure and response to the mental stress test [52] indicates that psychological stress in our laboratory elicit the same responses as a stress situation in real life like the military enlistment.

Duration of Stress Tests

One may speculate whether the duration of the cold pressor test and orthostatic test was too short to compare with 5 min mental stress. The cold pressor test lasted for 1 min in accordance with Hines and Brown, who introduced the test [61]. The peak response usually occurs within 30 s. Furthermore, an element of pain gradually dominates the test as the duration increases. Regarding the orthostatic test, Gehrking et al. have demonstrated a sensitivity of 88% for 1 min, and 99% for 2 min of head up tilt for detecting orthostatic hypotension [72]. All three stress tests had significant effects on blood pressure, heart rate, and catecholamines, indicating a satisfactory duration. Furthermore, the peak responses in heart rate, adrenaline and noradrenaline during mental stress were at 1 min. However, we cannot by certainty exclude group differences [52] if the cold pressor and orthostatic test had lasted longer.

33.5.1.3 Plasma Catecholamines as Measurements of Sympathoadrenal Activation

Plasma catecholamines are together with microneurography preferred tests for analyzing acute effects of stress tests on the sympathoadrenal system [73]. Arterial catecholamine measurements have previously been reported to be a more sensitive marker of overall sympathetic activity than venous sampling, and are superior to venous catecholamines in separating hypertensive and normotensive groups [24]. The sympathetic nervous system shows a differentiated activation pattern according to the situation, and there is uncertainty which part of the sympathetic nervous system may be the best determinant of weight development. Arterial samples reflect better the overall sympathetic activity including spillover from heart and kidney, while venous samples for a larger part reflect muscle sympathetic activity. Release from muscle sympathetic nerves contributes to approximately 50% of peripheral venous noradrenaline [74]. Thus, if sympathetic activity in muscle tissues is the most important determinant of future body fat, venous measurements would have been preferable, and could possibly explain the weak associations between noradrenaline activity and weight development compared to adrenaline that we found [54]. However, there are no indications that muscle sympathetic activity is crucial in this regard. Clinically, fat tends to deposit centrally and the sympathetic stimulation of visceral areas is better reflected through arterial sampling. Likewise, regarding the prediction of insulin resistance, venous samples could possibly have demonstrated an even better relationship between cold pressor responses and future insulin resistance than the findings of the present study, if one assumes that sympathetic activity to skeletal muscles is of most importance [55].

Regarding the adrenal medulla, arterial sampling is far better than venous when assessing the activity since about 50% of adrenaline is taken up by peripheral tissues. Arterial concentrations are thus higher and more precisely determined than venous (Fig. 33.12).

33.5.1.4 Insulin Resistance and Obesity

Insulin resistance was measured by HOMA-IR [55], in addition to fasting plasma glucose. HOMA-IR has been compared with the gold standard euglycemic hyperinsulinemic clamp, and was found to correlate in normal subjects ($r = 0.83, p < 0.01$) and even better in diabetic subjects ($r = 0.92, p < 0.0001$), indicating that HOMA-IR is valid also among diabetic subjects [58]. Unfortunately, at entry we only had information on fasting plasma glucose and were not able to determine HOMA-IR.

Traditionally, BMI has been used as a surrogate marker to assess the degree of obesity. Overweight and obesity is defined by the World Health Organization as BMI ≥ 25 and ≥ 30, respectively [75]. In recent years intra-abdominal adiposity, measured as waist circumference, has been shown to be an important risk factor for cardiovascular disease [76], and the health risk is increased compared to general obesity measured with BMI [77]. The third body fat parameter used [54] was triceps skinfold thickness, a measure of subcutaneous fat. Even though this examination is more dependent on the examiner than the two previous, we included all three parameters in our analyses in order to demonstrate the very consistent pattern of our findings.

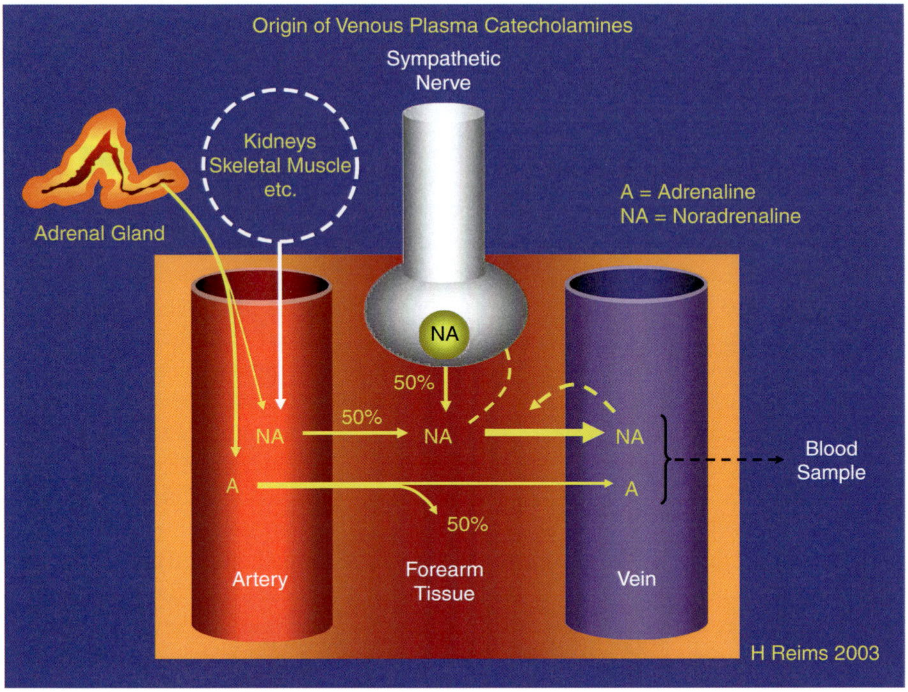

Fig. 33.12 Origin of plasma catecholamines; arterial concentrations represent a mixture of venous catecholamines effluents from all organs

33.5.1.5 Statistics

The major part of the statistical analyses [53–55] was based on parametric tests for normally distributed data. However, the subjects represented three separated groups representing significantly different blood pressures at military screening. One may thus question the use of linear regression analyses on this sample. It turned out, however, that the extreme blood pressure values at screening normalized when reexamined in the laboratory, probably due to regression to the mean. Resting systolic and diastolic blood pressure ended up as normally distributed, and we chose to analyze the sample as a continuous one.

A large number of statistical tests were performed mainly without any corrections for multiple testing, which may increase the risk of Type 1 error. However, the main purpose of the studies addressed a limited number of main hypotheses, and some of the additional statistical analyses were included in order to compare our studies with previous research. We used the Bonferroni correction on the univariate analyses [53]. We believe, however, that this procedure may have led to some Type 2 errors. As the significance level was very conservatively set to $p < 0.001$, several of the heart rate and catecholamine variables did not end up as significant predictors of future blood pressure, despite a consistent pattern between them.

33.5.2 Discussion of Results

33.5.2.1 Blood Pressure, Sympathoadrenal Activity, and Cardiovascular Risk Factors [52]

Due to a marked regression to the mean, there was in a previous study of ours a tendency that subjects with high screening blood pressure came close to normal when reexamined in laboratory [1]. To ensure differences in the resting blood pressure, the subjects underwent a second blood pressure examination, where we selected only the ones with extreme low and high blood pressure in addition to subjects with normal levels. Among these subjects, we found a clear relationship between resting blood pressure and arterial plasma catecholamine levels. Even though there are several reports of increased catecholamine levels in subjects with high blood pressure [78–81], this is the first study demonstrating an association between plasma catecholamines and blood pressure within the whole range of resting blood pressure, by showing that subjects with low blood pressure have decreased sympathetic tone compared to normotensives. While awareness of hypertension plays a role [30, 31, 56], it cannot explain the whole difference detected in cardiovascular and sympathoadrenal reactivity, as the associations demonstrated in our study were found in subjects unaware of their blood pressure status, indicating other explanations than mere awareness.

The original three screening groups showed a clear differentiation in cardiovascular and catecholamine responses to the mental stress test, in contrast to the cold pressor and orthostatic test where there were no such differences. There are several possible mechanisms explaining hyperreactivity to mental stress [60]: (1) Structural changes in the vascular wall or increased receptor sensitivity may amplify the pressor effect of catecholamines. However, one would have expected a similar hyperreactivity to the orthostatic and cold pressor test if vascular wall or receptor properties were the only explanation. (2) Hyperreactivity may be initiated in subcortical structures (hypothalamus and brain stem). The fact that we found differences not only in blood pressure and heart rate responses but also in catecholamine responses indicates a central origin. (3) The third option is mechanisms located in the cortical areas, as each subject has a different perception and reaction pattern. Some have described a "hypertensive personality," with a tendency to be submissive, to avoid confrontations and to suppress anger. We have previously demonstrated that stress reactivity is related to certain personality traits like muscular tension, irritability, and detachment [82].

The significant relationships between blood pressure and the cardiovascular risk factors triglycerides, HDL, HDL-total cholesterol ratio, fructosamine, and waist-hip ratio in our study demonstrate how blood pressure may represent a marker of other risk factors, even in young subjects below the age of 20. Likewise, the Tecumseh study showed a clear evidence of a worse cardiometabolic profile in young subjects with borderline hypertension compared to normotensives [83].

Thus, our data [52] suggests that resting blood pressure reflects both sympathetic activity and other cardiovascular risk factors. Furthermore, as high screening blood pressure also relates to mental stress responses, it is reasonable to question whether sympathoadrenal responses to mental stress are related to the development of cardiovascular risk factors.

33.5.2.2 Sympathoadrenal Activity and Development of Future Cardiovascular Risk Factors [53–55]

The subjects were reexamined in our laboratory 18 years after their first visit. It would have been of great interest to assess the predictive power of the initial catecholamine levels regarding future risk of angina pectoris, myocardial infarction, stroke, renal failure, diabetes, heart failure, and mortality, but as the mean age was 37 years at follow-up and organ damage often become evident at a later stage, we focused on elements of the metabolic syndrome, which may appear already at a young age. In addition to blood pressure, obesity, and insulin resistance, it would have been preferable to also present analyses on the association of future dyslipidemia, the last component of the metabolic syndrome [84]. However, due to the combination of nonsignificant results and insufficient power, we were not able to draw any firm conclusions.

Sympathoadrenal Activity During Rest Conditions Versus Stress Reactivity

Previous longitudinal studies have mainly examined resting plasma catecholamines [36, 38, 51] or urinary catecholamines [44] as predictors of future blood pressure, obesity, and insulin resistance. However, we did not find any significant associations during rest. One reason could be insufficient power, even though we had a larger sample size than two of the mentioned studies [36, 44]. Another possible explanation could be the different ethnicities represented in the various studies.

Anyhow, in contrast to these earlier studies, we found that catecholamines during stress were better predictors than the variables recorded at rest. Blood pressure at follow-up were markedly stronger related not only to catecholamine levels but also to blood pressure and heart rate during stress (especially mental stress) compared to rest [53]. Earlier findings have showed that casual office [85, 86] and ambulatory blood pressures [63, 87] are stronger predictors than the recommended standardized office measurements after several minutes of rest [28, 88], and measurements performed during situations involving elements of stress activation may be more useful as predictors of future blood pressure than standardized resting measurements [89, 90]. As for the prediction of weight gain [54] and insulin resistance [55], the strongest predictors were adrenaline response during mental stress and noradrenaline during cold pressor test, respectively.

The apparent importance of stress tests may be explained by the excellent ability to detect certain characteristics among subjects at risk, due to the special properties of the various tests. As an example, regarding weight development [54], mental stress is known to induce a more pronounced adrenaline release than the cold pressor test [60] and exerts its effects mainly through activation of β-receptors [48]. Thus, the association between mental stress reactivity and prediction of weight gain may indicate that reduced stimulation of β-adrenergic receptors plays an important role in the development of obesity. A low adrenaline response to mental stress in the laboratory possibly also reflects lower adrenaline reactivity during everyday life, including stressful daily activities, thus favoring less β-receptor stimulation and a lower metabolic turnover and subsequent weight gain. The cold pressor test, on the other hand, seems more appropriate in predicting future insulin resistance [55], as this test predominantly acts by increasing the sympathetic activity to peripheral arterioles in skeletal muscles and skin. Thus, subjects characterized by elevated sympathetic activity to these organs with subsequent vasoconstriction may develop insulin resistance through reduced glucose uptake in skeletal muscles [91].

The choice of stress test may also be important in predicting hypertension. A large proportion of young subjects prone to develop hypertension are characterized by a hyperkinetic circulation [29, 35]. Later, there is a transition from this early stage of hypertension development with increased cardiac output and nearly normal total peripheral resistance, to the later stage characterized by normalization of the cardiac output and increased total peripheral resistance [32, 60]. We found that responses to mental stress, which are predominantly β-mediated, may be better predictors than responses to the cold pressor test in our young cohort. Using the cold pressor test in longitudinal hypertension studies may be suboptimal in young subjects, as it elicits an α-adrenergic vascular response more than and a β-adrenergically mediated myocardial response [34, 92], and many of these young subjects prone to develop hypertension are characterized by the hyperkinetic circulation mediated by β-adrenergic receptors.

In contrast to studies on obesity and insulin resistance, much attention has been paid to stress testing and prediction of future development of hypertension in longitudinal studies. The reactivity hypothesis states that subjects characterized by elevated stress reactivity show increased cardiovascular risk [93]. One theory is that intermittent pressure elevations may lead to structural vascular changes, but attempts to produce irreversible, sustained blood pressure elevations purely as a consequence of transient elevations in dogs have not succeeded [94, 95]. Another possible link between hyperreactivity and development of hypertension is the direct effect of the catecholamines. Sympathetic stimulation has proven to be a trophic factor for vascular hypertrophy [96]. Thus, hyperreactive subjects with increased surges of catecholamine concentrations in the plasma may develop hypertrophy of smooth muscles in arterioles and increased total peripheral resistance, the hallmark of established essential hypertension [97].

Cause or Consequence of Increased Sympathoadrenal Activity?

The relationship between the individual components of the metabolic syndrome is complex, and to establish cause and effect in this enmeshed web is extremely difficult. As mentioned, most of the literature on associations between sympathoadrenal activity and blood pressure, obesity, and insulin resistance are based on cross-sectional studies, and long-term follow-up studies are preferable when exploring cause-and-effect relationships. However, it is important to emphasize that even though we have demonstrated that sympathoadrenal reactivity predicts certain features of the metabolic syndrome after 18 years, this is not evidence of a causal role in the development. Our findings only indicate in what order the events happen, and that there are significant associations between them. These associations could be explained by other unknown correlated factors. Another limitation is that we did not have plasma insulin measurements at entry [55], making it difficult to decide whether hyperreactive subjects at entry already had developed insulin resistance. Despite these limitations, the fact that the relationships remain significant after adjusting for several possible predictors strengthens the role of the sympathoadrenal system as a determinant of future blood pressure, obesity, and insulin resistance.

Apparently, some of the present findings may represent a paradox. Increased sympathoadrenal activity predispose to insulin resistance [55]. On the other hand, development of obesity seems to be related to a reduced activity in the adrenal medulla [54]. However, the association between obesity and insulin resistance has been known for many years, and these two cardiovascular risk factors are probably reinforcing each other [98]. Wouldn't it then be plausible that increased sympathoadrenal activity lead to both insulin resistance *and* obesity? It is important to note that adrenal medullary activity and overall sympathetic activity may show reciprocal alterations [8], and we believe that our findings are compatible with prior knowledge: reduced activity in the adrenal medulla may predict the development of obesity, with subsequent increase in sympathetic activity and development of insulin resistance (Fig. 33.4). It should be mentioned that noradrenaline tended to be a positive predictor of weight gain in the multiple regression analyses in our study [54], perhaps suggesting a more early role of obesity development than suggested in Figs. 33.4 and 33.13.

The Sympathoadrenal System and Blood Pressure [53]
The positive relationship in the present long-term study between plasma noradrenaline concentration during mental stress at entry and systolic blood pressure at follow-up independent of the initial blood pressure level strongly supports an important role of increased sympathetic nervous activity in early development of hypertension [29]. One may question the importance of our finding as the univariate correlation analyses of future blood pressure showed a much stronger relationship with blood pressure at entry compared to the catecholamine levels at entry in general. However,

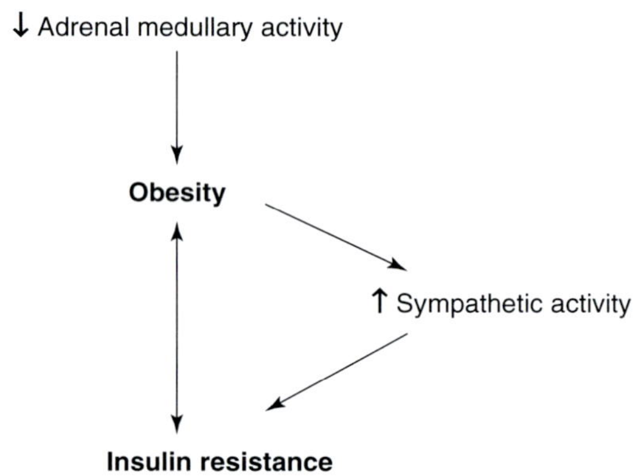

Fig. 33.13 Potential relation between adrenal medullary activity and metabolism

as shown in the multiple regression analyses, catecholamine levels may explain a remarkable high portion of the variance of future blood pressure after correcting for initial blood pressure and other known risk factors. Moreover, catecholamines after all are very indirect measures of true sympathoadrenal activity, thus one cannot expect too much from the analyses.

The catecholamines during mental stress seemed to have more importance in predicting future systolic blood pressure than diastolic blood pressure in the univariate analyses. This may be due to the fact that the β-adrenergic stimulation elicited by the mental stress test mostly affects the cardiac output and the systolic blood pressure, in contrast to diastolic blood pressure which is more affected by total peripheral resistance and plasma volume. However, since there are certain overlaps in confidence intervals of the correlation coefficients, we should be cautious to draw conclusions.

The underlying pathogenic mechanism behind the possible causal role of the sympathoadrenal activity may be that increased sympathoadrenal activity stimulates arteriolar remodeling, increasing the wall-to-lumen ratio, and thereby elevate the total peripheral resistance [99, 100]. Additionally, raised sympathetic activity is known to increase the blood viscosity [101], which again affects the peripheral resistance. Finally, elevated sympathetic tone to the kidneys will stimulate renin secretion, leading to the synthesis of angiotensin II and thereby promoting renal tubular reabsorption of sodium [11].

The Sympathoadrenal System and Obesity [54]

There is a clear relationship between obesity and the sympathoadrenal system. However, as mentioned earlier, the identification of cause and effect between the two of them is very difficult. Findings are heterogeneous, but a normal to high level of sympathetic activity is mostly seen in obesity [40]. Landsberg proposed that increased sympathetic activation and hypertension seen in obese subjects may be a consequence of insulin resistance and hyperinsulinemia [47]. On the other hand, *increased* sympathetic activity is shown to reduce β-adrenergic sensitivity [102, 103], thereby being a potential cause of obesity as hypothesized by Julius [104]. Representing a third option, there are reports suggesting the contrary, that *reduced* sympathoadrenal activity may be the predisposing factor. These apparently contradicting theories are confusing. However, our data [54] suggests that reduced activity only in the adrenal medulla may lead to increased weight, and this weight gain may perhaps then trigger a subsequent activation of the sympathetic nervous system (Fig. 33.4). In a setting with increased sympathetic tone, the β-responsiveness may decrease, leading to further weight gain and blood pressure elevation [104–106]. Reims et al. have previously found that BMI and waist circumference in borderline hypertensive subjects are independently associated with lower adrenaline levels [27]. Thus, as activity in the adrenal medulla and sympathetic nervous system reflect related but distinctive aspects of autonomic functions, they may act in a reciprocal manner regarding weight development.

The Sympathoadrenal System and Insulin Resistance [55]

Insulin resistance may be perhaps the most important feature of the metabolic syndrome. In obese subjects, insulin resistance is by many authors believed to result from increased fat mass [15]. The question remains, however, what causes insulin resistance in lean subjects. There are of course many factors involved, including genetic susceptibility and lifestyle. Some believe that a possible underlying determinant is the sympathetic nervous system [2, 107]. Previous cross-sectional studies in our group have shown positive relationships between insulin resistance and plasma catecholamine levels and heart rate [108].

Insulin resistance is inversely related to the number of open capillaries [49], and our finding thus supports the hemodynamic hypothesis of Julius et al., stating that pressure-induced restriction of the microcirculation limits nutritional flow and thereby impairs glucose uptake in the skeletal muscle [109], which is the major site of insulin resistance [110]. Furthermore, a previous study found a direct relationship between the number of sympathetic neural bursts to skeletal muscle tissue and HOMA-IR [111].

There are other possible mechanisms that may also explain how sympathetic overactivity could lead to insulin resistance. Catecholamines have a direct effect on the insulin action (not the secretion), thereby inhibiting the glucose uptake [112]. Moreover, β-adrenergic stimulation of skeletal muscle may promote a change to a higher proportion of poorly capillarized and insulin-resistant fast fibers [113]. Another possibility is that α-adrenergic vasoconstriction may contribute to raised hematocrit and whole blood viscosity [114, 115], thereby leading to increased peripheral vascular resistance and reduced nutritional flow [16, 17].

Long-Term Stability of Responses to the Stress Tests

Cardiovascular hyperreactivity to stress must be reasonably stable if it is considered to be important in the development of hypertension and cardiovascular disease. We also investigated long-term stability of blood pressure, heart rate, adrenaline, and noradrenaline responses to a cold pressor test and a mental arithmetic stress test (n = 81, two occasions 18 years apart) [116]. The 18-year correlations of the cardiovascular and adrenaline absolute responses during mental stress ranged from 0.6 to 0.8. The entry/follow-up correlation of systolic blood pressure during the mental stress test (95% CI: 0.69 to 0.86) was significantly higher than during the cold pressor test (95% CI: 0.30 to 0.65), and responses to mental stress overall appeared to be more stable than responses to the cold pressor test. Our study suggested that cardiovascular and sympathoadrenal reactivity, specifically to mental stress, are relatively stable individual characteristics. These results support one of the necessary preconditions to consider hyperreactivity involved in the development of hypertension and cardiovascular disease (Fig. 33.14).

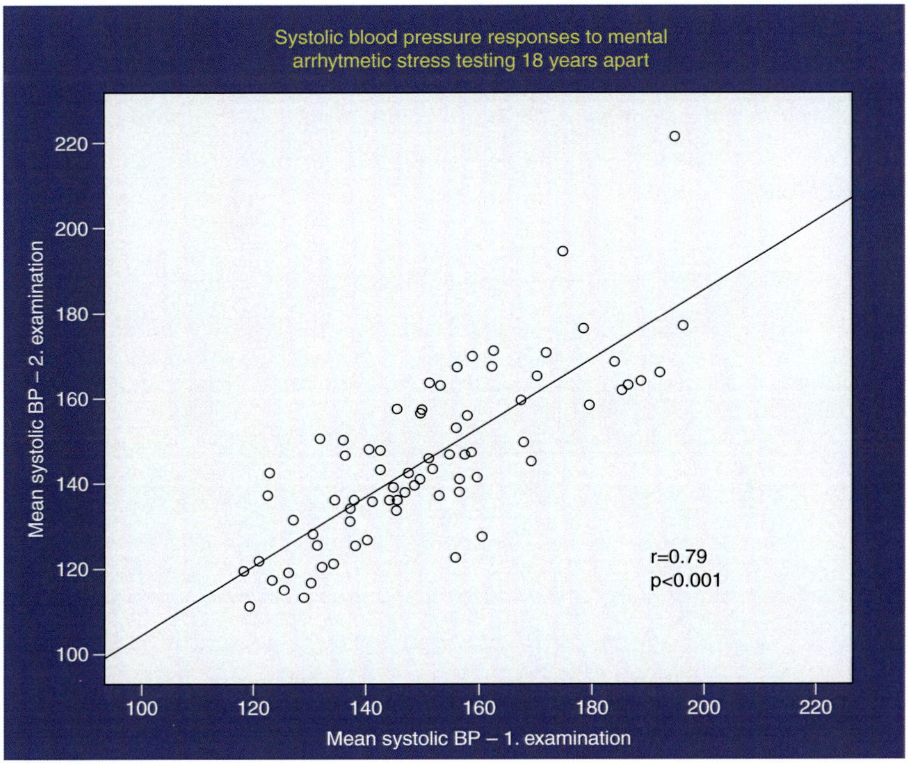

Fig. 33.14 Correlation between systolic blood pressures measured during mental arithmetic stress 18 years apart

Conclusions

We found that resting blood pressure was related to arterial plasma catecholamines, cardiovascular and sympathetic reactivity, and cardiovascular risk factors in a cross-sectional study in young men with low, normal, and high blood pressure who were unaware of their blood pressure status [52].

In a follow-up study over 18 years, initial sympathoadrenal reactivity to stress at the age of 19 was related to the development of future blood pressure [53], body fat [54], and indices of insulin resistance [55]. The responses to the cold pressor test and the mental stress test seemed to have different predictive impact on the development of these risk factors.

Partly due to resource-demanding procedures, there are little available data regarding the effect of the sympathoadrenal system on development of established cardiovascular morbidity and future mortality in follow-up studies. Blood pressure, heart rate, obesity, and insulin resistance, on the other hand, are well-known risk factors for cardiovascular diseases like stroke, coronary artery disease, heart failure, and peripheral vascular disease.

Acknowledgments This chapter is based on the PhD thesis that Arnljot Flaa, MD, defended at the University of Oslo in 2009. Though shortened the structure of the thesis has been maintained.

Conflict of interest: S.E. Kjeldsen reports modest honoraria from ABDiiBRAHiM, Bayer, MSD and Takeda. The other authors report no conflicts.

References

1. Rostrup M, Westheim A, Kjeldsen SE, Eide I. Cardiovascular reactivity, coronary risk factors, and sympathetic activity in young men. Hypertension. 1993;22(6):891–9.
2. Moan A, Nordby G, Rostrup M, Eide I, Kjeldsen SE. Insulin sensitivity, sympathetic activity, and cardiovascular reactivity in young men. Am J Hypertens. 1995;8(3):268–75.
3. Fossum E, Hoieggen A, Moan A, Rostrup M, Nordby G, Kjeldsen SE. Relationship between insulin sensitivity and maximal forearm blood flow in young men. Hypertension. 1998;32(5):838–43.
4. Shields RW Jr. Functional anatomy of the autonomic nervous system. J Clin Neurophysiol. 1993;10(1):2–13.
5. Goldstein DS. Peripheral catecholaminergic systems. Stress, catecholamines, and cardiovascular disease. New York: Oxford University Press; 1995. p. 103–63.
6. Lipworth BJ. Clinical pharmacology of beta 3-adrenoceptors. Br J Clin Pharmacol. 1996;42(3):291–300.
7. Gauthier C, Seze-Goismier C, Rozec B. Beta 3-adrenoceptors in the cardiovascular system. Clin Hemorheol Microcirc. 2007;37(1–2):193–204.
8. Young JB, Rosa RM, Landsberg L. Dissociation of sympathetic nervous system and adrenal medullary responses. Am J Phys. 1984;247(1 Pt 1):E35–40.
9. Levy RL, White PD, Stroud WD, Hillman CC. Transient tachycardia. Prognostic significance alone and in association with transient hypertension. JAMA. 1945;129(9):585–8.
10. Levy RL, Hillman CC, Stroud WD, White PD. Transient hypertension. Its significance in terms of later development of sustained hypertension and cardiovascular-renal diseases. JAMA. 1944;126(13):829–33.
11. Grassi G, Vailati S, Bertinieri G, et al. Heart rate as marker of sympathetic activity. J Hypertens. 1998;16(11):1635–9.
12. Seals DR, Dinenno FA. Collateral damage: cardiovascular consequences of chronic sympathetic activation with human aging. Am J Physiol Heart Circ Physiol. 2004;287(5):H1895–905.
13. Ernsberger P, Koletsky RJ, Friedman JE. Contribution of sympathetic nervous system overactivity to cardiovascular and metabolic disease. Rev Contemp Pharmacother. 1998;9(7):411–28.
14. Lakka HM, Laaksonen DE, Lakka TA, et al. The metabolic syndrome and total and cardiovascular disease mortality in middle-aged men. JAMA. 2002;288(21):2709–16.
15. Mancia G, Bousquet P, Elghozi JL, et al. The sympathetic nervous system and the metabolic syndrome. J Hypertens. 2007;25(5):909–20.
16. Expert Panel on Detection, Evaluation, and Treatment of High Blood Cholesterol in Adults. Executive summary of the third report of the National Cholesterol Education Program (NCEP) expert panel on detection, evaluation, and treatment of high blood cholesterol in adults (adult treatment panel III). JAMA. 2001;285(19):2486–97.
17. Alberti KGM, Zimmet P, Shaw J. The metabolic syndrome--a new worldwide definition. Lancet. 2005;366(9491):1059–62.
18. Esposito K, Giugliano D. The metabolic syndrome and inflammation: association or causation? Nutr Metab Cardiovasc Dis. 2004;14(5):228–32.
19. Siani A, Strazzullo P. Tackling the genetic bases of metabolic syndrome: a realistic objective? Nutr Metab Cardiovasc Dis. 2006;16(5):309–12.
20. Ritchie SA, Connell JM. The link between abdominal obesity, metabolic syndrome and cardiovascular disease. Nutr Metab Cardiovasc Dis. 2007;17(4):319–26.

21. Grassi G. Sympathetic overdrive and cardiovascular risk in the metabolic syndrome. Hypertens Res. 2006;29(11):839–47.
22. Grassi G, Quarti-Trevano F, Seravalle G, Dell'Oro R. Cardiovascular risk and adrenergic overdrive in the metabolic syndrome. Nutr Metab Cardiovasc Dis. 2007;17(6):473–81.
23. Beevers G, Lip GYH, O'Brien E. ABC of hypertension: the pathophysiology of hypertension. BMJ. 2001;322(7291):912–6.
24. Kjeldsen SE, Flaaten B, Eide I, Helgeland A, Leren P. Evidence of increased peripheral catecholamine release in patients with long-standing, untreated essential hypertension. Scand J Clin Lab Invest. 1982;42(3):217–23.
25. de Champlain J, Petrovich M, Gonzalez M, Lebeau R, Nadeau R. Abnormal cardiovascular reactivity in borderline and mild essential hypertension. Hypertension. 1991;17(4 Suppl):III22–8.
26. Kjeldsen SE, Zweifler AJ, Petrin J, Weder AB, Julius S. Sympathetic nervous system involvement in essential hypertension: increased platelet noradrenaline coincides with decreased beta-adrenoreceptor responsiveness. Blood Press. 1994;3(3):164–71.
27. Reims HM, Fossum E, Hoieggen A, Moan A, Eide I, Kjeldsen SE. Adrenal medullary overactivity in lean, borderline hypertensive young men. Am J Hypertens. 2004;17(7):611–8.
28. Julius S, Majahalme S. The changing face of sympathetic overactivity in hypertension. Ann Med. 2000;32(5):365–70.
29. Lund-Johansen P. Hemodynamic concepts of hypertension: cardiac output versus peripheral vascular resistance. In: Birkenhager WH, Robertson JIS, Zanchetti A, editors. Handbook of hypertension, Hypertension in the twentieth century: concepts and achievements, vol. 22. Amsterdam: Elsevier; 2004. p. 151–72.
30. Rostrup M, Kjeldsen SE, Eide IK. Awareness of hypertension increases blood pressure and sympathetic responses to cold pressor test. Am J Hypertens. 1990;3(12Pt1):912–7.
31. Rostrup M, Mundal HH, Westheim A, Eide I. Awareness of high blood pressure increases arterial plasma catecholamines, platelet noradrenaline and adrenergic responses to mental stress. J Hypertens. 1991;9(2):159–66.
32. Rostrup M, Ekeberg O. Awareness of high blood pressure influences on psychological and sympathetic responses. J Psychosom Res. 1992;36(2):117–23.
33. Cowley AW Jr. The concept of autoregulation of total blood flow and its role in hypertension. Am J Med. 1980;68(6):906–16.
34. Folkow B. Physiological aspects of primary hypertension. Physiol Rev. 1982;62(2):347–504.
35. Julius S. Transition from high cardiac output to elevated vascular resistance in hypertension. Am Heart J. 1988;116(2 Pt 2):600–6.
36. Bohm RO, van Baak MA, van Hooff ME, Mooy J, Rahn KH. A long-term study of plasma catecholamine levels and plasma renin activity in borderline hypertension. J Hypertens. 1987;5(6):655–61.
37. Perini C, Muller FB, Buhler FR. Suppressed aggression accelerates early development of essential hypertension. J Hypertens. 1991;9(6):499–503.
38. Masuo K, Kawaguchi H, Mikami H, Ogihara T, Tuck ML. Serum uric acid and plasma norepinephrine concentrations predict subsequent weight gain and blood pressure elevation. Hypertension. 2003;42(4):474–80.
39. Lefebvre PJ, Scheen AJ. Obesity: causes and new treatments. Exp Clin Endocrinol Diabetes. 2001;109(Suppl 2):S215–24.
40. Baak MA. The peripheral sympathetic nervous system in human obesity. Obes Rev. 2001;2(1):3–14.
41. Masuo K, Katsuya T, Fu Y, Rakugi H, Ogihara T, Tuck ML. Beta2- and beta3-adrenergic receptor polymorphisms are related to the onset of weight gain and blood pressure elevation over 5 years. Circulation. 2005;111(25):3429–34.
42. Eikelis N, Esler M. The neurobiology of human obesity. Exp Physiol. 2005;90(5):673–82.
43. Tentolouris N, Liatis S, Katsilambros N. Sympathetic system activity in obesity and metabolic syndrome. Ann N Y Acad Sci. 2006;1083:129–52.

44. Tataranni PA, Young JB, Bogardus C, Ravussin E. A low sympathoadrenal activity is associated with body weight gain and development of central adiposity in Pima Indian men. Obes Res. 1997;5(4):341–7.
45. Young JB, Landsberg L. Stimulation of the sympathetic nervous system during sucrose feeding. Nature. 1977;269(5629):615–7.
46. Landsberg L. Role of the sympathetic adrenal system in the pathogenesis of the insulin resistance syndrome. Ann N Y Acad Sci. 1999;892:84–90.
47. Landsberg L. Diet, obesity and hypertension: an hypothesis involving insulin, the sympathetic nervous system, and adaptive thermogenesis. QJM. 1986;61(3):1081–90.
48. Reaven GM, Lithell H, Landsberg L. Hypertension and associated metabolic abnormalities--the role of insulin resistance and the sympathoadrenal system. N Engl J Med. 1996;334(6):374–81.
49. Julius S, Gudbrandsson T, Jamerson K, Tariq SS, Andersson O. The hemodynamic link between insulin resistance and hypertension. J Hypertens. 1991;9(11):983–6.
50. Kaaja RJ, Poyhonen-Alho MK. Insulin resistance and sympathetic overactivity in women. J Hypertens. 2006;24(1):131–41.
51. Masuo K, Mikami H, Ogihara T, Tuck ML. Sympathetic nerve hyperactivity precedes hyperinsulinemia and blood pressure elevation in a young, nonobese Japanese population. Am J Hypertens. 1997;10(1):77–83.
52. Flaa A, Mundal HH, Eide IK, Kjeldsen SE, Rostrup M. Sympathetic activity and cardiovascular risk factors in young men in the low, normal, and high blood pressure ranges. Hypertension. 2006;47(3):396–402.
53. Flaa A, Kjeldsen SE, Eide IK, Rostrup M. Sympathoadrenal stress reactivity is a predictor of future blood pressure – an 18-year follow-up study. Hypertension. 2008;52(2):336–41.
54. Flaa A, Sandvik L, Kjeldsen SE, Eide IK, Rostrup M. Does sympathoadrenal activity predict changes in body fat? – An 18-year follow-up study. Am J Clin Nutr. 2008;87(6):1596–601.
55. Flaa A, Aksnes TA, Kjeldsen SE, Eide IK, Rostrup M. Increased sympathetic reactivity may predict insulin resistance – An 18-year follow-up study. Metabolism. 2008;57(10):1422–7.
56. Passon PG, Peuler JD. A simplified radioenzymatic assay for plasma norepinephrine and epinephrine. Anal Biochem. 1973;51:618–31.
57. Peuler JD, Johnson GA. Simultaneous single isotope radioenzymatic assay of plasma norepinephrine, epinephrine and dopamine. Life Sci. 1977;21(5):625–36.
58. Matthews DR, Hosker JP, Rudenski AS, Naylor BA, Treacher DF, Turner RC. Homeostasis model assessment: insulin resistance and beta-cell function from fasting plasma glucose and insulin concentrations in man. Diabetologia. 1985;28(7):412–9.
59. Brod J, FENCL V, HEJL Z, JIRKA J. Circulatory changes underlying blood pressure elevation during acute emotional stress (mental arithmetic) in normotensive and hypertensive subjects. Clin Sci. 1959;18:269–79.
60. Pickering TG, Gerin W. Area review: blood pressure reactivity: cardiovascular reactivity in the laboratory and the role of behavioral factors in hypertension: a critical review. Ann Behav Med. 1990;12(1):3–16.
61. Hines EA, Brown GE. A standard stimulus for measuring vasomotor reactions: its application in the study of hypertension. Mayo Clin Proc. 1932;7:332–5.
62. Hohnloser SH, Klingenheben T. Basic autonomic tests. In: Malik M, editor. Clinical guide to cardiac autonomic tests. Dordrecht: Kleuwer Academic Publishers; 1998. p. 51–65.
63. Mancia G, De Backer G, Dominiczak A, et al. Guidelines for the Management of Arterial Hypertension: the task force for the Management of Arterial Hypertension of the European Society of Hypertension (ESH) and of the European Society of Cardiology (ESC). J Hypertens. 2007;25(6):1105–87.
64. Eliasson K, Hjemdahl P, Kahan T. Circulatory and sympatho-adrenal responses to stress in borderline and established hypertension. J Hypertens. 1983;1(2):131–9.
65. Swain A, Suls J. Reproducibility of blood pressure and heart rate reactivity: a meta-analysis. Psychophysiology. 1996;33(2):162–74.

66. Kamarck TW, Lovallo WR. Cardiovascular reactivity to psychological challenge: conceptual and measurement considerations. Psychosom Med. 2003;65(1):9–21.
67. Floras JS, Hassan MO, Jones JV, Sleight P. Pressor responses to laboratory stresses and daytime blood pressure variability. J Hypertens. 1987;5(6):715–9.
68. Southard DR, Coates TJ, Kolodner K, Parker FC, Padgett NE, Kennedy HL. Relationship between mood and blood pressure in the natural environment: an adolescent population. Health Psychol. 1986;5(5):469–80.
69. Van Egeren LF, Sparrow AW. Laboratory stress testing to assess real-life cardiovascular reactivity. Psychosom Med. 1989;51(1):1–9.
70. Schneider RH, Julius S, Karunas R. Ambulatory blood pressure monitoring and laboratory reactivity in type A behavior and components. Psychosom Med. 1989;51(3):290–305.
71. van Doornen LJ, van Blokland RW. The relationship between cardiovascular and catecholamine reactions to laboratory and real-life stress. Psychophysiology. 1992;29(2):173–81.
72. Gehrking JA, Hines SM, Benrud-Larson LM, Opher-Gehrking TL, Low PA. What is the minimum duration of head-up tilt necessary to detect orthostatic hypotension? Clin Auton Res. 2005;15(2):71–5.
73. Grassi G, Seravalle G, Bolla G, et al. Heart rate as a sympathetic marker during acute adrenergic challenge. J Hypertens. 2008;26(1):70–5.
74. Kjeldsen SE, Schork NJ, Leren P, Eide IK. Arterial plasma norepinephrine correlates to blood pressure in middle-aged men with sustained essential hypertension. Am Heart J. 1989;118(4):775–81.
75. James PT, Leach R, Kalamara E, Shayeghi M. The worldwide obesity epidemic. Obes Res. 2001;9(Suppl 4):228S–33S.
76. Misra A, Vikram NK. Clinical and pathophysiological consequences of abdominal adiposity and abdominal adipose tissue depots. Nutrition. 2003;19(5):457–66.
77. Yusuf S, Hawken S, Ounpuu S, et al. Obesity and the risk of myocardial infarction in 27,000 participants from 52 countries: a case-control study. Lancet. 2005;366(9497):1640–9.
78. Clausen JO, Ibsen H, Dige-Petersen H, Borch-Johnsen K, Pedersen O. The importance of adrenaline, insulin and insulin sensitivity as determinants for blood pressure in young Danes. J Hypertens. 1995;13(5):499–505.
79. Julius S. The evidence for a pathophysiologic significance of the sympathetic overactivity in hypertension. Clin Exp Hypertens. 1996;18(3–4):305–21.
80. Mancia G. Bjorn Folkow Award Lecture. The sympathetic nervous system in hypertension. J Hypertens. 1997;15(12 Pt 2):1553–65.
81. Fossum E, Hoieggen A, Reims HM, et al. High screening blood pressure is related to sympathetic nervous system activity and insulin resistance in healthy young men. Blood Press. 2004;13(2):89–94.
82. Flaa A, Ekeberg O, Kjeldsen SE, Rostrup M. Personality may influence reactivity to stress. Biopsychosoc Med. 2007;1:5.
83. Julius S, Jamerson K, Mejia A, Krause L, Schork N, Jones K. The association of borderline hypertension with target organ changes and higher coronary risk. Tecumseh Blood Pressure study. JAMA. 1990;264(3):354–8.
84. LeBlanc J, Cote J, Jobin M, Labrie A. Plasma catecholamines and cardiovascular responses to cold and mental activity. J Appl Physiol. 1979;47(6):1207–11.
85. Georgiades A, de Faire U, Lemne C. Clinical prediction of normotension in borderline hypertensive men--a 10 year study. J Hypertens. 2004;22(3):471–8.
86. Jokiniitty JM, Majahalme SK, Kahonen MA, Tuomisto MT, Turjanmaa VM. Prediction of blood pressure level and need for antihypertensive medication: 10 years of follow-up. J Hypertens. 2001;19(7):1193–201.
87. Chobanian AV, Bakris GL, Black HR, et al. Seventh report of the Joint National Committee on prevention, detection, evaluation, and treatment of high blood pressure. Hypertension. 2003;42(6):1206–52.
88. Thomas CB, Duszynski KR. Blood pressure levels in young adulthood as predictors of hypertension and the fate of the cold pressor test. Johns Hopkins Med J. 1982;151(3):93–100.

89. Lovallo WR, Gerin W. Psychophysiological reactivity: mechanisms and pathways to cardiovascular disease. Psychosom Med. 2003;65(1):36–45.
90. Gudmundsdottir H, Strand A, Hoieggen A, et al. Do screening blood pressure and plasma catecholamines predict development of hypertension? Twenty-year follow-up of middle-aged men. Blood Press. 2008;17(2):94–103.
91. Egan BM. Neurohumoral, hemodynamic and microvascular changes as mechanisms of insulin resistance in hypertension: a provocative but partial picture. Int J Obes. 1991;15(Suppl 2):133–9.
92. Mancia G, Grassi G, Giannattasio C, Seravalle G. Sympathetic activation in the pathogenesis of hypertension and progression of organ damage. Hypertension. 1999;34(4 Pt 2):724–8.
93. Treiber FA, Kamarck T, Schneiderman N, Sheffield D, Kapuku G, Taylor T. Cardiovascular reactivity and development of preclinical and clinical disease states. Psychosom Med. 2003;65(1):46–62.
94. Julius S, Li Y, Brant D, Krause L, Buda AJ. Neurogenic pressor episodes fail to cause hypertension, but do induce cardiac hypertrophy. Hypertension. 1989;13(5):422–9.
95. Anderson DE, Kearns WD, Better WE. Progressive hypertension in dogs by avoidance conditioning and saline infusion. Hypertension. 1983;5(3):286–91.
96. Folkow B. Pathophysiology of hypertension: differences between young and elderly. J Hypertens Suppl. 1993;11(4):S21–4.
97. Rahn KH, Barenbrock M, Hausberg M. The sympathetic nervous system in the pathogenesis of hypertension. J Hypertens Suppl. 1999;17(3):S11–4.
98. Kahn BB, Flier JS. Obesity and insulin resistance. J Clin Invest. 2000;106(4):473–81.
99. Ross AE, Flaa A, Hoieggen A, Reims H, Eide IK, Kjeldsen SE. Gender specific sympathetic and hemorrheological responses to mental stress in healthy young subjects. Scand Cardiovasc J. 2001;35(5):307–12.
100. Reims HM, Sevre K, Hoieggen A, Fossum E, Eide I, Kjeldsen SE. Blood viscosity: effects of mental stress and relations to autonomic nervous system function and insulin sensitivity. Blood Press. 2005;14(3):159–69.
101. Esler M, Lambert G, Brunner-La Rocca HP, Vaddadi G, Kaye D. Sympathetic nerve activity and neurotransmitter release in humans: translation from pathophysiology into clinical practice. Acta Physiol Scand. 2003;177(3):275–84.
102. Lohse MJ. Molecular mechanisms of membrane receptor desensitization. Biochim Biophys Acta. 1993;1179(2):171–88.
103. Hausdorff WP, Caron MG, Lefkowitz RJ. Turning off the signal: desensitization of beta-adrenergic receptor function. FASEB J. 1990;4(11):2881–9.
104. Julius S, Valentini M, Palatini P. Overweight and hypertension: A 2-way street? Hypertension. 2000;35(3):807–13.
105. Seals DR, Bell C. Chronic sympathetic activation: consequence and cause of age-associated obesity? Diabetes. 2004;53(2):276–84.
106. Shibao C, Gamboa A, Diedrich A, et al. Autonomic contribution to blood pressure and metabolism in obesity. Hypertension. 2007;49(1):27–33.
107. Reims HM, Hoieggen A, Fossum E, Rostrup M, Eide I, Kjeldsen SE. Glucose disposal rates calculated from 60- to 90-minute isoglycemic hyperinsulinemic glucose clamp correlate with cardiovascular risk factors in borderline hypertensive young men. Metabolism. 2001;50(10):1175–80.
108. Nonogaki K. New insights into sympathetic regulation of glucose and fat metabolism. Diabetologia. 2000;43(5):533–49.
109. Natali A, Santoro D, Palombo C, Cerri M, Ghione S, Ferrannini E. Impaired insulin action on skeletal muscle metabolism in essential hypertension. Hypertension. 1991;17(2):170–8.
110. Grassi G, Dell'Oro R, Facchini A, Quarti TF, Bolla GB, Mancia G. Effect of central and peripheral body fat distribution on sympathetic and baroreflex function in obese normotensives. J Hypertens. 2004;22(12):2363–9.
111. Hamburg S, Hendler R, Sherwin RS. Influence of small increments of epinephrine on glucose tolerance in normal humans. Ann Intern Med. 1980;93(4):566–8.

112. Zeman RJ, Ludemann R, Easton TG, Etlinger JD. Slow to fast alterations in skeletal muscle fibers caused by clenbuterol, a beta 2-receptor agonist. Am J Phys. 1988;254(6 Pt 1):E726–32.
113. Cohn JN. Relationship of plasma volume changes to resistance and capacitance vessel effects of sympathomimetic amines and angiotensin in man. Clin Sci. 1966;30(2):267–78.
114. Hoieggen A, Fossum E, Moan A, Enger E, Kjeldsen SE. Whole-blood viscosity and the insulin-resistance syndrome. J Hypertens. 1998;16(2):203–10.
115. Hoieggen A, Fossum E, Nesbitt SD, Palmieri V, Kjeldsen SE. Blood viscosity, plasma adrenaline and fasting insulin in hypertensive patients with left ventricular hypertrophy. ICARUS, a LIFE Substudy. Insulin CARotids US Scandinavica. Blood Press. 2000;9(2–3):83–90.
116. Hassellund SS, Flaa A, Sandvik L, Kjeldsen SE, Rostrup M. Long-term stability of cardiovascular and catecholamine responses to stress tests: an 18-year follow-up study. Hypertension. 2010;55:131–6.

Part V

End Organ Damage in Prehypertension

Early Cardiovascular Dysfunction in Prehypertension

34

Ana Jelaković, Živka Dika, Vesna Herceg-Čavrak, Mario Laganović, Dragan Lović, and Bojan Jelaković

Prehypertension (PHT) is starting point in cardiovascular (CV) continuum and it should be considered as an intermediate phenotype between apparently health subjects and patients with sustained hypertension (HT). Although PHT in general is associated with higher risk for CV, cerebrovascular and renal morbidity and mortality, it is a heterogeneous group and subjects with PHT differ in mechanisms and pathways as well as in natural history, presence of CV dysfunction and risk classification (Fig. 34.1). It is of scientific interest but also of utmost pragmatical importance to identify PHT individuals with higher CV risk who are more likely to progress and who will mostly benefit from early interventions. Beside identification of different associated risk factors which cluster in PHT, for risk classification it is important to determine presence of subclinical target organ damages (TOD) and early CV dysfunction. Occurrence and characteristics of various early CV dysfunctions as well as differences in early CV dysfunction among age groups are presented and discussed in this chapter.

A. Jelaković · M. Laganović
Department of Nephrology, Hypertension, Dialysis and Transplantation, University Hospital Centre Zagreb, Zagreb, Croatia

Ž. Dika · B. Jelaković (✉)
Department of Nephrology, Hypertension, Dialysis and Transplantation, School of Medicine, University of Zagreb, University Hospital Centre Zagreb, Zagreb, Croatia

V. Herceg-Čavrak
Pediatric Clinic, Zagreb, Croatia

D. Lović
Clinic for Internal Medicine, Intermedica, Niš, Serbia

R. Zimlichman et al. (eds.), *Prehypertension and Cardiometabolic Syndrome*, Updates in Hypertension and Cardiovascular Protection,
https://doi.org/10.1007/978-3-319-75310-2_34

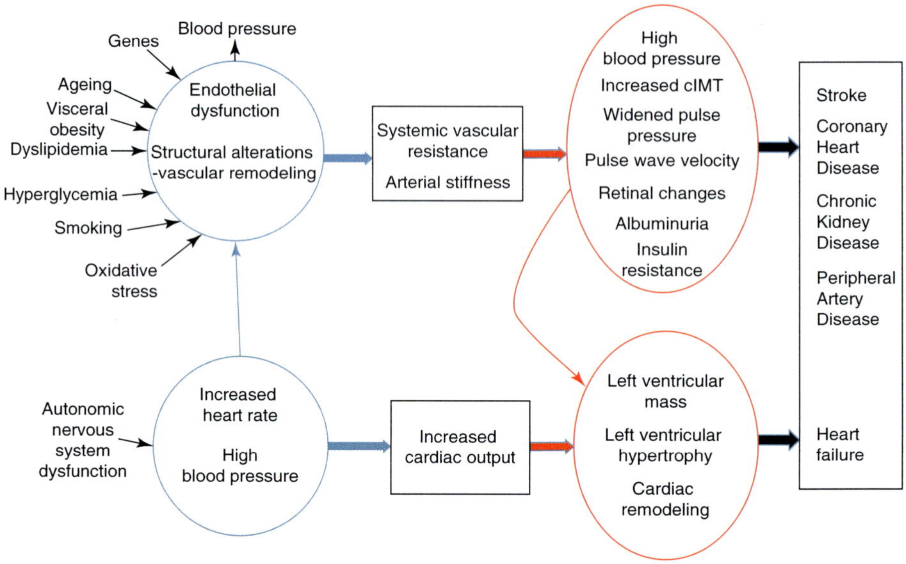

Fig. 34.1 Associated risk factors, general mechanisms, early cardiovascular dysfunction, and natural history in prehypertension

34.1 Changes in Systemic Hemodynamics and Arterial Stiffness

It was previously established that early stages of PHT are characterized with elevation of adrenergic tone typically evident by hyperkinetic status, i.e., increased heart rate (HR), cardiac volume (CV), cardiac output (CO), and cardiac index (CI), including total peripheral resistance (TPR) [1]. In studies presented in Table 34.1 HR was reported to be higher in PHT than in normotensives (NT) by most of the authors. Negative results were found in studies which enrolled small number of participants, in subjects from African descents and in older PHT. In all of studies pulse pressure (PP) was higher in PHT compared to NT counterparts. In the young-to-middle PHT (average age 43.2) Yano et al. observed higher systemic vascular resistance compared to NT, but no differences in left ventricular stroke volume. Interestingly, some racial differences were reported [2]. In the study conducted by Zhu et al., CO and CI were higher in American black youth PHT, while TPR, HR, and foot-pulse wave velocity (PWV) were higher in American white youth PHT [3]. Authors suggested that CV characteristics of PHT might be race-dependent proposing that PHT in young whites may be neurogenic, largely driven by excessive sympathetic tone while the observation that CO was increased in black PHT subjects could indicate the contribution of extracellular volume expansion indicating that PHT in black youth might be associated with salt sensitivity and sodium retention. In the Strong study Drukteinis et al. reported that TPR was higher in both the HT and PHT groups compared to NT but after adjustments the difference remained significant in only the HT group [4]. Abdelhammed et al. have evaluated hemodynamic characteristics of adult subjects with and without hypertension (HT), including those with PHT using impedance cardiography [5]. They found no difference in systemic vascular resistance index (SVRI = SVR × BSA) between PHT and subjects with optimal blood pressure (OBP), as well as between PHT and those with controlled HT (<120/80 mm Hg). A total of 22.2% of subjects with OBP and 50.0% of PHT showed vasoconstriction, as evidenced by high SVRI values. In HT group only 8.9% of subjects had SVRI in the normal range. As suggested by the authors, the transition from the normal state to the HT state may be bimodal among individuals with PHT—a group in which some individuals have elevated CO with low-to-normal SVR, whereas others have elevated SVR with low or normal CO. Subjects with PHT had a significantly lower total arterial compliance index (TACI = stroke index (SI)/pulse pressure (PP)) than those with OBP, while no difference was observed in SVRI between these groups.

Table 34.1 Association of early cardiovascular disease markers with prehypertension in children, adolescents, adults, and elderly

Early cardiovascular disease markers	Children and adolescents	Adults and elderly
Endothelial dysfunction	No evidence	Positive
Retinal changes	No association/negative	Positive *Blood pressure*
Albuminuria	Negative	Positive *Blood pressure* + *Associated clustered risk factors (glycemia, uric acid, obesity)*
Arterial stiffness	Positive *Blood pressure*	Positive *Blood pressure* + *Associated clustered risk factors (age, dyslipidemia)*
Carotid intima-media-thickness	Positive *Blood pressure* + *Obesity*	Positive *Blood pressure* + *Associated clustered risk factors (men, dyslipidemia, morning BP surge)*
Left ventricle Structure and geometry	Positive *Blood pressure* + *Obesity*	Positive *Blood pressure* + *Associated clustered risk factors (insulin resistance)*
Left ventricle Diastolic dysfunction	Positive *Blood pressure* + *Associated clustered risk factors*	Positive *Blood pressure* + *Associated clustered risk factors*
Left ventricle Systolic dysfunction	No association	Negative/positive[a] *Blood pressure* + *Metabolic abnormalities*

[a]Depending on imagining technique

The association of arterial stiffness with increased CV risk in PHT has not yet been fully clarified. Increased arterial stiffness was observed already in adolescents and children. Adolescents with HT and PHT have stiffer blood vessels and higher PWV than NT [6–10]. Stabouli et al. reported in the study of 124 children and adolescents 5–18 years of age that 24 h ABPM, daytime and nighttime PP levels were significantly higher in PHT and HT than in NT subjects [7]. It was proposed that increased aortic stiffness in children with high BP in the early stage could be explained by passive distension caused by arterial pressure and not primarily with intrinsic arterial wall changes [8]. Urbina et al. reported a graded increase in carotid-femoral PWV from NT to PHT and to HT youth aged 10–23 years (5.75 vs. 6.38 vs. 7.12 m/s) after adjusting for other CV risk factors [9]. A similar finding of a gradual increase in PWV in HT, PHT (high-normal BP) and HT children was also confirmed by Lurbe et al. in a group of children aged 8–18 [10]. In a twin cohort study of American youth (mean age 17.6) from Georgia Cardiovascular twin study, Zhu et al. found significant elevation of carotid-to-radial PWV and carotid-to-foot PWV from NT to PHT subjects after adjusting for age, gender, and BMI in white youths [3]. Garcia-Espinosa et al. analyzed vascular phenotype in 154 children (mean age 11; range 4–16 years) and observed that children with high BP exhibited higher aortic PWV, but the differences between NT and HT withdrew when normalizing for the BP levels and concluded that the differences are pressure-dependent and not related to early intrinsic aortic damage [8]. One large study in adolescents (10—23 years) showed a graded increase in AIx from NT to PHT and to HT (0.69 vs. 3.89 vs. 9.35%; $p < 0.0001$), even after adjusting for traditional CV risk factors [9]. On the contrary, in another survey of 121 adolescents 13–19 years of age no difference was found in AIx among the three BP categories, nor any significant correlation between AIx and peripheral SBP or DBP [11]. Authors explained this by shorter cumulative exposure to higher BP in adolescents as compared with adults. Drukteinis et al. reported higher pulse pressure/stroke volume index (assumed as markers of arterial stiffness) in a group of young PHT compared to NT [4]. In The San Antonio Heart Study Lorenzo et al. demonstrated that PHT is an independent predictor of all-cause and CV mortality in subjects free of diabetes and CV disease, but only if PP was widened [12]. PHT was not a risk factor for mortality if PP was narrow. They proposed that widened PP may select a group of individuals who are more susceptible to generalized vascular damage and atherosclerosis. Gedikli et al. found aortic PWV (10 ± 2.5 vs. 8.6 ± 1.7 m/s, $p = 0.004$) and AIx@75 (21 ± 8.3 vs. $10 \pm 9.1\%$, $p = 0.0001$) to be significantly higher in subjects with PHT than in NT [13]. In multiple linear regression analysis PHT was a significant predictor of aortic PWV ($b = 0.26, p = 0.009$) and AIx@75 ($b = 0.46, p = 0.0001$), suggesting that arterial functions were impaired in PHT. In a group of 1349 PHT (mean age 44 ± 9 years)after adjustments for confounding variables (age, gender, and mean blood pressure) the brachial-ankle PWV, but not the radial AI, was higher in subjects with PHT than in NT [14]. PWV and BMI > 25 were identified as significant predictors of the development of HT. These results suggested that increased arterial stiffness of the large to middle-sized arteries might be an independent risk factor for the new onset of HT in subjects with PHT. This is in line with results of Najjar et al. who demonstrated that a higher value of the carotid-femoral PWV was an independent risk factor for the new onset of

HT in 306 NT subjects [15]. In another analysis Tomiyama et al. revealed that the change of the brachial-ankle PWV during the follow-up period of 6 years was higher in the subjects with persistent PHT than in persistent NT and they concluded that PHT itself is a risk factor for increase of the arterial stiffness [16]. The annual increase of the brachial ankle PWV in elderly subjects (age > 60 years) with persistent PHT was higher than that in middle-aged subjects (age 40–59 years) with persistent PHT indicating that the accelerated progression of arterial stiffening caused by persistent PHT became more pronounced with advancing age. They observed that other CV risk factors may also augment the PHT-related progression of arterial stiffness. In a small group of young PHT men (mean age 34 years) Celik et al. observed that the mean aortic systolic and diastolic diameters of PHT were significantly higher than those in NT [17]. Aortic distensibility and strain indexes of PHT were found to be lower than those of NT while the mean aortic stiffness index beta of the PHT was significantly higher than that of the control group. Authors concluded that these findings suggested that arterial stiffness may develop prior to development of overt HT and increased arterial stiffness might be a mechanism in the initiation and/or progression of PHT to HT. Erdogan et al. demonstrated in the group of 60 PHT (mean age 43.6) that aortic distensibility was significantly lower and aortic stiffness index was significantly higher in both PHT and HT than those in NT and found impairment of aortic elasticity in PHT to be as severely as that in HT [18]. Authors concluded that the presence of PHT was significant predictor of impaired aortic elasticity. Proximal aortic impedance (Z_c) and aortic PWV were higher in PHT compared to NT while aortic compliance and distensibility were lower [2, 19]. Jia et al. even proposed that early detection of ascending aortic elasticity index changes, particularly aortic distensibility could be used for identification of high-risk PHT subjects [19]. Tiokka et al. also found lower aortic and carotid distensibilities in the PHT men (high-normal BP) than in NT [20]. In multivariate analysis, the differences in distensibilities between the groups disappeared when the values were adjusted for ox-LDL, thus they suggested that oxidative modification of LDL particles may play a pathophysiological role in the development of reduced arterial distensibility in HT.

Box 34.1 Arterial Stiffness as an Early Marker of Cardiovascular Dysfunction in PHT

1. Markers of arterial stiffness (pulse pressure, pulse wave velocity) are reported to be increased already in PHT children and adolescents. Widened pulse pressure may be considered as a biomarker of greater susceptibility to general vascular damage in PHT.
2. It was proposed that increased arterial stiffness in younger ages is blood pressure dependent and not related to early intrinsic changes in arterial wall.
3. Accelerating progression of arterial stiffness caused by persistent PHT is more pronounced with increasing aging. The role of other factors (age, glycemia, dyslipidemia) contributes to vascular wall changes.

4. PWV was identified as a significant predictor of the development of HT and arterial stiffness might be an independent risk factor development of overt HT.
5. It was proposed that widened pulse pressure and changes of aortic elasticity properties could be used for identification of high-risk subgroup of PHT subjects.

Gradual increase in arterial stiffness was observed from NT to PHT and HT. Further research is needed to clarify the chicken-egg question whether increased arterial stiffness is risk factor for PHT, or does PHT independently increases arterial stiffness. Nevertheless, it could be concluded that measurements of biomarkers of arterial stiffness (PP, carotid-femoral PWV, etc.) are valuable in identification of PHT subjects with higher CV risk.

34.2 Carotid Intima Media Thickness

It was demonstrated that carotid intima-to-media thickness (cIMT) is increased in subjects with borderline hypertension [2, 21], and some recent reports showed that PHT is also associated with increased cIMT. During childhood and adolescence cIMT correlates with age and with the increase in BP [22]. Most of these studies suggested an independent positive association between BP and cIMT in children and young people, even after adjustment for other CV risk factors. The correlation of PHT in children and adolescents and increased cIMT was observed in several studies. Urbina et al. presented an increased cIMT in PHT children and adolescents compared to the NT as independent determinant of target organ damage (TOD) [9]. Jourdan et al. reported thicker carotid and femoral IMT in young people who had systolic BP in the top 10th percentile of the distribution [23]. Stabouli et al. reported that obese children and adolescents have greater cIMT than nonobese subjects, independently of BP [24]. However, it is not clear whether higher cIMT values in PHT and HT children are of any clinical significance in adulthood. Manios et al. found that adult PHT and NT did not differ in common artery cIMT, but PHT with masked HT had higher cIMT than NT but also than PHT with normal daytime ABPM [25]. Alpaydin et al. reported that male gender, elevated mean platelet volume levels, and morning BP surge were independent predictors of greater cIMT in PHT [26]. Beside showing association of PHT with cIMT observations in both studies stressed the role of ABPM in determination of risk in PHT. According to the results of Hong et al. PHT correlated with thicker cIMT after adjustment for multiple risk factors. PHT had trend to have thicker cIMT but also significantly higher carotid plaque occurrence than NT [27]. Intensity of plaque formation in PHT was the same as in HT patients. In the PHT group they fail to observe any difference between subjects with high and high-normal BP. It was also reported that PHT subjects with thicker cIMT have also higher LVM than NT indicating that PHT increase risk for atherosclerosis and global CV risk [28]. The Multi-Ethnic Study of

Atherosclerosis (MESA) enrolled 6814 participants free of clinical cardiovascular disease and it was shown that in the group with high-normal BP cIMT was directly associated with systolic BP and inversely associated with diastolic BP, while LVM was directly related to SBP and DBP [29]. Karasek et al. analyzed dyslipidemic status in PHT and found that prevalence of PHT was the highest in hypertriglyceridemic persons [30]. In their study PHT subjects had thicker cIMT than NT in all dyslipidemic phenotypes (according to apolipoprotein B and triglycerides) suggesting that dyslipidemia and BP have cumulative effect on IMT in PHT. Femia et al. confirmed that PHT have thicker cIMT compared to NT, and the association between cIMT and PHT persists after adjustment for all known predictors [31]. However, in the follow-up period of 3.5 years they failed to observe difference in progression of cIMT between PHT and NT. Authors concluded that baseline measurements of cIMT reflects past log-term exposure to risk factors, whereas cIMT progression may be influenced by short-term changes in risk factor burden.

Box 34.2 Prehypertension and Carotid Intima-Media Thickness

1. Most of studies showed an independent positive association between PHT and cIMT starting from childhood and adolescence till the older ages.
2. In PHT other risk factors (i.e., dyslipidemia, morning BP surge, masked HT) additionally increase risk for thicker cIMT.
3. Presence of cIMT is associated with other target organ damages (i.e., LVH)
4. In addition to the presence of thicker cIMT it was also reported that intensity of atherosclerotic plaque formation in PHT is not different to HT.

Thicker cIMT is reported to be associated with PHT and could be considered as a determinant of early target organ damage.

34.3 Retinal Changes

Alternations in the structure and function of the microcirculation are one of the earliest changes in the pathogenesis of HT including enhanced vasoconstriction, reduced vasodilator responses, anatomic alterations, and rarefaction of arterioles or capillaries. Results of studies based on biopsies usually taken from subcutaneous fat tissue support the hypothesis that capillary rarefaction is an early hallmark of HT. Recently, new techniques and technologies in retinal photography have enabled investigations of microvascular structure and function in retina. Retinal vascular caliber can be noninvasively assessed from retinal photographs and computer-assisted approaches [32]. The noninvasive measurement of retinal vessel diameters of particular relevance are: the central retinal arteriolar equivalent (CRAE) and central retinal venular equivalent (CRVE), which, respectively, represent the average arteriolar and venular diameters in an eye. Noninvasive photographic measurement of retinal vessel diameters allows insights into microvascular alterations and their relation to CV risk factors [33–35]. Retinal arteriolar narrowing is strongly correlated with concurrent elevated BP levels, but retinal venular diameter may convey additional information. In some studies, NT persons with retinal arteriolar narrowing were more likely to develop HT. Increasing number of studies have shown that retinal vessel signs, that is, the narrowing of retinal arteriolar caliber and widening of venular caliber, have been associated with CV risk factors, systemic inflammation, and decreased renal function [36–39]. It has been suggested that generalized and focal narrowing of the retinal arterioles may be markers of a PHT because they predict the risk of HT in NT subjects [34, 40, 41]. The PHT group in the study by Murgan et al. had values of the CRAE equivalent to those of the HT group and significantly lower than those of the NT group [11]. Using qualitative and quantitative assessments of the retinal microcirculatory network via bilateral nonmydriatic retinography Grassi et al. found arteriolar-venular ratio in PHT to be below the normal values, i.e., greater than 0.92, indicating occurrence of an initial arteriolar narrowing process in the high-normal BP group [42]. They concluded that retinal arteriolar narrowing is an early phenomenon in PHT, and systolic BP and PP represent the major hemodynamic determinants of the retinal abnormalities in PHT. In the study of Murgan et al. no correlation was found of the retinal vascular parameters and the macrovascular parameter AIx in contrast to the findings of the Atherosclerosis Risk in Communities Study (ARIC) study, in which carotid arterial stiffness was strongly correlated with generalized retinal arteriolar narrowing [43]. The recent study in HT and PHT adolescents has shown negative correlation between CRAE and both peripheral (brachial) and central SBP, while no correlation was found in CRVE with BP [11]. This is consistent with the findings in studies of young adults and of small children, in which high BP had no influence on retinal venular diameter [40, 44, 45]. The plausible explanation of these findings could be the short cumulative exposure of the children and adolescents to high BP and the fact that the changes in vascular elasticity and pulse wave reflection that occur in HT occur at a later stage than does retinal arteriolar narrowing [46]. On the basis of baseline and the follow-up SBP measurements, each 20-μm decrease on retinal arteriolar caliber at baseline was associated with a 1.12 mmHg greater increase in SBP over 5 years [47]. Further, in Nagahama study the central BP was more closely associated with the narrowing of retinal arterioles (CRAE) than brachial BP, even in NT.

Box 34.3 Retinal Changes as an Early Marker of Cardiovascular Dysfunction in PHT

1. There is scarce evidence on retinal changes in PHT, however it was suggested that generalized and focal narrowing of the retinal arterioles may be early phenomenons and a markers of PHT because they predict the risk of HT in NT subjects.
2. It was reported that systolic BP and PP in PHT represent the major hemodynamic determinants of the retinal abnormalities, i.e., arteriolar narrowing.

3. Retinal vascular parameters do not correlate with the macrovascular parameter (i.e., Aix) what is in line with the fact that the changes in vascular elasticity of large arteries and pulse wave reflection occur at a later stage than does retinal arteriolar narrowing.
4. Negative correlation of retinal changes with BP was found in PHT adolescents and these findings could be due to the short cumulative exposure of the children and adolescents to high BP.

Obtained results suggest that retinal changes in PHT might be considered as an early sign of cardiovascular dysfunction, but further studies are needed.

34.4 Albuminuria as an Early Marker of Cardiovascular Dysfunction in PHT

It is well established that microalbuminuria (MA), which is considered a mirror of generalized endothelial damage, represents a marker not only of chronic kidney disease (CKD) but also of CV morbidity and mortality in diabetic patients, hypertensives nondiabetic and in general population [48]. MA is a useful test for the identification of people who are at high risk for CV events and who require more intensive therapy. Endothelial injury and dysfunction are thought to contribute to CV risk in PHT. Weil et al. reported on significantly lower forearm blood flow responses to acetylcholine (~30%) in PHT compared with NT and concluded that PHT is associated with impaired NO-mediated endothelium-dependent vasodilation [49]. Wang et al. observed association of elevated CRP and sICAM-1 with PHT suggesting that inflammation and endothelial dysfunction may have a role in the development of PHT and HT [50]. Nikolov et al. found that flow-mediated dilatation was reduced in PHT compared to NT group which was associated with increased ADMA and cVCAM-1 [51]. Vrdoljak, Jelaković et al. in a group of PHT who were free of CKD, diabetes, and previous CV incidents found that hepatocyte growth factor was significantly higher in subjects with high-normal BP than in those with OBP [52]. Hepatocyte growth factor which has antiapoptotic, anti-inflammatory, and antifibrotic properties was reported to be compensatory elevated in response to endothelial damage caused by HT, CKD, or diabetes. Keeping in mind high prevalence of PHT and the fact that PHT is very heterogenous group, it is of interest and importance to determine whether MA, as not only a marker of early kidney damage but also sign of systemic endothelial injury, can be used as a screening tool in adults with PHT to identify those at higher risk for CV disease or decline of renal function. It was observed in a NHANES III cohort (8751 non-hypertensive subjects) that high-normal BP and normal BP categories were significantly associated with increased OR of MA compared with OBP (OR = 2.13; 1.34, respectively) [53]. Analyzing NHANES data Ogunniyi et al. found that prevalence of MA was 4.5, 6.3, 12.4, and 25.3% in subjects with normal BP, PHT, stage 1 HT, and stage 2 HT, respectively [54]. In the group of middle-aged untreated subjects without diabetes

Tenekecioglu et al. observed the prevalence of MA to be 10, 25.9, and 33.9% in NT, PHT, and new-HT, respectively [55]. In PHT group subjects with MA had higher SBP, brain natriuretic peptide, LVMI and lower eGFR as compared to those with normal albumin excretion. In PHT MA was significantly correlated with SBP, LVMI, and brain natriuretic peptide. Vrdoljak, Jelaković et al. also found albumin-to-creatinine ratio (ACR) to have linear trend accords the BP categories being 4.08, 4.25, 5.05, and 5.77 mg/g in OBP, normal BP, high-normal BP, and untreated new-HT, respectively [52]. Kim et al. analyzed 2678 PHT subjects without a history of diabetes or hypertension and found that high-normal BP category had an independently significant association with MA (OR 1.692, 95% CI 1.097–2.611) [56]. Subjects with high-normal BP had higher ACR values than subjects with normal BP (11.06 ± 25.46 vs. 8.15 ± 20.43; $p = 0.006$). They suggested that the high prevalence of MA in the high-normal BP group with apparent normal renal function may reflect increased glomerular filtration pressure in response to elevated BP. In the group of 6771 subjects without diabetes and HT Lee et al. found MA in 4.0% of NT subjects and in 7.9% of PHT [57]. PHT subjects with MA had higher serum uric acid level than those with normoalbuminuria ($p = 0.006$) what was not observed in the NT group. In this cohort increased serum uric acid level was an independent factor for MA in the PHT group. They found that PHT subjects with MA had higher GFR levels than those with normoalbuminuria proposing that PHT might cause endothelial dysfunction and glomerular hypertension inducing glomerular hyperfiltration. In our group of non-treated subjects without diabetes and GFR > 60 ml/min prevalence of glomerular hyperfiltration was higher in PHT than in those with OBP and HT (25.5% vs. 21.8% vs. 18%, respectively) [52]. Subjects with glomerular hyperfiltration were younger, visceral obese, and had signs of sympathetic overactivity (higher leptin concentration and heart rate). During the 100 months follow-up period eGFR decreased significantly more in subjects with glomerular hyperfiltration compared to those with normal eGFR. This is in line with report of Okada et al. who found that the prevalence of glomerular hyperfiltration increased not only with increasing stage of prediabetes but also of PHT [58]. In the group of 1100 PHT and 2200 subjects with OBP Yi et al. found that prevalence of MA was 6.8% and 3.6%, respectively ($p < 0.0001$) [59]. In logistic regression it was shown that MA, brain natriuretic peptide, and serum uric level were significantly associated with the occurrence of PHT. After exclusion of patients with diabetes and hyperuricemia Peng et al. found in a group of subjects older than 30 years that persons with PHT are more likely to have MA than NT (OR 1.83 95% CI 1.12–2.99), and MA was positively associated with BP levels [60]. Ding et al. and Zhang et al. found that prevalence of MA in the group of 1796 women increases in parallel with BP category being 9.6%, 13.4%, and 27.6%, respectively, in NT, PHT, and HT [61, 62]. They also noticed dose-response relationship between ACR and the risk of PHT. In middle-aged NT subjects (622 PHT and 437 OBP) Wang et al. reported that prevalence of MA is rising with the increasing classification of glycemic level: normo, prediabetic, and diabetic, 14.8%, 18.3%, and 32.6%, respectively [63]. Statistically significant association between glycemic level and MA was present in PHT but not in OBP group. Urinary albumin excretion has been also reported as a predictor of developing HT and BP progression. A prospective study of 1499 nondiabetic, non-HT individuals has demonstrated that those in the highest quartile of the ACR had an adjusted OR of 1.93 for developing HT and 1.45 for BP progression [64]. Authors concluded that elevated ACR is associated with the development of HT in nondiabetic individuals who are not currently HT. Importantly, the increased risk of HT was evident at ACR values well below the conventional threshold for MA. Some authors failed to find MA in PHT subjects, but as authors themselves concluded this could be explained with younger age of subjects enrolled in those studies [4, 65]. During a median follow-up of 12.8 years Sehestedt et al. found in a population sample of 1968 untreated individuals without diabetes, prior stroke, or myocardial infarction that measuring two of PWV, atherosclerotic plaques or ACR was sufficient to significantly improve risk prediction in subjects with high-normal BP [66]. In our group of nondiabetic PHT with normal kidney function during the follow-up period of 100 months (IQ84–120), 11.337 person years of follow-up, incident HT was diagnosed in 48.2% of PHT with incident rate 7.53% per year. Beside age, systolic BP, and leptin, ACR was significant predictor of incident HT [67].

Aforementioned studies suggest that ACR might be a good biomarker and screening for MA may identify a subgroup of subjects who are at high risk for developing CV disease and renal impairment and could benefit from early therapy.

Box 34.4 Albuminuria as an Early Biomarker of Cardiovascular Dysfunction in PHT

1. Prevalence of MA is higher in PHT than in subjects with OBP, but lower than in non-treated hypertensives.
2. Subjects with PHT have higher risk for MA than those with normal BP.
3. Association of MA with PHT is present in diabetics but also in nondiabetics.
4. Prevalence of MA is increasing with the glycemic level.
5. Serum uric acid was reported by some authors to influence presence of MA in PHT subjects.
6. ACR is predictor of developing HT in nondiabetic PHT subjects.
7. It was proposed that MA in PHT subjects with normal global renal function may reflect glomerular hyperfiltration.

   It was also shown that renal function deteriorates more rapidly in PHT with glomerular hyperfiltration.
8. Negative results were observed in children and adolescents what could be explained with shorter period of exposition to higher values of BP.

It could be suggested that MA might be considered as a tool for identification of adult and elderly PHT subjects with additional high risk who may benefit from early treatment.

34.5 Changes of Left Ventricular Structure and Geometry

LV mass (LVM) was significantly elevated in PHT starting from childhood and adolescents [4, 9, 68]. DiBello et al. analyzed LV abnormalities in PHT with 2D-strain ECHO and found that LVM was significantly higher in PHT [69]. Ahnet al. found that LVMI was higher in both PHT men and PHT women ($p = 0.02$). Kim et al. evaluated the relationship between PHT and TOD using tissue Doppler imaging (TDI) and found that LVMI was significantly higher in PHT than in NT [71]. In the study conducted by Ahn et al. PHT subjects compared with NT had significantly higher Sokolow-Lyon and Cornell voltage for ECG left ventricular hypertrophy (LVH) [70]. PHT had higher prevalence of ECG LVH (men 16.9% vs. 5.9% men; 2.0% vs. 1.0% women). Using 2D mode ECHO Jung et al. in much larger cohort found that the proportion of LVH was 0.9%, 1.6%, 4.9%, and 3.4% in NT, PHT, controlled HT, and in newly diagnosed HT, respectively [72]. The fully adjusted ORs for LVH were 2.1 (95% CI 1.63–2.7) in all PHT, and 3.2 (95% CI 2.41–4.23) in nondiabetic PHT. In this study relative wall thickness (RWT) showed dose-response relationship order (NT, PHT, HT). The full adjusted ORs of increased RWT were 1.65 (95% CI 1.45–1.87) in PHT and 3.31 (95% CI 2.68–4.07) in newly diagnosed untreated HT. Changes in LV structure and geometry are registered already in children and adolescents with PHT [73–75]. Stabouli et al. reported the same prevalence of LVH of 20% in HT and PHT children. PHT children had higher LVMI than NT and similar to HT [7]. The combination of obesity and PHT increases the likelihood of LVH, as we found in the study of Falkner et al. [76]. In the African-American adolescent prevalence of LVH was 19% and 57% in normal weight and overweight adolescents, respectively. In PHT children, adolescents, and young adults (age range 10–23) Urbina et al. found no difference in concentric HT between PHT vs. NT while eccentric hypertrophy was slightly more prevalent (4.6 vs. 3.4%) [9]. It was found in the Strong study in young PHT (14–39 years of age) that after adjustment for covariates, both HT and PHT subjects had higher LV wall thickness (0.83 and 0.78 vs. 0.72 cm), LVM (182 and 161 vs. 137 g), and RWT (0.30 and 0.29 vs. 0.28 cm) and three- and twofold higher prevalence of LVH than their NT counterparts (all $p < 0.001$) [4]. They found minimally higher prevalence of concentric remodeling and threefold and twofold higher prevalence of eccentric LVH in the HT and PHT groups, respectively. In another study, it was found that PHT men and women have changes in LV geometry in the form of concentric remodeling (3.44 and 6.45%), eccentric hypertrophy (3.44 and 3.22%), and concentric hypertrophy (13.79 and 6.4%) [68]. In the same group posterior wall thickness (PWT), interventricular septum thickness (IVST), LVM, and RWT were raised but not statistically significant in both PHT men and women. Erdogan et al. found that IVS and PW thickness, left ventricular end-diastolic diameter (LVEDD), left ventricular end-systolic diameter (LVESD), ejection fraction (EF), left atrial (LA) diameter, and LVMI were similar between PHT and HT, and between PHT and NT [18]. This is in line with results from the study by Norton et al. who enrolled young-to-middle-aged subjects of African ancestry [65]. Before adjustment PHT was associated with LVMI, mean WT, PWV, early to late transmitral velocity, but not with other TOD (ACR, cIMT). However, after adjustments PHT was not independently associated with any TOD. Authors speculated that alternative risk factors may contribute to TOD and proposed that is possible that clustering of risk factors is principally responsible for TOD in PHT. On the contrary, Drukteinis et al. concluded that both the HT and PHT groups exhibited cardiac structural features associated with increased CV risk, including increased IVS, posterior wall, and RWT and higher LVM underlying that these data suggest parallels between CV effects of PHT and HT already in adolescents and young adults [4]. This is in agreement with observation and conclusion of Kim et al. who found that subtle alterations in CV structure were present in PHT [71]. As assessed by TDI-derived parameters, LV diastolic dysfunction appears to be an early manifestation of PHT subjects and precedes the development of LVH defined by current ECHO criteria indicating that PHT might be a potential contributor to the development of TOD. DiBello et al. demonstrated that PHT induces the same structural abnormalities of newly diagnosed, untreated HT patients, although in a milder manner [69]. However, they also found LV abnormalities to be associated not only with systolic ABPM and LVM but also with HOMA index. In elderly PHT, men had higher LV dimensions and LV wall thickness, while LVMI was similar to women. The LV filling pressure (E/E′) was higher in women. In PHT, the gender differences in cardiac structure were consistent with the constitutional differences between sexes and the higher filling pressure in women was similar to the findings in general population that may contribute to increased prevalence of Heart Failure with Preserved Ejection Fraction in women. Important and interesting data were collected in the 10-year follow-up study (MONICA/KORA Augsburg) where Markus et al. found that PHT displayed more pronounced aging-related increase in LV wall thickness and LV mass [77]. In addition, PHT was associated with a raised incidence of LV concentric remodeling (adjusted OR 10.7 CI 95% 2.82–40.4) and LVH (adjusted OR 5.3 CI 95% 1.58–17.9).

Box 34.5 Changes of Left Ventricular Structure and Geometry as an Early Sign of Cardiovascular Dysfunction in PHT

1. Left ventricular mass is higher in PHT men and women than in NT counterparts.
2. Changes in LV structure and geometry are presented already in PTH children and adolescents.
3. PHT subjects have two- to threefold higher risk and prevalence of LVH than NT.
4. PHT subjects displayed more pronounced aging-related changes in LV structure than NT.
5. PHT men were reported to have more eccentric and concentric hypertrophy, while PHT women had more concentric remodeling and higher LV filling pressure.
6. Some authors argued that associated risk factors and not PHT itself are principally responsible for LV structural changes.

Regardless changes in LV structure are independently related to PHT or they are associated with other risk factors observed abnormalities in structure and geometry in PHT subjects are similar to those in newly diagnosed, untreated HT patients, although in a milder manner.

34.6 Left Ventricular Diastolic Function

Data on left ventricular (LV) diastolic dysfunction in PHT are rare and there are just a few population-based studies on early changes in CV function. In the cohort of more than 52,000 adults in whom echocardiogram (ECHO) was performed Jung et al. found the presence of diastolic dysfunction in PHT. The adjusted mean E/E ratio, indicating increased filling pressure, was 7.89 (95% CI 7.85–7.94) in PHT who also had higher E/e ratio and LA diameter, while lower E/A ratio and septal e velocities [72]. This is accordant to the results of Bajpai et al. who observed active (E) and passive (A) transmitral peak velocities and their ratio (E/A ratio) to be decreased in PHT what is suggestive of compensatory diastolic dysfunction [68]. Ahn et al. reported that diastolic function was more decreased in PHT compared to NT (E/A men 1.14(0.6) vs. 1.3(0.4); women 1.11(0.6) vs. 1.25(0.5)) [70]. These results are in line with report of Celik et al. who found that PHT compared to NT had slower E velocity, faster A velocity, lower E/A ratio, longer deceleration time and IVRT (isovolumetric relaxation time) [17]. Using TDI (Tissue Doppler imaging), Kim et al. found that LV diastolic parameters/E/E ratio, TDI Ea velocity, E/Es ratio were impaired in PHT subjects [71]. In a large cohort of 4261 middle-aged adults Jang et al. observed that diastolic dysfunction grade 1 or 2 was significantly higher in PHT (31%) and HT (38%) compared to NT (19.1%) [78]. In men, the adjusted OR for diastolic dysfunction with PHT was 1.74 (CI 95% 1.44–2.04) for grade 1 and 1.31(CI 95% 0.84–2.04) for grade 2, while in females it was 1.32 (CI 95% 0.91–1.9) for grade 1 and 1.47(CI 95% 0.76–2.76) for grade 2. It was concluded that diastolic dysfunction appears to be significantly associated with PHT in apparently healthy middle-aged Korean population. These results are congruent with data obtained with 2D-strain ECHO. DiBello et al. found mild LV diastolic dysfunction in PHT, higher LVEDV (left ventricle end-diastolic volume) in PHT than in NT [69]. They found early and global LV diastolic dysfunction: peak E was progressively lower in PHT and HT. However, late diastolic LV functional phase appeared comparable among groups (PHT, HT, NT). Only the early phase of longitudinal function was impaired, essentially at the septum level. Prominently the E/e ratio showed a progressive and significant increase in PHT and HT compared to NT. It is interesting to analyze changes in LV function in various aging PHT subgroups. In the cohort of very young subjects (10–23 years) Urbina et al. found NT to be better than PHT for mitral E/A ratio, TDI Ea/Aa septal ratio, average septal/lateral Ea/Aa ratios, and E/average Ea/Aa TDI lateral and septal ratios [9]. In the Strong study which enrolled participants 14–39 years of age, mean mitral A velocity and atrial filling fraction were higher and the mean mitral E/A ratio was lower in both HT and PHT participants, even after covariate adjustment, but difference in mitral deceleration time did not remain significant after covariate adjustment [4]. IVRT was longer and the mean E velocity was slightly lower in HT and PHT participants, but the differences were not significant after adjustment for covariates. In elderly PHT (75 years of age) Santos et al. found that parameters of diastolic function (E/A, E′, and E/E′) were progressively worse in PHT and HT in comparison to subjects with OBP, and the adjusted prevalence of mild and moderate to severe diastolic dysfunction was higher in PHT (59%) as compared with OBP (44%) but lower than in HT (67%) [79]. They observed a tendency toward increasing LA size with higher BP but they failed to find statistically significant difference in LA size between PHT participants and those with OBP. Some authors failed to find PHT to be independently associated with LV dysfunction. Erdogan et al. found that compared to NT, PHT had significantly higher only IVRT, while the other diastolic parameters were just slightly different [18]. They concluded that LV diastolic function in PHT was not impaired as severely as that was in HT. In young-to-middle-aged PHT of African descent Norton et al. failed to prove PHT to be an independent predictor of TOD including diastolic dysfunction and suggested that early changes are largely attributed to associated risk factors that cluster with PHT [65]. However, in 10-year follow-up period Markus et al. observed that in subjects with persistent PHT the ratio of early and late diastolic peak transmitral flow velocities (E/A) decreased by 15.7% (compared to decrease of 7.7% in NT) [77]. The ratio of early diastolic peak myocardial relaxation velocities (E/EM) was higher and LA size was larger in PHT group. The adjusted OR for incident diastolic dysfunction was 2.52 (1.01–6.31) for the PHT group.

Box 34.6 Left Ventricular Diastolic Dysfunction and PHT

1. Diastolic function is more decreased in PHT than in NT, but not so severely as it was described in HT.
2. Impaired diastolic function is present not only in middle-aged and elderly PHT but also in young PHT and even in children and adolescents, indicating that this is one of the earliest manifestation of cardiovascular dysfunction in PHT.
3. In subjects with PHT compared to NT diastolic function decreased more rapidly.
4. Although majority of authors found PHT to be independently associated with diastolic dysfunction, some authors suggested that observed changes are more likely attributed to associated risk factors which cluster with PHT.

Left ventricular diastolic dysfunction is an early and prominent sign of cardiovascular dysfunction in PHT.

34.7 Left Ventricular Systolic Function in PHT

Contrary to LV diastolic dysfunction the overall LV systolic functions were reported to be normal in asymptomatic PHT subjects [68]. Even in elderly PHT authors failed to find differences in LV systolic function in PHT compared to subjects with OBP [79]. In the elderly PHT enrolled in the ARIC study neither EF nor circumferential strain significantly differed between NT and HT, and authors speculated that systolic abnormalities restricted to the subendocardial fibers might be present only in a more advanced HT status. In the Korean Genome study no statistically significant differences in LV systolic parameters, including EF and TDI systolic (Sa) velocity, were observed between PHT and NT [71]. Drukteinis et al. found that circumferential end-systolic stress was significantly elevated in both young-to-middle-aged HT and PHT compared to NT, but the circumferential end-systolic stress/end-systolic volume index, a load-adjusted measure of chamber contractility, did not differ among groups after adjustment [4]. Interestingly, 2D longitudinal systolic strain appeared significantly lower both at mid septum and mid lateral level in PHT according to the results of DiBello et al. [69]. Longitudinal 2D strain rate at septum level confirmed a progressive impairment in PHT and HT compared to NT, both of systolic and diastolic parameters. Instead, the radial and circumferential 2D systolic strain were comparable in all three groups and in all LV segments. Only longitudinal regional deformation (2D strain) appears altered in PHT and according to authors this could be related to an early abnormal systolic function limited to the subendocardial fibers. They observed the same even in PHT with normal LVMI. Using MRI technique Sironi et al. found that subjects with PHT as well as new-HT patients showed a graded reduction in systolic function, as documented by decreased LV shortening, despite normal ventricular volumes and pump function and similar values of wall stress [80]. The reduction in regional systolic function (LV circumferential shortening) was related to BP in a continuous fashion but as authors underlined, more interestingly, to metabolic abnormalities such as increased epicardial and visceral fat accumulation, triglyceride concentration, and insulin resistance. LV shortening was reduced in PHT and new-HT patients in all 3 of the regions (basal, middle, and apical LV segments) as compared with a control group of NT. However, it was shown in 10-year follow-up study that systolic function, contrary to diastolic function, did not display any substantial changes and Markus et al. suggested that this may indicate that persistent PHT does not affect contractility [77].

Box 34.7 Left Ventricular Systolic Function in PHT

1. In PHT there are even fewer data on LV systolic function than on diastolic dysfunction.
2. Using routine ECHO techniques LV systolic functions were reported by most of the authors to be normal in asymptomatic PHT subjects. It was observed even in elderly PHT subjects.
3. Interestingly, using more sophisticated methods (2D strain ECHO, MRI) early changes in systolic dysfunction were found.
4. Some authors raised the question whether PHT itself, i.e., BP values or metabolic abnormalities associated with PHT were significantly related to the reduction of LV systolic function in PHT.

Results on LV systolic dysfunction in PHT are controversial. More sophisticated techniques found early systolic dysfunction but the question whether this is independently related to PHT or is influenced with clustered metabolic abnormalities is still opened.

Table 34.2 Proposed test for detection of early cardiovascular dysfunction in prehypertensive subjects

Children and adolescents	Adults and elderly
Electrocardiogram	Electrocardiogram
Pulse wave velocity	Pulse wave velocity
	Microalbuminuria
Ambulatory BP monitoring	Ambulatory BP monitoring
Left ventricle ultrasound	Left ventricle ultrasound
Carotid intima-media thickness	Carotid intima-media thickness
	Optic fundus photography

Associations of early CV disease markers with PTH in children, adolescents, adults, and elderly are summarized in Table 34.2. In children and adolescents there is no evidence for endothelial dysfunction and lack of associations were observed between PHT and retinal changes, MA and left ventricle systolic dysfunction. BP is an independent risk factor for increased arterial stiffness, however, cIMT, changes in LV structure and geometry and LV dysfunction are attributed also to obesity and clustered risk factors. On the contrary, in adults and elderly there are data on positive association of endothelial dysfunction, retinal changes, and MA with PHT. Only retinal changes were reported to be independently associated with BP, while associated clustered risk factors were found, beside BP, to have impact on all other markers of early CV dysfunction. Proposed diagnostic tests for detection of early CV dysfunction are shown in Table 34.2. For risk stratification and planning intervention strategies ECG and PWV should be considered in all age groups, while MA could add information only in adults and elderly. PWV and MA were reported to be not only biomarkers of TOD but also to have prognostic value [66]. All other test could be suggested if they are available or more indicated (for instance ECHO in subjects with ECG determined LVH).

Early CV dysfunction is frequently present in PHT and early detection and identification of those individuals who are at higher global risk could enable us to start with more targeted interventions prior to occurrence of overt disease and nonfatal or fatal CV events.

References

1. Julius S, Nesbitt S. Sympathetic oveactivity in hypertension. A moving target. Am J Hypertens. 1996;9:113S–20S.
2. Yano Y, Neeland I, Ayers C, Peshock R, Berry J, Lloyd-Jones D, Greenland P, Mitchell G, Vongpatanasin W. Hemodynamic and mechanical properties of the proximal aorta in young and middle-aged adults with isolated systolic hypertension: the Dallas heart study. Hypertension. 2017;70:158–65.
3. Zhu H, Yan W, Ge D, Treiber FA, Harshfield GA, Kapuku G, Snieder H, Dong Y. Cardiovascular characteristics in American youth with prehypertension. Am J Hypertens. 2007;20:1051–7.
4. Drukteinis J, Roman M, Fabsitz R, Lee E, Best L, Rusell M, Devereux R. Cardia and systemic hemodynamic characteristics of hypertension and prehypertension in adolescets and young adults.The Strong Heart Study. Circulation. 2007;15:221–7.

5. Abdelhammed I, Smith R, Levy P, Smits G, Ferrario C. Noninvasive hemodynamic profiles in hypertensive subjects. Am J Hypertens. 2005;18:51S–9S.
6. Phillips AA, Chirico D, Coverdale NS, Fitzgibbon LK, Shoemaker JK, Wade TJ, Cairney J, O'Leary DD. The association between arterial properties and blood pressure in children. Appl Physiol Nutr Metab. 2015;40(1):72–8.
7. Stabouli S, Kotsis V, Rizos Z, Toumanidis S, Karagianni C, Constantopoulos A, Zakopoulos N. Left ventricular mass in normotensive, prehypertensive and hypertensive children and adolescents. Pediatr Nephrol. 2009;24(8):1545–51.
8. Garcia-Espinosa V, Curcio S, Marotta M, Castro JM, Arana M, Peluso G, Chiesa P, Giachetto G, Bia D, Zócalo Y. Changes in central aortic pressure levels, wave components and determinants associated with high peripheral blood pressure states in childhood: analysis of hypertensive phenotype. Pediatr Cardiol. 2016;37:1340–50.
9. Urbina EM, Khoury PR, McCoy C, Daniels SR, Kimball TR, Dolan LM. Cardiac and vascular consequences of pre-hypertension in youth. J Clin Hypertens (Greenwich). 2011;13:332–42.
10. Lurbe E, Torro I, Garcia-Vicent C, Alvarez J, Fernandez-Fornoso JA, Redon J. Blood pressure and obesity exert independent influences on pulse wave velocity in youth. Hypertension. 2012;60:550–5.
11. Murgan I, Beyer S, Kotliar KE, Weber L, Bechtold-Dalla Pozza S, Dalla Pozza R, Wegner A, Sitnikova D, Stock K, Heemann U, Schmaderer C, Baumann M. Arterial and retinal vascular changes in hypertensive and prehypertensive adolescents. Am J Hypertens. 2013;26:400–8.
12. Lorenzo C, Aung K, Stern M, Haffner S. Pulse pressure, prehypertension, and mortality: the San Antonio heart study. Am J Hypertens. 2009;22:1219–26.
13. Gedikli O, Kiris A, Ozturk S, Baltaci D, Karaman K, Durmus I, Baykan M, Celik S. Effects of prehypertension on arterial stiffness and wave reflections. Clin Exp Hypertens. 2010;32:84–9.
14. Tomiyama H, Matsumoto C, Yamada J, Yoshida M, OdairaM SK, Nagata M, Yamashina A. Predictors ofprogression from prehypertension to hypertension in Japanesemen. Am J Hypertens. 2009;22:630–6.
15. Najjar S, Scuteri A, Shetty V, Wright J, Muller FJ, Spurgeon H, Ferrucci L, Lakatta E. Pulse wave velocity is an independent predictor of the longitudinalincrease in systolic blood pressure and of incident hypertension inthe Baltimore Longitudinal Study of Aging. J Am Coll Cardiol. 2008;51:1377–83.
16. Tomiyama H, Hashimoto H, Matsumoto C, Odaira M, YoshidaM SK, Nagata M, Yamashina A, Doba N, Hinohara S. Effects of aging and persistent prehypertension on arterialstiffening. Atherosclerosis. 2011;217:130–4.
17. Celik T, Iyisoy A, Kursaklioglu H, Turhan H, CagdasYuksel U, Kilic S, Kutsi Kabul H, Genc C. Impaired aortic elasticproperties in young patients with prehypertension. Blood Press Monit. 2006;11:251–5.
18. Erdogan D, Caliskan M, Yildrim I, Gullu H, Baycan S, Ciftici O, Yildir A, Mederrisoglu H. Effects of normal blood pressure, prehypertension and hypertension on left ventricular diastolic function and aortic elastic properties. Blood Press. 2007;16:114–21.
19. Jia C, Jiang Y, Yang Z, Sun X, Yu Y, Wang H, Lu Y, Chen A, Wang Z. Ascending aortic elasticity and related risk factors study on prehypertension patients. Am J Hypertens. 2017;30:61–6.
20. Toikka J, Niemi P, Ahotupa M, Niinikoski H, Rönnemaa T, Viikari J, Hartiala J, Raitakari O. Decreased large artery distensibility in borderline hypertension is related to increased in vivo low-density lipoprotein oxidation. Scand J Clin Lab Invest. 2002;62:301–6.
21. Pauletto P, Palatini P, Da Ros S, Pagliara V, Santipolo N, Baccillieri S, Casiglia E, Mormino P, Pessina AC. Factors underlying the increase in carotid intima-media thickness in borderline hypertensives. Arterioscler Thromb Vasc Biol. 1999;19:1231–7.
22. Day TG, Park M, Kinra S. The association between blood pressure and carotid intima-media thickness in children: a systematic review. Cardiol Young. 2017:1–11.
23. Jourdan C, Wuhl E, Litwin M, Fahr K, Trelewicz J, Jobs K, Schenk JP, Grenda R, Mehls O, Tröger J, Schaefer F. Normative values for intima-media thickness and distensibility of large arteries in healthy adolescents. J Hypertens. 2005;23:1707–15.
24. Stabouli S, Kotsis V, Karagianni C, Zakopoulos N, Konstantopoulos A. Blood pressure and carotid artery intima-media thickness in children and adolescents: the role of obesity. Hell J Cardiol. 2012;53:41–7.

25. Manios E, Michas F, Tsivgoulis G, Stamatelopoulos K, Tsagalis G, Koroboki E, Alexaki E, Papamichael C, Vemmos K, Zakopoulos N. Impact of prehypertension on carotid artery intima-media thickening: actual or masked? Atherosclerosis. 2011;214:215–9.
26. Alpaydin S, Turan Y, Caliskan M, Caliskan Z, Aksu F, Ozyildirim S, Buyukterzi Z, Kostek O, Muderrisoglu H. Morning blood pressure surge is associated with carotid intima-media thickness in prehypertensive patients. Blood Press Monit. 2017;22:131–6.
27. Hong H, Wang H, Liao H. Prehypertension is associated with increased carotid atherosclerotic plaque in the community population of southern China. BMC Cardiovasc Disord. 2013;13:20–8.
28. Manios E, Tsivgoulis G, Koroboki E, Stamatelopoulos K, Papamichael C, Toumanidis S, Stamboulis E Vemmos K, Zakopoulos N. Impact of prehypertension on common carotid artery intima-media thickness and left ventricular mass. Stroke. 2009;40:1515–8.
29. Psaty BM, Arnold AM, Olson J, Saad MF, Shea S, Post W, Burke GL. Association between levels of blood pressure and measures of subclinical disease multi-ethnic study of atherosclerosis. Am J Hypertens. 2006;19:1110–7.
30. Karasek D, Vaaverkova H, Halenka M, Jackuliakova D, Frysak Z, Orsag J, Novotny D. Prehypertension in dyslipidemic individuals; relationship to metabolic parameters and intima-media thickness. Biomed Pap Med Fac Palacky Olomouc Czech Repub. 2013;157:41–9.
31. Femia R, Kozakova M, Nannipieri M, Gonzales-Villalpando C, Stern MP, Haffner SM, Ferrannini E. Carotid intima-media thickness in confirmed prehypertensive subjects predictors and progression. Arterioscler Thromb Vasc Biol. 2007;27:2244–9.
32. Liew G, Wang JJ, Mitchell P, Wong TY. Retinal vascular imaging: a new tool in microvascular disease research. Circ Cardiovasc Imaging. 2008;1:156–61.
33. Wong TY, Liew G, Tapp RJ, Schmidt MI, Wang JJ, Mitchell P, Klein R, Klein BE, Zimmet P, Shaw J. Relation between fasting glucose and retinopathy for diagnosis of diabetes: three population-based crosssectional studies. Lancet. 2008;371:736–43.
34. Wong TY, Klein R, Sharrett AR, Duncan BB, Couper DJ, Klein BEK, Hubbard LD, Nieto FJ. For the atherosclerosis risk in communities study. Retinal arteriolar diameter and risk for hypertension. Ann Intern Med. 2004;140:248–55.
35. Cuspidi C, Negri F, Giudici V, Sala C. Retinal changes and cardiac remodelling in systemic hypertension. Ther Adv Cardiovasc Dis. 2009;3:205–14.
36. Liew G, Sharrett AR, Wang JJ, Klein R, Klein BE, Mitchell P, Wong TY. Relative importance of systemic determinants of retinal arteriolar and venular caliber: the atherosclerosis risk in communities study. Arch Ophthalmol. 2008;126:1404–10.
37. Wong TY, Islam FM, Klein R, Klein BE, Cotch MF, Castro C, et al. Retinal vascular caliber, cardiovascular risk factors, and inflammation: the multiethnic study of atherosclerosis (MESA). Invest Ophthalmol Vis Sci. 2006;47:2341–50.
38. De Jong FJ, Ikram MK, Witteman JC, Hofman A, de Jong PT, Breteler MM. Retinal vessel diameters and the role of inflammation in cerebrovascular disease. Ann Neurol. 2007;61:491–5.
39. Sabanayagam C, Shankar A, Koh D, Chia KS, Saw SM, Lim SC, et al. Retinal microvascular caliber and chronic kidney disease in an Asian population. Am J Epidemiol. 2009;169:625–32.
40. Wang JJ, Mitchell P, Leung H, Rochtchina E, Wong TY, Klein R. Hypertensive retinal vessel wall signs in a general older population: the Blue Mountains eye study. Hypertension. 2003;42:534–41.
41. Wong TY, Klein R, Klein BEK, Tielsch J, Hubbard LD, Nieto FJ. Retinal microvascular abnormalities, and their relation to hypertension, cardiovascular diseases and mortality. Surv Ophthalmol. 2001;46:59–80.
42. Grassi G, Buzzi S, Dell Oro R, Mineo C, Dimitriadis K, Seravalle G, Lonati L, Cuspidi C. Structural alterations of the retinal microcirculation in the "prehypertensive" high-normal blood pressure state. Curr Pharm Des. 2013;19:2375–81.
43. Klein R, Sharrett AR, Klein BEK, Chambless L, Cooper S, Hubbard LD, Evans G. Are retinal arteriolar abnormalities related to atherosclerosis? The atherosclerosis risk in communities study. Arterioscler Thromb Vasc Biol. 2000;20:1644–50.
44. Sharrett AR, Hubbard LD, Cooper LS, Sorlie PD, Brothers RJ, Nieto FJ, Pinsky JL, Klein R. Retinal arteriolar diameters and elevated blood pressure: the atherosclerosis risk in communities study. Am J Epidemiol. 1999;150:263–70.

45. Mitchell P, Cheung N, de Haseth K, Taylor B, Rochtchina E, Islam FM, Wang JJ, Saw SM, Wong TY. Blood pressure and retinal arteriolar narrowing in children. Hypertension. 2007;49:1156–62.
46. Klein R, Klein BEK, Moss SE. The relation of systemic hypertension to changes in the retinal vasculature. The beaver dam eye study. Trans Am Ophthalmol Soc. 1997;95:329–50.
47. Dinga J, Wai KL, McGeechand K, Lkrama MK, Kawasaki R, Xie J, Klein R, Klein B BK, Frances Cotch M, Wang JJ, Mitchell P, Shaw JE, Takamasa K, Richey Sharrett A, Wonga TY, for the Meta-Eye Study Group. Retinal vascular caliber and the development of hypertension: a meta-analysis of individual participant data. J Hypertens. 2014;32:207–15.
48. Xia F, Liu G, Shi Y, Zhang Y. Impact of microalbuminuria on incident coronary heart disease, cardiovascular and all-cause mortality: a meta-analysis of prospective studies. Int J Clin Exp Med. 2015;8:1–9.
49. Weil BR, Stauffer BL, Greiner JJ, DeSouza CA. Prehypertension is associated with impaired nitric oxide-mediated endothelium-dependent vasodilation in sedentary adults. Am J Hypertens. 2011;24:976–81.
50. Wang G, Wang A, Tong W, Liu Y, Zhang Y. Association of elevated inflammatory and endothelial biomarkers with prehypertension among Mongolians in China. Hypertens Res. 2011;34:516–20.
51. Nikolov P, Nikolov J, Prbecova M, Deneva T, Vladimirova L, Atanasova P, Hrischev P, Gerogieva E, Nikolov F. Flow mediated vasodilatation and some biomarkers of endothelial activation in pre-hypertensive objects. 2015 Nov 24. pii: wimj.2015.033. https://doi.org/10.7727/wimj.2015.033.
52. Vrdoljak A, Ivković V, Karanović S, Dika Ž, Vuković I, Kos J, Laganović M, Željković Vrkić T, FištrekPrlić M, Pećin I, Jelaković B. Markers of early renal impairment in prehypertension. J Hypertension. 2016;34(Suppl 1. - ISH 2016 Abstract Book):e47.
53. Knight E, Kramer H, Curhan G. High normal blood pressure and microalbuminuria. Am J Kid Dis. 2003;41:588–95.
54. Ogunniyi MO, Croft JB, Greenlund KJ, Giles WH, Mensah GA. Racial/ethnic differences in microalbuminuria among adults with prehypertension and hypertension: National Health and nutrition examination survey (NHANES), 1999–2006. Am J Hypertens. 2010;23:859–64.
55. Tenekecioglu E, Yilmaz M, Yontar O, Karaagac K, Agca F, Tutuncu A, Kuzeytemiz M, Bekler A, Senturk M, Aydin U, Demir Ş. Microalbuminuria in untreated prehypertension and hypertension without diabetes. Int J Clin Exp Med. 2014;7:3420–9.
56. Kim B, Lee H, Sung K, Kim B, Kang J, Lee M, Park J. Comparison of microalbuminuria in 2 blood pressure categories of Prehypertensive subjects. Circ J. 2007;71:1283–128.
57. Lee J, Kim Y, Choi Y, Huh W, Kim D, Young H. Serum uric acid is associated with microalbuminuria in prehypertension. Hypertension. 2006;47:962–7.
58. Okada R, Yasuda Y, Tsushita K, Wakai K, Hamajima N, Matsuo S. Glomerular hyperfiltration in prediabetes and prehypertension. Nephrol Dial Transplant. 2012;27(5):1821.
59. Yi H, Zhang WZ, Zhang H, Chen YH, Zhou MC. Subclinical target organ damage in normotensive and prehypertensive patients. Minerva Cardioangiol. 2017;65:16–23.
60. Peng H, Ding J, Peng Y, Zhang Q, Xu Y, Chao X, Tian H, Zhang Y. Hyperuricemia and microalbuminuria are separately and independently associated with prehypertension among Chinese Han women. Metab Syndr Relat Disord. 2012;10:202–8.
61. Zhang Q, Peng H, Ding JS, Xu YY, Chao XQ, Tian HG, Zhang YH. Association between urinary albumin-to-creatinine ratio and prehypertension. Zhonghua Liu Xing Bing XueZaZhi. 2012;33:32–6.
62. Ding J, Peng H, Peng Y, Zhang Q, Xu Y, Chao X, Tian H, Zhang Y. Urinary albumin-to-creatinine ratio in a first-morning void urine and prehypertension among Chinese Han women. Blood Press. 2012;21:128–33.
63. Wang Q, Huang J, Sun Y, Zhang W, Gao Y, Yao W, Bian B, Li Y, Wu X, Niu K. Association of microalbuminuria with diabetes is stronger in people with prehypertension compared to those with ideal blood pressure. Nephrology (Carlton). 2017. https://doi.org/10.1111/nep.13082. [Epub ahead of print].

64. Wang T, Evans J, Meigs J, Rifai N, Fox C, D'Agostino R, Levy D, Vasan R. Low-grade albuminuria and the risks of hypertension and blood pressure progression. Circulation. 2005;111:1370–6.
65. Norton G, Maseko M, Libhaber E, Libhaber C, Majane O, Dessein P, Sareli P, Woodiwiss A. Is prehypertension an independent predictor of target organ changes in young-to-middle-aged persons of African descent? J Hypertens. 2008;26:2279–87.
66. Sehestedta T, Jeppesena J, Hansenb T, Rasmussene S, Wachtellf K, Ibseng H, Torp-Pedersenc C, Olsen M. Which markers of subclinical organ damage to measure in individuals with high normal blood pressure? J Hypertens. 2009;27:1165–71.
67. Ivkovic V, Parini A, Vrdoljak A, Karanovic S, Baric M, Abramovic M, Bachelli S, Cagnati M, Cicero A, D'Addato S, Esposti D, Fucek M, Grandi E, Kos J, Laganovic M, Rogic D, Rosticci M, Vukovic I, Borghi C, Jelakovic B. Predictors of incident hypertension in prehypertensives. J Hypertens. 2016;34:e127–8.
68. Bajpai J, Agarwal S, Garg B, Goel A. Impact of prehypertension on left ventricular structure, function and geometry. J Clin Diagn Res. 2014;8:BC07–10.
69. Di Bello V, Talini E, Gianno C, Dele Donne MG, Canale ML, Nardi C, Palagi C, Dini FL, Penno G, DelPrao S, Marzilli M, Pedrinelli R. Early left ventricular mechincs abnormalities in prehypertension: a two-dimensional strain echocardiography study. Am J Hypertens. 2010;23:405–12.
70. Ahn H-S, Kim S-J, Kim M-K, Choue C-W, Kim K-S, Song J-S, Bae J-H. The difference of left ventricular hypertrophy and the diastolic function between prehypertensives and normotensives. Korean Circulation J. 2006;36:437–42.
71. Kim S, Cho G-Y, Baik I, Lim S, Choi C, Lim H, Kim E, Park C, Kim J, Shin C. Early abnormalities of cardiovascular structure and function in middle-aged Korean adults with prehypertension; The Korean Genome Epidemiology Study. Am J Hypertens. 2011;24:218–24.
72. Jung J, Park S, Oh C-O, Kang J, Choi J-M, Ryoo J-H, Lee J-H. The influence of prehypertension, controlled and uncontrolled hypertension on left ventricular diastolic function and structure in the general Korean population. Hypertens Res. 2017;40:606–12.
73. Litwin M, Niemirska A, Sladowska J, Antoniewicz J, Daszkowska J, Wierzbicka A, Wawer Z, Grenda R. Left ventricular hypertrophy and arterial wall thickening in children with essential hypertension. Pediatr Nephrol. 2006;21:811–9.
74. Sorof JM, Turner J, Martin DS, Garcia K, Garami Z, Alexandrov AV, Wan F, Portman RJ. Cardiovascular risk factors and sequelae in hypertensive children identified by referral versus school-based screening. Hypertension. 2004;43:214–8.
75. McNiece KL, Gupta-Malhotra M, Samuels J, Bell C, Garcia K, Poffenbarger T, Sorof JM, Portman RJ, National High Blood Pressure Education Program Working Group. Left ventricular hypertrophy in hypertensive adolescents: analysis of risk by 2004 National High Blood Pressure Education Program Working Group staging criteria. Hypertension. 2007;50:392–5.
76. Falkner B, DeLoach S, Keith SW, Gidding SS. High risk blood pressure and obesity increase the risk for left ventricular hypertrophy in African-American adolescents. J Pediatr. 2013;162:94–100.
77. Markus M, Stritzke J, Lieb W, Mayer B, Luchner A, Doring A, Keil U, Hense H-W, Schunkert H. Implications of persistent prehypertension for ageing-related changes in left ventricular geometry and function: The MONICA/KORA Augsburg study. J Hypertens. 2008;26:2040–9.
78. Jang S, Kim S, Lee C, Cho E, Cho S, Lee S-C. Prehypertension and left ventricular dysfunction in middle-aged Koreans. Korean Circ J. 2016;46:536–41.
79. Santos A, Gupta D, Bello N, Gori M, Claggett B, Fuchs F, Shah A, Coresh J, Sharrett A, Cheng S, Solomon S. Prehypertension is associated with abnormalities of cardiac structure and function in the atherosclerosis risk in communities study. Am J Hypertens. 2016;29:568–74.
80. Sironi AM, Pingitore A, Ghione S, De Marchi D, Scattini B, Positano V, Muscelli E, Ciociaro D, Lombardi M, Ferrannini E, Gastaldelli A. Early hypertension is associated with reduced regional cardiac function, insulin resistance, epicardial, and visceral fat. Hypertension. 2008;51:282–8.

Part VI

Clinical Studies in Prehypertension

35 Neurogenic Mechanisms in Prehypertension and Pharmacologic Approaches to the Prevention and Treatment of Hypertension: Highlights of Professor Stevo Julius' Scientific Contributions

Brent M. Egan

Stevo Julius, MD, ScD, has served as Professor of Medicine at the University of Michigan Medical Center for more than 50 years where he continues as Professor Emeritus. During that time, he has made numerous original and important scientific contributions. His initial research centered on defining personality characteristics and autonomic mechanisms in the hemodynamic profile of individuals with borderline hypertension or prehypertension [1, 2]. Dr. Julius' early work was instrumental in defining a key primary role for the sympathetic nervous system in borderline and established hypertension [3–5].

In the middle phase of his scientific career, Dr. Julius and colleagues documented a key primary role for the sympathetic nervous system in the pathogenesis of hyperinsulinemia, insulin resistance, and the cardiometabolic syndrome [6–9]. All of the cardiometabolic phenomena were associated with increased heart rate, a marker of neurogenic activation. While an extensive body of research documents that excess caloric intake and obesity can drive the cardiometabolic syndrome [10], Dr. Julius demonstrated that elevated blood pressure was already present in young, normal weight children of hypertensive parents [8]. Excess weight gain and further elevation of blood pressure as well as multiple features of the cardiometabolic syndrome followed this early "prehypertensive" phase. Collectively, these data suggest that sympathetic activation with elevated blood pressure can precede the cardiometabolic syndrome.

B. M. Egan
Department of Medicine, University of South Carolina School of Medicine, Greenville, SC, USA

Care Coordination Institute, Greenville, SC, USA
e-mail: began@ccihealth.org

R. Zimlichman et al. (eds.), *Prehypertension and Cardiometabolic Syndrome*, Updates in Hypertension and Cardiovascular Protection,
https://doi.org/10.1007/978-3-319-75310-2_35

During the latter part of his still active career, Professor Julius has worked with longtime colleagues on pharmacological interventions for the prevention and treatment of hypertension [11–14]. The rational and provocative interpretation of the data from these trials has often challenged existing paradigms and stimulated critical thinking to enhance our understanding of hypertension-related risk and its mitigation. This review highlights several of Dr. Julius' original scientific contributions and the many clinically insightful and relevant applications of that work.

35.1 Borderline Hypertension—The Early Years

Personality characteristics associated with prehypertension and hypertension. In 1964, Harburg and Julius obtained blood pressures on 800 male undergraduate students at the University of Michigan who were waiting in line to register for classes. From this group, 74 white men were selected for having systolic blood pressure (BP, mmHg) values either in the upper or lower end of the distribution [1]. Students were classified as having high or low systolic BP according to their paired casual (screening and first follow-up visit), usual (self-measured home BP). Of 21 persons with a high paired casual SBP >140, 16 also had repeated home SBP readings >131. Among this group, 11 had high home BP readings, defined as sustained hypertension. The BP patterns of these young men were then related with self-ratings on the Cattell 16 Personality Factor Questionnaire.

Sustained elevation of systolic BP in male college students was associated with "submissiveness" and "sensitivity" as defined by Cattell's Questionnaire. Subjects with "high paired casual" systolic BP values described themselves as motivated to obtain social contacts, but in a "sensitive" and "anxious" manner. Subjects who were later selected for having a single high systolic BP on first entering the physician's office (second casual reading) tended more frequently to yield in an argument and then afterwards to change their private opinions toward agreement with partners who had an initially low systolic BP [1].

A subsequent study in 1986 by Professor Julius and coworkers utilized advances in questionnaire methodology to more thoroughly dissect personality characteristics of young college males with elevated BP in the screening, clinic and home environments [2]. The questionnaires included Spielberger's State-Trait Personality Inventory, the Anger Expression Scale, and the State Anger Reaction Scale [15]. As with the previous study [1], BP measurements were obtained on students waiting to register for their next semester classes. Undergraduate men in the upper end of the BP distribution were recalled to complete the questionnaires and to undergo self-measured home BP measurements. Two groups were identified. One group maintained high BP at home, and the second group had normal BP at home. Of interest, the group that maintained high BP at home reported greater intensity of anger and suppressed their anger to a greater extent than the group whose BP was normal at home.

The findings in this 1986 report were consistent with Alexander's original work and hypothesis [16] that inhibition of angry or hostile impulses can increase systemic BP. Moreover, the hypertensive personality has a long-term conflict between the need for passive dependence and the need for expressing hostile impulses. According to Alexander, it is this long-term conflict which can lead to sustained elevation of arterial BP or hypertension, evident among young men in the 1986 report [2].

Linkage of anger to sympathetic activation and parasympathetic withdrawal. Marci et al. studied autonomic and prefrontal cortex responses to autobiographical recall of emotions [17]. Of emotions studied, anger was the only one to show a significant increase in sympathetic activity, accompanied by a significant decrease in cardiac parasympathetic or vagal tone as measured by the high frequency component of heart rate variability. While the study by Marci and colleagues is not the first to show that anger induces sympathetic activation, it is among the clearest to show a reciprocal and concomitant reduction of cardiac vagal tone.

The role of sympathetic activation and parasympathetic inhibition in the hyperkinetic hemodynamic profile of borderline hypertension. Dr. Julius and colleagues published a series of papers on the hemodynamics of borderline hypertension in the prestigious American Heart Association Journal, Circulation in 1971. One report captured their work on sequential autonomic blockade of β-adrenoceptors with the nonselective blocker propranolol followed by parasympathetic inhibition using atropine [3]. Both autonomic blocking agents were administered intravenously at doses known to fully block the respective systems.

At baseline, individuals with hyperkinetic borderline hypertension had higher values than normotensive controls for cardiac output and heart rate (Fig. 35.1). β-Adrenoceptor blockade led to a larger fall of cardiac output and heart rate among

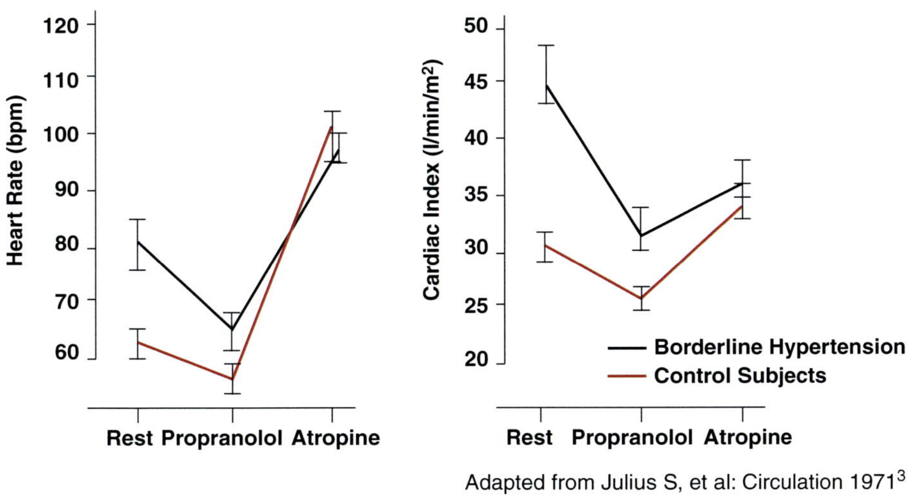

Fig. 35.1 At baseline, heart rate and cardiac index are higher in hyperkinetic borderline hypertensives than age- and sex-matched normal controls. After propranolol, heart rate and cardiac index decline more in the hyperkinetic than normal group, yet values remain higher in the former. With addition of atropine, heart rate and cardiac index increase less in the hyperkinetic than in the control group and significant between group differences were abolished

individuals with hyperkinetic borderline hypertension. These data were consistent with increased cardiac beta-adrenergic tone in the hyperkinetic group. Yet, cardiac output and heart rate remained significantly higher in the hyperkinetic borderline hypertensive group than in the normal controls. When atropine was administered while continuing beta-adrenergic blockade with propranolol, cardiac output and heart rate increased less in subjects with hyperkinetic borderline hypertension than in normal controls. The responses to atropine indicate that cardiac parasympathetic tone is lower in hyperkinetic borderline hypertension than in normal controls.

Only after total cardiac autonomic blockade with both propranolol and atropine were the differences in cardiac output and heart rate no longer significantly different between the group with hyperkinetic borderline hypertension and healthy controls. These data indicate that the hyperkinetic state of borderline hypertension reflects a reciprocal autonomic abnormality characterized both by increased sympathetic and reduced parasympathetic tone.

Transition from hyperkinetic borderline hypertension to normokinetic borderline and established essential hypertension. Research on borderline or prehypertension consistently identifies a hyperkinetic subset of young individuals with elevated cardiac output and a fast heart rate. Faster heart rates, even within the range of 60–100 beats/min, which are considered normal, are a strong predictor of future essential hypertension [18], and many hyperkinetic subjects appear to develop classical established hypertension [19]. However, the hyperkinetic state is much less common in adults with hypertension. Thus, transition from the hyperkinetic borderline hypertension to normokinetic, high-resistance hypertension almost certainly occurs and is supported by data from sequential hemodynamic studies [19].

In fact, Julius and colleagues provided further evidence that individuals with borderline hypertension and normal cardiac output may represent a later phase of the prior hyperkinetic state. More specifically, baseline heart rate was elevated less among individuals with borderline hypertension and normal cardiac output than in prior studies of the hyperkinetic subset with borderline hypertension. Following cardiac autonomic blockade with intravenous propranolol and atropine, their cardiac output was lower than normal controls [20]. Heart rate responses to the β-agonist isoproterenol were less in borderline hypertensives with normal cardiac output than in demographically matched normotensive controls. The borderline blood pressure elevation in subjects with normokinetic borderline hypertensive was maintained by an elevated vascular resistance. Compared to normokinetic group with borderline hypertension, the higher blood pressure in established hypertension reflects a further increase of vascular resistance as a normal cardiac out is maintained.

Of note, while hypertension in obesity was identified as a state of high cardiac output and normal vascular resistance, vascular resistance is elevated when compared to obese, demographically matched normal controls [21, 22]. The Ann Arbor group documented that forearm vasodilator responses to regional infusion of phentolamine were greater in overweight and obese than in leaner subjects, despite higher baseline flows with normal resistance in the obese group [23]. The inappropriately normal vascular resistance in obese subjects with elevated blood pressure is maintained by enhanced vascular alpha-adrenergic tone similar to the increased vascular α-adrenergic tone similar to that observed in neurogenic, high-renin hypertension [4, 5].

Mechanisms underlying the hemodynamic transition from hyperkinetic borderline hypertension to normokinetic hypertension. AUTOREGULATION. Dr. Arthur Guyton and colleagues demonstrated that volume expansion leads to increased cardiac output and tissue perfusion in excess of metabolic demands [24]. When this occurs, most organ systems increase vascular resistance to reestablish the balance between metabolic demands and supply, which raises arterial blood pressure. The phenomenon of matching blood flow to metabolic demands by varying vascular resistance is termed "autoregulation" [25].

Basis for an alternative explanation to autoregulation for the hemodynamic transition from hyperkinetic borderline to established hypertension with normal cardiac output. Studies in borderline hypertension provided two important pieces of evidence contrary to autoregulation as the mechanism for the hemodynamic transition. First, plasma volume was lower and not higher among borderline hypertensives than normal controls, when adjusted for body weight or when compared in weight-matched individuals with borderline hypertensive to healthy controls [26]. Second, in subjects with hyperkinetic borderline hypertension, higher cardiac output occurred together with greater total body oxygen consumption [27]. In fact, the regression line for cardiac output versus total body oxygen consumption was the same in subjects with borderline hypertension and demographically matched normal controls. The stimulus for autoregulation, based on whole body studies, was not apparent in hyperkinetic borderline hypertensives.

Neurogenic and vascular transformation. An alternative explanation for the hemodynamic transition from hyperkinetic borderline to normokinetic borderline and essential hypertension: Focus on decreased β-adrenergic sensitivity, cardiovascular remodeling and increased vascular α-adrenergic tone.

Cardiac changes. Sustained increases in cardiac sympathetic drive lead to decreased chronotropic and inotropic responses to β_1-adrenoceptor activation [20, 28, 29]. Furthermore, a decline in left ventricular compliance may contribute to lower stroke volume in patients with normokinetic mild hypertension [20, 30]. More specifically, Julius and colleagues documented that stroke volume in patients with mild hypertension was lower than in normotensive controls following cardiac autonomic blockade with propranolol and atropine. Stroke volume following cardiac autonomic blockade becomes largely dependent on end-diastolic volume. In these studies, cardiopulmonary blood volume was similar in hypertensive adults and normotensive controls, which suggests similar levels of preload [20, 30].

A stiffer, less compliant left ventricular in hypertensives could lead to lower ventricular volume end-diastole and a reduced stroke volume [28]. Decreased cardiac compliance, in turn, most likely reflects early cardiac restructuring in response to long-standing mild blood pressure elevation. Julius and coworker proposed that the combination of downregulation of cardiac β_1-adrenergic receptors with decreased chronotropic and inotropic responses to sympathetic drive together with decreased cardiac compliance and stroke volume contribute to the normalization of cardiac output in established hypertension [31].

Vascular changes. Concurrent structural vascular remodeling supports the progressive rise in vascular resistance. Sustained blood pressure elevation leads to remodeling of the arterial wall. Increased sympathetic stimulation is also well-documented vascular trophic factor [32, 33]. Thus, individuals with neurogenic borderline and established hypertension appear especially prone to cardiac and vascular remodeling. While medial smooth muscle hypertrophy with an increase in muscle wall mass can occur, the predominant change may reflect remodeling of the wall mass around a small vascular lumen based on anatomical studies in Denmark and physiologic studies in Ann Arbor [34, 35]. With either true hypertrophy with an increased vascular wall mass or remodeling of the vascular media with a normal wall mass surrounding a small lumen, the vascular wall:lumen ratio increases. In this setting, minimum vascular resistance is higher and vasoconstrictor responses are nonspecifically amplified. Folkow and colleagues were the pioneers in showing how an increased wall:lumen ratio contributes to hypertension by nonspecifically augmenting vascular resistance responses to vasoactive stimuli [36].

Subsequent studies by Dr. Julius and colleagues in relatively young subjects with Stage 1 hypertension compared to demographically and weight-matched normotensive controls were consistent with vascular remodeling as a nonspecific amplifier of arterial resistance in response to different vasoconstrictors (Fig. 35.2) [37]. Folkow's criteria for vascular remodeling as an amplifier of resistance responses were met in the Stage 1 hypertensive compared to matched controls including: (1) minimum forearm vascular resistance, an index of vascular remodeling, (2) vascular sensitivity to both vasoconstrictors, as estimated by the concentration required to induce 30% of the maximal vasoconstrictor response, was similar, (3) forearm vasoconstrictor responses to both norepinephrine and angiotensin were characterized by a

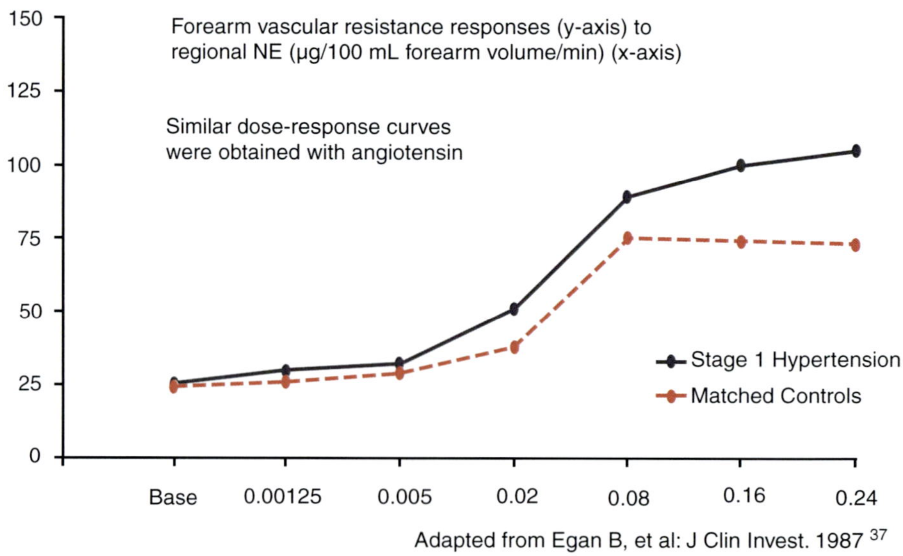

Fig. 35.2 Baseline forearm vascular resistance was slightly higher in Stage 1 hypertensives than matched normal controls. Note forearm resistance responses between the two groups diverge progressively with increasing doses of regional norepinephrine. Maximum forearm responses were also greater in hypertensives than in matched normotensive controls

steeper slope, and (4) greater maximum resistance responses. (5) forearm vascular responses to both vasoconstrictors were 'non-specifically' enhanced and also directly related to the minimum vascular resistance, a measure of vascular remodeling. Moreover, the vasodilator response to phentolamine was significantly greater in subjects with Stage 1 hypertension than in controls indicating greater vascular alpha-tone. The latter finding coincides with earlier studies by Drs. Esler, Julius and colleagues described next.

Neurogenic borderline and established essential hypertension. The investigative team then documented that adding systemic α-adrenergic blockade with phentolamine to cardiac autonomic blockade with propranolol and atropine normalized arterial blood pressure in approximately one-third of subjects with borderline hypertension (Fig. 35.3) [4, 5].

These subjects were characterized by high-renin values, which likely reflected increased sympathetic drive to β_1-receptors on the juxtaglomerular cells, which stimulate renin secretion. The fact that acute and total autonomic blockade normalized blood pressure by reducing vascular resistance suggested to the authors that angiotensin probably did not play a critical role in the elevated blood pressure of borderline hypertensive subjects with high plasma renin values.

The investigators subsequently extended their observations on high-renin and neurogenic hypertension to adults with established essential hypertension [5]. Subsequent studies using more contemporary methodologies including muscle sympathetic nerve activity and norepinephrine turnover documented sympathetic overactivity is present in a substantial proportion of adults with essential hypertension including those who are obese [38, 39].

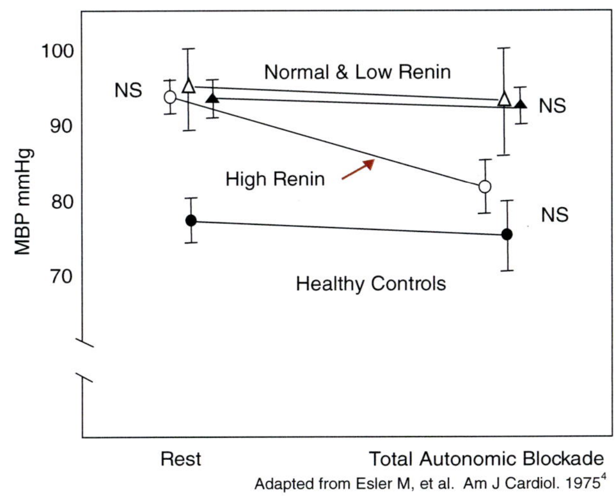

Fig. 35.3 Three groups of subjects with borderline hypertension were studied. The three groups included subjects with low renin (closed triangles), normal renin (open triangles), and high renin (open circles) borderline hypertension. All three groups with borderline hypertension had higher mean blood pressure (MBP, mmHg) at rest than healthy controls. Following total autonomic blockade with propranolol, atropine, and phentolamine, MBP fell only in the high renin group and was no longer significantly greater than MBP in normal controls (closed circles)

Renal norepinephrine spillover is increased in both obese hypertensives and normotensives, whereas cardiac norepinephrine spillover is higher only in obese hypertensives. The increased renal sympathetic activity likely supports the volume expansion with obesity and in obesity hypertension, while increased sympathetic drive to other organs including the heart appears to contribute to the elevated blood pressure. One might postulate that the increased systemic blood pressure should suppress renal and cardiac sympathetic activity in the hypertensive obese subset. The fact that renal sympathetic activity is increased and not suppressed in obese hypertensive adults indirectly supports the premise by Guyton and colleagues that factors intrinsic or extrinsic to the kidney that increase sodium-volume retention are required to sustain hypertension [24, 25].

Sympathetic activation and the cardiometabolic syndrome. In a population-based community sample in Tecumseh, Michigan, Dr. Julius and colleagues demonstrated that heart rate, a marker of sympathetic activation, correlated with several metabolic features of the cardiometabolic syndrome among young adults in the early phase of hypertension (Fig. 35.4) [40].

The relationship between heart rate and hyperinsulinemia was especially strong. The hyperinsulinemia most likely represents a compensatory response to insulin resistance as identified by the inverse relationship with HDL cholesterol and direct link with hypertriglyceridemia.

Skeletal muscle is a key target organ for insulin action [41]. Resistance to insulin-mediated glucose disposal, a dominant feature of the cardiometabolic syndrome, is exacerbated by increased vascular alpha-adrenergic tone [9, 42–44], a key feature of

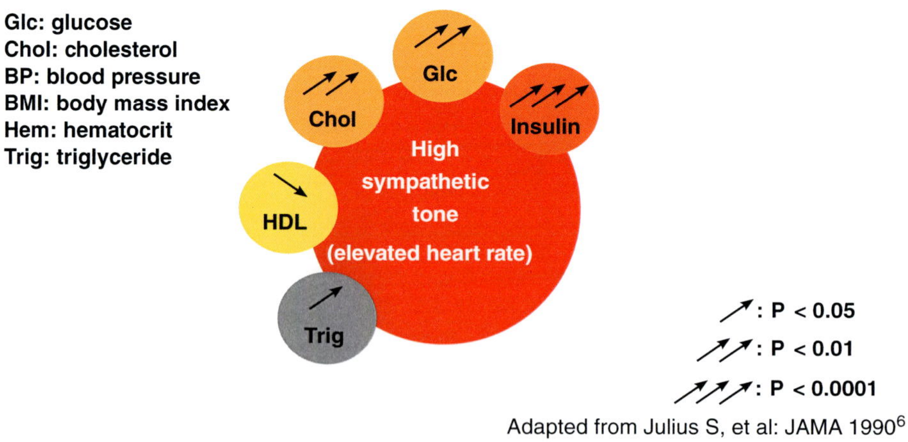

Fig. 35.4 Among young adults in Tecumseh, Michigan, Dr. Julius and colleagues documented that resting heart rate was highly correlated with plasma insulin, strongly correlated with fasting glucose (Glc) and total cholesterol (Chol), and modestly yet significantly with high-density lipoprotein cholesterol (HDL) and trigyclerides (Trig). Three arrows denotes significance at $p < 0.001$, two arrows $p < 0.01$, and a single arrow $p < 0.05$. Arrows pointing up and to the right indicate a positive association between heart rate and metabolic variables, whereas the arrow pointing down and to the left indicates a negative association

neurogenic hypertension [4, 5]. Drs. Jamerson and Julius demonstrated that insulin-mediated glucose disposal in the human forearm was acutely reduced in response to thigh-cuff inflation. Thigh-cuff inflation pools blood in the lower extremities, thereby unloading cardiopulmonary mechanoreceptors and inducing reflex forearm vasoconstriction [9]. In fact, reflex neurogenic vasoconstriction induced a greater degree of forearm insulin resistance than an intra-arterial norepinephrine infusion, which reduced forearm blood flow to the same extent as thigh cuff inflation [44]. Thus, reflex neurogenic vasoconstriction reduced glucose utilization by mechanisms in addition to reduced blood flow (Fig. 35.5) [44].

The authors cited studies indicating that reflex neurogenic vasoconstriction reduces the number of open capillaries in skeletal muscle. Moreover, capillary density in skeletal muscle is a major determinant of insulin-mediated glucose disposal in this tissue [45]. Their experimental data suggested that neurogenically mediated vasoconstriction [9, 44], observed in high-renin patients with borderline and established essential hypertension [4, 5], significantly diminishes insulin-mediated glucose disposal in skeletal muscle. This notion is consistent with studies showing that selective α_1-adrenoceptor antagonists improve insulin-mediate glucose disposal in hypertensive patients to a greater extent than renin-angiotensin system blockers [42, 43].

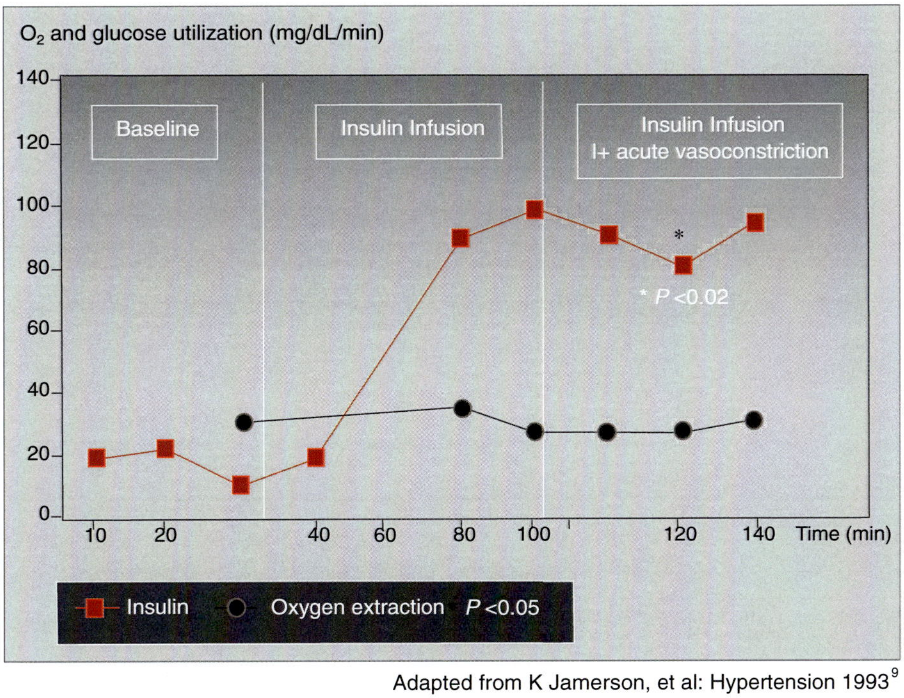

Fig. 35.5 After a 30-min baseline period, insulin was infused regionally to raise forearm insulin ~100 uU/mL for 90 min. Glucose utilization after 40–60 min of regional insulin rose 4–5-fold from baseline values. Thigh cuff inflation (beginning 60 min after the regional insulin infusion and continuing during thigh cuff inflation) minutes reduced forearm blood flow 19% and glucose utilization fell 23%, $p < 0.02$ [9]

Clinical importance of neurogenic effects on cardiometabolic variables. Effective antihypertensive therapy reduces stroke more than myocardial infarction [46, 47]. One potential explanation for the differential benefit of antihypertensive therapy is that hypertension is frequently associated with multiple other cardiovascular risk factors that raise the risk for myocardial infarction more than the risk for stroke. In fact, increased sympathetic tone may be involved in the genesis of multiple, pressure-independent coronary risk factors in hypertension [31].

Hypertension is frequently associated with hyperinsulinemia and insulin resistance [48]. Insulin resistance is frequently accompanied by a complex atherogenic dyslipidemia characterized by increased triglycerides, reduced HDL cholesterol, and an increased number of dense LDL cholesterol particles [49]. Julius and colleagues provided evidence that these cardiometabolic risk factors are related to increased sympathetic drive [9, 40]. They previously reported that increased sympathetic drive is associated with a relative resting tachycardia and elevated hematocrit [3, 26]. All of these factors (overweight/obesity, hyperinsulinemia, insulin resistance, dyslipidemia, tachycardia, higher hematocrit) are established risk factors for coronary heart disease and sudden death [31, 49–52].

Increased sympathetic drive and obesity: β-adrenoceptor downregulation and thermogenesis. Julius and colleagues documented that hyperkinetic borderline hypertension was characterized by increased cardiac output, which was matched to heightened oxygen consumptions [3, 27]. However, as noted previously, persistent excess sympathetic drive leads to desensitization or downregulation of β-adrenoceptors. The Ann Arbor group in collaboration with Italian colleagues explored the connection between downregulation of cardiac and thermogenic responses to the β-adrenoceptor agonist isoproterenol [53]. Subjects for this study included hypertensive adults and normal controls of comparable age but with lower body mass indices. The investigators documented that baseline heart rate was higher in the hypertensive group but that the responses of heart rate and oxygen consumption to isoproterenol were blunted in the hypertensive group. In fact, the chronotropic and thermogenic responses to isoproterenol were inversely related to urinary norepinephrine, an index of sympathetic drive.

Repeated neurogenic pressor episodes and future hypertension. A long-standing hypothesis posits that repeated neurogenic pressor episodes lead to sustained hypertension by inducing cardiovascular remodeling and renal injury [31]. Dr. Julius and colleagues described a reproducible hypertensive response to modest compression of both hind limbs in dogs using a fitted suit inflated to 30 mmHg [54]. While the inflation produced no discernible discomfort, systolic blood pressure rose approximately 30 mmHg 60–90 min after suit inflation and was maintained for the duration of 6-h hind limb compression. Heart rate also rose approximately 15 beats/min during hind limb compression. Over 9 weeks, 6 h of daily hind limb compression did not raise resting systolic blood pressure or heart rate but resulted in a 25–30% increase in left ventricular muscle mass. Thus, repeated neurogenic elevations of blood pressure sufficient to induce significant cardiac remodeling did not lead to sustained hypertension. While these experiments do not disprove the hypothesis that repeated neurogenic pressor episodes lead to sustained hypertension, the findings, nevertheless, raise questions.

In related studies, Julius and coworkers showed that the pressor responses to hind limb compression could be abolished by combined α- and β-adrenoceptor blockade but not by individual blockade of α- or β-adrenoceptors. In fact, in the presence of α-adrenoceptor blockade, dogs experienced the same hypertensive response to thigh cuff inflation mediated by a greater rise of cardiac output when neurogenic vasoconstriction was constrained. Conversely, during β-adrenoceptor blockade, the usual pressor response was mediated by a larger rise of vascular resistance when the increase of cardiac output was constrained. These and other observations led Julius and colleagues to consider the "pressure" seeking properties of the nervous system, which can be satisfied with variable contributions of flow and resistance [53].

Evidence of increased sympathetic tone in human hypertension has also been documented in human platelets. Kjeldsen and coworkers documented increased thromboglobulin, reflecting increased platelet turnover, and plasma epinephrine as well as a correlation between these two variables in hypertensive patients [55]. In subsequent studies in collaboration with the Ann Arbor group, Kjeldsen documented an inverse relationship between platelet noradrenaline, a marker for increased sympathetic drive, and decreased β-adrenoceptor responses [56]. The data suggest that increased sympathetic drive increases platelet turnover. Moreover, platelet norepinephrine, a long-term marker of sympathetic drive, is elevated in hypertension and is predictive of decreased β-receptor responses. These studies provide novel methodologic confirmation of excess sympathetic drive and downregulation of β-adrenoceptor responsiveness in hypertensive patients.

Summary of Dr. Julius work on increased sympathetic drive and multiple cardiovascular risk factors. As summarized in Fig. 35.6 [57], increased sympathetic drive, manifest as a faster heart rate, is strongly and positively correlated with blood pressure and hyperinsulinemia as well as glucose, triglycerides, cholesterol, hematocrit, and body mass index, and inversely correlated with HDL cholesterol. Moreover, suppressed anger appears to underlie the sympathetic activation and parasympathetic withdrawal, which unleash a cluster of risk factors for cardiovascular disease. During the next phase of his productive scientific career, Dr. Julius and colleagues focused efforts on preventing hypertension and its cardiovascular consequences.

Clinical trials to advance knowledge on preventing hypertension and its clinical consequences. Trial of Preventing Hypertension (TROPHY) [57]. In the more contemporary phase of his still active career, Professors Julius and colleagues conducted a landmark trial on preventing hypertension in subjects with prehypertension as defined by resting blood pressures in the 130–139/85–89 mmHg range. While blood pressure in this range has been defined as prehypertension since 1939 [58], the 2017 Hypertension Guideline developed by the American College of Cardiology and the American Heart Association now defines Stage 1 hypertension by blood pressure values of 130–139/80–89 mmHg [59]. Given this evolution in defining Stage 1 hypertension, TROPHY assumes even greater significance.

In TROPHY, approximately 800 subjects with repeating clinic blood pressure values in the 130–139/85–89 mmHg range were randomized to lifestyle

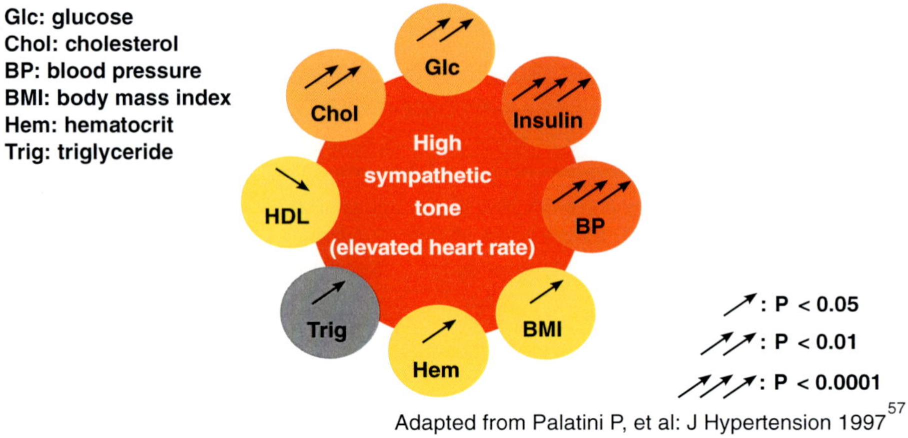

Fig. 35.6 High sympathetic tone as reflected by elevated heart rate, was very highly correlated with elevated blood pressure and insulin, strongly related to glucose and cholesterol and significantly related to HDL cholesterol, triglycerides, body mass index, and hematocrit

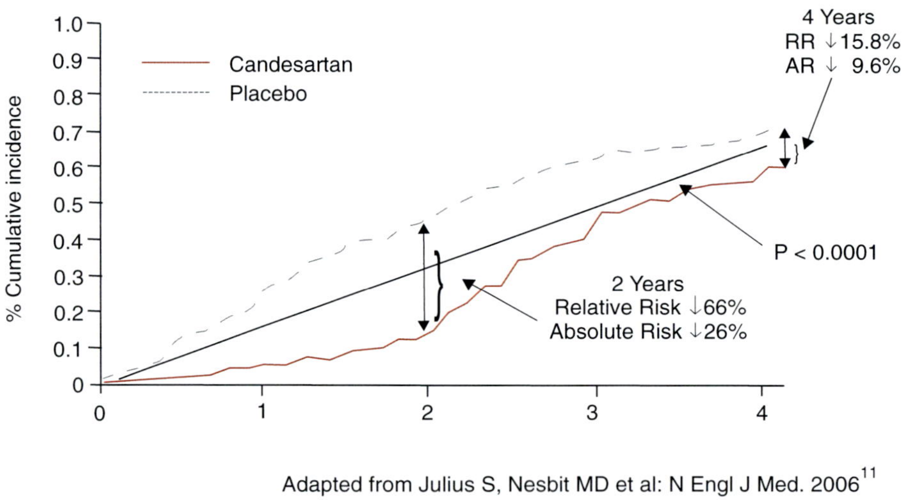

Fig. 35.7 Subjects with BP 130–139/85–89 randomized to candesartan (blue line) developed hypertension at 1/3 the rate of those on placebo during the 1st 2 years. While some "catch up" occurred in Years 3 and 4 when both groups received placebo, those initially on candesartan had a 15.8% relative reduction of incident hypertension at 4 years

intervention and the angiotensin receptor blocker, candesartan, or to lifestyle and placebo control [11]. After 2 years, candesartan was withdrawn and all subjects were followed for 2 additional years. As shown in Fig. 35.7, during the first 2 years, more subjects randomized to placebo developed hypertension than those randomized to candesartan, 40.4% versus 13.6%, $p < 0.001$. Thus, active treatment with candesartan reduced incident hypertension by two-thirds.

At 4 years, among subjects that had taken candesartan the first 2 years, 53.2% of them developed hypertension as compared to 63.0% in the placebo control group, $p < 0.001$, or a 15.6% relative reduction in incident hypertension [11]. It could be argued that most of the benefit for hypertension prevention was lost when candesartan was withdrawn. However, the 15.6% relative reduction of incident hypertension 2 years after candesartan was withdrawn is comparable to the reduction of incident hypertension seen with intensive and persistent lifestyle intervention over the same time period.

Given challenges with improving lifestyle patterns in the general population, pharmacotherapy provides a safe alternative for hypertension prevention. In fact, during the four years of TROPHY, serious adverse events occurred in 5.9% of patients assigned to the placebo group versus 3.5% among those randomized from the active treatment group. With the recent designation of Stage 1 hypertension as blood pressures in the 130–139/80–89 mmHg range, TROPHY is among the studies showing that blood pressure can be safely and effectively lowered in these individuals. More specifically, the 2017 ACC/AHA Hypertension Guideline recommends pharmacotherapy for Stage 1 hypertension when it occurs in conjunction with either clinical cardiovascular disease or a 10-year cardiovascular disease risk ≥10% [58].

Valsartan, amlodipine long-term evaluation (VALUE) study. **Importance of early blood pressure control** [12]. Professor Julius was a lead investigator on this important clinical trial, which generated some important and unexpected insights into preventing cardiovascular events in subjects at high risk. Among the important, unexpected insights, VALUE results indicated that differences in hypertension control during the first 3–6 months of the trial contributed to an excess of cardiovascular events. While conventional wisdom contends that it is important to "start low" and "go slow" when treating hypertension in an older, high-risk population, VALUE suggested that "starting too low" with pharmacotherapy, e.g., 80 mg valsartan, and "going too slow" in up-titrating doses and adding other classes of antihypertensive medications can lead to serious clinical cardiovascular events. Thus, it is important to balance the adverse effects of more rapid (aggressive) hypertension control with the benefit of fewer cardiovascular events.

Importance of the number of antihypertensive medications [13]. Another important and somewhat unexpected finding of VALUE was that among individuals requiring more than initial monotherapy in an attempt to control their hypertension, there was not a significant difference in clinical outcomes between those who did and did not attain hypertension control. The conventional wisdom is that the principal benefit of treating hypertension is mediated by blood pressure reduction, irrespective of the means by which control is attained. This iconoclastic finding in VALUE has been supported by a number of studies showing that blood pressure control among individuals with treatment resistant hypertension leads to less than expected benefits of blood pressure reduction. Individuals requiring more medications to achieve hypertension control may well be a higher-risk subset with greater degrees of insulin resistance and target organ damage [59]. Nevertheless, data that they do not attain more of the expected benefits of blood pressure reduction will hopefully lead to insights that improve their clinical management and outcomes.

Importance of heart rate in treated hypertensive patients Heart rate is long recognized as a cardiovascular risk factor [31, 57]. Heart rate reduction with β-blockers is linked to improved clinical outcomes in patients with coronary heart disease or with heart failure with reduced ejection fraction [60, 61]. Yet, the importance of heart rate as a predictor of outcomes in a high-risk group of treated hypertensive patients not selected specifically for coronary heart disease or chronic heart failure has not registered as a significant clinical topic prior to a re-analysis of VALUE trial data (Fig. 35.8) [14].

In this insightful analysis, Dr. Julius and coworkers showed that both blood pressure and heart rate significantly impacted the primary outcome of fatal and nonfatal heart disease and stroke. Within both the uncontrolled and the controlled subgroups of hypertensive patients in VALUE, those with resting heart rate of 80 bpm and higher had worse outcomes than those with lower resting heart rate values.

In summary, more than 50 years of research by Professor Julius and colleagues has documented a key role of high levels of anger and especially suppressed anger in the pathogenesis of elevated blood pressure. Evidence indicates that anger activates the sympathetic nervous system, while reduce parasympathetic tone. The Ann Arbor group showed that this reciprocal dysfunction of the two limbs of the autonomic nervous system underlies the hyperkinetic borderline hypertension and may be operative in neurogenic, high-renin hypertension. Dr. Julius and coworkers also documented a role for sympathetic activation in cardiometabolic risk and the cardiovascular continuum. In the most recent phase of research, attention has focused on national and multinational studies on the prevention and treatment of hypertension, which have yielded useful insights that have important implications for hypertension and cardiovascular disease prevention.

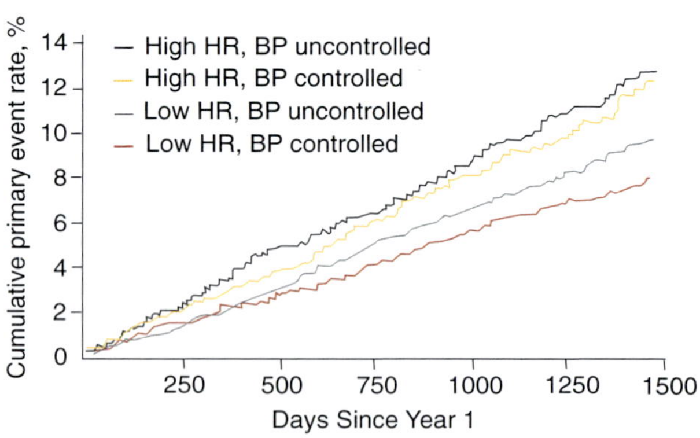

Adapted from Julius S, et al: Am J Cardioll 2012[14]

Fig. 35.8 Individuals in the upper quintile of resting heart rate (HR, ≥80 bpm) had more primary cardiovascular events than those with uncontrolled hypertension but resting HR in the lower four quintiles (<80 bpm). In multivariable hazards regression, among individuals with controlled hypertension those with faster heart rates had 53% more cardiovascular events (HR 1.53 [95% CI 1.26–1.85])

References

1. Harburg E, Julius S, McGinn NF, McLeod J, Hoobler SW. Personality traits and behavioral patterns associated with systolic blood pressure in college males. J Chronic Dis. 1964;17:405–14.
2. Schneider R, Egan B, Johnson EH, Drobney H, Julius S. Anger and anxiety in borderline hypertension. Psychosomatic Med. 1986;48:242–8.
3. Julius R, Pascual A, London R. Role of parasympathetic inhibition in the hyperkinetic type of borderline hypertension. Circulation. 1971;44:413–8.
4. Esler M, Julius S, Randall OS, Ellis CN, Kashima T. Relation of renin status to neurogenic vascular resistance in borderline hypertension. Am J Cardiol. 1975;36:708–15.
5. Esler M, Julius S, Zweifler A, Randall O, Harburg E, Gardiner H, et al. Mild high-renin essential hypertension: neurogenic human hypertension? N Engl J Med. 1977;296:405–11.
6. Julius S, Jamerson K, Mejia A, Krause L, Schork N, Jones K. The association of borderline hypertension with target organ changes and higher coronary risk. Tecumseh Blood Pressure Study. JAMA. 1990;264:354–8.
7. Julius S, Gudbrandsson T, Jamerson K, Andersson O. The interconnection between sympathetics, microcirculation, and insulin resistance in hypertension. Blood Press. 1992;1:9–19.
8. Julius S, Jamerson K. Sympathetics, insulin resistance and coronary risk in hypertension: the 'chicken-and-egg' question. J Hypertens. 1994;12:495–502.
9. Jamerson K, Julius S, Gudbrandsson T, Andersson O, Brant DO. Reflex sympathetic activation induces acute insulin resistance in the human forearm. Hypertension. 1993;21:618–23.
10. Wilson PWF, Meigs JB. Cardiometabolic risk: a Framingham perspective. Internat J Obes. 2008;32:S17–20.
11. Julius S, Nesbitt SD, Egan BM, Weber MA, Michelson EL, Kaciroti N, Black HR, Grimm RH Jr, Messerli FH, Oparil S, Schork MA. Feasibility of treating prehypertension with an angiotensin-receptor blocker. N Engl J Med. 2006;354:1685–97.
12. Julius S, Kjeldsen SE, Weber M, Brunner HR, Ekman S, Hansson L, Hau T, Laragh J, McInnes GT, Mitchell L, Plat F, Schork A, Smith B, Zanchetti A. Outcomes in hypertensive patients at high cardiovascular risk treated with regimens based on valsartan or amlodipine: The VALUE randomized trial. Lancet. 2004;363:2022–31.
13. Weber MA, Julius S, Kjedlsen SE, et al. Cardiovascular outcomes in hypertensive patients comparing single-agent therapy with combination therapy. J Hypertens. 2012;30:2213–22.
14. Julius S, Palatini P, Kjeldsen SE, Zanchetti A, Weber MA, McInnes GT, Brunner HR, Mancia G, Schork MA, Hua TA, Holzhauer B, Zappe D, Majahalme S, Jamerson K, Koylan N. Usefulness of heart rate to predict future cardiac events in treated patients with high-risk systemic hypertension. Am J Cardiol. 2012;109:685–92.
15. Spielberger CD, Johnson EH, Russell SF, Crane RJ, Jacobs GA, Worden TJ. The experience and expression of anger: construction and validation of an anger expression scale. In: Chesney MA, Rosenman RH, editors. Anger and hostility in cardiovascular and behavioral disorders. New York: Hemisphere/McGraw; 1985. p. 5–30.
16. Alexander F. Emotional factors in essential hypertension: presentation of a tentative hypothesis. Psychosom Med. 1939;1:175–9.
17. Marci CD, Glick DM, Loh R, Dougherty DD. Autonomic and prefrontal cortex responses to autobiographical recall of emotions. Cogn Affect Behav Neurosci. 2007;7:243–50.
18. Levy RL, White PD, Stroud WD. Transient tachycardia: prognostic significance alone and in association with transient hypertension. JAMA. 1945;129:585–8.
19. Lund-Johansen P. Hemodynamic alterations in early essential hypertension: recent advances. In: Gross F, Strassen, editors. Mild hypertension: recent advances. New York, NY: Raven Press; 1983. p. 237–49.
20. Julius S, Randall OS, Esler MD, Kashima T, Ellis C, Bennett J. Altered cardiac responsiveness and regulation in the normal cardiac output type of borderline hypertension. Circ Res. 1975;36(6 Suppl 1):199–207.

21. Messerli FH, Ventura HO, Resisin E, Dreslinski GR, Dunn FG, MacPhee AA, Frohlich ED. Borderline hypertension and obesity: two prehypertensive states with elevated cardiac output. Circulation. 1982;66:55–60.
22. Reisin E, Messerli FG, Ventura HO, Frohlich ED. Renal hemodynamic studies in obesity hypertension. J Hypertens. 1987;5:397–400.
23. Egan BM, Schork NJ, Weder AB. Regional hemodynamic abnormalities in overweight men. Focus on alpha-adrenergic vascular responses. Am J Hypertens. 1989;2(6 Part 1):428–34.
24. Guyton AC, Coleman TG. Quantitative analysis of the pathophysiology of hypertension. Circ Res. 1969;24(5 Suppl):1–19.
25. Guyton AC. Dominant role of the kidneys and accessory role of whole-body autoregulationin the pathogenesis of hypertension. Am J Hypertens. 1989;2:575–85.
26. Julius S, Pascual AV, Reilly K, London R. Abnormalities of plasma volume in borderline hypertension. Arch Intern Med. 1971;127:116–9.
27. Julius S, Conway J. Hemodynamic studies in patients with borderline blood pressure elevation. Circulation. 1968;38:282–8.
28. Cohn JN. Relationship of plasma volume changes to resistance and capacitance vessel effects of sympathomimetic amines and angiotensin in man. Clin Sci. 1966;30:267–78.
29. Kjeldsen SE, Moan A, Petrin J, Weder A, Julius S. Effects of increased arterial epinephrine on insulin, glucose and phosphate. Blood Press. 1996;5:27–31.
30. Julius R, Pascual A, Abbrecht P, London R. Effect of beta-adrenergic blockade on plasma volume in human subjects. Proc Soc Exp Biol Med. 1972;140:982–5.
31. Julius S, Majahalme S. The changing face of sympathetic overactivity in hypertension. Ann Med. 2000;32:365–70.
32. Hart MN, Heistad DD, Brody MJ. Effect of chronic hypertension and sympathetic denervation on wall/lumen ratio of cerebral vessels. Hypertension. 1980;2:419–28.
33. Bevan RD, Tsuru H, Bevan JH. Cerebral artery mass in the rabbit is reduced by chronic sympathetic denervation. Stroke. 1983;14:393–6.
34. Mulvany MJ. Small artery remodeling in hypertension. Basic Clin Pharm Toxicol. 2011;110:49–55.
35. Egan BM, Schork N, Panis R, Hinderliter A. Vascular structure enhances regional resistance responses in mild hypertension. J Hypertension. 1988;6(1):41–8.
36. Folkow B. Physiological aspects of primary hypertension. Physiol Rev. 1982;62:347–503.
37. Egan B, Panis R, Hinderliter A, Schork N, Julius S. Mechanism of increased alpha-adrenergic vasoconstriction in human essential hypertension. J Clin Invest. 1987;80:812–7.
38. Anderson EA, Sinkey CA, Lawton WJ, Mark AL. Elevated sympathetic nerve activity in borderline hypertensive humans: Evidence from direct intraneural recordings. Hypertension. 1989;14:177–83.
39. Esler M. The sympathetic system and hypertension. Am J Hypertens. 2000;13:99S–105S.
40. Julius S, Jamerson K, Mejia A, Krause L, Schork N, Jones K. The association of borderline hypertension with target orgnai changes and higher coronary risk. Tecumseh Blood Pressure Study. JAMA. 1990;264:354–8.
41. De Fronzo RA, Tripathy D. Skeletal muscle insulin resistance is the primary defect in type 2 diabetes. Diabetes Care. 2009;32(Suppl 2):S157–63.
42. Pollare T, Lithell H, Selinus I, Berne C. Application of prazosin is associated with an increase of insulin sensitivity in obese patients with hypertension. Diabetologia. 1988;31:415–20.
43. Berne C, Pollare T, Lithell H. Effects of antihypertensive treatment on insulin sensitivity with special reference to ACE inhibitors. Diabetes Care. 1991;14(Suppl 4):39–47.
44. Jamerson KA, Smith SD, Amerena JV, Grant E, Julius S. Vasoconstriction with norepinrphrine causes less forearm insulin resistance than a reflex sympathetic vasoconstriction. Hypertension. 1994;23(past 2):1006–11.
45. Lillioja S, Young AA, Culter CL, Ivy JL, Abbott WG, Zawadzki JK, Yki-Järvinen H, Christin L, Secomb TW, Bogardus C. Skeletal muscle capillary density and fiber type are possible determinants of in vivo insulin resistance in man. J Clin Invest. 1987;80:415–24.

46. MacMahon S, Peto R, Cutler J, Collins R, Sorlie P, Neaton J, Abbott R, Godwin J, Dyer A, Stamler J. Blood pressure, stroke, and coronary heart disease. Part I, Prolonged differences in blood pressure: prospective observational studies corrected for the regression dilution bias. Lancet. 1990;335:765–74.
47. Willey JZ, Moon YP, Kahn E, Rodriguez CJ, Rundek T, Cheung K, Sacco FL, Elkind MSV. Population attributable risks of hypertension and diabetes for cardiovascular disease and stroke in the Northern Manhattan Study. J Am Heart Assoc. 2014;3:e001106. https://doi.org/10.1161/JAHA.114.001106.
48. Hall JE, Brands MW, Zappe DH, Alonso GM. Insulin resistance, hyperinsulinemia, and hypertension: causes, consequences, or merely correlations? Proc Soc Exp Biol Med. 1994;208:317–29.
49. Howard BV. Insulin resistance and lipid metabolism. Am J Cardiol. 1990;84(Suppl 1A):28J–32J.
50. Pyorala K, Savolainen E, Kaukola S, Haapakoski J. Plasma insulin as a coronary heart disease risk factor: relationship to the other risk factors and predictive value during 9½ year follow-up of the Helsinki Policemen Study. Actu Med Stand Suppl. 1985;701:38–52.
51. Ducimetiere P, Eschwege E, Papoz L, Richard JL, Claude JR, Rosselin G. Relationship of plasma insulin levels to the incidence of myocardial infarction and coronary heart disease mortality in a middle-aged population. Diabetologia. 1980;19:205–10.
52. Palatini P, Benetos A, Grassi G, Julius S, Kjeldsen SE, Mancia G, Narkiewicz K, Parati G, Pessina AC, Ruilope LM, Zanchetti A. Identification and management of the hypertensive patient with elevated heart rate: Statement of a European Society of Hypertension Consensus Meeting. J Hypertens. 2006;24:603–10.
53. Valentini M, Julius S, Palatini P, Brook RD, Bard RL, Bisognano JD, Kaciroti N. Attenuation of haemodynamic, metabolic and energy expenditure responses to isoproterenol in patients with hypertension. J Hypertens. 2004;22:1999–2006.
54. Julius S, Li Y, Brant D, Krause L, Buda AJ. Neurogenic pressor episodes fail to cause hypertension, but do induce cardiac hypertrophy. Hypertension. 1989;13:422–9.
55. Kjeldsen SE, Gjesdal K, Eide I, Aakesson I, Amundsen R, Foss OP, et al. Increased beta-thromboglobulin in essential hypertension: interactions between arterial plasma adrenaline, platelet function and blood lipids. Actu Med Scund. 1983;213:369–73.
56. Kjeldsen SE, Zweifler AM, Petrin J, Wder AB, Julius S. Sympathetic nervous system involvement in essential hypertension: Increased platelet noradrenaline coincides with decreased β-adrenoreceptor responsiveness. Blood Press. 1994;3:164–71.
57. Palatini P, Julius S. Heart rate and the cardiovascular risk. J Hypertension. 1997;15:3–17.
58. Aronow WS, Casey DE, Collins KJ, et al. 2017 ACC/AHA/AAPA/ABC/ACPM/AGS/APhA/ASH/ASPC/NMA/PCNA guideline for the prevention, detection, evaluation, and management of high blood pressure in adults. Hypertension. 2017.
59. Rao A, Pandya V, Whaley-Connell A. Obesity and insulin resistance in resistant hypertension: Implications for the kidney. Adv Chron Kid Dis. 2015;22:211–7.
60. Kotecha D, Flather MD, Altman DG, et al. Heart rate and rhythm and the benefit of beta-blockers in patients with heart failure. J Am Coll Cardiol. 2017;69:2885–96.
61. Gheorghiade M, Goldstein S. β-blockers in the post-myocardial infarction patient. Circulation. 2002;106:394–8.

The PREVER Study

36

Sandra Costa Fuchs and Flávio Danni Fuchs

36.1 Introduction

Raised blood pressure (BP) has become the leading cause of non-transmissible chronic disease, particularly of cardiovascular disease. An aggregate analysis of 844 studies, conducted in 195 countries and territories, projected that in 2015, about 3.5 billion adults had systolic BP of at least 110 to 115 mm Hg and 874 million adults had systolic BP of 140 mm Hg or greater [1]. Projections from these data indicate that these levels BP exposed a large number of individuals to disability-adjusted life years (DALYs), mainly due to ischemic heart disease, followed by hemorrhagic stroke and ischemic stroke. Estimate based on data from World Health Organization regions found that about 62% of cerebrovascular disease and 49% of ischemic heart disease were attributable to SBP >115 mm Hg [2].

In the first decade of this century, there was an increase in the global discrepancies between the prevalence of hypertension and the control rate. There was a drop of 2.6% in prevalence in high-income countries, versus 7.7% raise in low- and middle-income countries. Similarly, controlled hypertension increased substantially in high-income countries (17.9–28.4%), and less in low- and middle-income countries (8.4–7.7%) [3]. The trends in Brazil are similar. A meta-analysis of population-based studies estimated a 28.7% (95% CI: 26.2–31.4%) prevalence of hypertension among adults [4], and 68.9% (95% CI: 64.1–73.3%) in elderlies [5], with less than one-third of patients having controlled BP (BP). In a cohort study conducted in

S. C. Fuchs (✉)
Graduate Program in Cardiology, School of Medicine, Universidade Federal do Rio Grande do Sul, Porto Alegre, Brazil

F. D. Fuchs
Division of Cardiology, Hospital de Clínicas de Porto Alegre, School of Medicine, Universidade Federal do Rio Grande do Sul, Porto Alegre, Brazil

R. Zimlichman et al. (eds.), *Prehypertension and Cardiometabolic Syndrome*, Updates in Hypertension and Cardiovascular Protection,
https://doi.org/10.1007/978-3-319-75310-2_36

southern Brazil, the risk attributed to hypertension on the incidence of cardiovascular events was 61% [6].

The epidemiological transition has already taken place in Brazil, and noncommunicable chronic diseases are already the main cause of morbidity and mortality. Brazilian health authorities prioritized hypertension among these problems, allocating resources to investigate strategies of reducing the consequences of hypertension. Among the projects funded by the Ministry of Health is the PREVER study. In this study, the same logistic was used to answer two questions of current interest in the prevention and management of hypertension: what is the effectiveness of an intervention to prevent the incidence of hypertension and what is the best drug option for the initiation of treatment initiation. The PREVER study consisted of two randomized, phase III, multicenter trials: the PREVENT-PREVENTION and PREVER-TREATMENT. The two studies are presented below.

36.2 PREVER Prevention Trial

36.2.1 Background and Aims

The risks of high BP are continuous and start at very low values, at least 115/75 mm Hg in adults [7]. This continuous risk of BP for cardiovascular events could not be used for clinical purposes, and a dichotomous definition of hypertension was therefore required. Older studies, with small samples, identified the risk when its absolute increase was high [8]. The values went progressively down, but 60 years ago were still set at 160/95 mm Hg [9]. In 1977, with diagnosis based mostly on diastolic BP, hypertension was diagnosed when diastolic BP was equal or higher than 100 mm Hg [10]. Interestingly, the risks of BP between 90 and 100 mm Hg, called borderline hypertension at that time, were already evident, both for cardiovascular mortality and morbidity, as for target organ damage [11]. Treatment was proposed for young individuals with other risk factors or evidences of target organ damage. Anticipating the modern methods of BP measurements, Stevo Julius and coworkers recommended the treatment when the average of 14 BP measurements, taken at home, were 140/90 mm Hg or higher, independently of the presence of risk factors or target organ damage [12].

When the risks of BP below 140/90 mm Hg became evident, the term prehypertension was coined. Prehypertension—SBP between 120 and 139 or diastolic BP between 80 and 89 mm Hg—was presented in the Seventh Report of the Joint National Committee (JNC 7), to identify an intermediate category of risk [13]. It was, somehow, equivalent to the old borderline definition for higher values. The higher precision in the identification of risk, accumulating evidences from dozens of cohort studies, and also from more precise methods of BP measurement, established, beyond reasonable doubt, that prehypertension carries on several risks and should be a focus of intervention.

In addition to being a risk factor for cardiovascular disease, prehypertension increases the risk of developing hypertension and promotes target organ damage. In a cohort study conducted in the city of Porto Alegre, Brazil, four out of five individuals with prehypertension developed hypertension in 10 years [14]. In the MONICA cohort, prehypertension was associated with risk for increasing left ventricular mass, compared to normal pressure [15]. A cohort study conducted in the Chinese population showed a similar pattern of cardiovascular deaths attributed to hypertension, 51.9% (95% CI 49.6–54.3) in men and 49.1% (95% CI 46.3–51.9) in women. In addition, it was established the attributable risk for prehypertension, ranging from 13.0% (95% CI 10.9–15.1) in men and 11.5% (95% CI 9.3–13.7) in women [16]. In the ARIC cohort, prehypertension increased LV remodeling and impaired diastolic function [17].

The consequences of prehypertension prompted to the development of two trials, which pioneering tested the efficacy of BP-lowering agents in prehypertension. In the first one, participants with prehypertension stage II—130 to 139 mm Hg of SBP or 85 to 89 mm Hg of diastolic BP—were randomly assigned to receive 2 years of candesartan or placebo, followed by 2 years of placebo for all [18]. Participants who developed stage 1 hypertension started treatment with BP-lowering agents. Both groups received recommendations for lifestyle changes. The 2-year results showed an incidence of hypertension of 13.6% in the candesartan arm versus 40.4% in the placebo group ($P < 0.001$), with a relative risk reduction of 66.3%. At the end of the four-year follow-up, 63.0% participants in the placebo group developed hypertension versus 53.2% of those in the candesartan group, with a relative risk reduction of 15.6%. The incidence of hypertension tended to approximate after 2 years of drug suspension. Treatment was well tolerated [18]. In the second trial, 1008 participants with office BP (either SBP 130–139 or DBP 85–89 mm Hg or both) were randomized to treatment with ramipril or a control group [19]. At the end of the 3-year follow-up, 30.7% in the ramipril group versus 42.9% in the control group did not develop hypertension, with a relative risk reduction of 34.4% [19].

Although there was strong evidence in favor of the effectiveness of pharmacological prevention of hypertension in individuals with high-normal BP, a clinical trial was lacking to assess whether the treatment was able to reduce the incidence of hypertension in individuals with the full spectrum of prehypertension and whether it could, also, prevent target organ damage. The PREVER-PREVENTION trial was designed to answer these questions [20]. The study aimed to investigate whether the drug treatment of individuals with prehypertension would reduce the incidence of hypertension and left ventricular mass, assessing the tolerability to the intervention.

36.2.2 Methods

PREVER-Prevention was a randomized placebo-controlled trial, with blinding and concealment, conducted at 21 academic medical centers in Brazil. Details of the study can be seen elsewhere [21].

The eligibility criteria included age between 30 and 70 years, prehypertension, for those who not taking BP-lowering agents. Before randomization, all study participants were enrolled in a 3-month lifestyle intervention. Advices were provided on weight loss, reduction in dietary intake of sodium, consumption of a DASH-type

(Dietary Approaches to Stop Hypertension) diet, and increase of physical activity. Participants whose mean BP was still within the prehypertension range after 3 months of lifestyle intervention were randomized to receive a combined pill containing 12.5 mg of chlorthalidone and 2.5 mg of amiloride or placebo, in a 1:1 ratio. Follow-up visits were done at 3, 6, 9, 12, 15, and 18 months after randomization.

The primary outcome was incidence of hypertension (systolic BP ≥140 mm Hg or diastolic BP ≥90 mm Hg), based on the average of 6 standardized BP measurements, performed in 3 clinic visits [13, 22]. Self-reported adverse events, development or worsening of microalbuminuria, changes in left ventricular mass (LVM), were secondary outcomes. Measurement of LVM was based on ECG recordings using Sokolow-Lyon and Cornell voltage and voltage-duration products [23, 24].

36.2.3 Main Results

A total of 730, out of 1433 participants included in the 3-month lifestyle intervention phase, fulfilled the eligibility criteria for enrollment in the PREVER-PREVENTION trial. Baseline characteristics and adherence to treatment participants to treatment were similar among the treatment arms. The incidence of hypertension was significantly lower in the chlorthalidone/amiloride group compared with placebo (hazard ratio 0.56; 95% CI 0.38–0.82; $P = 0.003$) (Fig. 36.1). The cumulative incidence of hypertension was 11.7% in the diuretic group compared with 19.5% in the placebo group ($P = 0.004$).

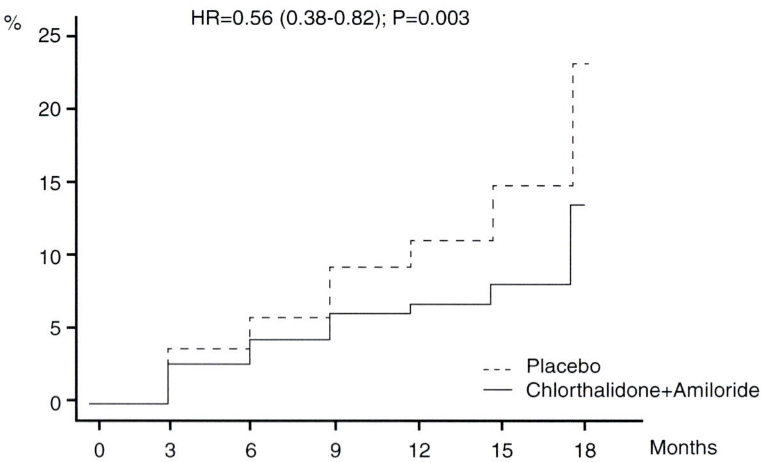

	0	3	6	9	12	15	18
Chlorthalidone + Amiloride (n)	372	326	283	253	242	240	312
Incidence (%)		2.8	2.1	2.4	0.4	1.7	4.5
Placebo (n)	358	316	280	260	235	225	290
Incidence (%)		3.8	2.1	3.5	2.6	4.4	8.6

Fig. 36.1 Incidence of hypertension according to treatment group during follow-up. HR indicates hazard ratio (reprinted with permission from the reference 20)

The Sokolow-Lyon voltage and voltage duration product reduced by a greater extent in patients allocated to the active intervention than to placebo.

36.2.4 Conclusions and Perspectives

The findings of the PREVER-PREVENTION, TROPHY, and PHARAO trials consistently documented the value of BP-lowering agents to prevent hypertension. The PREVER-PREVENTION showed this effect with a low dose of diuretics in the full range of prehypertension, and was the first to demonstrate beneficial effects on target organs. These studies added a piece of evidence supporting the view that prehypertension is already hypertension and should be a focus of interventions aiming to reduce the burden of cardiovascular diseases.

36.3 PREVER Treatment Trial

36.3.1 Background and Aims

Approximately 50% of patients with hypertension can have their BP (BP) controlled with one BP-lowering agent. Even those who need two or more drugs usually start with one agent. Therefore, the choice of the first option is a critical issue, and should be based in reliable evidences. The major guidelines converge in the recommendations of drug choice. Despite stating that the effectiveness to lower BP is the main reason for the choice of the agent, guidelines gave preference for antagonists of the renin-angiotensin system. The last European Guidelines indicate an ACE-inhibitor or an ARB for a long series of conditions, such as left ventricular hypertrophy, microalbuminuria renal dysfunction, atrial fibrillation, and diabetes mellitus, among others [25]. The NICE guidelines indicate ACE-inhibitors or ARB for patients younger than 55 years, despite the complete absence of evidences to support it [26]. The better tolerability of ARB (the ACE-inhibitors without cough) has given to this class the worldwide preference in the management of hypertension.

This preference is not aligned with the best evidence. The promotion of antihypertensive agents by pharmaceutical companies is sometimes based on trials with biased planning, presentation or interpretation of results [27]. Lisinopril, an ACE-inhibitor, was less efficacious than chlorthalidone in the prevention of strokes in black participants, and cardiovascular disease and heart failure independently of race in the ALLHAT trial [28].

Diuretics were the only class of BP-lowering drugs that showed consistent superiority over placebo in the prevention of stroke, coronary heart disease, heart failure, cardiovascular and all-cause mortality, as demonstrated in one report of the series of meta-analyses by Thomopoulos and coauthors [29]. The effect size was significantly higher with diuretics, even against events that were prevented by other classes of drugs.

The main concern, however, is with the effectiveness of ARB [30, 31]. In several clinical trials with patients with different criteria for enrollment, such as

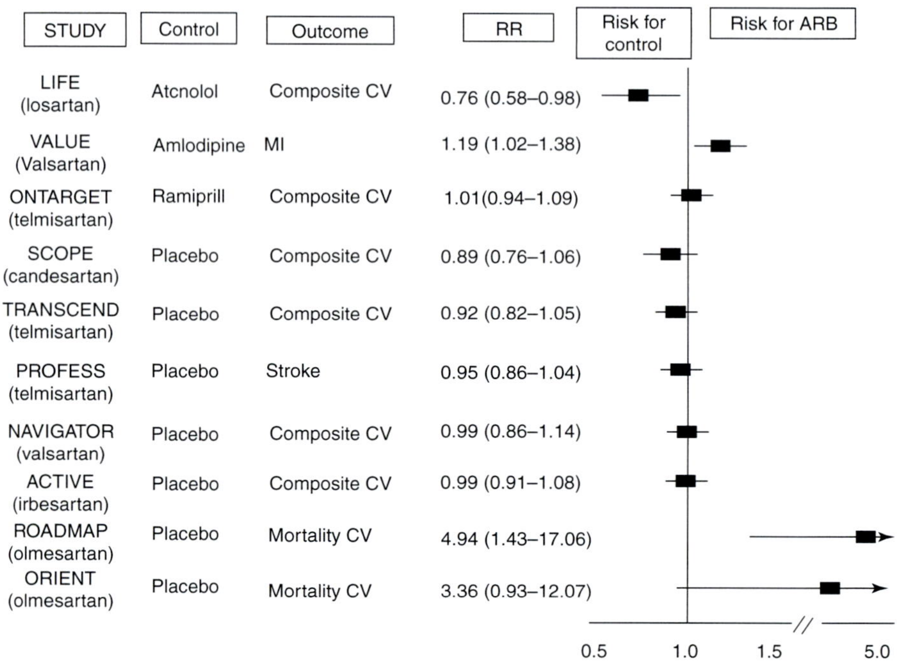

Fig. 36.2 Relative risks and 95% CIs for the occurrence of cardiovascular outcomes in clinical trials comparing angiotensin receptor blocker with other drugs or placebo in patients with hypertension or high cardiovascular risk [Reprinted with permission from 30] (references of the individual studies are cited in the text)

hypertension, heart failure, diabetes, stroke, atrial fibrillation, and others, ARB were not superior to placebo in the prevention of cardiovascular outcomes [32–38] (Fig. 36.2). Studies specifically designed to investigate the effectiveness of ARB in the prevention of incidence of recurrence of atrial fibrillation failed to demonstrate their effectiveness [36–41].

These and others clinical trials were included in several meta-analysis of studies comparing ARB to placebo and other drugs [42–46]. Among major outcomes, ARB were effective in the prevention of stroke and heart failure. In none, however, there was evidence that ARB were more efficacious than placebo to prevent myocardial infarction, cardiovascular and all-cause mortality.

Another relevant issue that argues against the effectiveness of ARB is the fraud committed in three major studies done with these agents, which were retracted from the literature [47–49].

There was no trial comparing the effectiveness of ARB with diuretics in the prevention of cardiovascular outcomes [50]. We could not find also a clinical trial comparing the BP-lowering effect of diuretics and ARB. Therefore we decided to compare these classes of BP drugs in regard to their BP effects and effects on surrogate outcomes, the main outcomes of the PREVER-treatment trial [51]. We chose the association of chlorthalidone with amiloride to compare with losartan. The preference for chlorthalidone was based on its superiority over hydrochlorothiazide in the prevention of cardiovascular events in a network meta-analysis [52], and on its higher and longer BP-lowering effect [53–55]. The association of amiloride aimed to antagonize the hypokalemia induced by chlorthalidone [56], which promotes a mild increase in blood glucose [57]. The Pathway-3 trial showed that the prevention of losses of potassium with amiloride prevented the increase in serum glucose in a glucose tolerance test, besides having a BP-lowering effect [58].

36.3.2 Methods

Details of the PREVER-TREATMENT trial were published on its protocol [59] and in the main report [51]. It was a randomized, double-blind, controlled trial, which included 655 participants who were followed for 18 months in 21 Brazilian academic centers. Trial participants were adult volunteers aged 30–70 years with stage I hypertension (BP 140–159 or 90–99 mm Hg), and no current use of BP-lowering medication. To be enrolled in the drug phase of the trial, participants should have uncontrolled BP after 3 months of a lifestyle intervention phase (recommendations for weight loss, dietary sodium reduction, adoption of a DASH-type diet, physical activity, and smoking cessation). Participants were randomized to 12.5/2.5 mg of chlorthalidone/amiloride ($N = 333$) or 50 mg of losartan ($N = 322$). If BP remained uncontrolled after 3 months, study medication dose was doubled, and if uncontrolled after 6 months, amlodipine (5 and 10 mg) and propranolol (40 and 80 mg BID) were added as open label drugs in a progressive fashion.

The primary outcome was difference in mean BP between the two treatment groups during follow-up. The proportion of patients with controlled hypertension, use of non-study BP-lowering medications, incidence of adverse events, development or worsening of microalbuminuria and left ventricular mass estimated by ECG criteria were additional outcomes. Fatal and nonfatal major cardiovascular events were secondary outcomes.

36.3.3 Main Results

The mean difference in systolic BP during 18 months of follow-up was 2.3 (95% CI: 1.2 to 3.3) mm Hg favoring chlorthalidone/amiloride. Compared to those randomized to diuretic, more participants allocated to losartan had their initial dose doubled and more of them used add-on antihypertensive medication (Fig. 36.3). Levels of blood glucose, glycosylated hemoglobin, and incidence of diabetes were no different between the two treatment groups. Serum potassium was lower and serum cholesterol was higher in the diuretic arm. Microalbuminuria tended to be higher in patients with diabetes allocated to losartan (28.5 ± 40.4 vs. 16.2 ± 26.7 mg, $P = 0.09$).

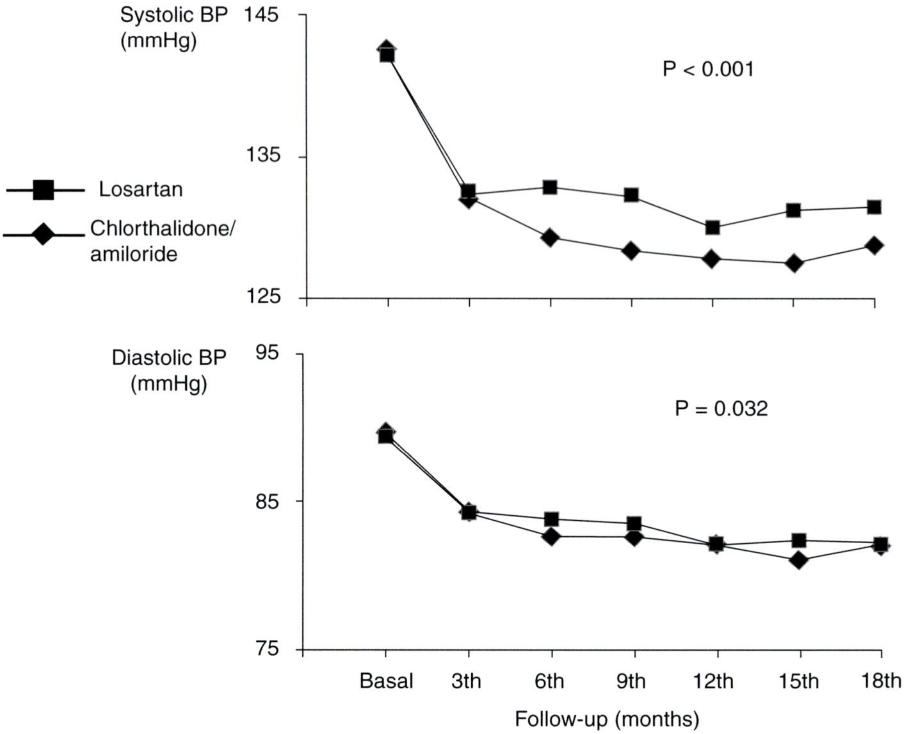

		Basal	3th	6th	9th	12th	15th	18th
Chlorthalidone/ amiloride (n)		333	304	288	278	270	269	310
	12.5/2.5		299	210	186	165	154	160
	25.0/5.0		4	77	92	106	118	126
Amlodipine	5.0			2	21	27	38	36
	10.0					9	11	19
Propranolol	40.0					1	4	5
	80.0					1	1	1
No trial drug (ITT)								27
Losartan (n)		322	298	275	266	260	247	299
	50		292	194	159	141	126	128
	100		6	80	106	120	122	140
Amlodipine	5.0		1	6	33	49	49	49
	10.0			2	5	9	14	23
Propranolol	40.0				1	6	10	10
	80.0						1	3
No trial drug (ITT)								31

Fig. 36.3 Systolic and diastolic BP values by study group during follow-up. The number of participants evaluated at each visit and the number who were treated with the higher dosage of their assigned study drug as well as the number that received a prescription for treatment with an open label drug is shown at each visit [reprinted with permission from the reference 51]

36.3.4 Perspectives

The greater reduction in BP with treatment based on a combination of chlorthalidone and amiloride compared to losartan, together with the superiority in the prevention of cardiovascular outcomes, recommend diuretics as the first option for the management of hypertension. Since effective treatments for hypertension are increasingly demanded, it is prudent to start antihypertensive treatment with more efficacious drugs [8].

Acknowledgments *Sources of Funding*: The Ministry of Health, Division of Science and Technology (DECIT), and Ministry of Science and Technology, Brazilian Innovation Agency (FINEP) (number 01080606/01), National Counsel of Technological and Scientific Development (CNPq), National Institute of Health Technology Assessment (IATS), and Hospital de Clinicas de Porto Alegre (FIPE-GPPG: 08621), RS, Brazil sponsored the PREVER study.

References

1. Forouzanfar MH, Liu P, Roth GA, Ng M, Biryukov S, Marczak L, et al. Global burden of hypertension and SBP of at least 110 to 115 mm hg, 1990–2015. JAMA. 2017;317:165–82.
2. World Health Report. Reducing risks, promoting healthy life. Geneva: World Health Organization; 2002. p. 2002.
3. Mills KT, Bundy JD, Kelly TN, Reed JE, Kearney PM, Reynolds K, Chen J, He J. Global disparities of hypertension prevalence and control: a systematic analysis of population-based studies from 90 countries. Circulation. 2016;134:441–50.
4. Picon RV, Fuchs FD, Moreira LB, Riegel G, Fuchs SC. Trends in prevalence of hypertension in Brazil: a systematic review with meta-analysis. PLoS One. 2012;7:e48255.
5. Picon RV, Fuchs FD, Moreira LB, Fuchs SC. Prevalence of hypertension among elderly persons in urban Brazil: a systematic review with meta-analysis. Am J Hypertens. 2013;26:541–8.
6. Moraes RS, Fuchs FD, Moreira LB, Wiehe M, Pereira GM, Fuchs SC. Risk factors for cardiovascular disease in a Brazilian population-based cohort study. Int J Cardiol. 2003;90:205–11.
7. Prospective Studies Collaboration. Age-specific relevance of usual BP to vascular mortality: a meta-analysis of individual data for one million adults in 61 prospective studies. Lancet. 2002;360:1903–13.
8. Fuchs FD. Essentials of hypertension. New York: Springer; 2017.
9. World Health Organization. Expert Committee on Cardiovascular Diseases and Hypertension & World Health Organization. Hypertension and coronary heart disease: classification and criteria for epidemiological studies, first report of the Expert Committee on Cardiovascular Diseases and Hypertension, Geneva, 13–18 October 1958. Geneva: World Health Organization; 1959. http://www.who.int/iris/handle/10665/4043.
10. Julius S. Classification of hypertension. In: Genest J, Koiw E, Kuchel O, editors. Hypertension. New York: McGraw-Hill; 1977. p. 9–12.
11. Julius S. Borderline hypertension. In: Genest J, Koiw E, Kuchel O, editors. Hypertension. New York: McGraw-Hill; 1977. p. 630–40.
12. Julius S, Ellis CN, Pascual AV, Matice M, Hansson L, Hunyor SN, et al. Home BP determination. Value in borderline ("labile") hypertension. JAMA. 1974;229:663–6.

13. Chobanian AV, Bakris GL, Black HR, Cushman WC, Green LA, Izzo JL Jr, et al. The seventh report of the joint National Committee on prevention, detection, evaluation, and treatment of high BP: the JNC 7 report. JAMA. 2003;289:2560–71.
14. Moreira LB, Fuchs SC, Wiehe M, Gus M, Moraes RS, Fuchs FD. Incidence of hypertension in Porto Alegre, Brazil: a population-based study. J Hum Hypertens. 2008;22:48–50.
15. Markus MR, Stritzke J, Lieb W, Mayer B, Luchner A, Döring A, et al. Implications of persistent prehypertension for ageing-related changes in left ventricular geometry and function: the MONICA/KORA Augsburg study. J Hypertens. 2008;26:2040–9.
16. He J, Gu D, Chen J, Wu X, Kelly TN, Huan J. Premature deaths attributable to BP in China: a prospective cohort study. Lancet. 2009;374:1765–72.
17. Santos AB, Gupta DK, Bello NA, Gori M, Claggett B, Fuchs FD, Shah AM, Coresh J, Sharrett AR, Cheng S, Solomon SD. Prehypertension is associated with abnormalities of cardiac structure and function in the atherosclerosis risk in communities study. Am J Hypertens. 2016;29:568–74.
18. Julius S, Nesbitt SD, Egan BM, Weber MA, Michelson EL, Kaciroti N, Black HR, Grimm RH Jr, Messerli FH, Oparil S, Schork MA, Trial of Preventing Hypertension (TROPHY) Study Investigators. Feasibility of treating prehypertension with an angiotensin-receptor blocker. N Engl J Med. 2006;354:1685–97.
19. Lüders S, Schrader J, Berger J, Unger T, Zidek W, Böhm M, Middeke M, Motz W, Lübcke C, Gansz A, Brokamp L, Schmieder RE, Trenkwalder P, Haller H, Dominiak P, PHARAO Study Group. The PHARAO study: prevention of hypertension with the angiotensin-converting enzyme inhibitor ramipril in patients with high-normal BP: a prospective, randomized, controlled prevention trial of the German Hypertension League. J Hypertens. 2008;26:1487–96.
20. Fuchs SC, Poli-de-Figueiredo CE, Figueiredo Neto JA, Scala LC, Whelton PK, Mosele F, de Mello RB, Vilela-Martin JF, Moreira LB, Chaves H, Mota Gomes M, de Sousa MR, Silva RP, Castro I, Cesarino EJ, Jardim PC, Alves JG, Steffens AA, Brandão AA, Consolim-Colombo FM, de Alencastro PR, Neto AA, Nóbrega AC, Franco RS, Sobral Filho DC, Bordignon A, Nobre F, Schlatter R, Gus M, Fuchs FC, Berwanger O, Fuchs FD. Effectiveness of Chlorthalidone Plus Amiloride for the prevention of hypertension: the PREVER-prevention randomized clinical trial. J Am Heart Assoc. 2016;5:e004248.
21. Fuchs FD, Fuchs SC, Moreira LB, Gus M, Nobrega AC, Poli-de-Figueiredo CE, Mion D, Bortoloto L, Consolim-Colombo F, Nobre F, Coelho EB, Vilela-Martin JF, Moreno H Jr, Cesarino EJ, Franco R, Brandão AA, de Sousa MR, Ribeiro AL, Jardim PC, Neto AA, Scala LC, Mota M, Chaves H, Alves JG, Filho DC, Pereira e Silva R, Neto JA, Irigoyen MC, Castro I, Steffens AA, Schlatter R, de Mello RB, Mosele F, Ghizzoni F, Berwanger O. Prevention of hypertension in patients with prehypertension: protocol for the PREVER-prevention trial. Trials. 2011;12:65.
22. ESH/ESC Task Force for the Management of Arterial Hypertension. 2013 Practice guidelines for the management of arterial hypertension of the European Society of Hypertension (ESH) and the European Society of Cardiology (ESC): ESH/ESC Task Force for the Management of Arterial Hypertension. J Hypertens. 2013;31:1925–38.
23. Sokolow M, Lyon TP. The ventricular complex in left ventricular hypertrophy as obtained by unipolar precordial and limb leads. Am Heart J. 1949;37:161–86.
24. Okin PM, Roman MI, Devereux BB, Borer JS, Kligtield P. Electrocardiographic diagnosis of left ventricular hypertrophy by the time-voltage integral of the QRS. J Am Coll Cardiol. 1994;23:133–40.
25. Mancia G, Fagard R, Narkiewicz K, Redon J, Zanchetti A, Böhm M, et al. ESH/ESC guidelines for the management of arterial hypertension. J Hypertens. 2013;2013(31):1281–57.
26. Krause T, Lovibond K, Caulfield M, McCormack T, Williams B. Guideline Development Group Management of hypertension: summary of NICE guidance. BMJ. 2011;343:d4891.
27. Fuchs FD. The corporate bias and the molding of prescription practices: the case of hypertension. Braz J Med Biol Res. 2009;42:224–8.

28. The Antihypertensive and Lipid-Lowering Treatment to Prevent Heart Attack Trial (ALLHAT). Major outcomes in high-risk hypertensive patients randomized to angiotensin-converting enzyme inhibitor or calcium channel blocker vs diuretic. JAMA. 2002;288:2981–97.
29. Thomopoulos C, Parati G, Zanchetti A. Effects of BP lowering on outcome incidence in hypertension: 4. Effects of various classes of antihypertensive drugs--overview and meta-analyses. J Hypertens. 2015;33:195–211.
30. Fuchs FD. The role of angiotensin receptor blockers in the prevention of cardiovascular and renal disease: time for reassessment? Evid Based Med. 2013;18:44–7.
31. Fuchs FD, DiNicolantonio JJ. Angiotensin receptor blockers for prevention of cardiovascular disease: where does the evidence stand? Open Heart. 2015;2:e000236.
32. Lithell H, Hansson L, Skoog I, Elmfeldt D, Hofman A, Olofsson B, et al., SCOPE Study Group. The Study on Cognition and Prognosis in the Elderly (SCOPE): principal results of a randomized double-blind intervention trial. J Hypertens. 2003;21:875–86.
33. Yusuf S, Sleight P, Anderson C, Teo K, Copland I, Ramos B, et al., TRANSCEND Investigators. Effects of the angiotensin-receptor blocker telmisartan on cardiovascular events in high-risk patients intolerant to angiotensin-converting enzyme inhibitors: a randomized controlled trial. Lancet. 2008;372:1174–83.
34. Yusuf S, Diener HC, Sacco RL, Cotton D, Ôunpuu S, Lawton WA, et al., PRoFESS Study Group. Telmisartan to prevent recurrent stroke and cardiovascular events. N Engl J Med. 2008;359:1225–37.
35. McMurray JJ, Holman RR, Haffner SM, Bethel A, Holzhauer B, Hua TA, et al., NAVIGATOR Study Group. Effect of valsartan on the incidence of diabetes and cardiovascular events. N Engl J Med. 2010;362:1477–90.
36. Yusuf S, Healey JS, Pogue J, Chrolavicius S, Flather M, Hart RG, et al., ACTIVE I Investigators. Irbesartan in patients with atrial fibrillation. N Engl J Med. 2011;364:928–38.
37. Haller H, Ito S, Izzo JL Jr, Januszewicz A, Katayama S, Menne J, et al., ROADMAP Trial Investigators. Olmesartan for the delay or prevention of microalbuminuria in type 2 diabetes. N Engl J Med. 2011;364:907–17.
38. Imai E, Chan JC, Ito S, Yamasaki T, Kobayashi F, Haneda H, et al. ORIENT study investigators. Effects of olmesartan on renal and cardiovascular outcomes in type 2 diabetes with overt nephropathy: a multicentre, randomised, placebo-controlled study. Diabetologia. 2011;54:2978–86.
39. Disertori M, Latini R, Barlera S, Franzosi MG, Staszewsky L, Maggioni AP, et al., GISSI-AF Investigators. Valsartan for prevention of recurrent atrial fibrillation. N Engl J Med. 2009;360:1606–17.
40. Goette A, Schön N, Kirchhof P, Breithardt G, Fetsch T, Häusler KG, et al. Angiotensin II-Antagonist in Paroxysmal Atrial Fibrillation (ANTIPAF)-Trial. Circ Arrhythm Electrophysiol. 2012;5:43–51.
41. Yamashita T, Inoue H, Okumura K, Kodama I, Aizawa Y, Atarashi H, et al. Randomized trial of angiotensin II-receptor blocker versus dihydropiridine calcium channel blocker in the treatment of paroxysmal atrial fibrillation with hypertension (J-RHYTHM II Study). Europace. 2011;13:473–9.
42. Bangalore S, Kumar S, Wetterslev J, Messerli FH. Angiotensin receptor blockers and risk of myocardial infarction: meta-analyses and trial sequential analyses of 147 020 patients from randomised trials. BMJ. 2011;342:d2234.
43. van Vark LC, Bertrand M, Akkerhuis KM, Brugts JJ, Fox K, Mourad JJ, Boersma E. Angiotensin-converting enzyme inhibitors reduce mortality in hypertension: a meta-analysis of randomized clinical trials of renin-angiotensin-aldosterone system inhibitors involving 158 998 patients. Eur Heart J. 2012;33:2088–97.
44. Cheng J, Zhang W, Zhang X, Han F, Li X, He X, Li Q, Chen J. Effect of angiotensin-converting enzyme inhibitors and angiotensin II receptor blockers on all-cause mortality, cardiovascular deaths, and cardiovascular events in patients with diabetes mellitus: a meta-analysis. JAMA Intern Med. 2014;174:773–85.

45. Elgendy IY, Huo T, Chik V, Pepine CJ, Bavry AA. Efficacy and safety of angiotensin receptor blockers in older patients: a meta-analysis of randomized trials. Am J Hypertens. 2015;28:576–85.
46. Bangalore S, Fakheri R, Wandel S, Toklu B, Wandel J, Messerli FH. Renin angiotensin system inhibitors for patients with stable coronary artery disease without heart failure: systematic review and meta-analysis of randomized trials. BMJ. 2017;356:j4.
47. Retraction. Combination treatment of angiotensin-II receptor blocker and angiotensin-converting-enzyme inhibitor in non-diabetic renal disease (COOPERATE): a randomised controlled trial. Lancet. 2009;374:1226.
48. Retraction. Valsartan in a Japanese population with hypertension and other cardiovascular disease (JIKEI HEART STUDY): a randomised, open-label, blinded endpoint morbidity-mortality study. Lancet. 2013;382:843.
49. Retraction. Effects of valsartan on morbidity and mortality in uncontrolled hypertensive patients with high cardiovascular risks: KYOTO HEART Study. Eur Heart J. 2013;34:1023.
50. Thomopoulos C, Parati G, Zanchetti A. Effects of BP lowering on outcome incidence in hypertension: 5. Head-to-head comparisons of various classes of antihypertensive drugs – overview and meta-analyses. J Hypertens. 2015;33:1321–41.
51. Fuchs FD, Scala LC, Vilela-Martin JF, Bandeira-de-Mello R, Mosele F, Whelton PK, et al. Effectiveness of chlorthalidone/amiloride versus losartan in patients with stage I hypertension: results from the PREVER-TREATMENT randomized trial. J Hypertens. 2016;34:798–806.
52. Roush GC, Holford TR, Guddati AK. Chlorthalidone compared with hydrochlorothiazide in reducing cardiovascular events: systematic review and network meta-analyses. Hypertension. 2012;59:1110–7.
53. Ernst ME, Carter BL, Goerdt CJ, Steffensmeier JJ, Phillips BB, Zimmerman MB, et al. Comparative antihypertensive effects of hydrochlorothiazide and chlorthalidone on ambulatory and office BP. Hypertension. 2006;47:352–8.
54. Peterzan MA, Hardy R, Chaturvedi N, Hughes AD. Meta-analysis of dose-response relationships for hydrochlorothiazide, chlorthalidone, and bendroflumethiazide on BP, serum potassium, and urate. Hypertension. 2012;59:1104–9.
55. Pareek AK, Messerli FH, Chandurkar NB, Dharmadhikari SK, Godbole AV, Kshirsagar PP, et al. Efficacy of low-dose chlorthalidone and hydrochlorothiazide as assessed by 24-h ambulatory BP monitoring. J Am Coll Cardiol. 2016;67:379–89.
56. Guerrero P, Fuchs FD, Moreira LM, Martins VM, Bertoluci C, Fuchs SC, et al. BP-lowering efficacy of amiloride versus enalapril as add-on drugs in patients with uncontrolled BP receiving hydrochlorothiazide. Clin Exp Hypertens. 2008;30:553–64.
57. Zillich AJ, Garg J, Basu S, Bakris GL, Carter BL. Thiazide diuretics, potassium, and the development of diabetes: a quantitative review. Hypertension. 2006;48:1–6.
58. Brown MJ, Williams B, Morant SV, Webb DJ, Caulfield MJ, Cruickshank JK, et al. Effect of amiloride, or amiloride plus hydrochlorothiazide, versus hydrochlorothiazide on glucose tolerance and BP (PATHWAY-3): a parallel-group, double-blind randomised phase 4 trial. Lancet Diabetes Endocrinol. 2016;4:136–47.
59. Fuchs FD, Fuchs SC, Moreira LB, Gus M, Nóbrega AC, Poli-de-Figueiredo CE, et al. A comparison between diuretics and angiotensin receptor blocker agents in patients with stage I hypertension (PREVER-treatment trial): study protocol for a randomized double blind controlled trial. Trials. 2011;12:53.

Part VII

Management of Prehypertension

Antihypertensive Drugs and Vascular Health

37

Alan C. Cameron, Giacomo Rossitto, Ninian N. Lang, and Rhian M. Touyz

Key Points

- Hypertension is characterised by structural remodelling and endothelial dysfunction
- Antihypertensive drugs that target vascular health appear to be most efficacious in reducing cardiovascular events
- New blood pressure lowering drugs may also promote vascular health

37.1 Introduction

Hypertension is the most important modifiable risk factor for cardiovascular disease [1, 2] and effective blood pressure (BP) control is a priority to prevent significant cardiovascular morbidity and mortality [2]. Hypertension is associated with structural, mechanical and functional changes of the vascular system that contribute to increased arterial stiffness, reduced elasticity, increased vascular tone and endothelial dysfunction [1, 3].

Hypertension-associated cardiovascular disease can be prevented or ameliorated by antihypertensive drugs through BP lowering and direct effects on target organs. Some antihypertensive drugs, such as angiotensin-converting enzyme (ACE) inhibitors (ACEIs), angiotensin II (Ang II) receptor blockers (ARBs) and some

A. C. Cameron · G. Rossitto · N. N. Lang · R. M. Touyz (✉)
Institute of Cardiovascular and Medical Sciences, British Heart Foundation Glasgow Cardiovascular Reserach Centre, University of Glasgow, Glasgow, UK
e-mail: rhian.touyz@glasgow.ac.uk

R. Zimlichman et al. (eds.), *Prehypertension and Cardiometabolic Syndrome*, Updates in Hypertension and Cardiovascular Protection,
https://doi.org/10.1007/978-3-319-75310-2_37

diuretics, particularly mineralocorticoid receptor antagonists (MRAs), may have a direct effect on cardiac, renal and vascular function. Accordingly, drugs that lower BP and are organ-protective may have added benefits. Targeting the vascular system may prevent or repair vascular damage and promote vascular health [3]. Here we highlight vascular changes that characterise hypertension and discuss potential benefits of targeting vascular health from a therapeutic viewpoint.

37.2 Vascular Biology of Hypertension

Hypertension is characterised by endothelial dysfunction, vascular remodelling, inflammation, calcification and arterial stiffness (Fig. 37.1) [1, 3]. These changes reduce the ability of arteries to adapt to tissue oxygen demands and culminate in target organ damage with associated ischaemia, infarction and injury [1]. The overall phenotype depends on interacting factors including genetics, physiological systems, diet, smoking, diabetes, dyslipidaemia and obesity [1, 4, 5]. When combined with pro-hypertensive factors there is vascular injury, arterial stiffening and early vascular ageing [1].

The pro-hypertensive phenotype involves activation of the renin-angiotensin-aldosterone system (RAAS), inflammation and oxidative stress, which contribute to

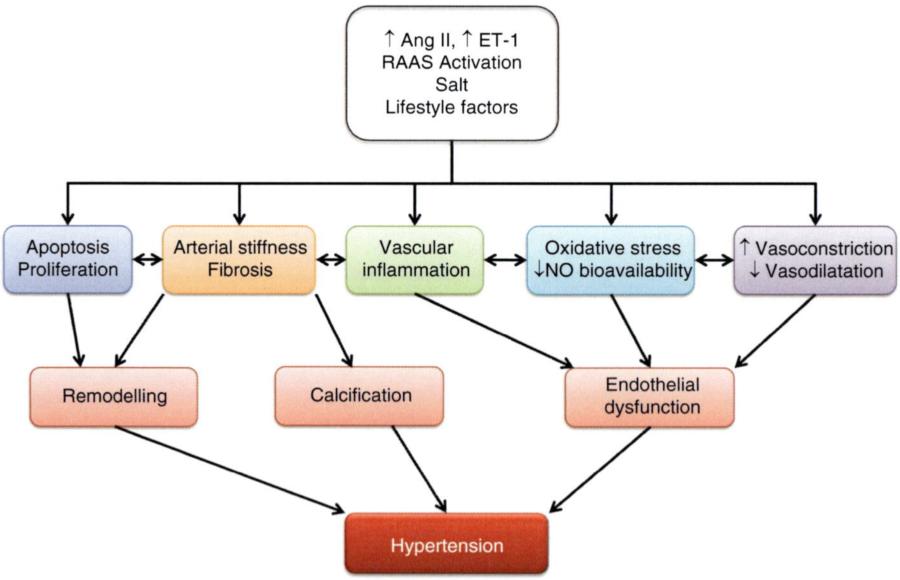

Fig. 37.1 Schematic of factors that can contribute to hypertension-associated vascular changes: pro-inflammatory, pro-fibrotic, redox-sensitive and growth/apoptotic pathways cause structural, functional and mechanical changes with remodelling, calcification and endothelial dysfunction. *RAAS* renin angiotensin aldosterone system, *Ang II* angiotensin II, *ET-1* endothelin-1, *NO* nitric oxide

vascular injury. Molecular and cellular mechanisms implicated in these effects include reduced nitric oxide (NO) production, increased ROS generation, pro-inflammatory and pro-fibrotic transcription factor activation, reduced collagen turnover, vascular calcification, smooth muscle cell proliferation and extracellular matrix (ECM) remodelling [1, 3]. This is exacerbated by increased Ang II, endothelin-1 (ET-1) and aldosterone, which stimulate pro-fibrotic and mitogenic signalling cascades. Increased p38mitogen-activated protein kinases (p38MAPK), extracellular signal regulated kinases 1/2 (ERK1/2) and transforming growth factor-β (TGF-β)/SMAD, galectin-3 and dysregulation of matrix metalloproteinases (MMPs) and tissue inhibitors of metalloproteinases (TIMPs) contribute to ECM remodelling and further vascular fibrosis [1].

37.2.1 The Extracellular Matrix and Vascular Fibrosis

The ECM is a fundamental component of connective tissue surrounding cells that maintains cellular and vascular integrity, as well as playing a critical role in cell signalling and regulation of cell-cell interactions. The relative quantities of collagen and elastin determine vascular biomechanical properties [1, 6, 7]. MMPs and TIMPs regulate the dynamic turnover of these components in the ECM and any imbalance leads to excess protein deposition, particularly collagen and fibronectin. Such deposition, along with calcification and collagen cross-linking by advanced glycation end-products [1], contributes to vascular fibrosis and stiffening (Fig. 37.2) [1]. Fibrosis initially occurs as a reversible and adaptive repair process, which progresses into the neighbouring interstitial spaces with progressive loss of elasticity [1]. Excessive fibrosis replaces parenchymal tissue, resulting in tissue fibrosis and target organ damage affecting the heart, brain and kidney. The major clinical consequences of these processes include heart failure, cerebrovascular disease, ischaemic heart disease and renal failure [1].

37.2.2 Oxidative Stress

Oxidative stress contributes to many molecular and cellular processes that evoke the vascular changes associated with hypertension. These include pro-inflammatory responses, oxidative modification of proteins, fibrosis and calcification, altered calcium homeostasis and redox-sensitive pro-inflammatory and pro-fibrotic transcription factor activation. A state of chronic, low-grade inflammation develops, which is regulated by enzyme systems that include NADPH oxidases (Nox) upregulation, endothelial nitric oxide synthase (eNOS) uncoupling and excessive O_2^- production by various Noxs and mitochondrial oxidases, resulting in endothelial dysfunction and vascular remodelling observed in hypertension [3, 8–11]. While xanthine oxidase also represents a source of ROS within the vasculature and may contribute to oxidative stress associated with hypertension, its precise role remains to be fully defined. [12]

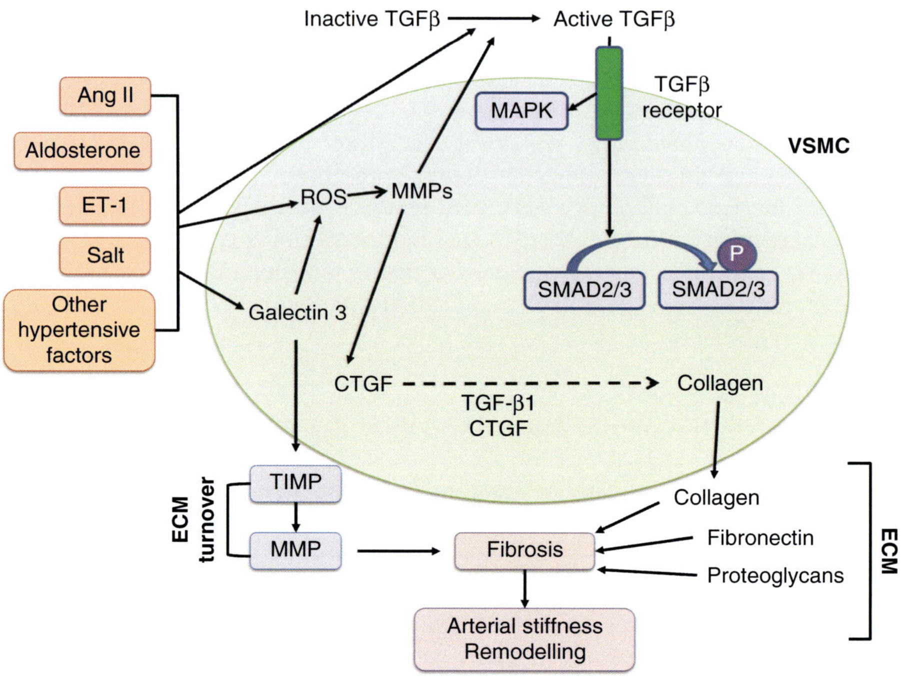

Fig. 37.2 Extracellular matrix (ECM) remodelling in hypertension. Angiotensin II (Ang II), aldosterone, endothelin-1 (ET-1), salt and other hypertensive factors promote ECM remodelling through activation of transforming growth factor-β (TGF-β), mitogen-activated protein kinase (MAPK) and SMAD pathways and reactive oxygen species (ROS). This leads to imbalance in tissue inhibitors of metalloproteinases (TIMP), matrix metalloproteinase (MMP) and connective tissue growth factor (CTGF) activation and upregulation of galectin-3. Collagen, fibronectin and proteoglycan deposition is increased, causing fibrosis, arterial stiffness and remodelling. Adapted from Harvey, et al. [1]

37.2.3 Salt and Inflammation

Animal models in which the "salt-sensitivity of blood pressure" trait[13] was inbred [14] led to identification of multiple key players in the compensatory pressure-natriuresis renal axis, including the RAAS, ET-1, and oxidative stress among many others, which have been reviewed elsewhere [15]. Beyond expansion of extracellular fluid volume, salt appears to exert a direct effect on vascular function, particularly via imbalance between pro-fibrotic TGF-β and NO availability [16, 17], generation of oxidative stress [17–20] and induction of vascular hypertrophy [21]. In line with such evidence, recent studies point to discrete accumulation of sodium in tissue microenvironments [22–25], thus suggesting a direct effect of local/perivascular sodium storage in promoting vascular dysfunction [26]. Moreover, excess salt activates multiple immune mediators [27] that have emerged as key determinants of vascular health and hypertension via pro-inflammatory and, ultimately, pro-fibrotic mediators [28, 29]. Accumulation of salt in microenvironments might amplify this pro-inflammatory effect [30].

37.3 Endothelial Function

The endothelium plays an essential role in vascular function through release of biologically active substances that influence vascular tone [3, 31]. NO is the best characterised relaxing factor and is derived via NOS which is constitutively active in endothelial cells [32–35]. NO is also released by neurohumoral mediators such as acetylcholine, bradykinin and by mechanical shear stress [31]. The endothelium also releases endogenous vasoconstrictors such as ET-1 [31, 36, 37]. The healthy endothelium has a vasodilator, anti-inflammatory and anti-thrombotic phenotype. However dysfunctional endothelium is pro-inflammatory, pro-thrombotic and has impaired vasodilator responses [3]. Consequently, endothelial dysfunction is central in the phenotypical changes associated with hypertension [38].

37.3.1 Assessing Endothelial Function

Endothelial function can be assessed by various methods including brachial artery flow-mediated dilatation (FMD) or venous occlusion plethysmography [38, 39]. These approaches measure vasomotor responses to pharmacological or mechanical stimuli [38]. NO and endothelium-derived hyperpolarising factor (EDHF) are fundamental mediators of endothelium-dependent vasodilatation [3, 38]. Reduced NO bioavailability is a key characteristic of endothelial dysfunction [3]. Endothelial dysfunction can also be examined at the cellular and molecular level by assessing endothelial cell proliferation, vascular permeability and leucocyte/endothelial cell interactions [40]. Endothelial microparticles have recently emerged as a novel biomarker of endothelial function [40]. Severity of hypertension correlates with impaired endothelial function and antihypertensive therapies which improve endothelial function appear to be associated with reduced cardiovascular risk [38, 41, 42].

37.3.2 Hypertension and Endothelial Dysfunction

As outlined, reduced NO bioavailability is central to the pathophysiology of hypertension-associated endothelial dysfunction, due in large part from reduced NO production and NO inactivation due to oxidative stress and vascular inflammation [38, 40, 43]. This promotes vasoconstriction and contributes to local inflammatory responses, leucocyte adhesion, vascular remodelling and arterial stiffness. Additional factors contributing to reduced NO bioavailability include elevated concentrations of endogenous NO inhibitors, eNOS uncoupling and altered signal transduction [40]. Deficiency in the substrate for NOS (L-arginine), as recently observed in association with increased urea synthesis in the context of a high salt diet [44], also limits NO production.

Vasoconstrictors such as ET-1 and Ang II may also contribute to endothelial dysfunction in hypertension [31]. An imbalance between NO and ET-1 systems may result in increased ET-1 activity and vasoconstriction [31, 45, 46], while Ang II interacts with the NO system to activate Noxs which contribute to oxidative stress [31, 47, 48]. ROS scavengers restore NO production and improve endothelial function in hypertension [40]. This supports the contribution of oxidative stress to hypertension-associated endothelial dysfunction and the benefits of targeting these changes with measures to restore antioxidant balance [40]. While antioxidant therapy has not yet been proven effective at reducing cardiovascular risk in patients, this may reflect the fact that most antioxidant approaches have focused on quenching ROS [49]. A more effective approach may be to target the source of ROS production, for example, inhibiting Nox activity.

37.3.3 Endothelial Dysfunction and Atherosclerosis

Endothelial dysfunction contributes to platelet aggregation, vascular smooth muscle cell proliferation and monocyte adhesion which are involved in the progression of atherosclerosis, plaque rupture and thrombosis [31, 50–53]. This is a key mechanism through which endothelial dysfunction can increase risk of myocardial infarction and stroke in patients with hypertension.

37.4 Vascular Remodelling

The remodelling of small arteries in hypertension is associated with increased media thickness and can be eutrophic or hypertrophic (Fig. 37.3). In eutrophic remodelling, which is generally found is essential (primary) hypertension, the media:lumen ratio is increased but the media cross-sectional area is not. Hypertrophic remodelling is typically found with secondary forms of hypertension and is characterised by an increase in both media:lumen ratio and media cross-sectional area [54]. Mechanisms contributing to eutrophic remodelling include expansion of the extracellular matrix with collagen deposition and low-grade inflammation that results in vascular fibrosis and increased arterial stiffening [54–60].

37.5 Arterial Stiffness

Hypertension-associated arterial stiffening is a result of altered vascular contraction and dilatation, fibrosis, ECM remodelling, cytoskeletal organisation, pro-inflammatory responses and oxidative stress [1]. Underlying processes involve dysregulation of endothelial and vascular smooth muscle cells, upregulation of adaptive immune responses, vascular smooth muscle cell growth and migration, changes in collagen:elastin ratio and vascular calcification [1, 3]. Structural changes result in reduced arterial compliance, elasticity and increased arterial stiffness. This demands greater force and further increases in BP which place an increased work load on the myocardium and result in left ventricular hypertrophy [3]. Methods to assess arterial stiffness include pulse wave velocity (PWV), pulse wave analysis, augmentation

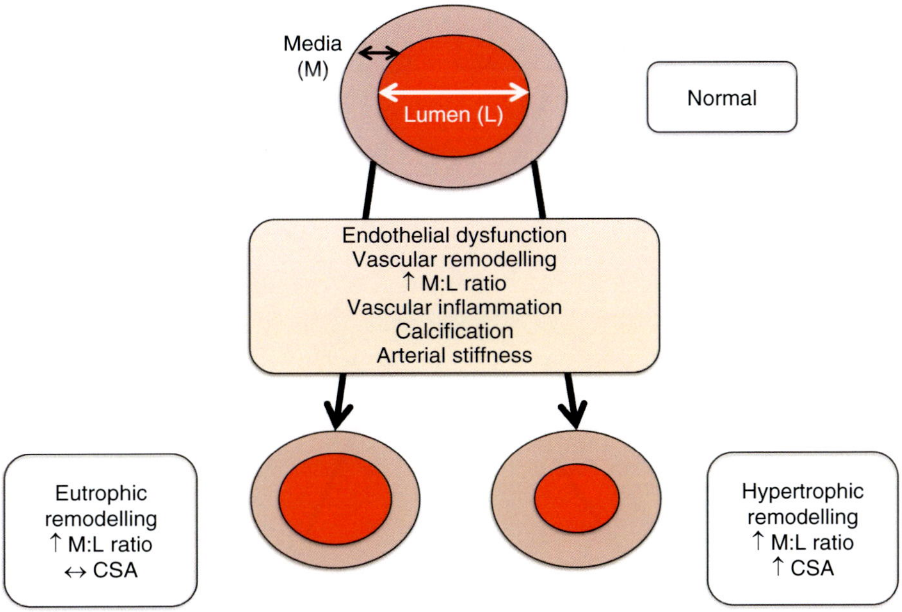

Fig. 37.3 Illustration of the changes that occur during hypertension-associated vascular remodelling: increased media-to-lumen ratio (M:L) and variable changes in cross-sectional area (CSA)

index (AIx), 24 h ambulatory BP monitoring and brachial artery FMD [1, 61]. Increased PWV occurs in the prehypertensive phase, suggesting that vascular changes may precede the onset of established hypertension [3] and PWV may be a useful tool to identify patients in the early prehypertensive phase.

37.6 Why Should We Target the Vascular System in the Treatment of Hypertension?

The endothelium is an important early target of hypertension and endothelial dysfunction is a risk marker for future cardiovascular events [40]. Targeting the vascular changes associated with hypertension should therefore be a focus of treatment, in addition to reducing BP (Fig. 37.4).[31, 40] Antihypertensive agents with the capacity to reverse endothelial dysfunction may reverse or prevent the progression of atherosclerosis and reduce the risk of cardiovascular disease [31].

ACEIs, ARBs and calcium channel blockers (CCBs) have all been shown to improve endothelial function with associated improvements in markers of oxidative stress [40]. ACEIs and ARBs reduce the production of ROS, while CCBs have antioxidant effects through improvements in the cellular redox and antioxidant state (Table 37.1) [31]. β-Blockers, despite lowering BP, generally do not improve endothelial function. Nebivolol and carvedilol are the exceptions, since nebivolol has NO donor properties and carvedilol may act as a scavenger of oxygen free radicals [31, 40].

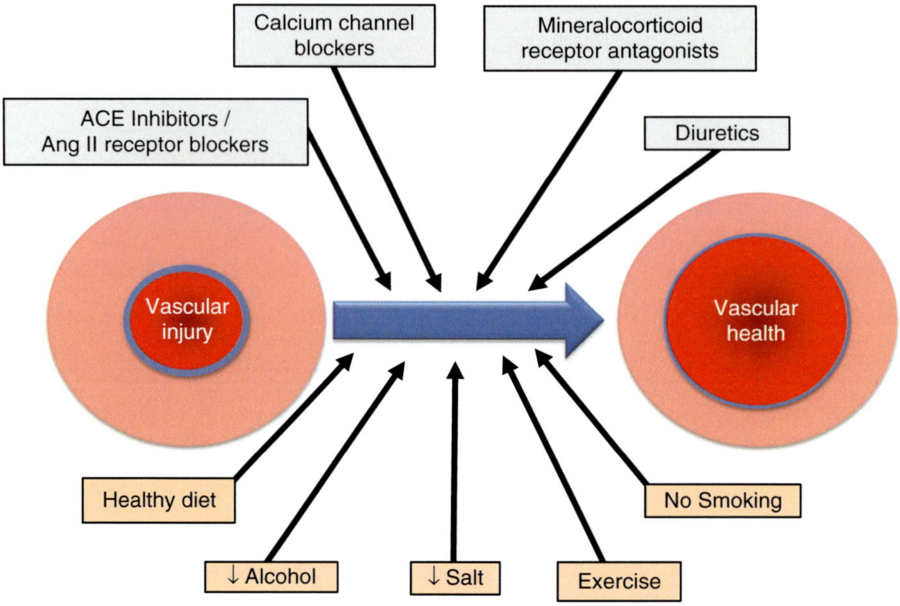

Fig. 37.4 Therapeutic approaches to promote vascular health: antihypertensive drugs and lifestyle modifications can ameliorate vascular damage and reduce target organ damage and cardiovascular complications

Table 37.1 Antihypertensive drugs and beneficial vascular effects

Drug class	Possible beneficial vascular effects
ACE inhibitors	Vasodilation Increased nitric oxide Anti-inflammatory Reduced reactive oxygen species
Angiotensin-II receptor blockers	Vasodilation Increased nitric oxide Anti-inflammatory Reduced reactive oxygen species
Calcium channel blockers	Improved cellular redox state
Diuretics	Reduced arterial stiffness Anti-inflammatory/fibrotic (via natriuresis)
Mineralocorticoid receptor antagonists	Anti-inflammatory Anti-fibrotic
β-Blockers	Increased nitric oxide Reactive oxygen species scavenger

Conclusive data on diuretics and diuretic-like agents on vascular health, particularly regarding oxidative stress and endothelial function, are scant compared to other classes and heterogeneous across different agents. Nevertheless, they appear to exert a beneficial effect on arterial stiffness [62–65] and, ultimately, in protecting against target organ damage (heart, kidneys, brain). This is particularly evident in salt-sensitive groups, such as blacks, elderly and patients with resistant hypertension, as endorsed by multiple guidelines [66, 67].

Mineralocorticoid receptor antagonists (MRA) combine the beneficial effects of the diuretic class with downstream blockade of the RAAS system, which is an important mediator of vascular remodelling through promotion of vascular hypertrophy, fibrosis, inflammation and oxidative stress. Chronic blockade of mineralocorticoid receptors reduces cardiovascular fibrosis in both animal models and human studies of hypertension [1, 68].

Some examples of how these beneficial effects of the different drug classes translated into robust cardiovascular outcomes in clinical trials are provided below. The Telmisartan versus Ramipril in renal ENdothelial Dysfunction (TRENDY) study demonstrated improved endothelial function in a diabetic population with hypertension and early-stage nephropathy treated with telmisartan and ramipril [69, 70]. The Losartan Intervention For Endpoint Reduction in Hypertension (LIFE) study compared losartan to atenolol-based therapy. Avoiding Cardiovascular Events through Combination Therapy in Patients Living with Systolic Hypertension (ACCOMPLISH) trial compared ACEI plus amlodipine versus ACEI plus a thiazide diuretic. As well as the Heart Outcomes Protection Evaluation (HOPE) study, these studies all showed superior clinical outcomes for treatment strategies with agents that improve endothelial function, such as RAAS blockers and CCBs [38, 71–74]. Overall, however, and at variance with β-blockers (atenolol) and α-blockers, diuretics do not fall short in terms of robust endpoints, i.e. cardiovascular events: this was shown in ALLHAT (Antihypertensive and Lipid-Lowering Treatment to Prevent Heart Attack Trial) [75] and recently reappraised by a systematic review and meta-analysis [76]. This might reflect a higher efficacy observed in salt-sensitive individuals, the benefit on arterial stiffness and/or other mechanisms, related to sodium balance and its local accumulation in tissues. BP lowering agents which improve vascular health may achieve the best reductions in cardiovascular risk and targeting the adverse vascular changes that contribute to the development of hypertension should be a priority when developing new antihypertensives.

37.7 Antihypertensive Drugs and Vascular Health

37.7.1 ACE Inhibitors and Angiotensin II Receptor Blockers

ACEIs improve endothelial function in animal models and clinical studies of hypertension [40], which may be due to direct vascular effects and to inhibition of bradykinin breakdown [31]. In clinical studies, ACEIs improve endothelial function as demonstrated by improved vascular responses to acetylcholine [31, 77–79] and improved FMD. This most likely relates to increased NO bioavailability and prevention of Ang II-induced oxidative stress [31, 80–85]. Most studies of ACEIs demonstrate greater lowering of central aortic than brachial artery BP [86, 87], which may relate to reduced oxidative stress and increased vasodilatation [86, 88]. ARBs may also have beneficial effects on endothelial function. The angiotensin type-1

(AT1) receptor antagonist losartan diminishes superoxide production, while blockade of AT1 receptors allows Ang II to bind to free angiotensin type-2 (AT2) receptors and subsequently stimulate AT2-receptor induced NO synthesis and release. This may be one of the mechanisms through which ARBs can restore NO bioavailability and improve endothelial function [31, 48, 89–91]. Losartan restores vasodilator responses to acetylcholine [31, 92] and has beneficial effects on FMD similar to those observed with ramipril [31, 81]. While ACEIs and ARBs have comparable BP-dependent reductions in cardiovascular risk, ACEIs also have BP-independent effects that have not been observed with ARBs [93].

37.7.2 Calcium Channel Blockers

CCBs, particularly dihydropyridine calcium channel antagonists such as amlodipine, improve endothelial function [40, 84, 94] by reducing intracellular Ca^{2+} concentration and possibly through antioxidant effects [31, 86]. Nifedipine reduces ET-1-induced vasoconstriction, improves endothelium-dependent vasodilation [95] and increases coronary vascular responses to acetylcholine [31]. Amlodipine increases basal NO release, while lacidipine increases vasodilator responses to acetylcholine and bradykinin [31, 96]. Endothelial cells do not express voltage-gated calcium channels and the improvements in endothelial function observed with CCBS are therefore unlikely to be calcium-dependent [31, 97]. Rather, CCBs appear to have antioxidant effects that may protect endothelial cells from oxygen free radicals, thus improving NO bioavailability and endothelial function [31, 98, 99]. Elderly patients are more likely to have isolated systolic hypertension with increased pulse pressure and increased arterial stiffness. Dihydropyridine CCBs have a more pronounced effect on central than brachial BP [86, 100] and may be the most appropriate antihypertensive drugs in elderly patients.

37.7.3 Diuretics

Often regarded as "renal" drugs, acting mostly on the volume component of hypertension, diuretic compounds were considered to have little or no effect on vascular health [63] and data with this regard are scant compared to other classes. Indeed, thiazide and thiazide-like diuretics (chlorthalidone, indapamide) appear as effective as CCBs and ARBs in reducing arterial stiffness and central pressure [62–64], although less than ACEIs [101] and MRAs [102]. Notably, the secondary increase in plasma aldosterone upon diuretic treatment might in part counteract the beneficial effects of the drugs [103], thereby supporting the use of diuretics as part of a combination strategy with RAAS blockers [104]. It is also interesting to note that the novel and highly effective neprilysin inhibitor/valsartan combination acts by coupling a natriuretic and a RAAS-blocking effect [105].

Classic thiazide diuretics do not reduce oxidative stress or improve endothelial function [106] and this reflects in a lack of benefit on endothelial-dependent vasodilation, compared to CCBs [107, 108]. However, a few reports suggest that indapamide has a vasodilatory activity mediated via free radical scavenging [109] and intrinsic Ca^{2+} antagonist effect [110]. Evidence, however, is much weaker than for other classes. Nevertheless, diuretics proved highly effective for prevention of cardiovascular events in the elderly [111] and, perhaps unsurprisingly, for prevention of heart failure in the general hypertensive population [2, 112]. Intriguingly, current trends in the understanding of heart failure pathophysiology, particularly for heart failure with preserved ejection fraction, point to (micro)vascular dysfunction as a primary culprit [113–116]. Whether diuretics or new drugs like sodium/glucose cotransporter 2 (SGLT2)-inhibitors [117] improve this microvascular dysfunction via modulation of (local) sodium balance, beyond an undisputable haemodynamic effect, is still a matter of speculation.

37.7.4 Mineralocorticoid Receptor Antagonists

Aldosterone exerts BP-elevating effects through interactions with the kidney that influence salt and water balance and may have additional direct effects on blood vessels [55, 118, 119]. Mineralocorticoid receptor activation may contribute to cardiovascular dysfunction, inflammation and fibrosis [55]. Therefore, beyond their diuretic properties, MRAs such as spironolactone and eplerenone have beneficial BP-independent effects on endothelial function and can reduce arterial stiffness. This may reflect blockade of aldosterone's pro-inflammatory and pro-fibrotic actions [86]. Spironolactone reduces PWV and augmentation index [120], while eplerenone reduces vascular stiffness, collagen/elastin ratio, pro-inflammatory mediators and systemic inflammatory markers in patients with hypertension. Because of all these addictive pleiotropic effects, it comes as no surprise that MRAs outperform other diuretics in improving arterial stiffness [102], FMD [121] or coronary flow reserve [122]. MRAs, including the highly promising novel selective non-steroidal finerenone 123, may therefore be an effective target to prevent vascular changes that occur in the development of hypertension, even out of the setting of resistant hypertension where MR antagonism was recently shown to be the strategy of choice [124].

37.7.5 β-Blockers

There is little evidence to suggest that β-blockers improve endothelial function. Atenolol may actually have a negative effect [31]. Nebivolol is a selective β_1-blocker which has vasodilator and NO donor properties that may improve endothelial function in patients with hypertension [31, 40, 125, 126]. Atenolol and nebivolol have similar reductions in brachial BP, while pulse pressure is significantly lower after nebivolol, suggesting nebivolol may have beneficial effects on arterial stiffness [86, 127]. Overall, the potential beneficial vascular effects of nebivolol appear most likely related to enhanced release of endothelium-derived NO with associated improvements in endothelial function and reduced arterial stiffness [86, 128]. Carvedilol is another selective β_1-blocker that has α1-adrenoceptor antagonistic properties as well as strong antioxidant effects that may improve endothelial function [31]. β-Blockers are less effective in improving endothelial function than RAAS blockers and CCBs [31].

37.8 Other Strategies to Improve Vascular Health in Hypertension

37.8.1 Smoking Cessation

Smoking acutely increases BP and can be associated with severe and malignant hypertension, although any chronic independent effects of smoking on BP appear small [129, 130]. However, smoking does contribute to the initiation and acceleration of vascular injury and atherosclerotic cardiovascular disease through endothelial dysfunction, oxidative stress, reduced NO bioavailability, vascular inflammation, increased arterial stiffness and a shift towards a pro-thrombotic state [131, 132]. Furthermore, smoking reduces brachial artery FMD in a dose-dependent manner, as a result of reduced NO bioavailability [132, 133]. This is particularly relevant in smokers who may be exposed to several periods of acute BP rises over the course of a day. Smoking exerts toxic effects on the endothelium which, combined with the adverse vascular effects of high BP, leads smoking and hypertension to have synergistic deleterious effects on vascular function and cardiovascular risk [129, 134]. Smoking cessation is therefore essential to reduce overall cardiovascular risk [2, 131, 135].

37.8.2 Exercise

Regular exercise can reduce BP [2, 135] and protect against arterial stiffness and endothelial dysfunction that occurs with advancing age [136]. Aerobic exercise reduces oxidative stress, inflammation and restores NO bioavailability [136]. Aerobic exercise improves forearm vascular responses to acetylcholine in older men [136, 137] that can be abolished by inhibition of eNOS, suggesting the benefits may be mediated by increased NO bioavailability [136, 138] Aerobic exercise also suppresses oxidative stress and may reduce vascular inflammation [136].

37.8.3 Diet and Weight Loss

Increased intake of fruit, vegetables and fish can reduce BP and improve endothelium-dependent forearm blood flow responses in patients with hypertension [139, 140]. This may be related to high polyphenol content in fruit and vegetables which can increase NO bioavailability [38, 139, 141, 142]. Increased consumption of fruit, vegetables and fish improves endothelial function, reduces BP and should be strongly encouraged [2, 135, 139].

Reducing salt intake can reduce systolic BP by as much as 5 mmHg [143, 144] and prevent hypertension [143, 145–149]. These improvements may be related to improved endothelial function, since the hypertensive effect of salt loading is linked to oxidative stress and reduced NO bioavailability [17, 38, 150–152], and beneficial impact on large elastic artery compliance, particularly in salt-sensitive patients, e.g. the elderly [153]. While it is still debated which is the optimal range of sodium intake for cardiovascular health [154, 155], there is general agreement that cutting down high sodium consumption below 5 g/day is beneficial [156, 157].

There is a dose-dependent relationship between reduction in alcohol intake and reduced BP [143, 158]. Light alcohol consumption may confer some protection against ischaemic heart disease and alcohol consumption should therefore be limited to $\leq$ 3 units per day for men and $\leq$ 2 units per day for women, while patients with hypertension who drink excessively should be strongly encouraged to reduce their alcohol intake [2, 135]. Weight loss reduces BP and even modest reductions can prevent hypertension by approximately 20% in individuals who are prehypertensive and overweight [143, 145].

37.9 Conclusions

Hypertension is characterised by vascular changes that include endothelial dysfunction, vasoconstriction, vascular remodelling, inflammation, fibrosis and arterial stiffness. These vascular processes work synergistically with high BP to increase cardiovascular risk. Hypertension is a growing public health burden with increases the risk of target organ damage and cardiovascular disease. Despite many antihypertensive drugs being available, optimal treatment remains a challenge. Antihypertensive drugs that promote vascular health, such as ACEIs, ARBs, CCBs, MRAs and, to some extent, diuretics, as well as newer cardiovascular drugs with natriuretic properties such as ARB-neprilysin inhibitors or SGLT2 inhibitors may positively influence vascular function. Lifestyle changes can also reduce the vascular effects of high BP and patients should be encouraged to reduce salt intake, exercise regularly, consume fish, fruit and vegetables, maintain a healthy weight, moderate their alcohol consumption and not smoke. New blood pressuring lowering drugs should target the vascular changes associated with hypertension. Advancing our understanding of the vascular mechanisms that cause high BP will facilitate discovery of drugs to reduce the burden of hypertension.

37.10 Compliance with Ethical Standards

Funding: No external funding was used in the preparation of this chapter.

Conflict of interest: Alan C. Cameron, Giacomo Rossitto, Ninian N. Lang, and Rhian M. Touyz declare that they have no conflict of interest that might be relevant to the contents of this chapter. The authors are supported by grants from the British Heart Foundation (RE/13/530177; RG/13/7/30099 and CH/4/29762).

References

1. Harvey A, Montezano AC, Lopes RA, Rios F, Touyz RM. Vascular fibrosis in aging and hypertension: molecular mechanisms and clinical implications. Can J Cardiol. 2016;32(5):659–68.
2. Touyz RM, Dominiczak AF. Hypertension guidelines: is it time to reappraise blood pressure thresholds and targets? Hypertension. 2016;67(4):688–9.
3. Taddei S, Virdis A, Ghiadoni L, Sudano I, Salvetti A. Effects of antihypertensive drugs on endothelial dysfunction: clinical implications. Drugs. 2002;62(2):265–84.
4. Harvey A, Montezano AC, Touyz RM. Vascular biology of ageing—implications in hypertension. J Mol Cell Cardiol. 2015;83(C):112–21.
5. Lopes RA, Neves KB, Tostes RC, Montezano AC, Touyz RM. Downregulation of nuclear factor erythroid 2-related factor and associated antioxidant genes contributes to redox-sensitive vascular dysfunction in hypertension. Hypertension. 2015;66(6):1240–50.
6. AlGhatrif M, Strait JB, Morrell CH, et al. Longitudinal trajectories of arterial stiffness and the role of blood pressure: the Baltimore longitudinal study of aging. Hypertension. 2013;62(5):934–41.
7. Lakatta EG, Levy D. Arterial and cardiac aging: major shareholders in cardiovascular disease enterprises: part I: aging arteries: a "set up" for vascular disease. Circulation. 2003;107(1):139–46.
8. Lakatta EG. The reality of aging viewed from the arterial wall. Artery Res. 2013;7(2):73–80.
9. Wind S, Beuerlein K, Armitage ME, et al. Oxidative stress and endothelial dysfunction in aortas of aged spontaneously hypertensive rats by NOX1/2 is reversed by NADPH oxidase inhibition. Hypertension. 2010;56(3):490–7.
10. Touyz RM, Briones AM, Sedeek M, Burger D, Montezano AC. NOX isoforms and reactive oxygen species in vascular health. Mol Interv. 2011;11(1):27–35.
11. Montezano AC, Touyz RM. Molecular mechanisms of hypertension--reactive oxygen species and antioxidants: a basic science update for the clinician. Can J Cardiol. 2012;28(3):288–95.
12. Montezano AC, Burger D, Ceravolo GS, Yusuf H, Montero M, Touyz RM. Novel Nox homologues in the vasculature: focusing on Nox4 and Nox5. Clin Sci. 2011;120(4):131–41.
13. Lee MY, Griendling KK. Redox signaling, vascular function, and hypertension. Antioxid Redox Signal. 2008;10(6):1045–59.
14. Weinberger MH, Miller JZ, Luft FC, Grim CE, Fineberg NS. Definitions and characteristics of sodium sensitivity and blood pressure resistance. Hypertension. 1986;8(6 Pt 2):II127–34.
15. Dahl LK, Heine M, Tassinari L. Role of genetic factors in susceptibility to experimental hypertension due to chronic excess salt ingestion. Nature. 1962;194:480–2.
16. Elijovich F, Weinberger MH, Anderson CAM, et al. Salt sensitivity of blood pressure: a scientific statement from the American Heart Association. Hypertension. 2016;68(3):e7–e46.
17. Chen PY, Sanders PW. L-arginine abrogates salt-sensitive hypertension in dahl/Rapp rats. J Clin Investig. 1991;88(5):1559–67.
18. Feng W, Ying W-Z, Aaron KJ, Sanders PW. Transforming growth factor-β mediates endothelial dysfunction in rats during high salt intake. Am J Physiol Renal Physiol. 2015;309(12):F1018–25.
19. Greaney JL, DuPont JJ, Lennon-Edwards SL, Sanders PW, Edwards DG, Farquhar WB. Dietary sodium loading impairs microvascular function independent of blood pressure in humans: role of oxidative stress. J Physiol Lond. 2012;590(21):5519–28.
20. Nurkiewicz TR, Boegehold MA. High salt intake reduces endothelium-dependent dilation of mouse arterioles via superoxide anion generated from nitric oxide synthase. Am J Physiol Regul Integr Comp Physiol. 2007;292(4):R1550–6.
21. Raffai G, Durand MJ, Lombard JH. Acute and chronic angiotensin-(1-7) restores vasodilation and reduces oxidative stress in mesenteric arteries of salt-fed rats. Am J Physiol Heart Circ Physiol. 2011;301(4):H1341–52.
22. Gu JW, Anand V, Shek EW, et al. Sodium induces hypertrophy of cultured myocardial myoblasts and vascular smooth muscle cells. Hypertension. 1998;31(5):1083–7.

23. Machnik A, Neuhofer W, Jantsch J, et al. Macrophages regulate salt-dependent volume and blood pressure by a vascular endothelial growth factor-C-dependent buffering mechanism. Nat Med. 2009;15(5):545–52.
24. Wiig H, Schröder A, Neuhofer W, et al. Immune cells control skin lymphatic electrolyte homeostasis and blood pressure. J Clin Invest. 2013;123(7):2803–15.
25. Kopp C, Linz P, Dahlmann A, et al. 23Na magnetic resonance imaging-determined tissue sodium in healthy subjects and hypertensive patients. Hypertension. 2013;61(3):635–40.
26. Titze J, Luft FC. Speculations on salt and the genesis of arterial hypertension. Kidney Int. 2017;91(6):1324–35.
27. Laffer CL, Scott RC, Titze JM, Luft FC, Elijovich F. Hemodynamics and salt-and-water balance link sodium storage and vascular dysfunction in salt-sensitive subjects. Hypertension. 2016;68(1):195–203.
28. Oh YS, Appel LJ, Galis ZS, et al. National Heart, Lung, and Blood Institute working group report on salt in human health and sickness: building on the current scientific evidence. Hypertension. 2016;68(2):281–8.
29. McMaster WG, Kirabo A, Madhur MS, Harrison DG. Inflammation, immunity, and hypertensive end-organ damage. Circ Res. 2015;116(6):1022–33.
30. Schiffrin EL. Immune mechanisms in hypertension and vascular injury. Clin Sci. 2014;126(4):267–74.
31. Foss JD, Kirabo A, Harrison DG. Do high-salt microenvironments drive hypertensive inflammation? Am J Physiol Regul Integr Comp Physiol. 2017;312(1):R1–4.
32. Furchgott RF, Zawadzki JV. The obligatory role of endothelial cells in the relaxation of arterial smooth muscle by acetylcholine. Nature. 1980;288(5789):373–6.
33. Palmer RM, Ferrige AG, Moncada S. Nitric oxide release accounts for the biological activity of endothelium-derived relaxing factor. Nature. 1987;327(6122):524–6.
34. Palmer RMJ, Ashton DS, Moncada S. Vascular endothelial cells synthesize nitric oxide from L-arginine. Nature. 1988;333(6174):664–6.
35. Bredt DS, Hwang PM, Glatt CE, Lowenstein C, Reed RR, Snyder SH. Cloned and expressed nitric oxide synthase structurally resembles cytochrome P-450 reductase. Nature. 1991;351(6329):714–8.
36. Yanagisawa M, Kurihara H, Kimura S, Goto K, Masaki T. A novel peptide vasoconstrictor, endothelin, is produced by vascular endothelium and modulates smooth muscle Ca2+ channels. J Hypertens Suppl. 1988;6(4):S188–91.
37. Inoue A, Yanagisawa M, Kimura S, et al. The human endothelin family: three structurally and pharmacologically distinct isopeptides predicted by three separate genes. Proc Natl Acad Sci U S A. 1989;86(8):2863–7.
38. Dharmashankar K, Widlansky ME. Vascular endothelial function and hypertension: insights and directions. Curr Hypertens Rep. 2010;12(6):448–55. https://doi.org/10.1007/s11906-010-0150-2.
39. Hamburg NM, Benjamin EJ. Assessment of endothelial function using digital pulse amplitude tonometry. Trends Cardiovasc Med. 2009;19(1):6–11.
40. Thuillez C, Richard V. Targeting endothelial dysfunction in hypertensive subjects. J Hum Hypertens. 2005;19:S21–5.
41. Modena MG, Bonetti L, Coppi F, Bursi F, Rossi R. Prognostic role of reversible endothelial dysfunction in hypertensive postmenopausal women. J Am Coll Cardiol. 2002;40(3):505–10.
42. Benjamin EJ, Larson MG, Keyes MJ, et al. Clinical correlates and heritability of flow-mediated dilation in the community: the Framingham heart study. Circulation. 2004;109(5):613–9.
43. Widlansky ME, Gokce N, Keaney JF, Vita JA. The clinical implications of endothelial dysfunction. J Am Coll Cardiol. 2003;42(7):1149–60.
44. Rakova N, Kitada K, Lerchl K, et al. Increased salt consumption induces body water conservation and decreases fluid intake. J Clin Invest. 2017;127(5):1932–43.
45. Haynes WG, Webb DJ. Endothelin as a regulator of cardiovascular function in health and disease. J Hypertens. 1998;16(8):1081–98.
46. Schiffrin EL. Role of Endothelin-1 in hypertension. Hypertension. 1999;34(4):876–81.

47. Griendling KK, Minieri CA, Ollerenshaw JD, Alexander RW. Angiotensin II stimulates NADH and NADPH oxidase activity in cultured vascular smooth muscle cells. Circ Res. 1994;74(6):1141–8.
48. Rajagopalan S, Kurz S, Münzel T, et al. Angiotensin II-mediated hypertension in the rat increases vascular superoxide production via membrane NADH/NADPH oxidase activation. Contribution to alterations of vasomotor tone. J Clin Investig. 1996;97(8):1916–23.
49. Myung S-K, Ju W, Cho B, et al. Efficacy of vitamin and antioxidant supplements in prevention of cardiovascular disease: systematic review and meta-analysis of randomised controlled trials. BMJ. 2013;346(jan18 1):f10.
50. Radomski MW, Palmer RM, Moncada S. Endogenous nitric oxide inhibits human platelet adhesion to vascular endothelium. Lancet. 1987;2(8567):1057–8.
51. Garg UC, Hassid A. Nitric oxide-generating vasodilators and 8-bromo-cyclic guanosine monophosphate inhibit mitogenesis and proliferation of cultured rat vascular smooth muscle cells. J Clin Investig. 1989;83(5):1774–7.
52. Kubes P, Suzuki M, Granger DN. Nitric oxide: an endogenous modulator of leukocyte adhesion. Proc Natl Acad Sci U S A. 1991;88(11):4651–5.
53. De Caterina R, Libby P, Peng HB, et al. Nitric oxide decreases cytokine-induced endothelial activation. Nitric oxide selectively reduces endothelial expression of adhesion molecules and proinflammatory cytokines. J Clin Investig. 1995;96(1):60–8.
54. Schiffrin EL. Vascular remodeling in hypertension: mechanisms and treatment. Hypertension. 2012;59(2):367–74.
55. Savoia C, Sada L, Zezza L, et al. Vascular inflammation and endothelial dysfunction in experimental hypertension. Int J Hypertens. 2011;2011(2 Suppl):1–8.
56. Blake GJ, Ridker PM. Novel clinical markers of vascular wall inflammation. Circ Res. 2001;89(9):763–71.
57. Sesso HD, Buring JE, Rifai N, Blake GJ, Gaziano JM, Ridker PM. C-reactive protein and the risk of developing hypertension. JAMA. 2003;290(22):2945–51.
58. Preston RA, Ledford M, Materson BJ, Baltodano NM, Memon A, Alonso A. Effects of severe, uncontrolled hypertension on endothelial activation: soluble vascular cell adhesion molecule-1, soluble intercellular adhesion molecule-1 and von Willebrand factor. J Hypertens. 2002;20(5):871–7.
59. Blake GJ, Rifai N, Buring JE, Ridker PM. Blood pressure, C-reactive protein, and risk of future cardiovascular events. Circulation. 2003;108(24):2993–9.
60. Thorand B, Löwel H, Schneider A, et al. C-reactive protein as a predictor for incident diabetes mellitus among middle-aged men: results from the MONICA Augsburg cohort study, 1984–1998. Arch Intern Med. 2003;163(1):93–9.
61. Van Bortel LM, Laurent S, Boutouyrie P, et al. Expert consensus document on the measurement of aortic stiffness in daily practice using carotid-femoral pulse wave velocity. J Hypertens. 2012;30(3):445–8.
62. Agnoletti D, Zhang Y, Borghi C, Blacher J, Safar ME. Effects of antihypertensive drugs on central blood pressure in humans: a preliminary observation. Am J Hypertens. 2013;26(8):1045–52.
63. Mackenzie IS, McEniery CM, Dhakam Z, Brown MJ, Cockcroft JR, Wilkinson IB. Comparison of the effects of antihypertensive agents on central blood pressure and arterial stiffness in isolated systolic hypertension. Hypertension. 2009;54(2):409–13.
64. Alem M, Milia P, Muir S, Lees K, Walters M. Comparison of the effects of diuretics on blood pressure and arterial stiffness in patients with stroke. J Stroke Cerebrovasc Dis. 2008;17(6):373–7.
65. Safar M, Laurent S, Safavian A, Pannier B, Asmar R. Sodium and large arteries in hypertension. Effects of indapamide. Am J Med. 1988;84(1B):15–9.
66. Roush GC, Sica DA. Diuretics for hypertension: a review and update. Am J Hypertens. 2016;29(10):1130–7.
67. Calhoun DA, Jones D, Textor S, et al. Resistant hypertension: diagnosis, evaluation, and treatment. A scientific statement from the American Heart Association professional

education Committee of the Council for high blood pressure research. Hypertension. 2008;51(6):1403–19.
68. Savoia C, Touyz RM, Amiri F, Schiffrin EL. Selective mineralocorticoid receptor blocker eplerenone reduces resistance artery stiffness in hypertensive patients. Hypertension. 2008;51(2):432–9.
69. Ruilope LM, Redón J, Schmieder R. Cardiovascular risk reduction by reversing endothelial dysfunction: ARBs, ACE inhibitors, or both? Expectations from the ONTARGET trial Programme. Vasc Health Risk Manag. 2007;3(1):1–9.
70. Schmieder RE, Delles C, Mimran A, Fauvel JP, Ruilope LM. Impact of telmisartan versus ramipril on renal endothelial function in patients with hypertension and type 2 diabetes. Diabetes Care. 2007;30(6):1351–6.
71. Dahlöf B, Devereux RB, Kjeldsen SE, et al. Cardiovascular morbidity and mortality in the losartan intervention for endpoint reduction in hypertension study (LIFE): a randomised trial against atenolol. Lancet. 2002;359(9311):995–1003.
72. Jamerson K, Weber MA, Bakris GL, et al. Benazepril plus amlodipine or hydrochlorothiazide for hypertension in high-risk patients. N Engl J Med. 2008;359(23):2417–28.
73. Hadi HAR, Carr CS, Suwaidi AJ. Endothelial dysfunction: cardiovascular risk factors, therapy, and outcome. Vasc Health Risk Manag. 2005;1(3):183–98.
74. Dagenais GR, Yusuf S, Bourassa MG, et al. Effects of ramipril on coronary events in high-risk persons: results of the heart outcomes prevention evaluation study. Circulation. 2001;104(5):522–6.
75. ALLHAT Officers and Coordinators for the ALLHAT Collaborative Research Group. The antihypertensive and lipid-lowering treatment to prevent heart attack trial. Major outcomes in high-risk hypertensive patients randomized to angiotensin-converting enzyme inhibitor or calcium channel blocker vs diuretic: the antihypertensive and lipid-lowering treatment to prevent heart attack trial (ALLHAT). JAMA. 2002;288(23):2981–97.
76. Fretheim A, Odgaard-Jensen J, Brørs O, et al. Comparative effectiveness of antihypertensive medication for primary prevention of cardiovascular disease: systematic review and multiple treatments meta-analysis. BMC Med. 2012;10:33.
77. Schiffrin EL. Correction of remodeling and function of small arteries in human hypertension by cilazapril, an angiotensin I-converting enzyme inhibitor. J Cardiovasc Pharmacol. 1996;27(Suppl 2):S13–8.
78. Schiffrin EL, Deng LY. Comparison of effects of angiotensin I-converting enzyme inhibition and beta-blockade for 2 years on function of small arteries from hypertensive patients. Hypertension. 1995;25(4 Pt 2):699–703.
79. Rizzoni D, Muiesan ML, Porteri E, et al. Effects of long-term antihypertensive treatment with lisinopril on resistance arteries in hypertensive patients with left ventricular hypertrophy. J Hypertens. 1997;15(2):197–204.
80. Mancini GB, Henry GC, Macaya C, et al. Angiotensin-converting enzyme inhibition with quinapril improves endothelial vasomotor dysfunction in patients with coronary artery disease. The TREND (trial on reversing ENdothelial dysfunction) study. Circulation. 1996;94(3):258–65.
81. Hornig B, Landmesser U, Kohler C, et al. Comparative effect of ace inhibition and angiotensin II type 1 receptor antagonism on bioavailability of nitric oxide in patients with coronary artery disease: role of superoxide dismutase. Circulation. 2001;103(6):799–805.
82. Antony I, Lerebours G, Nitenberg A. Angiotensin-converting enzyme inhibition restores flow-dependent and cold pressor test-induced dilations in coronary arteries of hypertensive patients. Circulation. 1996;94(12):3115–22.
83. Ghiadoni L, Virdis A, Magagna A, Taddei S, Salvetti A. Effect of the angiotensin II type 1 receptor blocker candesartan on endothelial function in patients with essential hypertension. Hypertension. 2000;35(1 Pt 2):501–6.
84. Taddei S, Virdis A, Ghiadoni L, Mattei P, Salvetti A. Effects of angiotensin converting enzyme inhibition on endothelium-dependent vasodilatation in essential hypertensive patients. J Hypertens. 1998;16(4):447–56.

85. Ghiadoni L, Magagna A, Versari D, et al. Different effect of antihypertensive drugs on conduit artery endothelial function. Hypertension. 2003;41(6):1281–6.
86. Dudenbostel T, Glasser SP. Effects of antihypertensive drugs on arterial stiffness. Cardiol Rev. 2012;20(5):259–63.
87. Protogerou AD, Stergiou GS, Vlachopoulos C, Blacher J, Achimastos A. The effect of antihypertensive drugs on central blood pressure beyond peripheral blood pressure. Part II: evidence for specific class-effects of antihypertensive drugs on pressure amplification. Curr Pharm Des. 2009;15(3):272–89.
88. Hirata K, Vlachopoulos C, Adji A, O'Rourke MF. Benefits from angiotensin-converting enzyme inhibitor "beyond blood pressure lowering": beyond blood pressure or beyond the brachial artery? J Hypertens. 2005;23(3):551–6.
89. Wiemer G, Schölkens BA, Wagner A, Heitsch H, Linz W. The possible role of angiotensin II subtype AT2 receptors in endothelial cells and isolated ischemic rat hearts. J Hypertens Suppl. 1993;11(5):S234–5.
90. Maeso R, Navarro-Cid J, Muñoz-García R, et al. Losartan reduces phenylephrine constrictor response in aortic rings from spontaneously hypertensive rats. Role of nitric oxide and angiotensin II type 2 receptors. Hypertension. 1996;28(6):967–72.
91. Seyedi N, Xu X, Nasjletti A, Hintze TH. Coronary kinin generation mediates nitric oxide release after angiotensin receptor stimulation. Hypertension. 1995;26(1):164–70.
92. Schiffrin EL, Park JB, Intengan HD, Touyz RM. Correction of arterial structure and endothelial dysfunction in human essential hypertension by the angiotensin receptor antagonist losartan. Circulation. 2000;101(14):1653–9.
93. Blood Pressure Lowering Treatment Trialists' Collaboration, Turnbull F, Neal B, et al. Blood pressure-dependent and independent effects of agents that inhibit the renin-angiotensin system. J Hypertens. 2007;25(5):951–8.
94. Taddei S, Virdis A, Ghiadoni L, Uleri S, Magagna A, Salvetti A. Lacidipine restores endothelium-dependent vasodilation in essential hypertensive patients. Hypertension. 1997;30(6):1606–12.
95. Sudano I, Virdis A, Taddei S, et al. Chronic treatment with long-acting Nifedipine reduces vasoconstriction to Endothelin-1 in essential hypertension. Hypertension. 2007;49(2):285–90.
96. Lyons D, Webster J, Benjamin N. The effect of antihypertensive therapy on responsiveness to local intra-arterial NG-monomethyl-L-arginine in patients with essential hypertension. J Hypertens. 1994;12(9):1047–52.
97. Himmel HM, Whorton AR, Strauss HC. Intracellular calcium, currents, and stimulus-response coupling in endothelial cells. Hypertension. 1993;21(1):112–27.
98. Lupo E, Locher R, Weisser B, Vetter W. In vitro antioxidant activity of calcium antagonists against LDL oxidation compared with alpha-tocopherol. Biochem Biophys Res Commun. 1994;203(3):1803–8.
99. Mak IT, Boehme P, Weglicki WB. Antioxidant effects of calcium channel blockers against free radical injury in endothelial cells. Correlation of protection with preservation of glutathione levels. Circ Res. 1992;70(6):1099–103.
100. Morgan T, Lauri J, Bertram D, Anderson A. Effect of different antihypertensive drug classes on central aortic pressure. Am J Hypertens. 2004;17(2):118–23.
101. Jiang X-J, O'Rourke MF, Zhang Y-Q, He X-Y, Liu L-S. Superior effect of an angiotensin-converting enzyme inhibitor over a diuretic for reducing aortic systolic pressure. J Hypertens. 2007;25(5):1095–9.
102. Ohta Y, Ishizuka A, Hayashi S, et al. Effects of a selective aldosterone blocker and thiazide-type diuretic on blood pressure and organ damage in hypertensive patients. Clin Exp Hypertens. 2015;37(7):569–73.
103. Matsui Y, Eguchi K, O'Rourke MF, Ishikawa J, Shimada K, Kario K. Association between aldosterone induced by antihypertensive medication and arterial stiffness reduction: the J-CORE study. Atherosclerosis. 2011;215(1):184–8.
104. Joannides R, Bellien J, Thurlure C, Iacob M, Abeel M, Thuillez C. Fixed combination of perindopril and Indapamide at low dose improves endothelial function in essential hypertensive patients after acute administration. Am J Hypertens. 2008;21(6):679–84.

105. Chrysant SG. Pharmacokinetic, pharmacodynamic, and antihypertensive effects of the neprilysin inhibitor LCZ-696: sacubitril/valsartan. J Am Soc Hypertens. 2017;11:461.
106. Zhou M-S, Schulman IH, Jaimes EA, Raij L. Thiazide diuretics, endothelial function, and vascular oxidative stress. J Hypertens. 2008;26(3):494–500.
107. Muiesan ML, Salvetti M, Monteduro C, et al. Effect of treatment on flow-dependent vasodilation of the brachial artery in essential hypertension. Hypertension. 1999;33(1 Pt 2):575–80.
108. Muiesan ML, Salvetti M, Belotti E, et al. Effects of barnidipine in comparison with hydrochlorothiazide on endothelial function, as assessed by flow mediated vasodilatation in hypertensive patients. Blood Press. 2011;20(4):244–51.
109. Vergely C, Walker MK, Zeller M, et al. Antioxidant properties of indapamide, 5-OH indapamide and hydrochlorothiazide evaluated by oxygen-radical absorbing capacity and electron paramagnetic resonance. Mol Cell Biochem. 1998;178(1–2):151–5.
110. Calder JA, Schachter M, Sever PS. Vasorelaxant actions of 5-OH-indapamide, a major metabolite of indapamide: comparison with indapamide, hydrochlorothiazide and cicletanine. Eur J Pharmacol. 1994;256(2):185–91.
111. Beckett NS, Peters R, Fletcher AE, et al. Treatment of hypertension in patients 80 years of age or older. N Engl J Med. 2008;358(18):1887–98.
112. Burnier M, Narkiewicz K, Kjeldsen SE. Prevention of heart failure mortality and hospitalizations in SPRINT, EMPA-REG, ALLHAT and HYVET: are diuretics the clue? Blood Press. 2017;26(4):193–4.
113. Waddingham MT, Paulus WJ. Microvascular paradigm in heart failure with preserved ejection fraction: a quest for proof of concept. Circ Heart Fail. 2017;10(6):e004179.
114. Paulus WJ, Tschöpe C. A novel paradigm for heart failure with preserved ejection fraction: comorbidities drive myocardial dysfunction and remodeling through coronary microvascular endothelial inflammation. J Am Coll Cardiol. 2013;62(4):263–71.
115. Mohammed SF, Hussain S, Mirzoyev SA, Edwards WD, Maleszewski JJ, Redfield MM. Coronary microvascular rarefaction and myocardial fibrosis in heart failure with preserved ejection fraction. Circulation. 2015;131(6):550–9.
116. Hwang S-J, Melenovsky V, Borlaug BA. Implications of coronary artery disease in heart failure with preserved ejection fraction. J Am Coll Cardiol. 2014;63(25 Pt A):2817–27.
117. Zinman B, Wanner C, Lachin JM, et al. Empagliflozin, cardiovascular outcomes, and mortality in type 2 diabetes. N Engl J Med. 2015;373(22):2117–28.
118. Schiffrin EL. Effects of aldosterone on the vasculature. Hypertension. 2006;47(3):312–8.
119. Williams GH. Cardiovascular benefits of aldosterone receptor antagonists: what about potassium? Hypertension. 2005;46(2):265–6.
120. de Souza F, Muxfeldt E, Fiszman R, Salles G. Efficacy of spironolactone therapy in patients with true resistant hypertension. Hypertension. 2010;55(1):147–52.
121. Yamanari H, Nakamura K, Miura D, Yamanari S, Ohe T. Spironolactone and chlorthalidone in uncontrolled elderly hypertensive patients treated with calcium antagonists and angiotensin II receptor-blocker: effects on endothelial function, inflammation, and oxidative stress. Clin Exp Hypertens. 2009;31(7):585–94.
122. Joffe HV, Kwong RY, Gerhard-Herman MD, Rice C, Feldman K, Adler GK. Beneficial effects of eplerenone versus hydrochlorothiazide on coronary circulatory function in patients with diabetes mellitus. J Clin Endocrinol Metab. 2007;92(7):2552–8.
123. Bärfacker L, Kuhl A, Hillisch A, et al. Discovery of BAY 94-8862: a nonsteroidal antagonist of the mineralocorticoid receptor for the treatment of cardiorenal diseases. ChemMedChem. 2012;7(8):1385–403.
124. Williams B, MacDonald TM, Morant S, et al. Spironolactone versus placebo, bisoprolol, and doxazosin to determine the optimal treatment for drug-resistant hypertension (PATHWAY-2): a randomised, double-blind, crossover trial. Lancet. 2015;386(10008):2059–68.
125. Cockcroft JR, Chowienczyk PJ, Brett SE, et al. Nebivolol vasodilates human forearm vasculature: evidence for an L-arginine/NO-dependent mechanism. J Pharmacol Exp Ther. 1995;274(3):1067–71.
126. Kubli S, Feihl F, Waeber B. Beta-blockade with nebivolol enhances the acetylcholine-induced cutaneous vasodilation. Clin Pharmacol Ther. 2001;69(4):238–44.

127. Dhakam Z, Yasmin MECM, et al. A comparison of atenolol and nebivolol in isolated systolic hypertension. J Hypertens. 2008;26(2):351–6.
128. Kampus P, Serg M, Kals J, et al. Differential effects of nebivolol and metoprolol on central aortic pressure and left ventricular wall thickness. Hypertension. 2011;57(6):1122–8.
129. Primatesta P, Falaschetti E, Gupta S, Marmot MG, Poulter NR. Association between smoking and blood pressure: evidence from the health survey for England. Hypertension. 2001;37(2):187–93.
130. Tuomilehto J, Elo J, Nissinen A. Smoking among patients with malignant hypertension. Br Med J (Clin Res Ed). 1982;284(6322):1086.
131. Virdis A, Giannarelli C, Fritsch Neves M, Taddei S, Ghiadoni L. Cigarette Smoking and Hypertension. Curr Pharm Des. 2010;16(23):2518–25.
132. Messner B, Bernhard D. Smoking and cardiovascular disease: mechanisms of endothelial dysfunction and early atherogenesis. Arterioscler Thromb Vasc Biol. 2014;34(3):509–15.
133. Celermajer DS, Sorensen KE, Gooch VM, et al. Non-invasive detection of endothelial dysfunction in children and adults at risk of atherosclerosis. Lancet. 1992;340(8828):1111–5.
134. Kannel WB. Importance of hypertension as a risk factor in cardiovascular disease. In: Hypertension: pathopsychology and treatment. New York, NY: McGraw-Hill; 1977. p. 888–910.
135. Williams B, Poulter NR, Brown MJ, et al. British hypertension society guidelines for hypertension management 2004 (BHS-IV): summary. BMJ. 2004;328(7440):634–40.
136. Santos-Parker JR, LaRocca TJ, Seals DR. Aerobic exercise and other healthy lifestyle factors that influence vascular aging. Adv Physiol Educ. 2014;38(4):296–307.
137. DeSouza CA, Shapiro LF, Clevenger CM, et al. Regular aerobic exercise prevents and restores age-related declines in endothelium-dependent vasodilation in healthy men. Circulation. 2000;102(12):1351–7.
138. Taddei S, Galetta F, Virdis A, et al. Physical activity prevents age-related impairment in nitric oxide availability in elderly athletes. Circulation. 2000;101(25):2896–901.
139. McCall DO, McGartland CP, McKinley MC, et al. Dietary intake of fruits and vegetables improves microvascular function in hypertensive subjects in a dose-dependent manner. Circulation. 2009;119(16):2153–60.
140. Appel LJ, Moore TJ, Obarzanek E, et al. A clinical trial of the effects of dietary patterns on blood pressure. DASH collaborative research group. N Engl J Med. 1997;336(16):1117–24.
141. Anter E, Thomas SR, Schulz E, Shapira OM, Vita JA, Keaney JF. Activation of endothelial nitric-oxide synthase by the p38 MAPK in response to black tea polyphenols. J Biol Chem. 2004;279(45):46637–43.
142. Widlansky ME, Duffy SJ, Hamburg NM, et al. Effects of black tea consumption on plasma catechins and markers of oxidative stress and inflammation in patients with coronary artery disease. Free Radic Biol Med. 2005;38(4):499–506.
143. Appel LJ, Brands MW, Daniels SR, et al. Dietary approaches to prevent and treat hypertension: a scientific statement from the American Heart Association. Hypertension. 2006;47(2):296–308.
144. He FJ, MacGregor GA. Effect of modest salt reduction on blood pressure: a meta-analysis of randomized trials. Implications for public health. J Hum Hypertens. 2002;16(11):761–70.
145. The Trials of Hypertension Prevention Collaborative Research Group. Effects of weight loss and sodium reduction intervention on blood pressure and hypertension incidence in overweight people with high-normal blood pressure. The trials of hypertension prevention, phase II. Arch Intern Med. 1997;157(6):657–67.
146. Langford HG, Blaufox MD, Oberman A, et al. Dietary therapy slows the return of hypertension after stopping prolonged medication. JAMA. 1985;253(5):657–64.
147. Whelton PK, Appel LJ, Espeland MA, et al. Sodium reduction and weight loss in the treatment of hypertension in older persons: a randomized controlled trial of nonpharmacologic interventions in the elderly (TONE). TONE collaborative research group. JAMA. 1998;279(11):839–46.

148. Weir MR, Hall PS, Behrens MT, Flack JM. Salt and blood pressure responses to calcium antagonism in hypertensive patients. Hypertension. 1997;30(3 Pt 1):422–7.
149. Appel LJ, Espeland MA, Easter L, Wilson AC, Folmar S, Lacy CR. Effects of reduced sodium intake on hypertension control in older individuals: results from the trial of nonpharmacologic interventions in the elderly (TONE). Arch Intern Med. 2001;161(5):685–93.
150. Kopkan L, Majid DSA. Superoxide contributes to development of salt sensitivity and hypertension induced by nitric oxide deficiency. Hypertension. 2005;46(4):1026–31.
151. Majid DSA, Kopkan L. Nitric oxide and superoxide interactions in the kidney and their implication in the development of salt-sensitive hypertension. Clin Exp Pharmacol Physiol. 2007;34(9):946–52.
152. Kopkan L, Castillo A, Navar LG, Majid DSA. Enhanced superoxide generation modulates renal function in ANG II-induced hypertensive rats. Am J Physiol Renal Physiol. 2006;290(1):F80–6.
153. Gates PE, Tanaka H, Hiatt WR, Seals DR. Dietary sodium restriction rapidly improves large elastic artery compliance in older adults with systolic hypertension. Hypertension. 2004;44(1):35–41.
154. Cogswell ME, Mugavero K, Bowman BA, Frieden TR. Dietary sodium and cardiovascular disease risk--measurement matters. N Engl J Med. 2016;375(6):580–6.
155. O'Donnell M, Mente A, Yusuf S. Sodium and cardiovascular disease. N Engl J Med. 2014;371(22):2137–8.
156. Mozaffarian D, Fahimi S, Singh GM, et al. Global sodium consumption and death from cardiovascular causes. N Engl J Med. 2014;371(7):624–34.
157. Mancia G, Oparil S, Whelton PK, et al. The technical report on sodium intake and cardiovascular disease in low- and middle-income countries by the joint working group of the world heart federation, the European Society of Hypertension and the European public health association. Eur Heart J. 2017;38(10):712–9.
158. Xin X, He J, Frontini MG, Ogden LG, Motsamai OI, Whelton PK. Effects of alcohol reduction on blood pressure: a meta-analysis of randomized controlled trials. Hypertension. 2001;38(5):1112–7.

Management of Prehypertension and Hypertension in Women of Childbearing Age

38

Agnieszka Olszanecka and Danuta Czarnecka

Cardiac disorders are the leading cause of deaths in women in developed countries [1, 2]. Hypertension is a major contributor to this mortality, potentially modifiable, but frequently undiagnosed or inadequately treated.

Gender-associated differences in the development of hypertension and cardiac diseases have been attributed to several factors, mainly the influence of estrogens on endothelial function. Although the exact mechanisms by which sex hormones influence the regulation of blood pressure are being investigated, there is increasing evidence that modulation of the activity of sympathetic nervous system and locally active hormones is of the major importance [3].

The gender differences in blood pressure appear during adolescence. Men have higher blood pressures compared with women at all ages. Hypertension is less common in women younger than 65 years of age, but after that higher percentage of women have hypertension compared with men. This difference in prevalence of hypertension in elderly will likely increase with continued aging of the female population [2]. The incidence of hypertension in women is also increasing in younger age groups, paralleling the epidemics of obesity. According to the data from National Health and Nutrition Examination Survey prevalence of hypertension increased between 1988 to 1994, 1999 to 2006, and 2007 to 2014 among non-Hispanic black males (37.5%, 39.5%, and 40.3%, respectively) and females (38.2%, 41.7%, and 42.9%, respectively), non-Hispanic white males (25.6%, 28.7%, and 30.4%, respectively) and females (22.9%, 27.8%, and 27.6%, respectively), and Mexican American females (25.0%, 26.1%, and 27.2%, respectively) [2]. In women in reproductive age based on NHANES 1999–2008 hypertension was found in 7.7%, an

A. Olszanecka (✉) · D. Czarnecka
First Department of Cardiology, Interventional Electrocardiology and Hypertension, Jagiellonian University Medical College, Cracow, Poland
e-mail: agnieszka.olszanecka@uj.edu.pl

R. Zimlichman et al. (eds.), *Prehypertension and Cardiometabolic Syndrome*, Updates in Hypertension and Cardiovascular Protection,
https://doi.org/10.1007/978-3-319-75310-2_38

estimated 4.9% of women of reproductive age used antihypertensive medication [4]. Latest reports show that in women between 20 and 34 years of age the prevalence of hypertension is 8% compared to 11% in men in the same age category [2]. In women aged 35–44, hypertension is diagnosed in 23% (vs. 23% in men), and in women aged 45–54, hypertension is detected in 33% (vs. 36% in men) [2].

As blood pressure shows linear correlation with cardiovascular mortality and incidence of stroke and myocardial infarction, the categories of prehypertension [5] or "normal and high-normal" blood pressure were extracted (in opposition to "optimal" blood pressure) [6] to identify subjects at higher risk of future cardiovascular events in whom some preventive strategies should be implemented.

Prevalence of prehypertension increased in last decades in both men and women [7]. The prevalence of prehypertension according to NHANES 1999–2000 in women and men by age group was 19.3% versus 44.7% (18–39 years) and 30.3% versus 38.7% (40–59 years) [7]. As compared with optimal blood pressure, high-normal blood pressure was associated with 2.5-fold increase of factor-adjusted hazard ratio for cardiovascular disease among women (95% CI 1.6–4.1) compared to 1.6 (95% CI 1.1–2.2) in men [8].

Although hypertension prevalence and absolute cardiovascular risk in young females is lower than in males and older women, this group of patients deserves special attention in terms of diagnostics and treatment. Relative risk of cardiovascular mortality for any given increase in blood pressure is much more pronounced in younger individuals. Hypertension and prehypertension management in the population of young women should focus of several age and gender-specific aspects as both diagnostics and therapy are limited by childbearing potential. Understanding the epidemiology and pathophysiology of hypertension in female in reproductive age may help clinicians identify important modifiable risk factors, which in turn may improve pregnancy outcomes and prevent cardiovascular disease in the future.

38.1 Diagnostics

Diagnostic process in hypertensive or prehypertensive subjects aims to:

1. Evaluate blood pressure values precisely, assess if the elevation in blood pressure is sustained
2. Calculate global cardiovascular risk by:
   (a) Assessment of hypertension-induced target-organ damage (including subclinical changes)
   (b) Assessment of classical cardiovascular risk factors
3. Assess probability and introduce diagnostics for secondary hypertension

A thorough history and physical examination as well as laboratory assessment are needed to identify subclinical or overt accompanying disease.

38.2 Patient's History

In reviewing the history key questions should focus on identification risk factors such as unhealthy diet, sedentary lifestyle, smoking, alcohol consumption, being obese, or overweight. The family history of premature cardiovascular incidents as well as family history of hypertension, diabetes, and obesity should be obtained. The irregular menstruations suggesting polycystic ovaries syndrome or use of oral contraceptive pills are important as this information may influence future diagnostic or therapeutic decisions.

The information about the previous blood pressure values or duration of established hypertensive disease, tolerance of medical treatment should be collected. The rare but characteristic for secondary hypertension symptoms should be identified—rapid blood pressure elevations with sweating, headache and tachycardia (pheochromocytoma), episodes of tetany, muscle weakness, polyuria (primary hyperaldosteronism), tachycardia, weight loss, anxiety (hyperthyroidism), irregular menstruations, polydypsia, polyuria, obesity (hypercortisolism), etc.

Gathering the data on concomitant chronic diseases may identify potential causes of blood pressure elevation or increase in total cardiovascular risk.

38.3 Physical Examination

38.3.1 Blood Pressure Measurement

Appropriate measurement and interpretation of the blood pressure value is essential in the diagnosis and management of hypertension. Technical issues include proper calibration of the validated device and appropriate cuff sizes-based setting. Despite the importance of office blood pressure measurement and its very widespread use, its value is compromised by phenomenon of blood pressure variability. Casual office readings are usually not sufficient to determine the status of an individual patient. To minimize the misdiagnosis—at least two readings should be taken at every visit, and as many as needed to obtain a stable level with less than a 5-mm Hg difference. During the first visit blood pressure should be measured on both arms. Moreover, at least two and, preferably, more sets of readings, weeks apart, should be taken unless the initial value is so high, e.g., greater than 180/120 mm Hg, indicating that immediate therapy is needed.

Out-of-office blood pressure measurements can be alternative to office blood pressure measurements and should be recommended to establish diagnosis and exclude white-coat hypertension. Home blood pressure measurements (HBPM) and 24 h ambulatory blood pressure monitoring (ABPM) can facilitate more reliable and reproducible estimations of blood pressure. European Society of Cardiology [6] and NICE [9] guidelines recommend HBPM and/or ABPM in the initial diagnostics of subjects with mild hypertension. The choice between these two methods depends on availability, costs of use, and patient preference.

As many as 32% of patients with hypertension diagnosed on the base of office blood pressure measurements have normal blood pressure at home or in ABPM, being reevaluated as "white-coat hypertensives" [10].

Women are more likely to have white-coat hypertension [11, 12], however this phenomenon is more pronounced in those older than 50 years and in pregnancy. Among predictors of white-coat hypertension, high perceived stress levels in women was shown to be associated with white-coat hypertension more than in men [13]. Women may experience a different stress response to clinic visits than men, as evidenced by their blood pressure measurements, and this might explain the high percentage of women experiencing white-coat hypertension in previous research. This issue is of special importance in pregnant females, in whom out-of-office blood pressure can optimize therapeutic decisions [14]. ABPM in pregnancy is the technique which best identifies hypertensive pregnant women at increased risk of adverse pregnancy outcomes [14, 15]. White-coat hypertension has been considered as benign condition, however recent analysis of IDACO database of 8582 subjects followed for over 10.6 years showed that the prognosis in white-coat hypertension strongly depends on age and on baseline cardiometabolic risk [16]. In subjects older than 60 years and with three or more cardiovascular risk factors at baseline, there was significantly more cardiovascular events during follow-up, than in normotensive individuals (adjusted hazard risk 2.19; 95% CI 1.09 to 4.37) [16]. In contrary, younger white-coat hypertensives with less than three cardiovascular risk factors exhibited similar cardiovascular morbidity/mortality as normotensive controls. The results did not differ according to sex [16].

Masked hypertension is the situation of discrepancy between office blood pressure measurements and ABPM, but with normal or high-normal blood pressure in the office and elevated blood pressure in ABPM. Masked hypertension—opposite to white-coat hypertension—more commonly affects men than women. The estimated frequency of masked hypertension in population-based trials was 13% [10]. The frequency of masked hypertension is higher if the office blood pressure remains in the categories of high-normal pressure. Masked hypertension is frequently associated with other cardiovascular risk factors and subclinical organ damage. The results of meta-analyses and prospective trials indicate that the risk of cardiovascular events is twofold higher in masked hypertensive patients than in true normotensives and is comparable to the risk of sustained hypertensives [10, 17, 18].

Except from proper blood pressure evaluation (including orthostatic blood pressure change), the canon of physical examination of hypertensive patient includes cardiac auscultation (detection of murmurs of aortic stenosis, aortic coarctation, etc.), auscultation of carotid and renal arteries, examination of the lungs (assessment of pulmonary congestion), abdominal palpation, examination of peripheral pulses, evaluation of peripheral edema, and measurement of ankle-brachial index. Attention should be paid to the presence of skin lesions (e.g., red striae in Cushing's syndrome, neurofibromas in Recklinghausen disease) or hirsutism.

Anthropometric measurements with body weight, height and waist circumference measurements are also included in the basics of physical examination.

According to the current recommendations [6] the basic tests in the diagnosis of each patient with elevated blood pressure include:

- Blood morphology
- Fasting glucose
- Potassium concentration
- Total cholesterol, HDL (high-density lipoproteins), and LDL (low-density lipoproteins) and triglycerides
- Creatinine concentration and glomerular filtration estimate
- Concentration of uric acid
- General urine test
- Electrocardiogram

In most patients, carefully collected medical history, thoughtful physical examination, and the abovementioned additional tests allow the assessment of the metabolic profile and the calculation of global cardiovascular risk, decide whether to initiate pharmacological treatment and, if necessary, suspect secondary hypertension.

38.4 Global Cardiovascular Risk

Conception of global cardiovascular risk evaluation in hypertensive or prehypertensive subjects was evolving from assessing traditional risk factors (e.g., hypercholesterolemia, obesity, diabetes mellitus, smoking) towards an integrated, multidisciplinary clinical approach, aimed at determining the total cardiovascular risk profile in each individual patient for planning early and effective strategies for cardiovascular prevention.

Hypertension and prehypertension is very rarely isolated problem, in vast majority it is associated with multiple risk factors and risk factor clustering is known to significantly increase the risk of cardiovascular mortality.

38.5 Female-Specific Cardiovascular Risk Factors

Gynecological and obstetric history including gestational hypertension, preeclampsia, gestational diabetes mellitus, preterm births, or birth of an infant small for gestational age is known to double the risk of future cardiovascular events [19, 20].

Recently in large prospective cohort study involving 116,430 women, the association between laparoscopically confirmed endometriosis and risk of hypertension was found [21]. Compared with women without endometriosis, relative risk for hypertension in endometriosis was 1.16 (95% CI 1.11–1.20) and for hypercholesterolemia 1.31 (95% CI 1.27–1.36). RRs for both hypercholesterolemia and hypertension were highest among women younger than 40 and decreased as age increased. Association between endometriosis and hypertension could be partly accounted for by hysterectomy/oophorectomy at earlier age, increased use of non-steroidal inflammatory drugs and hormonal therapy.

Among patients with systemic autoimmune diseases 78% are women [22]. Systemic autoimmune disorders including lupus erythematosus, psoriasis and psoriatic arthritis, and rheumatoid arthritis are associated with increased risk of coronary heart disease, independent of traditional risk factors [23]. In the report of Manzi and coworkers, women with systemic lupus erythematosus had a 5–6-fold increased risk of cardiovascular disease, while women aged 35–44 years were over 50 times more likely to have a myocardial infarction than were women of similar age in the Framingham Offspring Study [24].

Chronic inflammation, endothelial dysfunction and steroid therapy influencing blood pressure values and metabolic profile may partly explain cardiovascular burden in systemic diseases. It should be noted, however, that both hypertension and diabetes are more prevalent in patients with systemic lupus erythematosus compared to healthy age-matched controls [25].

Cigarette smoking in women is related with 25% higher risk of coronary heart disease compared with men [26]. From the practical point of view, health care professionals should strongly promote smoking cessation in all individuals, with special attention paid to female in childbearing age. Smoking during preconception and all stages of pregnancy increases the risk of low birth weights in infants (adjusted odds ratio 1.75, 95% CI 1.2–2.56) [27] and correlates with the risk of preterm delivery [28]. Women over 35 who smoke should be advised not to use oral contraceptives because of significant increase of thrombotic risk.

Epidemiological trials clearly show that the correlation exists between body weight and blood pressure in normal weight subjects and in overweight and obesity [29]. The associations of body weight with prehypertension and hypertension are stronger in women than in men [30]. According to NHANES trial, obesity was identified as the most significant modifiable risk factor for hypertension and prehypertension in women in reproductive age [4]. Obesity is not only related with the development of hypertension, but independently of blood pressure, increases the risk of subclinical organ damage like left ventricular hypertrophy and microalbuminuria [31]. Obese patients are at higher risk of stroke, coronary artery disease, congestive heart failure, cardiac arrhythmias (including atrial fibrillation), and sudden death [32, 33].

Obesity is a major component of the metabolic syndrome, a complex of interrelated risk factors for cardiovascular disease and diabetes, that arises from insulin resistance accompanying abnormal adipose tissue deposition and function. Although controversy exists regarding its pathogenesis and the appropriateness of considering it a distinct state, prospective observations indicate that metabolic syndrome has been reported to be a strong predictor of cardiovascular events, and cardiovascular risk in patients with metabolic syndrome is increased beyond the risk attributable to BMI [34]. Metabolic syndrome in women carries higher risk of coronary events than in men [35]. However, recent analyses found that this difference is mediated mainly by the role of overt diabetes in female, which triples the cardiovascular risk in women (while doubling it in men) [36].

Visceral adipose tissue is considered not only as energy storage, but is emerging as active endocrine organ secreting a number of hormone-like compounds termed adipokines, regulating many physiological processes. Visceral adipose tissue seems to link obesity with hypertension, diabetes, and atherosclerosis [37]. Leptin is an adipose tissue-derived hormone, which acts in the hypothalamus and regulates energy metabolism by decreasing appetite and increasing energy expenditure via sympathetic nerve activity in thermogenic and nonthermogenic tissues. In the rodent models of obesity, leptin loses its ability to suppress appetite but retains its sympathetic stimulation activity [38]. Leptin level was found to be higher in women than men at each level of BMI [39].

These observations underline the importance of the adipose tissue distribution rather than overall obesity as a key factor in predicting cardiovascular risk in women. Although body mass index and waist circumference have a high degree of collinearity, it should be noted that there is substantial heterogeneity of metabolic abnormalities in obese patients. From the point of view of everyday clinical practice a number of subjects have increased waist circumference being still in the group of normal or slightly increased BMI category. With this perspective waist circumference should become a routine measurement in the assessment of cardiovascular risk.

Abdominal visceral fat is associated with increased sympathetic overactivity that results in an increase in renin production, angiotensin 2 and aldosterone production, increased inflammatory mediators, oxidative stress, and decreased endothelial vasodilatation [40]. Sympathetic overactivity is one of the most important mechanisms—linking obesity to hypertension and hypertensive target-organ damage [41, 42].

38.6 Subclinical Organ Damage

The continuum of progression from elevated blood pressure towards clinically overt cardiovascular disease involves initially asymptomatic alterations in cardiac, vascular and renal function and structure. Detailed assessment of potential target-organ damage is of special importance in mild hypertensives and prehypertensive subjects.

Structural hypertension-induced changes in the heart are detectable even in children, adolescents, and young adults [43, 44]. Subanalysis of the Strong Heart Study cohort including 1940 participants younger than 40 years (mean age 26.8 ± 7.7 years; 57.5% of women) revealed that the prevalence of left ventricular hypertrophy was threefold higher in hypertensives and twofold higher in prehypertensives compared to their normotensive counterparts.

It has been documented that left ventricular hypertrophy predicts progression from prehypertension to hypertension independently of baseline blood pressure [45]. Echocardiographically determined left ventricular hypertrophy was diagnosed in 17% of 625 untreated prehypertensive participants of the Strong Heart Study [45]. The authors found that during 4 years of follow-up, 38% prehypertensives progressed to sustained arterial hypertension. Left ventricular mass and the presence of diabetes were the most important predictors of progression to hypertension.

It is of note that hypertensive women exhibit a greater prevalence of left ventricular hypertrophy than men for a similar degree of BP elevation [46–48]. Moreover, left ventricular hypertrophy is differently affecting prognosis in men and women, producing higher risk of coronary events [47] and stroke [49] in women. The mechanism by which LVH produces higher risk in women remains uncertain. Available data revealed that the changes in left ventricular mass in response to age and hypertrophic stimuli are different in men and women [50]. Women more often than men develop left ventricular concentric remodeling and have higher relative wall thickness. This pattern of left ventricular geometry contributes to imbalance between oxygen supply and oxygen demand in myocardial tissue, making women more susceptible to myocardial blood flow disturbances and ischemia [51].

Vascular changes in hypertension and prehypertension include increase in pulse wave velocity and structural changes in the vascular wall like increase in intima-media thickness (IMT) or presence of atherosclerotic plaques.

Prehypertension is associated with both increase in arterial stiffness assessed by measurement of pulse wave velocity and increase in carotid artery IMT [44].

In women age-related arterial stiffening was higher compared with men [52]. Increased arterial stiffness was associated with development of hypertension emergencies in pregnancy. Carotid-femoral pulse wave velocity was shown to be significantly higher in women who had history of preeclampsia than women with normotensive pregnancies [53]. Although it is unclear whether arterial stiffness is involved in the pathogenesis of preeclampsia or is only a marker of increased risk, assessment of arterial stiffness may be useful in predicting hypertensive emergencies in pregnancy and predict future cardiovascular complications in women with history of gestational hypertension.

Subclinical atherosclerosis defined as thickening of IMT or presence of atherosclerotic plaques was found in 63% participants of PESA (Progression of Early Subclinical Atherosclerosis) Trial [54]. In this large, asymptomatic middle-aged cohort ($n = 4570$; mean age 45.8 years) subclinical atherosclerosis was found more commonly in men than women (71 vs. 48%). Results of the other study proved that exposure to prehypertension before age 35 shows significant association with coronary calcium later in life [55], suggesting that young adulthood is a critical period in life when exposure to suboptimal blood pressure is particularly important.

Microalbuminuria—marker of subclinical renal damage—is a direct result of glomerular capillary permeability. Microalbuminuria correlates with future cardiovascular risk. In prehypertensives prevalence of microalbuminuria is higher than in normotensive population, even after exclusion of diabetic patients [56, 57].

Urine analysis in pregnancy is obligatory and detection of microalbuminuria may have prognostic value in prediction of adverse pregnancy outcome including preeclampsia and preterm delivery [58].

Retinopathy. Retinal microcirculation offers an opportunity to directly study the effects of hypertension on small vessels. Eye fundus examination is a primary study in patients with hypertensive urgencies and emergencies. In middle-aged subjects early changes in fundoscopy do not have prognostic significance being indistinguishable from age-related vascular thickening [59]. However in young patients, retinal arterioles narrowing and arteriovenous nicking indicate for chronic elevation of blood pressure and eye fundus examination may provide useful clues and facilitate decisions about implementation of antihypertensive treatment.

38.7 Secondary Hypertension

The prevalence of secondary hypertension and the most common etiologies vary by age group and gender. In young adults, particularly women, renal artery stenosis caused by fibromuscular dysplasia is one of the most important reasons of secondary hypertension.

Renal parenchymal diseases are dominant cause of hypertension in children and adolescents, with equal prevalence in both sexes. Coarctation of the aorta is second cause of hypertension in childhood, more common in men, but it affects up to 12% of women with Turner syndrome, which is 400 times higher than in general population [60]. The prevalence of primary hyperaldosteronism in young population is comparable in men and women [61], however it has to be remembered that diagnostic value of aldosterone-to-renin ratio may be compromised in women by the influence of estrogen and progesterone concentration changing in menstrual cycle, pregnancy, and during oral contraceptive use.

The most common endocrinopathy in female in reproductive age is polycystic ovaries syndrome (PCOS). PCOS is characterized by oligomenorrhea/amenorrhea, hyperandrogenaemia and polycystic ovaries and in the pathophysiology alterations in the secretion of gonadotropin-releasing hormone, defect in androgen synthesis and development of insulin resistance are underlined [62]. Insulin resistance, obesity, and metabolic syndrome coexisting with PCOS explain predisposition for arterial hypertension in these subjects [63]. In large community-based trial including 11,035 women with PCOS the risk of hypertension was 40% higher in PCOS compared to regularly menstruating controls (OR 1.41; 95% CI 1.31–1.51) [64]. Data on the influence of PCOS on long-term cardiovascular mortality and morbidity are not clear, and despite the increased prevalence of classical risk factors such as hypertension, diabetes, and dyslipidemia the prospective studies with hard endpoints failed to identify PCOS as a separate risk phenotype [65].

Hyper- and hypothyroidism may contribute to blood pressure changes due to the influence of thyroid hormones on vascular resistance and cardiac output. In women hyperthyroidism has more pronounced influence of cardiac performance [66], thus screening diagnostics of thyroid function is advised in this population.

Rare cause of secondary hypertension in young women is pheochromocytoma. As a significant contributor to maternal morbidity and mortality in pregnancy, pherchromocytoma should be excluded in women in childbearing age, if characteristic symptoms occur.

Separate issue in young females is drug-induced hypertension, among which oral contraceptive pill (OCP) use is the most important reason of blood pressure elevation. Pregnancy-induced hypertensive disorders will be discussed later in this article.

38.8 Fibromuscular Dysplasia

Fibromuscular dysplasia (FMD) is rare arterial pathology, defined as non-inflammatory non-atherosclerotic vascular disease, presenting anatomically in three different types, including "medial," "intimal," and "adventitial" fibroplasia. FMD affects to small and medium-sized arteries and leads to narrowing of arteries, which also become prone for dissections.

The exact prevalence of FMD in the general population and detailed etiology is not known. Disease predominantly affects young and middle-aged women. In the American registry of 447 patients with FMD, 91% were women in mean age 51.9 ± 13.4 years [67].

Dysplastic changes can be located in almost all arterial territories, but the most commonly FMD affects renal arteries (60–70% of patients, in 35% changes are located bilaterally) [68].

Narrowing of renal artery leads to renovascular hypertension, being the most common manifestation of the disease.

Second common localization of dysplastic arterial changes are carotid arteries (25–30%). Most subjects are asymptomatic, but both transient ischemic attacks and stroke incidents may be related with FMD. Carotid dysplastic changes may be accompanied by cerebral aneurysms, thus imaging of central nervous system vasculature is important in these patients.

New onset of arterial hypertension in young female and vascular bruit in epigastric area should raise the suspicion of FMD. FMD should also be considered in subjects with severe hypertension and headaches in the absence of obesity, use of contraceptives, and history of parenchymal renal disease.

Although catheter-based angiography remains the gold standard in the diagnostics of patients with FMD, initially noninvasive test should be performed—renal duplex scan, carotid ultrasound, computed tomography scans, and magnetic resonance imaging. Thoughtful early diagnostics is of special importance, as early treatment (percutaneous renal angioplasty with stent implantation) may lead to normalization or improvement in blood pressure control in majority of patients.

38.9 Oral Contraceptives

The use of oral contraceptives may be associated with an increase in blood pressure. Typically, the increase in blood pressure during oral contraception is low, but even 5% of women taking oral hormonal contraceptives may develop hypertension, especially after prolonged use [69, 70]. However, it has to be taken into account that abovementioned data are derived from studies that used contraception with significantly higher doses of both estradiol and progestogens then next generations pills. Currently used contraceptive pills contain lower doses of ethynylestradiol (20–25 μg) and lower doses of more selective progestogens (<1 mg). This has reduced the incidence of hypertension in second and third generation oral contraceptives users, although blood pressure in women using OCP is still higher than nonusers, even if blood pressure is in the normal range [71]. The primary mechanism of blood pressure elevation during use of OCP is thought to be increased hepatic synthesis of angiotensinogen, and subsequent salt and water retention.

Data on the effect of progestogens on blood pressure are ambiguous, the effect on blood pressure is rather small. Thus, according to some authors, a single compound containing only progestogen may be an alternative to a two-component contraceptive pill in women with a higher cardiovascular risk. In the longitudinal observation of over one million women, the use of progestin-only pills was not related to increase of the risk of thrombotic stroke and myocardial infarction [72]. Drospirenon is a synthetic progestogen, chemically related to spironolacton and possessing antimineralocorticoid properties, what might oppose the influence of estrogens on blood pressure. OCP based on combination of ethynylestradiol and drospirenon is not changing blood pressure, however in one, small prospective study the increase of heart rate was documented [73].

In most patients who develop hypertension during oral contraceptives, it is benign and resolves to 6 months after discontinuation of hormonal treatment.

Women with mild hypertension who use oral contraceptives may be offered: discontinuation of therapy and home self-monitoring, and reevaluation after few months (verification if hypertension is essential or drug-induced). The second method (especially if such are preferences of the patient) is the introduction of antihypertensive therapy (primarily diuretics) and continuation of oral contraceptives provided that blood pressure is controlled and patient has low total cardiovascular risk. In women with high cardiovascular risk and poor control of pressure, antihypertensive treatment and withdrawal of hormonal contraceptives are necessary.

38.10 Hypertensive Disorders in Pregnancy

Hypertensive disorders during pregnancy are significant concerns, they complicate 7–15% of all pregnancies and are one of the major causes of maternal and fetal mortality in developed countries [74]. Diagnosis of hypertension during pregnancy is based on absolute blood pressure values>140/90 mmHg recorded during two independent measurements at an interval of at least 6 h or when, even in a single measurement, blood pressure is >170/110 mmHg.

The classification of hypertension in pregnancy distinguishes the following categories:

- *Preexisting hypertension* (chronic hypertension—present before pregnancy or developing before the 20th week of pregnancy)
- *Gestational hypertension,* i.e., pregnancy-induced hypertension (develops after 20 weeks of gestation)
- *Preeclampsia,* i.e., gestational hypertension with proteinuria (>300 mg/L or 500 mg/24 h), eclampsia is diagnosed when seizures have occurred

- *Preexisting hypertension with superimposing proteinuria* (preeclampsia superimposing on chronic hypertension)
- *Unclassified hypertension* (diagnosed after 20 weeks of pregnancy, if previous pressure values are unknown)

It should be emphasized that preeclampsia and chronic hypertension in pregnancy should be considered as two different clinical entities.

Preeclampsia is a systemic disorder with generalized vascular endothelial malfunction, initialized by abnormal early trophoblastic implantation (insufficient migration to the persistent muscle structure of the central spiral artery). Thus, it can be divided into two stages: fetal stage—abnormal placental flow and maternal—systemic response with activation of inflammatory reaction, oxidative stress, and systemic endothelial dysfunction. Pathological changes in the course of this syndrome are therefore mainly ischemic and occur in the placenta, kidney, liver, and brain.

Chronic hypertension in pregnancy increases the risk of preeclampsia (which is 17–25% higher than in the general population), but in majority of patients the prognosis and pregnancy outcome are good. The problem of chronic hypertension in pregnancy is growing, with the current tendency to postpone motherhood decisions for a later life of a woman. Current statistics indicate that chronic hypertension is present in 1–5% of pregnant women (it is predicted that the incidence of obesity may increase due to the increasing obesity problem) [75].

The primary goal of treating pregnant women is to prevent maternal and fetal complications and carefully weigh the benefits of maternal treatment (risk of cardiovascular events) and the risk of its use to the fetus (teratogenic effects, placental hypoperfusion). It is important to realize that there are not many data on the safety of antihypertensive drugs in pregnancy.

Benefits of antihypertensive treatment were unquestionable only in patients with a pregnancy pressure of more than 160/110 mmHg, and they primarily concern the reduction of the risk of cerebrovascular complications in the mother, with no benefit from antihypertensive treatment for fetal development. In mild to moderate hypertension results of antihypertensive treatment are not clear. Meta-analysis of 49 trials comparing treatment versus no treatment on maternal and fetus outcome in mild and moderate pregnant hypertensives revealed that treatment did not result in either fetal benefit or harm [76]. Treatment also did not significantly reduce perinatal mortality or frequency of prematurity, preeclampsia, or abruptio placentae, but reduced the incidence of severe hypertension.

According to American guidelines blood pressure lowering treatment is required if blood pressure in pregnancy is >160/110 mmHg [77] and even>170/110 mmHg [78]. According to the ESC recommendations, pharmacological treatment may be introduced when the patient's pressure exceeds 140/90 mmHg in patients with hypertension in the presence of subclinical organ damage or coexisting diabetes or renal disease, and in uncomplicated hypertension when the blood pressure is above 150/95 mmHg [6, 79].

Despite the lack of data on blood pressure targets, most experts recommend that blood pressure should be maintained at 130–150/80–100 mmHg during antihypertensive treatment in pregnancy. The results of the CHIPS study (Control of Hypertension in pregnancy Study) provided that less-tight control of maternal hypertension (target diastolic blood pressure 100 mmHg) compared with tight control (target diastolic blood pressure 85 mmHg) resulted in no significant difference in the risk of perinatal outcomes, however tight control reduced the risk of severe hypertension [80].

The pharmacological options for effective antihypertensive treatment in pregnancy with acceptable safety profile in pregnancy include: *methyldopa* (250–500 mg po bid-qid, max 2 g/d), *labetalol* (100–400 mg po bid-tid, max 1200 mg/d), and *nifedipine* (slow-acting preparations, 20–60 mg po OD, max 120 mg/d) [6, 78, 81].

As during first semester of pregnancy physiological blood pressure reduction is observed, women with chronic hypertension who are normotensive or mildly hypertensive on medication may be considered to stop medication during early pregnancy, or continue medication with pregnancy-dedicated antihypertensive drugs, with close monitoring of the maternal blood pressure response. Due to high frequency of white-coat hypertension, ABPM use is recommended to estimate blood pressure values and guide therapy in pregnancy.

Recent report of the National Birth Defects Prevention Study revealed that early hypertensive treatment in pregnancy was associated with increased risk of fetal congenital heart diseases (aortic coarctation, pulmonary valve stenosis, Ebstein malformation, atrial septum defect 2, perimembranous ventricular septal defect) [82]. Nevertheless, except for Ebstein malformation, both untreated hypertension and late hypertension treatment were also associated with significantly increased risk of the same defects. The study had limited power to analyze the risk related to separate drug classes, but while methyldopa caused only modest increase in risk of congenital malformations, beta-blockers (including labetalol) use was significantly increasing the risk of congenital heart defects, similarly like renin-angiotensin-aldosterone system blockade. This observation rises some controversies and requires verification of the labetalol safety in pregnancy.

In each case, persistent blood pressure increase in a pregnant woman over 170/110 mmHg should be considered as urgency, requiring hospitalization and possibly extended diagnostics. The worsening of blood pressure control in chronic hypertension in pregnancy may indicate superimposing preeclampsia. The diagnosis can be challenging, as one or more factors used to diagnosed preeclampsia are already present in these subjects.

The definite treatment of preeclampsia is termination of pregnancy. Lowering blood pressure does not affect the course of preeclampsia, but should be implemented and optimized to prevent the maternal risk of vascular complications (stroke, acute heart failure, aortic dissection, etc.).

Emergent therapy for acute, severe blood pressure elevations in pregnancy includes—parenteral *labetalol* (starting from 20 mg intravenously over 2 min, with possible re-administration of the drug with doubling the dose in 10 min intervals, to cumulative dose 220 mg), *hydralazine* (starting from 5–10 mg intravenously over 2 min, with possible re-administration of the drug in 10 min intervals and increase of the dose to 20 mg, to cumulative dose 25 mg per h), and oral *nifedipine* (10 mg capsule, with possible re-administration of 20 mg tablet). In case of pulmonary edema iv *nitroglicerine* (5–10 μg/min) is recommended [81]. With abovementioned drug regimens in most patients blood pressure control can be achieved. Options for second-line therapy include *labetalol or nicardipine* by infusion pump. *Sodium nitroprusside* (0.25–5.0 μg/kg/min) is administered as a last resort with careful monitoring and avoidance of cyanide toxicity.

Current guidelines recommend the administration of low dose of aspirin from 12 weeks of pregnancy until the delivery in prevention of preeclampsia in women at high risk (history of preeclampsia, especially in accompanied by adverse outcome, multifetal gestation, chronic hypertension, type 1 or 2 diabetes, autoimmune disease such as systemic lupus erythematosus, or antiphospholipid syndrome, chronic kidney disease) [6, 81]. Aspirin might be considered in women with more than one moderate risk factor for preeclampsia (first pregnancy, age > 40 years, pregnancy interval of >10 years, BMI >35 kg/m^2 at first visit, family history of preeclampsia and multiple pregnancy), provided that they are at low risk of gastrointestinal hemorrhage.

Hypertensive mothers should not be discouraged from breastfeeding. Drugs which have no known adverse effects on babies receiving breast milk and appear to be safe during lactation are—labetalol, nifedipine, enalapril, captopril, and metoprolol [75].

38.11 Treatment of Prehypertension and Hypertension

38.11.1 Non-pharmacological Interventions in Hypertension and Prehypertension

Non-pharmacological treatment is necessary at every stage of hypertension and in all subjects defined as prehypertensives.

Its basic principles include diet, weight reduction, reduced salt intake, regular physical activity, reduced alcohol consumption, and smoking cessation. There was no clearly different effect of diet on the pressure in men and women; however, there was a trend towards greater reduction in systolic pressure in women using the DASH diet than in men [83].

The alcohol threshold for women is lower than for men, so women are not advised to consume more than 10–20 g of ethanol per day. Physical activity in women is associated not only with a significant reduction in blood pressure, but also with improved weight control, improved metabolic profile, and better quality of life.

Incorporation of lifestyle interventions and their persistent adherence is difficult to achieve in everyday practice. Multicomponent behavioral interventions were proven to reduce cardiovascular risk and cardiovascular morbidity [84, 85] and their implementation as a part of routine medical care may have a substantial impact on public health.

38.11.2 Pharmacological Treatment of Hypertension

Although current guidelines for management of hypertension do not differentiate gender-based therapeutic approaches, pathophysiological differences in female hypertension should be considered in clinical decisions and taken into account in individualization of therapy.

In young people, according to the NICE guidelines [9], the first choice drug should be angiotensin-converting enzyme inhibitors or angiotensin receptor antagonists, since hypertension often coexists with metabolic disorders and activation of sympathetic nervous system. Despite their obvious advantages, these drugs are not a preferred group for the pharmacotherapy of women of childbearing potential.

An alternative for women of childbearing potential, are calcium antagonists, thiazide-like diuretic, and in those with coexisting tachycardia and hyperkinetic circulation features—beta-blockers. Drugs in this group are not preferred in monotherapy for uncomplicated hypertension due to potential adverse effects on metabolic parameters such as insulin sensitivity or lipid profile. However, newer generations beta-adrenolytic, such as bisoprolol, nebivolol, or carvedilol, have more favorable profile.

Calcium antagonists are a metabolically neutral group of drugs, which are approved for use in pregnancy and therefore their use in women of childbearing potential is safe and may be a separate group of indications. The use of calcium antagonists is limited by the side effects—peripheral edema and facial flush, which are experienced in women twice as common as in men [86].

Diuretics are effective drugs but, as with beta-blockers, their use is limited by their metabolic profile, especially with high doses of thiazide. Diuretics are a valuable supplement to combination therapy, are the most commonly used second drug in combination therapy, and undoubtedly should be an indispensable part of triple therapy. Diuretic monotherapy, on the other hand, can also be considered in case of hypertension in young women in the course of oral contraception.

Pharmacological treatment of prehypertension has been investigated in several clinical trials. The prevention of prehypertension to hypertension was tested with the use of candesartan [87], ramipril [88], and low-dose chlortalidon-amilorid combination [89]. In all abovementioned studies, pharmacological intervention was associated with a significant reduction of developing hypertension. However, differences in the occurrence of cardiovascular events were not detected.

Based on the lack of long-term, prospective, randomized trials proving reduction in cardiovascular mortality and morbidity, current guidelines do not recommend implementation of pharmacotherapy in prehypertensive patients. However, detailed cardiovascular risk assessment should be performed in each individual with prehypertension, to exclude masked hypertension and to guide the decision of treatment schedule.

Early identification and treatment of cardiovascular risk factors in women is very important. Although women experience cardiovascular complications at an older age and at a lower rate than do men and absolute risk is lower in women than in men, the proportion of preventable cardiovascular complication is from 30 to 100% higher in women than in men. The lower absolute risk in women should therefore not be considered an excuse for therapeutic laxity [90].

References

1. Gholizadeh L, Davidson P. More similarities than differences: an international comparison of CVD mortality and risk factors in women. Health Care Women Int. 2008;29:3–22.
2. Benjami E, Blaha M, Chiuve S, Cushman M, Das S, Deo R, et al. Heart disease and stroke statistics – 2017 update a report from the American Heart Association. Circulation. 2017;135(10):e146–603.
3. dos Santos R, da Silva F, Ribeiro RJ, Stefanon I. Sex hormones in the cardiovascular system. Horm Mol Biol Clin Investig. 2014;18(2):89–103.
4. Bateman BT, Shaw KM, Kuklina EV, Callaghan WM, Seely EW, Herna S. Hypertension in women of reproductive age in the United States: NHANES 1999–2008. PLoS One. 2012;7(4):e36171.
5. Chobanian A, Bakris G, Black H, Cushman W, Green L, Izzo JJ, et al. The seventh report of the joint National Committee on prevention, detection, evaluation, and treatment of high blood pressure: the JNC 7 report. JAMA J Am Med Assoc. 2003;289(19):2560–72.
6. Mancia G, Fagard R, Narkiewicz K, Redon J, Zanchetti A, Böhm M, et al. 2013 ESH/ESC guidelines for the management of arterial hypertension: the task force for the management of arterial hypertension of the European Society of Hypertension (ESH) and of the European Society of Cardiology (ESC). Eur Heart J. 2013;34(28):2159–219.
7. Qureshi AI, Suri MFK, Kirmani JF, Divani AA. Prevalence and trends of prehypertension and hypertension in United States: National Health and nutrition examination surveys 1976 to 2000. Med Sci Monit. 2005;11(9):CR403–9. http://www.ncbi.nlm.nih.gov/pubmed/16127357; http://www.medscimonit.com/fulltxt.php?IDMAN=5896.
8. Conen D, Ridker PM, Buring JE, Glynn RJ. Risk of cardiovascular events among women with high normal blood pressure or blood pressure progression: prospective cohort study. BMJ. 2007;335(7617):432. http://www.pubmedcentral.nih.gov/articlerender.fcgi?artid=1962877&tool=pmcentrez&rendertype=abstract.
9. McManus RJ, Caulfield M, Williams B. NICE hypertension guideline 2011: evidence based evolution. BMJ. 2012;344(jan13 1):e181. https://doi.org/10.1136/bmj.e181.
10. Fagard RH, Cornelissen VA. Incidence of cardiovascular events in white-coat, masked and sustained hypertension versus true normotension: a meta-analysis. J Hypertens. 2007;25(11):2193–8. http://content.wkhealth.com/linkback/openurl?sid=WKPTLP:landingpage&an=00004872-200711000-00002.
11. Dolan E, Stanton A, Atkins N, Den Hond E, Thijs L, McCormack P, et al. Determinants of white-coat hypertension. Blood Press Monit. 2004;9(6):307–9. http://www.ncbi.nlm.nih.gov/pubmed/18927542.
12. James G, Marion R, Pickering T. White-coat hypertension and sex. Blood Press Monit. 1998;3(5):281–7. http://www.ncbi.nlm.nih.gov/pubmed/10212367.
13. Cobos B, Haskard-Zolnierek K, Howard K. White coat hypertension: improving the patient-health care practitioner relationship. Psychol Res Behav Manag. 2015;8:133–41. http://www.pubmedcentral.nih.gov/articlerender.fcgi?artid=4427265&tool=pmcentrez&rendertype=abstract.
14. Brown MA, Mangos G, Davis G, Homer C. The natural history of white coat hypertension during pregnancy. BJOG. 2005;112(5):601–6.
15. Hermida RC, Ayala DE. Prognostic value of office and ambulatory blood pressure measurements in pregnancy. Hypertension. 2002;40(3):298–303.
16. Franklin SS, Thijs L, Asayama K, Li Y, Hansen TW, Boggia J, et al. The cardiovascular risk of white-coat hypertension. J Am Coll Cardiol. 2016;68(19):2033–43.
17. Pierdomenico SD, Cuccurullo F. Prognostic value of white-coat and masked hypertension diagnosed by ambulatory monitoring in initially untreated subjects: an updated meta analysis. Am J Hypertens. 2011;24(1):52–8. https://academic.oup.com/ajh/article-lookup/doi/10.1038/ajh.2010.203.

18. Hänninen M-RA, Niiranen TJ, Puukka PJ, Johansson J, Jula AM. Prognostic significance of masked and white-coat hypertension in the general population. J Hypertens. 2012;30(4):705–12. http://content.wkhealth.com/linkback/openurl?sid=WKPTLP:landingpage&an=00004872-201204000-00016.
19. Bellamy L, Casas J-P, Hingorani AD, Williams DJ. Pre-eclampsia and risk of cardiovascular disease and cancer in later life: systematic review and meta-analysis. BMJ. 2007;335(7627):974. http://www.ncbi.nlm.nih.gov/pubmed/17975258; http://www.pubmedcentral.nih.gov/articlerender.fcgi?artid=PMC2072042.
20. Hermes W, Tamsma JT, Grootendorst DC, Franx A, van der Post J, van Pampus MG, et al. Cardiovascular risk estimation in women with a history of hypertensive pregnancy disorders at term: a longitudinal follow-up study. BMC Pregnancy Childbirth. 2013;13(1):126. http://bmcpregnancychildbirth.biomedcentral.com/articles/10.1186/1471-2393-13-126.
21. Mu F, Rich-Edwards J, Rimm EB, Spiegelman D, Forman JP, Missmer SA. Association between endometriosis and hypercholesterolemia or hypertension. Hypertension. 2017;70(1):59–65.
22. Fairweather D, Frisancho-Kiss S, Rose NR. Sex differences in autoimmune disease from a pathological perspective. Am J Pathol. 2008;173(3):600–9. http://linkinghub.elsevier.com/retrieve/pii/S0002944010616355.
23. Al Husain A, Bruce IN. Risk factors for coronary heart disease in connective tissue diseases. Ther Adv Musculoskelet Dis. 2010;2(3):145–53. http://tab.sagepub.com/cgi/doi/10.1177/1759720X10365301.
24. Manzi S, Meilahn E, Rairie J, Conte C, Medsger TJ, Jansen-McWilliams L, et al. Age-specific incidence rates of myocardial infarction and angina in women with systemic lupus erythematosus: comparison with the Framingham study. Am J Epidemiol. 1997;145(5):408–4015.
25. Bruce IN, Urowitz MB, Gladman DD, Ibanez D, Steiner G. Risk factors for coronary heart disease in women with systemic lupus erythematosus: the Toronto risk factor study. Arthritis Rheum. 2003;48(11):3159–67.
26. Huxley RR, Woodward M. Cigarette smoking as a risk factor for coronary heart disease in women compared with men: a systematic review and meta-analysis of prospective cohort studies. Lancet. 2011;378(9799):1297–305. https://doi.org/10.1016/S0140-6736(11)60781-2.
27. Jaddoe VWV, Troe E-JWM, Hofman A, Mackenbach JP, Moll HA, Steegers EAP, et al. Active and passive maternal smoking during pregnancy and the risks of low birthweight and preterm birth: the generation R study. Paediatr Perinat Epidemiol. 2008;22(2):162–71. https://doi.org/10.1111/j.1365-3016.2007.00916.x.
28. Ko T-J, Tsai L-Y, Chu L-C, Yeh S-J, Leung C, Chen C-Y, et al. Parental smoking during pregnancy and its association with low birth weight, small for gestational age, and preterm birth offspring: a birth cohort study. Pediatr Neonatol. 2014;55(1):20–7.
29. Dyer AR, Elliott P. The INTERSALT Study: relations of body mass index to blood pressure. INTERSALT co-operative research group. J Hum Hypertens. 1989;3(5):299–308. http://europepmc.org/abstract/MED/2810326.
30. Wakabayashi I. Stronger associations of obesity with prehypertension and hypertension in young women than in young men. J Hypertens. 2012;30(7):1423–9. http://www.ncbi.nlm.nih.gov/pubmed/22573123.
31. Poirier P, Giles TD, Bray GA, Hong Y, Stern JS, Pi-Sunyer FX, et al. Obesity and cardiovascular disease. Arterioscler Thromb Vasc Biol. 2006;26(5):968 LP–976. http://atvb.ahajournals.org/content/26/5/968.abstract.
32. Hubert HB, Feinleib M, McNamara PM, Castelli WP. Obesity as an independent risk factor for cardiovascular disease: a 26- year follow-up of participants in the Framingham heart study. Circulation. 1983;67(5):968–77. http://circ.ahajournals.org/cgi/doi/10.1161/01.CIR.67.5.968.
33. Romero-Corral A, Montori VM, Somers VK, Korinek J, Thomas RJ, Allison TG, et al. Association of bodyweight with total mortality and with cardiovascular events in coronary artery disease: a systematic review of cohort studies 5. Lancet. 2006;368(1474–547X (Electronic)):666–78.

34. Kip KE, Marroquin OC, Kelley DE, Johnson BD, Kelsey SF, Shaw LJ, et al. Clinical importance of obesity versus the metabolic syndrome in cardiovascular risk in women: a report from the Women's ischemia syndrome evaluation (WISE) study. Circulation. 2004;109(6):706–13.
35. Hunt KJ, Resendez RG, Williams K, Haffner SM, Stern MP. National Cholesterol Education Program versus World Health Organization metabolic syndrome in relation to all-cause and cardiovascular mortality in the San Antonio heart study. Circulation. 2004;110(10):1251–7.
36. Peters SAE, Huxley RR, Woodward M. Diabetes as risk factor for incident coronary heart disease in women compared with men: a systematic review and meta-analysis of 64 cohorts including 858,507 individuals and 28,203 coronary events. Diabetologia. 2014;57(8):1542–51.
37. Redón J, Cea-Calvo L, Moreno B, Monereo S, Gil-Guillén V, Lozano JV, et al. Independent impact of obesity and fat distribution in hypertension prevalence and control in the elderly. J Hypertens. 2008;26(9):1757–64.
38. Wang B, Chandrasekera PC, Pippin JJ. Leptin- and leptin receptor-deficient rodent models: relevance for human type 2 diabetes. Curr Diabetes Rev. 2014;10(2):131–45. http://www.ncbi.nlm.nih.gov/pubmed/24809394; http://www.pubmedcentral.nih.gov/articlerender.fcgi?artid=PMC4082168.
39. Ma D, Feitosa MF, Wilk JB, Laramie JM, Yu K, Leiendecker-Foster C, et al. Leptin is associated with blood pressure and hypertension in women from the National Heart, Lung, and Blood Institute family heart study. Hypertension. 2009;53(3):473–9.
40. Esler M, Straznicky N, Eikelis N, Masuo K, Lambert G, Lambert E. Mechanisms of sympathetic activation in obesity-related hypertension. Hypertension. 2006;48(5):787–96.
41. Lambert E, Straznicky N, Eikelis N, Esler M, Dawood T, Masuo K, et al. Gender differences in sympathetic nervous activity: influence of body mass and blood pressure. J Hypertens. 2007;25(7):1411–9. http://www.ncbi.nlm.nih.gov/pubmed/17563563.
42. Lambert E, Sari CI, Dawood T, Nguyen J, McGrane M, Eikelis N, et al. Sympathetic nervous system activity is associated with obesity-induced subclinical organ damage in young adults. Hypertension. 2010;56(3):351–8.
43. Daniels SR, Loggie JM, Khoury P, Kimball TR. Left ventricular geometry and severe left ventricular hypertrophy in children and adolescents with essential hypertension. Circulation. 1998;97(19):1907–11.
44. Urbina EM, Khoury PR, Mccoy C, Daniels SR, Kimball TR, Dolan LM. Cardiac and vascular consequences of pre-hypertension in youth. J Clin Hypertens. 2011;13(5):332–42.
45. De Marco M, De Simone G, Roman MJ, Chinali M, Lee ET, Russell M, et al. Cardiovascular and metabolic predictors of progression of prehypertension into hypertension: the strong heart study. Hypertension. 2009;54(5):974–80.
46. Okin PM, Gerdts E, Kjeldsen SE, Julius S, Edelman JM, Dahlöf B, et al. Gender differences in regression of electrocardiographic left ventricular hypertrophy during antihypertensive therapy. Hypertension. 2008;52(1):100–6.
47. Porthan K, Niiranen TJ, Varis J, Kantola I, Karanko H, Kähönen M, et al. ECG left ventricular hypertrophy is a stronger risk factor for incident cardiovascular events in women than in men in the general population. J Hypertens. 2015;33(6):1284–90. http://content.wkhealth.com/linkback/openurl?sid=WKPTLP:landingpage&an=00004872-201506000-00024.
48. Liebson PR, Grandits G, Prineas R, Dianzumba S, Flack JM, Cutler JA, et al. Echocardiographic correlates of left ventricular structure among 844 mildly hypertensive men and women in the treatment of mild hypertension study (TOMHS). Circulation. 1993;87(2):476–86. http://circ.ahajournals.org/content/87/2/476.abstract.
49. Antikainen RL, Grodzicki T, Palmer AJ, Beevers DG, Webster J, Bulpitt CJ. Left ventricular hypertrophy determined by Sokolow–Lyon criteria: a different predictor in women than in men? J Hum Hypertens. 2006;20(6):451–9. http://www.nature.com/doifinder/10.1038/sj.jhh.1002006.
50. Hayward CS, Webb CM, Collins P. Effect of sex hormones on cardiac mass. Lancet. 2001;357(9265):1354–6.
51. Truong Q, Toepker M, Mahabadi A, Bamberg F, Rogers I, Blankstein R, et al. Relation of left ventricular mass and concentric remodeling to extent of coronary artery disease by computed

tomography in patients without left ventricular hypertrophy: ROMICAT study. J Hypertens. 2010;27(12):2472–82.
52. Redfield MM, Jacobsen SJ, Borlaug BA, Rodeheffer RJ, Kass DA. Age- and gender-related ventricular-vascular stiffening: a community-based study. Circulation. 2005;112(15):2254–62.
53. Hausvater A, Giannone T, Sandoval Y-HG, Doonan RJ, Antonopoulos CN, Matsoukis IL, et al. The association between preeclampsia and arterial stiffness. J Hypertens. 2012;30(1):17–33. http://content.wkhealth.com/linkback/openurl?sid=WKPTLP:landingpage&an=00004872-201201000-00003.
54. Fernández-Friera L, Peñalvo JL, Fernández-Ortiz A, Ibañez B, López-Melgar B, Laclaustra M, et al. Prevalence, vascular distribution, and multiterritorial extent of subclinical atherosclerosis in a middle-aged cohort the PESA (progression of early subclinical atherosclerosis) study. Circulation. 2015;131(24):2104–13.
55. Pletcher MJ, Bibbins-Domingo K, Lewis CE, Wei GS, Sidney S, Carr JJ, et al. Prehypertension during young adulthood and coronary calcium later in life. Ann Intern Med. 2008;149(2):91–9.
56. Tenekecioglu E, Yilmaz M, Yontar OC, Karaagac K, Agca FV, Tutuncu A, et al. Microalbuminuria in untreated prehypertension and hypertension without diabetes. Int J Clin Exp Med. 2014;7(10):3420–9.
57. Lee JE, Kim YG, Choi YH, Huh W, Kim DJ, Oh HY. Serum uric acid is associated with microalbuminuria in prehypertension. Hypertension. 2006;47(5):962–7. http://graphics.tx.ovid.com/ovftpdfs/FPDDNCDCKFHCAH00/fs046/ovft/live/gv023/00004268/00004268-200605000-00027.pdf.
58. Jayaballa M, Sood S, Alahakoon I, Padmanabhan S, Cheung NW, Lee V. Microalbuminuria is a predictor of adverse pregnancy outcomes including preeclampsia. Pregnancy Hypertens. 2015;5(4):303–7.
59. Cuspidi C, Meani S, Salerno M, Fusi V, Severgnini B, Valerio C, et al. Retinal microvascular changes and target organ damage in untreated essential hypertensives. J Hypertens. 2004;22(11):2095–102. http://www.ncbi.nlm.nih.gov/pubmed/15480092.
60. Wong S, Burgess T, Cheung M, Zacharin M. The prevalence of turner syndrome in girls presenting with coarctation of the aorta. J Pediatr. 2014;164(2):259–63.
61. Noilhan C, Barigou M, Bieler L, Amar J, Chamontin B, Bouhanick B. Causes of secondary hypertension in the young population: a monocentric study. Ann Cardiol Angeiol. 2016;65(3):159–64.
62. Wang H-S, Wang T-H. Polycystic ovary syndrome (PCOS), insulin resistance and insulin-like growth factors (IGfs)/IGF-binding proteins (IGFBPs). Chang Gung Med J. 2003;26(8):540–53.
63. Bentley-Lewis R, Seely E, Dunaif A. Ovarian hypertension: polycystic ovary syndrome. Endorinol Metab Clin North Am. 2011;40(2):433–49. http://www.pubmedcentral.nih.gov/articlerender.fcgi?artid=2867586&tool=pmcentrez&rendertype=abstract.
64. Lo JC, Feigenbaum SL, Yang J, Pressman AR, Selby JV, Go AS. Epidemiology and adverse cardiovascular risk profile of diagnosed polycystic ovary syndrome. J Clin Endocrinol Metab. 2006;91(4):1357–63. http://www.ncbi.nlm.nih.gov/pubmed/16434451.
65. Wild S, Pierpoint T, McKeigue P, Jacobs H. Cardiovascular disease in women with polycystic ovary syndrome at long-term follow-up: a retrospective cohort study. Clin Endocrinol. 2000;52(5):595–600.
66. Pearce EN, Yang Q, Benjamin EJ, Aragam J, Vasan RS. Thyroid function and left ventricular structure and function in the Framingham heart study. Thyroid. 2010;20(4):369–73. http://www.pubmedcentral.nih.gov/articlerender.fcgi?artid=2867586&tool=pmcentrez&rendertype=abstract.
67. Olin JW, Froehlich J, Gu X, Michael Bacharach J, Eagle K, Gray BH, et al. The United States registry for fibromuscular dysplasia: results in the first 447 patients. Circulation. 2012;125(25):3182–90.
68. Persu A, Giavarini A, Touzé E, Januszewicz A, Sapoval M, Azizi M, et al. European consensus on the diagnosis and management of fibromuscular dysplasia. J Hypertens. 2014;32(7):1367–78. http://content.wkhealth.com/linkback/openurl?sid=WKPTLP:landingpage&an=00004872-201407000-00003.

69. Dong W, Colhoun HM, Poulter NR. Blood pressure in women using oral contraceptives: results from the health survey for England 1994. J Hypertens. 1997;15(10):1063–8. http://www.ncbi.nlm.nih.gov/pubmed/9350579.
70. Chasan-Taber L, Willett W, Manson J, Spiegelman D, Hunter D, Curhan G, et al. Prospective study of oral contraceptives and hypertension among women in the United States [Internet]. Circulation. 1996;94:483–9. http://ovidsp.ovid.com/ovidweb.cgi?T=JS&PAGE=reference&D=emed7&NEWS=N&AN=26266136.
71. Williamson PM, Buddle ML, Brown MA, Whitworth JA. Ambulatory blood pressure monitoring (ABPM) in the normal menstrual cycle and in women using oral contraceptives. Comparison with conventional blood pressure measurement. Am J Hypertens. 1996;9(10 Pt 1):953–8.
72. Lidegaard Ø, Løkkegaard E, Jensen A, Skovlund CW, Keiding N. Thrombotic stroke and myocardial infarction with hormonal contraception. N Engl J Med. 2012;366(24):2257–66. http://www.ncbi.nlm.nih.gov/pubmed/22693997.
73. Cagnacci A, Ferrari S, Napolitano A, Piacenti I, Arangino S, Volpe A. Combined oral contraceptive containing drospirenone does not modify 24-h ambulatory blood pressure but increases heart rate in healthy young women: prospective study. Contraception. 2013;88(3):413–7.
74. Magee LA, Von Dadelszen P, Chan S, Gafni A, Gruslin A, Helewa M, et al. The control of hypertension in pregnancy study pilot trial. BJOG. 2007;114(6):770.
75. Visintin C, Mugglestone MA, Almerie MQ, Nherera LM, James D, Walkinshaw S. Management of hypertensive disorders during pregnancy: summary of NICE guidance. BMJ. 2010;341(September):c2207.
76. Abalos E, Duley L, Steyn D. Antihypertensive drug therapy for mild to moderate hypertension during pregnancy. Cochrane Database Syst Rev. 2014;2:CD002252. https://doi.org/10.1002/14651858. PREG.
77. American College of Obstetricians and Gynecologists, Task Force on Hypertension in Pregnancy. Hypertension in pregnancy. Report of the American College of Obstetricians and Gynecologists' Task Force on Hypertension in Pregnancy. Obstet Gynecol. 2013;122(5):1122–31. http://www.ncbi.nlm.nih.gov/pubmed/24150027, http://linkinghub.elsevier.com/retrieve/pii/S0733865112000562%5Cnhttp://www.ncbi.nlm.nih.gov/pubmed/24150027.
78. Magee LA, Bc V, Helewa M, Mb W, Rey E, Qc M, et al., Sogc Clinical Practice Guideline. Diagnosis, evaluation, and management of the hypertensive disorders of pregnancy: executive summary. J Obstet Gynaecol Can. 2014;36(5):416–38.
79. Regitz-Zagrosek V, Blomstrom Lundqvist C, Borghi C, Cifkova R, Ferreira R, Foidart JM, et al. ESC Guidelines on the management of cardiovascular diseases during pregnancy. Eur Heart J. 2011;32(24):3147–97.
80. Magee LA, Von Dadelszen P, Rey E, Ross S, Asztalos E, Murphy KE, et al. Less-tight versus tight control of hypertension in pregnancy. N Engl J Med. 2015;372(24):2367–8.
81. Committee on Obstetric Practice. Emergent therapy for acute-onset, severe hypertension during pregnancy and the postpartum period. Obstet Gynecol. 2013;122(5):1122–31.
82. Fisher S, Van Zutphen A, Werler M, Lin A, Romitti P, Druschel C, et al. Maternal antihypertensive medication use and congenital heart defects. Updated results from the National Birth Defects Prevention Study. Hypertension. 2017;69(5):798–805.
83. Harrington JM, Fitzgerald AP, Kearney PM, McCarthy VJC, Madden J, Browne G, et al. DASH diet score and distribution of blood pressure in middle-aged men and women. Am J Hypertens. 2013;26(11):1311–20.
84. Maruthur NM, Wang N-Y, Appel LJ. Lifestyle interventions reduce coronary heart disease risk: results from the PREMIER trial. Circulation. 2009;119(15):2026–31.
85. Cook NR, Cutler JA, Obarzanek E, Buring JE, Rexrode KM, Kumanyika SK, et al. Long term effects of dietary sodium reduction on cardiovascular disease outcomes: observational follow-up of the trials of hypertension prevention (TOHP). BMJ. 2007;334(7599):885. http://www.bmj.com/cgi/doi/10.1136/bmj.39147.604896.55.
86. Rodenburg EM, Stricker BH, Visser LE. Sex differences in cardiovascular drug-induced adverse reactions causing hospital admissions. Br J Clin Pharmacol. 2012;74(6):1045–52.

87. Julius S, Nesbitt SD, Egan BM, Weber MA, Michelson EL, Kaciroti N, et al. Feasibility of treating prehypertension with an angiotensin-receptor blocker. N Engl J Med. 2006;354(16):1685–97. http://www.ncbi.nlm.nih.gov/pubmed/16537662.
88. Luders S, Schrader J, Berger J, Unger T, Zidek W, Bohm M, et al. The PHARAO study: prevention of hypertension with angiotensin-converting enyme inhibitor ramipril in patients with high normal blood pressure: a prospective, randomized, controlled prevention trial of the German Hypertension League. J Hypertens. 2008;26(7):1487–96.
89. Fuchs SC, Poli-de-Figueiredo CE, Figueiredo Neto JA, Scala LCN, Whelton PK, Mosele F, et al. Effectiveness of chlorthalidone plus amiloride for the prevention of hypertension: The PREVER-prevention randomized clinical trial. J Am Heart Assoc. 2016;5(12):e004248.
90. Boggia J, Thijs L, Hansen TW, Li Y, Kikuya M, Björklund-Bodegård K, et al. Ambulatory blood pressure monitoring in 9357 subjects from 11 populations highlights missed opportunities for cardiovascular prevention in women. Hypertension. 2011;57(3):397–405.

Non-pharmacologic Approaches for the Management of Prehypertension

39

Reuven Zimlichman

For many years there has been a dispute regarding which goal levels of blood pressure (BP) are considered normal, optimal, and abnormal. Generally, the definition gradually decreases, being based upon risk calculations and consequently, the recommendation for non-pharmacological and pharmacologic treatment change accordingly.

The relationship between BP and cardiovascular (CV) risk is linear, beginning at a BP of 115/75 mmHg, cardiovascular risk doubles for each increase of 20/10 mmHg. Thus, even individuals with prehypertension have an increased risk of stroke, myocardial infarction, and total CV events [1].

Therapeutic decisions are based upon cost benefit ratio. The costs to be considered are financial expenses by the patients and the general population as well as nonfinancial aspects, as the commitment to comply with a therapeutic approach. The benefit is estimated by the measured risk reduction, frequently by surrogate endpoints and optimally by reduction in morbidity and mortality. The success in reducing morbidity and mortality is determined by choosing the appropriate intervention and by both the feasibility and success of the intervention.

In this chapter I will review the basic concepts of the therapeutic approach to prehypertension, the evidence for its success, who is to be treated, and how. I will assess also the feasibility of the interventions.

Of course the main proof of treatment success is reduction of morbidity and mortality but its effect on quality of life should be evaluated as well.

R. Zimlichman
Medicine and Hypertension Institute, Wolfson Medical Center, Holon, Israel

Brunner Institute for Cardiovascular Research, Sackler Faculty of Medicine, Tel-Aviv University, Tel Aviv-Yafo, Israel

Institute for Quality in Medicine, Israeli Medical Association, Ramat Gan, Israel
e-mail: zimlich@post.tau.ac.il

R. Zimlichman et al. (eds.), *Prehypertension and Cardiometabolic Syndrome*, Updates in Hypertension and Cardiovascular Protection,
https://doi.org/10.1007/978-3-319-75310-2_39

Hypertension is a progressive disease. BP measurements in populations are Gaussian and reflect the wide distribution in the population as a whole. Similar patterns of distribution exist in patient subgroups according to age, gender, and concomitant disease. While tracking BP levels in specific populations the curves will still be of Gaussian shape when converted to logarithmic scale.

The gradual increase in BP is associated with aging. Structural changes in blood vessels cause gradual stiffening of the arterial walls increasing the systolic blood pressure (SBP). The rate of arterial stiffening differs in patients and is determined by genetic factors, concomitant diseases, lifestyle change, etc. The interrelation between BP level and arterial stiffening creates a vicious cycle; arterial stiffening causes increase in BP and increased BP further enhances the arterial stiffening and increases BP. Enhanced rate of arterial stiffening with the resulting increase in SBP is termed early vascular aging (EVA).

39.1 Epidemiology of Prehypertension

While considering epidemiological aspects of prehypertension the majority of information exists from population studies performed mainly in the USA. The prevalence of prehypertension is 31% while hypertension and normotension are 23% and 39%, respectively. Thus, about 60% of the adult US population has prehypertension or hypertension [2]. The age-adjusted prevalence of prehypertension is greater in men than in women at 39% versus 23.1%, respectively [3].

The risk of developing hypertension in individuals that are 75 years old in the USA is approximately 90% and thus methods to prevent progression from prehypertension to hypertension should by studied [4]. Patients with stage 2 prehypertension (BP of 130–139/85–89 mm Hg) are at threefold or greater risk for progression to hypertension, while in those with stage 1 prehypertension (BP of 120–129/80–84 mm Hg) the risk of progression to hypertension is roughly half of this value. Progression from prehypertension to hypertension is affected and accompanied by obesity, hyperinsulinemia, insulin resistance, hypertriglyceridemia, reduced LDL cholesterol, and elevated amount of small, dense LDL particles.

Compared with normotensives, prehypertensives are more likely to be overweight and obese. They have more concomitant CV risk factors and thus a higher risk to develop cardiovascular disease (CVD).

Moreover, prehypertensives have additional risk factors, as high levels of fibrinogen, plasminogen activator inhibitor-1 (PAI-1), adipokines, inflammatory cytokines and endothelial dysfunction, left ventricular hypertrophy, diastolic dysfunction and decreased coronary flow reserve [5]. The accepted therapeutic approach in patients with hypertension and prehypertension is "The high risk strategy, in which high risk patients, those with 10-year coronary heart disease risk of ≥20%, have to be treated." However, we should also consider the population attributable risk, which estimates the number of CV events in those at lower risk. In fact, the number of CV events in individuals at low risk is still considerable and probably no less in total than of those with high CV risk [6].

The group of patients with prehypertension defined as having BP level of 120–139/80–89 is non-homogenous, the CV risk increases gradually with BP levels and with the presence of other CV risk factors.

39.2 Risk of Cardiovascular Disease

Several recent meta-analyses on prehypertension and the relative risk for coronary disease, stroke, and total CVD included information about office BP measurements and most of the included patients were without previous CVD. The findings of these meta-analyses confirm that prehypertension increases the risk of CVD; moreover, the risk of fatal and nonfatal events was higher in stage 2 prehypertension than in stage 1 prehypertension [7–10]. In these meta-analyses the relative risk ratios after adjustment for risk factors, as smoking, gender, age, and dyslipidemia, averaged about 4.3% with estimated 10-year rate of 43% [11].

Individuals with heart failure or coronary artery disease were at even higher risk.

The Strong Heart Study revealed that individuals with prehypertension alone were almost twice as likely to develop CVD, while those with diabetes alone were almost three times as likely to develop CVD. Moreover, patients with both prehypertension and diabetes were nearly four times more likely to develop CVD.

Since prehypertension is extremely prevalent, about one-third of CV events in the global population occur in patients with prehypertension. Generally, patients with prehypertension have an annual absolute excess of CVD of 0.31–0.61% with an average of 0.5% approximately. If about 30 million subjects in the USA have stage 2 prehypertension, this population will include about 150,000 excess CV events annually [11, 12].

39.3 Non-pharmacological Interventions

Lifestyle modification includes interventions such as weight loss, dietary alternation, exercise, cessation of smoking, and relaxation methods. Dietary intervention includes multiple variables, among these are weight loss, change in dietary habits, including reduced sodium content and moderation of alcohol consumption, and additional dietary components that are sometimes difficult to isolate by their specific effects in total lifestyle intervention, therefore resulting in somewhat inconsistent evidence. Nonetheless, all of these lifestyle modifications have been shown beneficiary, not only in hypertensive patients but also in diabetics, obese, and other groups with increased CV risk.

A review published in 1978 stated that exercise should be recommended to mildly hypertensive patients as well as to the entire public for its long-term benefit in weight control in a sedentary society [13].

Many studies have since shown enthusiastic results regarding lifestyle intervention benefits; however, these beneficial results as reducing BP and CV risk have been shown in randomized clinical trials. Beyond the strict experimental condition, the results are less convincing and sometimes questionable, especially in long-term studies. Changing lifestyle is not easy and frequently fails [14], thus results of such studies are inconsistent and not always convincing.

The evidence regarding non-pharmacologic treatment of prehypertension and hypertension is based on several types of evidence. Epidemiological evidence proves the relationship between BP levels and the intervention. This approach does not prove a causal relationship and is mainly of suggestive nature. Non-pharmacological intervention may act as a marker for the physiological phenomena. The non-pharmacological intervention could imply to a direct or indirect causal relationship but does not prove it.

Physiological understanding may suggest the causal effect of non-pharmacological intervention. However, there is no accepted mechanistic hypothesis that can explain the influence of non-pharmacological intervention on BP reduction. Also concluding from similar interventions in animals is problematic, because the mechanisms of experimental hypertension in various animal models differ from the mechanisms in human hypertension. Thus, research in this field has to rely on properly conducted interventional studies in humans. Several major obstacles in such studies are proper blinding of study participants, creation of large groups of subjects, and defining a limited number of variables in the intervention studied [15].

39.4 Weight Reduction

A direct positive relation has been found between body weight or body mass and BP. The Intersalt study that included 52 communities worldwide found that with the exception of age, weight had the strongest and most consistent correlation with BP level [16]. Also, individuals with central or upper body obesity with higher waist-to-hip ratio are more likely to have higher BP and increased risk to develop CV morbidity and mortality [17]. European and US guidelines state that the lowest all-cause mortality rates are at BMI range of 20–25 kg/m^2 [18, 19].

The exact optimal body composition is disputed in the literature. Practically weighing the patient or determining his weight does not enable to determine the fat/muscle composition; these data can be useful in identifying subjects that will benefit from weight loss. Achieving a loss of 6–8% of body weight can lead to 5 and 4 mm Hg decrease in systolic blood pressure (SBP) and diastolic blood pressure (DBP), respectively, and weight loss of about 10 kg may lower SBP by 5–20 mm Hg [20].

In another study it has been shown that weight reduction lowers BP, even while sodium and potassium dietary content are kept constant. A weight loss of about 5 kg was associated with decline of 5.4/2.4 mm Hg and an addition of sodium restriction to weight loss was associated with additional BP decline [21].

The mechanism of increased BP in obese subjects is not entirely clear.

The sympathetic nervous system activity which is increased in obesity most probably plays a role in the pathogenetic mechanism, with activation of the plasma renin-angiotensin-aldosterone system, expansion of plasma volume, hyperinsulinemia and increased inflammatory markers.

It has been shown that weight reduction lowers BP. When sodium and potassium intake was constant during the follow-up, a weight loss of about 5 Kg was associated with a BP decline of 5.4/4.2 mmHg and when sodium restriction was added it further enhanced the BP decline [21].

Weight loss in overweight subjects not only lowers BP, it has been shown to lower total cholesterol, to correct insulin resistance, to lower plasma renin activity, and to diminish cardiac output. However, these changes were not associated with cardiovascular and all-cause mortality. Both National Health and Nutrition Examination Survey (NHANES) and Multiple Risk Factor Intervention Trial (MRFIT) studies have shown increased cardiovascular and all-cause mortality [22].

Despite the evidence of the obesity paradox in CVD, weight loss is a well-accepted and proven method to lower BP in patients with hypertension. Moreover, it was suggested that the adverse effect was limited only to lean subjects and weight loss should be recommended for obese individuals.

A well-accepted concept during the years is that weight loss as well as other lifestyle interventions should be adopted in order to replace or augment effects of drug therapy, in all patients with hypertension. This approach is especially rewarding in subjects with prehypertension and mild hypertension, in which lifestyle modification and especially weight loss may obviate the need to begin pharmacological treatment. In a prospective study, placebo control subjects who lost 4.5 kg had a BP decline similar to that achieved by chlorthalidone or atenolol [23].

39.4.1 The Efficacy of Lifestyle Interventions

Several studies have evaluated the impact of lifestyle interventions on BP levels and on progression to hypertension. Trials of hypertension prevention (TOHP II) was an intensive long-term study of lifestyle interventions. 2382 participants with DBP of 83–89 mmHg and SBP of <140 mmHg were randomized to usual care, weight loss, and sodium restriction or a combination of the latter two [24]. Over 4 years 44.4% of the usual care group developed hypertension compared to 38.5% (RR = 0.87, *P*-0.06) of the weight loss group. 38.1% of the sodium restriction group and 37.6% (RR = 0.85, $P = 0.01$) of the combined group developed hypertension—in this study hypertension diagnosis was based upon a single BP measurement. This intensive lifestyle modification caused absolute reduction of 6–7% and relative reduction of 13–15% in the development of hypertension [5].

The Oslo diet and Anti-Smoking trial included 1234 men 40–50 years old which were in the upper quartile of risk, based on total cholesterol, smoking, and BP. Participants with SBP higher than 150 mmHg were excluded. Participants in the intervention group reduced intake of fat calories from 28 to 44% ($p < 0.01$), increased the ratio of polyunsaturated fat to saturated fat intake from 1.01 to 0.39 ($p < 0.01$), raised fiber consumption from 4.4 to 6.0 g/day ($p < 0.05$), lowered total cholesterol from 341 to 263 mg/dl ($p < 0.01$), decreased cigarette use from 10 to 6 per day, and lost weight of 3.7 versus 0.6 kg in the control group [25, 26].

Together the Oslo Diet and Smoking study and the TOHP II studies have shown that lifestyle intervention can prevent and/or delay the onset of hypertension and of CV events in subjects at risk. Additional studies in the field mostly confirmed these findings but these were more limited due to difficulties in standardization, participant compliance, and the presence of multiple confounders which limited isolation of specific components of the intervention.

Based on the concept of the efficacy of lifestyle interventions, a trend to improve lifestyle was seen in the USA. It has been shown that during the years 1963 to 1975 consumption of salt, saturated fat, and smoking declined [27]. However, evidence of contradictory trends in the recent years show a growing epidemic of obesity and the associated increase in diabetes which leads to trends of increased rates of hypertension and concomitant risk of CVD.

Most individuals with prehypertension have at least one concomitant condition associated with increased CV risk. The NHANES and the NHANES II mortality studies showed that more than 90% of individuals with prehypertension have one or more CV risk factors, i.e., dyslipidemia, early family history of CVD, smoking, obesity, hyperinsulinemia with insulin resistance, impaired fasting glucose, prothrombotic state, endothelial dysfunction, and increased vascular stiffness.[28]

The lifestyle intervention arm of the Diabetes Prevention Program (DPP) enrolled 1079 subjects with impaired glucose tolerance. The goal of this study was a minimum of 7% weight loss and a minimum of 150 minutes of physical activity per week with a moderate caloric restriction (500–700 less calories per day) engaging in physical activity of moderate intensity. After a 2.8-year follow-up, the intervention showed a 58% reduction in the incidence of diabetes [29]. In addition, the study showed a decreased need for antihypertensive medications, and less occurrences of new cases of hypertension.

In the DPP study the prevalence of hypertension was about 30% in the comparison groups. After 3 years of follow-up it was about 40% in the placebo and metformin arms but remained about 30% in the intensive lifestyle arm, representing a risk reduction of 33% in the development of hypertension in the intensive lifestyle intervention group compared with placebo and metformin arms [30].

39.5 Dietary Modification

Nutrition habits and their correlation to BP have been examined in several studies. The European Prospective Investigation into Cancer and Nutrition (EPIC) study demonstrated that in 7061 non-hypertensive women (35–64 years) body weight, waist circumference, body mass index (BMI), and consumption of processed meat, wine, and potatoes directly correlated with BP levels. This study also demonstrated that increasing consumption of vegetables, eggs, and yoghurt decreased SBP and DBP [31].

The recent NutriNet–Sante study reported a similar relationship between nutrition and BP levels in 8670 healthy volunteers and an inverse association between BP and fruit and vegetable consumption [32].

The dietary approaches to stop hypertension (DASH) were a landmark study in the field of dietary lifestyle modification which affected nutrition patterns worldwide.

The DASH diet includes low fat dairy products with high intake of fruits, vegetables, and fiber. It is difficult to define which specific nutrients exerted the beneficiary effect of the DASH diet intervention, and most probably a combination of several of its components contribute to the favorable outcomes [33].

The DASH Diet lowered BP in all subgroups; these effects were more pronounced in African Americans with BP reduction effects being stronger in hypertensive than non-hypertensive subjects [34]. The DASH study has shown significant reduction in both SBP and DBP with magnitudes to pharmacotherapy for mild hypertension. Despite the limited evidence on the long-term effects of the DASH diet it is recommended, with weight loss and physical activity, for prevention and management of BP [19].

The Exercise and Nutrition interventions for CardiOvasculaR hEalth (ENCORE) study evaluated the long-term effects of the DASH study. The participants were followed for 8 months after the completion of 16-week intervention. The results showed beneficiary effects; nonetheless, methods that will ensure long-term compliance with intervention should be developed [35].

Improvement of dietary habits can reduce BP levels, postpone or even prevent progression to hypertension if practiced over a long period. A study published in 1950 reported that Cretan population has lower prevalence of hypertension, CVD as myocardial infarction and stroke and even some types of cancer [36]. This study stimulated the research on benefits of living in the Mediterranean area. One of the major determinants studied was the differences in the diet in the Mediterranean region defined as the "Mediterranean diet." The characteristics of this diet are—high content of monosaturated fatty acids (MUFA) and polyunsaturated fatty acids (PUFA). Other characteristics are moderate consumption of alcohol and dairy products, increased intake of fruits and vegetables, and low intake of red meat and processed red meat products. The Mediterranean diet is rich in fiber, phenols, flavonoids, isoflavones, phytosterols, other plant acids, and phytochemicals which probably have beneficial effects on oxidative stress and mainly on the cardiovascular and nervous systems [37].

The SUN study evaluated 9408 subjects followed up for 6 years consuming the Mediterranean diet. The intervention was associated with decrease in SBP and DBP levels. Moderate implementation of the diet was associated with a decrease of 2.4/1.3 mmHg while strict implication decreased BP further (3.1/1.0 mmHg). In addition, adoption of the diet in patients with very high CV risk resulted in SBP reduction of 7.1 mmHg [38].

In the ATTICA study, 1188 subjects without CVD but with BP levels at prehypertensive range adopted the Mediterranean diet and were followed up for 5 years for development of hypertension. Among 798 subjects that returned during the 5-year follow-up period, 18.7% of the men and 24.6% of the women were diagnosed as hypertensive [39].

The mechanisms of effect of the Mediterranean diet on BP reduction are most probably multifactorial and are not fully understood. It appears that the diet has beneficiary effects on BP and CV event reduction but physical activity and other measures probably play a role in this effect.

In a recent meta-analysis involving 50 studies and 534,906 subjects it has been shown that the Mediterranean diet lowered BP levels and the incidence of the metabolic syndrome and its components [40].

39.6 Sodium Intake

Change in the consumed diet with accompanying weight reduction is always associated with changes in dietary constituents, while many of these are suggested as of specific influence on BP. It is well accepted that excess sodium intake is a key driver of high BP across age, sex, and ethnic groups [41].

Current clinical guidelines limit sodium intake to a maximum of 2400 mg/day in prehypertensive patients and as a complimentary approach to pharmacological therapy in hypertensive subjects [41]. The main justification of this approach was provided in the global sodium consumption survey of 66 countries [18].

In another study the DASH diet lowered BP at all three different sodium levels. Changing from the intermediate to low sodium diet resulted in additional BP reduction [42].

There is strong evidence for sodium depletion associated with BP decline. Moreover, sodium depletion enhances the BP response to antihypertensive treatment and especially to angiotensin-converting enzyme (ACE) inhibitors and angiotensin-receptor blockers (ARBs). The mechanisms of sodium-induced effect on BP are not entirely clear. Sodium is involved with the renin-angiotensin-aldosterone system in controlling volume and blood vessel constriction and maintaining blood flow and blood pressure. Nonetheless, it cannot be excluded that other dietary associated changes, in this type of diet, affect BP levels. Moreover, the exclusion of other confounding factors as body weight, alcohol consumption, etc. weaken the scope and significance of BP decrease [17]. Studies have shown that migration from a low to high sodium environment was accompanied by BP increase, but it is clear that additional lifestyle changes exist in migration of populations.

It has been found that individuals differ in their response to salt, thus two groups were defined—salt-sensitive and salt-resistant subjects.

It is widely accepted that dietary sodium restriction should be recommended, and when reduced will lower BP in some, but not all normotensive, prehypertensive and hypertensive subjects. The dietary sodium in various populations is usually between 100 and 200 mmol/day and sodium content of more than 200 mmol/day should be strongly discouraged. Severe sodium restriction, as shown in several short-term studies, is efficacious but impractical in the long run. Low compliance with sodium reduced diets is always a limiting factor in the practical dietary approach. It has been show that assistance of dietary consulting by nutritionist improves dietary compliance.

Optimally dietary salt content of about 70–90 mmol/day should be advised. It has been suggested that a threshold dietary reduction of more than 50 mmol/d must be practiced in order to significantly induce BP decrease [43].

In order to significantly reduce dietary salt levels, abstinence from processed fast foods and a total change in dietary habits is required. Interventions to lower dietary sodium content should not be limited to sodium alone, they should by multifaceted and include the whole range intervention of complete lifestyle changes of which sodium restriction is important but only one of many components. The response to salt reduction is inconsistent, it should be evaluated in all subjects. In some patients with prehypertension it may prevent and delay beginning of pharmacological treatment and may delay the appearance of hypertension.

Other nutritional factors in the non-pharmacological approach to treat prehypertension and hypertension have been discussed in the literature. The effect of potassium on BP in intervention trials is inconsistent. Observational studies suggested that individuals with greater intake of potassium have lower incidence of stroke [44]. However, it is not clear whether the effect is of potassium alone or other different constituents of the diet are responsible for this change.

Magnesium is a vasodilator and was traditionally used to control BP in eclampsia and preeclampsia, but there is absolutely no evidence in population studies to justify its use in the treatment of prehypertension and hypertension. Reduced dietary content of calcium was associated with increased BP in population studies but the results of calcium supplementation were inconsistent [45]. Increased dietary polyunsaturated fat and reduction in saturated fat have been suggested but not confirmed as hypotensive agents.

39.7 Alcohol Restriction

Alcohol consumption and its association with several cardiovascular diseases follows a J-shaped curve. Light alcohol consumption protects from CVD compared to nondrinkers while overconsumption exponentially increases the risk of CVD and CV events [46]. Acute excess of alcohol (binge drinking) causes multiple cardiovascular deleterious effects. A study that evaluated the effect of one or more episodes of binge drinking per week found excess of prehypertension prevalence in both men and women [47].

Chronic excess of alcohol increases the risk of hypertension in a dose-dependent manner and increases the risk of stroke and myocardial infarction [48].

A meta-analysis that evaluated mainly observational studies in the field noted significant reduction in SBP (−3.3 mmHg) and DBP (−2.0 mmHg) in response to intervention counseling programs [49].

Despite the observational evidence of cardio-protective effect of light to moderate drinking (up to one drink per day in women and up to two drinks in men), this recommendation in nondrinkers should not be adopted since excess drinking and alcoholism can develop at later stages of life.

39.8 Physical Exercise

Physical exercise is recommended by all guidelines for the whole population—normotensives, prehypertensives, and hypertensives. The higher the CV risk, the stronger the recommendation. Observational data suggest that active and fit individuals have lower BP and lower CV mortality and morbidity [17].

Although many interventional clinical trials of exercise training have been performed, not all were controlled, and excluded multiple confounding factors to enable reaching conclusive results.

Exercise is characterized by several categories. Dynamic aspects of physical activity are considered isotonic and refer to joint and large muscle movement in contrast to isometric exercise, which includes contraction of muscles without movement of joints. The consideration of aerobic exercise includes changes in availability and use of oxygen for energy production and muscle contraction [50]. It is speculated that exercise provides cardio-protection of the vascular wall and that repeated bouts of sheer stress confer a vascular conditioning effect, increase in endothelial nitric oxide, a vasodilator that reduces BP. Repeated bouts of exercise may induce resetting of the baroreceptors lowering resting BP [51].

A large number of studies have been performed to evaluate the effects of aerobic and resistance BP in normotensive, prehypertensive, and hypertensive subjects.

A recent review confirmed that exercise lowered BP independent of weight loss. Generally, studies using conventional measurements of BP were more consistent than ambulatory BP measurements. In meta-analysis that included 54 randomized controlled studies, including aerobic intervention, a significant reduction of BP (3.8/2/6 mmHg) was found [52].

Another meta-analysis examined resistance exercise and showed a BP decrease of $3^{+}/^{-}3/3^{+}/^{-}2$ mmHg in studies that lasted ≥4 weeks [53].

However, resistance exercise has been shown to increase arterial stiffness and is not recommended as antihypertensive treatment. The data regarding increasing arterial stiffness were not confirmed in women and future studies are needed in this field.

39.9 Biofeedback, Stress and Coping in Prehypertension and Hypertension

It is well accepted that an acute episode of stress will cause BP elevation. This change will be for a limited time period. BP increases in response to surrounding events are seen in normotensive, prehypertensive, as well in hypertensive subjects. It is less obvious whether repeated episodes of stress and/or chronic stress will induce chronic increase in BP to prehypertensive and hypertensive levels. A major factor that complicates the issue further is the fact that different subjects respond differently to similar degrees of stress. This response is affected by genetic and possible prenatal factors, but clearly and mainly by environmental and constitutional factors. Moreover, BP response to stress is further complicated as it is influenced by additional factors as arterial stiffness which also affects the BP response to stress (the stiffer the arteries, the greater the increase in BP).

Multiple methods have been suggested for coping with stress. One of them is Biofeedback-assisted relaxation therapy. Several studies found that psychological intervention reduces BP. These studies were relatively short (around 10 week program) in which subjects received psychological treatment or biofeedback [54].

In another study the resperate device was used to achieve slow, deep breathing in order to achieve relaxation response. A significant decrease in BP was achieved after 8 weeks of using the device [55]. Additional studies confirmed these findings.

Additional stress reduction programs have been suggested and achieved success in BP reduction. These included breathing, meditation, and relaxation interventions. The possible mechanisms of relaxation and biofeedback approaches are involved with the balance between the sympathetic and parasympathetic nervous systems. Generally, stimulation of parasympathetic nervous system activity reduces BP.

Since patients with prehypertension are usually treated with non-pharmacological measures, this is the ideal target population for stress reduction approach as well. Several points should be highlighted while estimating the value of stress reduction programs. The efficacy of stress reduction will be higher in stressed, tense subjects, therefore these subjects should be selected for this type of intervention. The likelihood of response is associated with adherence to medical recommendation, willingness, and ability to follow instructions, for home and workplace relaxation sessions [54].

It should be remembered that selection of proper patients for this type of intervention is important. Although several short-term studies showed the effectiveness of this intervention, long-term compliance is essential and will determine the long-term effect of the intervention.

Conclusions

BP and the risk of CVD correlate throughout the BP range. Since hypertension is a progressive disease correlated best with age but also with CV risk factors gradual increase in BP is accompanied by proportional increase in arterial stiffness and CV events. Interventional procedures along this continuum will depend upon cost/benefit ratio, generally the higher the BP, the higher the risk and higher the benefit of the intervention.

Prehypertensives are more likely to be obese and have additional CV risk factors and are more likely to progress to overt hypertension. Thus, it is justified to make every effort to prevent progression to hypertension, with its concomitant consequences. While the question of pharmacological treatment in prehypertensive patients is debated there is no doubt that non-pharmacological treatment should be practiced in these subjects.

Dietary modification, weight loss, regular physical activity, moderation of alcohol intake, and other lifestyle changes have been shown to reduce BP, prevent or delay progression to hypertension, and reduce CV events. Also these interventions can diminish the need for pharmacological treatment. Lifestyle modification is important for the prehypertensive population but is also equally important for the healthy population. Education and practice of a healthy lifestyle should be pursued by all.

References

1. Guo X, Zhang X, Guo L, et al. Association between pre-hypertension and cardiovascular outcomes: a systematic review and meta-analysis of prospective studies. Curr Hypertens Rep. 2013;15:703–16.
2. Chobanian AV, Bakris GL, Black HR, et al. The seventh report of the joint national committee on prevention, detection, evaluation, and treatment of high blood pressure: the JNC 7 report. JAMA. 2003;289:2560–71.
3. Greenlund KJ, Croft JB, Mensah GA. Prevalence of heart disease and stroke risk factors in persons with prehypertension in the United States, 1999–2000. Arch Intern Med. 2004;164:2113–8.
4. Nesbitt SD. Treatment options for prehypertension. Curr Opin Nephrol Hypertens. 2007;16:250–5.
5. Egan BM, Nesbitt SD, Julius S. Prehypertension: should we be treating with pharmacologic therapy? Ther Adv Cardiovasc Dis. 2008;2:305–14.
6. Rose G. Strategy of prevention: lessons from cardiovascular disease. Br Med J (Clin Res Ed). 1981;282:1847.
7. Huang Y, Cai X, Li Y, et al. Prehypertension and the risk of stroke a meta-analysis. Neurology. 2014;82:1153–61.
8. Huang Y, Su L, Cai X, et al. Association of all-cause and cardiovascular mortality with prehypertension: a meta-analysis. Am Heart J. 2014;167:160–8.
9. Huang Y, Wang S, Cai X, et al. Prehypertension and incidence of cardiovascular disease: a meta-analysis. BMC Med. 2013;11:177.
10. Guo X, Zhang X, Zheng L, et al. Prehypertension is not associated with all-cause mortality: a systematic review and meta-analysis of prospective studies. PLoS One. 2013;8:e61796.
11. Egan BM, Stevens-Fabry S. Prehypertension [mdash] prevalence, health risks, and management strategies. Nat Rev Cardiol. 2015;12:289–300.
12. Zhang Y, Lee ET, Devereux RB, et al. Prehypertension, diabetes, and cardiovascular disease risk in a population-based sample. Hypertension. 2006;47:410–4.
13. Blackburn H. Non-pharmacologic treatment of hypertension. Ann N Y Acad Sci. 1978;304:236–42.
14. Fuchs FD. Prehypertension: the rationale for early drug therapy. Cardiovasc Ther. 2010;28:339–43.
15. Swales JD. Non-pharmacological antihypertensive therapy. Eur Heart J. 1988;9:45–52.
16. Rose G, Stamler J, Stamler R, et al. Intersalt: an international study of electrolyte excretion and blood pressure. Results for 24 hour urinary sodium and potassium excretion. Br Med J. 1988;297:319–28.
17. Alderman MH. Non-pharmacological treatment of hypertension. Lancet. 1994;344:307–11.
18. Mozaffarian D, Fahimi S, Singh GM, et al. Global sodium consumption and death from cardiovascular causes. N Engl J Med. 2014;371:624–34.
19. Van Horn L. Dietary sodium and blood pressure: how low should we go? Prog Cardiovasc Dis. 2015;58:61–8.
20. McLaren L, Sumar N, Barberio AM, et al. Population-level interventions in government jurisdictions for dietary sodium reduction. Cochrane Database Syst Rev. 2016;9:CD010166.
21. Reisin E, Abel R, Modan M, et al. Effect of weight loss without salt restriction on the reduction of blood pressure in overweight hypertensive patients. N Engl J Med. 1978;298:1–6.
22. Dahl LK. Possible role of salt intake in the development of essential hypertension. Int J Epidemiol. 2005;34:967–72.
23. Wassertheil-Smoller S, Blaufox MD, Oberman AS, et al. The trial of antihypertensive interventions and management (TAIM) study: adequate weight loss, alone and combined with drug therapy in the treatment of mild hypertension. Arch Intern Med. 1992;152:131–6.
24. Lasser VI, Raczynski JM, Stevens VJ, et al. Trials of hypertension prevention, phase II structure and content of the weight loss and dietary sodium reduction interventions. Ann Epidemiol. 1995;5:156–64.

25. Hjermann I, et al. Smoking and diet intervention in healthy coronary high risk men. Methods and 5-year-follow-up of risk factors in a randomized trial. The Oslo Study. J Oslo City Hosp. 1980;30:3–17.
26. Hjermann I, Holme I, Byre KV, et al. Effect of diet and smoking intervention on the incidence of coronary heart disease: report from the Oslo Study Group of a randomised trial in healthy men. Lancet. 1981;318:1303–10.
27. Moser M. A decade of progress in the management of hypertension. Hypertension. 1983;5:808–13.
28. Mainous AG, Everett CJ, Liszka H, et al. Prehypertension and mortality in a nationally representative cohort. Am J Cardiol. 2004;94:1496–500.
29. Knowler WC, Diabetes Prevention Program Research Group. Reduction in the incidence of type 2 diabetes with lifestyle intervention or metformin. N Engl J Med. 2002;346:393–403.
30. Dagogo-Jack S, Egbuonu N, Edeoga C. Principles and practice of nonpharmacological interventions to reduce cardiometabolic risk. Med Princ Pract. 2010;19:167.
31. Reddy KS, Katan MB. Diet, nutrition and the prevention of hypertension and cardiovascular diseases. Public Health Nutr. 2004;7:167–86.
32. Lelong H, Galan P, Kesse-Guyot E, et al. Relationship between nutrition and blood pressure: a cross-sectional analysis from the NutriNet-sante study, a French web-based cohort study. Am J Hypertens. 2015;28:362–71.
33. Fung TT, Rimm EB, Spiegelman D, et al. Association between dietary patterns and plasma biomarkers of obesity and cardiovascular disease risk. Am J Clin Nutr. 2001;73:61–7.
34. Vollmer WM, Sacks FM, Ard J, et al. Effects of diet and sodium intake on blood pressure: subgroup analysis of the DASH-sodium trial. Ann Intern Med. 2001;135:1019–28.
35. Hinderliter AL, Sherwood A, Craighead LW, et al. The long-term effects of lifestyle change on blood pressure: one-year follow-up of the ENCORE study. Am J Hypertens. 2013;27:734–41.
36. Allbaugh L. Food and nutrition. In: Crete: a case study of an underdeveloped area. Princeton, NJ: Princeton University Press; 1953. p. 97–135.
37. Vamvakis A, Gkaliagkousi E, Triantafyllou A, et al. Beneficial effects of nonpharmacological interventions in the management of essential hypertension. JRSM Cardiovasc Dis. 2017;6:2048004016683891.
38. Estruch R, Martinez-González MA, Corella D, et al. Effects of a Mediterranean-style diet on cardiovascular risk factors: a randomized trial. Ann Intern Med. 2006;145:1–11.
39. Pitsavos C, Chrysohoou C, Panagiotakos DB, et al. Abdominal obesity and inflammation predicts hypertension among prehypertensive men and women: the ATTICA study. Heart Vessel. 2008;23:96–103.
40. Kastorini C-M, Milionis HJ, Esposito K, et al. The effect of Mediterranean diet on metabolic syndrome and its components: a meta-analysis of 50 studies and 534,906 individuals. J Am Coll Cardiol. 2011;57:1299–313.
41. Davy BM, Halliday TM, Davy KP. Sodium intake and blood pressure: new controversies, new labels... New guidelines? J Acad Nutr Diet. 2015;115:200–4.
42. Sacks FM, Svetkey LP, Vollmer WM, et al. Effects on blood pressure of reduced dietary sodium and the dietary approaches to stop hypertension (DASH) diet. N Engl J Med. 2001;344:3–10.
43. MacGregor GA, Sagnella GA, Markandu ND, et al. Double-blind study of three sodium intakes and long-term effects of sodium restriction in essential hypertension. Lancet. 1989;334:1244–7.
44. Khaw K-T, Barrett-Connor E. Dietary potassium and stroke-associated mortality. N Engl J Med. 1987;316:235–40.
45. Luft FC. Putative mechanism of blood pressure reduction induced by increases in dietary calcium intake. Am J Hypertens. 1990;3:156S–60S.
46. O'Keefe JH, Bhatti SK, Bajwa A, et al. Alcohol and cardiovascular health: the dose makes the poison… or the remedy. Mayo Clin Proc. 2014;89:382–93.
47. Piano MR, Mazzuco A, Kang M, et al. Cardiovascular consequences of binge drinking: an integrative review with implications for advocacy, policy, and research. Alcohol Clin Exp Res. 2017;41:487–96.

48. Ozemek C, Phillips SA, Popovic D, et al. Nonpharmacologic management of hypertension: a multidisciplinary approach. Curr Opin Cardiol. 2017;32:381–8.
49. Xue X, Jiang H, Frontini MG, et al. Effects of alcohol reduction on blood pressure: a meta-analysis of randomised controlled trials. Hypertension. 2001;38:1112–7.
50. Lackland DT, Voeks JH. Metabolic syndrome and hypertension: regular exercise as part of lifestyle management. Curr Hypertens Rep. 2014;16:492.
51. Collier SR, Landram MJ. Treatment of prehypertension: lifestyle and/or medication. Vasc Health Risk Manag. 2012;8:613.
52. Whelton SP, Chin A, Xin X, et al. Effect of aerobic exercise on blood pressure: a meta-analysis of randomized, controlled trials. Ann Intern Med. 2002;136:493–503.
53. Kelley GA, Kelley KS. Progressive resistance exercise and resting blood pressure. Hypertension. 2000;35:838–43.
54. McGrady A. The effects of biofeedback in diabetes and essential hypertension. Cleve Clin J Med. 2010;77:S68–71.
55. Elliott WJ, Izzo JL, White WB, et al. Graded blood pressure reduction in hypertensive outpatients associated with use of a device to assist with slow breathing. J Clin Hypertens. 2004;6:553–9.

Prehypertension: A Case in Favor of Early Use of Diuretics

40

Flávio Danni Fuchs and Sandra Costa Fuchs

The diagnosis of hypertension has faced extraordinary and controversial developments. Guidelines [1–5] are going in opposite directions in the establishment of blood pressure (BP) thresholds for diagnosis and goals of treatment. This chapter makes a case in favor of leaving behind the diagnosis of prehypertension, which should be promoted to true hypertension. Diuretics are natural candidates to start drug therapy in patients who do not respond to nondrug interventions, with preference for more efficacious agents associated with a potassium-sparing agent.

40.1 Risks of Prehypertension

The uncovering of the risks of blood pressure elevation with age, together with the identification of their causes and the development of effective strategies for its prevention and treatment, are among the outstanding achievements of humankind. Businesspersons from life insurance companies firstly noted the risks of high blood pressure in 1911 [6]. In the thirties of the last century, however, Paul White still stated, on his classic book of heart disease [7], that hypertension could be an important compensatory mechanism, which should not be tampered. Dozens of cohort studies conducted between the fourth and the ninth decades of the last century, with large samples, established beyond any reasonable doubt that high BP was a major

F. D. Fuchs (✉)
Division of Cardiology, Hospital de Clínicas de Porto Alegre, School of Medicine, Universidade Federal do Rio Grande do Sul, Porto Alegre, Brazil
e-mail: ffuchs@hcpa.edu.br

S. C. Fuchs
Graduate Program in Cardiology, School of Medicine, Universidade Federal do Rio Grande do Sul, Porto Alegre, Brazil

R. Zimlichman et al. (eds.), *Prehypertension and Cardiometabolic Syndrome*, Updates in Hypertension and Cardiovascular Protection,
https://doi.org/10.1007/978-3-319-75310-2_40

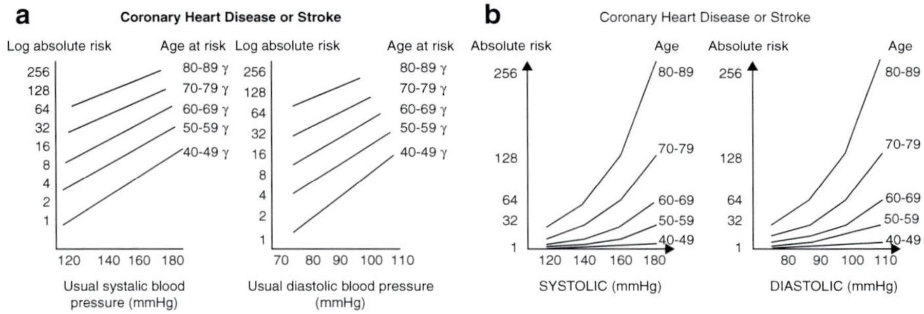

Fig. 40.1 Absolute risk for coronary heart disease or stroke by BP levels, stratified by age groups; (**a**) vertical axis log-transformed; (**b**) real axis (Reprinted with permission from reference [8] (**a**) and [9] (**b**))

cardiovascular risk factor. The thresholds for the starting of risk, however, were evident at high blood pressure values, because the low absolute incidence of cardiovascular events at lower BP values conferred low statistical power in individual studies.

The Prospective Studies Collaboration compiled the individual data of more than one million individuals, who were followed for 15 years in 61 cohort studies, with 56,000 deaths from cardiovascular events [8]. The risk of elevated BP for cardiovascular events increased steadily from 75 and 115 mmHg of diastolic and systolic pressures, respectively, doubling every 10 mmHg of diastolic or 20 mmHg of systolic BP (Fig. 40.1a). Figure 40.1b, with real intervals on the vertical axis, demonstrated that at lower BP levels the absolute incidence of events was low, particularly at younger ages. Duplication of low risks have less absolute impact, with more significant increase (inflection of the curve) when the previous absolute risks were already high. Points of higher inflection were employed to define the thresholds for diagnosis of hypertension in the past.

The increase in the precision to identify BP thresholds for cardiovascular risks led to diagnostic values progressively down, from 160/95 mmHg in old guidelines to 140/90 mmHg in the current ones. There are solid evidences, however, that they should be lower, at least 120/80 mmHg.

Besides CHD and stroke, high systolic or diastolic BP are the major cause of many other cardiovascular and non-cardiovascular consequences, such as hypertensive cardiomyopathy, heart failure, aortic valve stenosis, aortic syndromes, peripheral arterial disease, atrial fibrillation, chronic kidney disease, dementias, diabetes, age-related macular degeneration, and erectile dysfunction [9].

The risks for these outcomes start at prehypertension levels. Besides, prehypertension is a risk for development of full hypertension and target organ damage. In a cohort study conducted in Porto Alegre, Brazil, four among five individuals with prehypertension developed hypertension in 10 years [10] (Fig. 40.2). Similar incidence has been shown in other populations, such as in a nationwide Japanese cohort [11].

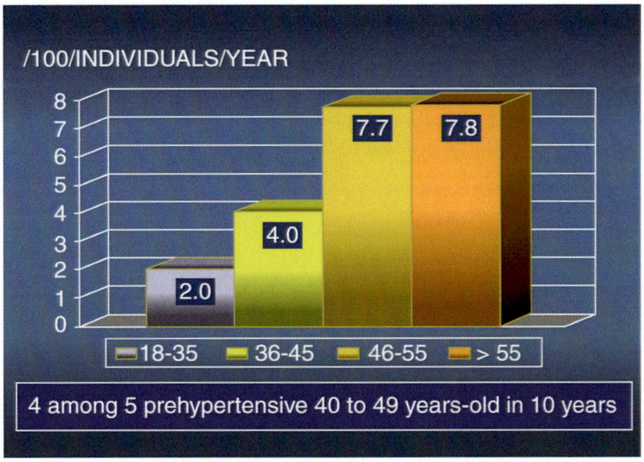

Fig. 40.2 Incidence of hypertension in population-based cohort in Porto Alegre, Brazil (reprinted with permission from the reference [9])

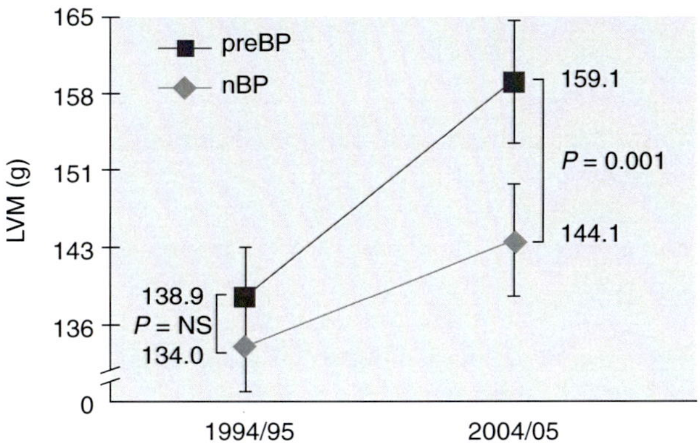

Fig. 40.3 Increase of left ventricular mass in participants with prehypertension and optimal BP in the MONICA cohort (reprinted with permission from the reference [12])

Target organ damage in individuals with prehypertension has been demonstrated in several studies. For instance, in the MONICA cohort, prehypertension was a risk for increasing left ventricular mass compared to individuals with normal BP [12] (Fig. 40.3). Findings from the ARIC cohort showed that prehypertension was associated with heart abnormalities in structure and function in elderly individuals [13]. The risks of prehypertension for the development of chronic kidney disease were demonstrated in the Kaiser Permanente [14] and Ohasama cohorts [15].

40.1.1 Benefits of Treating Prehypertension

The evidence that treating patients with prehypertension leads to substantial reduction of cardiovascular outcomes was available for many years, but was restricted to patients with cardiovascular disease. Several randomized clinical trials, which enrolled patients with coronary heart disease, heart failure, stroke, and diabetes,

Table 40.1 Beneficial effects of BP-lowering drugs in patients with normal BP and cardiovascular disease

Clinical condition	Studies (reference)	Active treatment	Primary outcome	RRR (95% CI)
Diabetes mellitus	Micro-HOPE [16]	Ramipril	MI, stroke, CV death	25% (12 to 36)
Any evidence of atherosclerosis	HOPE [17]	Ramipril	MI, stroke, CV death	22% (14 to 30)
	EUROPA [18]	Perindopril	MI, CV death, or cardiac arrest	20% (9 to 29)
Recovery from stroke	PROGRESS [19]	Indapamide plus perindopril	Stroke	42% (19 to 58)
Asymptomatic heart failure	SOLVED [20]	Enalapril	CV deaths	12% (−3 to 26)
Overt heart failure	SOLVED [21]	Enalapril	CV deaths	18% (6 to 28)
	SAVE [22]	Captopril		21% (5 to 35)
Class IV heart failure	CONSENSUS [23]	Enalapril	Total mortality	40% ($P = 0.002$)

RRR relative risk reduction

showed the prevention of cardiovascular outcomes with active treatment compared to placebo [16–23] (Table 40.1). The interpretation of the authors of these trials was that the benefit was due to pleiotropic effects of the drugs employed in the trials, mostly beta-blockers and ACE inhibitors, and only in one trial, diuretics. The blood pressure-lowering effect, however, could explain the beneficial effect of drugs in the clinical conditions presented on Table 40.1 [24]. This view was confirmed in two meta-analyses that included patients with and without hypertension [25, 26]. We postulated that drug treatment should be offered to patients with prehypertension, which is a window of opportunity to reduce the consequences of high BP [27, 28].

Most authors, who considered that the clinical conditions were confounders of the benefit of blood pressure-lowering drugs, disdained the evidences obtained in patients with cardiovascular disease. Moreover, the possibility that excessive blood pressure reduction could increase the incidence of cardiovascular events, particularly in patients with coronary artery disease (the J-shape phenomenon), was accepted by experts and guidelines.

Nonetheless, the J-shape phenomenon should not be a reason for concern in the treatment of high BP [29]. The evidences in favor of the existence of the J-shape phenomenon came from cohort studies and from post hoc analyses of randomized controlled trials. These analyses of randomized trials compared the incidence of events in patients with low and high BP achieved during the trial, independently of the original randomized group. As in cohort studies, the apparent higher intensity of BP lowering may be secondary to the development of subclinical disease or frailty. These patients would benefit from further BP reduction [29]. A remarkable example is the CONSENSUS trial [23]. Patients randomized to the active treatment arm had baseline blood pressure of 118/74 mmHg, and received 18.4 mg per day on average of enalapril (target dose 40 mg per day). All-cause mortality was 40% lower in the active treatment group.

Recent meta-analyses have provided evidences against the existence of a clinically relevant J-shape phenomenon, particularly when they include trials with participants with cardiovascular disease [30], and compared more and less intensive strategies to lower BP [31]. This benefit was not so evident in a meta-analysis that excluded trials with participants with previous cardiovascular disease [32].

There is no trial comparing the effectiveness of drugs to prevent cardiovascular disease in patients with prehypertension without cardiovascular disease. The low absolute incidence of cardiovascular events in these individuals would require a very large sample to reject the null hypothesis. The SPRINT trial [33] provided an indirect evidence that individuals with prehypertension benefit from the attempt to reduce blood pressure below 120 mmHg. Despite the high cardiovascular risk, few participants of SPRINT had previous cardiovascular disease and none had diabetes or a previous cerebrovascular event. The consistent effectiveness in the prevention of more than 30% of cardiovascular events and all-cause mortality in individuals older than 75 years, free of cardiovascular disease and diabetes, was an impressive finding [34].

The first meta-analysis that maintained participants on their original group of randomization was recently published [35]. The lowest risk for cardiovascular disease and all-cause mortality was at BP between 120 and 124 mmHg (there was insufficient statistical power for participants with BP below 120 mmHg). Comparing with BP higher than 160 mmHg, participants that reached BP between 120 and 124 mmHg had a hazard ratio of 0.36 (95% CI, 0.26–0.51) for the incidence of major cardiovascular events.

Besides the evidences that drug treatment reduces the incidence of cardiovascular events, there are evidences that drug treatment reduces the incidence of hypertension and target organ damage.

Two randomized trials enrolled participants with high-normal BP to assess the efficacy of candesartan [36] and ramipril [37] to prevent the development of full hypertension. In the TROPHY study [36], there was a reduction of 66.3% in the incidence of hypertension in 2 years for patients treated with average doses of candesartan. In the study PHARAO, ramipril lowered by 34.4% the incidence of hypertension [37].

The PREVER-prevention trial evaluated the effectiveness of a combined pill of chlorthalidone (12.5 mg) with amiloride (2.5 mg) to prevent hypertension and target organ damage in patients with prehypertension [38]. During a follow-up of 18 months, individuals under diuretic treatment achieved 46% of prevention in the incidence of hypertension in comparison with participants allocated to placebo (Fig. 40.4, left). This trial was the first to demonstrate that drug treatment of individuals with prehypertension prevented the progression of target organ damage. Participants allocated to active treatment had reduction of left ventricular mass estimated by electrocardiogram (Fig. 40.4, right).

The evidence reviewed here supports the recommendation to initiate drug therapy in individuals with prehypertension who do not respond to lifestyle-change recommendations.

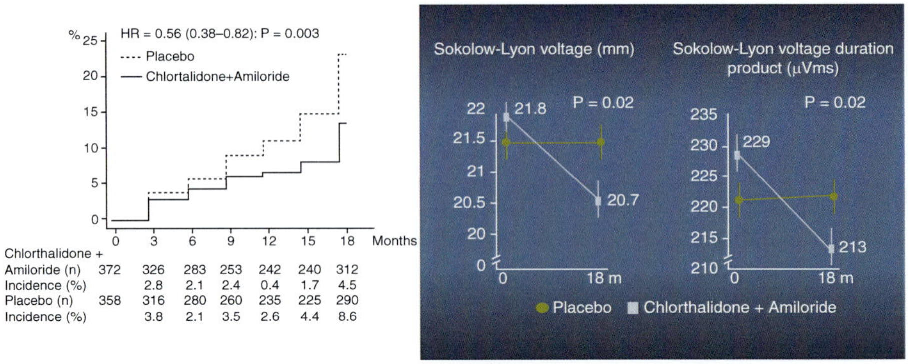

Fig. 40.4 The effect of diuretic treatment on the prevention of hypertension (*left*) and on ECG indexes of left ventricular hypertrophy (*right*) in patients with prehypertension: The PREVER-prevention trial (reprinted with permission from reference [38] (*left*) and [9] (*right*))

40.1.2 Drug Preference in the Management of Prehypertension

Placebo-controlled trials demonstrated the effectiveness of drug therapy to prevent cardiovascular events and death in patients with prehypertension and cardiovascular disease. Trials with patients with heart failure employed ACE inhibitors [20–23] and beta-blockers [39, 40]. The meta-analyses of several trials [25] demonstrated that beta-blockers are the more efficacious agents in patients recovered from myocardial infarction. Indapamide prevented the recurrence of stroke [19]. ACE inhibitors reduced the incidence of cardiovascular events in patients with chronic coronary artery disease and diabetes [16–18].

Diuretics were tested exclusively in the post-stroke trial [19], but are part of the management of heart failure. They were highly effective in preventing heart failure in several trials, such as the SHEP [41], HYVET [42], and ALLHAT [43] trials. Angiotensin-receptor blockers (ARB) were inert in the prevention of cardiovascular events in several trials of secondary prevention or in patients with high cardiovascular risk [44–50]. These and other studies were included in meta-analyses that failed to demonstrate the effectiveness of ARB in the prevention of myocardial infarction and all-cause mortality [51–56]. Moreover, three large positive trials of ARB were retracted because of fraud [57–59]. These evidences suggest that ARB are not the best option for patients with hypertension [60, 61] and therefore for patients with prehypertension.

In face of the absence of comparative trials of drugs in prehypertension, it is valid to consider the mechanism of action of drugs—biological plausibility—one of the criteria of causality of Bradford-Hill. The soundest hypothesis on pathogenesis of the elevation of BP with age is the maladaptation to chronic sodium overload [9]. Individuals with kidneys efficient to retain sodium need higher renal perfusion pressures to excrete the unnatural sodium overload, leading to chronic increase of BP.

Diuretics would circumvent this efficiency, promoting the excretion of sodium without increasing BP. Tobian, who proposed the concept of pressure natriuresis, demonstrated in an experiment that diuretics prevented the increase of blood pressure in experimental [62]. If diuretics were discovered nowadays, they would probably count with the sympathy of the pharmaceutical industry and doctors at all, and would be eventually pointed as the cure of hypertension.

Another postulate of Bradford-Hill—evidence from analogous models—supports the preference for diuretics in the management of prehypertension. The results of randomized controlled trials with patients with hypertension will likely be reproduced in prehypertension. Despite the worldwide preference for ARB and other groups, diuretics, in particular chlorthalidone, are the more effective agents in the prevention of many cardiovascular events in patients with hypertension. They were the only group that showed consistent superiority over placebo in the prevention of stroke, coronary heart disease, heart failure, cardiovascular and all-cause mortality, as demonstrated in one of the series of meta-analyses by Thomopoulos and coauthors [56]. The effect size was significantly higher with diuretics, even in events that were prevented by other classes. ARB, again, had the worst record, and did not avoid the occurrence of coronary heart disease, cardiovascular and all-cause mortality.

The largest and best-designed randomized clinical trial that compared four classes of drugs was the ALLHAT trial [63, 64]. The incidence of heart failure, identified by hospitalization or death, was 35% higher in patients treated with amlodipine compared to those treated with chlorthalidone. Several outcomes were more frequent in patients treated with lisinopril compared to patients treated with chlorthalidone: 15% more strokes, 10% more cardiovascular disease, and 19% more cases of heart failure, among others. Figure 40.5 shows the comparison of efficacy of chlorthalidone with amlodipine and with lisinopril in the prevention of major cardiovascular outcomes.

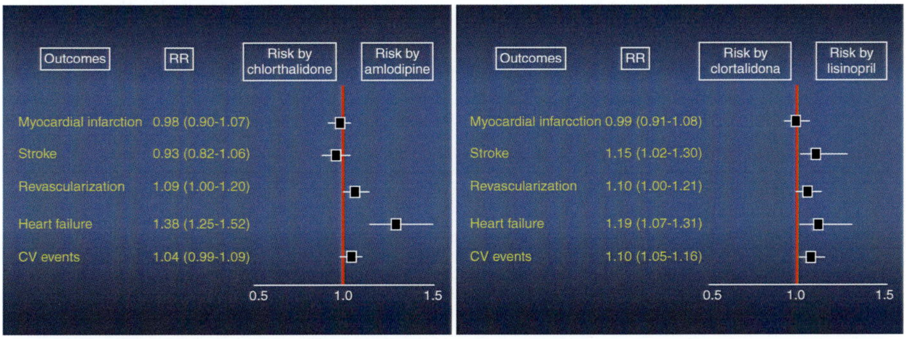

Fig. 40.5 Relative risk (RR) for incidence of cardiovascular outcomes in patients allocated to chlorthalidone and amlodipine (*left*) and chlorthalidone and lisinopril (*right*) in the ALLHAT study (reprinted with permission from [9])

40.1.3 Why Chlorthalidone Associated with Potassium-Sparing Diuretics?

There are no head-to-head trials with hard outcomes comparing different diuretics. An old network meta-analysis showed equivalence between different agents, but there were few studies available for comparison [65]. Another network meta-analysis included comparisons of chlorthalidone and hydrochlorothiazide with other active treatments, in addition to the comparison with placebo [66]. Chlorthalidone was superior to hydrochlorothiazide in the prevention of cardiovascular events despite the similar effects over office BP.

In a retrospective analysis of the MRFIT trial [67], the incidence of cardiovascular events was lower during the periods of treatment with chlorthalidone than hydrochlorothiazide.

Studies compared directly and indirectly the BP-lowering effectiveness of chlorthalidone, hydrochlorothiazide, and other diuretics. In a randomized crossover clinical trial, chlorthalidone (25 mg) had a more intense effect over nightly ambulatory blood pressure than hydrochlorothiazide (50 mg) [68]. In a meta-analysis of clinical trials with short duration [69], the BP-lowering efficacy of hydrochlorothiazide was equivalent to that of other antihypertensives only when used at a dose of 50 mg. Another meta-analysis compared the BP-lowering effect of hydrochlorothiazide in 26 trials, chlorthalidone in three trials, and bendroflumethiazide in one trial [70]. The estimated dose of each drug predicted to reduce systolic BP by 10 mm Hg was 1.4, 8.6, and 26.4 mg, respectively, for bendroflumethiazide, chlorthalidone, and hydrochlorothiazide. The only parallel, head-to-head comparison of chlorthalidone and hydrochlorothiazide was reported in a small randomized and parallel clinical trial with ABP monitoring [71]. There was higher BP-lowering effect of chlorthalidone (6.25 mg) than hydrochlorothiazide (12.5 mg) (Fig. 40.6).

Hypokalemia induced by diuretics may lessen their beneficial effect. In a post hoc analysis of the SHEP trial [72], participants of the active treatment arm with serum potassium below 3.5 mEq/L did not present the beneficial effects of chlorthalidone. The reduction in serum potassium also promotes a mild increase in

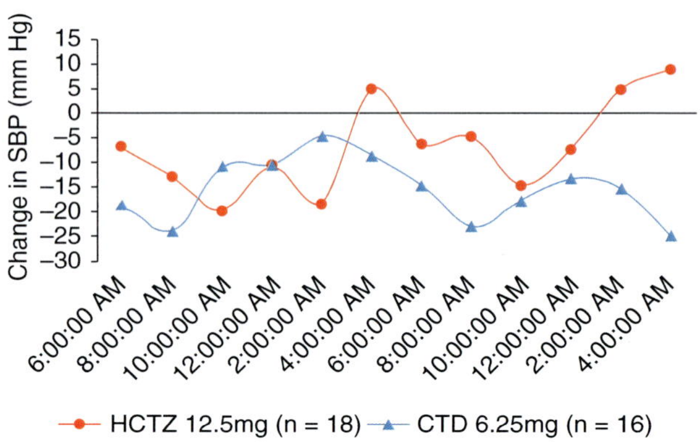

Fig. 40.6 Effects of chlorthalidone versus hydrochlorothiazide on 24 h ABP monitoring (Reprinted with permission from [71])

blood glucose observed in patients treated with thiazide diuretics [73]. Old uncontrolled studies identified the potassium-sparing effect of amiloride, triamterene, and spironolactone. Contemporaneous randomized trials confirmed this effect. We showed that amiloride corrected the serum levels of potassium in patients treated with hydrochlorothiazide in the same intensity than enalapril, and had a BP-lowering effect as well [74]. The elegant Pathway-3 trial showed that the prevention of loss of potassium with amiloride in patients treated with hydrochlorothiazide prevented the increase in serum glucose in a glucose tolerance test (Fig. 40.7), besides having a BP-lowering effect [75].

The association of hydrochlorothiazide with amiloride was compared with other options and placebo in two randomized controlled trials with hard outcomes. In the MRC trial of older adults, the association was superior to placebo and atenolol in the prevention of stroke, coronary events, and all cardiovascular events [76]. In the study INSIGHT [77], patients treated with this association had lower incidence of myocardial infarction and heart failure than participants treated with a long-acting preparation of nifedipine. The PREVER-prevention trial was the only that tested the association of chlorthalidone and amiloride over blood pressure and target organ damage [38].

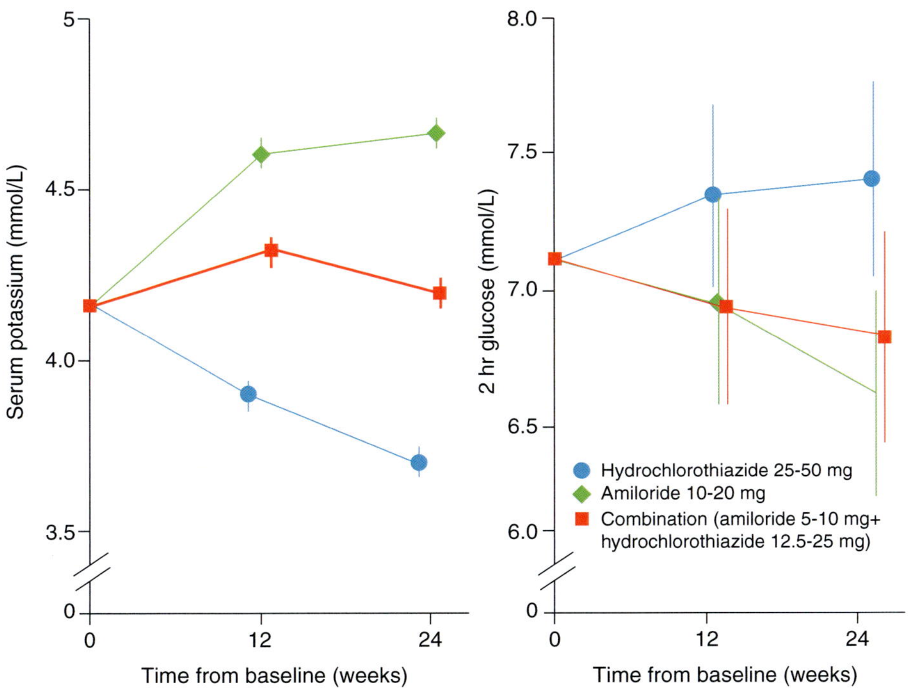

Fig. 40.7 Serum potassium (*left*) and 2-H glucose test (*right*) after treatment with hydrochlorothiazide, amiloride, and the combination of them (Reprinted with permission from [75])

Conclusion

The coming years will see a profound shift in the definition of hypertension. The focus on early diagnosis and treatment, not waiting for the full development of advanced stages of hypertension, may eradicate the consequences of high blood pressure. Chlorthalidone associated with amiloride may have preference to start treatment in individuals who do not respond to recommendations to change their lifestyle.

References

1. James PA, Oparil S, Carter BL, Cushman WC, Dennison-Himmelfarb C, Handler J, et al. 2014 evidence-based guideline for the management of high BP in adults: report from the panel members appointed to the Eighth Joint National Committee (JNC 8). JAMA. 2014;311:507–20.
2. Mancia G, Fagard R, Narkiewicz K, Redon J, Zanchetti A, Böhm M, et al. ESH/ESC Guidelines for the management of arterial hypertension. J Hypertens. 2013;2013(31):1281–57.
3. Qaseem A, Wilt TJ, Rich R, Humphrey LL, Frost J, Forciea MA, Clinical Guidelines Committee of the American College of Physicians and the Commission on Health of the Public and Science of the American Academy of Family Physicians. Pharmacologic treatment of hypertension in adults aged 60 years or older to higher versus lower blood pressure targets: a clinical practice guideline from the American College of Physicians and the American Academy of Family Physicians. Ann Intern Med. 2017;166(6):430–7.
4. Leung AA, Nerenberg K, Daskalopoulou SS, McBrien K, Zarnke KB, Dasgupta K, et al. Hypertension Canada's 2016 Canadian hypertension education program guidelines for blood pressure measurement, diagnosis, assessment of risk, prevention, and treatment of hypertension. Can J Cardiol. 2016;32(5):569–88.
5. Gabb GM, Mangoni AA, Anderson CS, Cowley D, Dowden JS, Golledge J, et al. Guideline for the diagnosis and management of hypertension in adults – 2016. Med J Aust. 2016;205(2):85–9.
6. Fisher JW. The diagnostic value of the sphygmomanometer in examinations for life insurance. JAMA. 1914;63:1752–4.
7. White P. Heart disease. 2nd ed. New York, NY: McMillan Co; 1937. p. 326.
8. Prospective Studies Collaboration. Age-specific relevance of usual BP to vascular mortality: a meta-analysis of individual data for one million adults in 61 prospective studies. Lancet. 2002;360:1903–13.
9. Fuchs FD. Essentials of hypertension. New york: Springer; 2017.
10. Moreira LB, Fuchs SC, Wiehe M, Gus M, Moraes RS, Fuchs FD. Incidence of hypertension in Porto Alegre, Brazil: a population-based study. J Hum Hypertens. 2008;22:48–50.
11. Takashima N, Ohkubo T, Miura K, Okamura T, Murakami Y, Fujiyoshi A, et al., NIPPON DATA80 Research Group. Long-term risk of BP values above normal for cardiovascular mortality: a 24-year observation of Japanese aged 30 to 92 years. J Hypertens. 2014;32:236–44.
12. Markus MR, Stritzke J, Lieb W, Mayer B, Luchner A, Döring A, et al. Implications of persistent prehypertension for ageing-related changes in left ventricular geometry and function: the MONICA/KORA Augsburg study. J Hypertens. 2008;26:2040–9.
13. Santos AB, Gupta DK, Bello NA, Gori M, Claggett B, Fuchs FD, et al. Prehypertension is associated with abnormalities of cardiac structure and function in the atherosclerosis risk in communities study. Am J Hypertens. 2016;29:568–74.
14. Hsu CY, McCulloch CE, Darbinian J, Go AS, Iribarren C. Elevated blood pressure and risk of end-stage renal disease in subjects without baseline kidney disease. Arch Intern Med. 2005;165(8):923–8.
15. Kanno A, Kikuya M, Ohkubo T, Hashimoto T, Satoh M, Hirose T, et al. Pre-hypertension as a significant predictor of chronic kidney disease in a general population: the Ohasama Study. Nephrol Dial Transplant. 2012;27:3218–23.

16. The Heart Outcomes Prevention Evaluation Study Investigators. Effects of ramipril on cardiovascular and microvascular outcomes in people with diabetes mellitus: results of the HOPE study and MICRO-HOPE substudy. Lancet. 2000;355:253–9.
17. The Heart Outcomes Prevention Evaluation Study Investigators. Effects of an angiotensin-converting-enzyme inhibitor, ramipril, on cardiovascular events in high-risk patients. N Engl J Med. 2000;342:145–53.
18. Fox KM, EURopean trial on reduction of cardiac events with Perindopril in stable coronary Artery disease Investigators. Efficacy of perindopril in reduction of cardiovascular events among patients with stable coronary artery disease: randomised, double-blind, placebo-controlled, multicentre trial (the EUROPA study). Lancet. 2003;362:782–8.
19. PROGRESS Collaborative Group. Randomised trial of a perindopril-based blood-pressure-lowering regimen among 6105 individuals with previous stroke or transient ischaemic attack. Lancet. 2001;358:1033–41.
20. The SOLVD investigators. Effect of enalapril on mortality and development of heart failure in asymptomatic patients with reduced left ventricular ejection fractions. N Engl J Med. 1992;327:685–91.
21. The SOLVD investigators. Effect of enalapril on survival in patients with reduced left ventricular ejection fractions and congestive heart failure. N Engl J Med. 1991;325:669–77.
22. Pfeffer MA, Braunwald E, Moye LA, Basta L, Brown EJ Jr, Cuddy TE, et al. Effect of captopril on mortality and morbidity in patients with left ventricular dysfunction after myocardial infarction: results of the survival and ventricular enlargement trial. The SAVE Investigators. N Eng J Med. 1992;327:669–77.
23. The CONSENSUS Trial Study Group. Effects of enalapril on mortality in severe congestive heart failure. N Engl J Med. 1987;316:1429–35.
24. Fuchs FD. Blood pressure-lowering drugs: essential therapy for some patients with normal BP. Expert Rev Cardiovasc Ther. 2004;2:771–5.
25. Law MR, Morris JK, Wald NJ. Use of BP lowering drugs in the prevention of cardiovascular disease: meta-analysis of 147 randomised trials in the context of expectations from prospective epidemiological studies. BMJ. 2009;338:B1665.
26. Thompson AM, Hu T, Eshelbrenner CL, Reynolds K, He J, Bazzano LA. Antihypertensive treatment and secondary prevention of cardiovascular disease events among persons without hypertension: a meta-analysis. JAMA. 2011;305:913–22.
27. Fuchs FD. Prehypertension: the rationale for early drug therapy. Cardiovasc Ther. 2010;28:339–43.
28. Fuchs FD, de Mello RB, Fuchs SC. Preventing the progression of prehypertension to hypertension: role of antihypertensives. Curr Hypertens Rep. 2015;17:505.
29. Fuchs FD, Fuchs SC. Blood pressure targets in the treatment of high BP: a reappraisal of the J-shaped phenomenon. J Hum Hypertens. 2014;28:80–4.
30. Ettehad D, Emdin CA, Kiran A, Anderson SG, Callender T, Emberson J, et al. Blood pressure lowering for prevention of cardiovascular disease and death: a systematic review and meta-analysis. Lancet. 2016;387:957–67.
31. Xie X, Atkins E, Lv J, Bennett A, Neal B, Ninomiya T, et al. Effects of intensive BP lowering on cardiovascular and renal outcomes: updated systematic review and meta-analysis. Lancet. 2016;387:43543.
32. Thomopoulos C, Parati G, Zanchetti A. Effects of BP lowering on outcome incidence in hypertension: 7. Effects of more vs. less intensive BP lowering and different achieved BP levels updated overview and meta-analyses of randomized trials. J Hypertens. 2016;34:613–22.
33. SPRINT Research Group, Wright JT Jr, Williamson JD, Whelton PK, Snyder JK, Sink KM, Rocco MV, et al. A randomized trial of intensive versus standard blood-pressure control. N Engl J Med. 2015;373:2103–16.
34. Williamson JD, Supiano MA, Applegate WB, Berlowitz DR, Campbell RC, Chertow GM, et al. Intensive vs standard BP control and cardiovascular disease outcomes in adults aged ≥75 years: a randomized clinical trial. JAMA. 2016;315:2673–82.

35. Bundy JD, Li C, Stuchlik P, Bu X, Kelly TN, Mills KT, et al. Systolic blood pressure reduction and risk of cardiovascular disease and mortality. JAMA Cardiol. 2017;2(7):775–81.
36. Julius S, Nesbitt SD, Egan BM, Weber MA, Michelson EL, Kaciroti N, et al., Trial of Preventing Hypertension (TROPHY) Study Investigators. Feasibility of treating prehypertension with an angiotensin-receptor blocker. N Engl J Med. 2006;354:1685–97.
37. Lüders S, Schrader J, Berger J, Unger T, Zidek W, Böhm M, et al., PHARAO Study Group. The PHARAO study: prevention of hypertension with the angiotensin-converting enzyme inhibitor ramipril in patients with high-normal BP – a prospective, randomized, controlled prevention trial of the German Hypertension League. J Hypertens. 2008;26:1487–96.
38. Fuchs SC, Poli-de-Figueiredo Carlos E, Figueiredo-Neto JA, Scala LC, Whelton PK, Mosele F, et al. Effectiveness of chlorthalidone plus amiloride for the prevention of hypertension: The PREVER PREVENTION Randomized Clinical Trial. J Am Heart Assoc. 2016;e004248:5.
39. MERIT-HF Study Group. Effect of metoprolol CR/XL in chronic heart failure. Metoprolol CR/XL Randomised Intervention Trial in Congestive Heart Failure (MERIT-HF). Lancet. 1999;353:2001–7.
40. Poole-Wilson PA, Swedberg K, Cleland JG, Di Lenarda A, Hanrath P, Komajda M, et al. Comparison of carvedilol and metoprolol on clinical outcomes in patients with chronic heart failure in the Carvedilol Or Metoprolol European Trial (COMET): randomised controlled trial. Lancet. 2003;362:7–13.
41. SHEP Cooperative Research Group. Prevention of stroke by antihypertensive drug treatment in older persons with isolated systolic hypertension. JAMA. 1991;265:3255–64.
42. Beckett NS, Peters R, Fletcher AE, Staessen JA, Liu L, Dumitrascu D, et al., HYVET Study Group. Treatment of hypertension in patients 80 years of age or older. N Engl J Med. 2008;358(18):1887–98.
43. Davis BR, Kostis JB, Simpson LM, Black HR, Cushman WC, Einhorn PT, et al. Heart failure with preserved and reduced left ventricular ejection fraction in the antihypertensive and lipid-lowering treatment to prevent heart attack trial. Circulation. 2008;118(22):2259–67.
44. Lithell H, Hansson L, Skoog I, Elmfeldt D, Hofman A, Olofsson B, et al., SCOPE Study Group. The Study on Cognition and Prognosis in the Elderly (SCOPE): principal results of a randomized double-blind intervention trial. J Hypertens. 2003;21(5):875–86.
45. Yusuf S, Sleight P, Anderson C, Teo K, Copland I, Ramos B, et al., TRANSCEND Investigators. Effects of the angiotensin-receptor blocker telmisartan on cardiovascular events in high-risk patients intolerant to angiotensin-converting enzyme inhibitors: a randomized controlled trial. Lancet. 2008;372(9644):1174–83.
46. Yusuf S, Diener HC, Sacco RL, Cotton D, Ôunpuu S, Lawton WA, et al., PRoFESS Study Group. Telmisartan to prevent recurrent stroke and cardiovascular events. N Engl J Med. 2008;359(12):1225–37.
47. McMurray JJ, Holman RR, Haffner SM, Bethel A, Holzhauer B, Hua TA, et al., NAVIGATOR Study Group. Effect of valsartan on the incidence of diabetes and cardiovascular events. N Engl J Med. 2010;362(16):1477–90.
48. Yusuf S, Healey JS, Pogue J, Chrolavicius S, Flather M, Hart RG, et al., ACTIVE I Investigators. Irbesartan in patients with atrial fibrillation. N Engl J Med. 2011;364(10):928–38.
49. Haller H, Ito S, Izzo JL Jr, Januszewicz A, Katayama S, Menne J, et al., ROADMAP Trial Investigators. Olmesartan for the delay or prevention of microalbuminuria in type 2 diabetes. N Engl J Med. 2011;364(10):907–17.
50. Imai E, Chan JC, Ito S, Yamasaki T, Kobayashi F, Haneda H, et al., ORIENT study investigators. Effects of olmesartan on renal and cardiovascular outcomes in type 2 diabetes with overt nephropathy: a multicentre, randomised, placebo-controlled study. Diabetologia. 2011;54(12):2978–86.
51. Bangalore S, Kumar S, Wetterslev J, Messerli FH. Angiotensin receptor blockers and risk of myocardial infarction: meta-analyses and trial sequential analyses of 147 020 patients from randomised trials. BMJ. 2011;342:d2234.
52. van Vark LC, Bertrand M, Akkerhuis KM, Brugts JJ, Fox K, Mourad JJ, Boersma E. Angiotensin-converting enzyme inhibitors reduce mortality in hypertension: a

meta-analysis of randomized clinical trials of renin-angiotensin-aldosterone system inhibitors involving 158 998 patients. Eur Heart J. 2012;33:2088–97.
53. Cheng J, Zhang W, Zhang X, Han F, Li X, He X, Li Q, Chen J. Effect of angiotensin-converting enzyme inhibitors and angiotensin II receptor blockers on all-cause mortality, cardiovascular deaths, and cardiovascular events in patients with diabetes mellitus: a meta-analysis. JAMA Intern Med. 2014;174:773–85.
54. Elgendy IY, Huo T, Chik V, Pepine CJ, Bavry AA. Efficacy and safety of angiotensin receptor blockers in older patients: a meta-analysis of randomized trials. Am J Hypertens. 2015;28:576–85.
55. Bangalore S, Fakheri R, Wandel S, Toklu B, Wandel J, Messerli FH. Renin angiotensin system inhibitors for patients with stable coronary artery disease without heart failure: systematic review and meta-analysis of randomized trials. BMJ. 2017;356:j4.
56. Thomopoulos C, Parati G, Zanchetti A. Effects of blood pressure lowering on outcome incidence in hypertension: 4. Effects of various classes of antihypertensive drugs--overview and meta-analyses. J Hypertens. 2015;33(2):195–211.
57. Retraction. Combination treatment of angiotensin-II receptor blocker and angiotensin-converting-enzyme inhibitor in non-diabetic renal disease (COOPERATE): a randomised controlled trial. Lancet. 2009;374(9697):1226.
58. Retraction. Valsartan in a Japanese population with hypertension and other cardiovascular disease (JIKEI HEART STUDY): a randomised, open-label, blinded endpoint morbidity-mortality study. Lancet. 2013;382(9895):843.
59. Retraction. Effects of valsartan on morbidity and mortality in uncontrolled hypertensive patients with high cardiovascular risks: KYOTO HEART Study. Eur Heart J. 2013;34(14):1023.
60. Fuchs FD. The role of angiotensin receptor blockers in the prevention of cardiovascular and renal disease: time for reassessment? Evid Based Med. 2013;18:44–7.
61. Fuchs FD, DiNicolantonio JJ. Angiotensin receptor blockers for prevention of cardiovascular disease: where does the evidence stand? Open Heart. 2015;2:e000236.
62. Tobian L. Evidence for Na-retaining humoral agents and vasoconstrictor humoral agents in hypertension-prone Dahl ‘S’ rats. Prevention of NaCl-induced hypertension in Dahl ‘S’ rats with thiazide. Horm Res. 1979;11(6):277–91.
63. ALLHAT Officers. Major cardiovascular events in hypertensive patients randomized to doxazosin vs. chlorthalidone. JAMA. 2000;283:1967–75.
64. The Antihypertensive and Lipid-Lowering Treatment to Prevent Heart Attack Trial (ALLHAT). Major outcomes in high-risk hypertensive patients randomized to angiotensin-converting enzyme inhibitor or calcium channel blocker vs diuretic. JAMA. 2002;288(23):2981–97.
65. Psaty BM, Lumley T, Furberg CD. Meta-analysis of health outcomes of chlorthalidone-based vs non-chlorthalidone-based low-dose diuretic therapies. JAMA. 2004;292(1):43–4.
66. Roush GC, Holford TR, Guddati AK. Chlorthalidone compared with hydrochlorothiazide in reducing cardiovascular events: systematic review and network meta-analyses. Hypertension. 2012;59:1110–7.
67. Dorsch MP, Gillespie BW, Erickson SR, Bleske BE, Weder AB. Chlorthalidone reduces cardiovascular events compared with hydrochlorothiazide: a retrospective cohort analysis. Hypertension. 2011;57:689–94.
68. Ernst ME, Carter BL, Goerdt CJ, Steffensmeier JJ, Phillips BB, Zimmerman MB, et al. Comparative antihypertensive effects of hydrochlorothiazide and chlorthalidone on ambulatory and office blood pressure. Hypertension. 2006;47(3):352–8.
69. Messerli FH, Makani H, Benjo A, Romero J, Alviar C, Bangalore S. Antihypertensive efficacy of hydrochlorothiazide as evaluated by ambulatory blood pressure monitoring: a meta-analysis of randomized trials. J Am Coll Cardiol. 2011;57(5):590–600.
70. Peterzan MA, Hardy R, Chaturvedi N, Hughes AD. Meta-analysis of dose-response relationships for hydrochlorothiazide, chlorthalidone, and bendroflumethiazide on blood pressure, serum potassium, and urate. Hypertension. 2012;59:1104–9.
71. Pareek AK, Messerli FH, Chandurkar NB, Dharmadhikari SK, Godbole AV, Kshirsagar PP, et al. Efficacy of low-dose chlorthalidone and hydrochlorothiazide as assessed by 24-h ambulatory blood pressure monitoring. J Am Coll Cardiol. 2016;67(4):379–89.

72. Franse LV, Pahor M, Di Bari M, Somes GW, Cushman WC, Applegate WB. Hypokalemia associated with diuretic use and cardiovascular events in the systolic hypertension in the elderly program. Hypertension. 2000;35(5):1025–30.
73. Zillich AJ, Garg J, Basu S, Bakris GL, Carter BL. Thiazide diuretics, potassium, and the development of diabetes: a quantitative review. Hypertension. 2006;48(2):1–6.
74. Guerrero P, Fuchs FD, Moreira LM, Martins VM, Bertoluci C, Fuchs SC, et al. Blood pressure-lowering efficacy of amiloride versus enalapril as add-on drugs in patients with uncontrolled blood pressure receiving hydrochlorothiazide. Clin Exp Hypertens. 2008;30(7):553–64.
75. Brown MJ, Williams B, Morant SV, Webb DJ, Caulfield MJ, Cruickshank JK, et al. Effect of amiloride, or amiloride plus hydrochlorothiazide, versus hydrochlorothiazide on glucose tolerance and blood pressure (PATHWAY-3): a parallel-group, double-blind randomised phase 4 trial. Lancet Diabetes Endocrinol. 2016;4(2):136–47.
76. MRC Working Party. Medical Research Council trial of treatment of hypertension in older adults: principal results. Br Med J. 1992;304:405–12.
77. Brown MJ, Palmer CR, Castaigne A, Leew PW, Mancia G, Rosenthal T, et al. Morbidity and mortality in patients randomised to double-blind treatment with a long-acting calcium-channel blocker or diuretic in the International Nifedipine GITS study (INSIGHT). Lancet. 2000;356(9227):366–72.

41 Prehypertension in the Era of Personalized Medicine in 2017

Pavel Hamet, Mounsif Haloui, and Johanne Tremblay

41.1 Introduction

Still a recent history, but with enough hope, hype and rebound that we may ask ourselves where *personalized medicine* is going. It actually started at the dawn of Modern medicine with Hippocrates of Kos in fourth century BC when he stated, "It is more important to know who has the disease than to know which disease the person has." The subsequent evolution is called *observational medicine* with Avicenna and Claude Bernard to William Osler and many others cumulating in *evidence based medicine* started in last century by epidemiologists-methodologists such as David Sacket, Suzan and Robert Fletcher and Elvan Feinstein. This is still a gold standard in setting guidelines based mainly on large randomized clinical trials. Several weaknesses include selection bias and limited relevance to "real-life" situations. Simply stated, any treatments which are effective as a mean in 10,000 subjects without significant side effects can and should be approved and used in everybody, based on evidence from trials. Only rarely the notion of prevalence of responders in a given population has been considered. And we have only recently realized that most medications used to treat common chronic diseases such as type 2 diabetes, hypertension, osteoporosis, depression, and others are effective in only 40 to 60 percent of subjects [1]. In current practice, we are adding successively different classes of medication until improvement or control without withdrawing the first or second drug that has no beneficial effect, resulting in high cost and potential unjustified side effects.

P. Hamet (✉) · M. Haloui · J. Tremblay
University of Montreal, Montreal, QC, Canada
e-mail: pavel.hamet@umontreal.ca

R. Zimlichman et al. (eds.), *Prehypertension and Cardiometabolic Syndrome*, Updates in Hypertension and Cardiovascular Protection,
https://doi.org/10.1007/978-3-319-75310-2_41

41.2 Initial Strategies in Genomic Exploration

Initial genomic-based selection of drugs came from candidate gene approaches for pharmacodynamics or metabolizing genes for pharmacokinetics [2]. This approach is clearly limited in prediction, prevention and therapy of complex, polygenic traits and diseases such as blood pressure and so-called "essential" hypertension, while in monogenic forms of hypertension (Liddle syndrome, glucocorticoid remediable hypertension, etc.) drugs are usually both causally selected and clearly different from our common armamatum in hypertension.

Several strategies are now aimed at improving the selection of initial medication based on individual's genomic profile, i.e., *personalized health care* [3]. This is now made possible by the complete sequencing of human genome and cataloging the list of millions of variants that exist between individuals, races and diseases and most importantly the capacity to detect on a single chip or array most of them being frequent (more than 1%) or rare (less than 1%) in populations. Currently, mathematical process of imputation that takes into account linkage disequilibrium of up to ten million variants can be derived from single chip or array. This progress is followed by a rapid decrease in costs that recently resulted in an explosion of Genome-wide Association Study (GWAS) results in hundreds of diseases and conditions.

41.3 GWAS, Their Benefits and Limits

The current (as of June 15, 2017) *GWAS catalogue* includes a list of single nucleotide polymorphisms (SNP) that are considered significantly associated at genome-wide (with $p < 5 \times 10^{-8}$) threshold with traits or diseases. For instance, 373 SNPs are associated with cardiovascular diseases and 487 are associated with cardiovascular traits; 1182 SNPs are associated to immune system and 682 for nervous system, etc. [4]. For hypertension, the initial results were deceiving, when the early GWAS of Welcome Trust, that was successful in reporting many significant associations for several diseases, claimed that no association could be observed for hypertension [5]. Careful reading of the methodology immediately pointed to an important problem: the phenotype, blood pressure was not recorded or not asked in subjects included in the "control sample" diluting any association gradient of such a frequent condition as hypertension with ~30% prevalence in general population. Only later, using carefully phenotyped cohorts and with over 120,000 subjects analyzed, 29 SNPs were found to be associated with hypertension [6]. More importantly, the SNPs that were associated with hypertension were also determining its main complications, such as stroke and coronary artery disease, but somewhat surprisingly they were not associated with chronic kidney disease or albuminuria. Potential reasons for this will be discussed below.

GWAS represented a significant investment in funding but yielded an impressive amount of data that improved the understanding of complex diseases, at least for its genetic component. The whole field was and is still frequently criticized for its lack of resolution of a significant proportion of effect size of a phenotype, typically limited to 5–10% of the variance being explained by the sum of its genetic variants.

Furthermore, it is argued that "clinical traditional risk factors" account for a similar degree of phenotype variance. We argue that this is not surprising considering how it is approached: when LDL, blood pressure, BMI, and diabetes are used as risk factors, they may even outperform the genomic determinants, since their intrinsic genomic and environmental determinants are both included in the model. Thus, genomic contribution to hypertension is also included in BMI, insulin resistance, and dyslipidemia. We have recently reflected on the importance to position of the *clinical utility* of genomics in an Editorial comment "Missing heritability or need for reality check of clinical utility in genomic testing?" [7].

Our argument is that if genomic determinants have a predictive power as good as "traditional risk factors," this is an important improvement, providing that the timing of genetic testing is correct since genomic determinants are present from conception, allowing for early detection even in pre-symptomatic phase, and prevention can be considered. For instance, about 40% of patients with T2D are at risk of developing diabetic nephropathy, yet there is no indication for use of medications such as angiotensin converting enzyme inhibitors (ACEi) in spite of their demonstrated ability to prevent the development of microalbuminuria in ADVANCE [8] and BENEDICT [9]. Problem is that the capacity to prevent is not in itself an indication to administer medications such as ACEi to all T2D patients. However, if a genetic risk can detect, say, 75% risk probability, it should be easy to apply health economic criteria and demonstrate whether a test, followed by medication, is of value in preventing/retarding a condition such as albuminuria, well demonstrated to be associated with cardiovascular mortality in a convincing set of over 600,000 subjects [10]. Moreover, it is conceivable that other conditions should be considered, since microalbuminuria may be present in prediabetes in context of metabolic syndrome and hyperuricemia [11].

It should be however expected that situation be rather complex for several reasons. It is recognized that in polygenic disorders the impact of the vast majority of individual alleles is very small. Furthermore, their localization is generally outside of transcribed sequence, in intronic segments and often completely outside of genes, where they are expected to impact transcription via interactions with regulatory elements. The latter situation made the causality of gene more difficult to unravel and the former results in requirement of multiple genomic components to be considered simultaneously. Figure 41.1 from our unpublished initial genomic exploration of ADVANCE trial (Hamet, Tremblay, ADVANCE 2017 unpublished data, see methods [12]) illustrate that when comparing "cases" of combined macro- and microvascular complications, which was the primary endpoint in ADVANCE with "controls," diabetic subjects from ADVANCE, without any complication at baseline or during the trial, recruited simply for long duration of T2D or old age, more than one hundred alleles of such genes involved in systems such as immunity, inflammation, and cardiovascular regulation are needed to separate cases from controls while respecting the direction of effect on risk and protection. It is apparent from this figure that while in the middle of the allelic distribution there is overlap between cases and controls, the first and last quarters can be clearly stratified into normal and risk groups.

An additional complication in allelic based prediction of outcomes is gene pleiotropy and gene × gene as well as gene × environment interactions. A good example

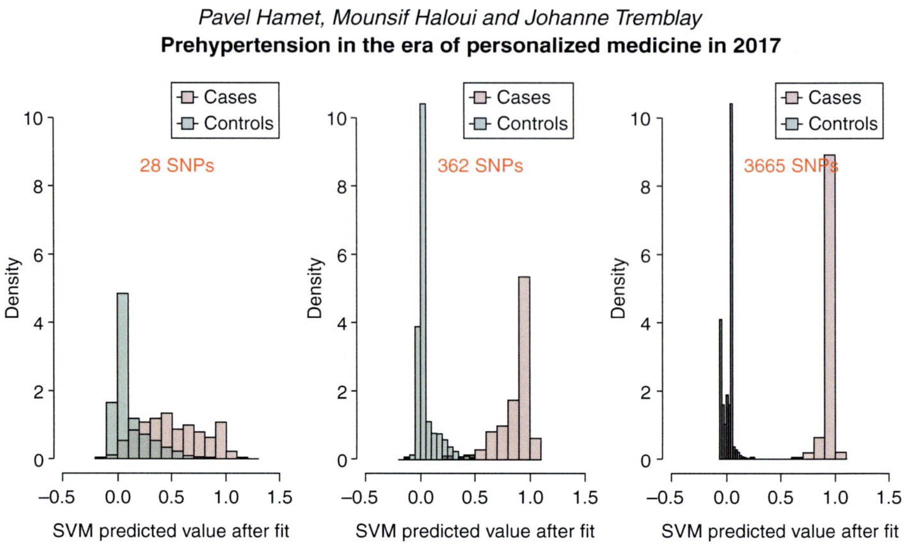

Fig. 41.1 Relationship between number of SNPs and prediction of MACE (major adverse cardiac events)

of the former is the uromodulin gene, well-studied gene in the pathogenesis of hypertension and kidney disease with frequent contradictory results. This gene is causally involved in an autosomal dominant form of disease of familial interstitial nephropathy, a rare genetic condition. Multiple mutations were described in affected families, all of them located in coding sequence leading to anomalies of gene product secretion or function. Distinct is its impact on glomerular filtration rate and even microalbuminuria, with abnormal urinary quantity of *uromodulin* which is the most abundant protein of urine (call initially the Tamm and Horsfall's mucoprotein) as a result of large set of SNPs, 95% of them being in noncoding regions of the gene as a part of polygenic determinants of glomerular filtration decline [13]. In this context, the impact of associated SNPs is an order of magnitude more important for nephropathy in nondiabetic and in diabetic patients. Yet an additional implication of the same gene appears to be in pathogenesis of hypertension, potentially implicating uric acid and sodium reabsorption [14].

An example of how environment can significantly alter our capacity to evaluate gene implication in a disease comes from the analysis of the impact of the FTO gene. We have initially described several metabolic phenotypes (including triglyceride levels, systolic and diastolic blood pressure and epinephrine levels clustering in a single locus on chromosome 16 in our set of 120 multigenerational founder families of French Canadians from North–East of Quebec, Canada [15, 16]. This locus has been later described and confirmed by many GWAS to be one of the most significant locus for obesity, and its association modulated by exercise [17]. Surprisingly, we were the only group that observed also hypertension determinants at that same locus [16]. Our further analyses revealed that the associations with systolic and diastolic blood pressures were significant only when and if antihypertensive medication was withdrawn during a period of 4 weeks, as we did in our study. This is a seminal observation, as antihypertensive agents are almost never withdrawn particularly not in studies of obesity and thus the important association with hypertension was completely overlooked (see Fig. 2. in 18).

From this observation, it is clear that presence of medication, which modifies significantly the studied phenotype, as an "environment," completely overshadows an existing genetic association.

41.4 AGE and SEX as Confounders

In most epidemiological studies, age and sex are considered significant covariates and results are usually appropriately adjusted for these confounders. Our studies in French-Canadian families demonstrated that in families with genetic predisposition to hypertension (increased familial prevalence comparatively to general population), its penetrance is early compared to general population, i.e., genetic impact accelerates penetrance, while the environmental impact occurs later and is determined by life-long environmental exposure. The effect size of this is not negligible: in hypertensive families the probability of being hypertensive, if your siblings are, is twice than that of general population after the age of 50, but it is tenfold higher if you are less than 25 year old. This fact is particularly relevant for "prehypertension" in young subjects, as we can expect a much stronger genetic impact, easier to detect even before clinical symptoms.

Age can be also counterintuitively involved: a set of genes, which include CASZ1 gene (intronic rs880315), were demonstrated to be associated with the increase of blood pressure in young subjects (20–40 years old) and the same allele is associated with decrease of systolic blood pressure after age of 60 [19]. This age-dependent physiological impact modification is attributable to epigenetics, since CASH1 gene is an important target of epigenetic modulation [20]. Somewhat analogous situation is present when comparing micro- and macro-vascular outcomes in ADVANCE trial. The incidence of macro-vascular events, MI, and stroke increases with age and diabetes duration, while the susceptibility to renal events is highest when diabetes is diagnosed before age of 50 and declines thereafter [21]. From those studies, it is evident that "adjustment for age," assuming unidirectional increase of risk with advancing age may obscure the reality. These considerations are relevant when studying different ages, and separation by age strata may offer superior approach to simple "adjustment."

Our studies in French-Canadian hypertensive families demonstrated age- and sex-specific loci. 25% of all loci were identified as age-specific and another 25% as sex-specific loci, i.e., not detectable when age or sex were adjusted. As an example we can mention a locus on chromosome 12 (rs575121) of which GG genotype is associated with highest blood pressure in man, while being associated with lowest blood pressure in women, though brothers and sisters within same families [22]. Winkler et al. [23] illustrated in a meta-analysis of over 300,000 subjects the importance of interactions of gene × sex × age effects where many loci of BMI were missed initially and revealed only by studying strata by age and sex separately.

41.5 Gene × Disease Interaction

The impact of the presence of disease "environment" may yet be another challenge in interpreting genomic determinants of an outcome. An example is the *RAB38* gene, demonstrated to be associated with albuminuria in diabetic but not in nondiabetic patients carrying the same rs649529T allele (present in 45% of subjects) [24]. Our studies of CKDGen demonstrated that in experimental diabetes the knockout of this gene had no effect on blood pressure or glycemia or albuminuria. When diabetes was induced experimentally by injections of streptozotocin, diabetes appeared in both control and K/O animals and only animals without *rab38* gene developed albuminuria within few weeks. It thus takes a gene defect and the presence of diabetes for phenotypic penetrance. We propose that the negative results of GWAS of hypertension may represent an analogous situation where renal impairment needs another risk factor in addition to hypertension to reveal its genetic associations [6].

41.6 Impact of Geoethnicity

The differences among different racial groups in prevalence of cardiovascular complications are well documented and recognized [25]. Thus, for instance renal impairment and stoke are known to be more prevalent in Asians than in Caucasians and their genetic bases is usually underlined by different alleles. We have recently demonstrated that differences in both phenotypic presentation and allelic structure are present between Caucasians of Balto-Slavic versus Germano-Celtic origins [12]. We have identified shared and distinct loci associated to age of onset of T2D in patients from these two geo-ethnic groups. PROX1/PROX1-AS1 genes (rs340841) has the highest effect size on age of onset of T2D. SNP rs340841 homozygous CC genotype is associated with 2 years earlier onset of T2D in Slavic patients living in either Slavic or Celtic countries. This locus is also associated with GFR decline in Slavic, with macroalbuminuria and hypertension in all ADVANCE subjects of Caucasian origin and with Interleukin-6 levels at baseline. In a recent literature search, we found that PROX1 gene has been associated with abnormal glucose metabolism and risk of diabetes with variations depending on ethnicity. We concluded that fine granularity of distinction in geo-ethnic background assists in resolution of clinically relevant genetic contribution to cardiovascular complication in T2D.

41.7 *Genetic Risk Scores* (GRS) and Clinical Utility

Major challenge in recognition of clinical utility of personalized genomics is the widespread recognition of limited impact of individual alleles as discussed above.

Novel paradigm uses an algorithm that combines several alleles according to diverse models. Usually alleles are simply added into a genetic risk score (GRS), but improvement is often demonstrated when weighted for their effect size, or beta values. The difference in number of alleles incorporated into a GRS for a specific phenotype is compensated by correction for the number of alleles used. From initial 5 to 10 allele reports, recent publications use poly-alleles, into so-called polyGRS with hundreds or even thousands of alleles. A major departure from dogma of significance in genomics, following Bonferroni genome-wide significance of 5×10^{-8}, is being recently replaced by inclusion of nominally significant SNPs, with same direction of risk, providing that this is resulting in improvement of C-statistic or even better net reclassification index. Initially, this approach was applied in exploration of shared genomic impact for a phenotype. Thus, Holliday et al. [26] was able to demonstrate the relationship between kidney function and atherosclerotic stroke with polygenic GRS of decline of eGFR and increase of albumin/creatinine ratio sharing genomic determinants with specific types of stroke.

An important study from heath economic point of view was the exploration of statin administration as a function of genetic risk score of myocardial infarction. Using data from the largest statin trials, 27 genome-wide significant SNPs were included in a weighted GRS and subjects were stratified into low, intermediate, and high GRS groups of incident and recurrent coronary heart disease outcome categories. The study demonstrated a significant gradient in relative risk reduction from 13, 29 to 48% in these categories and absolute risk reduction resulted in threefold gradient of number needed to treat (NNT) between categories [27]. The rationale for detecting this high risk category by GRS and not simply by cholesterol levels is thus open to exploration.

Another study of significant health economic impact is the much discussed relevance of total prostatectomy. Prostate cancer is frequently neglected for its "benign outcomes," yet it is the number one killer in males. Nora Pashayan [28] developed a GRS for prostate cancer and demonstrated the potential of its application: in low risk score category, 50% of interventions appeared unnecessary, but this number decreased to only 2% in patients with high GRS. Indeed, GRS require validation in additional cohorts, but with such potential, are clearly deserving attention.

Table 41.1 included here illustrates some examples of clinical utility of GRS and polyGRS. Generally, AUC and impact on stratification (NRI) improved with increasing number of SNPs, yet we have observed in literature that the limit is phenotype-specific and related to biological relationship of genomic regions as well as requiring at least minimal evidence of phenotype/genotype association.

The future is to develop simple algorithms to execute and interpret polyGRS, test them prospectively for their clinical utility and assess their health economic value. We are not there yet, but we can say with confidence that when appropriately targeted for time and disease, polyGRS are solid future values for treatment decisions with strong accent on prevention.

Table 41.1 Examples of five studies evaluating the relationship between unweighted, weighted, and polygenetic risk scores and some cardiovascular outcomes or traits which proved their clinical utility

Reference (first author, year)[a]	Outcome/Trait[b]	Sample[c]	Source of SNPs for GRS	GRS (n of SNPs, Weights)	Effect estimate[d]	Clinical utility[d]
Läll et al., 2017 [29]	Incident T2D, CVD mortality, all-cause mortality	1181 T2D cases 9092 controls	T2D, multiple sources [30]	65, 600, 2100, W 800, 1000, 1400, dW	For GRS quintile 5 vs. 1 I-T2D, HR = 3.45 (2.31–5.17) For GRS quintile 5 vs. 1–4 I-T2D, HR = 1.95 (1.52–2.51) CVD mortality, HR = 1.27 (1.10–1.64) All-cause mortality, HR = 1.14 (1.02–1.27)	ΔC index = 0.012 (p (LRT) = 2.01×10^{-11}) NRI for T2D = 0.324
Belsky et al., 2013 [31]	Obesity-related phenotypes, mortality	ARIC study 10,745 participants 55% female 77% white 23% AA	BMI, obesity, weight, waist circumference, adiposity (16 sources) [31]	32, uW, W	White ARIC: Obesity increase by 19.35% per uW-GRS SD ($p < 10^{-18}$) Obesity increase by 20.51% per W-GRS SD ($p < 10^{-18}$) AA ARIC: Obesity increase by 3.54% per uW-GRS SD ($p = 0.059$) Obesity increase by 4.92% per W-GRS SD ($p = 0.017$) Mortality, HR = 1.12 (1.04–1.15)	White ARIC: ΔAUC = 0.048 (0.031–0.066), $p<10^{-7}$ IDI = 0.006, $p = 7.81 \times 10^{-13}$ AA ARIC: ΔAUC = 0.005 (0.005–0.015), $p = 0.30$ IDI = 0.001, $p = 0.055$

Reference (first author, year)[a]	Outcome/Trait[b]	Sample[c]	Source of SNPs for GRS	GRS (n of SNPs, Weights)	Effect estimate[d]	Clinical utility[d]
Ehret et al., 2011 [6]	Hypertension/SBP, DBP	23,294 (women)	SBP, DBP	29, W	OR = 1.23 (1.19–1.28) per GRS SD SBP: $\beta = 1.65$ (0.10) mmHg per GRS SD ($p = 6.5 \times 10^{-63}$) DBP: $\beta = 1.06$ (0.07) mmHg per GRS SD ($p = 8.4 \times 10^{-57}$)	
Hachiya et al., 2017 [32]	Incident ischemic stroke (I-IS) Large-vessel disease (LVD), small-vessel disease (SVD), cardioembolic stroke (CE)	3 sets from BioBank Japan project (derivative dataset, 26,470 controls & 13,214 IS) KyushuU & JPJM (predictive ability datasets, 1433 controls & 1433 IS)	IS, multiple sources (see supplementary Tables I & II from reference [32]	5, W 12, 49, 565 …537,999 polyGRS	For WGRS quintile 5 vs. 1 KyushuU: I-IS, OR = 1.17 (0.89–1.54) $p = 0.313$ JPJM: I-IS, OR = 1.45 (0.87–2.42) $p = 0.172$ For PolyGRS quintile 5 vs. 1 KyushuU: I-IS, OR = 1.75 (1.33–2.31) $p < 0.001$ JPJM: I-IS, OR = 1.99 (1.19–3.33) $p = 0.033$ I-IS, OR = 1.17 (1.08–1.27) per PolyGRS SD, $p < 0.001$ For KyushuU, quintile 5 vs. 1 LVD, OR = 1.26 (1.09–1.47) per PolyGRS SD, $p = 0.002$ SVD, OR = 1.18 (1.04–1.34) per PolyGRS SD, $p = 0.012$ CE, OR = 1.28 (1.00–1.62) per PolyGRS SD, $p = 0.047$	For polyGRS, KyushuU, IS: ΔCindex = 0.045, $p = 0.007$ NRI = 0.176 (0.095–0.262), $p < 0.001$ IDI = 0.008 (0.004–0.012), $p < 0.001$ LVD: ΔCindex = 0.054, $p = 0.066$ NRI = 0.206 (0.060–0.351), $p = 0.006$ IDI = 0.013 (0.004–0.021), $p = 0.004$ SVD: ΔCindex = 0.049, $p = 0.044$ NRI = 0.185 (0.060–0.310), $p = 0.003$ IDI = 0.007 (0.002–0.012), $p = 0.011$ CE: Not significant

(continued)

Table 41.1 (contiued)

Reference (first author, year)[a]	Outcome/Trait[b]	Sample[c]	Source of SNPs for GRS	GRS (n of SNPs, Weights)	Effect estimate[d]	Clinical utility[d]
Van Setten et al., 2015 [33]	Coronary artery calcification	2599	T2D [30], CAD/MI [34], LDL [35], TC [35], BMI [36]	T2D: 55, W CAD/MI: 8918, W LDL: 58, W TC: 72, W BMI: 31, W	PVE = 0.25% for GRS_{T2D} ($p = 4.0 \times 10^{-2}$) PVE = 1.50% for $GRS_{CAD/MI}$ ($p = 1.6 \times 10^{-11}$) PVE = 0.25% for GRS_{LDL} ($p = 1.6 \times 10^{-3}$) PVE = 0.15% for GRS_{TC} ($p = 8.5 \times 10^{-3}$) PVE = 0.25% for GRS_{BMI} ($p = 2.6 \times 10^{-2}$)	

SNP single nucleotide polymorphism, *GRS* genetic risk score, *W* weighted, *uW* unweighted, *dW* double weighted, *PolyGRS* Poly genetic risk score, *Δ* change, *LRT* Likelihood ratio test, *NRI* net reclassification improvement index, *SD* standard deviation, *AUC* area under the receiver-operator curve, *IDI* integrated discrimination index, *HR* hazard ratio, *CVD* cardiovascular disease, *I-T2D* incident type 2 diabetes, *BMI* body mass index, *SBP* systolic blood pressure, *DBP* diastolic blood pressure, *AA* African American, *JPJM* Japan public health center and Japan multi-institutional collaborative cohort studies, *KyushuU* Kyushu university

[a]Only selected GRS analyses are reported

[b]Cardiovascular outcome or specific trait tested for association with GRS

[c]Refers to the sample used for evaluating the association between CVD outcome or trait and GRS

[d]The adjustment variables are specific for each outcome/trait (see appropriate reference)

Acknowledgments The authors would like to acknowledge the participation of thousands of subjects in their studies, their collaborations with colleagues from ADVANCE trial, CKDGen Consortium and Clinpradia studies and financial help from public sources (Genome Quebec, CIHR, MESI) as well as private partners Les Laboratoires Servier and Servier Canada, Omnimed and Affymetrix, Medpharmgene Inc and OPTI-THERA Inc.

References

1. Spear BB, Heath-Chiozzi M, Huff J. Clinical application of pharmacogenetics. Trends Mol Med. 2001;7(5):201–4.
2. Motulsky AG, King MC. The great adventure of an American human geneticist. Annu Rev Genomics Hum Genet. 2016;17:1–15.
3. Topol EJ. Individualized medicine from prewomb to tomb. Cell. 2014;157(1):241–53.
4. Hindorff LA, MacArthur J, Morales J, Junkins HA, Hall PN, Klemm AK, Manolio TA. A catalog of published genome-wide association studies. http://www.genome.gov/gwastudies/. Accessed 15 June 2017.
5. Burton PR, Clayton DG, Cardon LR, Craddock N, Deloukas P, Duncanson A, Kwiatkowski DP, McCarthy MI, Ouwehand WH, Samani NJ, Todd JA, Donnelly P, Barrett JC, Burton PR, Davison D, Donnelly P, Easton D, Evans D, Leung HT, Marchini JL, Morris AP, Spencer CC, Tobin MD, Cardon LR, Clayton DG, Attwood AP, Boorman JP, Cant B, Everson U, Hussey JM, Jolley JD, Knight AS, Koch K, Meech E, Nutland S, Prowse CV, Stevens HE, Taylor NC, Walters GR, Walker NM, Watkins NA, Winzer T, Todd JA, Ouwehand WH, Jones RW, McArdle WL, Ring SM, Strachan DP, Pembrey M, Breen G, St Clair D, Caesar S, Gordon-Smith K, Jones L, Fraser C, Green EK, Grozeva D, Hamshere ML, Holmans PA, Jones IR, Kirov G, Moskvina V, Nikolov I, O'Donovan MC, Owen MJ, Craddock N, Collier DA, Elkin A, Farmer A, Williamson R, McGuffin P, Young AH, Ferrier IN, Ball SG, Balmforth AJ, Barrett JH, Bishop DT, Iles MM, Maqbool A, Yuldasheva N, Hall AS, Braund PS, Burton PR, Dixon RJ, Mangino M, Suzanne S, Tobin MD, Thompson JR, Samani NJ, Bredin F, Tremelling M, Parkes M, Drummond H, Lees CW, Nimmo ER, Satsangi J, Fisher SA, Forbes A, Lewis CM, Onnie CM, Prescott NJ, Sanderson J, Mathew CG, Barbour J, Mohiuddin MK, Todhunter CE, Mansfield JC, Ahmad T, Cummings FR, Jewell DP, Webster J, Brown MJ, Clayton DG, Lathrop GM, Connell J, Dominczak A, Samani NJ, Marcano CA, Burke B, Dobson R, Gungadoo J, Lee KL, Munroe PB, Newhouse SJ, Onipinla A, Wallace C, Xue M, Caulfield M, Farrall M, Barton A, Bruce IN, Donovan H, Eyre S, Gilbert PD, Hider SL, Hinks AM, John SL, Potter C, Silman AJ, Symmmons DP, Thomson W, Worthington J, Clayton DG, Dunger DB, Nutland S, Stevens HE, Walker NM, Widmer B, Todd JA, Frayling TA, Freathy RM, Lango H, Perry JR, Shields BM, Weedon MN, Hattersley AT, Hitman GA, Walker M, Elliott KS, Groves CJ, Lindgren CM, Rayner NW, Timpson NJ, Zeggini E, McCarthy MI, Newport M, Sirugo G, Lyons E, Vannberg F, Hill AV, Bradbury LA, Farrar C, Pointon JJ, Wordsworth P, Brown MA, Franklyn JA, Heward JM, Simmonds MJ, Gough SC, Seal S, Stratton MR, Rahman N, Ban M, Goris A, Sawcer SJ, Compston A, Conway D, Jallow M, Newport M, Sirugo G, Rockett KA, Kwiatowski DP, Bumpstead SJ, Chaney A, Downes K, Ghori MJ, Gwilliam R, Hunt SE, Inouye M, Keniry A, King E, McGinnis R, Potter S, Ravindrarajah R, Whittaker P, Widden C, Withers D, Deloukas P, Leung HT, Nutland S, Stevens HE, Walker NM, Todd JA, Easton D, Clayton DG, Burton PR, Tobin MD, Barrett JC, Evans D, Morris AP, Cardon LR, Cardin NJ, Davison D, Ferreira T, Pereira-Gale J, Hallgrimsdottir IB, Howie BN, Marchini JL, Spencer CC, Su Z, Teo YY, Vukcevic D, Donnelly P, Bentley D, Brown MA, Gordon LR, Caulfield M, Clayton DG, Compston A, Craddock N, Deloukas P, Donnelly P, Farrall M, Gough SC, Hall AS, Hattersley AT, Hill AV, Kwiatkowski DP, Mathew C, McCarthy MI, Ouwehand WH, Parkes M, Pembrey M, Rahman N, Samani NJ, Stratton MR, Todd JA, Worthington J. Genome-wide association study of 14,000 cases of seven common diseases and 3,000 shared controls Wellcome Trust Case Control Consortium. Nature. 2007;447(7145):661–78.

6. International Consortium for Blood Pressure Genome-Wide Association Studies, Ehret GB, Munroe PB, Rice KM, Bochud M, Johnson AD, Chasman DI, Smith AV, Tobin MD, Verwoert GC, Hwang SJ, Pihur V, Vollenweider P, O'Reilly PF, Amin N, Bragg-Gresham JL, Teumer A, Glazer NL, Launer L, Zhao JH, Aulchenko Y, Heath S, Sõber S, Parsa A, Luan J, Arora P, Dehghan A, Zhang F, Lucas G, Hicks AA, Jackson AU, Peden JF, Tanaka T, Wild SH, Rudan I, Igl W, Milaneschi Y, Parker AN, Fava C, Chambers JC, Fox ER, Kumari M, Go MJ, van der Harst P, Kao WH, Sjögren M, Vinay DG, Alexander M, Tabara Y, Shaw-Hawkins S, Whincup PH, Liu Y, Shi G, Kuusisto J, Tayo B, Seielstad M, Sim X, Nguyen KD, Lehtimäki T, Matullo G, Wu Y, Gaunt TR, Onland-Moret NC, Cooper MN, Platou CG, Org E, Hardy R, Dahgam S, Palmen J, Vitart V, Braund PS, Kuznetsova T, Uiterwaal CS, Adeyemo A, Palmas W, Campbell H, Ludwig B, Tomaszewski M, Tzoulaki I, Palmer ND, CARDIoGRAM Consortium, CKDGen Consortium, KidneyGen Consortium, EchoGen Consortium, CHARGE-HF Consortium, Aspelund T, Garcia M, Chang YP, O'Connell JR, Steinle NI, Grobbee DE, Arking DE, Kardia SL, Morrison AC, Hernandez D, Najjar S, McArdle WL, Hadley D, Brown MJ, Connell JM, Hingorani AD, Day IN, Lawlor DA, Beilby JP, Lawrence RW, Clarke R, Hopewell JC, Ongen H, Dreisbach AW, Li Y, Young JH, Bis JC, Kähönen M, Viikari J, Adair LS, Lee NR, Chen MH, Olden M, Pattaro C, Bolton JA, Köttgen A, Bergmann S, Mooser V, Chaturvedi N, Frayling TM, Islam M, Jafar TH, Erdmann J, Kulkarni SR, Bornstein SR, Grässler J, Groop L, Voight BF, Kettunen J, Howard P, Taylor A, Guarrera S, Ricceri F, Emilsson V, Plump A, Barroso I, Khaw KT, Weder AB, Hunt SC, Sun YV, Bergman RN, Collins FS, Bonnycastle LL, Scott LJ, Stringham HM, Peltonen L, Perola M, Vartiainen E, Brand SM, Staessen JA, Wang TJ, Burton PR, Soler Artigas M, Dong Y, Snieder H, Wang X, Zhu H, Lohman KK, Rudock ME, Heckbert SR, Smith NL, Wiggins KL, Doumatey A, Shriner D, Veldre G, Viigimaa M, Kinra S, Prabhakaran D, Tripathy V, Langefeld CD, Rosengren A, Thelle DS, Corsi AM, Singleton A, Forrester T, Hilton G, McKenzie CA, Salako T, Iwai N, Kita Y, Ogihara T, Ohkubo T, Okamura T, Ueshima H, Umemura S, Eyheramendy S, Meitinger T, Wichmann HE, Cho YS, Kim HL, Lee JY, Scott J, Sehmi JS, Zhang W, Hedblad B, Nilsson P, Smith GD, Wong A, Narisu N, Stančáková A, Raffel LJ, Yao J, Kathiresan S, O'Donnell CJ, Schwartz SM, Ikram MA, Longstreth WT Jr, Mosley TH, Seshadri S, Shrine NR, Wain LV, Morken MA, Swift AJ, Laitinen J, Prokopenko I, Zitting P, Cooper JA, Humphries SE, Danesh J, Rasheed A, Goel A, Hamsten A, Watkins H, Bakker SJ, van Gilst WH, Janipalli CS, Mani KR, Yajnik CS, Hofman A, Mattace-Raso FU, Oostra BA, Demirkan A, Isaacs A, Rivadeneira F, Lakatta EG, Orru M, Scuteri A, Ala-Korpela M, Kangas AJ, Lyytikäinen LP, Soininen P, Tukiainen T, Würtz P, Ong RT, Dörr M, Kroemer HK, Völker U, Völzke H, Galan P, Hercberg S, Lathrop M, Zelenika D, Deloukas P, Mangino M, Spector TD, Zhai G, Meschia JF, Nalls MA, Sharma P, Terzic J, Kumar MV, Denniff M, Zukowska-Szczechowska E, Wagenknecht LE, Fowkes FG, Charchar FJ, Schwarz PE, Hayward C, Guo X, Rotimi C, Bots ML, Brand E, Samani NJ, Polasek O, Talmud PJ, Nyberg F, Kuh D, Laan M, Hveem K, Palmer LJ, van der Schouw YT, Casas JP, Mohlke KL, Vineis P, Raitakari O, Ganesh SK, Wong TY, Tai ES, Cooper RS, Laakso M, Rao DC, Harris TB, Morris RW, Dominiczak AF, Kivimaki M, Marmot MG, Miki T, Saleheen D, Chandak GR, Coresh J, Navis G, Salomaa V, Han BG, Zhu X, Kooner JS, Melander O, Ridker PM, Bandinelli S, Gyllensten UB, Wright AF, Wilson JF, Ferrucci L, Farrall M, Tuomilehto J, Pramstaller PP, Elosua R, Soranzo N, Sijbrands EJ, Altshuler D, Loos RJ, Shuldiner AR, Gieger C, Meneton P, Uitterlinden AG, Wareham NJ, Gudnason V, Rotter JI, Rettig R, Uda M, Strachan DP, Witteman JC, Hartikainen AL, Beckmann JS, Boerwinkle E, Vasan RS, Boehnke M, Larson MG, Järvelin MR, Psaty BM, Abecasis GR, Chakravarti A, Elliott P, van Duijn CM, Newton-Cheh C, Levy D, Caulfield MJ, Johnson T. Genetic variants in novel pathways influence blood pressure and cardiovascular disease risk. Nature. 2011;478(7367):103–9.
7. Hamet P. Missing heritability or need for reality check of clinical utility in genomic testing? J Hypertens. 2014;32(7):1395–6.
8. de Galan BE, Perkovic V, Ninomiya T, Pillai A, Patel A, Cass A, Neal B, Poulter N, Harrap S, Mogensen CE, Cooper M, Marre M, Williams B, Hamet P, Mancia G, Woodward M, Glasziou P, Grobbee DE, MacMahon S, Chalmers J, ADVANCE Collaborative Group. Lowering blood pressure reduces renal events in type 2 diabetes. J Am Soc Nephrol. 2009;20(4):883–92.

9. Ruggenenti P, Perna A, Ganeva M, Ene-Iordache B, Remuzzi G, BENEDICT Study Group. Impact of blood pressure control and angiotensin-converting enzyme inhibitor therapy on new-onset microalbuminuria in type 2 diabetes: a post hoc analysis of the BENEDICT trial. J Am Soc Nephrol. 2006;17(12):3472–81.
10. Matsushita K, Coresh J, Sang Y, Chalmers J, Fox C, Guallar E, Jafar T, Jassal SK, Landman GW, Muntner P, Roderick P, Sairenchi T, Schöttker B, Shankar A, Shlipak M, Tonelli M, Townend J, van Zuilen A, Yamagishi K, Yamashita K, Gansevoort R, Sarnak M, Warnock DG, Woodward M, Ärnlöv J, CKD Prognosis Consortium. Estimated glomerular filtration rate and albuminuria for prediction of cardiovascular outcomes: a collaborative meta-analysis of individual participant data. Lancet Diabetes Endocrinol. 2015;3(7):514–25.
11. Krajcoviechova A, Tremblay J, Wohlfahrt P, Bruthans J, Tahir MR, Hamet P, Cifkova R. The impact of blood pressure and visceral adiposity on the association of serum uric acid with albuminuria. Am J Hypertens. 2016;29:1335–42.
12. Hamet P, Haloui M, Harvey F, Marois-Blanchet FC, Sylvestre MP, Tahir MR, Simon PH, Kanzki BS, Raelson J, Long C, Chalmers J, Woodward M, Marre M, Harrap S, Tremblay J. PROX1 gene CC genotype as a major determinant of early onset of type 2 diabetes in Slavic participants from ADVANCE study. J Hypertens. 2017;35(Suppl 1):S24–32.
13. Gorski M, Tin A, Garnaas M, McMahon GM, Chu AY, Tayo BO, Pattaro C, Teumer A, Chasman DI, Chalmers J, Hamet P, Tremblay J, Woodward M, Aspelund T, Eiriksdottir G, Gudnason V, Harris TB, Launer LJ, Smith AV, Mitchell BD, O'Connell JR, Shuldiner AR, Coresh J, Li M, Freudenberger P, Hofer E, Schmidt H, Schmidt R, Holliday EG, Mitchell P, Wang JJ, de Boer IH, Li G, Siscovick DS, Kutalik Z, Corre T, Vollenweider P, Waeber G, Gupta J, Kanetsky PA, Hwang SJ, Olden M, Yang Q, de Andrade M, Atkinson EJ, Kardia SL, Turner ST, Stafford JM, Ding J, Liu Y, Barlassina C, Cusi D, Salvi E, Staessen JA, Ridker PM, Grallert H, Meisinger C, Müller-Nurasyid M, Krämer BK, Kramer H, Rosas SE, Nolte IM, Penninx BW, Snieder H, Fabiola Del Greco M, Franke A, Nöthlings U, Lieb W, Bakker SJ, Gansevoort RT, van der Harst P, Dehghan A, Franco OH, Hofman A, Rivadeneira F, Sedaghat S, Uitterlinden AG, Coassin S, Haun M, Kollerits B, Kronenberg F, Paulweber B, Aumann N, Endlich K, Pietzner M, Völker U, Rettig R, Chouraki V, Helmer C, Lambert JC, Metzger M, Stengel B, Lehtimäki T, Lyytikäinen LP, Raitakari O, Johnson A, Parsa A, Bochud M, Heid IM, Goessling W, Köttgen A, Kao WH, Fox CS, Böger CA. Genome-wide association study of kidney function decline in individuals of European descent. Kidney Int. 2015;87(5):1017–29.
14. Graham LA, Padmanabhan S, Fraser NJ, Kumar S, Bates JM, Raffi HS, Welsh P, Beattie W, Hao S, Leh S, Hultstrom M, Ferreri NR, Dominiczak AF, Graham D, McBride MW. Validation of uromodulin as a candidate gene for human essential hypertension. Hypertension. 2014;63(3):551–8.
15. Hamet P, Merlo E, Seda O, Broeckel U, Tremblay J, Kaldunski M, Gaudet D, Bouchard G, Deslauriers B, Gagnon F, Antoniol G, Pausová Z, Labuda M, Jomphe M, Gossard F, Tremblay G, Kirova R, Tonellato P, Orlov SN, Pintos J, Platko J, Hudson TJ, Rioux JD, Kotchen TA, Cowley AW Jr. Quantitative founder-effect analysis of French Canadian families identifies specific loci contributing to metabolic phenotypes of hypertension. Am J Hum Genet. 2005;76(5):815–32.
16. Pausova Z, Syme C, Abrahamowicz M, Xiao Y, Leonard GT, Perron M, Richer L, Veillette S, Smith GD, Seda O, Tremblay J, Hamet P, Gaudet D, Paus T. A common variant of the FTO gene is associated with not only increased adiposity but also elevated blood pressure in French Canadians. Circ Cardiovasc Genet. 2009;2(3):260–9.
17. Andreasen CH, Stender-Petersen KL, Mogensen MS, Torekov SS, Wegner L, Andersen G, Nielsen AL, Albrechtsen A, Borch-Johnsen K, Rasmussen SS, Clausen JO, Sandbaek A, Lauritzen T, Hansen L, Jørgensen T, Pedersen O, Hansen T. Low physical activity accentuates the effect of the FTO rs9939609 polymorphism on body fat accumulation. Diabetes. 2008;57(1):95–101.
18. Simon PH, Sylvestre MP, Tremblay J, Hamet P. Key considerations and methods in the study of gene-environment interactions. Am J Hypertens. 2016;29(8):891–9.

19. Simino J, Shi G, Bis JC, Chasman DI, Ehret GB, Gu X, Guo X, Hwang SJ, Sijbrands E, Smith AV, Verwoert GC, Bragg-Gresham JL, Cadby G, Chen P, Cheng CY, Corre T, de Boer RA, Goel A, Johnson T, Khor CC, LifeLines Cohort Study, Lluís-Ganella C, Luan J, Lyytikäinen LP, Nolte IM, Sim X, Sõber S, van der Most PJ, Verweij N, Zhao JH, Amin N, Boerwinkle E, Bouchard C, Dehghan A, Eiriksdottir G, Elosua R, Franco OH, Gieger C, Harris TB, Hercberg S, Hofman A, James AL, Johnson AD, Kähönen M, Khaw KT, Kutalik Z, Larson MG, Launer LJ, Li G, Liu J, Liu K, Morrison AC, Navis G, Ong RT, Papanicolau GJ, Penninx BW, Psaty BM, Raffel LJ, Raitakari OT, Rice K, Rivadeneira F, Rose LM, Sanna S, Scott RA, Siscovick DS, Stolk RP, Uitterlinden AG, Vaidya D, van der Klauw MM, Vasan RS, Vithana EN, Völker U, Völzke H, Watkins H, Young TL, Aung T, Bochud M, Farrall M, Hartman CA, Laan M, Lakatta EG, Lehtimäki T, Loos RJ, Lucas G, Meneton P, Palmer LJ, Rettig R, Snieder H, Tai ES, Teo YY, van der Harst P, Wareham NJ, Wijmenga C, Wong TY, Fornage M, Gudnason V, Levy D, Palmas W, Ridker PM, Rotter JI, van Duijn CM, Witteman JC, Chakravarti A, Rao DC. Gene-age interactions in blood pressure regulation: a large-scale investigation with the CHARGE, Global BPgen, and ICBP Consortia. Am J Hum Genet. 2014;95(1):24–38.
20. Igarashi J, Muroi S, Kawashima H, Wang X, Shinojima Y, Kitamura E, Oinuma T, Nemoto N, Song F, Ghosh S, Held WA, Nagase H. Quantitative analysis of human tissue-specific differences in methylation. Biochem Biophys Res Commun. 2008;376(4):658–64.
21. Zoungas S, Woodward M, Li Q, Cooper ME, Hamet P, Harrap S, Heller S, Marre M, Patel A, Poulter N, Williams B, Chalmers J, ADVANCE Collaborative Group. Impact of age, age at diagnosis and duration of diabetes on the risk of macrovascular and microvascular complications and death in type 2 diabetes. Diabetologia. 2014;57(12):2465–74.
22. Seda O, Tremblay J, Gaudet D, Brunelle PL, Gurau A, Merlo E, Pilote L, Orlov SN, Boulva F, Petrovich M, Kotchen TA, Cowley AW Jr, Hamet P. Systematic, genome-wide, sex-specific linkage of cardiovascular traits in French Canadians. Hypertension. 2008;51(4):1156–62.
23. Winkler TW, Justice AE, Graff M, Barata L, Feitosa MF, Chu S, Czajkowski J, Esko T, Fall T, Kilpeläinen TO, Lu Y, Mägi R, Mihailov E, Pers TH, Rüeger S, Teumer A, Ehret GB, Ferreira T, Heard-Costa NL, Karjalainen J, Lagou V, Mahajan A, Neinast MD, Prokopenko I, Simino J, Teslovich TM, Jansen R, Westra HJ, White CC, Absher D, Ahluwalia TS, Ahmad S, Albrecht E, Alves AC, Bragg-Gresham JL, de Craen AJ, Bis JC, Bonnefond A, Boucher G, Cadby G, Cheng YC, Chiang CW, Delgado G, Demirkan A, Dueker N, Eklund N, Eiriksdottir G, Eriksson J, Feenstra B, Fischer K, Frau F, Galesloot TE, Geller F, Goel A, Gorski M, Grammer TB, Gustafsson S, Haitjema S, Hottenga JJ, Huffman JE, Jackson AU, Jacobs KB, Johansson Å, Kaakinen M, Kleber ME, Lahti J, Mateo Leach I, Lehne B, Liu Y, Lo KS, Lorentzon M, Luan J, Madden PA, Mangino M, McKnight B, Medina-Gomez C, Monda KL, Montasser ME, Müller G, Müller-Nurasyid M, Nolte IM, Panoutsopoulou K, Pascoe L, Paternoster L, Rayner NW, Renström F, Rizzi F, Rose LM, Ryan KA, Salo P, Sanna S, Scharnagl H, Shi J, Smith AV, Southam L, Stančáková A, Steinthorsdottir V, Strawbridge RJ, Sung YJ, Tachmazidou I, Tanaka T, Thorleifsson G, Trompet S, Pervjakova N, Tyrer JP, Vandenput L, van der Laan SW, van der Velde N, van Setten J, van Vliet-Ostaptchouk JV, Verweij N, Vlachopoulou E, Waite LL, Wang SR, Wang Z, Wild SH, Willenborg C, Wilson JF, Wong A, Yang J, Yengo L, Yerges-Armstrong LM, Yu L, Zhang W, Zhao JH, Andersson EA, Bakker SJ, Baldassarre D, Banasik K, Barcella M, Barlassina C, Bellis C, Benaglio P, Blangero J, Blüher M, Bonnet F, Bonnycastle LL, Boyd HA, Bruinenberg M, Buchman AS, Campbell H, Chen YD, Chines PS, Claudi-Boehm S, Cole J, Collins FS, de Geus EJ, de Groot LC, Dimitriou M, Duan J, Enroth S, Eury E, Farmaki AE, Forouhi NG, Friedrich N, Gejman PV, Gigante B, Glorioso N, Go AS, Gottesman O, Gräßler J, Grallert H, Grarup N, Gu YM, Broer L, Ham AC, Hansen T, Harris TB, Hartman CA, Hassinen M, Hastie N, Hattersley AT, Heath AC, Henders AK, Hernandez D, Hillege H, Holmen O, Hovingh KG, Hui J, Husemoen LL, Hutri-Kähönen N, Hysi PG, Illig T, De Jager PL, Jalilzadeh S, Jørgensen T, Jukema JW, Juonala M, Kanoni S, Karaleftheri M, Khaw KT, Kinnunen L, Kittner SJ, Koenig W, Kolcic I, Kovacs P, Krarup NT, Kratzer W, Krüger J, Kuh D, Kumari M, Kyriakou T, Langenberg C, Lannfelt L, Lanzani C, Lotay V, Launer LJ, Leander K, Lindström J, Linneberg A, Liu YP, Lobbens S, Luben R, Lyssenko V, Männistö S, Magnusson PK, Mcardle WL, Menni C,

Merger S, Milani L, Montgomery GW, Morris AP, Narisu N, Nelis M, Ong KK, Palotie A, Pérusse L, Pichler I, Pilia MG, Pouta A, Rheinberger M, Ribel-Madsen R, Richards M, Rice KM, Rice TK, Rivolta C, Salomaa V, Sanders AR, Sarzynski MA, Scholtens S, Scott RA, Scott WR, Sebert S, Sengupta S, Sennblad B, Seufferlein T, Silveira A, Slagboom PE, Smit JH, Sparsø TH, Stirrups K, Stolk RP, Stringham HM, Swertz MA, Swift AJ, Syvänen AC, Tan ST, Thorand B, Tönjes A, Tremblay A, Tsafantakis E, van der Most PJ, Völker U, Vohl MC, Vonk JM, Waldenberger M, Walker RW, Wennauer R, Widén E, Willemsen G, Wilsgaard T, Wright AF, Zillikens MC, van Dijk SC, van Schoor NM, Asselbergs FW, de Bakker PI, Beckmann JS, Beilby J, Bennett DA, Bergman RN, Bergmann S, Böger CA, Boehm BO, Boerwinkle E, Boomsma DI, Bornstein SR, Bottinger EP, Bouchard C, Chambers JC, Chanock SJ, Chasman DI, Cucca F, Cusi D, Dedoussis G, Erdmann J, Eriksson JG, Evans DA, de Faire U, Farrall M, Ferrucci L, Ford I, Franke L, Franks PW, Froguel P, Gansevoort RT, Gieger C, Grönberg H, Gudnason V, Gyllensten U, Hall P, Hamsten A, van der Harst P, Hayward C, Heliövaara M, Hengstenberg C, Hicks AA, Hingorani A, Hofman A, Hu F, Huikuri HV, Hveem K, James AL, Jordan JM, Jula A, Kähönen M, Kajantie E, Kathiresan S, Kiemeney LA, Kivimaki M, Knekt PB, Koistinen HA, Kooner JS, Koskinen S, Kuusisto J, Maerz W, Martin NG, Laakso M, Lakka TA, Lehtimäki T, Lettre G, Levinson DF, Lind L, Lokki ML, Mäntyselkä P, Melbye M, Metspalu A, Mitchell BD, Moll FL, Murray JC, Musk AW, Nieminen MS, Njølstad I, Ohlsson C, Oldehinkel AJ, Oostra BA, Palmer LJ, Pankow JS, Pasterkamp G, Pedersen NL, Pedersen O, Penninx BW, Perola M, Peters A, Polašek O, Pramstaller PP, Psaty BM, Qi L, Quertermous T, Raitakari OT, Rankinen T, Rauramaa R, Ridker PM, Rioux JD, Rivadeneira F, Rotter JI, Rudan I, den Ruijter HM, Saltevo J, Sattar N, Schunkert H, Schwarz PE, Shuldiner AR, Sinisalo J, Snieder H, Sørensen TI, Spector TD, Staessen JA, Stefania B, Thorsteinsdottir U, Stumvoll M, Tardif JC, Tremoli E, Tuomilehto J, Uitterlinden AG, Uusitupa M, Verbeek AL, Vermeulen SH, Viikari JS, Vitart V, Völzke H, Vollenweider P, Waeber G, Walker M, Wallaschofski H, Wareham NJ, Watkins H, Zeggini E, CHARGE Consortium, DIAGRAM Consortium, GLGC Consortium, Global-BPGen Consortium, ICBP Consortium, MAGIC Consortium, Chakravarti A, Clegg DJ, Cupples LA, Gordon-Larsen P, Jaquish CE, Rao DC, Abecasis GR, Assimes TL, Barroso I, Berndt SI, Boehnke M, Deloukas P, Fox CS, Groop LC, Hunter DJ, Ingelsson E, Kaplan RC, MI MC, Mohlke KL, O'Connell JR, Schlessinger D, Strachan DP, Stefansson K, van Duijn CM, Hirschhorn JN, Lindgren CM, Heid IM, North KE, Borecki IB, Kutalik Z, Loos RJ. The influence of age and sex on genetic associations with adult body size and shape: a large-scale genome-wide interaction study. PLoS Genet. 2015;11(10):e1005378.

24. Teumer A, Tin A, Sorice R, Gorski M, Yeo NC, Chu AY, Li M, Li Y, Mijatovic V, Ko YA, Taliun D, Luciani A, Chen MH, Yang Q, Foster MC, Olden M, Hiraki LT, Tayo BO, Fuchsberger C, Dieffenbach AK, Shuldiner AR, Smith AV, Zappa AM, Lupo A, Kollerits B, Ponte B, Stengel B, Krämer BK, Paulweber B, Mitchell BD, Hayward C, Helmer C, Meisinger C, Gieger C, Shaffer CM, Müller C, Langenberg C, Ackermann D, Siscovick D, DCCT/EDIC, Boerwinkle E, Kronenberg F, Ehret GB, Homuth G, Waeber G, Navis G, Gambaro G, Malerba G, Eiriksdottir G, Li G, Wichmann HE, Grallert H, Wallaschofski H, Völzke H, Brenner H, Kramer H, Mateo Leach I, Rudan I, Hillege HL, Beckmann JS, Lambert JC, Luan J, Zhao JH, Chalmers J, Coresh J, Denny JC, Butterbach K, Launer LJ, Ferrucci L, Kedenko L, Haun M, Metzger M, Woodward M, Hoffman MJ, Nauck M, Waldenberger M, Pruijm M, Bochud M, Rheinberger M, Verweij N, Wareham NJ, Endlich N, Soranzo N, Polasek O, van der Harst P, Pramstaller PP, Vollenweider P, Wild PS, Gansevoort RT, Rettig R, Biffar R, Carroll RJ, Katz R, Loos RJ, Hwang SJ, Coassin S, Bergmann S, Rosas SE, Stracke S, Harris TB, Corre T, Zeller T, Illig T, Aspelund T, Tanaka T, Lendeckel U, Völker U, Gudnason V, Chouraki V, Koenig W, Kutalik Z, O'Connell JR, Parsa A, Heid IM, Paterson AD, de Boer IH, Devuyst O, Lazar J, Endlich K, Susztak K, Tremblay J, Hamet P, Jacob HJ, Böger CA, Fox CS, Pattaro C, Köttgen A. Genome-wide association studies identify genetic loci associated with albuminuria in diabetes. Diabetes. 2016;65(3):803–17.

25. Nadkarni GN, Horowitz CR. Genomics in CKD: is this the path forward? Adv Chronic Kidney Dis. 2016;23(2):120–4.

26. Holliday EG, Traylor M, Malik R, Bevan S, Maguire J, Koblar SA, Sturm J, Hankey GJ, Oldmeadow C, McEvoy M, Sudlow C, Rothwell PM, Coresh J, Hamet P, Tremblay J, Turner ST, de Andrade M, Rao M, Schmidt R, Crick PA, Robino A, Peralta CA, Jukema JW, Mitchell P, Rosas SE, Wang JJ, Scott RJ, Dichgans M, Mitchell BD, Kao WH, Fox CS, Levi C, Attia J, Markus HS, CKDGen Consortium and the International Stroke Genetics Consortium. Polygenic overlap between kidney function and large artery atherosclerotic stroke. Stroke. 2014;45(12):3508–13.
27. Mega JL, Stitziel NO, Smith JG, Chasman DI, Caulfield MJ, Devlin JJ, Nordio F, Hyde CL, Cannon CP, Sacks FM, Poulter NR, Sever PS, Ridker PM, Braunwald E, Melander O, Kathiresan S, Sabatine MS. Genetic risk, coronary heart disease events, and the clinical benefit of statin therapy: an analysis of primary and secondary prevention trials. Lancet. 2015;385(9984):2264–71.
28. Pashayan N, Duffy SW, Neal DE, Hamdy FC, Donovan JL, Martin RM, Harrington P, Benlloch S, Amin Al Olama A, Shah M, Kote-Jarai Z, Easton DF, Eeles R, Pharoah PD. Implications of polygenic risk-stratified screening for prostate cancer on overdiagnosis. Genet Med. 2015;17(10):789–95.
29. Läll K, Mägi R, Morris A, Metspalu A, Fischer K. Personalized risk prediction for type 2 diabetes: the potential of genetic risk scores. Genet Med. 2017;19(3):322–9.
30. Morris AP, Voight BF, Teslovich TM, Ferreira T, Segrè AV, Steinthorsdottir V, Strawbridge RJ, Khan H, Grallert H, Mahajan A, Prokopenko I, Kang HM, Dina C, Esko T, Fraser RM, Kanoni S, Kumar A, Lagou V, Langenberg C, Luan J, Lindgren CM, Müller-Nurasyid M, Pechlivanis S, Rayner NW, Scott LJ, Wiltshire S, Yengo L, Kinnunen L, Rossin EJ, Raychaudhuri S, Johnson AD, Dimas AS, Loos RJ, Vedantam S, Chen H, Florez JC, Fox C, Liu CT, Rybin D, Couper DJ, Kao WH, Li M, Cornelis MC, Kraft P, Sun Q, van Dam RM, Stringham HM, Chines PS, Fischer K, Fontanillas P, Holmen OL, Hunt SE, Jackson AU, Kong A, Lawrence R, Meyer J, Perry JR, Platou CG, Potter S, Rehnberg E, Robertson N, Sivapalaratnam S, Stančáková A, Stirrups K, Thorleifsson G, Tikkanen E, Wood AR, Almgren P, Atalay M, Benediktsson R, Bonnycastle LL, Burtt N, Carey J, Charpentier G, Crenshaw AT, Doney AS, Dorkhan M, Edkins S, Emilsson V, Eury E, Forsen T, Gertow K, Gigante B, Grant GB, Groves CJ, Guiducci C, Herder C, Hreidarsson AB, Hui J, James A, Jonsson A, Rathmann W, Klopp N, Kravic J, Krjutškov K, Langford C, Leander K, Lindholm E, Lobbens S, Männistö S, Mirza G, Mühleisen TW, Musk B, Parkin M, Rallidis L, Saramies J, Sennblad B, Shah S, Sigurðsson G, Silveira A, Steinbach G, Thorand B, Trakalo J, Veglia F, Wennauer R, Winckler W, Zabaneh D, Campbell H, van Duijn C, Uitterlinden AG, Hofman A, Sijbrands E, Abecasis GR, Owen KR, Zeggini E, Trip MD, Forouhi NG, Syvänen AC, Eriksson JG, Peltonen L, Nöthen MM, Balkau B, Palmer CN, Lyssenko V, Tuomi T, Isomaa B, Hunter DJ, Qi L, Wellcome Trust Case Control Consortium, Meta-Analyses of Glucose and Insulin-related traits Consortium (MAGIC) Investigators, Genetic Investigation of ANthropometric Traits (GIANT) Consortium, Asian Genetic Epidemiology Network–Type 2 Diabetes (AGEN-T2D) Consortium, South Asian Type 2 Diabetes (SAT2D) Consortium, Shuldiner AR, Roden M, Barroso I, Wilsgaard T, Beilby J, Hovingh K, Price JF, Wilson JF, Rauramaa R, Lakka TA, Lind L, Dedoussis G, Njølstad I, Pedersen NL, Khaw KT, Wareham NJ, Keinanen-Kiukaanniemi SM, Saaristo TE, Korpi-Hyövälti E, Saltevo J, Laakso M, Kuusisto J, Metspalu A, Collins FS, Mohlke KL, Bergman RN, Tuomilehto J, Boehm BO, Gieger C, Hveem K, Cauchi S, Froguel P, Baldassarre D, Tremoli E, Humphries SE, Saleheen D, Danesh J, Ingelsson E, Ripatti S, Salomaa V, Erbel R, Jöckel KH, Moebus S, Peters A, Illig T, de Faire U, Hamsten A, Morris AD, Donnelly PJ, Frayling TM, Hattersley AT, Boerwinkle E, Melander O, Kathiresan S, Nilsson PM, Deloukas P, Thorsteinsdottir U, Groop LC, Stefansson K, Hu F, Pankow JS, Dupuis J, Meigs JB, Altshuler D, Boehnke M, McCarthy MI, DIAbetes Genetics Replication And Meta-analysis (DIAGRAM) Consortium. Large-scale association analysis provides insights into the genetic architecture and pathophysiology of type 2 diabetes. Nat Genet. 2012;44(9):981–90.
31. Belsky DW, Moffitt TE, Sugden K, Williams B, Houts R, McCarthy J, Caspi A. Development and evaluation of a genetic risk score for obesity. Biodemography Soc Biol. 2013;59(1):85–100.

32. Hachiya T, Kamatani Y, Takahashi A, Hata J, Furukawa R, Shiwa Y, Yamaji T, Hara M, Tanno K, Ohmomo H, Ono K, Takashima N, Matsuda K, Wakai K, Sawada N, Iwasaki M, Yamagishi K, Ago T, Ninomiya T, Fukushima A, Hozawa A, Minegishi N, Satoh M, Endo R, Sasaki M, Sakata K, Kobayashi S, Ogasawara K, Nakamura M, Hitomi J, Kita Y, Tanaka K, Iso H, Kitazono T, Kubo M, Tanaka H, Tsugane S, Kiyohara Y, Yamamoto M, Sobue K, Shimizu A. Genetic predisposition to ischemic stroke: a polygenic risk score. Stroke. 2017;48(2):253–8.
33. van Setten J, Išgum I, Pechlivanis S, Tragante V, de Jong PA, Smolonska J, Platteel M, Hoffmann P, Oudkerk M, de Koning HJ, Nöthen MM, Moebus S, Erbel R, Jöckel KH, Viergever MA, Mali WP, de Bakker PI. Serum lipid levels, body mass index, and their role in coronary artery calcification: a polygenic analysis. Circ Cardiovasc Genet. 2015;8(2):327–33.
34. CARDIoGRAMplusC4D Consortium, Deloukas P, Kanoni S, Willenborg C, Farrall M, Assimes TL, Thompson JR, Ingelsson E, Saleheen D, Erdmann J, Goldstein BA, Stirrups K, König IR, Cazier JB, Johansson A, Hall AS, Lee JY, Willer CJ, Chambers JC, Esko T, Folkersen L, Goel A, Grundberg E, Havulinna AS, Ho WK, Hopewell JC, Eriksson N, Kleber ME, Kristiansson K, Lundmark P, Lyytikäinen LP, Rafelt S, Shungin D, Strawbridge RJ, Thorleifsson G, Tikkanen E, Van Zuydam N, Voight BF, Waite LL, Zhang W, Ziegler A, Absher D, Altshuler D, Balmforth AJ, Barroso I, Braund PS, Burgdorf C, Claudi-Boehm S, Cox D, Dimitriou M, Do R, DIAGRAM Consortium, CARDIOGENICS Consortium, Doney AS, El Mokhtari N, Eriksson P, Fischer K, Fontanillas P, Franco-Cereceda A, Gigante B, Groop L, Gustafsson S, Hager J, Hallmans G, Han BG, Hunt SE, Kang HM, Illig T, Kessler T, Knowles JW, Kolovou G, Kuusisto J, Langenberg C, Langford C, Leander K, Lokki ML, Lundmark A, McCarthy MI, Meisinger C, Melander O, Mihailov E, Maouche S, Morris AD, Müller-Nurasyid M, MuTHER Consortium, Nikus K, Peden JF, Rayner NW, Rasheed A, Rosinger S, Rubin D, Rumpf MP, Schäfer A, Sivananthan M, Song C, Stewart AF, Tan ST, Thorgeirsson G, van der Schoot CE, Wagner PJ, Wellcome Trust Case Control Consortium, Wells GA, Wild PS, Yang TP, Amouyel P, Arveiler D, Basart H, Boehnke M, Boerwinkle E, Brambilla P, Cambien F, Cupples AL, de Faire U, Dehghan A, Diemert P, Epstein SE, Evans A, Ferrario MM, Ferrières J, Gauguier D, Go AS, Goodall AH, Gudnason V, Hazen SL, Holm H, Iribarren C, Jang Y, Kähönen M, Kee F, Kim HS, Klopp N, Koenig W, Kratzer W, Kuulasmaa K, Laakso M, Laaksonen R, Lee JY, Lind L, Ouwehand WH, Parish S, Park JE, Pedersen NL, Peters A, Quertermous T, Rader DJ, Salomaa V, Schadt E, Shah SH, Sinisalo J, Stark K, Stefansson K, Trégouët DA, Virtamo J, Wallentin L, Wareham N, Zimmermann ME, Nieminen MS, Hengstenberg C, Sandhu MS, Pastinen T, Syvänen AC, Hovingh GK, Dedoussis G, Franks PW, Lehtimäki T, Metspalu A, Zalloua PA, Siegbahn A, Schreiber S, Ripatti S, Blankenberg SS, Perola M, Clarke R, Boehm BO, O'Donnell C, Reilly MP, März W, Collins R, Kathiresan S, Hamsten A, Kooner JS, Thorsteinsdottir U, Danesh J, Palmer CN, Roberts R, Watkins H, Schunkert H, Samani NJ. Large-scale association analysis identifies new risk loci for coronary artery disease. Nat Genet. 2013;45(1):25–33.
35. Global Lipids Genetics Consortium, Willer CJ, Schmidt EM, Sengupta S, Peloso GM, Gustafsson S, Kanoni S, Ganna A, Chen J, Buchkovich ML, Mora S, Beckmann JS, Bragg-Gresham JL, Chang HY, Demirkan A, Den Hertog HM, Do R, Donnelly LA, Ehret GB, Esko T, Feitosa MF, Ferreira T, Fischer K, Fontanillas P, Fraser RM, Freitag DF, Gurdasani D, Heikkilä K, Hyppönen E, Isaacs A, Jackson AU, Johansson A, Johnson T, Kaakinen M, Kettunen J, Kleber ME, Li X, Luan J, Lyytikäinen LP, Magnusson PK, Mangino M, Mihailov E, Montasser ME, Müller-Nurasyid M, Nolte IM, O'Connell JR, Palmer CD, Perola M, Petersen AK, Sanna S, Saxena R, Service SK, Shah S, Shungin D, Sidore C, Song C, Strawbridge RJ, Surakka I, Tanaka T, Teslovich TM, Thorleifsson G, Van den Herik EG, Voight BF, Volcik KA, Waite LL, Wong A, Wu Y, Zhang W, Absher D, Asiki G, Barroso I, Been LF, Bolton JL, Bonnycastle LL, Brambilla P, Burnett MS, Cesana G, Dimitriou M, Doney AS, Döring A, Elliott P, Epstein SE, Eyjolfsson GI, Gigante B, Goodarzi MO, Grallert H, Gravito ML, Groves CJ, Hallmans G, Hartikainen AL, Hayward C, Hernandez D, Hicks AA, Holm H, Hung YJ, Illig T, Jones MR, Kaleebu P, Kastelein JJ, Khaw KT, Kim E, Klopp N, Komulainen P, Kumari M, Langenberg C, Lehtimäki T, Lin SY, Lindström J, Loos RJ, Mach F, McArdle WL, Meisinger C, Mitchell BD, Müller G, Nagaraja R, Narisu N, Nieminen TV, Nsubuga RN, Olafsson I, Ong KK, Palotie A,

Papamarkou T, Pomilla C, Pouta A, Rader DJ, Reilly MP, Ridker PM, Rivadeneira F, Rudan I, Ruokonen A, Samani N, Scharnagl H, Seeley J, Silander K, Stancáková A, Stirrups K, Swift AJ, Tiret L, Uitterlinden AG, van Pelt LJ, Vedantam S, Wainwright N, Wijmenga C, Wild SH, Willemsen G, Wilsgaard T, Wilson JF, Young EH, Zhao JH, Adair LS, Arveiler D, Assimes TL, Bandinelli S, Bennett F, Bochud M, Boehm BO, Boomsma DI, Borecki IB, Bornstein SR, Bovet P, Burnier M, Campbell H, Chakravarti A, Chambers JC, Chen YD, Collins FS, Cooper RS, Danesh J, Dedoussis G, de Faire U, Feranil AB, Ferrières J, Ferrucci L, Freimer NB, Gieger C, Groop LC, Gudnason V, Gyllensten U, Hamsten A, Harris TB, Hingorani A, Hirschhorn JN, Hofman A, Hovingh GK, Hsiung CA, Humphries SE, Hunt SC, Hveem K, Iribarren C, Järvelin MR, Jula A, Kähönen M, Kaprio J, Kesäniemi A, Kivimaki M, Kooner JS, Koudstaal PJ, Krauss RM, Kuh D, Kuusisto J, Kyvik KO, Laakso M, Lakka TA, Lind L, Lindgren CM, Martin NG, März W, McCarthy MI, McKenzie CA, Meneton P, Metspalu A, Moilanen L, Morris AD, Munroe PB, Njølstad I, Pedersen NL, Power C, Pramstaller PP, Price JF, Psaty BM, Quertermous T, Rauramaa R, Saleheen D, Salomaa V, Sanghera DK, Saramies J, Schwarz PE, Sheu WH, Shuldiner AR, Siegbahn A, Spector TD, Stefansson K, Strachan DP, Tayo BO, Tremoli E, Tuomilehto J, Uusitupa M, van Duijn CM, Vollenweider P, Wallentin L, Wareham NJ, Whitfield JB, Wolffenbuttel BH, Ordovas JM, Boerwinkle E, Palmer CN, Thorsteinsdottir U, Chasman DI, Rotter JI, Franks PW, Ripatti S, Cupples LA, Sandhu MS, Rich SS, Boehnke M, Deloukas P, Kathiresan S, Mohlke KL, Ingelsson E, Abecasis GR. Discovery and refinement of loci associated with lipid levels. Nat Genet. 2013;45(11):1274–83.

36. Speliotes EK, Willer CJ, Berndt SI, Monda KL, Thorleifsson G, Jackson AU, Lango Allen H, Lindgren CM, Luan J, Mägi R, Randall JC, Vedantam S, Winkler TW, Qi L, Workalemahu T, Heid IM, Steinthorsdottir V, Stringham HM, Weedon MN, Wheeler E, Wood AR, Ferreira T, Weyant RJ, Segrè AV, Estrada K, Liang L, Nemesh J, Park JH, Gustafsson S, Kilpeläinen TO, Yang J, Bouatia-Naji N, Esko T, Feitosa MF, Kutalik Z, Mangino M, Raychaudhuri S, Scherag A, Smith AV, Welch R, Zhao JH, Aben KK, Absher DM, Amin N, Dixon AL, Fisher E, Glazer NL, Goddard ME, Heard-Costa NL, Hoesel V, Hottenga JJ, Johansson A, Johnson T, Ketkar S, Lamina C, Li S, Moffatt MF, Myers RH, Narisu N, Perry JR, Peters MJ, Preuss M, Ripatti S, Rivadeneira F, Sandholt C, Scott LJ, Timpson NJ, Tyrer JP, van Wingerden S, Watanabe RM, White CC, Wiklund F, Barlassina C, Chasman DI, Cooper MN, Jansson JO, Lawrence RW, Pellikka N, Prokopenko I, Shi J, Thiering E, Alavere H, Alibrandi MT, Almgren P, Arnold AM, Aspelund T, Atwood LD, Balkau B, Balmforth AJ, Bennett AJ, Ben-Shlomo Y, Bergman RN, Bergmann S, Biebermann H, Blakemore AI, Boes T, Bonnycastle LL, Bornstein SR, Brown MJ, Buchanan TA, Busonero F, Campbell H, Cappuccio FP, Cavalcanti-Proença C, Chen YD, Chen CM, Chines PS, Clarke R, Coin L, Connell J, Day IN, den Heijer M, Duan J, Ebrahim S, Elliott P, Elosua R, Eiriksdottir G, Erdos MR, Eriksson JG, Facheris MF, Felix SB, Fischer-Posovszky P, Folsom AR, Friedrich N, Freimer NB, Fu M, Gaget S, Gejman PV, Geus EJ, Gieger C, Gjesing AP, Goel A, Goyette P, Grallert H, Grässler J, Greenawalt DM, Groves CJ, Gudnason V, Guiducci C, Hartikainen AL, Hassanali N, Hall AS, Havulinna AS, Hayward C, Heath AC, Hengstenberg C, Hicks AA, Hinney A, Hofman A, Homuth G, Hui J, Igl W, Iribarren C, Isomaa B, Jacobs KB, Jarick I, Jewell E, John U, Jørgensen T, Jousilahti P, Jula A, Kaakinen M, Kajantie E, Kaplan LM, Kathiresan S, Kettunen J, Kinnunen L, Knowles JW, Kolcic I, König IR, Koskinen S, Kovacs P, Kuusisto J, Kraft P, Kvaløy K, Laitinen J, Lantieri O, Lanzani C, Launer LJ, Lecoeur C, Lehtimäki T, Lettre G, Liu J, Lokki ML, Lorentzon M, Luben RN, Ludwig B, MAGIC, Manunta P, Marek D, Marre M, Martin NG, Mcardle WL, Mccarthy A, Mcknight B, Meitinger T, Melander O, Meyre D, Midthjell K, Montgomery GW, Morken MA, Morris AP, Mulic R, Ngwa JS, Nelis M, Neville MJ, Nyholt DR, O'Donnell CJ, O'Rahilly S, Ong KK, Oostra B, Paré G, Parker AN, Perola M, Pichler I, Pietiläinen KH, Platou CG, Polasek O, Pouta A, Rafelt S, Raitakari O, Rayner NW, Ridderstråle M, Rief W, Ruokonen A, Robertson NR, Rzehak P, Salomaa V, Sanders AR, Sandhu MS, Sanna S, Saramies J, Savolainen MJ, Scherag S, Schipf S, Schreiber S, Schunkert H, Silander K, Sinisalo J, Siscovick DS, Smit JH, Soranzo N, Sovio U, Stephens J, Surakka I, Swift AJ, Tammesoo ML, Tardif JC, Teder-Laving M, Teslovich TM, Thompson JR, Thomson B, Tönjes A, Tuomi T, van Meurs JB, van Ommen GJ, Vatin V, Viikari J, Visvikis-Siest S, Vitart V, Vogel CI, Voight

BF, Waite LL, Wallaschofski H, Walters GB, Widen E, Wiegand S, Wild SH, Willemsen G, Witte DR, Witteman JC, Xu J, Zhang Q, Zgaga L, Ziegler A, Zitting P, Beilby JP, Farooqi IS, Hebebrand J, Huikuri HV, James AL, Kähönen M, Levinson DF, Macciardi F, Nieminen MS, Ohlsson C, Palmer LJ, Ridker PM, Stumvoll M, Beckmann JS, Boeing H, Boerwinkle E, Boomsma DI, Caulfield MJ, Chanock SJ, Collins FS, Cupples LA, Smith GD, Erdmann J, Froguel P, Grönberg H, Gyllensten U, Hall P, Hansen T, Harris TB, Hattersley AT, Hayes RB, Heinrich J, Hu FB, Hveem K, Illig T, Jarvelin MR, Kaprio J, Karpe F, Khaw KT, Kiemeney LA, Krude H, Laakso M, Lawlor DA, Metspalu A, Munroe PB, Ouwehand WH, Pedersen O, Penninx BW, Peters A, Pramstaller PP, Quertermous T, Reinehr T, Rissanen A, Rudan I, Samani NJ, Schwarz PE, Shuldiner AR, Spector TD, Tuomilehto J, Uda M, Uitterlinden A, Valle TT, Wabitsch M, Waeber G, Wareham NJ, Watkins H, Procardis Consortium, Wilson JF, Wright AF, Zillikens MC, Chatterjee N, McCarroll SA, Purcell S, Schadt EE, Visscher PM, Assimes TL, Borecki IB, Deloukas P, Fox CS, Groop LC, Haritunians T, Hunter DJ, Kaplan RC, Mohlke KL, O'Connell JR, Peltonen L, Schlessinger D, Strachan DP, van Duijn CM, Wichmann HE, Frayling TM, Thorsteinsdottir U, Abecasis GR, Barroso I, Boehnke M, Stefansson K, North KE, MI MC, Hirschhorn JN, Ingelsson E, Loos RJ. Association analyses of 249,796 individuals reveal 18 new loci associated with body mass index. Nat Genet. 2010;42(11):937–48.

Treatment of High-Normal Blood Pressure in the Guidelines

42

Jana Brguljan and Giuseppe Ambrosio

42.1 Introduction

Hypertension is the most important treatable risk factor in cardiovascular disease prevention. The number of people affected by hypertension has raised in all regions of the world from 2000 to 2015, reflecting not only the growing and ageing of global population, but also that more than 80% of the world is doomed to develop hypertension. As a consequence of the predicted increase of about 10% in the global prevalence of hypertension, between 2000 and 2025 an estimated 560 million extra people will be affected by hypertension [1]. This prospect is daunting, given that in 2010 high blood pressure was already the biggest single contributor to the global burden of disease and to worldwide mortality, leading to 9.4 million deaths each year [2].

The relation between cardiovascular outcome and blood pressure (BP) is log-linear, without a critical level above which the risk sharply increases [3]. However, for the diagnosis and management of hypertension, clinicians need operational thresholds [4, 5]. Therefore, guidelines propose classification and treatment based on conventional, home, and ambulatory blood pressure measurements. In the world there exist differences among nations due to genetic and environment influence. This is why also differences exist in blood pressure definitions. The Joint National Committee on the Prevention, Detection, Evaluation and Treatment of High Blood Pressure (JNC8) [6], and the World Health Organization and the International Society of Hypertension (WHO-ISH) [4] proposed a classification of blood pressure

J. Brguljan
Division of Hypertension, Internal Department, University Medical Center Ljubljana, Ljubljana, Slovenia

G. Ambrosio (✉)
Division of Cardiology, University of Perugia School of Medicine, Perugia, Italy
e-mail: giuseppe.ambrosio@ospedale.perugia.it

R. Zimlichman et al. (eds.), *Prehypertension and Cardiometabolic Syndrome*, Updates in Hypertension and Cardiovascular Protection,
https://doi.org/10.1007/978-3-319-75310-2_42

based on conventional measurement into normal, prehypertensive, and hypertensive levels. The estimate prevalence of prehypertensive in a general population varies from 31% [7] to 33% [8].

The definition of "high-normal" blood pressure is shared by ESC/ESH [9] and Canadian Hypertension guidelines [10], all based on office blood pressure measurement defining optimal, normal, high-normal, and hypertension in ESC/ESH 2013 guidelines.

42.2 Choice of Thresholds

In 2003, the USA Joint National Committee Guidelines (JNC7) on hypertension decided to unify normal and high-normal blood pressure categories into a single entity termed 'prehypertension'. This was based on evidence from the Framingham study that in such individuals the chance of developing hypertension is higher than in those with a blood pressure < 120/80 mmHg (termed 'normal' blood pressure) at all ages. In the 1997 categories were optimal, normal, high-normal, and hypertension stages 1, 2, and 3.

In contrast, the ESH/ESC Committee has decided not to use this terminology for the following reasons: (1) even in the Framingham study the risk of developing hypertension was definitely higher in subjects with high-normal (130–139/85–89 mmHg) than in those with normal blood pressure (120–129/80–84 mmHg) and therefore there is little reason to combine the two groups together; (2) given the ominous significance of the word hypertension for the laypeople, the term 'prehypertension' may create anxiety and request for unnecessary medical support and examinations in many subjects; (3) most importantly, although lifestyle changes recommended by the 2003 JNC7 Guidelines for all prehypertensive individuals may be a valuable population strategy, in practice this category is a highly differentiated one, with the extremes consisting of subjects in no need of any intervention (e.g. an elderly individual with a blood pressure of 120/80 mmHg) as opposed to subjects with a high or very high-risk profile (e.g. after stroke or with diabetes) in whom drug treatment is required [11]. There were no additional evidences from randomized clinical trials to change this statement also in guidelines published in 2013, except for starting point of medical treatment. The same classification is used for all adults, whereas different criteria, based on percentiles, are adopted for children and adolescents [12].

Canada is a country with the greatest achievement of controlled blood pressure. In their new 2017 guidelines giving guideless for hypertension patient treatment, they used also automatic unattended (i.e. non-observed AOBP) blood pressure technique, but high-normal blood pressure was defined only based on non-AOBP. When using non-AOBP, a mean SBP 140 mm Hg or DBP 90 mm Hg is high, and an SBP between 130 and 139 mm Hg and/or a DBP between 85 and 89 mm Hg is high-normal [10].

Limits of high-normal blood pressure are only defined based upon office blood pressure measurements, whereas limits for high-normal blood pressure when using home or ambulatory techniques are not defined.

42.3 Definition in Different Guidelines

Guidelines	Definition (OBPM)	SBP/DBP (mmHg)
ESH/ESC 2013 [9]	High-normal BP	130–139 and/or 85–89
2014 Report From the Panel Members Appointed to the Eighth Joint National Committee (JNC 8) [13]	Prehypertension	120–139 and/or 80–89
Hypertension Canada's Guidelines 2017 [10]	High-normal BP	130–139 and/or 85–89

42.4 Size of the Problem

There are few facts which confirm the important role of high-normal blood pressure or prehypertension and stage 1 hypertension, because they are the forms of high blood pressure that contribute most to mortality. Based on cardiovascular mortality data for 164,685 men with prehypertension and hypertension, fully 79% of deaths over a 15-year period were among men with systolic blood pressure that showed either prehypertension or stage 1 (140–159 mm Hg) hypertension [14, 15].

In the Framingham Study [16] the 4-year progression rate from prehypertension to hypertension was 37% in subjects below age 65 years, and 50% in older participants. In a European Flemish population study, the progression rates over 10 years' follow-up were 25% in persons below 50 years and 50% in those aged 50 years or older [17]. Looking from the population perspective we can see that prehypertension is a precursor of hypertension.

Besides, prehypertension is associated with numerous abnormalities that increase cardiovascular risk independent of BP. Based on the TECUMSEH BP Study, for example, Dr. Julius and colleagues reported that individuals with borderline hypertension were significantly more likely to have high total cholesterol, low HDL, higher levels of triglycerides, insulin, and glucose, and to weight more (all $p < 0.001$ versus normotensive study participants) [18]. Furthermore, an association of prehypertension with other cardiovascular risk factors has been established [19].

It was pointed out that the term prehypertension was coined in 1939 in the context of earlier studies that linked high blood pressure recorded during physical examination for life insurance proposes to subsequent morbidity and mortality. These individuals had an increased risk of hypertension, cardiovascular disease, and early death from cardiovascular causes [20].

In a trial of subjects with high-normal BP, 40% of subjects in the placebo arm developed hypertension within 2 years and 63% within 4 years [21]. This is consistent with observational data, indicating that these individuals exhibit higher four-year rates of progression to overt hypertension [16]. In addition, the 10-year risk of incident cardiovascular disease was greater in both men (hazard ratio 1.6; 95% CI 1.1 to 2.3) and women (hazard ratio 1.8; 95% CI 1.0 to 3.1) with high-normal BP than in subjects with BP levels lower than 120/80 mm Hg [22]. Those older than 65 years of age with high-normal BP levels had the highest risk of progression to hypertension and development of cardiovascular disease. In this group, the crude incidence rate of cardiovascular events per 1000 patient years was 20 in women and 28 in men. These data indicate that patients with high-normal blood pressure have: (a) a higher risk of progression to overt hypertension and (b) worse prognosis than patients with optimal blood pressure levels. Therefore, although antihypertensive therapy is not recommended, close surveillance in the form of annual blood pressure checks is recommended [10].

Prehypertension and masked hypertension carry a great risk of developing hypertension. In the Flemish Study on Environment, Genes and Health Outcomes (FLEMENGHO) [17], the 4-year progression rates from prehypertension to hypertension were 17.9 and 26.3% in participants younger than 50 years or older, respectively. In the Copenhagen Monitoring of Trends and Determinants in Cardiovascular Disease [23], the progression rate over 10 years was 37.3%. By multivariable-adjusted analysis, progression to prehypertension or to hypertension was associated with 10-year cardiovascular risks of 11.1% and 13.9%, respectively.

42.5 Importance of Blood Pressure Measurements and Masked Hypertension

Blood pressure changes with time and conditions of measurement. Estimation of CV risk is largely based on conventional office blood pressure. Until quite recently the diagnosis of hypertension relied entirely on clinic blood pressure measurement. Accumulating evidence favours measuring blood pressure with 24 h ambulatory blood pressure (ABPM), or if not possible with home blood pressure monitoring [24]. In some people, BP is abnormally elevated when measured at doctor's office. This is called "white-coat" hypertension. Opposite to white-coat hypertension, in some people BP is elevated when measured outside not inside the clinic, and this is called masked hypertension. In several observational studies it was confirmed that people with masked hypertension are at higher cardiovascular risk and people with white-coat hypertension should not be treated for hypertension [25]. These phenomena were also observed in people within the high-normal blood pressure group or prehypertension. At subject-level data IDACO meta-analysis included 7826 people randomly recruited from 11 populations, not treated with blood pressure-lowering drugs and covered on average over 11.3 years of follow-up. Using the daytime ABPM in our current study out of the office blood pressure revealed masked hypertension in 29.3% of participants with prehypertension. Compared to normotensive group, where only about 7% of people had masked hypertension, about 29% have masked hypertension in prehypertension group. These subjects were at a 2 times higher risk of developing a cardiovascular event and 3 times higher to developing stroke than those within the real prehypertensive group, and thus need to be treated, but with the usually used clinical blood pressure measurement technique they would be overlooked and exposed to the risk of experiencing an early cardiovascular event. Diabetic patients, smokers, alcohol consumers, men, and individuals with increased cholesterol (≥5.7 mmol/L) are at increased risk of having masked hypertension [26].

Manios and co-workers [27] enrolled 807 referred patients, whose office blood pressure was less than 140 mm Hg systolic and 90 mm Hg diastolic. Prevalence of pure prehypertension and prehypertension with masked hypertension was 59.9% and 19.7%, respectively. After adjustments, prehypertensive patients with masked hypertension had higher ($P < 0.01$) carotid intima-media thickness than either prehypertensive patients without masked hypertension or normotensive subjects (712 vs. 649 vs. 655 μm). Shimbo and colleagues [28] studied 813 untreated participants recruited from a worksite-based population, from whom they obtained 9 blood pressure readings (3 at each of 3 visits over 3 weeks). Among 482 normotensive (<120/<80 mm Hg) and 287 prehypertensive (120–139/80–85 mm Hg) participants, the prevalence of masked hypertension was 3.9% and 34.1%, respectively. By multivariable-adjusted models, participants with prehypertension or masked hypertension (awake blood pressure ≥ 135/≥85 mm Hg) had a greater left ventricular mass index than those with normotension (60.8 vs. 64.2 g/m^2; $P < 0.01$), but left ventricular mass index was not different among prehypertensive participants without and with masked hypertension (66.1 vs. 68.6 g/m^2; $P = 0.19$).

42.6 Could Development of Hypertension Be Prevented?

Two randomized clinical trials explored whether antihypertensive drug treatment can prevent progression from prehypertension to hypertension. In TROPHY (Trial of Preventing Hypertension) [21], prehypertensive participants (130–139/85–89 mm Hg) were randomly assigned to be treated for 2 years with candesartan ($n = 391$) or placebo ($n = 381$), followed by 2 years on placebo for all ($n = 772$). During the first 2 years, hypertension developed in 154 participants in the placebo group and 53 in the candesartan group (relative risk reduction [RRR], 66%; CI, 56–75%; $P < 0.001$). After 4 years, hypertension (office blood pressure, 140/90 mm Hg) had developed in 240 and 208 participants in the placebo and candesartan group, respectively (RRR, 16%; CI, $P < 0.007$). However, the proportion of participants requiring antihypertensive drug treatment during follow-up (placebo vs. candesartan, 12.6 vs. 11.5%; RRR, 0.91; CI, 0.62–1.34), or having hypertension at 4 years (1.3 vs. 1.5%; RRR, 1.17; CI, 0.36–3.80), was similar in both groups.

In PHARAO (Prevention of Hypertension with the Angiotensin-Converting Enzyme Inhibitor Ramipril in Patients with High-Normal Blood) [29], 1008 subjects with high-normal blood pressure (130–139/85–89 mm Hg) were randomized to ramipril 5 mg daily or placebo. Over 3 years of follow-up, the RRR for the incidence of hypertension was 34% (CI, 19–47%; $P = 0.0001$). Ramipril also proved to be more effective in reducing the incidence of manifest office hypertension in patients with baseline daytime ambulatory blood pressure within the high-normal range (125–134/80–84 mm Hg). The incidence of cerebrovascular and cardiovascular events showed no statistically significant differences between the two groups.

Clinicians should also think beyond BP therapy for patients with high-normal BP. Since prehypertension usually occurs in the presence of one or more other major risk factors, Jan Östergren, MD, PhD, Karolinska University Hospital, Stockholm

(Sweden), recommends combining effective BP and dyslipidemia therapy. The additive effect of cholesterol and BP has been known since at least the 1992 publication of data from MRFIT [15] and the additional risk associated with multiple risk factors is recognized in the 2007 update of the ESH guidelines for treating hypertension [30].

Evidence certainly suggests that optimal risk reduction is achieved when both BP and cholesterol are targeted, benefits being more than just additive. Recent studies suggest a synergy between statin therapy and antihypertensive therapy, such as the ASCOT trial reported by Dr. Östergren and colleagues. Given the evidence, Dr. Östergren said, the polypill concept could increase compliance and efficacy of treatment.

Finally, based on the vascular protective actions of renin-angiotensin system blockade, Prof. Thomas Unger, Chair of Pharmacology and Director of the Institute of Pharmacology at the Charité—Universitätsmedizin Berlin (Germany), recommends considering these agents in patients with prehypertension and multiple risk factors [31].

42.7 Importance of the Overall Risk Profile

In 2007 ESH/ESC guidelines it was suggested to initiate drug treatment in high-normal blood pressure range in high-risk patient having diabetes, renal diseases, or concomitant CV diseases. However, it was pointed out in 2009 that evidences are scanty. For diabetes recommendations is based on results of the 'normotensive' component of the ABCD trial [32], which however has important limitations: 'normotension' was defined as a SBP less than 160 mmHg, the trial size was small, the primary endpoint was the change in creatinine clearance (with no statistically significant difference between treatments), and a statistically significant reduction of cardiovascular events in the group randomized to more intensive treatment was limited to the incidence of stroke but did not extend to other cardiovascular events. Recommendations also derive from subgroup analyses of two other large trials, like MICROHOPE [33] and ADVANCE [34]. However, in MICROHOPE, normotension was defined by history, entry BP values were not mentioned, and the statistical significance of cardiovascular event reduction in the 'normotensive group' was not reported; in ADVANCE, the benefit of antihypertensive treatment was significant in patients with an entry SBP 140 mmHg or more, but not in those in whom it was below this value. Similar findings were obtained when stratification was based on the presence or absence of a history of hypertension.

Lowering blood pressure always shows beneficial effect on stroke. In PROGRESS trial, in patients with a previous stroke or transient ischemic attack BP, lowering was accompanied by a marked reduction in the incidence of recurrent stroke and cardiovascular events in both hypertensive and normotensive patients. However, in that study, hypertension was defined by SBP values of 160 mmHg or more, and in a subsequent analysis, a significant reduction in recurrent stroke with treatment was only observed when entry SBP was 140 mmHg or more [90]. Furthermore, entry BP values in PROGRESS were reported irrespective of background treatment present in 50% of patients [35, 36], and therefore they cannot be used to take decisions on initiation of treatment in untreated patients. In PATS study [37], where reduction of CV events was shown in patients with previous stroke, only 16% of normotensive were included.

In most of trials with coronary artery disease randomized drugs were added on a background of antihypertensive drugs, therefore we cannot define them as normotensive [38]. Same consideration applies to recent large meta-analyses showing the benefits of BP-lowering therapy also in individuals with baseline SBP above and below 140 mmHg, since the great majority of the individuals had been involved in trials in which antihypertensive agents were present at baseline [9].

Even though TROPHY and PHARAO study have shown that administration of antihypertensive drugs can slower the progression of hypertension, it is not clear how far this benefit goes, whether it lasts and really delays events, and if it is cost-effective.

Based on all these data, the last 2013 ESH/ESC [9] guidelines state that unless necessary evidence is obtained it is not recommended to initiate antihypertensive drug therapy at high-normal blood pressure. It is strongly recommended to undergo lifestyle changes.

42.8 Phenotype of People with High-Normal Blood Pressure (Adolescents, Pregnant Women)

Discussing about group of people in high-normal blood pressure range we would certainly need to distinguish between different phenotype groups, because predication, development, and consequence of hypertension would not be the same considering adolescent or an elderly person. We shall follow up adolescents really closely to prevent the consequences on target organ damage and progression to hypertension [39]. With respect to pregnant women, there is no definition of high-normal blood pressure in this group.

42.9 Recommended Treatment

Guidelines are usually production of group of specialists and reviewers who among recognized and published studies suggest diagnostic and therapeutic aspects of hypertension.

In all of the guidelines, regardless of how these category of population are defined, only lifestyle changes are recommended. In our daily practice we can see that instructions to these recommendations are hard to follow, and even more to retain, yet they can still be very effective.

One of the most effective one is *weight reduction*. In a meta-analysis by Neter et al. twenty-five randomized, controlled trials were included, with a total of 4874 participants. A net weight reduction of −5.1 kg (95% confidence interval [CI], −6.03 to −4.25) by means of caloric restriction, increased physical activity, or both, reduced systolic blood pressure by −4.44 mm Hg (95% CI, −5.93 to −2.95) and diastolic blood pressure by −3.57 mm Hg (95% CI, −4.88 to −2.25). Blood pressure reductions were −1.05 mm Hg (95% CI, −1.43 to −0.66) systolic and −0.92 mm Hg (95% CI, −1.28 to −0.55) diastolic when expressed per kilogram of weight loss [40].

Subsequent meta-analyses in patients with hypertension confirmed the blood pressure-lowering effect of weight reduction by weight reducing diet, in comparison with control. Weighted mean differences in weight and systolic/diastolic blood pressure: −4.1 kg; −6.3/−3.4 mmHg [41] and −4.0 kg; −4.5/−3.2 mmHg in the one described by Siebenhofer et al. [42].

Effective *weight loss* will only go coupled with increased regular exercise. We can distinguish between dynamic aerobic endurance training, which involves large muscle groups in dynamic activities, designed specifically to increase aerobic endurance performance, and resistance training, which involves strength, weight, static and/or isometric training, designed specifically to increase muscular strength, power and/or endurance. In meta-analyses done by Cornelissen and Fagard 71 studies were included, ~57% men, age median 47 years; range 21–83 years. Dynamic aerobic endurance training decreased resting systolic and diastolic blood pressure by −3.0 and −2.4 and daytime ambulatory systolic and diastolic by −3.3 and −3.5 mmHg [43]. Aerobic interval training has also been shown to reduce BP [44].

Impact of *resistance training* on blood pressure and other cardiovascular risk factors in a meta-analysis of randomized controlled trials analysing 1012 subjects resulted in −3.5 and −3.2 change in systolic and diastolic BP [45]. Dynamic resistance training was followed by significant BP reduction, as well as improvement in other metabolic parameters, and performance of resistance exercises on 2–3 days per week can be advised. Isometric exercises are not recommended, since data from only a few studies are available. People should be advised to participate in at least 30 min of moderate-intensity dynamic aerobic exercise (walking, jogging, cycling, or swimming) on 5–7 days per week [46].

Third recommended point is *salt restriction*. There are doubts about actual positive effect of this measure, but it is known overall that average intake of salt in population is too high, and the truth is that not all the people are salt-sensitive. But there is causal relationship between salt intake and BP in most of population. On the other hand, there is no evidence that reducing salt intake causes harm.

In one of the meta-analyses including 17 randomized trials in hypertensives (n = 734) and 11 trials in normotensives (n = 2220) [47] it was shown that modest reduction in salt intake, from a usual intake of »10 to »5 g of salt per day over a more prolonged period of time resulted in the pooled estimates of blood pressure fall of 4.96/2.73 ± 0.40/0.24 mmHg in hypertensives ($P < 0.001$ for both systolic and diastolic) and 2.03/0.97 ± 0.27/0.21 mmHg in normotensives ($P < 0.001$ for both systolic and diastolic). Advice should be given to avoid salted products like bread and conserved products because there is high salt content. A daily intake of 5–6 g of salt is thus recommended in general population.

Other recommended lifestyle changes would include moderation in alcohol consumption, eating Mediterranean diet, and smoking cessation.

Meta-analysis of 40 RCTs showed that *calcium supplementation* (approximately 1 g/day) may significantly reduce systolic BP by 1.9 mm Hg and diastolic BP by 1.0 mm Hg. The BP effect tended to be more pronounced in populations with a habitually low calcium intake (2.6/1.3 mm Hg). Blood pressure showed no further decrease when calcium doses exceeded 1 g/day [48].

Randomized controlled trials of *magnesium supplementation* in normotensive and hypertensive subjects were included in the meta-analysis of Jee et al. where 20 trials were included 1220 participants, 85 weeks median duration and 15.4 mmol of daily doses of magnesium resulted in overall weighted net change in blood pressure systolic −0.6(−2.2; +1.0), diastolic −0.8(−2.1; +0.5) with the tests for heterogeneity: $P < 0.001$ [49].

It was demonstrated in TOHP Ii and Oslo Diet and Smoking intervention that rigorously applied lifestyle interventions can prevent, or at least delay, the onset of hypertension and cardiovascular events in at-risk subjects [50] Recomended lifestyle changes are listed in Table 42.1.

Another interesting point for clinicians would be how to follow these high-normal people. In ESH/ESC guidelines they are considered as low-risk population unless more risk factors or symptomatic cardiovascular disease or chronic kidney disease more the stage 4 or diabetes with organ damage is present, when they are considered as very high-risk population. But nevertheless only lifestyle changes and no blood pressure intervention is recommended.

Considering recommendation how often to control blood pressure in these specific group of population and not to miss the moment when medical therapy should be considered, in Canadian guidelines it is recommended that if at the visit 1 OBPM

Table 42.1 Adoption of lifestyle changes [9]

Recommendations	Class[a]	Level[b,d]	Level[b,e]
Salt restriction to 5–6 g per day is recommended.	I	A	B
Moderation of alcohol consumption to no more than 20–30 g of ethanol per day in men and to no more than 10–20 g of ethanol per day in women is recommended.	I	A	B
Increased consumption of vegetables, fruits, and low-fat dairy products is recommended.	I	A	B
Reduction of weight to BMI of 25 kg/m^2 and of waist circumference to <102 cm in men and <88 cm in women is recommended, unless contraindicated.	I	A	B
Regular exercise, i.e. at least 30 min of moderate dynamic exercise on 5–7 days per week is recommended.	I	A	B
It is recommended to give all smokers advice to quit smoking and to offer assistance.	I	A	B

BMI body mass index
[a]Class of recommendation
[b]Level of evidence
[c]Reference(s) supporting levels of evidence
[d]Based on the effect on BP and/or CV risk profile
[e]Based on outcome studies

is high-normal annual follow-up is recommended. In ESH/ESC guidelines there is no specific time recommendation, but high-normal blood pressure in the office is one of the clinical indications for out-of-office blood pressure measurements for diagnostic purposes.

Conclusion

High-normal blood pressure individuals are at higher risk to develop hypertension and cardiovascular events. Considering the high prevalence of masked hypertension in this group, first masked hypertension should be excluded, preferably by ABMP.

Even though in the past guidelines from 2007 they were not recognized as a homogenous group, later in 2013 it was corrected that there is no additional value of pharmacological treatment in this group of population even thought having concomitant diseases. Upon the later guidelines they shall undergo to the lifestyle modifications and regular follow-up of blood pressure measurements. Lifestyle changes should include losing excess weight, becoming physically active, limiting alcoholic beverages, and following a heart-healthy eating plan, including cutting back on salt and other forms of sodium. Smoking cessation is strongly recommended. If they have other risk factors they should be followed closely.

References

1. Kearney PM, Whelton M, Reynolds K, Muntner P, Whelton PK, He J. Global burden of hypertension: analysis of worldwide data. Lancet. 2005;365:217–23.
2. Lim SS, Vos T, Flaxman AD, Danaei G, et al. A comparative risk assessment of burden of disease and injury attributable to 67 risk factors and risk factor clusters in 21 regions, 1990–2010: a systematic analysis for the Global Burden of Disease Study 2010. Lancet. 2012;380:2224–60.
3. Lewington S, Clarke R, Qizilbash N, Peto R, Collins R, Prospective Studies Collaboration. Age-specific relevance of usual blood pressure to vascular mortality: a meta-analysis of individual data for one million adults in 61 prospective studies. Lancet. 2002;360(9349):1903–13.
4. Whitworth JA, World Health Organization ISoHWG. 2003 World Health Organization (WHO)/International Society of Hypertension (ISH) statement on management of hypertension. J Hypertens. 2003;21(11):1983–92.
5. Chobanian AV, Bakris GL, Black HR, Cushman WC, Green LA, Izzo JL Jr, Jones DW, Materson BJ, Oparil S, Wright JT Jr, Roccella EJ, the National High Blood Pressure Education Program Coordinating Committee. Seventh report of the Joint National Committee on prevention, detection, evaluation, and treatment of high blood pressure. Hypertension. 2003;42(6):1206–52.
6. James PA, Oparil S, Carter BL, Cushman WC, Dennison-Himmelfarb C, Handler J, Lackland D, LeFevre ML, MacKenzie TD, Ogedegbe O, Smith SC Jr, Svetkey LP, Taler SJ, Townsend RR, Wright JT Jr, Narva AS, Ortiz E. 2014 evidence-based guideline for the management of high blood pressure in adults: report from the panel members appointed to the Eighth Joint Committee (JNC 8). JAMA. 2014;311:507–20.
7. Mainous AG III, Everett CJ, Liszka H, King DE, Egan BM. Prehypertension and mortality in a nationally representative cohort. Am J Cardiol. 2004;94:1496–500.
8. Liszka HA, Mainous AG III, King DE, Everett CJ, Egan BM. Prehypertension and cardiovascular morbidity. Ann Fam Med. 2005;3:294–9.

9. Mancia G, Fagard R, Narkiewicz K, Redón J, Zanchetti A, Böhm M, Christiaens T, Cifkova R, De Backer G, Dominiczak A, Galderisi M, Grobbee DE, Jaarsma T, Kirchhof P, Kjeldsen SE, Laurent S, Manolis AJ, Nilsson PM, Ruilope LM, Schmieder RE, Sirnes PA, Sleight P, Viigimaa M, Waeber B, Zannad F. 2013 ESH/ESC Guidelines for the management of arterial hypertension: the task force for the management of arterial hypertension of the European Society of Hypertension (ESH) and of the European Society of Cardiology (ESC). Eur Heart J. 2013;34:2159–219.
10. Leung AA, Daskalopoulou SS, Dasgupta K, McBrien K, Butalia S, Zarnke KB, Nerenberg K, Harris KC, Nakhla M, Cloutier L, Gelfer M, Lamarre-Cliche M, Milot A, Bolli P, Tremblay G, McLean D, Tobe SW, Ruzicka M, Burns KD, Vallée M, Prasad GVR, Gryn SE, Feldman RD, Selby P, Pipe A, Schiffrin EL, McFarlane PA, Oh P, Hegele RA, Khara M, Wilson TW, Penner SB, Burgess E, Sivapalan P, Herman RJ, Bacon SL, Rabkin SW, Gilbert RE, Campbell TS, Grover S, Honos G, Lindsay P, Hill MD, Coutts SB, Gubitz G, Campbell NRC, Moe GW, Howlett JG, Boulanger JM, Prebtani A, Kline G, Leiter LA, Jones C, Côté AM, Woo V, Kaczorowski J, Trudeau L, Tsuyuki RT, Hiremath S, Drouin D, Lavoie KL, Hamet P, Grégoire JC, Lewanczuk R, Dresser GK, Sharma M, Reid D, Lear SA, Moullec G, Gupta M, Magee LA, Logan AG, Dionne J, Fournier A, Benoit G, Feber J, Poirier L, Padwal RS, Rabi DM. Hypertension Canada's 2017 Guidelines for diagnosis, risk assessment, prevention, and treatment of hypertension in adults. Can J Cardiol. 2017;33(5):557–76.
11. Mancia G, De Backer G, Dominiczak A, Cifkova R, Fagard R, Germano G, Grassi G, Heagerty AM, Kjeldsen SE, Laurent S, Narkiewicz K, Ruilope L, Rynkiewicz A, Schmieder RE, Boudier HA, Zanchetti A, Vahanian A, Camm J, De Caterina R, Dean V, Dickstein K, Filippatos G, Funck-Brentano C, Hellemans I, Kristensen SD, McGregor K, Sechtem U, Silber S, Tendera M, Widimsky P, Zamorano JL, Erdine S, Kiowski W, Agabiti-Rosei E, Ambrosioni E, Lindholm LH, Viigimaa M, Adamopoulos S, Agabiti-Rosei E, Ambrosioni E, Bertomeu V, Clement D, Erdine S, Farsang C, Gaita D, Lip G, Mallion JM, Manolis AJ, Nilsson PM, O'Brien E, Ponikowski P, Redon J, Ruschitzka F, Tamargo J, van Zwieten P, Waeber B, Williams B, Management of Arterial Hypertension of the European Society of Hypertension, European Society of Cardiology. 2007 Guidelines for the Management of Arterial Hypertension: the task force for the Management of Arterial Hypertension of the European Society of Hypertension (ESH) and of the European Society of Cardiology (ESC). J Hypertens. 2007;25(6):1105–87.
12. Lurbe E, Cifkova R, Cruickshank JK, Dillon MJ, Ferreira I, Invitti C, et al. Management of high blood pressure in children and adolescents: recommendations of the European Society of Hypertension. J Hypertens. 2009;27:1719–42.
13. James PA, Oparil S, Carter BL, Cushman WC, Dennison-Himmelfarb C, Handler J, Lackland DT, LeFevre ML, MacKenzie TD, Ogedegbe O, Smith SC Jr, Svetkey LP, Taler SJ, Townsend RR, Wright JT Jr, Narva AS, Ortiz E. 2014 evidence-based guideline for the management of high blood pressure in adults: report from the panel members appointed to the Eighth Joint National Committee (JNC 8). JAMA. 2014;311(5):507–20.
14. http://www.eshonline.org/annual-meeting-posts/to-treat-or-not-to-treat-what-to-do-for-high-normal-bp/.
15. Terry PD, Abramson JL, Neaton JD, MRFIT Research Group. Blood pressure and risk of death from external causes among men screened for the multiple risk factor intervention trial. Am J Epidemiol. 2007;165(3):294–301.
16. Vasan RS, Larson MG, Leip EP, Kannel WB, Levy D. Assessment of frequency of progression to hypertension in non-hypertensive participants in the Framingham Heart Study: a cohort study. Lancet. 2001;358(9294):1682–6.
17. Zhang H, Thijs L, Kuznetsova T, Fagard RH, Li X, Staessen JAJ. Progression to hypertension in the non-hypertensive participants in the Flemish Study on environment, genes and health outcomes. Hypertension. 2006;24(9):1719–27.
18. Julius S, Majahalme S, Nesbitt S, Grant E, Kaciroti N, Ombao H, Vriz O, Valentini MC, Amerena J, Gleiberman L. A "gender blind" relationship of lean body mass and blood pressure in the Tecumseh study. Am J Hypertens. 2002;15(3):258–63.

19. Xu T, Liu J, Zhu G, Liu J, Han S. Prevalence of prehypertension and associated risk factors among Chinese adults from a large-scale multi-ethnic population survey. BMC Public Health. 2016;16(1):775.
20. Pimenta E, Oparil S. Prehypertension: epidemiology, consequences and treatment. Nat Rev Nephrol. 2010;6(1):21–30.
21. Julius S, Nesbitt SD, Egan BM, et al., Trial of Preventing Hypertension (TROPHY) Study Investigators. Feasibility of treating prehypertension with an angiotensin-receptor blocker. N Engl J Med. 2006;354:1685–97.
22. Vasan RS, Larson MG, Leip EP, Evans JC, O'Donnell CJ, Kannel WB, Levy D. Impact of high-normal blood pressure on the risk of cardiovascular disease. N Engl J Med. 2001;345(18):1291–7.
23. Hansen TW, Staessen JA, Zhang H, Torp-Pedersen C, Rasmussen S, Thijs L, Ibsen H, Jeppesen J. Cardiovascular outcome in relation to progression to hypertension in the Copenhagen MONICA cohort. Am J Hypertens. 2007;20(5):483–91.
24. Staessen JA, Li Y, Hara A, Asayama K, Dolan E, O'Brien E. Blood pressure measurement anno 2016. Am J Hypertens. 2017;30(5):453–63.
25. Celis H, Fagard RH. White-coat hypertension: a clinical review. Eur J Intern Med. 2004;15(6):348–57.
26. Brguljan-Hitij J, Thijs L, Li Y, Hansen TW, Boggia J, Liu YP, Asayama K, Wei FF, Bjorklund-Bodegard K, Gu YM, Ohkubo T, Jeppesen J, Torp-Pedersen C, Dolan E, Kuznetsova T, Katarzyna SS, Tikhonoff V, Malyutina S, Casiglia E, Nikitin Y, Lind L, Sandoya E, Kawecka-Jaszcz K, Filipovsky J, Imai Y, Wang J, O'Brien E, Staessen JA, on behalf of the International Database on Ambulatory blood pressure in relation to Cardiovascular Outcome Investigators. Risk stratification by ambulatory blood pressure monitoring across JNC classes of conventional blood pressure. Am J Hypertens. 2014;27(7):956–65.
27. Manios E, Michas F, Tsivgoulis G, Stamatelopoulos K, Tsagalis G, Koroboki E, Alexaki E, Papamichael C, Vemmos K, Zakopoulos N. Impact of prehypertension on carotid artery intima-media thickening: actual or masked? Atherosclerosis. 2011;214(1):215–9.
28. Shimbo D, Newman JD, Schwartz JE. Masked hypertension and prehypertension: diagnostic overlap and interrelationships with left ventricular mass: the Masked Hypertension Study. Am J Hypertens. 2012;25(6):664–71.
29. Lüders S, Schrader J, Berger J, et al. The PHARAO study: prevention of hypertension with the angiotensin-converting enzyme inhibitor ramipril in patients with high-normal blood pressure – a prospective, randomized, controlled prevention trial of the German Hypertension League. J Hypertens. 2008;26:1487–96.
30. Mancia G, De Backer G, Dominiczak A, et al. Guidelines for the management of arterial hypertension: the task force for the management of arterial hypertension of the European Society of Hypertension (ESH) and of the European Society of Cardiology (ESC). Eur Heart J. 2007;28:1462–536.
31. Sever P, Dahlöf B, Poulter N, et al. Potential synergy between lipid-lowering and blood-pressure-lowering in the Anglo-Scandinavian cardiac outcomes trial. Eur Heart J. 2006;27:2982–8.
32. Schrier RW, Estacio RO, Esler A, Mehler P. Effects of aggressive blood pressure control in normotensive type 2 diabetic patients on albuminuria, retinopathy and strokes. Kidney Int. 2002;61:1086–97.
33. Heart Outcomes Prevention Evaluation (HOPE) Study Investigators. Effects of ramipril on cardiovascular and microvascular outcomes in people with diabetes mellitus: results of the HOPE study and MICROHOPE substudy. Lancet. 2000;355:253–9.
34. ADVANCE Collaborative Group. Effects of a fixed combination of perindopril and indapamide on macrovascular and microvascular outcomes in patients with type 2 diabetes mellitus (the ADVANCE trial): a randomised controlled trial. Lancet. 2007;370:829–40.
35. PROGRESS Collaborative Study Group. Randomised trial of perindopril based blood pressure-lowering regimen among 6108 individuals with previous stroke or transient ischaemic attack. Lancet. 2001;358:1033–41.

36. Arima H, Chalmers J, Woodward M, Anderson C, Rodgers A, Davis S, MacMahon S, Neal B, for the PROGRESS Collaborative Group. Lower target blood pressures are safe and effective for the prevention of recurrent stroke: the PROGRESS trial. J Hypertens. 2006;24:1201–8.
37. PATS Collaborating Group. Poststroke antihypertensive treatment study. A preliminary result. Chin Med J. 1995;108:710–7.
38. Zanchetti A, Grassi G, Mancia G. When should antihypertensive drug treatment be initiated and to what levels should systolic blood pressure be lowered? A critical re-appraisal. J Hypertens. 2009;27:923–34.
39. Aglony M, Acevedo M, Ambrosio G. Hypertension in adolescents. Expert Rev Cardiovasc Ther. 2009;7(12):1595–603.
40. Neter JE, Stam BE, Kok FJ, Grobbee DE, Geleijnse JM. Influence of weight reduction on blood pressure: a meta-analysis of randomized controlled trials. Hypertension. 2003;42:878–84.
41. Horvath K, Jeitler K, Siering U, Stich AK, Skipka G, Gratzer TW, Siebenhofer A. Long-term effects of weight-reducing interventions in hypertensive patients: systematic review and meta-analysis. Arch Intern Med. 2008;168(6):571–80.
42. Siebenhofer A, Jeitler K, Berghold A, Waltering A, Hemkens LG, Semlitsch T, Pachler C, Strametz R, Horvath K. Long-term effects of weight-reducing diets in hypertensive patients. Cochrane Database Syst Rev. 2011;9:CD008274.
43. Cornelissen VA, Fagard RH. Effects of endurance training on blood pressure, blood pressure-regulating mechanisms, and cardiovascular risk factors. Hypertension. 2005;46:667–75.
44. Molmen-Hansen HE, Stolen T, Tjonna AE, Aamot IL, Ekeberg IS, Tyldum GA, et al. Aerobic interval training reduces blood pressure and improves myocardial function in hypertensive patients. Eur J Prev Cardiol. 2012;19:151–60.
45. Cornelissen VA, Fagard RH, Coeckelberghs E, Vanhees L. Impact of resistance training on blood pressure and other cardiovascular risk factors: a meta-analysis of randomized, controlled trials. Hypertension. 2011;58:950–8.
46. Fagard RH. Exercise therapy in hypertensive cardiovascular disease. Prog Cardiovasc Dis. 2011;53:404–11.
47. He FJ, McGregor GA. Effect of modest salt reduction on blood pressure: a meta-analysis of randomized trials. Implications for public health. J Hum Hypertens. 2002;16:761–70.
48. van Mierlo LA, Arends LR, Streppel MT, Zeegers MP, Kok FJ, Grobbee DE, Geleijnse JM. Blood pressure response to calcium supplementation: a meta-analysis of randomized controlled trials. J Hum Hypertens. 2006;20(8):571–80.
49. Jee SH, Miller ER 3rd, Guallar E, Singh VK, Appel LJ, Klag MJ. The effect of magnesium supplementation on blood pressure: a meta-analysis of randomized clinical trials. Am J Hypertens. 2002;15(8):691–6.
50. Egan BM, Nesbitt SD, Julius S. Prehypertension: should we be treating with pharmacologic therapy? Ther Adv Cardiovasc Dis. 2008;2(4):305–14.